Contents

General Chapters

Mission and Preface
USP 41–NF 36 and *Supplements*

This section provides background information on the United States Pharmacopeial Convention (USP), as well as general information about the 41st revision of the *United States Pharmacopeia* (*USP 41*) and the 36th edition of the *National Formulary* (*NF 36*) and their *Supplements*. Unless otherwise noted, the text in *USP 41–NF 36* is official May 1, 2018, the text in the *First Supplement to USP 41–NF 36* is official August 1, 2018, and the text in the *Second Supplement* to *USP 41–NF 36* is official December 1, 2018.

MISSION STATEMENT

USP–NF is published in continuing pursuit of the mission of USP: *To improve global health through public standards and related programs that help ensure the quality, safety, and benefit of medicines and foods.*

HISTORY

USP has a rich history, dating back to 1820, when 11 physicians met in the Senate Chamber of the U.S. Capitol building to establish a pharmacopeia for the United States. Learn more about USP's history and major milestones on the USP website (https://www.usp.org/about/usp-timeline).

CONTENT OF *USP–NF*

USP–NF contains official substance (ingredient) and product monographs for official articles recognized in *USP–NF* (see *General Notices 2.20 Official Articles*). *USP–NF* also includes monographs for compounded preparations. With few exceptions, such as articles covered by *Global Health* monographs, all articles for which monographs are provided in *USP–NF* are legally marketed in the United States or are contained in legally marketed articles. *Global Health* monographs are provided for articles that are not approved or legally marketed in the United States, but that have been approved by a stringent regulatory authority [as defined by the World Health Organization (WHO)] and are used for essential purposes in other parts of the world.

A *USP–NF* monograph for an official substance, product, or preparation may consist of various components, including the article's name; definition; packaging, storage, and other requirements; and a specification. General chapters provide frequently cited procedures, sometimes with acceptance criteria, in order to compile into one location repetitive information that is applicable to many monographs. See *General Notices 3.10 Applicability of Standards* for more information about standards contained in *USP–NF* monographs and general chapters.

New and revised monographs and general chapters and omitted monographs from this edition are indicated in the *Admissions* section.

USP–NF Organization—The *USP–NF* is published online as the *USP–NF Online*. *USP–NF* is also printed as a five-vol-ume set. To facilitate convenient use and reference, all five volumes include the combined index, as well as the *USP General Notices* and the *Guide to General Chapters*. *Volume 1* includes front matter (*Mission and Preface, People,* governance pages and websites, and *Admissions/Annotations*) and *USP* monographs A–I. *Volume 2* includes *USP* monographs J–Z. *Volume 3* includes *Global Health* monographs, *Dietary Supplements* monographs, *NF Admissions/Annotations, Excipients,* and *NF* monographs. *Volume 4* includes general chapters numbered below 1000 (*General Tests and Assays*—including chapter charts), *Reagents,* and *Reference Tables*. *Volume 5* includes general chapters numbered above 1000 (*General Information*) and *Dietary Supplements* general chapters. General chapters specific to dietary supplements are included in numerical order with the rest of the general chapters in *USP*. Excipient monographs are usually presented in *NF* but also may appear in *USP* with suitable cross-referencing when they are also drug substances. The *Excipients* section (*Volume 3*) presents a tabulation of excipients by functional category.

Supplements—*Supplements* to *USP–NF* follow a standard schedule each year: the *First Supplement* is published in February and becomes official August 1. The *Second Supplement* is published in June and becomes official December 1. Users of USP print products must retain *Supplements* and check the "Official Text" section of USP's website to have up-to-date official text. The *USP–NF Online* is updated with each *Supplement* or annual revision. Each time a new edition or *Supplement* is released during the subscription period, a new electronic version is issued. The *Index* in each *Supplement* is cumulative and includes citations to the annual revision and, for the *Second Supplement*, citations to the *First Supplement*. The contents of the two *Supplements* are integrated into the annual edition of the following year, along with new official revisions that have been adopted since the *Second Supplement* to the previous compendia.

Revisions to USP–NF—*USP–NF* is continuously revised by an exceptional process of public involvement and substantial interaction between USP and its stakeholders, both domestically and internationally. Revisions are presented annually in the *USP–NF* and in twice-yearly *Supplements*, and as *Accelerated Revisions* on USP's website [*Errata, Interim Revision Announcements (IRAs),* and *Revision Bulletins*].

Standard Revisions—USP's standard revision process calls for publication of a proposed revision in the *Pharmacopeial Forum (PF)* for a 90-day notice and comment period and, after the revision is approved by the relevant USP Expert Committee, publication in the next *USP–NF* or *Supplement,* as applicable.

Accelerated Revisions—The *Accelerated Revision* process is used to make revisions to *USP–NF* official more quickly than through USP's *Standard Revision* process. Learn more about *Revision Bulletins, Interim Revision Announcements (IRA), Errata,* and the criteria for and implementation of each on the USP website (http://www.uspnf.com/official-text).

Modification of Compendial References—USP and its Expert Committees periodically deem it necessary to modify general chapter titles or similar text that may be referenced in other standards throughout the *USP–NF*. When this occurs, USP staff undertake a rigorous process for identifying and updating such references. These updates may occur through a routine revision, or, in cases in which an update appears to present no significant change in the affected standard, through a direct update of the reference in that standard without providing an opportunity for notice and comment. In all cases, USP will publish on its website a notice indicating the source change, any resulting references, and whether those references will be updated through a routine revision or a direct update.

Updating Chemical Information—Updates to the Chemical Information section at the beginning of monographs occur on an ongoing basis and are not identified with revision symbols. Chemical names and molecular weights are updated when a monograph undergoes revision to match the official source, *United States Adopted Names* (*USAN*). Chemical structures are updated on a continuous basis.

Chemical names typically reflect the naming conventions at the time of the monograph development or revision. If the nomenclature rules of CAS or IUPAC are significantly changed, the chemical names can be revised or added to implement those rules. Molecular weights are derived from the chemical formula and are based on the table of atomic weights. Atomic weights are recommended by the IUPAC and reflect the isotopic composition of normal terrestrial material. When the IUPAC recommended values are changed, it is understood that the changes in molecular weights will be made in due course.

Graphical representation of the chemical compound structures is intended as a visual aid to help establish chemical identity and is understood to represent one of many possible ways to depict the molecule. Addition of a graphical representation or changes in such representation, that result in the same chemical information, e.g., a flipped chiral molecule or adding a molecule structure, may be introduced outside of the revision process. It is also understood that in the case of tautomerism, the molecule depicted may be one of the tautomers, but it is intended to represent all isomers in equilibrium. Stereogenic centers depicted with plain bonds imply mixtures of pertinent stereomers—enantiomer, diastereomers, epimers (anomers), etc.

Depending on the timing of these updates, users may see a difference in a chemical structure between the publications in *PF* and *USP–NF*, and between the *USP–NF* and the *USP–NF Online*.

Shading and Symbols—Shading is used to identify text that has been modified, added, or deleted since it was last published. Symbols identify the beginning and end of each revision or nonharmonized text. The following table summarizes the types of symbols and the associated subscripts used in USP publications:

Revision Type	Symbol	Subscript
Interim Revision Announcement	•new text• (IRA 1-Jul-2018)	(IRA 1-Jul-2018)*
Revision Bulletin	•new text• (RB 1-Jan-2018)	(RB 1-Jan-2018)*
Text deletion	•(IRA 1-Jul-2018) or	(IRA 1-Jul-2018)*
	■1S (USP41) or	1S (USP41)*
	▲▲(USP41)	USP41**
Adopted in Supplement	■new text■1S (USP41)	1S or 2S (USP annual edition)*
Adopted in USP–NF	▲new text▲ (USP41)	USP annual edition**
Harmonization	◆residual national text or nonharmonized text◆	

* A subscript number or date indicates the *IRA*, *Revision Bulletin*, or *Supplement* in which the revision first appeared.
** An example of a revision that was officially adopted in the *USP–NF* would be ▲USP41.

Revision Type	Symbol	Subscript
Errata	•new text• (ERR 1-Jul-2018)	(ERR 1-Jul-2018)
Chapter references	•new text• (CN 1-May-2018)	(CN 1-May-2018)
	•new text• (Official 1-Dec-2018)	(Official 1-Dec-2018)

* A subscript number or date indicates the *IRA*, *Revision Bulletin*, or *Supplement* in which the revision first appeared.
** An example of a revision that was officially adopted in the *USP–NF* would be ▲USP41.

The following table shows symbols and official dates for *IRAs* and *Supplements* to *USP 41–NF 36*.

IRAs and *Supplements* to *USP 41–NF 36*
Official Dates and Symbols

Supplement	Proposed IRA	Official Date	Symbols
	44(1)	July 1, 2018	•and• (IRA 1-Jul-2018)
1		Aug. 1, 2018	■and■1S (USP41)
	44(2)	Sept. 1, 2018	•and• (IRA 1-Sep-2018)
	44(3)	Nov. 1, 2018	•and• (IRA 1-Nov-2018)
2		Dec. 1, 2018	■and■2S (USP41)
	44(4)	Jan. 1, 2019	•and• (IRA 1-Jan-2019)
	44(5)	Mar. 1, 2019	•and• (IRA 1-Mar-2019)
USP 42–NF 37	44(6)	May 1, 2019	•and• (IRA 1-May-2019)

Also, in the *USP–NF Online*, monographs and general chapters that have been revised but not yet published in the *USP–NF* or its *Supplements* (e.g., as *Accelerated Revisions*) will contain icons that will link to the page on the USP website where the new official text can be viewed. These icons will link to *Accelerated Revisions* (*Revision Bulletins, Interim Revision Announcements*, and *Errata*) and *Stage 6 Harmonization* (see *Harmonization Activities* below).

Commentary—For revisions that are published for public review and comment in *PF*, the proposal may advance to official status or be republished in *PF* for further notice and comment. If comments are received, they are considered and incorporated as appropriate by the Expert Committee(s). In cases where proposals advance to official status without republication in *PF*, a summary of comments received and the appropriate Expert Committee's responses are published in the *Commentary* section of the USP website at the time the revision is published.

The *Commentary* is not part of the official text and is not intended to be enforceable by regulatory authorities. Rather, it explains the basis of the Expert Committee's response to public comments. If there is a difference between the contents of the *Commentary* and the official text, the official text prevails. In case of a dispute or question of interpretation, the language of the official text, alone and independent of the *Commentary*, shall prevail.

Print and Electronic Presentations—See *General Notices 2.10 Official Text* for more information about *USP–NF* product formats.

USP–NF Translations—Translations of the *USP–NF* are available in Spanish, Russian, and Chinese. The Spanish translation is current; other translations are based on previous revisions of the *USP–NF*.

USP Reference Standards—The use of USP Reference Standards promotes uniform quality of drugs and supports reliability and consistency by those performing compliance testing and other users of *USP–NF*, including manufacturers, buyers, and regulatory authorities. USP Reference Standards are referenced in specific procedures in both monographs and general chapters. USP advances this material via careful characterization studies and collaborative testing, followed by review and approval of the compendial use of the reference material by Expert Committees of the Council of Experts. The *USP Catalog*, which lists the collection of USP

Reference Standards, and more information about use and storage, can be accessed on USP's website (http://www.usp.org/reference-standards). This program benefits from the widespread voluntary contribution of suitable materials and test data from pharmaceutical manufacturers.

USP GOVERNING, STANDARDS-SETTING, AND ADVISORY BODIES

USP's governing, standards-setting, and advisory bodies include the USP Convention, the Board of Trustees, the Council of Experts and its Expert Committees, Expert Panels, Subcommittees, Joint Standard-Setting Subcommittees, and staff. Additional volunteer bodies include Stakeholder Forums and Project Teams, which offer stakeholders the opportunity to contribute, through advice and recommendations, to the advancement of USP's standards and processes. Learn about the composition and work of the USP Convention, Board of Trustees, Expert Committees, and Expert Panels on the USP website (http://www.usp.org/about/convention-membership). Learn more about Stakeholder Forums and Project Teams on the USP website (https://www.usp.org/get-involved/provide-input/stakeholder-forums). A listing of all current Voting Delegates of the USP Convention and members and Government Liaisons to the Council of Experts and its Expert Committees and Expert Panels is included in the *People* section.

Working with the Food and Drug Administration—USP works with the Secretary of the Department of Health and Human Services, and the principal agency in the Department for this work is the Food and Drug Administration (FDA). USP works in many ways with the agency, but the primary interaction is through the Government Liaison Program. The Government Liaison Program allows representatives of FDA and other government agencies to participate in Expert Committee and Expert Panel meetings, enabling interactions between government staff and Expert Committees. Staff in the FDA Centers who are responsible for review of compendial activities provide specific links and opportunities for exchange of comments. The Office of Policy for Pharmaceutical Quality in the Center for Drug Evaluation and Research provides a primary compendial point of contact between FDA and USP.

RULES AND PROCEDURES

Governing Documents—*USP–NF* standards are recognized widely because they are authoritative and science-based and are established by a transparent and credible process. See the *Articles of Incorporation* section in this book; the Bylaws (https://www.usp.org/about/convention-membership/bylaws), and the *Rules and Procedures of the Council of Experts* (https://www.usp.org/about/leadership/policies-rules). Collectively, these documents serve USP volunteers and staff as the governing principles for USP's standards-setting activities.

LEGAL RECOGNITION

Recognition of *USP–NF*—*USP–NF* is recognized by law and custom in many countries throughout the world. In the United States, the Federal Food, Drug, and Cosmetic Act (FD&C Act) defines the term "official compendium" as the official *USP*, the official *NF*, the official *Homeopathic Pharmacopeia of the United States*, or any supplement to them. *USP–NF* standards play a role in the adulteration and misbranding provisions of the FD&C Act, which apply as well to biologics, a subset of drugs, under the Public Health Service Act (see *General Notices 2.30 Legal Recognition*).

FDA requires that names for articles that are not official must be clearly distinguished and differentiated from any name recognized in an official compendium. Drugs with a name recognized in *USP–NF* also will be considered misbranded unless they meet compendial standards for packaging and labeling (see *General Notices 3.10.10 Applicability of Standards to Drug Products, Drug Substances, and Excipients* for more information).

Drugs—USP's goal is to have substance and drug product monographs in *USP–NF* for FDA-approved drugs in the United States, including chemical and biologic medicines, and their ingredients. USP also provides monographs in *USP–NF* for legally marketed therapeutic products not approved by FDA, e.g., pre-1938 drugs, over-the-counter (OTC) drugs marketed under FDA's OTC Monograph system, dietary supplements, and compounded preparations. The *Global Health* section of *USP–NF* contains monographs for articles that are not approved or legally marketed in the United States, but that have been approved by a stringent regulatory authority (as defined by WHO) and are used for essential purposes in other parts of the world. Conformance with a *USP–NF* monograph, if applicable, is required at all times in the life of an article from production to expiration.

Biologics—In the United States, biologics are considered to be a subset of drugs, whether they are approved by FDA under the FD&C Act [and receive a new drug application (NDA)] or under the Public Health Service Act [PHS Act, where they receive a biologics license application (BLA)]. As a result, all PHS Act biologics are subject to the applicable drug regulatory requirements of the FD&C Act, which means they are required to comply with the adulteration and misbranding provisions of the FD&C Act, including *USP–NF* compendial requirements, to the extent that such requirements apply to a particular biologic product. This is equally so for biologics approved under the long-standing PHS Act "351(a)" pathway, as well as the new "351(k)" pathway for biosimilars added by the 2010 healthcare reform legislation (Biologics Price Competition and Innovation Act, Title VII, Subtitle A of the Patient Protection and Affordable Care Act, Public Law 111-148).

Dietary Supplements—The Dietary Supplement Health and Education Act of 1994 amendments to the FD&C Act provide that a dietary supplement may be deemed a misbranded food if it is covered by the specifications of an official compendium (e.g., *USP–NF*), is represented as conforming to the specifications of an official compendium, and fails to so conform. This contrasts with pharmaceutical products, wherein conformance to applicable compendial standards is mandatory, whether or not the product claims to conform.

Compounding—USP provides general chapters and monographs for compounded preparations, as well as monographs for bulk substances used in compounding. USP standards are recognized in various provisions of the FD&C Act and such provisions do not differentiate between manufactured and compounded medicines. Moreover, the FD&C Act and the 2013 Drug Quality and Security Act specifically reference USP standards for compounding. Learn more about compounding on the USP website (http://www.usp.org/compounding).

Medical Devices—Section 201(h) of the FD&C Act defines a device as an instrument, apparatus, similar article, or component thereof recognized in *USP–NF*. Section 502(e) of the FD&C Act defines the established name of a device in the absence of an FDA designation of the official name as the official title in an official compendium. Despite these statutory provisions, there is no comparable recognition of USP's role in establishing compendial standards for medical devices as exists for drugs and biologics. Under authority granted by the Food and Drug Administration Modernization Act of 1997, the Center for Devices and Radiological Health recognizes national and international standards, including some *USP* tests and assays, for medical devices.

Nomenclature—For information on the nomenclature development process, the Nomenclature and Labeling Expert Committee, and USP's work with United States Adopted Names (USAN), see the USP website (https://www.usp.org/expert-committees/nomenclature-and-labeling-expert-committee-work-plan).

Chemical Names and CAS Registry Numbers—Chemical subtitles given in the monographs are index names used by the Chemical Abstracts Service (CAS) of the American Chemical Society. They are provided only in monographs in which the titles specify substances that are definable chemical entities. The first subtitle is the inverted form of the systematic chemical name developed by CAS for the purpose of the Collective Index (CI). The second subtitle, given in uninverted form, is a preferred IUPAC name (PIN) sanctioned and used by the International Union of Pure and Applied Chemistry (IUPAC). Preferred IUPAC names also are used by the WHO. Occasionally a third subtitle is supplied for historical reasons or when the synonym uses an alternative, but equivalent, naming convention. Monographs with chemical subtitles also generally carry CAS registry numbers. These bracketed numbers function independently of nomenclature as invariant numerical designators of unique, unambiguous chemical substances in the CAS registry, and thus are convenient and widely used.

HARMONIZATION ACTIVITIES

USP participates in several collaborative activities with global pharmacopeias in both bilateral and multilateral settings. Examples of USP's current activities include the following.

Pharmacopeial Discussion Group—USP harmonizes pharmacopeial excipient monographs and general chapters through the Pharmacopeial Discussion Group (PDG), which includes representatives from the European, Japanese, and United States pharmacopeias, and WHO (as an observer). According to the PDG definition, "a pharmacopeial general chapter or other pharmacopeial document is harmonized when a pharmaceutical substance or product tested by the document's harmonized procedure yields the same results, and the same accept/reject decision is reached." Information regarding PDG, including history, the PDG working procedure, a glossary, and lists of monographs and general chapters that have completed stages 1–6 of the pharmacopeial harmonization process, resulting in an approved USP Stage 6 Harmonization text, is available on USP's website (https://www.usp.org/harmonization-standards/pdg/stage-6-notices).

International Meeting of the World Pharmacopeias—USP works with WHO and global pharmacopeial partners on the strategy and establishment of Good Pharmacopoeial Practices (GPhP) as a set of guiding principles for the appropriate establishment of pharmacopeial standards.

Adopt/Adapt Agreements—USP grants the rights to copy and/or adapt USP standards for use in other pharmacopeias through this formal mechanism.

Bilateral Agreements—USP partners with pharmacopeias for the joint development of pharmacopeial standards using this informal process.

USP Exchange Programs—USP regularly welcomes the exchange of scientific personnel through this program, with the goal of sharing scientific knowledge among global organizations involved in standards setting and the effective use of standards.

OTHER USP COMPENDIA

USP Compounding Compendium—The *USP Compounding Compendium* is an electronic compendium that includes all compounding-related general chapters from the *USP–NF* as well as the supporting general chapters that are referenced in the compounding general chapters and in *USP–NF General Notices*. The purpose of the *USP Compounding Compendium* is to provide compounding practitioners with convenient access to associated general chapters.

USP Herbal Medicines Compendium—The *USP Herbal Medicines Compendium (HMC)* is an online compendium that helps ensure the quality of the herbal ingredients used in herbal medicines. *HMC* monographs provide quality specifications—tests, procedures, and acceptance criteria—with validated analytical procedures and allied reference materials that aid in conformity assessment. *HMC* can help ingredient manufacturers, herbal product manufacturers, regulatory agencies, and other stakeholders to assess conformance of herbal medicinal ingredients with independent public standards and to control the quality of articles moving in international commerce. The *HMC* is available at https://hmc.usp.org.

USP Dietary Supplements Compendium—The *Dietary Supplements Compendium* combines, in a two-volume set, *USP–NF* standards for dietary supplements, standards and information from the *Food Chemicals Codex*, regulatory and industry documents, and other tools and resources. It is published every three years as a hardcover print edition.

Food Chemicals Codex—The *Food Chemicals Codex (FCC)* is a compendium of internationally recognized monograph standards and tests for the purity and quality of food ingredients, e.g., preservatives, flavorings, colorings, and nutrients. *FCC* is published every two years, with supplements every six months, and is available in print and electronic formats. Proposed revisions to *FCC* are available for public viewing and comment through the *FCC Forum*. The *FCC Forum* can be accessed free of charge at forum.foodchemicalscodex.org.

OTHER USP RESOURCES

Chromatographic Columns—This comprehensive reference, previously titled *Chromatographic Reagents*, provides detailed information needed to conduct chromatographic procedures found in *USP–NF*. *Chromatographic Columns* lists the brand names of the column reagents cited in every proposal for new or revised gas- or liquid-chromatographic analytical procedures that have been published in *PF* since 1980. *Chromatographic Columns* also helps to track which column reagents were used to validate analytical procedures that have become official. The branded column reagents list is updated bimonthly and maintained on USP's website.

USP Dictionary—The *USP Dictionary of USAN and International Drug Names* provides, in a single volume, the most up-to-date United States Adopted Names of drugs; official *USP–NF* names; nonproprietary, brand, and chemical names; graphic formulas; molecular formulas and weights; CAS registry numbers and code designations; drug manufacturers; and pharmacologic and therapeutic categories. The *Dictionary* helps to ensure the accuracy of the following: product labeling; reports, articles, and correspondence; FDA regulatory filings; and pharmaceutical package inserts. It is published annually. For more information about the *Dictionary* see the USP website (https://www.usp.org/products/usp-dictionary).

People

2015–2020 Revision Cycle

Officers of the USP Convention, Board of Trustees, and the Council of Experts, Expert Committees, and Expert Panels

Officers (2015–2020)

Jesse L. Goodman, M.D., M.P.H.
President
Washington, DC
Timothy R. Franson, B.S. Pharm., M.D.
Past President
Indianapolis, IN
John E. Courtney, Ph.D.
Treasurer
Bethesda, MD
Susan S. de Mars, J.D.
Secretary
Rockville, MD

Board of Trustees (2015–2020)

Thomas R. Temple, B.S. Pharm., M.S., F.A. Ph.A.
Chair
Trustee At-Large
Des Moines, IA
Gregory E. Amidon, Ph.D.
Trustee Representing the Pharmaceutical Sciences
Ann Arbor, MI
Laura Herman, M.B.A., M.A.
Trustee Representing the Public
New Canaan, CT
Robert J. Meyer, M.D.
Trustee Representing the Medical Sciences
Charlottesville, VA
Marilyn K. Speedie, Ph.D.
Trustee Representing the Pharmaceutical Sciences
Minneapolis, MN
Stephen P. Spielberg, M.D., Ph.D.
Trustee Representing the Medical Sciences
Upper Gwynedd, PA
Gail R. Wilensky, Ph.D.
Trustee At-Large
Bethesda, MD
Susan C. Winckler, R.Ph., J.D.
Trustee At-Large
Alexandria, VA
Ron T. Piervincenzi, Ph.D.
Chief Executive Officer, February 2014–present
(ex-officio)
Rockville, MD

Council of Experts (2015–2020)

Jaap Venema, Ph.D.
Chair, Council of Experts
Rockville, MD
Richard A. Blessing, M.S.
Chair, Chemical Medicines Monographs 1
North Chicago, IL
Edward K. Chess, Ph.D.
Chair, Biologics Monographs 3—Complex Biologics
McHenry, IL
Stephanie Y. Crawford, Ph.D., M.P.H.
Chair, Nomenclature and Labeling
Chicago, IL
Gigi S. Davidson, B.S. Pharm., DICVP
Chair, Compounding
Raleigh, NC
Michael R. De Felippis, Ph.D.
Chair, Biologics Monographs 1—Peptides
Indianapolis, IN
James E. De Muth, Ph.D., R.Ph.
Chair, General Chapters—Dosage Forms
Madison, WI
Jonathan W. DeVries, Ph.D.
Chair, Food Ingredients
Golden Valley, MN
Dennis E. Doherty, M.D., FCCP
Chair, Healthcare Quality
Lexington, KY
Reinhard Walter, Ph.D.
Chair, Chemical Medicines Monographs 6
Morristown, NJ
Mary G. Foster, Pharm.D., BFA
Chair, General Chapters—Packaging and Distribution
Blue Bell, PA
Dennis K.J. Gorecki, B.S.P., Ph.D.
Chair, Non-Botanical Dietary Supplements
Saskatoon, Saskatchewan, Canada
Xiaorong He, Ph.D.
Chair, General Chapters—Physical Analysis
Ridgefield, CT
Mary C. Houck, Ph.D.
Chair, Excipient Monographs 2
Norman, OK

David Hussong, Ph.D.
Chair, General Chapters—Microbiology
Kensington, MD
Kim C. Huynh-Ba, M.S.
Chair, Chemical Medicines Monographs 4
Newark, DE
Amy J. Karren, B.Sc.
Chair, Chemical Medicines Monographs 5
Flagstaff, AZ
Nancy Lewen, B.Sc.
Chair, General Chapters—Chemical Analysis
Indianapolis, IN
Robin J. Marles, B.Sc., M.Sc., Ph.D.
Chair, Botanical Dietary Supplements and Herbal Medicines
Ottawa, Ontario, Canada
Michael G. Mulkerrin, Ph.D.
Chair, Biologics Monographs 2—Proteins
Hillsborough, CA
Eric Jon Munson, Ph.D.
Chair, Excipient Monographs 1
Lexington, KY
Bernard A. Olsen, Ph.D.
Chair, Chemical Medicines Monographs 3
Wake Forest, NC
Ernest Parente, Ph.D.
Chair, Chemical Medicines Monographs 2
Saint Louis, MO
Robert R. Singer, M.S.
Chair, General Chapters—Statistics
Union City, CA
Reinhard Walter, Ph.D.
Chair, Chemical Medicines Monographs 6
Whippany, NJ
Wesley E. Workman, Ph.D.
Chair, General Chapters—Biological Analysis
Saint Charles, MO

Expert Committees (2015–2020)

[Note—The following listing of Expert Committees includes the Expert Panels that serve in an advisory capacity to the specific Expert Committee. The listing of Expert Panels and their membership represents those that have been fully formed and approved as of July 2015. Expert Panels are continuously formed and concluded throughout the USP revision cycle, and other membership listings will appear in the future.]

Expert Panels for the Council of Experts Executive Committee

Spanish Translation Expert Panel
OSCAR QUATTROCCHI, M.SC., *Chair*
Peggy Casanova, M.Sc.; Ofelia Espejo, Ph.D.; Lidiette Fonseca González, M.Sc.; José Juárez Eyzaguirre, Ph.D.; Monica I. Hirschhorn, M.Sc.; Francisco Kuribrena; Pilar Pais, Ph.D.; José María Parisi, M.Sc.; Luisa Fernanda Ponce D'León Quiroga, Ph.D.; Mauricio A. Seigelchifer, Ph.D.; Ofelia Villalva-Rojas; Caroline R. Weinstein-Oppenheimer, Ph.D.

Expert Committees for the *United States Pharmacopeia*

Nomenclature and Labeling
STEPHANIE Y. CRAWFORD, PH.D., M.P.H., *Chair*
Mary B. Baker, Pharm.D.; Dawn M. Boothe, D.V.M., Ph.D.; Mike Cohen, M.S.; Elizabeth Igne Ferreira, Ph.D.; Karen Hauda, J.D., M.S.; Kent Johnson, M.Pharm.; Armen Melikian, Ph.D.; Ajay Parashar, M.S.; Ginette A. Pepper, R.N., Ph.D., FAAN; Thomas Reinders, Pharm.D.; Joanne G. Schwartzberg, M.D.; Maged Sharaf, Ph.D.; Eric Sheinin, Ph.D.; Thomas Tice, Ph.D.; Claudia Vincenzi, Ph.D., Pharm.D.; Gillian Woollett, Ph.D.

Pronunciation Expert Panel
WILLIAM M. HELLER, PH.D., *Chair*
Mary B. Baker, Pharm.D.; Stephanie Y. Crawford, Ph.D.; Doreen J. Elston, Pharm.D.; Kent Johnson, M. Pharm.; David F. Long, Ph.D.; Joan C. May, Ph.D.; Anthony Palmieri, Ph.D.; Ginette A. Pepper, R.N., Ph.D., FAAN; Thomas P. Reinders, Pharm.D.

Healthcare Quality
DENNIS DOHERTY, M.D., FCCP, *Chair*
Timothy Albertson, Ph.D.; Phil Ayers, Pharm.D.; Danial Edwin Baker, Pharm.D.; Mark Decerbo, Pharm.D.; Peter Glassman, M.B.B.S.; Roy Guharoy, Pharm.D., M.B.A.; Raymond Hohl, M.D.; Duane Kirking, Ph.D.; Raymond Love, Pharm.D.; Marcus Reidenberg, M.D.; Melody Ryan, Pharm.D.; Joanne Schwartzberg, M.D.; Patricia Sokol, J.D.; J. Russell Teagarden, D.M.H.; Jeanne Tuttle, B.S. Pharm.; Terri Warholak, Ph.D.; Hsiang Shonna Yin, M.S.

Drug Allergy and Intolerance Classification Expert Panel
RAYMOND LOVE, PHARM.D., *Chair*
Gay Dolin, M.S.N.; Roy Guharoy, Pharm.D., M.B.A.; Robert Hausam, M.D.; Russell Leftwich, M.D.; Robert McClure, M.D.; Gerald McEvoy, Pharm.D.; Tejal Patel, Pharm.D.; Seth Powsner, Ph.D.; George Allen Robinson, B.S. Pharm; Shelly Spiro, B.S. Pharm

Health Literacy Expert Panel
JOANNE G. SCHWARTZBERG, M.D., *Chair*
Cindy Brach, MPP; Joseph Chebli, Pharm.D.; Nicole Cook, Ph.D.; Terry Davis, Ph.D.; Radhika Devraj, Ph.D.; Gerald McEvoy, Pharm.D.; Juliet Nguyen, Pharm.D.; Ruth Parker, M.D.; Seth Powsner, Ph.D.; N. Lee Rucker; Patricia Sokol, J.D.; Charity Strothers, Pharm.D.; J. Russell Teagarden, D.M.H.; Keith Trettin, B.S. Pharm

Model Guidelines for All Marketed Products Expert Panel
DUANE M. KIRKING, PH.D., *Chair*
Daniel E. Baker, Pharm.D.; Lauren Hoffman, Pharm.D.; Gerald McEvoy, Pharm.D.; Seth Powsner, Ph.D.; N. Lee Rucker; Brian Solow, M.D.; J. Russell Teagarden, D.M.H.; Jeanne Tuttle, B.S. Pharm; Dennis West, Ph.D.

Parenteral Nutrition Safety Expert Panel
PHIL AYERS, PHARM.D., *Chair*
Mary B. Baker, Pharm.D.; Elizabeth Bobo, M.S.; Denise Bohrer, Ph.D.; Joseph Boullata, Pharm.D.; Mark Decerbo, Pharm.D.; Kathleen M. Gura, Pharm.D.; Deborah Houston, Pharm.D.; Matthew T. Jenkins, M.S.; Gordon Scott Sacks, Pharm.D.; Maureen Schanck, Pharm.D.; David Seres, M.D.; Connie Rae Sullivan, B.S. Pharm; Patricia Worthington, M.S.N.

Chemical Medicines Monographs 1
RICHARD A. BLESSING, M.S., *Chair*
Gennady Ananchenko, Ph.D.; Elizabeth (Betsy) Cariello; Alain Duguet, Ph.D.; Leslie Furr, M.S.; Rupa Iyer, M.S.; Monika Jain, Ph.D.; Greg Kaster, M.S.; Jasmina Novakovic, Ph.D.; Naidu Petla, Ph.D.; Jeff Rohrer, Ph.D.; David Schuck, Ph.D.; Nilesh Shinde, M.S.; Jan Srbek, Ph.D.; Giordano Trazzi, Ph.D.

Chemical Medicines Monographs 2
ERNEST PARENTE, PH.D., *Chair*
Mahmoud Al Omari, Ph.D.; Allan Bokser, Ph.D.; Matthew Borer, Ph.D.; Jama Elmi, Ph.D.; Michael Koberda, Ph.D.; Joan C. May, Ph.D.; Beth Minter; Maria Ines Santoro, Ph.D.; Jeff Schwartzenhauer, M.S.; Dennis Stephens, Ph.D.; Sumathi V. Rao, Ph.D.; Luciano Virgili, Ph.D.; Zhenyu Wang, Ph.D.; Joseph Yakupkovic, Ph.D.; Patrick Yat, Ph.D.

Chemical Medicines Monographs 3
BERNARD A. OLSEN, PH.D., *Chair*
Samuel Akapo, Ph.D.; Bianca Avramovitch, Ph.D.; Amy Barker, Ph.D.; Lynn Blessing, M.S.; Thomas Broadbent, Ph.D.; Ian Chung, Ph.D.; Debashis Das, Ph.D.; Jeffrey Fleitman, Ph.D.; Yuri Goldberg, Ph.D.; Qamrul Islam, M.S.; Eric Kesslen, Ph.D.; Pauline Lacroix, M.S.; Donald Parsons, Ph.D.; David Reed, M.B.A.; Murugan Saravanan, M.S.; Joseph Stowell, Ph.D.

Chemical Medicines Monographs 4
KIM C. HUYNH-BA, M.S., *Chair*
Josep Maria de Ciurana Gay, M.S.; Simona Dragan, Ph.D.; Natalia Borisovna Epshtein, Pharm.D., M.S.N.; Quanyin Gao, Ph.D.; Jerome M. Lewis, Ph.D.; Oscar Liu, Ph.D.; Annarapu Malleswara, Ph.D.; Mariann Neverovitch, M.S.; Patrick Noland, M.S.; James A. Ponto, M.S.; Hemant Kumar Sharma, Ph.D.; William Taraszewski, Ph.D.; Martin Williamson, Ph.D.; Min Xia, Ph.D.; Steve S. Zigler, Ph.D.

⟨821⟩ Identification and Assay of Radionuclides and ⟨1821⟩ Radioactivity Theory and Practice and ⟨1823⟩ Drugs for Positron Emission Tomography Expert Panel—CONCLUDED
SALLY W. SCHWARZ, M.S., *Chair*
Cathy Sue Cutler, Ph.D.; Jonathan M. Fitzsimmons, Ph.D.; Paula M. Jacobs, Ph.D.; Thijs Kroon, Pharm.D.; Jerome M. Lewis, Ph.D.; Roger Moroney, M.S.; James A. Ponto, M.S.; Duann V. Thistlethwaite, B.S.; Steven S. Zigler, Ph.D.

⟨825⟩ Radiopharmaceuticals Compounding Chapter
VACANT, *Chair*
David Barnes, B.S. Pharm; Allegra DePietro, M.S.; Wendy Galbraith, Pharm.D.; Fred Patrick Gattas, Pharm.D.; Richard Lewis Green, B.S. Pharm; Brenda Sue Jensen, M.A.; Patricia C. Kienle, M.P.A.; Vivian Sue Loveless, Pharm.D.; Paul Barry Mahan, B.S. Pharm; Rezaul H. Mannan, Ph.D.; James Ponto, M.S.; Steve Zigler, Ph.D.

Non-Radioactive Imaging Agents Expert Panel
JEROME M. LEWIS, PH.D., *Chair*
Francisco Aguilar-Parrilla, Ph.D.; James Walter Brodack, Ph.D.: Dilip R. Choudhury, Ph.D.; Francette Delaloge, Ph.D.; Joseph Louis Glajch, Ph.D.; Ernest Victor Groman, Ph.D.; Gordon Craig Hill, Ph.D.; Aurelie Mieze-Richard, Pharm.D.; Patrick Noland, M.S.; Scott Roberts

Radioactive Drugs Expert Panel
JAMES A. PONTO, M.S., *Chair*
Corinne Bensimon, Ph.D.; Jonathan M. Fitzsimmons, Ph.D.; Umesh Gangadharmath, Ph.D.; Thijs Kroon, Pharm.D.; Adrian Nunn, Ph.D.; David Pipes, Ph.D.; Kara

Weatherman, Pharm.D.; Martin Williamson, Ph.D.; Steve Zigler, Ph.D.

Chemical Medicines Monographs 5
AMY J. KARREN, *Chair*
D.J. Doan, M.S; Sushil Gangwal, Ph.D.; Assad Kazeminy, Ph.D.; Min Li, Ph.D.; Judy Lin, M.S.; Pauline McGregor, Ph.D.; Marian Meyer, Ph.D., M.B.A.; Jonathan Parks; Justin Pennington, Ph.D.; Vijaya Ramesh, B.Pharm.; Gurvinder Singh Rekhi, Ph.D.; Iffaaz Salahudeen, Ph.D.; Mary W. Seibel; Hameraj Singh, Ph.D.; Michael Skibic, M.S.

Chemical Medicines Monographs 6
REINHARD WALTER, PH.D., *Chair*
Seamus Boland; Robert Graham Buice, Ph.D., M.B.A.; Timothy Gilmor, Ph.D.; Carmen Gonzalez, Ph.D.; John Joseph Herries, Ph.D.; Todd Lewis, M.S.; William Long, Ph.D.; Phil Nethercote, Ph.D.; Raphael Ornaf, Ph.D.; David Hitchcock Rogers, Ph.D.; Thomas Rosanske, Ph.D.; Christina Szabo, Ph.D.; Reinhard Walter, Ph.D.; Xiaoping Wang, Ph.D.; Kylen Whitaker, Ph.D.; Zeena Williams, Ph.D.

Acetaminophen OTC Expert Panel—CONCLUDED
KYLEN WHITAKER, PH.D., *Chair*
Tina M. Engel, Ph.D.; David A. Fay, Ph.D.; Saulius A. Gylys; Michael T. Rankin, M.S.; David H. Rogers, Ph.D.; Gregory K. Webster, Ph.D.; Jonathan Zeszotarski, Ph.D.

Biologics Monographs 1—Peptides
MIKE DE FELIPPIS, PH.D., *Chair*
Wilfried Arz, Ph.D.; Chaim Eidelman, Ph.D.; Gyongyi Gratzl, Ph.D.; Gerhard Haas, Ph.D.; Morten Hach, M.S.; Marion King, Ph.D.; Peter Larson; Jean-Marc Poudrel, Ph.D.; Harold Rode, Ph.D.; Raimon Rubires, Ph.D.; Zachary Shriver, Ph.D.; Ved Srivastava, Ph.D.; Michael Verlander, Ph.D.

Glatiramer Expert Panel
GYONGYI GRATZL, PH.D., *Chair*
Joseph Louis Glajch, Ph.D.; Satyanarayana Kota, Ph.D.; Barbara Mulloy, Ph.D.; Todd A. Osiek, Ph.D.; Marcia Cecilia Rusjan; Rakesh Singh Shekhawat, Ph.D.; Zachary Shriver, Ph.D.; Rene Thuermer, Ph.D.; Patrick Vallano, Ph.D.; Michael Verlander, Ph.D; Vera Weinstein, Ph.D.

Glucagon Expert Panel
HAROLD RODE, PH.D., *Chair*
Jan Amstrup, Ph.D.; Matthew W. Borer, Ph.D.; Gerhard Manfred Haas, Ph.D.; Anne Munk Jespersen, Ph.D.; Elizabeth Kramer, Ph.D.

Insulin Expert Panel
NED MOZIER, PH.D., *Chair*
Jan Amstrup, Ph.D.; Wilfried Arz, Ph.D.; Heather Boux, Ph.D.; Chris Burns, Ph.D.; Jill Crouse-Zeineddini, Ph.D.; Morten Hach, M.S.; Elizabeth Kramer, Ph.D.; Karthik Ramani, Ph.D.; Harold Rode, Ph.D.

Biologics Monographs 2—Proteins
MICHAEL MULKERRIN, PH.D., *Chair*
Gregory Beck, Ph.D.; Heather Boux, Ph.D.; Chris Burns, Ph.D.; Frédéric Carrière, Ph.D.; Michel Girard, Ph.D.; Anne Munk Jespersen; Sridevi Khambhampaty, Ph.D.; Robert Mayer, Ph.D.; Ned Mozier, Ph.D.; Dhananjay Patankar, Ph.D.; Mauricio Seigelchifer, Ph.D.; Jill Crouse-Zeineddini, Ph.D.

Enzyme Expert Panel
FRÉDÉRIC CARRIÈRE, PH.D., *Chair*
Gregory Beck, Ph.D.; Francis Dwulet, Ph.D.; Olaf Friedrich, Ph.D.; Luigi Giovanni Ghidorsi; Christopher

Hosty, M.S.; Vincent Jannin; Andreas Koerner, Ph.D.; Thomas K. Langdon, B.Sc.

Fc Function Assays Expert Panel
JILL CROUSE-ZEINEDDINI, PH.D., *Chair*
Shan Chung, Ph.D.; Marina Feschenko, Ph.D.; Scott Kuhns, Ph.D.; LeeAnn Machiesky, M.S.; Veena Pai Raiker, Ph.D.; Bhavin Parekh, Ph.D.; Teresa Surowy, Ph.D.; Max Tejada, Ph.D.

Biologics Monographs 3—Complex Biologics
EDWARD K. CHESS, PH.D., *Chair*
Mehrshid Alai, Ph.D.; Pascal Anger, Ph.D.; Parastoo Azadi, Ph.D.; Svetlana Bergelson, Ph.D.; Barbara Blum, Ph.D., M.P.H.; Mirella Ezban, Ph.D.; Elaine Gray, Ph.D.; Donald MacLean, Ph.D.; Nicole Provost, Ph.D.; Elizabeth I. Read, M.D.; Peter Vandeberg, Ph.D.; Christian Viskov, Ph.D.; Darin Weber, Ph.D.

Bovine Unfractionated Heparin Expert Panel— CONCLUDED
WESLEY E. WORKMAN, PH.D., *Chair*
Tania Andrade, B.S. Pharm.; Irene Bartoli, B.Sc.; Maria Leticia Bertot, Pharm.D.; Elaine Gray, Ph.D.; Marco Guerrini, Pharm.D.; Kristian Johansen, Ph.D.; Robert Linhardt, Ph.D.; Barbara Mulloy, Ph.D.; Marilene Nuss Rangel; Zachary Shriver, Ph.D.; Pearle Torralba, Ph.D.; Christian Viskov, Ph.D.

CD-34 Positive Cells Expert Panel—CONCLUDED
NICOLE M. PROVOST, PH.D., *Chair*
Ruud Hulspas, Ph.D.; Elizabeth I. Read, M.D.; Michael D. Rosu-Myles, Ph.D.; Luisa Saraiva, Ph.D.; Richard J. Stebbings, Ph.D.; D. Robert Sutherland, M.Sc.; Lili Wang, Ph.D.; Albertus W. Wognum, Ph.D.

Low Molecular Weight Heparins Expert Panel
ELAINE GRAY, PH.D., AND EDWARD K. CHESS, PH.D., *Co-Chairs*
Nicolas C.R. Amiot, Ph.D.; Christopher P. Bryant, Ph.D.; Ishan Capila, Ph.D.; Venkatesan S. Chidambaram, Ph.D.; Gyongyi S. Gratzl, Ph.D.; Kristian Johansen, Ph.D.; Annarapu Malleswara, Ph.D.; Barbara Mulloy, Ph.D.; Anna K.Y. Nordin; Bruna Parma, M.Sc.; Zachary Shriver, Ph.D.; Christian Viskov, Ph.D.

Low Molecular Weight Heparins Expert Panel
ELAINE GRAY, PH.D., AND EDWARD K. CHESS, PH.D., *Co-Chairs*
Nicolas C.R. Amiot, Ph.D.; Christopher P. Bryant, Ph.D.; Ishan Capila, Ph.D.; Venkatesan S. Chidambaram, Ph.D.; Gyongyi S. Gratzl, Ph.D.; Kristian Johansen, Ph.D.; Annarapu Malleswara, Ph.D.; Barbara Mulloy, Ph.D.; Anna K.Y. Nordin; Bruna Parma, M.Sc.; Zachary Shriver, Ph.D.; Christian Viskov, Ph.D.

Biologics Monographs 4—Antibiotics
PASCAL ANGER, PH.D., *Chair*
Elizabeth (Betsy) Bruce Cariello, B.A.; Sheila Deneau, B.Sc.; Colleen Guthrie, B.Sc.; Robert Klasson, M.S.; Mark G. Papich, M.S.; Cindy Reid, B.Sc.; Jennifer Jaye Schimmel, M.D.; Jonathan A. Stewart, B.Sc.; Yaozuo Yuan, Ph.D.

General Chapters—Biological Analysis
WESLEY E. WORKMAN, PH.D., *Chair*
Robert Bell, Ph.D.; Mahesh Bhalgat, Ph.D.; Christopher Jones, Ph.D.; Jeremy Kunkel, Ph.D.; Huijuan Li, Ph.D.; Kenneth Miller, Ph.D.; Anthony Mire-Sluis, Ph.D.; Anthony A.G. Ridgway, Ph.D.; Wendy Saffell-Clemmer, M.S.; Martin Vanderlaan, Ph.D.; Teruhide Yamaguchi, Ph.D.; Earl Zablackis, Ph.D.

Bioassay General Chapter
DAVID LANSKY, PH.D., *Chair*
Jan Amstrup, Ph.D.; Walter Hauck, Ph.D.; Bhavin Parekh, Ph.D.; Andrew Rugaiganisa, M.S.; Perceval Sondag, M.S.; Ralf Stegmann, Ph.D.; Ryan Yamagata, M.S.; Lingmin Zeng, Ph.D.

Biologics Stability Expert Panel
ANTHONY MIRE-SLUIS, PH.D., *Chair*
Kimberly Cheung, M.S.; Nila Das, Ph.D.; Stephanie Ferrari, M.S.; Jens Krogh Rasmussen, M.S.; Joseph Kutza, Ph.D.; Lori A. McCaig, Ph.D.; Cornelia Nickenig; Nausheen Rahman, Ph.D.; Camilla Santos, Ph.D.; Michael Walsh, M.S.; Allison Wolf, M.S.

Cell Banking Expert Panel
ROBERT BELL, PH.D., *Chair*
Jeri Ann Bosse, Ph.D.; Sunil Gairola, Ph.D.; Anne Gondran, Ph.D.; Luhong He, Ph.D.; Ruud Hulspas, Ph.D.; Jette Dina Kreiberg, Ph.D.; Michael Laird, Ph.D.; Lye Theng Lock, Ph.D.; Archie Lovatt, Ph.D.; Sam Yaghmour, M.S.; Earl Zablackis, Ph.D.

Residual DNA in Biotechnology-Derived Products Expert Panel
WESLEY E. WORKMAN, PH.D., *Chair*
Pascal R. Anger, Ph.D.; Jon R. Borman; Scott Kuhns, Ph.D.; Weihong Wang, Ph.D.; Judith Zhu-Shimoni, Ph.D.

Vaccine Polysaccharide NMR Identity Testing Expert Panel
CHRISTOPHER JONES, PH.D., *Chair*
Yves Aubin, Ph.D.; Francesco Berti, Ph.D.; Cristiana Campa, Ph.D.; Thomas P. Jacques, Ph.D.; Michael T. Jones, Ph.D.; Jeremy P. Kunkel, Ph.D.; Neil Ravenscroft, Ph.D.; Philippe Talaga, Ph.D.; Earl Zablackis, Ph.D.

Validation of Commercial Test Kits Expert Panel
KENNETH MILLER, PH.D., *Chair*
Heather Boux, Ph.D.; David Good, M.S.; Wendy Saffell-Clemmer, M.S.; Linda Starr-Spires, Ph.D.

Viral Vaccines Expert Panel
EARL ZABLACKIS, PH.D., *Chair*
Lopa Adhikary, Ph.D.; Luca Benetti, Ph.D.; Sunil Gairola, Ph.D.; Lucy Gisonni-Lex, M.S.; Keith Howard, Ph.D.; Christopher Jones, Ph.D.; Archie Lovatt, Ph.D.; Brij Patel, Ph.D.; Silke Schepelmann, Ph.D.; Vaneet Sharma, Ph.D.; Mark Van Ooij, Ph.D.

General Chapters—Chemical Analysis
NANCY LEWEN, B.SC., *Chair*
Anthony Bevilacqua, Ph.D.; Christopher Burgess, Ph.D.; Robert Cambron, Ph.D.; Thomas DiFeo, Ph.D.; John Dolan, Ph.D.; Joseph Louis Glajch, Ph.D.; John Hammond; John Hinshaw, Ph.D.; Brent Kleintop, Ph.D.; Steven Leinbach, M.S.; Gregory Martin, M.S.; Nuno Matos, B.Sc.; Oscar Quattrocchi, M.Sc.; Helmut Rockstroh, Ph.D.; Mark Schweitzer, Ph.D.; Timothy Shelbourn, M.S.; Rostyslaw O. Slabicky, B.Sc.; Teri Soli, Ph.D.; Kevin A. Swiss, Ph.D.; Timothy J. Wozniak, Ph.D.

Analytical Methodologies Based on the Light Scattering Phenomena Expert Panel
KEVIN SWISS, PH.D., *Chair*
Emilia Byrne, M.S.; Nila Das, Ph.D.; Joseph Louis Glajch, Ph.D.; Thomas Gonyon, B.Sc.; John Peter Hammond; Stephen Hussey; Chris Jones, Ph.D.; Jonathan Kingsbury, Ph.D.; Richard Meury, B.Sc.; Helmut Rockstroh, Ph.D.; Jack Saad, B.Sc.; William F. Weiss, Ph.D.; Eloise Welfare, Ph.D.; Earl Zablackis, Ph.D.

Chemometrics Expert Panel—CONCLUDED

PEI CHEN, PH.D., AND NUNO MATOS, *Co-Chairs*

Chunsheng Cai, Ph.D.; Robert Tom Cambron, Ph.D.; Peter de B. Harrington, Ph.D.; Mark J. Henson, Ph.D.; Yang (Angela) Liu, Ph.D.; Zhenqi (Pete) Shi, Ph.D.; Yvan C.D. Vander Heyden, Ph.D.; Stanislav O. Zakharkin, Ph.D.; Lin Zhang, Ph.D.

Elemental Impurities Expert Panel

NANCY LEWEN, B.SC., *Chair*

Charles Barton, Ph.D., DABT; Courtney M. Callis, M.P.H., DABT; Steven J. Dentali, Ph.D.; Anna M. Fan, Ph.D., DABT; Edward James Fletcher; Bruce A. Fowler, Ph.D., A.T.S.; Roland Frotschl; Assad J. Kazeminy, Ph.D.; Richard Ko, Pharm.D., Ph.D.; Timothy L. Shelbourn, M.B.A., M.S.

Good Documentation Practices Expert Panel—CONCLUDED

KIM C. HUYNH-BA, M.S., *Chair*

Kathleen V. Brady, B.S.; Frank J. Diana, Ph.D.; Lisa Ann Fink, M.B.A.; Craig Hamilton, Ph.D.; Judy Lin, M.S.; Anjan K. Mittal, M.Pharm.; Kevin A. Swiss, Ph.D.

Modernization of Identification Tests Expert Panel

NANCY LEWEN, B.SC., *Chair*

Anthony C. Bevilacqua, Ph.D.; Geoffrey P.R. Carr, Ph.D.; Pei Chen, Ph.D.; Jonathan W. DeVries, Ph.D.; Maryna Dmitriieva, Ph.D.; Michael Hornig, Ph.D.; Bernard A. Olsen, Ph.D.; Jeffrey S. Rohrer, Ph.D.

⟨467⟩ Residual Solvents Expert Panel

OSCAR A. QUATTROCCHI, M.SC., *Chair*

Coleman C. Chasteen, M.S.; John Connelly, Ph.D.; Jeffrey Fleitman, Ph.D.; John V. Hinshaw, Ph.D.; Bruce P. Johnson, Ph.D.; Eric C. Kesslen, Ph.D.; Brent Kleintop, Ph.D.; Elizabeth Kovacs; Paul W. Lockwood, M.S.; Gregory P. Martin, M.S.; Kevin A. Swiss, Ph.D.; Yuwen Wang, Ph.D.

Quality Standards for Pharmaceutical Continuous Manufacturing Expert Panel

NUNO MATOS, B.SC., *Chair*

Shaukat Ali, Ph.D.; Ahmad Almaya; Brian Carlin, Ph.D.; Thomas Garcia, Ph.D.; Douglas Hausner, Ph.D.; Eric Jayjock, Ph.D.; Keith Jensen, Ph.D.; Johannes Khinast; Pramod Kotwal; Marcus Krumme, Ph.D.; Kim Lamey, Ph.D.; Fernando Muzzio, Ph.D.; William Randolph, Ph.D.; Mark Schweitzer, Ph.D.; Raymond Skwierczynski, Ph.D.; Kelly Swinney, Ph.D.; Bernhardt Tout, Ph.D.; Amy Walia, M.A.

Validation and Verification Expert Panel

GREGORY P. MARTIN, M.S., *Chair*

Kimber L. Barnett, Ph.D.; Christopher Burgess, Ph.D.; Paul D. Curry, Ph.D.; Gyongyi S. Gratzl, Ph.D.; John P. Hammond, FRSC; Elizabeth Kovacs; David J. LeBlond, Ph.D.; Rosario LoBrutto, Ph.D.; Pauline L. McGregor, Ph.D.; Phil Nethercote, Ph.D.; Allen C. Templeton, Ph.D.; David P. Thomas, Ph.D.; M.L. Jane Weitzel

Water for Analytical and Pharmaceutical Purposes Expert Panel

TERI C. SOLI, PH.D., *Chair*

Anthony C. Bevilacqua, Ph.D.; Lucia Clontz, D.H.Sc., M.Sc.; Max S. Lazar; Nancy Lewen, B.Sc.; Bruno Rossi, M.S.; Rostyslaw O. Slabicky, B.Sc.

General Chapters—Physical Analysis

XIAORONG HE, PH.D., *Chair*

Shaukat Ali, Ph.D.; Lawrence H. Block, Ph.D.; Geoff Carr, Ph.D.; Martin Coffey, Ph.D.; Tim Freeman; David J. Goldfarb, Ph.D.; Bruno Hancock, Ph.D.; Stephen Hoag, Ph.D.; Mario Hubert, Ph.D.; Richard Meury; Matthew Mullarney, M.S.; Prabu Nambiar, Ph.D.; Myke Scoggins, Ph.D.; Changquan Sun, Ph.D.; Zhigang Sun, Ph.D.; Allen Templeton, Ph.D.; Eloise Welfare, Ph.D.; Dale Wurster, Ph.D.; Bing-Shiou Yang, Ph.D.; Geoff Zhang, Ph.D.

Impurities in Drug Substance and Drug Products Expert Panel

PRABU NAMBIAR, PH.D., M.B.A., *Chair*

Shaukat Ali, Ph.D.; Steven W. Baertschi, Ph.D.; Judy P. Boehlert, Ph.D.; Robert G. Buice, Ph.D.; Greg J. Davies; Xiaorong He, Ph.D., M.B.A.; Kim C. Huynh-Ba, M.S.; Michael Koberda, Ph.D.; Robert E. Osterberg, R.Ph., Ph.D., Fellow-ATS; Ernest Parente, Ph.D.; Oscar Quattrocchi, M.Sc.; David H. Rogers, Ph.D.; Mark Schweitzer, Ph.D.; Mary W. Seibel; Rostyslaw O. Slabicky, B.Sc.; Teri C. Soli, Ph.D.; Kevin A. Swiss, Ph.D.

General Chapters—Dosage Forms

JAMES E. DE MUTH, PH.D., *Chair*

Emmanuel Akala, Ph.D.; Ilgaz Akseli, Ph.D.; Scott Aldrich; Susan Cady, M.S.; Paul Curry, Ph.D.; Mario González, Ph.D.; Vivian A. Gray, B.S.; Ralph Heasley, Ph.D.; Anthony Hickey, Ph.D.; Michael Houghton; Munir A. Hussain, Ph.D.; Johannes Krämer, Ph.D.; Stefan Leiner, Ph.D.; David Long, Ph.D.; John Mauger, Ph.D.; Colin Minchom, Ph.D.; Jolyon Mitchell, Ph.D.; Muller Pierre-Alain, Ph.D.; Guirag Poochikian, Ph.D.; Chetan Pujara, Ph.D.; Shobhan Sabnis, Ph.D.; John Shabushnig, Ph.D.; Raymond D. Skwierczynski, Ph.D.; Jason Suggett, Ph.D., M.B.A.; Monica Tejwani, Ph.D.; Thomas Tice, Ph.D.; Kevin Warner, Ph.D.; Mehran Yazdanian, Ph.D.

⟨771⟩ Ophthalmic Preparation Expert Panel

ASHIM K. MITRA, PH.D., *Chair*

Dale S. Aldrich, Ph.D.; Martin Coffey, Ph.D.; Paul Curry, Ph.D.; Jeffrey S. Fleitman, Ph.D.; John Mauger, Ph.D.; Seshadri Neervannan, Ph.D.; Stacey M. Platzer; Chetan Pujara, Ph.D.; Satish K. Singh, Ph.D.; Monica Tejwani, Ph.D.; Thomas R. Tice, Ph.D.

⟨788⟩ Particulate Matter in Injections Expert Panel

DALE S. ALDRICH, PH.D., *Chair*

Dan Berdovich; Mary Lee Ciolkowski, Ph.D.; Kevin Dahl, Ph.D.; Linda Narhi, Ph.D.; Kent A. Peterson; Dean Ripple, Ph.D.

Liquid-Filled Capsules Expert Panel

VIVIAN A. GRAY, B.S., *Chair*

Joe Fotso, Ph.D.; Munir A. Hussain, Ph.D.; Stephen C. Tindal; Madhusudan Vudathala, M.Pharm., M.B.A.

Performance Test for Semisolid Dosage Forms Expert Panel

KAILAS THAKKER, PH.D., *Chair*

Bryan Crist; James E. De Muth, Ph.D.; Geoffrey N. Grove, Ph.D.; L. Thomas Hall, Ph.D.; John S. Heaney; Patricia L. Lee, M.S.; Patrick C. Mahn; William M. Rosenthal; Steve W. Shaw

Solubility Criteria for Veterinary Drugs Expert Panel

SUSAN CADY M.S., *Chair*

Bryan Crist; Mario A. Gonzalez, Ph.D.; Mark G. Papich, M.S., D.V.M.; Alan F. Parr, Pharm.D., Ph.D.; Monica Tejwani, Ph.D.

Sutures Expert Panel

JAMES E. DE MUTH, PH.D., *Chair*

Edwin Anderson, M.S.; John C. Chen; Frank Corniello; Nomi Steen

Use of Enzymes in the Dissolution Testing of Gelatin Capsules Expert Panel

VIVIAN A. GRAY, B.S., *Chair*

Ewart Cole, Ph.D.; Luigi Ghidorsi; Jian-Hwa Guo, Ph.D.; Feixue Han, Ph.D.; Jian-Hwa Han, Ph.D.; Christopher T.

Hosty; Jianmei D. Kochling, Ph.D.; Johannes Krämer, Ph.D.; Thomas Langdon; Steven R. Leinbach; Stefan Leiner, Ph.D.; Gregory P. Martin, M.S.; Steven M. Meyerhoffer, Ph.D.; Richard C. Moreton, Ph.D.; Krishnaswamy S. Raghavan, Ph.D.; Edward Shneyvas, Ph.D.; Jason A. Suggett, Ph.D.; Stephen C. Tindal; Madhusudan Vudathala, M.Pharm., M.B.A.; Hu Wang, M.S.

Visual Inspection of Parenterals Expert Panel
RUSSELL E. MADSEN, M.S., *Chair*
Dale S. Aldrich, Ph.D.; John D. Ayres, M.D., J.D.; Roy Cherris; John G. Shabushnig, Ph.D.; Deborah Shnek, Ph.D.

General Chapters—Microbiology
DAVID HUSSONG, PH.D., *Chair*
James Agalloco, M.S.; James Akers, Ph.D.; Dilip Ashtekar, Ph.D.; Anthony Cundell, Ph.D.; Dennis Guilfoyle, Ph.D.; Rajesh Gupta, Ph.D.; Russell Madsen, M.S.; Karen McCullough, M.S.; Robert Mello, Ph.D.; David Roesti, Ph.D.; Donald Singer, M.S.; Paul Stinavage, Ph.D.; Edward Tidswell, Ph.D.

Modern Microbiological Methods Expert Panel
ANTHONY CUNDELL, PH.D., AND EDWARD TIDSWELL, PH.D., *Co-Chairs*
Thierry Bonnevay, Ph.D.; Ralph Breton, B.S. Pharm.; Claudio Denoya, Ph.D.; Gary du Moulin, Ph.D.; John Duguid, B.Sc.; Rajesh Gupta, Ph.D.; David Hussong, Ph.D.; Matthew Jenkins, M.S.; Amy Lynn McDaniel, Ph.D.; Michael Miller, Ph.D.; Felix Montero Julian, Ph.D.; David Newon, Ph.D.; Kuldip Patel; Steven Richter, Ph.D.; David Roesti, Ph.D.; Yongqiang Zhang, Ph.D.; Steve S. Zigler, Ph.D.

General Chapters—Packaging and Distribution
MARY G. FOSTER, PHARM.D., BFA, *Chair*
Chris Anderson, M.A.; Bettine Boltres, Ph.D.; Glaucia Braga, Ph.D.; Jeffrey Carrico, Pharm.D.; Chris Chandler, Pharm.D.; Michael N. Eakins, Ph.D.; Dana Guazzo, Ph.D.; Renaud Janssen, Ph.D.; Dennis Jenke, Ph.D.; Wendy Mach, B.Sc.; Dan Malinowski; Daniel Norwood, Ph.D.; Devinder Pal, M.Pharm.; Diane Paskiet, M.S.; Robert Seevers, Ph.D.; Cheryl Stults, Ph.D.; Li Xiong, Ph.D.; Gao Yonghua, B.S.Pharm.

⟨381⟩ Elastomeric Closure for Injections Expert Panel
DIANE M. PASKIET, M.S., AND RENAUD JANSSEN, PH.D., *Co-Chairs*
Douglas J. Ball, M.S., DABT; Michael N. Eakins, Ph.D.; Dana Guazzo, Ph.D.; Dennis R. Jenke, Ph.D.; Douglas Kiehl, M.S., B.S.; Heinz Kirchmeyer, Ph.D.; Philippe LeGall, M.S.; Daniel L. Norwood, Ph.D.; Michael A. Ruberto, Ph.D.; Lisa M. Yoest, M.S.

⟨659⟩ Packaging and Storage Requirements Expert Panel—CONCLUDED
CHRIS CHANDLER, PHARM.D., *Chair*
Glaucia Braga, B.Sc.; Jeffrey Carrico, Pharm.D.; Mary G. Foster, Pharm.D. BFA; Eleanor Freeman, B.S.; Wendy Mach, B.Sc.; Devinder Pal, M.Pharm.; Robert H. Seevers, Ph.D.; Gao Yonghua, B.S. Pharm; Li Xiong, Ph.D.

⟨660⟩ Containers—Glass Expert Panel
BETTINE BOLTRES, PH.D., AND MICHAEL EAKINS, PH.D., *Co-Chairs*
Michael E. Akers, B.A.; Alberto Biavati, Ph.D.; Juan Cerdan-Diaz; Carol Rea Flynn, M.S.; Emanuel Guadagnino, M.D.; Daniel Edward Haines, Ph.D.; Kelly Murphy, Ph.D.; Volker Rekowski; Jennifer Martell Roark, B.Sc.; Holger Roehl, Ph.D.; Gao Yonghua, B.S. Pharm.; Jingwei Zhang, Ph.D.

Biocompatibility of Materials Used in Packaging Systems, Medical Devices, and Implants Expert Panel
DANIEL L. NORWOOD, PH.D., *Chair*
Douglas J. Ball, M.S.; Stephen A. Barat, Ph.D.; William P. Beierschmitt, Ph.D.; Denise Bohrer, Ph.D.; Tage C.G. Carlson, Ph.D.; Michael N. Eakins, Ph.D.; Jill A. Glosson, B.A.; John Iannone, B.Sc.; Renaud Janssen, Ph.D.; Douglas E. Kiehl, M.Sc.; Wendy Mach, B.Sc.; Robert Przygoda; Anita Y. Sawyer, M.S.; Cheryl Stults, Ph.D.

Clinical Trial Materials (GDP) Expert Panel—CONCLUDED
MARY G. FOSTER, PHARM.D., BFA, *Chair*
Christopher Anderson, M.A.; Rafik H. Bishara, Ph.D.; Glaucia K. Braga, Ph.D.; Jeffrey Carrico, Pharm.D.; Steven A. Jacobs, M.B.A.; Martin Jeiven, M.S.; Claude Jolicoeur, B.S.; Gao Yonghua, B.S. Pharm.

⟨661.3⟩ Plastic Systems Used for Manufacturing Pharmaceutical Products Expert Panel
DENNIS R. JENKE, PH.D., *Chair*
Weibing Ding, Ph.D.; Michael N. Eakins, Ph.D.; Mary G. Foster, Pharm.D., BFA; James Hathcock, Ph.D.; Jerold (Jerry) M. Martin, M.S.; Diane M. Paskiet, M.S.; Robert Steininger; Cheryl L.M. Stults, Ph.D.; Ken M. Wong, M.Sc.

⟨662⟩ Metal Packaging Components and Systems
CHERYL STULTS, PH.D., *Chair*
Peter Claessens; Benjamin Jeyaretnam, Ph.D.; Ralph Lessor, Ph.D.; Gaby Reckzuegel; John Willenbrock, B.Sc.

General Chapters—Statistics
ROBERT R. SINGER, M.S., *Chair*
Bruno Boulanger, Ph.D.; Richard Burdick, Ph.D.; David Christopher, M.S.; David Lansky, Ph.D.; Dave LeBlond, Ph.D.; Juris Meija, Ph.D.; Anthony Okinczyc, M.P.H.; Peter Rigsby, M.S.; Dennis Sandell, Ph.D.; Timothy Schofield, M.A.; Charles Tan, Ph.D.; Edwin van den Heuvel, Ph.D.; Jane Weitzel; Harry Yang, Ph.D.

Content Uniformity with Large Sample Sizes Expert Panel
DENNIS SANDELL, PH.D., *Chair*
Ilgaz Akseli; James S. Bergum, Ph.D.; Paul Curry, Ph.D.; Walter Hauck, Ph.D.; Jeffrey Hofer, M.S.; Gregory L. Larner, M.S.; Raymond Skwierczynski, Ph.D.

Expert Committees for the *National Formulary*

Excipients Monographs 1
ERIC MUNSON, PH.D., *Chair*
Thiago Carvalho, Ph.D.; Brian Carlin, Ph.D.; Richard Cawthorne, Ph.D.; Richard Creekmore, Ph.D.; Vivek Dave, Ph.D.; Felicitas Guth; Otilia Koo, Ph.D.; Phil Merrell, Ph.D.; Dominic Moore; Chris Moreton, Ph.D.; Jasmine Musakhanian, M.S.; Charles Vesey, M.S.; Richard Wendt, Ph.D.; Jin Zhao, Ph.D.

⟨1059⟩ Chapter Excipient Performance Expert Panel
GREGORY AMIDON, PH.D., AND RICHARD MORETON, PH.D., *Co-Chairs*
Ilgaz Akseli; Shaukat Ali, Ph.D.; Lawrence Block, Ph.D.; Thiago Cardoso Carvalho, Ph.D.; Brian Carlin, Ph.D.; Richard Creekmore, Ph.D.; Stephen Hoag, Ph.D.; Johannes Khinast; Jasmine Musakhanian, M.S.; Natarajan Rajagopalan, Ph.D.; Hiroko Shibata, Ph.D.; Jiasheng Tu, Ph.D.; Katherine Ulman, B.Sc.; Maureen Taylor Vander Fliet, M.S.; John Wang, Ph.D.

⟨1059⟩ Excipient Performance Expert Panel—CONCLUDED
ERIC A. SCHMITT, PH.D., *Chair*
> Abdullah M. Al-Mohizea, Ph.D.; Shaukat Ali, Ph.D.; Lawrence H. Block, Ph.D.; Patrick Deluca, Ph.D.; Carl Frey, M.S.; Xiaorong He, Ph.D., M.B.A.; Stephen W. Hoag, Ph.D.; Michelle A. Long, Ph.D.; Richard C. Moreton, Ph.D.; Prabu Nambiar, Ph.D., M.B.A.; James A. Ponto, M.S.; Kent Sternitzke, Ph.D.; Kevin A. Swiss, Ph.D.; Sean V. Taylor, Ph.D.

⟨1197⟩ Good Distribution Practices for Bulk Pharmaceutical Excipients Expert Panel—CONCLUDED
RICHARD C. MORETON, PH.D., *Chair*
> Lawrence H. Block, Ph.D.; William Dale Carter, M.S.; Zak T. Chowhan, Ph.D.; Marc Fages; Elizabeth Ferguson-Brown; Mary G. Foster, Pharm.D., BFA; Linda A. Herzog, M.B.A.; Ashok V. Katdare, Ph.D.; Zakiya Kurdi, Ph.D.; Edward G. Malawer, Ph.D., CQA; Frank Milek, Ph.D.; Becca Mitchell; Dwight Mutchler; Garnet E. Peck, Ph.D.; Mike Schultz, R.Ph.; Alexa Smith, M.S.; Glenn Sokoloski; Kelly Taylor; Jiasheng Tu, Ph.D.

Excipients Monographs 2
MARY C. HOUCK, PH.D., *Chair*
> Lawrence H. Block, Ph.D.; Andrew Bluj; Tim Cabelka, Ph.D.; Arya Jayatilaka, Ph.D.; Russell Maus, Ph.D.; Robert E. Osterberg, R.Ph., Ph.D., Fellow-ATS; Julie Warner Pier, M.S.; Anisul Quadir, Ph.D.; Gwen Rucker; Barbara Serr, Ph.D.; Huimin Sun, Ph.D.; Jiasheng Tu, Ph.D.; Jacqueline Tordik; Fan Wu, Ph.D.; Timothy Yasika

Glycerin Expert Panel
TIM B. CABELKA, PH.D., *Chair*
> Frances K. Byrne, M.S.; Ian A. Duncan, Ph.D.; Tanja Natterer; Marian J. Rinken, Ph.D.; Gwen E. Rucker, B.S.; David A. Sharknas, B.S.; Hong Zhou, Ph.D.

Povidones Expert Panel—CONCLUDED
BERNHARD D. FUSSNEGGER, PH.D., AND CARL PERINI, M.S., *Co-Chairs*
> Feng Chen, Ph.D.; David J. Fillar, M.B.A.; Edward G. Malawer, Ph.D.; Syed A.A. Rizvi, Ph.D.; John W. Spink, Ph.D.; Fan Wu, Ph.D.

Talc Methods Expert Panel
JULIE WARNER PIER, M.S., AND MARTIN RUTSTEIN, PH.D., *Co-Chairs*
> Daniel Crane; Sean M. Fitzgerald, B.Sc.; Mickey E. Gunter, Ph.D.; Don Halterman, M.S.; Mary C. Houck, Ph.D.; Lee Poye, B.Sc.; Matthew S. Sanchez, Ph.D.; Alan M. Segrave, B.Sc.; Gary P. Tomanino, B.Sc.; Drew R. Van Ordern, M.A.; James Webber, Ph.D.

Expert Committees for the *USP* and the *Dietary Supplements Compendium*

Botanical Dietary Supplements and Herbal Medicines
ROBIN J. MARLES, PH.D., *Chair*
> Nana Fredua Bafi-Yeboa, M.S.; Thomas Brendler, B.A.; Josef A. Brinckmann; Paula Naomi Brown, Ph.D.; Angela Calderon, Ph.D.; Steven Dentali, Ph.D.; Edward Fletcher, B.A.; Stefan Gafner, Ph.D.; Joerg Gruenwald, Ph.D.; De-an Guo, Ph.D.; Sukhdev Swami Handa, M.Pharm., Ph.D.; James Harnly, Ph.D.; Craig Hopp, Ph.D.; Scott A. Jordan, Ph.D.; Ikhlas Khan, Ph.D.; Richard Ko, Pharm.D.; Tieraona Low Dog, M.D.; Mirtha Navarro, Ph.D.; Pilar Pais, Ph.D.; Guido Pauli, Pharm.D., Ph.D.; Eike Reich, Ph.D.; Paul Schiff, Ph.D.; Shangmei Shi, B.Sc.

Green Tea Extract Hepatotoxicity Expert Panel
RICHARD KO, PHARM.D., *Chair*
> Amy Lynne Roe, Ph.D.; Joseph M. Betz, Ph.D.; Bill Gurley, Ph.D.; Kan He, Ph.D.; Scott Jordan, Ph.D.; Mahendra P. Kapoor, Ph.D.; Tieraona Low Dog, M.D.; Robin James Marles, Ph.D.; Victor Navarro, M.D.

Herbal Medicines Compendium (HMC) East Asia Expert Panel
DE-AN GUO, PH.D., *Chair*
> Yuan-shiun Chang, Ph.D.; ShiLin Chen, Ph.D.; Takashi Hakamatsuka, Ph.D.; Shen Ji, Ph.D.; Yeong Shik Kim, Ph.D.; Hwee-Ling Koh, Ph.D.; Clara Bik San Lau, Ph.D; Ping Li, Ph.D.; Qing Li, Ph.D.; Shuangcheng Ma, Ph.D.; Shangmei Shi; Viet Hung Tran, Ph.D.; Pengfei Tu, Ph.D.; Wanying Wu, Ph.D.; Zhongzhen Zhao, Ph.D.

Herbal Medicines Compendium (HMC) South Asia Expert Panel
SUKHDEV S. HANDA, PH.D., FNAIM, FNA.SC, *Chair*
> Amit Agarwal, Ph.D.; Rasadah Mat Ali, Ph.D.; Mohamed Zahir Mohammed Farhad; C.K. Katiyar, Ph.D.; Ami Fazlin Syed Mohamed, Ph.D.; A. Nagarajan, Ph.D.; D.G. Naik, Ph.D.; Sankaran Natarajan, Ph.D.; M.K. Raina, Ph.D.; J.L.N. Sastry, Ph.D.; Rajeev Kr. Sharma, Ph.D.; R. Sundaram, Ph.D.; Neeraj Tandon, Ph.D.; Surapote Wongyai, Ph.D.

Dietary Supplements Safety Modeling—CONCLUDED
MARY L. HARDY, M.D., *Chair*
> V.A. Shiva Ayyadurai, Ph.D.; Mary A. Fox, Ph.D., M.P.H.; Scott A. Jordan, Ph.D.; Mkaya Mwamburi, M.D., MA (Econ); Diane R. Mould, Ph.D.; Robert E. Osterberg, R.Ph., Ph.D., Fellow-ATS; Charlie Yoe, Ph.D.

Cannabis Expert Panel
IKHLAS A. KHAN, PH.D., *Chair*
> Paula N. Brown, Ph.D.; Lawrence Deyton, M.D.; Mahmoud A. Elsohly, Ph.D.; Sytze Elzinga, M.S.; Philippe Henry, Ph.D.; Christopher Hudalla, Ph.D.; Holly Johnson, Ph.D.; Robin Marles, Ph.D.; Jeremy Melanson, Ph.D.; Rao S. Rapaka, Ph.D.; Roy Upton; Gordon Vrdoljak, Ph.D.; Joshua Wurzer, B.Sc.

Non-Botanical Dietary Supplements
DENNIS K.J. GORECKI, B.S.P., PH.D., *Chair*
> Joseph Betz, Ph.D.; Michael Bradley, M.S.; James Brooks, Ph.D.; Bill Gurley, Ph.D.; Chung Hyun, M.S.; Joy Joseph, M.S.; Raimar Löbenberg, Ph.D.; Richard Myers, Ph.D.; James Neal-Kababick, B.Sc.; Peter Rice, Pharm.D., Ph.D.; Amy Roe, Ph.D.; Aniko Solyom, Ph.D.; Karunakar Sukuru, Ph.D.; Darryl Sullivan, Ph.D.; Edward Waysek, Ph.D.

⟨2251⟩ Adulteration of Dietary Supplements with Drugs and Drug Analogs Expert Panel
DENNIS K.J. GORECKI, B.S.P., PH.D., *Chair*
> Joseph M. Betz, Ph.D.; Pei Chen, Ph.D.; Hans Geyer, Ph.D.; Jana B. Hildreth, B.A.; Hwee-Ling Koh, Ph.D.; Ikhlas A. Khan, Ph.D.; Cynthia L. Morris-Kukoski, Pharm.D., DABAT, FAACT; James Neal-Kababick, B.Sc.; Olivier Rabin, Ph.D.; John Spink, Ph.D.; Darryl Sullivan, Ph.D.; Nicole Vu, Ph.D.; Kate Yu, Ph.D.

Extended-Release Dietary Supplements Expert Panel—CONCLUDED
JOY A. JOSEPH, M.S., *Chair*
> Charles Barton, Ph.D., DABT; Joseph F. Borzelleca, Ph.D.; Michael S. Bradley, M.S.; James R. Brooks, Ph.D.; Marion Ehrich, Ph.D.; Vivian A. Gray, B.S.; Carol Johnston, Ph.D., RD; Raimar Löbenberg, Ph.D.; Alexander G. Schauss, Ph.D., FACN; Elizabeth A. Yetley, Ph.D.

Probiotics Expert Panel
MARY ELLEN SANDERS, *Chair*
Mike Bradley, M.S.; James Brooks, Ph.D.; Pierre Burguiere, Ph.D.; Scott Jackson, Ph.D.; David Keller; Marco Pane, M.S.; Amy Roe, Ph.D.; Jean Schoeni, Ph.D.; Bufy Stahl, B.Sc.; Christina Skovgaard Vegge, Ph.D.

Expert Committees for the *Food Chemicals Codex*

Food Ingredients
JONATHAN W. DEVRIES, PH.D., *Chair*
Richard C. Cantrill, Ph.D.; Junshi Chen, M.D.; Hwei-Fang Cheng, Ph.D.; Henry Chin, Ph.D.; Grady Chism, Ph.D.; Robin Churchill, Ph.D.; Roger Clemens, DrPH; John Clos, Ph.D.; Helen Darling, Ph.D.; Andrew Ebert, Ph.D.; Jaap Evers, Ph.D.; Carl Frey, M.S.; Einat Haleva, Ph.D.; Lori Klopf, Ph.D.; Hemant G. Koshia, Ph.D.; Dana Krueger, B.Sc.; Diane McColl, J.D.; Bert Popping, Ph.D.; Yoko Uematsu, Ph.D.; Yongning Wu, Ph.D.; Liangli Yu, Ph.D.

Food Adulteration Expert Panel
HENRY CHIN, PH.D., *Chair*
Grant Abernethy, Ph.D.; David Bolliet; Richard C. Cantrill, Ph.D.; Christophe Cavin, Ph.D.; Robin Churchill, Ph.D.; Helen Darling, Ph.D.; Jonathan W. DeVries, Ph.D.; Andrew Ebert, Ph.D.; Kim Huynh-Ba, M.S.; Shaun Kennedy; Dana Krueger, B.Sc.; Michele Lees, Ph.D.; Fernando Antunes Lopes; Bert Popping, Ph.D.; Lars Reimann, M.S.; Roman Romero, Ph.D.; Thomas Tarantelli, B.Sc.; Yoko Uematsu, Ph.D.; Saskia van Ruth, Ph.D.; Carl Winter, Ph.D.; Yongning Wu, Ph.D.

Food Adulterants Hazard Identification Expert Panel
HENRY CHIN, PH.D., *Chair*
Andrew Ebert, Ph.D.; Richard Lane, Ph.D.; Diane McColl, J.D.; Bert Popping, Ph.D.; Joseph Scimeca; Carl Winter, Ph.D.

Non-Targeted Methods for Milk Ingredients Expert Panel—CONCLUDED
ROBERT MAGALETTA, PH.D., *Chair*
Sned Bhandari, Ph.D.; Jonathan W. DeVries, Ph.D.; Gerard Downey, Ph.D.; Stephen Ellison, Ph.D.; James M. Harnly, Ph.D.; Elizabeth Hobbs; Steven Holroyd, Ph.D.; Gregory A. Israelson, B.Sc.; Joseph Katzenmeyer; Andrew Mackey, Ph.D.; Benjamin B. Perston, Ph.D.; Jianwei Qin, Ph.D.; Roman Romero, Ph.D.; Paul Wehling; Thomas Wheat, Ph.D.; Steven Zbylut, Ph.D.

Olive Oil Authenticity and Quality Expert Panel
RICHARD C. CANTRILL, PH.D., *Chair*
Diego Luis Garcia-Gonzalez, Ph.D.; Claudia Guillaume, M.Sc.; Zohar Kerem, Ph.D.; Paul H. Miller, B.A.; Agusti Jordi Romero, Ph.D.; Selina Wang, Ph.D.

Expert Committees for the *USP* and *USP on Compounding*

Compounding
GIGI S. DAVIDSON, B.S. PHARM., DICVP, *Chair*
Lisa Ashworth, B.S. Pharm., R.Ph.; Gus Bassani, Pharm.D.; Edmund J. Elder, Jr., Ph.D.; Ryan Forrey, Pharm.D., M.S.; Deborah Houston, Pharm.D.; Brenda Jensen, M.A.; Patricia C. Kienle, M.P.A.; William A. Mixon, M.S.; John Musil, Pharm.D.; David Newton,

Ph.D.; Alan Parr, Pharm.D., Ph.D.; Abby Roth; Robert Shrewsbury, Ph.D.; Connie Rae Sullivan, B.S. Pharm.; James T. Wagner; Brenda Yuzdepski, B.S. Pharm.

Compounding with Hazardous Drugs Expert Panel—CONCLUDED
PATRICIA C. KIENLE, M.P.A., *Chair*
Thomas H. Connor, Ph.D.; Eric Kastango, M.B.A., B.S. Pharm.; Melissa A. McDiarmid, M.D., M.P.H.; Kenneth R. Mead, Ph.D.; Martha Polovich, Ph.D.; Lucille A. Power; James T. Wagner

Government Liaisons to Expert Committees and Expert Panels

Jibril Abdus-Samad, Ph.D.; Eileen Abt, Ph.D.; Rajiv Agarwal, Ph.D.; Mohammed Ahmed, M.S.; Om Anand, Ph.D.; Shalini Anand, Ph.D.; Kristen Anderson, Ph.D.; Matthew Barlow, RN, BSN; Julie N. Barrows, Ph.D.; Jacinta Batson, M.B.A.; Eden Bermingham, DVM, M.S., DACVCP; Ashwinkumar Bhirde, Ph.D.; Jonathan Bray, B.S.; Michael Brent; Michael Brewer, Ph.D.; Daniel Brown, Janice Brown, M.S.; Bruney Lana, Ph.D.; Lucinda Buhse, Ph.D.; Teresa Cain, Ph.D.; Steven Casper, Ph.D.; Wiley Chambers, M.D.; Jane Chang, Ph.D.; Anissa Cheung, Ph.D.; Donna Christner, Ph.D.; John Cipollo, Ph.D.; David Claffey, Ph.D.; Maegen Colehour, M.S.; Celia Noemi Cruz, Ph.D.; Mike Darj, Ph.D.; Swapan De, Ph.D.; Ian DeVeau, Ph.D., Ph.D.; Julie Dohm, Ph.D.; Zedong Dong, Ph.D.; Jason Dreabit, M.A.; Stephanie Emory, Ph.D.; Okponanabofa Eradiri, Ph.D.; Cory Evans, Ph.D.; Raafat Fahmy, Ph.D.; Adam Fisher, Ph.D.; Daniel Folmer, Ph.D.; Rick Friedman, M.S.; Michael Furness, M.S.; Christopher Galliford, Ph.D.; Zongming Gao, Ph.D.; Mary Papa Ghods, RPh; Mohamed Ghorab, Ph.D.; Tapash Ghosh, Ph.D.; Devinder Gill, Ph.D.; Gurpreet Gill-Sangha, Ph.D.; Lillie Golson, Pharm.D.; Jennifer Goode, Ph.D.; Edisa Gozun, Pharm.D.; Yin Guo, Ph.D.; William Hallett, Ph.D.; Blake Hamann, Ph.D.; Bruce Harris, Ph.D.; Danielle Marie Harris, Pharm.D.; Joel Hathaway, Ph.D.; Mohammad Heidaran, Ph.D.; William Hess, B.S. Pharm; Yong Hu, Ph.D.; Gloria Huang, Ph.D.; Laura Huffman, M.S.; Gregory Hunter, Ph.D.; Latiff Hussain, Ph.D.; Mai Huynh, Ph.D.; Robert Iser, M.S.; Karthik Iyer, Ph.D.; Edwin Jao, Ph.D.; Young Jhon; Ravindra Kasliwal, Ph.D.; David Keire, Ph.D.; Michael Kennedy, Ph.D.; James Kenney, Ph.D.; Saeed Khan, Ph.D.; Erin Kim, Ph.D.; Kathryn E. King, Ph.D.; Bogdan Kurtyka, Ph.D.; David Lau, M.A.; Hyoung S. Lee, Ph.D.; Sau Lee, Ph.D.; David Lewis, Ph.D.; Xihao Li; Jing Li, Ph.D.; Jennifer Liang, Ph.D.; June Liang, Ph.D.; Tsai-Lien Lin, Ph.D.; Ewa Marszal, Ph.D.; Marilyn Martinez, Ph.D.; Timothy McGovern, Ph.D.; Jeffrey Medwid, Ph.D.; Randa Melhem, Ph.D.; John Metcalfe, Ph.D.; Yana Mille, B.S. Pharm; Adil Mohammad, Ph. D.; Magdi Mossoba, Ph.D.; Laura Moussa, Ph.D.; Karunakar Neelam, Ph.D.; Nina Ni, Ph.D.; Pallavi Nithyanandan, Ph.D.; Scott Edward Norris, Ph.D.; Rachel Novak, Ph.D.; Sarai Obando, Ph.D.; Thomas O'Connor, Ph.D.; Steven Oh, Ph.D.; Andrea Ottesen, Ph.D.; Frank Perrella, Ph.D.; Erika Pfeiler, Ph.D.; Laura Pogue, Ph.D.; Zhihao Peter Qiu, Ph.D.; Radhika Rajagopalan, Ph.D.; Muthukumar Ramaswamy, Ph.D.; Sam G. Raney, Ph.D.; Ashutosh Rao, Ph.D.; Shahnaz Read, Ph.D.; Bhagwant Rege, Ph.D.; James Rice, Ph.D.; Jason Rodriguez, Ph.D.; Sara Rothman; Allen Rudman, Ph.D.; R.D. Satzger, Ph.D.; Zuben Erach Sauna, Ph.D.; Deborah Schmiel; Ph.D.; Suzanne Sechen, Ph.D.; Hamid Shafiei, Ph.D.; Rakhi Shah, Ph.D.; Balajee Shanmugam, Ph.D.; Meiyu Shen, Ph.D.; Xiaobin Shen, Ph.D.; Akhtar Siddiqui, Ph.D.; Mark Skasko, Ph.D.; Cynthia Sommers, Ph.D., Fenhong Song, Ph.D.; Charudharshini Srinivasan, Ph.D.; Jannavi Srinivasan, Ph.D.; Benjamin Stevens, M.P.H.; Marla Stevens-Riley, Ph.D.; Ann Stohlman, V.M.D.; Yichun Sun, Ph.D.; Zhigang Sun, Ph.D.; Jennifer Swisher, Ph.D.; Frank Switzer, Ph.D.; Neeru Takiar, M.S.; Carmen Tartera, Ph.D.; Jennifer Thomas, Ph.D.; Yiying Tsai, Pharm.D.; Saleh Turujman, Ph.D.; Katherine Tyner,

Ph.D.; John Whyte, Ph.D.; Steve Wolfgang, Ph.D.; Bingyuan Wu, Ph.D.; Geoffrey Wu, Ph.D.; Larisa Wu, Ph.D.; Jo Wyeth, Pharm.D.; Xiaoming Xu, Ph.D.; Yuda Zong, Ph.D.

Other Government Liaisons

Agency for Healthcare Research and Quality
Diane D. Cousins, R.Ph.

U.S. Centers for Disease Control and Prevention
Joseph Perz, Ph.D.; Nadine Shehab, Pharm.D., M.P.H.; Melissa Schaefer, M.D.

Health Canada
Victoria Kyeyune, Ph.D.; Jessica Priem, M.S.

National Administration of Medicines, Foods and Medical Technology (ANMAT)
Carolina Abba, Pharm.D.

National Institutes of Health
Kwangmoon Lee, Ph.D.; Rao Rapaka, Ph.D.; Cynthia Dyann Davis, Ph.D.

Saudi Food and Drug Authority
Ali Mohammed Alhomaidan, Ph.D.; Ali M. Alsamil, Ph.D.

In Memoriam

USP would like to acknowledge the following Expert Volunteers and Government Liaisons who have passed away during the 2015–2020 Cycle:
Stefan Christians, Ph.D. (Biologics Monographs 2—Proteins)
Scott V.W. Sutton, Ph.D. (General Chapters—Microbiology Expert Committee)

Admissions

New Articles Appearing in This Supplement

GENERAL CHAPTERS

⟨198⟩ Nuclear Magnetic Resonance Spectroscopy Identity
  Testing of Bacterial Polysaccharides Used in Vaccine
  Manufacture

USP 41

Acamprosate Calcium
Amlodipine and Atorvastatin Tablets
Brimonidine Tartrate
Calcium Citrate Malate
Cholecalciferol Tablets
Prasugrel Hydrochloride

Raltegravir Tablets
Raltegravir Chewable Tablets
Rosuvastatin Calcium
Rosuvastatin Tablets
Tranexamic Acid Injection

DIETARY SUPPLEMENTS

Ascorbic Acid Chewable Gels
Cholecalciferol Chewable Gels
Coffee Fruit Dry Extract
Coix Seed

Coix Seed Powder
Menaquinone-4
Valerian Root Dry Extract Capsules
Valerian Root Powder Capsules

NF 36

Glyceryl Tricaprylate

Isopropyl Isostearate

ANNOTATED LIST

Monographs, General Chapters, Reagents, and Tables Affected by Changes Appearing in This Supplement

Page citations refer to the pages of this Supplement. Note—In the lists below, if a section is new or if a subsection is added to or deleted from an existing section, it is labeled as such in parentheses after the section or subsection name. Items on this list that appear without the designation "new", "added", or "deleted" are items in which changes have been made to existing official text.

General Chapters

General Tests and Assays

Biological Tests and Assays
⟨123⟩ Glucagon Bioidentity Tests, 8627
Introduction and *Procedure*
Chemical Tests and Assays
⟨198⟩ Nuclear Magnetic Resonance Spectroscopy Identity Testing of Bacterial Polysaccharides Used in Vaccine Manufacture (new), 8633
Physical Tests and Determinations
⟨724⟩ Drug Release, 8637
General Drug Release Standards
⟨741⟩ Melting Range or Temperature, 8644

General Information

⟨1151⟩ Pharmaceutical Dosage Forms, 8648
⟨1231⟩ Water for Pharmaceutical Purposes, 8674
Waters Used for Pharmaceutical Manufacturing and Testing Purposes; Validation and Qualification of Water Purification, Storage, and Distribution Systems; Design and Operation of Purified Water and Water for Injection Systems; Sampling; Chemical Evaluations; Microbial Evaluations; and *Alert and Action Levels and Specifications*

Dietary Supplements

⟨2040⟩ Disintegration and Dissolution of Dietary Supplements, 8712
Dissolution

Reagents, Indicators, and Solutions

Reagent Specifications
Ammonium Hydrogen Difluoride (new), 8499
Benzil (new), 8499
Blood Group A₁ Red Blood Cells and Blood Group B Red Blood Cells (deleted), 8500
Cadmium Nitrate, 8500
2-Chlorobenzophenone (new), 8500
2-Chloroethylamine Monohydrochloride, 8500
Cupric Nitrate Hydrate (deleted), 8500
3-Cyclohexylpropionic Acid (new), 8500
L-Cystine, 8500
Deschloroclotrimazole (new), 8500
N,N'-Diisopropylethylenediamine (new), 8500
Dimethylcarbonate (new), 8500
Dimidium Bromide (new), 8500

2-Ethylhexanoic Acid (new), 8500
(±)-1-(9-Fluorenyl)ethanol (new), 8500
(+)-1-(9-Fluorenyl)ethyl Chloroformate Solution (new), 8500
Fluoroandrostadiene Carboxylic Acid (new), 8501
Gadolinium Sulfate, 8501
25% Hydrochloric Acid (new), 8501
Isopropyl Stearate (new), 8501
Isostearic Acid (new), 8501
Lithium Sulfate, 8501
3-Mercaptopropionic Acid (new), 8501
Methyl Isobutyrate (new), 8501
3-Methyl-2-pentanone (new), 8502
4-Morpholine Propane Sulfonic Acid (new), 8502
Nitric Acid, Ultratrace (new), 8502
Petroleum Ether (new), 8502
Phenylacetic Acid (new), 8502
Sodium Phosphate (new), 8502
Sulfan Blue (new), 8502
Sulfuric Acid, Diluted, 8502
1,1,3,3-Tetramethylbutylamine (new), 8502
Tetramethylethylenediamine (new), 8502
n-Tricosane (deleted), 8502
Water, Ammonia-Free, 8502
Test Solutions
4 N Hydrochloric Acid TS (new), 8502
0.1 M Monobasic Sodium Phosphate TS (new), 8502
0.05 M Monobasic Sodium Phosphate TS (new), 8502
0.1 N Sodium Chloride TS (new), 8502
10 N Sulfuric Acid TS (new), 8502
Volumetric Solutions
0.1 N Ceric Sulfate VS, 8503
0.01 M Sodium Thiosulfate VS, 8503
0.02 N Sulfuric Acid VS (new), 8503
Chromatographic Columns
L52, 8503
L86, 8503
L107 (new), 8503
L110 (new), 8503
L112 (new), 8504

Reference Tables

Container Specifications for Capsules and Tablets
Amlodipine and Atorvastatin Tablets (new), 8505
Cholecalciferol Tablets (new), 8507
Raltegravir Tablets (new), 8513
Raltegravir Tablets, Chewable (new), 8513
Rosuvastatin Tablets (new), 8513
Tocainide Hydrochloride Tablets (deleted), 8514
Valerian Root Dry Extract Capsules (new), 8514
Valerian Root Powder Capsules (new), 8514
Description and Relative Solubility of USP and NF Articles
Acamprosate Calcium (new), 8516

Monographs (USP 41)

IMPURITIES
Limit of Methanol and Dichloromethane
Eszopiclone Tablets, 8335
PERFORMANCE TESTS
Dissolution
IMPURITIES
ADDITIONAL REQUIREMENTS
Labeling (added)
Glycine, 8337
IMPURITIES
Related Compounds (added)
ADDITIONAL REQUIREMENTS
Hydrocortisone Acetate Ophthalmic Ointment
(deleted), 8339
Hydroxyzine Pamoate Oral Suspension (deleted),
8339
Isoleucine, 8340
IMPURITIES
Related Compounds
ADDITIONAL REQUIREMENTS
USP Reference Standards
Levocarnitine, 8341
IDENTIFICATION
Test B (added)
IMPURITIES
Enantiomeric Purity (added)
SPECIFIC TESTS
Optical Rotation, Specific Rotation (deleted)
ADDITIONAL REQUIREMENTS
Packaging and Storage
Lidocaine, 8343
IDENTIFICATION
Infrared Absorption, Test A
ASSAY
IMPURITIES
Organic Impurities (added)
SPECIFIC TESTS (deleted)
ADDITIONAL REQUIREMENTS
USP Reference Standards
Lidocaine Hydrochloride Oral Topical Solution,
8344
IDENTIFICATION
Infrared Absorption, Test A
ASSAY
IMPURITIES
ADDITIONAL REQUIREMENTS
USP Reference Standards
Lidocaine Hydrochloride Topical Solution, 8346
IDENTIFICATION
Infrared Absorption, Test A
IMPURITIES
ADDITIONAL REQUIREMENTS
USP Reference Standards
Mebendazole Tablets, 8347
IDENTIFICATION
ASSAY
PERFORMANCE TESTS
Uniformity of Dosage Units
IMPURITIES (added)
ADDITIONAL REQUIREMENTS
USP Reference Standards
Meloxicam Oral Suspension, 8349
IDENTIFICATION
Test A
ASSAY
IMPURITIES
ADDITIONAL REQUIREMENTS
USP Reference Standards
Metaproterenol Sulfate Inhalation Aerosol (deleted), 8351
Methotrexate Injection, 8352
IDENTIFICATION
Test B (added)
ASSAY
IMPURITIES (added)

ADDITIONAL REQUIREMENTS
Miconazole Nitrate, 8353
IDENTIFICATION
ASSAY
IMPURITIES
Organic Impurities
SPECIFIC TESTS
Optical Rotation, Specific Rotation (added)
ADDITIONAL REQUIREMENTS
Miconazole Nitrate Topical Powder, 8355
IDENTIFICATION
ASSAY
IMPURITIES (added)
ADDITIONAL REQUIREMENTS
Minocycline Hydrochloride, 8357
IDENTIFICATION
IMPURITIES
Organic Impurities
Montelukast Sodium Oral Granules, 8358
PERFORMANCE TESTS
Dissolution
IMPURITIES
Moxifloxacin Hydrochloride, 8361
IMPURITIES
Enantiomeric Purity
Naproxen Sodium Tablets, 8363
ASSAY
IMPURITIES
Nicotine Transdermal System, 8365
DEFINITION
IDENTIFICATION
Test B (added)
ASSAY
PERFORMANCE TESTS
Drug Release
IMPURITIES (added)
ADDITIONAL REQUIREMENTS
USP Reference Standards
Nifedipine Extended-Release Tablets, 8369
PERFORMANCE TESTS
Dissolution
Norelgestromin, 8376
ASSAY
IMPURITIES
Organic Impurities
Octinoxate, 8377
IDENTIFICATION
ASSAY
IMPURITIES
ADDITIONAL REQUIREMENTS
USP Reference Standards
Octisalate, 8378
DEFINITION
IDENTIFICATION
Octocrylene, 8379
IDENTIFICATION
Olmesartan Medoxomil Tablets, 8380
ASSAY
PERFORMANCE TESTS
Dissolution
ADDITIONAL REQUIREMENTS
Labeling (added)
Omega-3-Acid Ethyl Esters, 8382
ADDITIONAL REQUIREMENTS
Labeling
Omega-3-Acid Ethyl Esters Capsules, 8385
ADDITIONAL REQUIREMENTS
Labeling
Oxybutynin Chloride Extended-Release Tablets,
8387
PERFORMANCE TESTS
Dissolution
Pantoprazole Sodium, 8392
IDENTIFICATION
Infrared Absorption, Test A

ASSAY
IMPURITIES
SPECIFIC TESTS
Pentazocine, 8394
  DEFINITION
  IDENTIFICATION
  ASSAY
  IMPURITIES
    Ordinary Impurities (deleted) and *Organic Impurities* (added)
  SPECIFIC TESTS
    Melting Range or Temperature (deleted) and *Bacterial Endotoxins Test* (added)
  ADDITIONAL REQUIREMENTS
    Labeling (added)
Perphenazine Injection (deleted), 8396
Perphenazine Oral Solution (deleted) 8396
Perphenazine Syrup (deleted), 8397
Phenoxybenzamine Hydrochloride Capsules, 8397
  IMPURITIES
Pilocarpine Hydrochloride Tablets, 8399
  IDENTIFICATION
  ASSAY
  PERFORMANCE TESTS
  IMPURITIES
Pralidoxime Chloride, 8401
  CHEMICAL INFORMATION
  IDENTIFICATION
    Infrared Absorption, Test A
  ASSAY
  IMPURITIES
    Organic Impurities (added)
  SPECIFIC TESTS
    Melting Range or Temperature (deleted)
Pralidoxime Chloride for Injection, 8402
  IDENTIFICATION
    Infrared Absorption, Test A
  ASSAY
  IMPURITIES
  SPECIFIC TESTS
    Completeness of Solution (deleted)
Prasugrel Hydrochloride (new), 8403
Pravastatin Sodium, 8406
  IDENTIFICATION
    Identification Tests—General, Test B and *Test C* (added)
  ASSAY
  IMPURITIES
  SPECIFIC TESTS
    Limit of Alcohol
  ADDITIONAL REQUIREMENTS
    USP Reference Standards
Pyridostigmine Bromide Tablets, 8408
  IMPURITIES
Raltegravir Tablets (new), 8409
Raltegravir Chewable Tablets (new), 8411
Rizatriptan Benzoate Orally Disintegrating Tablets, 8413
  IDENTIFICATION
    Test B (added)
  ASSAY
  PERFORMANCE TESTS
    Dissolution
  IMPURITIES
Rosuvastatin Calcium (new), 8415
Rosuvastatin Tablets (new), 8417
Salmeterol Xinafoate, 8419
  ASSAY
  IMPURITIES
    Organic Impurities
  ADDITIONAL REQUIREMENTS
    USP Reference Standards
Scopolamine Hydrobromide, 8420
  DEFINITION
  IDENTIFICATION

    Test C (added)
  ASSAY
  IMPURITIES
  ADDITIONAL REQUIREMENTS
    USP Reference Standards
Sodium Fluoride Oral Solution, 8422
  IDENTIFICATION
    Test A
  ASSAY
  ADDITIONAL REQUIREMENTS
    USP Reference Standards
Sodium Fluoride and Acidulated Phosphate Topical Solution, 8423
  IDENTIFICATION
  ASSAY
  SPECIFIC TESTS
    Other Requirements (deleted)
  ADDITIONAL REQUIREMENTS
    Labeling and *USP Reference Standards*
Somatropin, 8424
  IMPURITIES
    Limit of High Molecular Weight Proteins
  SPECIFIC TESTS
    Total Protein Content
Sumatriptan Nasal Spray, 8426
  IDENTIFICATION
    Test B (added)
  ASSAY
  IMPURITIES
  ADDITIONAL REQUIREMENTS
    USP Reference Standards
Taurine, 8428
  CHEMICAL INFORMATION
  IDENTIFICATION
    Test B (added)
  ASSAY
Terbutaline Sulfate Inhalation Aerosol (deleted), 8429
Tetracycline, 8430
  IMPURITIES
Tetrahydrozoline Hydrochloride Ophthalmic Solution, 8431
  IDENTIFICATION
  ASSAY
  IMPURITIES (added)
  ADDITIONAL REQUIREMENTS
    Packaging and Storage
Tiamulin, 8433
  IDENTIFICATION
    Infrared Absorption, Test A
  ASSAY
  IMPURITIES
    Limit of Alcohol and Toluene
Tiamulin Fumarate, 8434
  IDENTIFICATION
    Infrared Absorption, Test A
  ASSAY
  IMPURITIES
    Limit of Residual Solvents (deleted) and *Organic Impurities*
  SPECIFIC TESTS
    Melting Range or Temperature (deleted)
Tocainide Hydrochloride (deleted), 8436
Tocainide Hydrochloride Tablets (deleted), 8436
Tolterodine Tartrate, 8437
  IMPURITIES
    Organic Impurities
Tranexamic Acid Injection (new), 8439
Tranylcypromine Tablets, 8440
  IDENTIFICATION
  ASSAY
  PERFORMANCE TESTS
    Dissolution
  IMPURITIES
Trazodone Hydrochloride Tablets, 8442

IDENTIFICATION
  Test A
ASSAY
PERFORMANCE TESTS
  Dissolution
IMPURITIES
Triamterene, 8444
  CHEMICAL INFORMATION
  IDENTIFICATION
  ASSAY
  IMPURITIES
  ADDITIONAL REQUIREMENTS
    USP Reference Standards
Verapamil Hydrochloride Extended-Release Tablets, 8446
  IDENTIFICATION
  ASSAY
  PERFORMANCE TESTS
    Dissolution
  IMPURITIES
  ADDITIONAL REQUIREMENTS
    Packaging and Storage and *USP Reference Standards*
Xylazine, 8450
  IDENTIFICATION
    Infrared Absorption, Test A and *Thin-Layer Chromatographic Identification Test, Test C* (deleted)
  IMPURITIES
    Limit of Acetone and Isopropyl Alcohol and *Organic Impurities*
  SPECIFIC TESTS
    Melting Range or Temperature (deleted)

Monographs (Dietary Supplements)

Ascorbic Acid Chewable Gels (new), 8453
Cholecalciferol Chewable Gels (new), 8454
Coffee Fruit Dry Extract (new), 8455
Coix Seed (new), 8457

Coix Seed Powder (new), 8460
Flax Seed Oil, 8462
  DEFINITION
  SPECIFIC TESTS
    Fats and Fixed Oils, Peroxide Value; Fats and Fixed Oils, Iodine Value; Fats and Fixed Oils, Saponification Value; and *Fats and Fixed Oils, Unsaponifiable Matter*
Menaquinone-4 (new), 8462
Methylcobalamin, 8463
  ASSAY
  IMPURITIES
Methylcobalamin Tablets, 8464
  STRENGTH
Salix Species Bark, 8465
Salix Species Bark Dry Extract, 8467
Salix Species Bark Powder, 8469
Valerian Root Dry Extract Capsules (new), 8471
Valerian Root Powder Capsules (new), 8472

Monographs (NF 36)

Ethylcellulose, 8485
  DEFINITION
  IDENTIFICATION
  ASSAY
  ADDITIONAL REQUIREMENTS
    Labeling and *USP Reference Standards*
Glyceryl Tricaprylate (new), 8487
Isopropyl Isostearate (new), 8489
Methyl Salicylate, 8490
  DEFINITION
  ASSAY
Polydextrose, 8491
  IDENTIFICATION
    Chromatographic Identity, Test E (added)
  ASSAY
Squalane, 8494
  DEFINITION
  ADDITIONAL REQUIREMENTS
    Labeling (added)

General Notices and Requirements

Applying to Standards, Tests, Assays, and Other Specifications of the United States Pharmacopeia

GENERAL NOTICES AND REQUIREMENTS

The *General Notices and Requirements* section (the *General Notices*) presents the basic assumptions, definitions, and default conditions for the interpretation and application of the *United States Pharmacopeia* (*USP*) and the *National Formulary* (*NF*).

Requirements stated in these *General Notices* apply to all articles recognized in the *USP* and *NF* (the "compendia") and to all general chapters unless specifically stated otherwise.

1. TITLE AND REVISION

The full title of this publication (consisting of five volumes and including its *Supplements*), is *The Pharmacopeia of the United States of America*, Forty-First Revision and the *National Formulary*, Thirty-Sixth Edition. These titles may be abbreviated to *USP 41*, to *NF 36*, and to *USP 41–NF 36*. The *United States Pharmacopeia*, Forty-First Revision, and the *National Formulary*, Thirty-Sixth Edition, supersede all earlier revisions. Where the terms "*USP*," "*NF*," or "*USP–NF*" are used without further qualification during the period in which these compendia are official, they refer only to *USP 41*, *NF 36*, and any *Supplement(s)* thereto. The same titles, with no further distinction, apply equally to print or electronic presentation of these contents. Although *USP* and *NF* are published under one cover and share these *General Notices*, they are separate compendia.

This revision is official beginning May 1, 2018 unless otherwise indicated in specific text.

Supplements to *USP* and *NF* are published periodically.

Accelerated Revisions, published periodically on the *Official Text* section of USP's website (http://www.usp.org/uspnf/official-text), are designed to make revisions official more quickly than through the routine process for publishing standards in the *USP–NF*. *Interim Revision Announcements* are Accelerated Revisions to *USP* and *NF* that contain official revisions and their effective dates.

Revision Bulletins are Accelerated Revisions to official text or postponements that require expedited publication. They generally are official immediately unless otherwise specified in the *Revision Bulletin*.

Errata are Accelerated Revisions representing corrections to items erroneously published. Announcements of the availability of new USP Reference Standards and announcements of tests or procedures that are held in abeyance pending availability of required USP Reference Standards are also available on the "Official Text" tab of USP's website.

2. OFFICIAL STATUS AND LEGAL RECOGNITION

2.10. Official Text

Official text of the *USP* and *NF* is published in the *USP–NF Online* (www.uspnf.com) in the edition identified as "CURRENTLY OFFICIAL" and in Accelerated Revisions that supersede the *USP–NF Online* as described below.

Routine revisions are published in the *USP–NF Online* and become official on the date indicated, usually six months after publication. Accelerated Revisions supersede the *USP–NF Online* and become official on the date indicated. Links to Accelerated Revisions on the USP website can be found in any superseded monograph or general chapter in the *USP–NF Online*.

Print and USB flash drive versions of the *USP* and *NF* also are available. Routine revisions are provided with the same timing as the *USP–NF Online*. Official text published in *Supplements* supersedes that in the previously published print or USB flash drive versions of *USP–NF*. These versions also are superseded by Accelerated Revisions as described above.

In the event of any disparity between the print or USB flash drive versions and the *USP–NF Online*, the *USP–NF Online* will be deemed to apply.

2.20. Official Articles

An *official article* is an article that is recognized in *USP* or *NF*. An article is deemed to be recognized and included in a compendium when a monograph for the article is published in the compendium and an official date is generally or specifically assigned to the monograph.

The title specified in a monograph is the *official title* for such article. Other names considered to be synonyms of the official titles may not be used as substitutes for official titles.

Official articles include both *official substances* and *official products*. An *official substance* is a drug substance, excipient, dietary ingredient, other ingredient, or component of a finished device for which the monograph title includes no indication of the nature of the finished form.

An *official product* is a drug product, dietary supplement, compounded preparation, or finished device for which a monograph is provided.

2.30. Legal Recognition

The *USP* and *NF* are recognized in the laws and regulations of many countries throughout the world. Regulatory authorities may enforce the standards presented in the *USP* and *NF*, but because recognition of the *USP* and *NF* may vary by country, users should understand applicable laws and regulations. In the United States under the Federal Food, Drug, and Cosmetic Act (FDCA), both *USP* and *NF* are recognized as official compendia. A drug with a name recognized in *USP–NF* must comply with compendial identity standards or be deemed adulterated, misbranded, or both. See, e.g., FDCA § 501(b) and 502(e)(3)(b); also FDA regulations, 21 CFR § 299.5(a&b). To avoid being deemed adulterated, such drugs must also comply with compendial standards for strength, quality, and purity, unless labeled to show all respects in which the drug differs. See, e.g., FDCA § 501(b) and 21 CFR § 299.5(c). In addition, to avoid being deemed misbranded, drugs recognized in *USP–NF* must also be packaged and labeled in compliance with compendial standards. See FDCA § 502(g).

A dietary supplement represented as conforming to specifications in *USP* will be deemed a misbranded food if it fails to so conform. See FDCA § 403(s)(2)(D).

Enforcement of *USP* standards is the responsibility of FDA and other government authorities in the U.S. and elsewhere. USP has no role in enforcement.

Change to read:

3. CONFORMANCE TO STANDARDS

3.10. Applicability of Standards

Standards for an article recognized in the compendia (*USP–NF*) are expressed in the article's monograph, applicable general chapters, and *General Notices*. The identity, strength, quality, and purity of an article are determined by the official tests, procedures, and acceptance criteria, and other requirements incorporated in the monograph, in applicable general chapters, or in the *General Notices*. "Applicable general chapters" means general chapters numbered below 1000 or above 2000 that are made applicable to an article through reference in *General Notices*, a monograph, or another applicable general chapter numbered below 1000. Where the requirements of a monograph differ from the requirements specified in these *General Notices* or an applicable general chapter, the monograph requirements apply and supersede the requirements of the *General Notices* or applicable general chapters, whether or not the monograph explicitly states the difference.

General chapters numbered 1000 to 1999 are for informational purposes only. They contain no mandatory tests, assays, or other requirements applicable to any official article, regardless of citation in a general chapter numbered below 1000, a monograph, or these *General Notices*. General chapters numbered above 2000 apply only to articles that are intended for use as dietary ingredients and dietary supplements. General chapter citations in *NF* monographs refer to *USP* general chapters.

Early adoption of revised standards in advance of the official date is allowed by USP unless specified otherwise at the time of publication. Where revised standards for an existing article have been published as final approved "official text" (as approved in section *2.10 Official Text*) but have not yet reached the official date (six months after publication, unless otherwise specified; see "official date", section *2.20. Official Articles*), compliance with the revised standard shall not preclude a finding or indication of conformance with compendial standards, unless USP specifies otherwise by prohibiting early adoption in a particular standard.

The standards in the relevant monograph, general chapter(s), and *General Notices* apply at all times in the life of the article from production to expiration. It is also noted that the manufacturer's specifications, and manufacturing practices (e.g., Quality by Design, Process Analytical Technology, and Real Time Release Testing initiatives), generally are followed to ensure that the article will comply with compendial standards until its expiration date, when stored as directed. Every compendial article in commerce shall be so constituted that when examined in accordance with these assays and test procedures, it meets all applicable pharmacopeial requirements (*General Notices*, monographs, and general chapters). Thus, any official article is expected to meet the compendial standards if tested, and any official article actually tested as directed in the relevant monograph must meet such standards to demonstrate compliance.

Some tests, such as those for *Dissolution* and *Uniformity of Dosage Units*, require multiple dosage units in conjunction with a decision scheme. These tests, albeit using a number of dosage units, are in fact one determination. These procedures should not be confused with statistical sampling plans. The similarity to statistical procedures may seem to suggest an intent to make inference to some larger group of units, but in all cases, statements about whether the compendial standard is met apply only to the units tested. Repeats, replicates, statistical rejection of outliers, or extrapolations of results to larger populations, as well as the necessity and appropriate frequency of batch testing, are neither specified nor proscribed by the compendia; such decisions are based on the objectives of the testing. Frequency of testing and sampling are left to the preferences or direction of those performing compliance testing, and other users of *USP–NF*, including manufacturers, buyers, or regulatory authorities.

Official products are prepared according to recognized principles of good manufacturing practice and from ingredients that meet *USP* or *NF* standards, where standards for such ingredients exist (for dietary supplements, see section *3.10.20 Applicability of Standards to Medical Devices, Dietary Supplements, and Their Components and Ingredients*).

Official substances are prepared according to recognized principles of good manufacturing practice and from ingredients complying with specifications designed to ensure that the resultant substances meet the requirements of the compendial monographs.

3.10.10. Applicability of Standards to Drug Products, Drug Substances, and Excipients

The applicable *USP* or *NF* standard applies to any article marketed in the United States that (1) is recognized in the compendium and (2) is intended or labeled for use as a drug or as an ingredient in a drug. Such articles (drug products, drug substances, and excipients) include both human drugs (whether dispensed by prescription, "over the counter," or otherwise), as well as animal drugs. The applicable standard applies to such articles whether or not the added designation "USP" or "NF" is used. The standards apply equally to articles bearing the official titles or names derived by transposition of the definitive words of official titles or transposition in the order of the names of two or more ▲drug substances▲USP41 in official titles, or where there is use of synonyms with the intent or effect of suggesting a significant degree of identity with the official title or name.

3.10.20. Applicability of Standards to Medical Devices, Dietary Supplements, and Their Components and Ingredients

An article recognized in *USP* or *NF* shall comply with the compendial standards if the article is a medical device, component intended for a medical device, dietary supplement, dietary ingredient, or other ingredient that is intended for incorporation into a dietary supplement, and is labeled as conforming to the *USP* or *NF*.

Generally, dietary supplements are prepared from ingredients that meet *USP*, *NF*, or *Food Chemicals Codex* standards. Where such standards do not exist, substances may be used in dietary supplements if they have been shown to be of acceptable food grade quality using other suitable procedures.

3.10.30. Applicability of Standards to the Practice of Compounding (New)

USP compounding practice standards, *Pharmaceutical Compounding—Nonsterile Preparations* ⟨795⟩ and *Pharmaceutical Compounding—Sterile Preparations* ⟨797⟩, as appropriate, apply to compounding practice or activity regardless of whether a monograph exists for the compounded preparation or these chapters are referenced in such a monograph. In the United States, ⟨795⟩ and ⟨797⟩ are not applicable to drugs compounded by entities registered with FDA as outsourcing facilities as defined by FDCA § 503B, because such facilities are required to comply with FDA's current good manufacturing practice requirements. Compounded preparations, including drug products compounded by outsourcing facilities, may also be subject to applicable monographs; see section *2.20 Official Articles* and section *4.10 Monographs*.

3.20. Indicating Conformance

A drug product, drug substance, or excipient may use the designation "USP" or "NF" in conjunction with its official title or elsewhere on the label only when (1) a monograph is provided in the specified compendium and (2) the article complies with the identity prescribed in the specified compendium.

When a drug product, drug substance, compounded preparation, or excipient differs from the relevant *USP* or *NF* standard of strength, quality, or purity, as determined by the application of the tests, procedures, and acceptance criteria set forth in the relevant compendium, its difference shall be plainly stated on its label.

When a drug product, drug substance, compounded preparation, or excipient fails to comply with the identity prescribed in *USP* or *NF* or contains an added substance that interferes with the prescribed tests and procedures, the article shall be designated by a name that is clearly distinguishing and differentiating from any name recognized in *USP* or *NF*.

A medical device, dietary supplement, or ingredient or component of a medical device or dietary supplement may use the designation "USP" or "NF" in conjunction with its official title or elsewhere on the label only when (1) a monograph is provided in the specified compendium and (2) the article complies with the monograph standards and other applicable standards in that compendium.

The designation "USP" or "NF" on the label may not and does not constitute an endorsement by USP and does not represent assurance by USP that the article is known to comply with the relevant standards. USP may seek legal redress if an article purports to be or is represented as an official article in one of USP's compendia and such claim is determined by USP not to be made in good faith.

The designation "USP–NF" may be used on the label of an article provided that the label also bears a statement such as "Meets *NF* standards as published by USP," indicating the particular compendium to which the article purports to apply.

When the letters "USP," "NF," or "USP–NF" are used on the label of an article to indicate compliance with compendial standards, the letters shall appear in conjunction with the official title of the article. The letters are not to be enclosed in any symbol such as a circle, square, etc., and shall appear in capital letters.

If a dietary supplement does not comply with all applicable compendial requirements but contains one or more dietary ingredients or other ingredients that are recognized in *USP* or *NF*, the individual ingredient(s) may be designated as complying with *USP* or *NF* standards or being of *USP* or *NF* quality provided that the designation is limited to the individual ingredient(s) and does not suggest that the dietary supplement complies with *USP* standards.

4. MONOGRAPHS AND GENERAL CHAPTERS

4.10. Monographs

Monographs set forth the article's name, definition, specification, and other requirements related to packaging, storage, and labeling. The specification consists of tests, procedures, and acceptance criteria that help ensure the identity, strength, quality, and purity of the article. For general requirements relating to specific monograph sections, see section *5 Monograph Components*.

Because monographs may not provide standards for all relevant characteristics, some official substances may conform to the *USP* or *NF* standard but differ with regard to nonstandardized properties that are relevant to their use in specific preparations. To assure substitutability in such instances, users may wish to ascertain functional equivalence or determine such characteristics before use.

4.10.10. Applicability of Test Procedures

A single monograph may include more than one test, procedure, and/or acceptance criterion for the same attribute. Unless otherwise specified in the monograph, all tests are requirements. In some cases, monograph instructions allow the selection of tests that reflect attributes of different manufacturers' articles, such as different polymorphic forms, impurities, hydrates, and dissolution. Monograph instructions indicate the tests, procedures, and/or acceptance criteria to be used and the required labeling.

The order in which the tests are listed in the monograph is based on the order in which they are approved by the relevant Expert Committee for inclusion in the monograph. Test 1 is not necessarily the test for the innovator or for the reference product. Depending on monograph instructions, a labeling statement is not typically required if Test 1 is used.

4.10.20. Acceptance Criteria

The acceptance criteria allow for analytical error, for unavoidable variations in manufacturing and compounding, and for deterioration to an extent considered acceptable under practical conditions. The existence of compendial acceptance criteria does not constitute a basis for a claim that an official substance that more nearly approaches 100% purity "exceeds" compendial quality. Similarly, the fact that an article has been prepared to tighter criteria than those specified in the monograph does not constitute a basis for a claim that the article "exceeds" the compendial requirements.

An official product shall be formulated with the intent to provide 100% of the quantity of each ingredient declared on the label. Where the minimum amount of a substance present in a dietary supplement is required by law to be higher than the lower acceptance criterion allowed for in the monograph, the upper acceptance criterion contained in the monograph may be increased by a corresponding amount.

The acceptance criteria specified in individual monographs and in the general chapters for compounded preparations are based on such attributes of quality as might be expected to characterize an article compounded from suitable bulk drug substances and ingredients, using the procedures provided or recognized principles of good compounding practice, as described in these compendia.

4.20. General Chapters

Each general chapter is assigned a number that appears in angle brackets adjacent to the chapter name (e.g., *Chromatography* ⟨621⟩). General chapters may contain the following:

- Descriptions of tests and procedures for application through individual monographs,
- Descriptions and specifications of conditions and practices for pharmaceutical compounding,
- General information for the interpretation of the compendial requirements,
- Descriptions of general pharmaceutical storage, dispensing, and packaging practices, or
- General guidance to manufacturers of official substances or official products.

When a general chapter is referenced in a monograph, acceptance criteria may be presented after a colon.

Some chapters may serve as introductory overviews of a test or of analytical techniques. They may reference other general chapters that contain techniques, details of the procedures, and, at times, acceptance criteria.

Change to read:

5. MONOGRAPH COMPONENTS

5.10. Molecular Formula

The use of the molecular formula for the ▲official substance(s)▲*USP41* named in defining the required strength of a compendial article is intended to designate the chemical entity or entities, as given in the complete chemical name of the article, having absolute (100%) purity.

5.20. Added Substances

Added substances are presumed to be unsuitable for inclusion in an official article and therefore prohibited, if their presence impairs the bioavailability, therapeutic efficacy, or safety of the official article; or they interfere with the assays and tests prescribed for determining compliance with the compendial standards (see section *3.20 Indicating Conformance*).

The air in a container of an official article may, where appropriate, be evacuated or be replaced by carbon dioxide, helium, argon, or nitrogen, or by a mixture of these gases. The use of such gas need not be declared in the labeling.

5.20.10. Added Substances in Official Substances

Official substances may contain only the specific added substances that are permitted by the individual monograph. Such added substances shall not exceed the quantity required for providing their intended effect. Where such addition is permitted, the label shall indicate the name(s) and amount(s) of any added substance(s).

5.20.20. Added Substances (Excipients and Ingredients) in Official Products

Suitable substances and excipients such as antimicrobial agents, pharmaceutical bases, carriers, coatings, flavors, preservatives, stabilizers, and vehicles may be added to an official product to enhance its stability, usefulness, or elegance, or to facilitate its preparation, unless otherwise specified in the individual monograph.

Added substances and excipients employed solely to impart color may be incorporated into official products other than those intended for parenteral or ophthalmic use, in accordance with the regulations pertaining to the use of colors issued by the U.S. Food and Drug Administration (FDA), provided such added substances or excipients are otherwise appropriate in all respects. (See also *Injections and Implanted Drugs Products* ⟨1⟩, *Product Quality Tests Common to Parenteral Dosage Forms, Specific Tests, Vehicles and added substances, Added substances.*)

The proportions of the substances constituting the base in ointment and suppository products and preparations may be varied to maintain a suitable consistency under different climatic conditions, provided that the concentrations of ▲drug substances▲*USP41* are not varied and provided that the bioavailability, therapeutic efficacy, and safety of the preparation are not impaired.

5.20.20.1. In Compounded Preparations

Compounded preparations for which a complete composition is given shall contain only the ingredients named in the formulas unless specifically exempted herein or in the individual monograph. Deviation from the specified processes or methods of compounding, although not from the ingredients or proportions thereof, may occur provided that the finished preparation conforms to the relevant standards and to preparations produced by following the specified process.

Where a monograph for a compounded preparation calls for an ingredient in an amount expressed on the dried basis, the ingredient need not be dried before use if due allowance is made for the water or other volatile substances present in the quantity taken.

Specially denatured alcohol formulas are available for use in accordance with federal statutes and regulations of the Internal Revenue Service. A suitable formula of specially denatured alcohol may be substituted for Alcohol in the manufacture of official preparations intended for internal or topical use, provided that the denaturant is volatile and does not remain in the finished product. A preparation that is intended for topical application to the skin may contain specially denatured alcohol, provided that the denaturant is either a usual ingredient in the preparation or a permissible added substance; in either case the denaturant shall be identified on the label of the topical preparation. Where a process is given in the individual monograph, any preparation compounded using denatured alcohol shall be identical to that prepared by the monograph process.

5.20.20.2. In Dietary Supplements

Additional ingredients may be added to dietary supplement products provided that the additional ingredients: (1) comply with applicable regulatory requirements; and (2) do not interfere with the assays and tests prescribed for determining compliance with compendial standards.

5.30. Description and Solubility

Only where a quantitative solubility test is given in a monograph and is designated as such is it a test for purity.

A monograph may include information regarding the article's description. Information about an article's "description and solubility" also is provided in the reference table *Description and Relative Solubility of USP and NF Articles.* The reference table merely denotes the properties of articles that comply with monograph standards. The reference table is intended primarily for those who use, prepare, and dispense drugs and/or related articles. Although the information provided in monographs and the information in the reference table may indirectly assist in the preliminary evaluation of an article, it is not intended to serve as a standard or test for purity.

The approximate solubility of a compendial substance is indicated by one of the following descriptive terms:

Descriptive Term	Parts of Solvent Required for 1 Part of Solute
Very soluble	Less than 1
Freely soluble	From 1 to 10
Soluble	From 10 to 30
Sparingly soluble	From 30 to 100
Slightly soluble	From 100 to 1,000
Very slightly soluble	From 1,000 to 10,000
Practically insoluble, or Insoluble	Greater than or equal to 10,000

5.40. ▲Identification▲*USP41*

A compendial test titled ▲▲*USP41* *Identification* is provided as an aid in verifying the identity of articles as they are purported to be, e.g., those taken from labeled containers, and to establish whether it is the article named in *USP–NF*. The ▲▲*USP41* *Identification* test for a particular article may consist of one or more procedures. When a compendial ▲▲*USP41* *Identification* ▲test▲*USP41* is undertaken, all requirements of all specified procedures in the test must be met to satisfy the requirements of the test. Failure of an article to meet all the requirements of a prescribed ▲▲*USP41* *Identification* test (i.e., failure to meet the requirements of all of the specified procedures that are components of that test) indicates that the article is mislabeled and/or adulterated.

5.50. Assay

Assay tests for compounded preparations are not intended for evaluating a compounded preparation before dispensing, but instead are intended to serve as the official test in the event of a question or dispute regarding the preparation's conformance to official standards.

5.50.10. Units of Potency (Biological)

For substances that cannot be completely characterized by chemical or physical means or that need confirmation of functionality or tertiary structure, it may be necessary to express quantities of biological activity in units of biological potency, each defined by an authoritative, designated reference standard. In cases where international reference materials have been discontinued, international units of potency may be defined in terms of molecular mass, such as in the cases of vitamins A, D, and E.

Where available, World Health Organization (WHO) international biological standards define the International Units (IU). *USP* monographs refer to the units assigned by USP Reference Standards either directly as International Units (IU) or as "USP Units." For some biological products, units of potency are value assigned against a corresponding U.S. Standard established by FDA, whether or not International Units or USP Units have been defined (see *Biologics* ⟨1041⟩). Note that product-related labeling, e.g., on containers, need not use the full phrase "USP [product name] Units" that appears in many *USP* monograph labeling sections. The term "USP Units" can be used on product labeling consistent with USP compendial requirements, provided it is clear from the context that the ▲potency▲*USP41* is stated in terms of USP [product name] Units. In such circumstances it should be clear that "USP Units" and "USP [product name] Units" share the same meaning.

5.60. Impurities and Foreign Substances

Tests for the presence of impurities and foreign substances are provided to limit such substances to amounts that are unobjectionable under conditions in which the article is customarily employed (see also *Impurities in Drug Substances and Drug Products* ⟨1086⟩).

Nonmonograph tests and acceptance criteria suitable for detecting and controlling impurities that may result from a change in the processing methods or that may be introduced from external sources should be employed in addition to the tests provided in the individual monograph, where the presence of the impurity is inconsistent with applicable good manufacturing practices or good pharmaceutical practices.

5.60.10. Other Impurities in *USP* and *NF* Articles

If a *USP* or *NF* monograph includes an assay or organic impurity test based on chromatography, other than a test for residual solvents, and that monograph procedure does not detect an impurity present in the substance, the amount and identity of the impurity, where both are known, shall be stated in the labeling (certificate of analysis) of the official substance, under the heading *Other Impurity(ies)*.

The presence of any unlabeled other impurity in an official substance is a variance from the standard if the content is 0.1% or greater. The sum of all *Other Impurities* combined with the monograph-detected impurities may not exceed 2.0% (see *Ordinary Impurities* ⟨466⟩), unless otherwise stated in the monograph.

The following categories of drug substances are excluded from *Other Impurities* requirements:
- Fermentation products and semi-synthetics derived therefrom,
- Radiopharmaceuticals,
- Biologics,
- Biotechnology-derived products,
- Peptides,
- Herbals, and
- Crude products of animal or plant origin.

Any substance known to be toxic shall not be listed under *Other Impurities*.

5.60.20. Residual Solvents in *USP* and *NF* Articles

All *USP* and *NF* articles are subject to relevant control of residual solvents, even when no test is specified in the individual monograph. If solvents are used during production, they must be of suitable quality. In addition, the toxicity and residual level of each solvent shall be taken into consideration, and the solvents limited according to the principles defined and the requirements specified in *Residual Solvents* ⟨467⟩, using the general methods presented therein or other suitable methods.

5.60.30. Elemental Impurities in USP Drug Products and Dietary Supplements

▲△USP41 Elemental impurities ▲△USP41 in official drug products ▲are controlled△USP41 according to the principles defined and requirements specified in *Elemental Impurities—Limits* ⟨232⟩. ▲△USP41 Elemental contaminants ▲△USP41 in official dietary supplements ▲are controlled△USP41 according to the principles defined and requirements specified in *Elemental Contaminants in Dietary Supplements* ⟨2232⟩. ▲△USP41

5.70. Performance Tests

Where content uniformity determinations have been made using the same analytical methodology specified in the *Assay*, with appropriate allowances made for differences in sample preparation, the average of all of the individual content uniformity determinations may be used as the *Assay* value.

5.80. USP Reference Standards

USP Reference Standards are authentic specimens that have been approved as suitable for use as comparison standards in *USP* or *NF* tests and assays. (See *USP Reference Standards* ⟨11⟩.) Where *USP* or *NF* tests or assays call for the use of a USP Reference Standard, only those results obtained using the specified USP Reference Standard are conclusive. Where a procedure calls for the use of a compendial article rather than for a USP Reference Standard as a material standard of reference, a substance meeting all of the compendial monograph requirements for that article shall be used. If any new *USP* or *NF* standard requires the use of a new USP Reference Standard that is not yet available, that portion of the standard containing the requirement shall not be official until the specified USP reference material is available.

Unless a Reference Standard label bears a specific potency or content, assume the Reference Standard is 100.0% pure in the official application. Unless otherwise directed in the procedure in the individual monograph or in a general chapter, USP Reference Standards are to be used in accor-

dance with the instructions on the label of the Reference Standard.

6. TESTING PRACTICES AND PROCEDURES

6.10. Safe Laboratory Practices

In performing compendial procedures, safe laboratory practices shall be followed, including precautionary measures, protective equipment, and work practices consistent with the chemicals and procedures used. Before undertaking any procedure described in the compendia, the analyst should be aware of the hazards associated with the chemicals and the techniques and means of protecting against them. These compendia are not designed to describe such hazards or protective measures.

6.20. Automated Procedures

Automated and manual procedures employing the same basic chemistry are considered equivalent ▲provided the automated system is properly qualified as being suitable to execute the compendial manual method and the analytical procedure is verified under the new equipment conditions. △USP41

6.30. Alternative and Harmonized Methods and Procedures

▲An alternative method or procedure is defined as any method or procedure other than the compendial method or procedure for the article in question. The alternative method or procedure must be fully validated (see *Validation of Compendial Procedures* ⟨1225⟩) and must produce comparable results to the compendial method or procedure within allowable limits established on a case-by-case basis. Alternative methods or procedures can be developed for any one of a number of reasons not limited to simplification of sample preparation, enhanced precision and accuracy, improved (shortened) run time, or being better suited to automation than the compendial method or procedure.△USP41 Only those results obtained by the methods and procedures given in the compendia are conclusive.

▲For evaluation as a potential replacement or addition to the standard,△USP41 alternative ▲methods and△USP41 procedures should be submitted to USP ▲△USP41 (see section *4.10. Monographs*).

Certain general chapters contain a statement that the text in question is harmonized with the corresponding text of the *European Pharmacopoeia* and/or the *Japanese Pharmacopoeia* and that these texts are interchangeable. Therefore, if a substance or preparation is found to comply with a requirement using an interchangeable method or procedure from one of these pharmacopeias, it should comply with the requirements of the *USP–NF*. When a difference appears, or in the event of dispute, only the result obtained by the method and/or procedure given in the *USP–NF* is conclusive.

6.40. Dried, Anhydrous, Ignited, or Solvent-Free Basis

All calculations in the compendia assume an "as-is" basis unless otherwise specified.

Test procedures may be performed on the undried or unignited substance and the results calculated on the dried, anhydrous, or ignited basis, provided a test for *Loss on Drying*, or *Water Determination*, or *Loss on Ignition*, respectively, is given in the monograph. Where the presence of moisture or other volatile material may interfere with the procedure, previous drying of the substance is specified in the individual monograph and is obligatory.

The term "solvent-free" signifies that the calculation shall be corrected for the presence of known solvents as determined using the methods described in ⟨467⟩ unless a test for limit of organic solvents is provided in the monograph.

The term "previously dried" without qualification signifies that the substance shall be dried as directed under *Loss on Drying* ⟨731⟩ or *Water Determination* ⟨921⟩ (gravimetric determination).

Where drying in vacuum over a desiccant is directed, a vacuum desiccator, a vacuum drying pistol, or other suitable vacuum drying apparatus shall be used.

6.40.10. Ignite to Constant Weight

"Ignite to constant weight" means that ignition shall be continued at $800 \pm 25°$, unless otherwise indicated, until two consecutive weighings, the second of which is taken after an additional period appropriate to the nature and quantity of the residue, do not differ by more than 0.50 mg per g of substance taken.

6.40.20. Dried to Constant Weight

"Dried to constant weight" means that drying shall be continued until two consecutive weighings, the second of which is taken after an additional drying period appropriate to the nature and quantity of the residue, do not differ by more than 0.50 mg per g of substance taken.

6.50. Preparation of Solutions

6.50.10. Filtration

Where a procedure gives direction to "filter" without further qualification, the liquid shall be passed through suitable filter paper or equivalent device until the filtrate is clear. Due to the possibility of filter effects, the initial volumes of a filtrate may be discarded.

6.50.20. Solutions

Unless otherwise specified, all solutions shall be prepared with Purified Water. Solutions for quantitative measures shall be prepared using accurately weighed or accurately measured analytes (see section *8.20 About*).

An expression such as "(1 in 10)" means that 1 part *by volume* of a liquid shall be diluted with, or 1 part *by weight* of a solid shall be dissolved in, a sufficient quantity of the diluent or solvent to make the volume of the finished solution 10 parts *by volume*. ▲For example, a 1 in 10 solution is prepared by diluting 1 mL of a liquid or dissolving 1 g of a solid in sufficient solvent to make 10 mL of the solution. ▲*USP41* An expression such as "(20:5:2)" means that the respective numbers of parts, by volume, of the designated liquids shall be mixed, unless otherwise indicated.

6.50.20.1. Adjustments to Solutions

When a specified concentration is called for in a procedure, a solution of other normality or molarity may be used, provided that allowance is made for the difference in concentration and that the change does not increase the error of measurement.

Proportionately larger or smaller quantities than the specified weights and volumes of assay or test substances and Reference Standards may be taken, provided the measurement is made with at least equivalent accuracy.

Unless otherwise indicated, analyte concentrations shall be prepared to within ten percent (10%) of the indicated value. In the case in which a procedure is adapted to the working range of an instrument, solution concentrations may differ from the indicated value by more than ten percent (10%), with appropriate changes in associated calculations. Any changes shall fall within the validated range of the instrument.

When adjustment of pH is indicated with either an acid or base and the concentration is not indicated, appropriate concentrations of that acid or base may be used.

6.50.20.2. Test Solutions

Information on Test Solutions (TS) is provided in the *Test Solutions* portion of the *Reagents, Indicators, and Solutions* section of the *USP–NF*. Use of an alternative Test Solution or a change in the Test Solution used may require validation.

6.50.20.3. Indicator Solutions

Where a procedure specifies the use of an indicator TS, approximately 0.2 mL, or 3 drops, of the solution shall be added unless otherwise directed.

6.60. Units Necessary to Complete a Test

Unless otherwise specified, a sufficient number of units to ensure a suitable analytical result shall be taken.

6.60.10. Tablets

Where the procedure of a Tablet monograph directs to weigh and finely powder not fewer than a given number of Tablets, a counted number of Tablets shall be weighed and reduced to a powder. The portion of the powdered Tablets taken shall be representative of the whole Tablets and shall, in turn, be weighed accurately.

6.60.20. Capsules

Where the procedure of a Capsule monograph gives direction to remove, as completely as possible, the contents of not fewer than a given number of the Capsules, a counted number of Capsules shall be carefully opened and the contents quantitatively removed, combined, mixed, and weighed accurately. The portion of mixed Capsules contents taken shall be representative of the contents of the Capsules and shall, in turn, be weighed accurately.

6.70. Reagents

The proper conduct of the compendial procedures and the reliability of the results depend, in part, upon the quality of the reagents used in the performance of the procedures. Unless otherwise specified, reagents conforming to the specifications set forth in the current edition of *Reagent Chemicals* published by the American Chemical Society (ACS) shall be used. Where such ACS reagent specifications are not available or where the required purity differs, compendial specifications for reagents of acceptable quality are provided (see the *Reagents, Indicators, and Solutions* section of the *USP–NF*). Reagents not covered by any of these specifications should be of a grade suitable to the proper performance of the method of assay or test involved.

Listing of these reagents, including the indicators and solutions employed as reagents, in no way implies that they have therapeutic utility; furthermore, any reference to *USP* or *NF* in their labeling shall include also the term "reagent" or "reagent grade." USP may supply reagents if they otherwise may not be generally commercially available.

6.80. Equipment

Unless otherwise specified, a specification for a definite size or type of container or apparatus in a procedure is given solely as a recommendation. Other dimensions or types may be used if they are suitable for the intended use.

6.80.10. Apparatus for Measurement

Where volumetric flasks or other exact measuring, weighing, or sorting devices are specified, this or other equipment of at least equivalent accuracy shall be employed.

6.80.10.1. Pipet/Pipette

Where a pipet/pipette is specified, a suitable buret may be substituted. Where a "to contain" pipet/pipette is specified, a suitable volumetric flask may be substituted.

6.80.10.2. Light Protection

Where low-actinic or light-resistant containers are specified, either containers specially treated to protect contents from light or clear containers that have been rendered opaque by application of a suitable coating or wrapping may be used.

6.80.20. Instrumental Apparatus

An instrument may be substituted for the specified instrument if the substitute uses the same fundamental principles of operation and is of equivalent or greater sensitivity and accuracy. These characteristics shall be qualified as appropriate. Where a particular brand or source of a material, instrument, or piece of equipment, or the name and address of a manufacturer or distributor, is mentioned (ordinarily in a footnote), this identification is furnished solely for informational purposes as a matter of convenience, without implication of approval, endorsement, or certification.

6.80.20.1. Chromatographic Tubes and Columns

The term "diameter" refers to internal diameter (ID).

6.80.20.2. Tubing

The term "diameter" refers to outside diameter (OD).

6.80.20.3. Steam Bath

Where use of a steam bath is directed, use actively flowing steam or another regulated heat source controlled at an equivalent temperature.

6.80.20.4. Water Bath

A water bath requires vigorously boiling water unless otherwise specified.

6.80.30. Temperature Reading Devices

Temperature reading devices suitable for pharmacopeial tests conform to specifications that are traceable to a National Institute of Standards and Technology (NIST) standard or equivalent. Temperature reading devices may be of the liquid-in-glass type or an analog or digital temperature indicator type, such as a resistance temperature device, thermistor, or thermocouple. Standardization of thermometers is performed on an established testing frequency with a temperature standard traceable to NIST. For example, refer to the current issue of American Society of Testing and Materials (ASTM) standards E1 for liquid-in-glass thermometers.

7. TEST RESULTS

7.10. Interpretation of Requirements

Analytical results observed in the laboratory (or calculated from experimental measurements) are compared with stated acceptance criteria to determine whether the article conforms to compendial requirements.

The reportable value, which often is a summary value for several individual determinations, is compared with the acceptance criteria. The reportable value is the end result of a completed measurement procedure, as documented.

Where acceptance criteria are expressed numerically herein through specification of an upper and/or lower limit, permitted values include the specified values themselves, but no values outside the limit(s). Acceptance criteria are considered significant to the last digit shown.

7.10.5. Nominal Concentrations in Equations

Where a "nominal concentration" is specified, calculate the concentration based on the label claim. In assay procedures, water correction is typically stated in the Definition and on the label of the USP Reference Standard. For other procedures, correction for assayed content, potency, or both is made prior to using the concentration in the equation provided in the monograph.

7.10.10. Equivalence Statements in Titrimetric Procedures

The directions for titrimetric procedures conclude with a statement of the weight of the analyte that is equivalent to each mL of the standardized titrant. In such an equivalence statement, the number of significant figures in the concentration of the titrant should be understood to correspond to the number of significant figures in the weight of the analyte. Corrections to calculations based on the blank determination are to be made for all titrimetric assays where appropriate (see *Titrimetry* ⟨541⟩).

7.20. Rounding Rules

The observed or calculated values shall be rounded off to the number of decimal places that is in agreement with the limit expression. Numbers should not be rounded until the final calculations for the reportable value have been completed. Intermediate calculations (e.g., slope for linearity) may be rounded for reporting purposes, but the original (not rounded) value should be used for any additional required calculations. Acceptance criteria are fixed numbers and are not rounded.

When rounding is required, consider only one digit in the decimal place to the right of the last place in the limit expression. If this digit is smaller than 5, it is eliminated and the preceding digit is unchanged. If this digit is equal to or greater than 5, it is eliminated and the preceding digit is increased by 1.

8. TERMS AND DEFINITIONS

8.10. Abbreviations

- RS refers to a USP Reference Standard.
- CS refers to a Colorimetric Solution.
- TS refers to a Test Solution.
- VS refers to a Volumetric Solution that is standardized in accordance with directions given in the individual monograph or in the *Reagents, Indicators, and Solutions* section of *USP–NF*.

8.20. About

"About" indicates a quantity within 10%.

If the measurement is stated to be "accurately measured" or "accurately weighed," follow the statements in *Volumetric Apparatus* ⟨31⟩ and *Balances* ⟨41⟩, respectively.

8.30. Alcohol Content

Percentages of alcohol, such as those under the heading *Alcohol Content*, refer to percentage by volume of C_2H_5OH at 15.56°. Where a formula, test, or assay calls for alcohol, ethyl alcohol, or ethanol, the *USP* monograph article Alcohol shall be used. Where reference is made to "C_2H_5OH," absolute (100%) ethanol is intended. Where a procedure calls for dehydrated alcohol, alcohol absolute, or anhydrous alcohol, the *USP* monograph article Dehydrated Alcohol shall be used.

8.40. Atomic Weights

Atomic weights used in computing molecular weights and the factors in the assays and elsewhere are those established by the IUPAC Commission on Isotopic Abundances and Atomic Weights.

8.50. Blank Determinations

Where it is directed that "any necessary correction" be made by a blank determination, the determination shall be conducted using the same quantities of the same reagents treated in the same manner as the solution or mixture containing the portion of the substance under assay or test, but with the substance itself omitted.

Illustration of Rounding Numerical Values for Comparison with Requirements			
Compendial Requirement	**Unrounded Value**	**Rounded Result**	**Conforms**
Assay limit ≥98.0%	97.96%	98.0%	Yes
	97.92%	97.9%	No
	97.95%	98.0%	Yes
Assay limit ≤101.5%	101.55%	101.6%	No
	101.46%	101.5%	Yes
	101.45%	101.5%	Yes
Limit test ≤0.02%	0.025%	0.03%	No
	0.015%	0.02%	Yes
	0.027%	0.03%	No
Limit test ≤3 ppm	3.5 ppm	4 ppm	No
	3.4 ppm	3 ppm	Yes
	2.5 ppm	3 ppm	Yes

8.60. Concomitantly

"Concomitantly" denotes that the determinations or measurements are to be performed in immediate succession.

8.70. Desiccator

The instruction "in a desiccator" indicates use of a tightly closed container of suitable size and design that maintains an atmosphere of low moisture content by means of a suitable desiccant such as anhydrous calcium chloride, magnesium perchlorate, phosphorus pentoxide, or silica gel. See also section *8.220 Vacuum Desiccator*.

8.80. Logarithms

Logarithms are to the base 10.

8.90. Microbial Strain

A microbial strain cited and identified by its American Type Culture Collection (ATCC) catalog number shall be used directly or, if subcultured, shall be used not more than five passages removed from the original strain.

8.100. Negligible

"Negligible" indicates a quantity not exceeding 0.50 mg.

8.110. NLT/NMT

"NLT" means "not less than." "NMT" means "not more than."

8.120. Odor

"Odorless," "practically odorless," "a faint characteristic odor," and variations thereof indicate evaluation of a suitable quantity of freshly opened material after exposure to the air for 15 minutes. An odor designation is descriptive only and should not be regarded as a standard of purity for a particular lot of an article.

8.130. Percent

"Percent" used without qualification means:
- For mixtures of solids and semisolids, percent weight in weight;
- For solutions or suspensions of solids in liquids, percent weight in volume;
- For solutions of liquids in liquids, percent volume in volume;
- For solutions of gases in liquids, percent weight in volume.

For example, a 1 percent solution is prepared by dissolving 1 g of a solid or semisolid, or 1 mL of a liquid, in sufficient solvent to make 100 mL of the solution.

8.140. Percentage Concentrations

Percentage concentrations are expressed as follows:
- *Percent Weight in Weight* (w/w) is defined as the number of g of a solute in 100 g of solution.
- *Percent Weight in Volume* (w/v) is defined as the number of g of a solute in 100 mL of solution.
- *Percent Volume in Volume* (v/v) is defined as the number of mL of a solute in 100 mL of solution.

8.150. Pressure

Pressure is determined by use of a suitable manometer or barometer calibrated in terms of the pressure exerted by a column of mercury of the stated height.

8.160. Reaction Time

Reaction time is 5 minutes unless otherwise specified.

8.170. Specific Gravity

Specific gravity is the weight of a substance in air at 25° divided by the weight of an equal volume of water at the same temperature.

8.180. Temperatures

Temperatures are expressed in centigrade (Celsius) degrees, and all measurements are made at 25° unless otherwise indicated. Where moderate heat is specified, any temperature not higher than 45° (113° F) is indicated.

8.190. Time

Unless otherwise specified, rounding rules, as described in section *7.20 Rounding Rules*, apply to any time specified.

8.200. Transfer

"Transfer" indicates a quantitative manipulation.

8.210. Vacuum

"Vacuum" denotes exposure to a pressure of less than 20 mm of mercury (2.67 kPas), unless otherwise indicated.

8.220. Vacuum Desiccator

"Vacuum desiccator" indicates a desiccator that maintains a low-moisture atmosphere at a reduced pressure of not more than 20 mm of mercury (2.67 kPas) or at the pressure designated in the individual monograph.

8.230. Water

8.230.10. Water as an Ingredient in an Official Product

As an ingredient in an official product, water meets the requirements of the appropriate water monograph in *USP* or *NF*.

8.230.20. Water in the Manufacture of Official Substances

When used in the manufacture of official substances, water shall meet the requirements for drinking water as set forth in the U.S. Environmental Protection Agency National Primary Drinking Water Regulations or in the drinking water regulations of the European Union or of Japan, or in the World Health Organization's Guidelines for Drinking Water Quality. Additional specifications may be required in monographs.

8.230.30. Water in a Compendial Procedure

When water is called for in a compendial procedure, the *USP* monograph article Purified Water shall be used unless otherwise specified. Definitions for other types of water are provided in *Reagents, Indicators, and Solutions* and in *Water for Pharmaceutical Purposes* ⟨1231⟩.

8.240. Weights and Measures

In general, weights and measures are expressed in the International System of Units (SI) as established and revised by the *Conférence générale des poids et mesures*. For compendial purposes, the term "weight" is considered to be synonymous with "mass."

Molality is designated by the symbol m preceded by a number that represents the number of moles of the designated solute contained in 1 kilogram of the designated solvent.

Molarity is designated by the symbol M preceded by a number that represents the number of moles of the designated solute contained in an amount of the designated solvent that is sufficient to prepare 1 liter of solution.

Normality is designated by the symbol N preceded by a number that represents the number of equivalents of the designated solute contained in an amount of the designated solvent that is sufficient to prepare 1 liter of solution.

The symbol for degrees (°) without a qualifying unit of measure represents degrees Celsius.

Chart of Symbols and Prefixes commonly employed for SI metric units and other units:

	Units	Symbol	Notes
Length			
	meter	m	
	centimeter	cm	
	millimeter	mm	
	micrometer	μm	Previously referred to as a micron
	nanometer	nm	Previously the symbol mμ (for millimicron) was used
	Ångström	Å	Equal to 0.1 nm
Mass			
	kilogram	kg	
	gram	g	
	milligram	mg	

	Units	Symbol	Notes
	microgram	µg	The symbol µg is used in the *USP* and *NF* to represent micrograms, but micrograms may be represented as "mcg" for labeling and prescribing purposes. The term "gamma," symbolized by γ, frequently is used to represent micrograms in biochemical literature.
	nanogram	ng	
	picogram	pg	
	dalton	Da	Also referred to as the unified atomic mass unit and is equal to 1/12 times the mass of the free carbon 12 atom.
	kilodalton	kDa	
Time			
	second	s	
	minute	min	
	hour	h	
Volume			
	liter	L	1 L is equal to 1000 cm³ (cubic centimeters)
	deciliter	dL	
	milliliter	mL	1 mL is equal to 1 cm³, sometimes referred to as cc
	microliter	µL	
Temperature			
	Celsius	°C	
Amount of Substance			
	mole	mol	Historically referred to as gram-molecular weight or gram-atomic weight
	millimole	mmol	
	micromole	µmol	
	femtomole	fmol	
	equivalent	Eq	Also referred to as gram-equivalent weight. It is used in the calculation of substance concentration in units of normality. This unit is no longer preferred for use in analytical chemistry or metrology.
	milli equivalent	mEq	
	osmole	Osmol	Osmotic pressure of a solution, related to substance concentration.
	milliosmole	mOsmol	
Pressure			
	pascal	Pa	
	kilopascal	kPa	

	Units	Symbol	Notes
	pounds per square inch	psi	
	millimeter of mercury	mmHg	Equal to 133.322 Pa
Electrical units			
	ampere	A	
	volt	V	
	millivolt	mV	
	hertz	Hz	Unit of frequency
	kilohertz	kHz	
	megahertz	MHz	
	electron volt	eV	
	kilo-electron volt	keV	
	mega-electron volt	MeV	
Radiation			
	becquerel	Bq	SI unit of activity for radionuclides
	kilobecquerel	kBq	
	megabecquerel	MBq	
	gigabecquerel	GBq	
	curie	Ci	Non-SI unit of activity for radionuclides
	millicurie	mCi	
	microcurie	µCi	
	nanocurie	nCi	
Other			
	acceleration due to gravity	g	Used to express rate of centrifugation
	revolutions per minute	rpm	Used to express rate of centrifugation

Selected SI Prefixes

Name	Symbol	Factor
giga	G	10^9
mega	M	10^6
kilo	k	10^3
deci	d	10^{-1}
centi	c	10^{-2}
milli	m	10^{-3}
micro	µ	10^{-6}
nano	n	10^{-9}
pico	p	10^{-12}
femto	f	10^{-15}

9. PRESCRIBING AND DISPENSING
9.10. Use of Metric Units

Prescriptions for compendial articles shall be written to state the quantity and/or strength desired in metric units unless otherwise indicated in the individual monograph [see also section *5.50.10 Units of Potency (Biological)* above]. If an amount is prescribed by any other system of measurement, only an amount that is the metric equivalent of the prescribed amount shall be dispensed. Abbreviations for the terms "Units" or "International Units" shall not be used for labeling or prescribing purposes. Apothecary unit designations on labels and labeling shall not be used.

9.20. Changes in Volume

In the dispensing of prescription medications, slight changes in volume owing to variations in room temperatures may be disregarded.

10. PRESERVATION, PACKAGING, STORAGE, AND LABELING

10.10. Packaging and Storage

All articles in *USP* or *NF* are subject to the packaging and storage requirements specified in *Packaging and Storage Requirements* ⟨659⟩, unless different requirements are provided in an individual monograph.

10.20. Labeling

All articles in *USP* or *NF* are subject to the labeling requirements specified in *Labeling* ⟨7⟩, unless different requirements are provided in an individual monograph.

Official Monographs for USP 41

Add the following:

▪Acamprosate Calcium

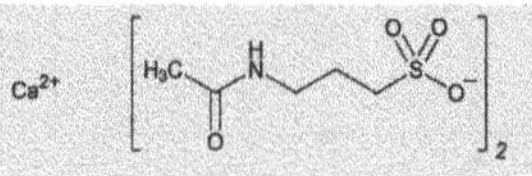

$C_{10}H_{20}CaN_2O_8S_2$ 400.48

1-Propanesulfonic acid, 3-(acetylamino)-, calcium salt (2:1);
Calcium 3-(acetylamino)propane-1-sulfonate [77337-73-6].

DEFINITION
Acamprosate Calcium contains NLT 98.0% and NMT 102.0% of acamprosate calcium ($C_{10}H_{20}CaN_2O_8S_2$), calculated on the dried basis.

IDENTIFICATION
- **A. INFRARED ABSORPTION ⟨197K⟩**
- **B.** The retention time of the major peak of the *Sample solution* corresponds to that of the *Standard solution*, as obtained in the *Assay*.
- **C. IDENTIFICATION TESTS—GENERAL ⟨191⟩**, *Chemical Identification Tests, Calcium*: Meets the requirements

ASSAY
- **PROCEDURE**
  Mobile phase: Add 5.0 mL of triethylamine per 1 L of water and adjust with phosphoric acid to a pH of 4.0.
  System suitability solution: 10 mg/mL of USP Acamprosate Calcium RS and 0.005 mg/mL each of USP Acamprosate Related Compound B RS and glacial acetic acid in water. Sonication may be used to aid in dissolution.
  Standard solution: 0.3 mg/mL of USP Acamprosate Calcium RS in water. Sonication may be used to aid in dissolution.
  Sample solution: 0.3 mg/mL of Acamprosate Calcium in water. Sonication may be used to aid in dissolution.
  Chromatographic system
  (See *Chromatography ⟨621⟩, System Suitability*.)
  Mode: LC
  Detector: UV 210 nm
  Column: 4.6-mm × 25-cm; 5-µm packing L1
  Flow rate: 0.7 mL/min
  Injection volume: 20 µL
  Run time: NLT 2 times the retention time of the acamprosate peak
  System suitability
  Samples: *System suitability solution* and *Standard solution*
  [NOTE—See *Table 1* for the relative retention times.]
  Suitability requirements
  Resolution: NLT 1.5 between acetic acid and acamprosate related compound B; NLT 1.3 between acamprosate related compound B and acamprosate, *System suitability solution*
  Tailing factor: NMT 2.0, *Standard solution*
  Relative standard deviation: NMT 0.73%, *Standard solution*

Analysis
  Samples: *Standard solution* and *Sample solution*
  Calculate the percentage of acamprosate calcium ($C_{10}H_{20}CaN_2O_8S_2$) in the portion of Acamprosate Calcium taken:

$$Result = (r_U/r_S) \times (C_S/C_U) \times 100$$

r_U = peak response from the *Sample solution*
r_S = peak response from the *Standard solution*
C_S = concentration of USP Acamprosate Calcium RS in the *Standard solution* (mg/mL)
C_U = concentration of Acamprosate Calcium in the *Sample solution* (mg/mL)

Acceptance criteria: 98.0%–102.0% on the dried basis

IMPURITIES
- **LIMIT OF ACAMPROSATE RELATED COMPOUND A**
  Solution A: 5 g/L of fluorescamine in acetonitrile. Use within 24 h of preparation.
  Buffer: 13.8 g/L of monobasic sodium phosphate prepared as follows. Transfer a suitable amount of monobasic sodium phosphate to a volumetric flask. Dissolve in 90% of the final flask volume of water. Adjust with 10 N sodium hydroxide TS or phosphoric acid to a pH of 6.5. Dilute with water to volume.
  Mobile phase: Acetonitrile, methanol, and *Buffer* (10:10:80)
  Diluent: 24.6 g/L of boric acid prepared as follows. Transfer a suitable amount of boric acid to an appropriate volumetric flask. Dissolve in 90% of the final flask volume of water. Adjust with 10 N sodium hydroxide TS to a pH of 10.4. Dilute with water to volume.
  Standard stock solution A: 250 µg/mL of USP Acamprosate Related Compound A RS in water
  Standard stock solution B: 1 µg/mL of USP Acamprosate Related Compound A RS from *Standard stock solution A* in *Diluent*
  Standard solution: Transfer 3.0 mL of *Standard stock solution B* to an appropriate container. Add 0.15 mL of *Solution A* and shake vigorously for 30 s. Heat in a water bath at 50° for 30 min. Cool under a stream of cold water, centrifuge, and pass the supernatant through a suitable membrane filter.
  Sample stock solution A: 20 mg/mL of Acamprosate Calcium in water
  Sample stock solution B: 2000 µg/mL of Acamprosate Calcium from *Sample stock solution A* in *Diluent*
  Sample solution: Transfer 3.0 mL of *Sample stock solution B* to an appropriate container. Add 0.15 mL of *Solution A* and shake for 30 s. Heat in a water bath at 50° for 30 min. Cool under a stream of cold water, centrifuge, and pass the supernatant through a suitable membrane filter.
  Chromatographic system
  (See *Chromatography ⟨621⟩, System Suitability*.)
  Mode: LC
  Detector: UV 261 nm
  Column: 4.6-mm × 15-cm; 3- or 5-µm packing L1
  Flow rate: 1 mL/min
  Injection volume: 20 µL
  Run time: NLT 2 times the retention time of acamprosate related compound A

System suitability
Sample: *Standard solution*
[NOTE—The relative retention times for fluorescamine and acamprosate related compound A are about 0.5 and 1.0, respectively. Acamprosate calcium is not detected by this chromatographic system.]
Suitability requirements
Resolution: NLT 2.0 between fluorescamine and acamprosate related compound A
Relative standard deviation: NMT 5.0% for acamprosate related compound A
Analysis
Samples: *Standard solution* and *Sample solution*
Calculate the percentage of acamprosate related compound A in the portion of Acamprosate Calcium taken:

$$\text{Result} = (r_U/r_S) \times (C_S/C_U) \times 100$$

r_U = peak response from the *Sample solution*
r_S = peak response from the *Standard solution*
C_S = concentration of USP Acamprosate Calcium Related Compound A RS in the *Standard solution* (µg/mL)
C_U = concentration of Acamprosate Calcium in the *Sample solution* (µg/mL)
Acceptance criteria: NMT 0.05%
• **ORGANIC IMPURITIES**
Mobile phase: Add 5.0 mL of triethylamine per 1 L of water and adjust with phosphoric acid to a pH of 4.0.
System suitability solution: 10 mg/mL of USP Acamprosate Calcium RS and 0.005 mg/mL each of USP Acamprosate Related Compound B RS and glacial acetic acid in water. Sonication may be used to aid in dissolution.
Standard solution: 0.005 mg/mL of USP Acamprosate Calcium RS in water. Sonication may be used to aid in dissolution.
Sample solution: 10 mg/mL of Acamprosate Calcium in water. Sonication may be used to aid in dissolution.
Chromatographic system
(See *Chromatography* ⟨621⟩, *System Suitability*.)
Mode: LC
Detector: UV 210 nm
Column: 4.6-mm × 25-cm; 5-µm packing L1
Flow rate: 0.7 mL/min
Injection volume: 20 µL
Run time: NLT 6 times the retention time of the acamprosate peak
System suitability
Samples: *System suitability solution* and *Standard solution*
[NOTE—The relative retention time for acetic acid is 0.7; see *Table 1* for the other relative retention times.]
Suitability requirements
Resolution: NLT 1.5 between acetic acid and acamprosate related compound B; NLT 1.3 between acamprosate related compound B and acamprosate, *System suitability solution*
Tailing factor: NMT 1.5 for acamprosate, *Standard solution*
Relative standard deviation: NMT 15.0% for acetic acid, *System suitability solution*; NMT 5% for acamprosate, *Standard solution*
Analysis
Samples: *Standard solution* and *Sample solution*
Calculate the percentage of each impurity in the portion of Acamprosate Calcium taken:

$$\text{Result} = (r_U/r_S) \times (C_S/C_U) \times 100$$

r_U = peak response of each impurity from the *Sample solution*
r_S = peak response of acamprosate from the *Standard solution*

C_S = concentration of USP Acamprosate Calcium RS in the *Standard solution* (mg/mL)
C_U = concentration of Acamprosate Calcium in the *Sample solution* (mg/mL)
Acceptance criteria: See *Table 1*.

Table 1

Name	Relative Retention Time	Acceptance Criteria, NMT (%)
Calcium[a]	0.4	—
Acamprosate related compound B	0.8	0.05
Acamprosate	1.0	—
N-Methyl acamprosate[b]	1.9	0.05
Any individual unspecified impurity	—	0.05
Total impurities[c]	—	0.5

[a] Included for identification only. This peak is due to the calcium counter-ion and hence is not an impurity.
[b] 3-(N-Methylacetamido)propane-1-sulfonate.
[c] The sum of acamprosate related compound A from the *Limit of Acamprosate Related Compound A* test and all impurities from the test for *Organic Impurities*.

SPECIFIC TESTS
• **PH ⟨791⟩**
Sample solution: 0.05 g/mL of Acamprosate Calcium in carbon dioxide-free water
Acceptance criteria: 5.5–7.0
• **LOSS ON DRYING ⟨731⟩**
Analysis: Dry at 105° for 3 h.
Acceptance criteria: NMT 0.4%

ADDITIONAL REQUIREMENTS
• **PACKAGING AND STORAGE:** Store in tight containers.
• **USP REFERENCE STANDARDS ⟨11⟩**
USP Acamprosate Calcium RS
USP Acamprosate Related Compound A RS
3-Aminopropane-1-sulfonic acid.
$C_3H_9NO_3S$ 139.17
USP Acamprosate Related Compound B RS
Calcium 3-formamidopropane-1-sulfonate.
$C_8H_{16}CaN_2O_8S_2$ 372.42

■1S *(USP41)*

Acetaminophen Oral Suspension

DEFINITION
Acetaminophen Oral Suspension is a suspension of Acetaminophen in a suitable aqueous vehicle. It contains NLT 90.0% and NMT 110.0% of the labeled amount of acetaminophen ($C_8H_9NO_2$).

IDENTIFICATION
• **A. INFRARED ABSORPTION ⟨197K⟩**
Sample: Transfer a volume of Oral Suspension, equivalent to 240 mg of acetaminophen, to a separator. Add 50 mL of ethyl acetate, and shake. Filter the ethyl acetate extract through a funnel containing glass wool and 10 g of anhydrous sodium sulfate. Collect the filtrate in a beaker, and evaporate on a steam bath to dryness. Dry the residue under vacuum over silica gel.
Acceptance criteria: The crystals so obtained meet the requirements.

Add the following:

■• **B.** The retention time of the acetaminophen peak of the *Sample solution* corresponds to that of the *Standard solution*, as obtained in the *Assay*.■1S (*USP41*)

ASSAY

Change to read:

• **PROCEDURE**
  ■**Solution A:** Acetonitrile, trifluoroacetic acid, and water (14: 0.1: 86)
  Solution B: Acetonitrile, trifluoroacetic acid, and water (90: 0.1: 10)
  Mobile phase: See *Table 1*.

Table 1

Time (min)	Solution A (%)	Solution B (%)
0.0	100	0
4.0	100	0
5.0	0	100
6.0	100	0
10.0	100	0

Diluent: Methanol, phosphoric acid, and water (50: 0.1: 50)
Standard stock solution: 1.6 mg/mL of USP Acetaminophen RS in *Diluent*
Standard solution: 0.064 mg/mL of USP Acetaminophen RS in *Solution A*, from *Standard stock solution*
Sample stock solution: Nominally 1.6 mg/mL of acetaminophen prepared as follows. Transfer a quantity equivalent to about 160 mg of acetaminophen from a volume of Oral Suspension, previously well shaken, to a 100-mL volumetric flask. Add 60 mL of *Diluent*, and shake by mechanical means for 30 min. Dilute with *Diluent* to volume. Mix well. Allow the sample to settle, or centrifuge.
Sample solution: Nominally 0.064 mg/mL of acetaminophen in *Solution A*, from *Sample stock solution*
Chromatographic system
  (See *Chromatography* ⟨621⟩, *System Suitability*.)
  Mode: LC
  Detector: UV 214 nm
  Column: 4.6-mm × 15-cm; 3.5-μm packing L11
  Flow rate: 1 mL/min
  Injection volume: 30 μL
System suitability
  Sample: *Standard solution*
  Suitability requirements
    Tailing factor: NMT 2.0
    Relative standard deviation: NMT 2.0%
Analysis
  Samples: *Standard solution* and *Sample solution*
  Calculate the percentage of the labeled amount of acetaminophen ($C_8H_9NO_2$) in the portion of Oral Suspension taken:

$$Result = (r_U/r_S) \times (C_S/C_U) \times 100$$

r_U = peak response of acetaminophen from the *Sample solution*
r_S = peak response of acetaminophen from the *Standard solution*
C_S = concentration of USP Acetaminophen RS in the *Standard solution* (mg/mL)
C_U = nominal concentration of acetaminophen in the *Sample solution* (mg/mL)■1S (*USP41*)

Acceptance criteria: 90.0%–110.0%

PERFORMANCE TESTS
• **UNIFORMITY OF DOSAGE UNITS** ⟨905⟩
  For single-unit containers: Meets the requirements
• **DELIVERABLE VOLUME** ⟨698⟩
  For multiple-unit containers: Meets the requirements

IMPURITIES

Delete the following:

■• 4-**AMINOPHENOL IN ACETAMINOPHEN-CONTAINING DRUG PRODUCTS** ⟨227⟩: Meets the requirements■1S (*USP41*)

Add the following:

■• **ORGANIC IMPURITIES**
  Solution A: 0.2% trifluoroacetic acid in water
  Solution B: 0.2% trifluoroacetic acid in acetonitrile
  Mobile phase: See *Table 2*.

Table 2

Time (min)	Solution A (%)	Solution B (%)
0.0	98	2
1.0	98	2
8.0	80	20
9.0	5	95
10.0	5	95
10.5	98	2
13.0	98	2

Buffer: 10 mM sodium citrate dihydrate, with a pH of 4.0, prepared by adding 1.1 g of sodium citrate dihydrate and 1.3 g of citric acid monohydrate to a 1-L volumetric flask, dissolving, and diluting with water to volume. Adjust with sodium citrate dihydrate to increase the pH or with citric acid monohydrate to decrease the pH, if necessary, to achieve a pH of 4.0.
Diluent: Acetonitrile and *Buffer* (10:90)
Sensitivity solution: 0.16 μg/mL of USP Acetaminophen RS and 0.08 μg/mL of USP 4-Aminophenol RS in *Diluent*
Standard solution: 1.6 μg/mL each of USP Acetaminophen RS and USP 4-Aminophenol RS in *Diluent*
Sample solution: Nominally 1.6 mg/mL of acetaminophen in *Diluent* prepared as follows. Transfer a quantity equivalent to about 160 mg of acetaminophen from a volume of Oral Suspension, previously well shaken, to a 100-mL volumetric flask. Add 60 mL of *Diluent*, and shake by mechanical means for 1 h. Dilute with *Diluent* to volume. Mix well. Pass a portion of this solution through a suitable filter.
Chromatographic system
  (See *Chromatography* ⟨621⟩, *System Suitability*.)
  Mode: LC
  Detector: UV 272 nm
  Column: 2.1-mm × 15-cm; 1.8-μm packing L1
  Column temperature: 40°
  Flow rate: 0.5 mL/min
  Injection volume: 2.5 μL
System suitability
  Samples: *Sensitivity solution* and *Standard solution*
  [NOTE—See *Table 3* for relative retention times.]
  Suitability requirements
    Tailing factor: NMT 2.0 for acetaminophen and 4-aminophenol, *Standard solution*
    Relative standard deviation: NMT 5.0% for acetaminophen and 4-aminophenol, *Standard solution*
    Signal-to-noise ratio: NLT 10 for acetaminophen and 4-aminophenol, *Sensitivity solution*

Analysis
Samples: *Standard solution* and *Sample solution*
Calculate the percentage of 4-aminophenol in the portion of Oral Suspension taken:

$$Result = (r_U/r_S) \times (C_S/C_U) \times 100$$

r_U = peak response of 4-aminophenol from the *Sample solution*
r_S = peak response of 4-aminophenol from the *Standard solution*
C_S = concentration of USP 4-Aminophenol RS in the *Standard solution* (mg/mL)
C_U = nominal concentration of acetaminophen in the *Sample solution* (mg/mL)

Calculate the percentage of acetaminophen dimer or any unspecified impurity in the portion of Oral Suspension taken:

$$Result = (r_U/r_S) \times (C_S/C_U) \times 100$$

r_U = peak response of acetaminophen dimer or any unspecified impurity from the *Sample solution*
r_S = peak response of acetaminophen from the *Standard solution*
C_S = concentration of USP Acetaminophen RS in the *Standard solution* (mg/mL)
C_U = nominal concentration of acetaminophen in the *Sample solution* (mg/mL)

Acceptance criteria: See *Table 3*. The reporting threshold is 0.05% for any impurities.

Table 3

Name	Relative Retention Time	Acceptance Criteria, NMT (%)
4-Aminophenol	0.28	0.15
Acetaminophen	1.0	—
Acetaminophen dimer[a]	1.57	0.15
Any unspecified impurity	—	0.15
Total impurities	—	2.0

[a] N,N'-(6,6'-Dihydroxy-[1,1'-biphenyl]-3,3'-diyl)diacetamide.

■1S (USP41)

SPECIFIC TESTS
• **pH ⟨791⟩:** 4.0–6.9

ADDITIONAL REQUIREMENTS
• **PACKAGING AND STORAGE:** Preserve in tight containers, and store at controlled room temperature.
• **USP REFERENCE STANDARDS ⟨11⟩**
  USP Acetaminophen RS
  USP 4-Aminophenol RS

Acetaminophen Tablets

DEFINITION
Acetaminophen Tablets contain NLT 90.0% and NMT 110.0% of the labeled amount of acetaminophen ($C_8H_9NO_2$).

IDENTIFICATION
• **A.** The retention time of the acetaminophen peak of the *Sample solution* corresponds to that of the *Standard solution*, as obtained in the *Assay*.

■• **B. THIN-LAYER CHROMATOGRAPHIC IDENTIFICATION TEST ⟨201⟩**
Sample solution: Nominally 1 mg/mL of acetaminophen prepared as follows. Triturate 50 mg of acetaminophen from powdered Tablets in 50 mL of methanol, and filter. Use the clear filtrate.
Chromatographic system
Developing solvent system: Methylene chloride and methanol (4:1)
Acceptance criteria: Meet the requirements■1S (USP41)

■• **B.** The UV spectrum of the acetaminophen peak of the *Sample solution* corresponds to that of the *Standard solution*, as obtained in the *Assay*.■1S (USP41)

ASSAY

• **PROCEDURE**
■**Solution A:** 1% (v/v) glacial acetic acid in water
Solution B: Methanol
Mobile phase: See *Table 1*. Return to original conditions and re-equilibrate the system for 4 min.

Table 1

Time (min)	Solution A (%)	Solution B (%)
0.0	90	10
4.0	90	10
4.1	20	80
6.0	20	80

Diluent: Methanol and water (10:90)
Standard solution: 0.01 mg/mL of USP Acetaminophen RS in *Diluent*
Sample stock solution: Nominally 0.1 mg/mL of acetaminophen in *Diluent* prepared as follows. Transfer an appropriate amount of acetaminophen from NLT 10 Tablets to a suitable volumetric flask and dilute with *Diluent* to volume. Centrifuge or pass a portion of this solution through a suitable filter. [NOTE—Sonication or shaking may be necessary.]
Sample solution: Nominally 0.01 mg/mL of acetaminophen in *Diluent* from the *Sample stock solution*. Pass a portion of this solution through a suitable filter.
Chromatographic system
(See *Chromatography ⟨621⟩, System Suitability*.)
Mode: LC
Detector: UV 243 nm. For *Identification B*, use a diode array detector in the range of 220–400 nm.
Column: 3.0-mm × 10-cm; 3.5-µm packing L1
Column temperature: 40°
Flow rate: 0.5 mL/min
Injection volume: 10 µL
System suitability
Sample: *Standard solution*
Suitability requirements
Tailing factor: NMT 2.0
Relative standard deviation: NMT 2.0%
Analysis
Samples: *Standard solution* and *Sample solution*
Calculate the percentage of the labeled amount of acetaminophen ($C_8H_9NO_2$) in the portion of Tablets taken:

$$Result = (r_U/r_S) \times (C_S/C_U) \times 100$$

r_U = peak response of acetaminophen from the *Sample solution*

r_S = peak response of acetaminophen from the *Standard solution*

C_S = concentration of USP Acetaminophen RS in the *Standard solution* (mg/mL)

C_U = nominal concentration of acetaminophen in the *Sample solution* (mg/mL)∎1S (USP41)

Acceptance criteria: 90.0%–110.0%

PERFORMANCE TESTS
- **Dissolution ⟨711⟩**
 Medium: pH 5.8 phosphate buffer (see *Reagents, Indicators, and Solutions—Buffer Solutions*); 900 mL
 Apparatus 2: 50 rpm
 Time: 30 min
 Standard solution: A known concentration of USP Acetaminophen RS in *Medium*
 Sample solution: A filtered portion of the solution under test, suitably diluted with *Medium* to obtain a concentration similar to that of the *Standard solution*
 Instrumental conditions
 Mode: UV
 Analytical wavelength: Maximum absorbance at about 243 nm
 Analysis
 Samples: *Standard solution* and *Sample solution*
 Calculate the percentage of the labeled amount of acetaminophen ($C_8H_9NO_2$) dissolved.
 Tolerances: NLT 80% (Q) of the labeled amount of acetaminophen ($C_8H_9NO_2$) is dissolved.
 For Tablets labeled as chewable
 Medium: pH 5.8 phosphate buffer (see *Reagents, Indicators, and Solutions—Buffer Solutions*); 900 mL
 Apparatus 2: 75 rpm
 Time: 45 min
 Standard solution, Sample solution, Instrumental conditions, and **Analysis:** Proceed as directed above.
 Tolerances: NLT 75% (Q) of the labeled amount of acetaminophen ($C_8H_9NO_2$) is dissolved.
- **Uniformity of Dosage Units ⟨905⟩:** Meet the requirements

IMPURITIES

Delete the following:

■• **4-Aminophenol in Acetaminophen-Containing Drug Products ⟨227⟩:** Meet the requirements∎1S (USP41)

Add the following:

■• **Organic Impurities**
 It is suggested to protect all solutions containing acetaminophen or 4-aminophenol from light.
 Buffer: Dissolve 1.9 g of ammonium formate in 1 L of water. Add 1.0 mL of formic acid.
 Solution A: Dissolve 3.1 g of ammonium acetate in 1 L of water. Add 1.0 mL of trifluoroacetic acid.
 Solution B: Acetonitrile, methanol, and water (10:75:15)
 Solution C: Dissolve 3.1 g of ammonium acetate in 1000 mL of *Solution B*. Add 1.0 mL of trifluoroacetic acid.
 Mobile phase: See *Table 2*. Return to original conditions and re-equilibrate the system for 4 min.

Table 2

Time (min)	Solution A (%)	Solution C (%)
0	97	3
5	70	30

Table 2 (Continued)

Time (min)	Solution A (%)	Solution C (%)
10	10	90
11	10	90

Diluent: Methanol and *Buffer* (5:95)

Sensitivity solution: 0.000175 mg/mL of USP 4-Aminophenol RS in *Diluent*. Sonicate to dissolve, if necessary.

Standard solution: 0.00175 mg/mL of USP 4-Aminophenol RS and 0.0035 mg/mL of USP Acetaminophen RS in *Diluent*. Sonicate to dissolve, if necessary.

Sample stock solution: Nominally 5 mg/mL of acetaminophen in *Diluent* from NLT 10 Tablets. [NOTE—It is recommended to shake on a flat bed at low speed (180 oscillations/min) to dissolve, if necessary.]

Sample solution: Nominally 3.5 mg/mL of acetaminophen in *Diluent* prepared as follows. Pass a portion of the *Sample stock solution* through a suitable filter of 0.2-μm pore size. Discard the first 2 mL of the filtrate. Dilute a suitable volume of the filtrate with *Diluent* to volume.

Chromatographic system
(See *Chromatography ⟨621⟩, System Suitability*.)
Mode: LC
Detector: UV 272 nm. For *Identification B*, use a diode array detector in the range of 200–400 nm.
Column: 4.6-mm × 15-cm; 3-μm packing L1
Column temperature: 40°
Flow rate: 0.9 mL/min
Injection volume: 25 μL
System suitability
Samples: *Sensitivity solution* and *Standard solution*
Suitability requirements
Relative standard deviation: NMT 5.0% for 4-aminophenol and acetaminophen, *Standard solution*
Signal-to-noise ratio: NLT 10 for 4-aminophenol, *Sensitivity solution*
Analysis
Samples: *Standard solution* and *Sample solution*
Calculate the percentage of 4-aminophenol in the portion of Tablets taken:

$$Result = (r_U/r_S) \times (C_S/C_U) \times 100$$

r_U = peak response of 4-aminophenol from the *Sample solution*

r_S = peak response of 4-aminophenol from the *Standard solution*

C_S = concentration of USP 4-Aminophenol RS in the *Standard solution* (mg/mL)

C_U = nominal concentration of acetaminophen in the *Sample solution* (mg/mL)

Calculate the percentage of any unspecified impurity in the portion of Tablets taken:

$$Result = (r_U/r_S) \times (C_S/C_U) \times 100$$

r_U = peak response of any unspecified impurity from the *Sample solution*

r_S = peak response of acetaminophen from the *Standard solution*

C_S = concentration of USP Acetaminophen RS in the *Standard solution* (mg/mL)

C_U = nominal concentration of acetaminophen in the *Sample solution* (mg/mL)

Acceptance criteria: See *Table 3*.

Table 3

Name	Relative Retention Time	Acceptance Criteria, NMT (%)
4-Aminophenol	0.53	0.15
Acetaminophen	1.0	—
Any unspecified impurity	—	0.15
Total impurities	—	0.60

■1S (USP41)

ADDITIONAL REQUIREMENTS
- **PACKAGING AND STORAGE:** Preserve in tight containers, and store at controlled room temperature.
- **LABELING:** Label Tablets that must be chewed to indicate that they are to be chewed before swallowing.

Change to read:

- **USP REFERENCE STANDARDS ⟨11⟩**
  USP Acetaminophen RS
  ■USP 4-Aminophenol RS
  4-Aminophenol.
  C_6H_7NO　　109.13■1S (USP41)

Amitriptyline Hydrochloride

$C_{20}H_{23}N \cdot HCl$　　　　　　　　　　　313.86

1-Propanamine, 3-(10,11-dihydro-5*H*-dibenzo[*a*,*d*]cyclohepten-5-ylidene)-*N*,*N*-dimethyl-, hydrochloride;
10,11-Dihydro-*N*,*N*-dimethyl-5*H*-dibenzo[*a*,*d*]cycloheptene-$\Delta^{5,\gamma}$-propylamine hydrochloride [549-18-8].

DEFINITION
Amitriptyline Hydrochloride contains NLT 98.0% and NMT 102.0% of amitriptyline hydrochloride ($C_{20}H_{23}N \cdot HCl$), calculated on the dried basis.

IDENTIFICATION

Change to read:

- **A. INFRARED ABSORPTION** ■⟨197⟩: [NOTE—Methods described in ⟨197K⟩ or ⟨197A⟩ may be used.]■1S (USP41)
- **B.** The retention time of the major peak of the *Sample solution* corresponds to that of the *Standard solution*, as obtained in the *Assay*.
- **C. IDENTIFICATION TESTS—GENERAL ⟨191⟩**, *Chemical Identification Tests, Chloride*: Meets the requirements

ASSAY

Change to read:

- **PROCEDURE**
  ■1S (USP41)
  Buffer: ■1.4 g/L of anhydrous dibasic sodium phosphate■1S (USP41) in water, adjusted with ■1.5 M phosphoric acid TS■1S (USP41) to a pH of 7.7

Mobile phase: Methanol and *Buffer* ■(70:30)■1S (USP41)
System suitability stock solution A: 1 mg/mL of USP Amitriptyline Related Compound A RS in methanol
System suitability stock solution B: 0.4 mg/mL of USP Amitriptyline Hydrochloride RS, 0.6 mg/mL each of USP Amitriptyline Related Compound B RS, USP Cyclobenzaprine Hydrochloride RS, and USP Nortriptyline Hydrochloride RS in *Mobile phase*
Standard solution: 0.2 mg/mL of USP Amitriptyline Hydrochloride RS in *Mobile phase*
System suitability solution: ■0.5 µg/mL of USP Amitriptyline Related Compound A RS, 1 µg/mL of USP Amitriptyline Hydrochloride RS, and 1.5 µg/mL each of USP Amitriptyline Related Compound B RS, USP Cyclobenzaprine Hydrochloride RS, and USP Nortriptyline Hydrochloride RS■1S (USP41) from suitable volumes of *Standard solution, System suitability stock solution A*, and *System suitability stock solution B* in *Mobile phase*
Sample solution: 0.2 mg/mL of Amitriptyline Hydrochloride in *Mobile phase*
Chromatographic system
(See *Chromatography ⟨621⟩, System Suitability*.)
Mode: LC
Detector: UV 215 nm
Column: 4.6-mm × 25-cm; 5-µm packing L7
Column temperature: 45°
Flow rate: 1.5 mL/min
Injection volume: 20 µL
Run time: ■NLT■1S (USP41) 1.5 times the retention time of amitriptyline
System suitability
Samples: *Standard solution* and *System suitability solution*
[NOTE—For relative retention times, see *Table 1*.]
Suitability requirements
Resolution: NLT 1.5 between amitriptyline related compound B and nortriptyline, *System suitability solution*
Relative standard deviation: ■NMT 0.73%■1S (USP41) for amitriptyline, *Standard solution*
Analysis
Samples: *Standard solution* and *Sample solution*
Calculate the percentage of amitriptyline hydrochloride ($C_{20}H_{23}N \cdot HCl$) in the portion of Amitriptyline Hydrochloride taken:

$$\text{Result} = (r_U/r_S) \times (C_S/C_U) \times 100$$

r_U = peak response from the *Sample solution*
r_S = peak response from the *Standard solution*
C_S = concentration of USP Amitriptyline Hydrochloride RS in the *Standard solution* (mg/mL)
C_U = concentration of Amitriptyline Hydrochloride in the *Sample solution* (mg/mL)
Acceptance criteria: 98.0%–102.0% on the dried basis

IMPURITIES
- **RESIDUE ON IGNITION ⟨281⟩:** NMT 0.1%

Delete the following:

- ●**HEAVY METALS**, *Method II* ⟨231⟩: NMT 10 ppm● (Official 1-Jan-2018)

Change to read:

- **ORGANIC IMPURITIES**
  ■1S (USP41) **Buffer, Mobile phase, Chromatographic system,** and **System suitability:** Proceed as directed in the *Assay*.
  Standard solution: Use the *System suitability solution*, prepared as directed in the *Assay*.

Sample solution: 1000 µg/mL of Amitriptyline Hydrochloride in *Mobile phase*

Analysis

Samples: *Standard solution* and *Sample solution*

Calculate the percentages of ■amitriptyline related compound A, amitriptyline related compound B, and nortriptyline hydrochloride■1S (USP41) in the portion of Amitriptyline Hydrochloride taken:

$$\text{Result} = (r_U/r_S) \times (C_S/C_U) \times 100$$

r_U = peak response of ■amitriptyline related compound A, amitriptyline related compound B, or nortriptyline■1S (USP41) from the *Sample solution*

r_S = peak response of ■amitriptyline related compound A, amitriptyline related compound B, or nortriptyline■1S (USP41) from the *Standard solution*

C_S = concentration of ■USP Amitriptyline Related Compound A RS, USP Amitriptyline Related Compound B RS, or USP Nortriptyline Hydrochloride RS■1S (USP41) in the *Standard solution* (µg/mL)

C_U = concentration of Amitriptyline Hydrochloride in the *Sample solution* (µg/mL)

■Calculate the percentage of cyclobenzaprine in the portion of Amitriptyline Hydrochloride taken:

$$\text{Result} = (r_U/r_S) \times (C_S/C_U) \times (M_{r1}/M_{r2}) \times 100$$

r_U = peak response of cyclobenzaprine from the *Sample solution*

r_S = peak response of cyclobenzaprine from the *Standard solution*

C_S = concentration of USP Cyclobenzaprine Hydrochloride RS in the *Standard solution* (µg/mL)

C_U = concentration of Amitriptyline Hydrochloride in the *Sample solution* (µg/mL)

M_{r1} = molecular weight of cyclobenzaprine, 275.39

M_{r2} = molecular weight of cyclobenzaprine hydrochloride, 311.85■1S (USP41)

Calculate the percentage of each unspecified impurity in the portion of Amitriptyline Hydrochloride taken:

$$\text{Result} = (r_U/r_S) \times (C_S/C_U) \times 100$$

r_U = peak response of any unspecified impurity from the *Sample solution*

r_S = peak response of USP Amitriptyline Hydrochloride RS from the *Standard solution*

C_S = concentration of USP Amitriptyline Hydrochloride RS in the *Standard solution* (µg/mL)

C_U = concentration of Amitriptyline Hydrochloride in the *Sample solution* (µg/mL)

■1S (USP41)

Acceptance criteria: See *Table 1*. ■Do not include any peak with a relative retention time less than 0.22.

■1S (USP41)

Table 1

Name	Relative Retention Time	Acceptance Criteria, NMT (%)
Amitriptyline related compound A	0.35	0.05
Amitriptyline related compound B	0.52	0.15
Nortriptyline	0.60	0.15
Cyclobenzaprine	0.76	0.15
Amitriptyline	1.0	—

Table 1 (Continued)

Name	Relative Retention Time	Acceptance Criteria, NMT (%)
Any individual unspecified impurity	—	0.10
Total impurities	—	1.0

SPECIFIC TESTS

Change to read:

- **pH ⟨791⟩**
  Sample: 10 mg/mL in water
  Acceptance criteria: 5.0–6.0 ■1S (USP41)

Change to read:

- **LOSS ON DRYING ⟨731⟩**
  Analysis: Dry ■1S (USP41) at a pressure not exceeding 5 mm of mercury at 60° to constant weight.
  Acceptance criteria: NMT 0.5%

ADDITIONAL REQUIREMENTS

- **PACKAGING AND STORAGE:** Preserve in well-closed containers.
- **USP REFERENCE STANDARDS ⟨11⟩**
  USP Amitriptyline Hydrochloride RS
  USP Amitriptyline Related Compound A RS
    10,11-Dihydro-5H-dibenzo[a,d]cyclohepten-5-one;
    Also known as Dibenzosuberone.
    $C_{15}H_{12}O$ 208.26
  USP Amitriptyline Related Compound B RS
    5-[3-(Dimethylamino)propyl]-10,11-dihydro-5H-dibenzo[a,d]-cyclohepten-5-ol;
    Also known as Amitriptynol.
    $C_{20}H_{25}NO$ 295.42
  USP Cyclobenzaprine Hydrochloride RS
  USP Nortriptyline Hydrochloride RS

Delete the following:

■Amitriptyline Hydrochloride Injection

DEFINITION

Amitriptyline Hydrochloride Injection is a sterile solution of Amitriptyline Hydrochloride in Water for Injection. It contains NLT 90.0% and NMT 110.0% of the labeled amount of amitriptyline hydrochloride ($C_{20}H_{23}N \cdot HCl$).

IDENTIFICATION

- **A.**
  Sample solution: Pipet 1 mL of Injection into a 125-mL separator containing 10 mL of water and 1 mL of 1 N sodium hydroxide, mix, extract with two 10-mL portions of methylene chloride, and evaporate the extracts on a steam bath just to dryness. Dissolve the residue in methanol, add 1 mL of 1.2 N hydrochloric acid, and then add methanol to make 100 mL. Dilute 10 mL of this solution with methanol to 100 mL.
  Acceptance criteria: The UV absorption spectrum of this solution exhibits a maximum at the same wavelength as that of a similar solution of USP Amitriptyline Hydrochloride RS, concomitantly measured.

- **B.** The retention time of the major peak of the *Sample solution* corresponds to that of the *Standard solution*, as obtained in the *Assay*.

ASSAY
- **PROCEDURE**
  Buffer: Dissolve 11.04 g of monobasic sodium phosphate in 900 mL of water, adjust with phosphoric acid to a pH of 2.5 ± 0.5, and dilute with water to 1000 mL.
  Mobile phase: Acetonitrile and *Buffer* (42:58)
  Standard solution: 0.2 mg/mL of USP Amitriptyline Hydrochloride RS in water
  Sample solution: Nominally 0.2 mg/mL of amitriptyline hydrochloride from a suitable volume of the Injection in water
  Chromatographic system
  (See *Chromatography* ⟨621⟩, *System Suitability*.)
  Mode: LC
  Detector: UV 254 nm
  Column: 4-mm × 30-cm; packing L1
  Flow rate: 2 mL/min
  Injection volume: 20 µL
  System suitability
  Sample: *Standard solution*
  Suitability requirements
  Column efficiency: NLT 800 theoretical plates
  Tailing factor: NMT 2.0
  Relative standard deviation: NMT 2.0%
  Analysis
  Samples: *Standard solution* and *Sample solution*
  Calculate the percentage of the labeled amount of amitriptyline hydrochloride ($C_{20}H_{23}N \cdot HCl$) in the portion of Injection taken:

$$Result = (r_U/r_S) \times (C_S/C_U) \times 100$$

r_U = peak response from the *Sample solution*
r_S = peak response from the *Standard solution*
C_S = concentration of USP Amitriptyline Hydrochloride RS in the *Standard solution* (mg/mL)
C_U = nominal concentration of amitriptyline hydrochloride in the *Sample solution* (mg/mL)
  Acceptance criteria: 90.0%–110.0%

SPECIFIC TESTS
- **PYROGEN TEST** ⟨151⟩
  Sample: Amitriptyline Hydrochloride Injection, diluted with Sodium Chloride Injection containing 0.9% of sodium chloride to a concentration of 2.5 mg of amitriptyline hydrochloride/mL
  Acceptance criteria: Meets the requirements for a test dose of 1 mL/kg
- **PH** ⟨791⟩: 4.0–6.0
- **OTHER REQUIREMENTS:** Meets the requirements in *Injections and Implanted Drug Products* ⟨1⟩

ADDITIONAL REQUIREMENTS
- **PACKAGING AND STORAGE:** Preserve in single-dose or multiple-dose containers, preferably of Type I glass.
- **USP REFERENCE STANDARDS** ⟨11⟩
  USP Amitriptyline Hydrochloride RS
  ■1S *(USP41)*

Add the following:

■Amlodipine and Atorvastatin Tablets

DEFINITION
Amlodipine and Atorvastatin Tablets contain an amount of amlodipine besylate equivalent to NLT 90.0% and NMT 110.0% of the labeled amount of amlodipine ($C_{20}H_{25}ClN_2O_5$) and an amount of atorvastatin calcium equivalent to NLT 94.5% and NMT 105.0% of the labeled amount of atorvastatin ($C_{33}H_{34}FN_2O_5$). It may contain suitable antioxidants.

IDENTIFICATION
- **A.** The UV spectrum of the major peaks of the *Sample solution* exhibits maxima and minima at the same wavelengths as that of the *Standard solution*, as obtained in the *Assay*.
- **B.** The retention times of the major peaks of the *Sample solution* correspond to those of the *Standard solution*, as obtained in the *Assay*.

ASSAY
- **PROCEDURE**
  Solution A: Dissolve 1.54 g of ammonium acetate in 1000 mL of water and add 2 mL of triethylamine. Adjust with acetic acid to a pH of 5.0.
  Mobile phase: Acetonitrile, methanol, and *Solution A* (38:15:47)
  Buffer: Transfer 7 mL of triethylamine to a 1000-mL volumetric flask containing 900 mL of water and mix. Adjust with dilute phosphoric acid (1 in 100) to a pH of 3.0 and dilute with water to volume.
  Diluent: Acetonitrile, methanol, and *Buffer* (3:7:10)
  Standard stock solution 1: 0.35 mg/mL of USP Amlodipine Besylate RS in methanol
  Standard stock solution 2: 0.44 mg/mL of USP Atorvastatin Calcium RS in methanol
  Standard solution: Prepare solutions of USP Amlodipine Besylate RS and USP Atorvastatin Calcium RS in *Mobile phase* at concentrations given in *Table 1* from *Standard stock solution 1* and *Standard stock solution 2*.

Table 1

Strength of Tablet Amlodipine/ Atorvastatin (mg/mg)	Concentration of Amlodipine Besylate (mg/mL)	Concentration of Atorvastatin Calcium (mg/mL)
2.5/10, 5/20, 10/40	0.028	0.088
2.5/20, 5/40, 10/80	0.014	0.088
5/10, 10/20	0.028	0.044
2.5/40, 5/80	0.014	0.176
10/10	0.028	0.022

  Sample solution: Transfer NLT 10 Tablets to a suitable volumetric flask. Add about 20% of the final volume of the volumetric flask size in *Diluent* and sonicate to disperse the Tablets. Add about 40% of the final volume of the volumetric flask size in *Diluent*, sonicate for 20 min, and dilute with *Diluent* to volume. Centrifuge and transfer a suitable quantity of the supernatant to an appropriate suitable volumetric flask. Dilute with *Mobile phase* to volume to obtain the nominal concentrations of amlodipine and atorvastatin similar to that of the *Standard solution*.
  Chromatographic system
  (See *Chromatography* ⟨621⟩, *System Suitability*.)
  Mode: LC
  Detector: UV 237 nm. For *Identification A*, use a diode array detector in the range of 200–400 nm.

Column: 4.6-mm × 15-cm; 5-µm packing L1
Column temperature: 35°
Flow rate: 1 mL/min
Injection volume: 20 µL
Run time: NLT 3.5 times the retention time of amlodipine
System suitability
  Sample: *Standard solution*
  Suitability requirements
    Tailing factor: NMT 2.0 for both peaks
    Relative standard deviation: NMT 2.0% for both peaks
Analysis
  Samples: *Standard solution* and *Sample solution*
Calculate the percentage of the labeled amount of amlodipine ($C_{20}H_{25}ClN_2O_5$) in the portion of Tablets taken:

$$\text{Result} = (r_U/r_S) \times (C_S/C_U) \times (M_{r1}/M_{r2}) \times 100$$

r_U = peak response of amlodipine from the *Sample solution*
r_S = peak response of amlodipine from the *Standard solution*
C_S = concentration of USP Amlodipine Besylate RS in the *Standard solution* (mg/mL)
C_U = nominal concentration of amlodipine in the *Sample solution* (mg/mL)
M_{r1} = molecular weight of amlodipine, 408.88
M_{r2} = molecular weight of amlodipine besylate, 567.05

Calculate the percentage of the labeled amount of atorvastatin ($C_{33}H_{34}FN_2O_5$) in the portion of Tablets taken:

$$\text{Result} = (r_U/r_S) \times (C_S/C_U) \times [M \times (M_{r1}/M_{r2})] \times 100$$

r_U = peak response of atorvastatin from the *Sample solution*
r_S = peak response of atorvastatin from the *Standard solution*
C_S = concentration of USP Atorvastatin Calcium RS in the *Standard solution* (mg/mL)
C_U = nominal concentration of atorvastatin in the *Sample solution* (mg/mL)
M = number of moles of atorvastatin per mole of atorvastatin calcium, 2
M_{r1} = molecular weight of atorvastatin, 558.64
M_{r2} = molecular weight of atorvastatin calcium, 1209.39

Acceptance criteria
  Amlodipine: 90.0%–110.0%
  Atorvastatin: 94.5%–105.0%

PERFORMANCE TESTS

- **DISSOLUTION ⟨711⟩**
Solution A, Mobile phase, Standard stock solution 1, Standard stock solution 2, Chromatographic system, and **System suitability:** Proceed as directed in the *Assay*.
Medium: 0.1% polysorbate 80 in pH 6.8 phosphate buffer; 900 mL
Apparatus 2: 75 rpm
Time: 20 min
Standard solution: (L_1/900) mg/mL of amlodipine and (L_2/900) mg/mL of atorvastatin in *Medium* from *Standard stock solution 1* and *Standard stock solution 2*, where L_1 is the label claim of amlodipine in mg/Tablet, and L_2 is the label claim of atorvastatin in mg/Tablet
Sample solution: Centrifuge the solution under test and use the supernatant.

Analysis
  Samples: *Standard solution* and *Sample solution*
Calculate the percentage of the labeled amount of amlodipine ($C_{20}H_{25}ClN_2O_5$) dissolved:

$$\text{Result} = (r_U/r_S) \times C_S \times V \times (M_{r1}/M_{r2}) \times (1/L) \times 100$$

r_U = peak response of amlodipine from the *Sample solution*
r_S = peak response of amlodipine from the *Standard solution*
C_S = concentration of USP Amlodipine Besylate RS in the *Standard solution* (mg/mL)
V = volume of *Medium*, 900 mL
M_{r1} = molecular weight of amlodipine, 408.88
M_{r2} = molecular weight of amlodipine besylate, 567.05
L = label claim of amlodipine (mg/Tablet)

Calculate the percentage of the labeled amount of atorvastatin ($C_{33}H_{34}FN_2O_5$) dissolved:

$$\text{Result} = (r_U/r_S) \times C_S \times V \times [M \times (M_{r1}/M_{r2})] \times (1/L) \times 100$$

r_U = peak response of atorvastatin from the *Sample solution*
r_S = peak response of atorvastatin from the *Standard solution*
C_S = concentration of USP Atorvastatin Calcium RS in the *Standard solution* (mg/mL)
V = volume of *Medium*, 900 mL
M = number of moles of atorvastatin per mole of atorvastatin calcium, 2
M_{r1} = molecular weight of atorvastatin, 558.64
M_{r2} = molecular weight of atorvastatin calcium, 1209.39
L = label claim of atorvastatin (mg/Tablet)

Tolerances: NLT 80% (Q) of the labeled amount of amlodipine ($C_{20}H_{25}ClN_2O_5$) and atorvastatin ($C_{33}H_{34}FN_2O_5$) are dissolved.

- **UNIFORMITY OF DOSAGE UNITS ⟨905⟩:** Meet the requirements

IMPURITIES

- **ORGANIC IMPURITIES RELATED TO AMLODIPINE**
Buffer 1: Add 7 mL of triethylamine in 1000 mL of water and adjust with phosphoric acid to a pH of 2.5. Add 1.8 g of tetrabutylammonium hydrogen sulfate and mix well.
Solution A: Methanol and *Buffer 1* (40:60)
Solution B: Acetonitrile, methanol, and *Buffer 1* (40:40:20)
Mobile phase: See *Table 2*.

Table 2

Time (min)	Solution A (%)	Solution B (%)
0	90	10
2	90	10
7	75	25
16	70	30
18	55	45
24	25	75
30	10	90
31	0	100
35	0	100
36	90	10
40	90	10

Buffer 2: Add 7 mL of triethylamine in 1000 mL of water. Adjust with phosphoric acid to a pH of 3.0.

Diluent 1: Methanol and water (50:50)
Diluent 2: Methanol and *Buffer 2* (50:50)
Standard stock solution: 0.7 mg/mL of USP Amlodipine Besylate RS in *Diluent 2*, prepared as follows. Transfer a suitable amount of USP Amlodipine Besylate RS to a suitable volumetric flask and dissolve in a quantity of methanol, about 20% of the volume of the flask. Dilute with *Diluent 2* to volume.
Standard solution 1: 5 µg/mL of USP Amlodipine Related Compound A RS in *Diluent 1*
Standard solution 2: 3.5 µg/mL of USP Amlodipine Besylate RS from *Standard stock solution* in *Diluent 2*
Sample solution: Nominally 0.5 mg/mL of amlodipine in *Diluent 2*, prepared as follows. Finely powder NLT 25 Tablets and transfer a portion of the powder, equivalent to 50 mg of amlodipine to a 100-mL volumetric flask. Add about 40 mL of methanol, shake to disperse, and sonicate for 15 min. Add about 40 mL of *Buffer 2* and sonicate for another 10 min. Dilute with *Diluent 2* to volume, centrifuge, and use the supernatant. Pass a portion of the solution through a suitable filter of 0.22-µm pore size. Prepare this solution fresh.
Chromatographic system
(See *Chromatography* ⟨621⟩, *System Suitability*.)
Mode: LC
Detector: UV 270 nm for amlodipine related compound A; 360 nm for all other impurities
Column: 2.1-mm × 15-cm; 1.8-µm packing L1
Column temperature: 40°
Flow rate: 0.3 mL/min
Injection volume: 5 µL
System suitability
Sample: *Standard solution 2*
Suitability requirements
Tailing factor: NMT 2.0
Relative standard deviation: NMT 5.0%
Analysis
Samples: *Standard solution 1, Standard solution 2,* and *Sample solution*
Calculate the percentage of amlodipine related compound A in the portion of Tablets taken:

$$Result = (r_U/r_S) \times (C_S/C_U) \times (M_{r1}/M_{r2}) \times 100$$

r_U = peak response of amlodipine related compound A from the *Sample solution*
r_S = peak response of amlodipine related compound A from *Standard solution 1*
C_S = concentration of USP Amlodipine Related Compound A RS in *Standard solution 1* (mg/mL)
C_U = nominal concentration of amlodipine in the *Sample solution* (mg/mL)
M_{r1} = molecular weight of amlodipine related compound A free base, 406.86
M_{r2} = molecular weight of amlodipine related compound A fumarate, 522.94

Calculate the percentage of atorvastatin–amlodipine adduct or any unspecified degradation product in the portion of Tablets taken:

$$Result = (r_U/r_S) \times (C_S/C_U) \times (M_{r1}/M_{r2}) \times (1/F) \times 100$$

r_U = peak response of each degradation product from the *Sample solution*
r_S = peak response of amlodipine from *Standard solution 2*
C_S = concentration of USP Amlodipine Besylate RS in *Standard solution 2* (mg/mL)
C_U = nominal concentration of amlodipine in the *Sample solution* (mg/mL)
M_{r1} = molecular weight of amlodipine, 408.88
M_{r2} = molecular weight of amlodipine besylate, 567.05
F = relative response factor (see *Table 3*)

Acceptance criteria: See *Table 3*. Disregard peaks at the relative retention times of 2.18, 2.47 (atorvastatin), and 2.79 min.

Table 3

Name	Relative Retention Time	Relative Response Factor	Acceptance Criteria, NMT (%)
Amlodipine related compound A	0.59	—	0.50
Amlodipine	1.00	—	—
Atorvastatin–amlodipine adduct[a]	3.49	0.47	0.50
Any unspecified degradation product	—	1.0	0.20
Total degradation products for amlodipine	—	—	1.0

[a] 3-Ethyl 5-methyl 4-(2-chlorophenyl)-2-[(2-{(3R,5R)-7-[2-(4-fluorophenyl)-5-isopropyl-3-phenyl-4-(phenylcarbamoyl)-1H-pyrrol-1-yl]-3,5-dihydroxyheptanamido}ethoxy)methyl]-6-methyl-1,4-dihydropyridine-3,5-dicarboxylate.

- **ORGANIC IMPURITIES RELATED TO ATORVASTATIN**
Buffer 1: Dissolve 6.8 g of potassium dihydrogen phosphate in 1000 mL of water and adjust with dilute phosphoric acid (1 in 10) to a pH of 3.4.
Buffer 2: Dissolve 6.8 g of potassium dihydrogen phosphate in 1000 mL of water and adjust with triethylamine to a pH of 7.0.
Solution A: Tetrahydrofuran, acetonitrile, and *Buffer 1* (5:25:70)
Solution B: Tetrahydrofuran, acetonitrile, and *Buffer 2* (5:70:25)
Mobile phase: See *Table 4*.

Table 4

Time (min)	Solution A (%)	Solution B (%)
0	85	15
30	75	25
70	40	60
75	25	75
80	25	75
85	85	15
90	85	15

Diluent: Acetonitrile and water (50:50)
System suitability solution: Heat a suitable amount of USP Atorvastatin Calcium RS at 60° for 1 h for degradation; 0.55 mg/mL of degraded USP Atorvastatin Calcium RS, 3 µg/mL each of USP Atorvastatin Related Compound A RS, USP Atorvastatin Related Compound B RS, USP Atorvastatin Related Compound C RS, and USP Atorvastatin Related Compound H RS in *Diluent*. Sonication may be necessary for complete dissolution.
Standard solution: 2.7 µg/mL of USP Atorvastatin Calcium RS in *Diluent*
Sample solution: Nominally 0.5 mg/mL of atorvastatin in *Diluent*, prepared as follows. Transfer an amount equivalent to 50 mg of atorvastatin from a portion of NLT 20 finely powdered Tablets to a 100-mL volumetric flask. Add about 10 mL of acetonitrile, shake to disperse, and sonicate for 5 min. Add about 70 mL of *Diluent* and sonicate for another 20 min. Dilute with *Diluent* to volume and centrifuge. Prepare this solution fresh.

Chromatographic system
(See *Chromatography* ⟨621⟩, *System Suitability.*)
Mode: LC
Detector: UV 246 nm
Column: 4.6-mm × 25-cm; 4-µm packing L11
Column temperature: 45°
Flow rate: 1.2 mL/min
Injection volume: 20 µL
System suitability
Samples: *System suitability solution* and *Standard solution*
Suitability requirements
Resolution: NLT 1.0 between atorvastatin pyrrolidone analog and atorvastatin related compound A, *System suitability solution*
Relative standard deviation: NMT 5.0%, *Standard solution*
Analysis
Samples: *Standard solution* and *Sample solution*
Calculate the percentage of each atorvastatin specified or unspecified degradation product in the portion of Tablets taken:

$$Result = (r_U/r_S) \times (C_S/C_U) \times [M \times (M_{r1}/M_{r2})] \times (1/F) \times 100$$

r_U = peak response of each atorvastatin degradation product from the *Sample solution*
r_S = peak response of atorvastatin from the *Standard solution*
C_S = concentration of USP Atorvastatin Calcium RS in the *Standard solution* (mg/mL)
C_U = nominal concentration of atorvastatin in the *Sample solution* (mg/mL)
M = number of moles of atorvastatin per mole of atorvastatin calcium, 2
M_{r1} = molecular weight of atorvastatin, 558.64
M_{r2} = molecular weight of atorvastatin calcium, 1209.39
F = relative response factor (see *Table 5*)
Acceptance criteria: See *Table 5*. Disregard any impurity peaks less than 0.05% and the peaks from amlodipine related impurities.

Table 5

Name	Relative Retention Time	Relative Response Factor	Acceptance Criteria, NMT (%)
Atorvastatin pyrrolidone analog[a]	0.86	0.67	0.45
Atorvastatin related compound A[b]	0.91	—	—

[a] (3R,5R)-7-[5-(4-Fluorophenyl)-3-isopropyl-2-oxo-4-phenyl-3-(phenyl-carbamoyl)-2,3-dihydro-1H-pyrrol-1-yl]-3,5-dihydroxyheptanoic acid.
[b] Process impurity included in the table for identification only. Process impurities are controlled in the drug substance, and are not to be reported or included in the total impurities for the drug product.
[c] 4-{6-(4-Fluorophenyl)-7,8-epoxy-6-hydroxy-8a-isopropyl-7-phenyl-8-(phenylcarbamoyl)hexahydro-2H-pyrrolo[2,1-b][1,3]oxazin-2-yl}-3-hydroxybutanoic acid.
[d] (3R)-4-(1b-(4-Fluorophenyl)-7-hydroxy-7-isopropyl-1a-phenyl-7a-(phenylcarbamoyl)hexahydro-1aH-oxireno[2′,3′:3,4]pyrrolo[2,1-b][1,3]oxazin-3-yl)-3-hydroxybutanoic acid.
[e] 4-(4-Fluorophenyl)-2,4-dihydroxy-2-isopropyl-N,5-diphenyl-3,6-dioxabicyclo[3.1.0]hexane-1-carboxamide.
[f] 3-(4-Fluorobenzoyl)-2-isobutyryl-N,3-diphenyloxirane-2-carboxamide.
[g] Sum of atorvastatin epoxy tetrahydrofuran analog and atorvastatin oxirane.
[h] (3R,5R)-tert-Butyl 7-(2-(4-fluorophenyl)-5-isopropyl-3-phenyl-4-(phenylcarbamoyl)-1H-pyrrol-1-yl)-3,5-dihydroxyheptanoate.
[i] Sum of the total degradation products for amlodipine from the test for *Organic Impurities Related to Amlodipine* and the total degradation products for atorvastatin from the test for *Organic Impurities Related to Atorvastatin.*

Table 5 (Continued)

Name	Relative Retention Time	Relative Response Factor	Acceptance Criteria, NMT (%)
Atorvastatin related compound B[b]	0.95	—	—
Atorvastatin	1.00	—	—
Atorvastatin related compound C[b]	1.04	—	—
Atorvastatin epoxy pyrrolooxazin 6-hydroxy analog[c]	1.35	0.39	0.5
Atorvastatin epoxy pyrrolooxazin 7-hydroxy analog[d]	1.40	0.52	0.5
Atorvastatin related compound H	1.78	1.0	1.0
Atorvastatin epoxy tetrahydrofuran analog[e]	1.96	0.63	
Atorvastatin oxirane[f]	2.23	1.0	0.5[g]
Atorvastatin tert-butyl ester[b,h]	2.55	—	—
Any unspecified degradation product	—	—	0.20
Total degradation products for atorvastatin	—	—	2.0
Total degradation products[i]	—	—	3.0

[a] (3R,5R)-7-[5-(4-Fluorophenyl)-3-isopropyl-2-oxo-4-phenyl-3-(phenyl-carbamoyl)-2,3-dihydro-1H-pyrrol-1-yl]-3,5-dihydroxyheptanoic acid.
[b] Process impurity included in the table for identification only. Process impurities are controlled in the drug substance, and are not to be reported or included in the total impurities for the drug product.
[c] 4-{6-(4-Fluorophenyl)-7,8-epoxy-6-hydroxy-8a-isopropyl-7-phenyl-8-(phenylcarbamoyl)hexahydro-2H-pyrrolo[2,1-b][1,3]oxazin-2-yl}-3-hydroxybutanoic acid.
[d] (3R)-4-(1b-(4-Fluorophenyl)-7-hydroxy-7-isopropyl-1a-phenyl-7a-(phenylcarbamoyl)hexahydro-1aH-oxireno[2′,3′:3,4]pyrrolo[2,1-b][1,3]oxazin-3-yl)-3-hydroxybutanoic acid.
[e] 4-(4-Fluorophenyl)-2,4-dihydroxy-2-isopropyl-N,5-diphenyl-3,6-dioxabicyclo[3.1.0]hexane-1-carboxamide.
[f] 3-(4-Fluorobenzoyl)-2-isobutyryl-N,3-diphenyloxirane-2-carboxamide.
[g] Sum of atorvastatin epoxy tetrahydrofuran analog and atorvastatin oxirane.
[h] (3R,5R)-tert-Butyl 7-(2-(4-fluorophenyl)-5-isopropyl-3-phenyl-4-(phenylcarbamoyl)-1H-pyrrol-1-yl)-3,5-dihydroxyheptanoate.
[i] Sum of the total degradation products for amlodipine from the test for *Organic Impurities Related to Amlodipine* and the total degradation products for atorvastatin from the test for *Organic Impurities Related to Atorvastatin.*

ADDITIONAL REQUIREMENTS
• **PACKAGING AND STORAGE:** Preserve in well-closed containers. Store at controlled room temperature.
• **USP REFERENCE STANDARDS** ⟨11⟩
USP Amlodipine Besylate RS
USP Amlodipine Related Compound A RS
3-Ethyl 5-methyl [2-(2-aminoethoxymethyl)-4-(2-chlorophenyl)-6-methyl-3,5-pyridinedicarboxylate] fumarate.
$C_{20}H_{23}ClN_2O_5 \cdot C_4H_4O_4$ 522.94
USP Atorvastatin Calcium RS
USP Atorvastatin Related Compound A RS
Calcium (3R,5R)-7-[2-isopropyl-4,5-diphenyl-3-(phenylcarbamoyl)-1H-pyrrol-1-yl]-3,5-dihydroxyheptanoate (1:2).
$C_{66}H_{70}CaN_4O_{10}$ 1119.38

USP Atorvastatin Related Compound B RS
(3S,5R)-7-[3-(Phenylcarbamoyl)-5-(4-fluorophenyl)-2-iso-
propyl-4-phenyl-1H-pyrrol-1-yl]-3,5-dihydroxyhepta-
noic acid calcium salt.
$C_{66}H_{68}CaF_2N_4O_{10}$ 1155.34
USP Atorvastatin Related Compound C RS
Calcium (3R,5R)-7-[2,3-Bis(4-fluorophenyl)-5-isopropyl-
4-(phenylcarbamoyl)-1H-pyrrol-1-yl]-3,5-dihydrox-
yheptanoate (1:2).
$C_{66}H_{66}CaF_4N_4O_{10}$ 1191.34
USP Atorvastatin Related Compound H RS
5-(4-Fluorophenyl)-1-{2-[(2R,4R)-4-hydroxy-6-oxote-
trahydro-2H-pyran-2-yl]ethyl}-2-isopropyl-N,4-diphenyl-
1H-pyrrole-3-carboxamide.
$C_{33}H_{33}FN_2O_4$ 540.62

■1S *(USP41)*

Amlodipine and Valsartan Tablets

DEFINITION
Amlodipine and Valsartan Tablets contain NLT 90.0% and
NMT 110.0% of the labeled amount of amlodipine
($C_{20}H_{25}ClN_2O_5$) and valsartan ($C_{24}H_{29}N_5O_3$).

IDENTIFICATION
- **A.** The UV absorption spectra of the major peaks of *Sam-
  ple solution A* and *Sample solution B* and those of the
  Standard solution exhibit maxima and minima at the
  same wavelengths, as obtained in the *Assay*.
- **B.** The retention times of the major peaks of *Sample solu-
  tion A* and *Sample solution B* correspond to those of the
  Standard solution, as obtained in the *Assay*.

ASSAY
- **PROCEDURE**
  Solution A: Water and triethylamine (1000:10). Adjust
    with phosphoric acid to a pH of 2.8.
  Solution B: Methanol and acetonitrile (700:300)
  Mobile phase: See *Table 1*.

Table 1

Time (min)	Solution A (%)	Solution B (%)
0	50	50
3	50	50
15	30	70
20	30	70
20.1	50	50
25	50	50

  Diluent: *Solution A* and *Solution B* (50:50)
  Standard solution: 0.14 mg/mL of USP Amlodipine
    Besylate RS and 0.16 mg/mL of USP Valsartan RS. Add
    methanol to 5% of the final volume to dissolve, and
    dilute with *Diluent* to volume.
  Sample stock solution: Transfer NLT 10 Tablets into a
    suitable volumetric flask. Initially add water to 10% of
    the final volume, and sonicate to disperse as needed.
    Add *Diluent*, using about 70% of the final volume, and
    shake for up to 45 min to disperse. Following disper-
    sion, sonicate for 15 min, and shake for 30 min. Dilute
    with *Diluent* to volume to obtain a solution containing
    known nominal concentrations of 0.1–0.2 mg/mL of
    amlodipine and 1.6–6.4 mg/mL of valsartan. Centrifuge
    the solution for about 10 min at 3000 rpm.
  Sample solution A: Nominally equivalent to 0.1 mg/mL
    of amlodipine in *Diluent* from the *Sample stock solution*
  Sample solution B: Nominally equivalent to 0.16 mg/
    mL of valsartan in *Diluent* from the *Sample stock solution*

Chromatographic system
(See *Chromatography* ⟨621⟩, *System Suitability*.)
  Mode: LC
  Detector: UV 237 nm. For *Identification A*, use a diode
    array detector in the range of 200–400 nm.
  Column: 3.9-mm × 15-cm; 5-µm packing L1
  Temperatures
    Autosampler: 10°
    Column: 30°
  Flow rate: 1.0 mL/min
  Injection volume: 10 µL
System suitability
  Sample: *Standard solution*
  Suitability requirements
    Tailing factor: NMT 1.5 for both amlodipine and
      valsartan
    Relative standard deviation: NMT 2.0% for
      amlodipine and valsartan
Analysis
  Samples: *Standard solution, Sample solution A*, and
    Sample solution B
  Calculate the percentage of the labeled amount of
    amlodipine ($C_{20}H_{25}ClN_2O_5$) in the portion of Tablets
    taken:

$$Result = (r_U/r_S) \times (C_S/C_U) \times (M_{r1}/M_{r2}) \times 100$$

r_U	= peak response of amlodipine from *Sample solution A*
r_S	= peak response of amlodipine from the *Standard solution*
C_S	= concentration of USP Amlodipine Besylate RS in the *Standard solution* (mg/mL)
C_U	= nominal concentration of amlodipine in *Sample solution A* (mg/mL)
M_{r1}	= molecular weight of amlodipine, 408.88
M_{r2}	= molecular weight of amlodipine besylate, 567.05

  Calculate the percentage of the labeled amount of
    valsartan ($C_{24}H_{29}N_5O_3$) in the portion of Tablets taken:

$$Result = (r_U/r_S) \times (C_S/C_U) \times 100$$

r_U	= peak response of valsartan from *Sample solution B*
r_S	= peak response of valsartan from the *Standard solution*
C_S	= concentration of USP Valsartan RS in the *Standard solution* (mg/mL)
C_U	= nominal concentration of valsartan in *Sample solution B* (mg/mL)

  Acceptance criteria: 90.0%–110.0%

PERFORMANCE TESTS

Change to read:

- **DISSOLUTION** ⟨711⟩
  Test 1
  Buffer: Dissolve 6.805 g of monobasic potassium
    phosphate and 0.896 g of sodium hydroxide in water,
    and dilute with water to 1000 mL. Adjust with 0.2 N
    sodium hydroxide or 1 M phosphoric acid to a pH of
    6.8.
  Medium: *Buffer*, 1000 mL
  Apparatus 2: 75 rpm
  Time: 30 min
  Mobile phase: Acetonitrile, water, and trifluoroacetic
    acid (500:500:2)
  Diluent: 1 mg/mL of polysorbate 80 in *Buffer*
  System suitability solution: 0.4 mg/mL each of USP
    Amlodipine Besylate RS and USP Valsartan RS, pre-
    pared as follows. Initially dissolve in methanol to 40%
    of the total volume, and dilute with *Buffer* to volume.

Standard stock solution A: 0.072 mg/mL of USP Amlodipine Besylate RS, prepared as follows. Initially dissolve in methanol to 4% of the final volume, and dilute with *Diluent* to volume.

Standard stock solution B: 2.2 mg/mL of USP Valsartan RS in methanol

Standard solution: (L_1/1000) mg/mL of amlodipine and (L_2/1000) mg/mL of valsartan in *Diluent* from *Standard stock solution A* and *Standard stock solution B*, where L_1 is the label claim of amlodipine in mg/Tablet, and L_2 is the label claim of valsartan in mg/Tablet

Sample solution: Pass a portion of the solution under test through a suitable filter of 0.45-μm pore size. Discard the first 10 mL of the filtrate.

Chromatographic system
(See *Chromatography* ⟨621⟩, *System Suitability*.)
Mode: LC
Detector: UV 230 nm
Column: 4.6-mm × 15-cm; 4-μm packing L11
Column temperature: 40°
Flow rate: 1.2 mL/min
Injection volume: 10 μL
Run time: NLT 2 times the retention time of amlodipine

System suitability
Samples: *System suitability solution* and *Standard solution*
Suitability requirements
Resolution: NLT 2.0 between amlodipine and valsartan, *System suitability solution*
Tailing factor: NMT 2.0 for amlodipine and valsartan, *Standard solution*
Relative standard deviation: NMT 2.0% for amlodipine and valsartan, *Standard solution*

Analysis
Samples: *Standard solution* and *Sample solution*
Calculate the percentage of the labeled amount of amlodipine ($C_{20}H_{25}ClN_2O_5$) dissolved:

$$\text{Result} = (r_U/r_S) \times C_S \times V \times (M_{r1}/M_{r2}) \times (1/L_1) \times 100$$

r_U = peak response of amlodipine from the *Sample solution*
r_S = peak response of amlodipine from the *Standard solution*
C_S = concentration of USP Amlodipine Besylate RS in the *Standard solution* (mg/mL)
V = volume of *Medium*, 1000 mL
M_{r1} = molecular weight of amlodipine, 408.88
M_{r2} = molecular weight of amlodipine besylate, 567.05
L_1 = label claim of amlodipine (mg/Tablet)

Calculate the percentage of the labeled amount of valsartan ($C_{24}H_{29}N_5O_3$) dissolved:

$$\text{Result} = (r_U/r_S) \times C_S \times V \times (1/L_2) \times 100$$

r_U = peak response of valsartan from the *Sample solution*
r_S = peak response of valsartan from the *Standard solution*
C_S = concentration of USP Valsartan RS in the *Standard solution* (mg/mL)
V = volume of *Medium*, 1000 mL
L_2 = label claim of valsartan (mg/Tablet)

Tolerances: NLT 80% (*Q*) of the labeled amount of amlodipine ($C_{20}H_{25}ClN_2O_5$) and valsartan ($C_{24}H_{29}N_5O_3$) is dissolved.

Test 2: If the product complies with this test, the labeling indicates that the product meets USP *Dissolution Test 2*.
Medium and **Time:** Proceed as directed in *Dissolution Test 1*; 1000 mL.

Apparatus 2: 50 rpm
Buffer: Mix 7.0 mL of triethylamine with 1000 mL of water. Adjust with phosphoric acid to a pH of 3.0.
Solution A: Acetonitrile and *Buffer* (10:90)
Solution B: Acetonitrile and *Buffer* (90:10)
Mobile phase: See *Table 2*.

Table 2

Time (min)	Solution A (%)	Solution B (%)
0	80	20
7	30	70
8	80	20
10	80	20

Standard stock solution A: 0.14 mg/mL of USP Amlodipine Besylate RS, prepared as follows. Initially dissolve in 10% of the final volume of methanol, and dilute with *Medium* to volume.

Standard stock solution B: 1.6 mg/mL of USP Valsartan RS in methanol

Standard solution: (L_1/1000) mg/mL of amlodipine and (L_2/1000) mg/mL of valsartan in •*Medium*• (IRA 1-Nov-2017) from *Standard stock solution A* and *Standard stock solution B*, where L_1 is the label claim of amlodipine in mg/Tablet, and L_2 is the label claim of valsartan in mg/Tablet

Sample solution: Pass a portion of the solution under test through a suitable filter of 1-μm pore size.

Chromatographic system
(See *Chromatography* ⟨621⟩, *System Suitability*.)
Mode: LC
Detector: UV 237 nm
Column: 4.6-mm × 15-cm; 5-μm packing L1
Temperatures
Autosampler: 10°
Column: 50°
Flow rate: 1.5 mL/min
Injection volume: 20 μL

System suitability
Sample: *Standard solution*
Suitability requirements
Tailing factor: NMT 2.0 for amlodipine and valsartan
Relative standard deviation: NMT 2.0% for amlodipine and valsartan

Analysis
Samples: *Standard solution* and *Sample solution*
Calculate the percentage of the labeled amount of amlodipine ($C_{20}H_{25}ClN_2O_5$) dissolved:

$$\text{Result} = (r_U/r_S) \times C_S \times V \times (M_{r1}/M_{r2}) \times (1/L_1) \times 100$$

r_U = peak response of amlodipine from the *Sample solution*
r_S = peak response of amlodipine from the *Standard solution*
C_S = concentration of USP Amlodipine Besylate RS in the *Standard solution* (mg/mL)
V = volume of *Medium*, 1000 mL
M_{r1} = molecular weight of amlodipine, 408.88
M_{r2} = molecular weight of amlodipine besylate, 567.05
L_1 = label claim of amlodipine (mg/Tablet)

Calculate the percentage of the labeled amount of valsartan ($C_{24}H_{29}N_5O_3$) dissolved:

$$\text{Result} = (r_U/r_S) \times C_S \times V \times (1/L_2) \times 100$$

r_U = peak response of valsartan from the *Sample solution*
r_S = peak response of valsartan from the *Standard solution*

C_S = concentration of USP Valsartan RS in the *Standard solution* (mg/mL)
V = volume of *Medium*, 1000 mL
L_2 = label claim of valsartan (mg/Tablet)
  Tolerances: NLT 75% (*Q*) of the labeled amount of amlodipine ($C_{20}H_{25}ClN_2O_5$) is dissolved and NLT 80% (*Q*) of the labeled amount of valsartan ($C_{24}H_{29}N_5O_3$) is dissolved.
Test 3: If the product complies with this test, the labeling indicates that the product meets USP *Dissolution Test 3*.
  Medium, Apparatus 2, and **Time:** Proceed as directed in *Dissolution Test 1*.
  Solution A: Acetonitrile, trifluoroacetic acid, and water (10: 0.1: 90)
  Solution B: Acetonitrile, trifluoroacetic acid, and water (90: 0.1: 10)
  Mobile phase: See *Table 3*.

Table 3

Time (min)	Solution A (%)	Solution B (%)
0.01	90	10
2.5	10	90
3.0	90	10
5.0	90	10

  Diluent: Acetonitrile and water (50:50)
  Standard stock solution A: 0.14 mg/mL of USP Amlodipine Besylate RS, prepared as follows. Initially dissolve in *Diluent* about 4% of the final volume, and dilute with *Medium* to volume.
  Standard stock solution B: 1.6 mg/mL of USP Valsartan RS, prepared as follows. Initially dissolve in about 20% of the final volume of *Diluent*, and dilute with *Medium* to volume.
  Standard solution: (L_1/1000) mg/mL of amlodipine and (L_2/1000) mg/mL of valsartan in *Medium* from *Standard stock solution A* and *Standard stock solution B*, where L_1 is the label claim of amlodipine in mg/Tablet, and L_2 is the label claim of valsartan in mg/Tablet
  Sample solution: Pass a portion of the solution under test through a suitable filter of 0.45-µm pore size and discard the first few milliliters of the filtrate.
  Chromatographic system
  (See *Chromatography* ⟨621⟩, *System Suitability*.)
   Mode: LC
   Detector: UV 237 nm for amlodipine and UV 270 nm for valsartan
   Column: 4.6-mm × 10-cm; 5-µm packing L1
   Flow rate: 1.5 mL/min
   Injection volume: 10 µL
  System suitability
   Sample: *Standard solution*
   Suitability requirements
    Tailing factor: NMT 2.0 for amlodipine and valsartan
    Relative standard deviation: NMT 2.0% for amlodipine and valsartan
  Analysis
   Samples: *Standard solution* and *Sample solution*
   Calculate the percentage of the labeled amount of amlodipine ($C_{20}H_{25}ClN_2O_5$) dissolved:

$$\text{Result} = (r_U/r_S) \times C_S \times V \times (M_{r1}/M_{r2}) \times (1/L_1) \times 100$$

r_U = peak response of amlodipine from the *Sample solution*
r_S = peak response of amlodipine from the *Standard solution*
C_S = concentration of USP Amlodipine Besylate RS in the *Standard solution* (mg/mL)
V = volume of *Medium*, 1000 mL
M_{r1} = molecular weight of amlodipine, 408.88

M_{r2} = molecular weight of amlodipine besylate, 567.05
L_1 = label claim of amlodipine (mg/Tablet)
  Calculate the percentage of the labeled amount of valsartan ($C_{24}H_{29}N_5O_3$) dissolved:

$$\text{Result} = (r_U/r_S) \times C_S \times V \times (1/L_2) \times 100$$

r_U = peak response of valsartan from the *Sample solution*
r_S = peak response of valsartan from the *Standard solution*
C_S = concentration of USP Valsartan RS in the *Standard solution* (mg/mL)
V = volume of *Medium*, 1000 mL
L_2 = label claim of valsartan (mg/Tablet)
  Tolerances: NLT 75% (*Q*) of the labeled amount of amlodipine ($C_{20}H_{25}ClN_2O_5$) is dissolved and NLT 80% (*Q*) of the labeled amount of valsartan ($C_{24}H_{29}N_5O_3$) is dissolved.
• **UNIFORMITY OF DOSAGE UNITS** ⟨905⟩: Meet the requirements

IMPURITIES

Change to read:

• **ORGANIC IMPURITIES**
  Mobile phase, Diluent, Sample solution A, Sample solution B, and **Chromatographic system:** Proceed as directed in the *Assay*.
  Standard stock solution A: Prepare as directed for the *Standard solution* in the *Assay*.
  System suitability solution: Dissolve a suitable quantity of USP Valsartan Related Compound B RS in *Standard stock solution A* to obtain a solution containing 0.08 mg/mL of USP Valsartan Related Compound B RS, 0.14 mg/mL of USP Amlodipine Besylate RS, and 0.16 mg/mL of USP Valsartan RS.
  Sensitivity solution: 0.14 µg/mL of USP Amlodipine Besylate RS and 0.16 µg/mL of USP Valsartan RS in *Diluent* from *Standard stock solution A*
  Standard stock solution B: 0.1 mg/mL of USP Amlodipine Related Compound A RS as free base, prepared as follows. Add methanol to 5% of the final volume to dissolve, and dilute with *Diluent* to volume.
  Standard solution: 0.0005 mg/mL of USP Amlodipine Related Compound A RS as free base, and 0.0003 mg/mL each of USP Amlodipine Besylate RS and USP Valsartan RS in *Diluent* from *Standard stock solution A* and *Standard stock solution B*, respectively
  System suitability
   Samples: *System suitability solution, Sensitivity solution,* and *Standard solution*
   Suitability requirements
    Resolution: More than 4.0 between amlodipine and valsartan related compound B and more than 4.0 between valsartan related compound B and valsartan, *System suitability solution*
    Relative standard deviation: NMT 5.0% for amlodipine related compound A, amlodipine, and valsartan, *Standard solution*
    Signal-to-noise ratio: NLT 10 for amlodipine and valsartan, *Sensitivity solution*
  Analysis
   Samples: *Sample solution A, Sample solution B,* and *Standard solution*
   Calculate the percentage of amlodipine related compound A free base in the portion of Tablets taken:

$$\text{Result} = (r_U/r_S) \times (C_S/C_U) \times (M_{r1}/M_{r2}) \times 100$$

r_U = peak response of amlodipine related compound A from *Sample solution A*

r_S = peak response of amlodipine related compound A from the *Standard solution*

C_S = concentration of USP Amlodipine Related Compound A RS in the *Standard solution* (mg/mL)

C_U = nominal concentration of amlodipine in *Sample solution A* (mg/mL)

M_{r1} = molecular weight of amlodipine related compound A free base, 406.86

M_{r2} = molecular weight of amlodipine related compound A fumarate, 522.93

Calculate the percentage of valsartan related degradation •products other than valsartan related compound A• (IRA 1-Nov-2017) in the portion of Tablets taken:

$$\text{Result} = (r_U/r_S) \times (C_S/C_U) \times 100$$

r_U = peak response of valsartan related degradation product from *Sample solution B*

r_S = peak response of valsartan from the *Standard solution*

C_S = concentration of USP Valsartan RS in the *Standard solution* (mg/mL)

C_U = nominal concentration of valsartan in *Sample solution B* (mg/mL)

Calculate the percentage of each unspecified degradation product in the portion of Tablets taken:

$$\text{Result} = (r_U/r_S) \times (C_S/C_U) \times (M_{r1}/M_{r2}) \times 100$$

r_U = peak response of each unspecified degradation product from *Sample solution A*

r_S = peak response of amlodipine from the *Standard solution*

C_S = concentration of USP Amlodipine Besylate RS in the *Standard solution* (mg/mL)

C_U = nominal concentration of amlodipine in *Sample solution A* (mg/mL)

M_{r1} = molecular weight of amlodipine, 408.88

M_{r2} = molecular weight of amlodipine besylate, 567.05

Acceptance criteria: See *Table 4*. Disregard valsartan related compound B, the benzenesulfonic acid peak at relative retention time 0.19, and any peaks below 0.1%.

Table 4

Name	Relative Retention Time	Acceptance Criteria, NMT (%)
Devaleryl valsartan[a]	0.24	0.2
Amlodipine related compound A[b]	0.50	0.5

[a] N-{[2'-(1H-Tetrazole-5-yl)biphenyl-4-yl]methyl}-L-valine.

[b] 3-Ethyl 5-methyl [2-(2-aminoethoxymethyl)-4-(2-chlorophenyl)-6-methyl-3,5-pyridinedicarboxylate].

[c] These are specified unidentified degradation products. No information is available about chemical structures or chemical names for these impurities.

[d] N-Butyryl-N-{[2'-(1H-tetrazole-5-yl)biphenyl-4-yl]methyl}-L-valine.

[e] N-Valeryl-N-{[2'-(1H-tetrazole-5-yl)biphenyl-4-yl]methyl}-L-valine ethyl ester.

•[f] If valsartan related compound A is a potential degradation product, the total degradation products limit does not include valsartan related compound A and amlodipine related compound A.• (IRA 1-Nov-2017)

Table 4 (Continued)

Name	Relative Retention Time	Acceptance Criteria, NMT (%)
Valsartan related degradation product 1[c]	0.54	0.2
Valsartan related degradation product 2[c]	0.81	0.2
Amlodipine	1.00	—
Valsartan related compound B[d]	1.34	—
Valsartan related degradation product 3[c]	1.44	0.2
Valsartan	1.74	—
Valsartan related degradation product 4[c]	2.06	0.2
Valsartan ethyl ester[e]	2.32	0.2
Any other unspecified degradation product	—	0.2
Total degradation products •[f] (IRA 1-Nov-2017)	—	1.2; •2.0, if valsartan related compound A is a potential degradation product• (IRA 1-Nov-2017)

[a] N-{[2'-(1H-Tetrazole-5-yl)biphenyl-4-yl]methyl}-L-valine.

[b] 3-Ethyl 5-methyl [2-(2-aminoethoxymethyl)-4-(2-chlorophenyl)-6-methyl-3,5-pyridinedicarboxylate].

[c] These are specified unidentified degradation products. No information is available about chemical structures or chemical names for these impurities.

[d] N-Butyryl-N-{[2'-(1H-tetrazole-5-yl)biphenyl-4-yl]methyl}-L-valine.

[e] N-Valeryl-N-{[2'-(1H-tetrazole-5-yl)biphenyl-4-yl]methyl}-L-valine ethyl ester.

•[f] If valsartan related compound A is a potential degradation product, the total degradation products limit does not include valsartan related compound A and amlodipine related compound A.• (IRA 1-Nov-2017)

Add the following:

•• **LIMIT OF VALSARTAN RELATED COMPOUND A**

[NOTE—Valsartan related compound A is a process impurity and a formulation-specific degradation product.]

Mobile phase: n-Hexane, 2-propanol, and trifluoroacetic acid (850:150:1)

System suitability solution: 0.04 mg/mL each of USP Valsartan Related Compound A and USP Valsartan RS in *Mobile phase*

Standard solution: 0.001 mg/mL of USP Valsartan Related Compound A RS in *Mobile phase*

Sample solution: Nominally 0.5 mg/mL of valsartan in *Mobile phase* from a suitable amount of finely crushed powder from NLT 20 Tablets. Sonication may be necessary for complete dissolution. Pass through a suitable filter of 0.45-μm pore size.

Chromatographic system
(See *Chromatography* ⟨621⟩, *System Suitability*.)
Mode: LC
Detector: UV 230 nm
Column: 4.6-mm × 25-cm; 5-µm packing L40
Temperatures
Autosampler: 10°
Column: 30°
Flow rate: 0.8 mL/min
Injection volume: 20 µL
Run time: NLT 3.5 times the retention time of valsartan related compound A
System suitability
Samples: *System suitability solution* and *Standard solution*
[NOTE—The relative retention times for valsartan related compound A and valsartan are about 0.7 and 1.0, respectively.]
Suitability requirements
Resolution: NLT 2.0 between valsartan and valsartan related compound A, *System suitability solution*
Relative standard deviation: NMT 5.0% for valsartan related compound A, *Standard solution*
Analysis
Samples: *Standard solution* and *Sample solution*
Calculate the percentage of valsartan related compound A in the portion of Tablets taken:

$$\text{Result} = (r_U/r_S) \times (C_S/C_U) \times 100$$

r_U = peak response of valsartan related compound A from the *Sample solution*
r_S = peak response of valsartan related compound A from the *Standard solution*
C_S = concentration of USP Valsartan Related Compound A RS in the *Standard solution* (mg/mL)
C_U = nominal concentration of valsartan in the *Sample solution* (mg/mL)
Acceptance criteria: NMT 1.0%• (IRA 1-Nov-2017)

ADDITIONAL REQUIREMENTS

- **PACKAGING AND STORAGE:** Store at controlled room temperature, in tight containers, and in a dry place.
- **LABELING:** When more than one *Dissolution* test is given, the labeling states the *Dissolution* test used only if *Test 1* is not used.

Change to read:

- **USP REFERENCE STANDARDS** ⟨11⟩
  USP Amlodipine Besylate RS
  USP Amlodipine Related Compound A RS
  3-Ethyl 5-methyl [2-(2-aminoethoxymethyl)-4-(2-chlorophenyl)-6-methyl-3,5-pyridinedicarboxylate] fumarate.
  $C_{20}H_{23}ClN_2O_5 \cdot C_4H_4O_4$ 522.93
  USP Valsartan RS
  •USP Valsartan Related Compound A RS
  N-Valeryl-*N*-{[2'-(1*H*-tetrazole-5-yl)biphenyl-4-yl]methyl}-D-valine.
  $C_{24}H_{29}N_5O_3$ 435.52• (IRA 1-Nov-2017)
  USP Valsartan Related Compound B RS
  N-Butyryl-*N*-{[2'-(1*H*-tetrazole-5-yl)biphenyl-4-yl]methyl}-L-valine.
  $C_{23}H_{27}N_5O_3$ 421.49

Amlodipine, Valsartan, and Hydrochlorothiazide Tablets

DEFINITION
Amlodipine, Valsartan, and Hydrochlorothiazide Tablets contain NLT 92.5% and NMT 107.5% each of the labeled amounts of amlodipine ($C_{20}H_{25}ClN_2O_5$), valsartan ($C_{24}H_{29}N_5O_3$), and hydrochlorothiazide ($C_7H_8ClN_3O_4S_2$).

IDENTIFICATION
- **A.** The UV absorption spectra of the amlodipine, valsartan, and hydrochlorothiazide peaks of *Sample solution A*, *Sample solution B*, and *Sample solution C*, and those of the *Standard solution* exhibit maxima and minima at the same wavelengths, as obtained in the *Assay*.
- **B.** The retention times of the amlodipine, valsartan, and hydrochlorothiazide peaks of *Sample solution A*, *Sample solution B*, and *Sample solution C* correspond to those of the *Standard solution*, as obtained in the *Assay*.

ASSAY
- **PROCEDURE**
  Use amber glassware for all solutions containing drug substances.
  Solution A: Acetonitrile, water, and phosphoric acid (50:950:1)
  Solution B: Acetonitrile, water, and phosphoric acid (950:50:1)
  Mobile phase: See *Table 1*.

Table 1

Time (min)	Solution A (%)	Solution B (%)
0	95	5
3	50	50
6	40	60
10	5	95
10.1	95	5
15	95	5

Diluent: Acetonitrile and water (500:500)
0.1% Phosphoric acid: Water and phosphoric acid (1000:1)
Standard solution: 0.14 mg/mL of USP Amlodipine Besylate RS, 0.064 mg/mL of USP Valsartan RS, and 0.025 mg/mL of USP Hydrochlorothiazide RS in *Diluent*
Sample stock solution: Transfer NLT 10 Tablets into a suitable volumetric flask. Add *0.1% Phosphoric acid* to 4% of the total volume to disperse the Tablets. Sonicate for 10 min. Add 4% of the total volume of acetonitrile, swirl to mix, and add 60% of the total volume of *Diluent*. Sonicate for 20 min. Dilute with *Diluent* to volume to obtain solutions of nominal concentrations stated in *Table 2*. Centrifuge, and use the clear supernatant.

Table 2

Tablet Strength Amlodipine/ Valsartan/ Hydrochlorothiazide (mg/mg/ mg)	Nominal Concentration of Amlodipine (mg/mL)	Nominal Concentration of Valsartan (mg/mL)	Nominal Concentration of Hydrochlorothiazide (mg/mL)
5/160/12.5	0.1	3.2	0.25
10/160/12.5	0.2	3.2	0.25
5/160/25	0.1	3.2	0.5
10/160/25	0.2	3.2	0.5
10/320/25	0.1	3.2	0.25

Sample solution A: Nominally equivalent to 0.1 mg/mL of amlodipine in *Diluent* from *Sample stock solution*
Sample solution B: Nominally equivalent to 0.064 mg/mL of valsartan in *Diluent* from *Sample stock solution*
Sample solution C: Nominally equivalent to 0.025 mg/mL of hydrochlorothiazide in *Diluent* from *Sample stock solution*
Chromatographic system
(See *Chromatography* ⟨621⟩, *System Suitability*.)
Mode: LC
Detector: UV 225 nm. For *Identification A*, use a diode array detector in the range of 200–400 nm.
Column: 4.6-mm × 15-cm; 3-μm packing L1
Column temperature: 40°
Flow rate: 1.5 mL/min
Injection volume: 10 μL
System suitability
Sample: *Standard solution*
Suitability requirements
Tailing factor: NMT 2.0 for amlodipine, valsartan, and hydrochlorothiazide
Relative standard deviation: NMT 2.0% for amlodipine, valsartan, and hydrochlorothiazide
Analysis
Samples: *Standard solution, Sample solution A, Sample solution B,* and *Sample solution C*
Calculate the percentage of the labeled amount of amlodipine ($C_{20}H_{25}ClN_2O_5$) in the portion of Tablets taken:

$$\text{Result} = (r_U/r_S) \times (C_S/C_U) \times (M_{r1}/M_{r2}) \times 100$$

r_U = peak response of amlodipine from *Sample solution A*
r_S = peak response of amlodipine from the *Standard solution*
C_S = concentration of USP Amlodipine Besylate RS in the *Standard solution* (mg/mL)
C_U = nominal concentration of amlodipine in *Sample solution A* (mg/mL)
M_{r1} = molecular weight of amlodipine, 408.88
M_{r2} = molecular weight of amlodipine besylate, 567.05

Calculate the percentage of the labeled amount of valsartan ($C_{24}H_{29}N_5O_3$) in the portion of Tablets taken:

$$\text{Result} = (r_U/r_S) \times (C_S/C_U) \times 100$$

r_U = peak response of valsartan from *Sample solution B*
r_S = peak response of valsartan from the *Standard solution*
C_S = concentration of USP Valsartan RS in the *Standard solution* (mg/mL)
C_U = nominal concentration of valsartan in *Sample solution B* (mg/mL)

Calculate the percentage of the labeled amount of hydrochlorothiazide ($C_7H_8ClN_3O_4S_2$) in the portion of Tablets taken:

$$\text{Result} = (r_U/r_S) \times (C_S/C_U) \times 100$$

r_U = peak response of hydrochlorothiazide from *Sample solution C*
r_S = peak response of hydrochlorothiazide from the *Standard solution*
C_S = concentration of USP Hydrochlorothiazide RS in the *Standard solution* (mg/mL)
C_U = nominal concentration of hydrochlorothiazide in *Sample solution C* (mg/mL)

Acceptance criteria: 92.5%–107.5%

PERFORMANCE TESTS

Change to read:

- **DISSOLUTION ⟨711⟩**
  Test 1
  Buffer: Dissolve 6.805 g of monobasic potassium phosphate and 0.896 g of sodium hydroxide in 1000 mL of water. Adjust with 0.2 N sodium hydroxide or 1 M phosphoric acid to a pH of 6.8.
  Medium: *Buffer;* 900 mL
  Apparatus 2
  For 5/160/12.5, 10/160/12.5, 5/160/25, and 10/160/25 (mg/mg/mg) of Tablet strengths (amlodipine/valsartan/hydrochlorothiazide): 50 rpm
  For 10/320/25 (mg/mg/mg) of Tablet strengths (amlodipine/valsartan/hydrochlorothiazide): 55 rpm
  Time: 30 min
  Solution A: Acetonitrile, water, and phosphoric acid (50:950:1)
  Solution B: Acetonitrile, water, and phosphoric acid (950:50:1)
  Mobile phase: See *Table 3*.

Table 3

Time (min)	Solution A (%)	Solution B (%)
0.00	67	33
2.50	23	77
2.51	67	33
4.00	67	33

Diluent: 1 mg/mL of polysorbate 80 in *Buffer*
Standard stock solution A: 0.07 mg/mL of USP Amlodipine Besylate and 0.124 mg/mL of USP Hydrochlorothiazide RS. Initially dissolve with 4% of the total volume of methanol, and dilute with *Diluent* to volume.
Standard stock solution B: 3.2 mg/mL of USP Valsartan RS in methanol
Standard solution: 0.014 mg/mL of USP Amlodipine Besylate RS, 0.16 mg/mL of USP Valsartan RS, and 0.0248 mg/mL of USP Hydrochlorothiazide RS in *Diluent* from *Standard stock solution A* and *Standard stock solution B*, respectively
Sample solution: Pass a portion of the solution under test through a suitable filter of 0.45-μm pore size. Discard at least the first 10 mL of the filtrate.
Chromatographic system
(See *Chromatography* ⟨621⟩, *System Suitability*.)
Mode: LC
Detector: UV 250 nm
Column: 4.6-mm × 5-cm; 3-μm packing L1
Column temperature: 30°
Flow rate: 1.5 mL/min
Injection volume
For 10/320/25 (mg/mg/mg) of Tablet strengths (amlodipine/valsartan/hydrochlorothiazide): 5 μL
For 5/160/12.5, 10/160/12.5, 5/160/25, and 10/160/25 (mg/mg/mg) of Tablet strengths (amlodipine/valsartan/hydrochlorothiazide): 10 μL
System suitability
Sample: *Standard solution*
Suitability requirements
Resolution: NLT 3.0 between amlodipine and valsartan
Tailing factor: NMT 2.0 for amlodipine, valsartan, and hydrochlorothiazide

Relative standard deviation: NMT 2.0% for amlodipine, valsartan, and hydrochlorothiazide
Analysis
Samples: *Standard solution* and *Sample solution*
Calculate the percentage of the labeled amount of amlodipine ($C_{20}H_{25}ClN_2O_5$) dissolved:

$$\text{Result} = (r_U/r_S) \times C_S \times V \times (M_{r1}/M_{r2}) \times (1/L_1) \times 100$$

r_U = peak response of amlodipine from the *Sample solution*
r_S = peak response of amlodipine from the *Standard solution*
C_S = concentration of USP Amlodipine Besylate RS in the *Standard solution* (mg/mL)
V = volume of *Medium*, 900 mL
M_{r1} = molecular weight of amlodipine, 408.88
M_{r2} = molecular weight of amlodipine besylate, 567.05
L_1 = label claim of amlodipine (mg/Tablet)
Calculate the percentage of the labeled amount of valsartan ($C_{24}H_{29}N_5O_3$) dissolved:

$$\text{Result} = (r_U/r_S) \times C_S \times V \times (1/L_2) \times 100$$

r_U = peak response of valsartan from the *Sample solution*
r_S = peak response of valsartan from the *Standard solution*
C_S = concentration of USP Valsartan RS in the *Standard solution* (mg/mL)
V = volume of *Medium*, 900 mL
L_2 = label claim of valsartan (mg/Tablet)
Calculate the percentage of the labeled amount of hydrochlorothiazide ($C_7H_8ClN_3O_4S_2$) dissolved:

$$\text{Result} = (r_U/r_S) \times C_S \times V \times (1/L_3) \times 100$$

r_U = peak response of hydrochlorothiazide from the *Sample solution*
r_S = peak response of hydrochlorothiazide from the *Standard solution*
C_S = concentration of USP Hydrochlorothiazide RS in the *Standard solution* (mg/mL)
V = volume of *Medium*, 900 mL
L_3 = label claim of hydrochlorothiazide (mg/Tablet)
Tolerances: NLT 75% (*Q*) of the labeled amount of amlodipine ($C_{20}H_{25}ClN_2O_5$) is dissolved, NLT 80% (*Q*) of the labeled amount of valsartan ($C_{24}H_{29}N_5O_3$) is dissolved, and NLT 80% (*Q*) of the labeled amount of hydrochlorothiazide ($C_7H_8ClN_3O_4S_2$) is dissolved.
Test 2: If the product complies with this test, the labeling indicates that the product meets USP *Dissolution Test 2.*
Medium: Proceed as directed under *Dissolution Test 1*; 900 mL.
Apparatus 2
For Tablets labeled to contain amlodipine/valsartan/hydrochlorothiazide, 5/160/12.5, 10/160/12.5, 5/160/25, 10/160/25, and 5/80/12.5 (mg/mg/mg): 50 rpm
For Tablets labeled to contain amlodipine/valsartan/hydrochlorothiazide, 10/320/25 (mg/mg/mg): 55 rpm
Times
For valsartan and hydrochlorothiazide: 30 min
For amlodipine: 45 min
Buffer: Mix 7.0 mL of triethylamine with 1000 mL of water. Adjust with phosphoric acid to a pH of 3.0.
Solution A: Acetonitrile and *Buffer* (10:90)
Solution B: Acetonitrile and *Buffer* (90:10)
Mobile phase: See *Table 4.*

Table 4

Time (min)	Solution A (%)	Solution B (%)
0	90	10
7	30	70
8	90	10
15	90	10

Standard stock solution A: 0.35 mg/mL of USP Amlodipine Besylate RS, prepared as follows. Initially dissolve in 10% of the final volume of methanol and dilute with *Medium* to volume.
Standard stock solution B: 1.6 mg/mL of USP Valsartan RS in methanol
Standard stock solution C: 0.7 mg/mL of USP Hydrochlorothiazide RS, prepared as follows. Initially dissolve in 25% of the final volume of methanol and dilute with *Medium* to volume.
Standard solution: (L_1/1000) mg/mL of amlodipine, (L_2/1000) mg/mL of valsartan, and (L_3/1000) mg/mL of hydrochlorothiazide in •*Medium*• (IRA 1-Nov-2017) from *Standard stock solution A, Standard stock solution B,* and *Standard stock solution C,* where L_1 is the label claim of amlodipine in mg/Tablet, L_2 is the label claim of valsartan in mg/Tablet, and L_3 is the label claim of hydrochlorothiazide in mg/Tablet
Sample solution: Pass a portion of the solution under test through a suitable filter of 1-μm pore size.
Chromatographic system
(See *Chromatography ⟨621⟩, System Suitability.*)
Mode: LC
Detector: UV 237 nm
Column: 4.6-mm × 15-cm; 5-μm packing L1
Temperatures
Autosampler: 10°
Column: 50°
Flow rate: 1.5 mL/min
Injection volume: 20 μL
System suitability
Sample: *Standard solution*
Suitability requirements
Tailing factor: NMT 2.0 for each peak
Relative standard deviation: NMT 2.0% for each peak
Analysis
Samples: *Standard solution* and *Sample solution*
Calculate the percentage of the labeled amount of amlodipine ($C_{20}H_{25}ClN_2O_5$) dissolved:

$$\text{Result} = (r_U/r_S) \times C_S \times V \times (M_{r1}/M_{r2}) \times (1/L_1) \times 100$$

r_U = peak response of amlodipine from the *Sample solution*
r_S = peak response of amlodipine from the *Standard solution*
C_S = concentration of USP Amlodipine Besylate RS in the *Standard solution* (mg/mL)
V = volume of *Medium*, 900 mL
M_{r1} = molecular weight of amlodipine, 408.88
M_{r2} = molecular weight of amlodipine besylate, 567.05
L_1 = label claim of amlodipine (mg/Tablet)
Calculate the percentage of the labeled amount of valsartan ($C_{24}H_{29}N_5O_3$) dissolved:

$$\text{Result} = (r_U/r_S) \times C_S \times V \times (1/L_2) \times 100$$

r_U = peak response of valsartan from the *Sample solution*
r_S = peak response of valsartan from the *Standard solution*
C_S = concentration of USP Valsartan RS in the *Standard solution* (mg/mL)
V = volume of *Medium*, 900 mL

L_2 = label claim of valsartan (mg/Tablet)
Calculate the percentage of the labeled amount of hydrochlorothiazide ($C_7H_8ClN_3O_4S_2$) dissolved:

$$Result = (r_U/r_S) \times C_S \times V \times (1/L_3) \times 100$$

r_U = peak response of hydrochlorothiazide from the *Sample solution*
r_S = peak response of hydrochlorothiazide from the *Standard solution*
C_S = concentration of USP Hydrochlorothiazide RS in the *Standard solution* (mg/mL)
V = volume of *Medium*, 900 mL
L_3 = label claim of hydrochlorothiazide (mg/Tablet)

Tolerances: NLT 75% (*Q*) of the labeled amount of amlodipine ($C_{20}H_{25}ClN_2O_5$) is dissolved, NLT 80% (*Q*) of the labeled amount of valsartan ($C_{24}H_{29}N_5O_3$) is dissolved, and NLT 80% (*Q*) of the labeled amount of hydrochlorothiazide ($C_7H_8ClN_3O_4S_2$) is dissolved.

Test 3: If the product complies with this test, the labeling indicates that the product meets USP *Dissolution Test 3*.

Medium: Dissolve 6.80 g of monobasic potassium phosphate in 1000 mL of water. Adjust with 10% sodium hydroxide solution to a pH of 6.8; 1000 mL for valsartan and hydrochlorothiazide; 900 mL for amlodipine.

Apparatus 2
For valsartan and hydrochlorothiazide: 50 rpm
For amlodipine in Tablets labeled to contain amlodipine/valsartan/hydrochlorothiazide, 10/320/25 (mg/mg/mg): 55 rpm
For amlodipine in Tablets labeled to contain amlodipine/valsartan/hydrochlorothiazide, 5/160/12.5, 10/160/12.5, 5/160/25, 10/160/25, and 5/80/12.5 (mg/mg/mg): 50 rpm

Times
For valsartan and hydrochlorothiazide: 30 min
For amlodipine: 45 min

Solution A: Acetonitrile, trifluoroacetic acid and water (10: 0.1: 90)
Solution B: Acetonitrile, trifluoroacetic acid and water (90: 0.1: 10)
Mobile phase: See *Table 5*.

Table 5

Time (min)	Solution A (%)	Solution B (%)
0.01	90	10
2.5	10	90
3.0	90	10
5.0	90	10

Diluent: Acetonitrile and water (50:50)
Standard stock solution A: 0.15 mg/mL of USP Amlodipine Besylate RS in *Medium*, prepared as follows. Initially dissolve and sonicate in 5% of the final volume of *Diluent*, and dilute with *Medium* to volume.
Standard stock solution B: 1.6 mg/mL of USP Valsartan RS in *Medium*, prepared as follows. Initially dissolve and sonicate in 20% of the final volume of *Diluent*, and dilute with *Medium* to volume.
Standard stock solution C: 0.25 mg/mL of USP Hydrochlorothiazide RS in *Medium*, prepared as follows. Initially dissolve and sonicate in 10% of the final volume of *Diluent*, and dilute with *Medium* to volume.
Standard solution: (L_1/1000) mg/mL of amlodipine, (L_2/1000) mg/mL of valsartan, and (L_3/1000) mg/mL of hydrochlorothiazide in *Diluent* from *Standard stock solution A*, *Standard stock solution B*, and *Standard stock solution C*, where L_1 is the label claim of amlodipine in mg/Tablet, L_2 is the label claim of valsartan in mg/Tablet, and L_3 is the label claim of hydrochlorothiazide in mg/Tablet

Sample solution: Pass a portion of the solution under test through a suitable filter of 0.45-µm pore size. Discard at least the first few milliliters of the filtrate.

Chromatographic system
(See *Chromatography* ⟨621⟩, *System Suitability*.)
Mode: LC
Detectors
For amlodipine: UV 237 nm
For valsartan and hydrochlorothiazide: UV 270 nm
Column: 4.6-mm × 10-cm; 5-µm packing L1
Flow rate: 1.5 mL/min
Injection volume: 10 µL
System suitability
Sample: *Standard solution*
Suitability requirements
Tailing factor: NMT 2.0 for each peak
Relative standard deviation: NMT 2.0% for each peak
Analysis
Samples: *Standard solution* and *Sample solution*
Calculate the percentage of the labeled amount of amlodipine ($C_{20}H_{25}ClN_2O_5$) dissolved:

$$Result = (r_U/r_S) \times C_S \times V \times (M_{r1}/M_{r2}) \times (1/L_1) \times 100$$

r_U = peak response of amlodipine from the *Sample solution*
r_S = peak response of amlodipine from the *Standard solution*
C_S = concentration of USP Amlodipine Besylate RS in the *Standard solution* (mg/mL)
V = volume of *Medium*, 900 mL
M_{r1} = molecular weight of amlodipine, 408.88
M_{r2} = molecular weight of amlodipine besylate, 567.05
L_1 = label claim of amlodipine (mg/Tablet)

Calculate the percentage of the labeled amount of valsartan ($C_{24}H_{29}N_5O_3$) dissolved:

$$Result = (r_U/r_S) \times C_S \times V \times (1/L_2) \times 100$$

r_U = peak response of valsartan from the *Sample solution*
r_S = peak response of valsartan from the *Standard solution*
C_S = concentration of USP Valsartan RS in the *Standard solution* (mg/mL)
V = volume of *Medium*, 1000 mL
L_2 = label claim of valsartan (mg/Tablet)

Calculate the percentage of the labeled amount of hydrochlorothiazide ($C_7H_8ClN_3O_4S_2$) dissolved:

$$Result = (r_U/r_S) \times C_S \times V \times (1/L_3) \times 100$$

r_U = peak response of hydrochlorothiazide from the *Sample solution*
r_S = peak response of hydrochlorothiazide from the *Standard solution*
C_S = concentration of USP Hydrochlorothiazide RS in the *Standard solution* (mg/mL)
V = volume of *Medium*, 1000 mL
L_3 = label claim of hydrochlorothiazide (mg/Tablet)

Tolerances
For Tablets labeled to contain amlodipine/valsartan/hydrochlorothiazide, 5/160/12.5, 10/160/12.5, 5/160/25, and 10/160/25 (mg/mg/mg): NLT 75% (*Q*) of the labeled amount of amlodipine ($C_{20}H_{25}ClN_2O_5$) is dissolved, NLT 80% (*Q*) of the labeled amount of valsartan ($C_{24}H_{29}N_5O_3$) is dissolved, and NLT 80% (*Q*) of the labeled amount of hydrochlorothiazide ($C_7H_8ClN_3O_4S_2$) is dissolved.
For Tablets labeled to contain amlodipine/valsartan/hydrochlorothiazide, 5/160/25, and 10/320/25 (mg/mg/mg): NLT 70% (*Q*) of the labeled

amount of amlodipine ($C_{20}H_{25}ClN_2O_5$) is dissolved, NLT 80% (*Q*) of the labeled amount of valsartan ($C_{24}H_{29}N_5O_3$) is dissolved, and NLT 80% (*Q*) of the labeled amount of hydrochlorothiazide ($C_7H_8ClN_3O_4S_2$) is dissolved.

- **UNIFORMITY OF DOSAGE UNITS ⟨905⟩:** Meet the requirements

IMPURITIES

Change to read:

- **ORGANIC IMPURITIES**
  Use amber glassware for all solutions containing drug substances.
  Mobile phase, Diluent, Sample solution A, Sample solution B, Sample solution C, and **Chromatographic system:** Proceed as directed in the *Assay.*
  System suitability solution: 0.02 mg/mL each of USP Benzothiadiazine Related Compound A RS and USP Valsartan Related Compound B RS, 0.005 mg/mL of USP Amlodipine Related Compound A RS, 0.14 mg/mL of USP Amlodipine Besylate RS, 0.064 mg/mL of USP Valsartan RS, and 0.025 mg/mL of USP Hydrochlorothiazide RS in *Diluent*
  Sensitivity solution: 0.14 µg/mL of USP Amlodipine Besylate RS, 0.064 µg/mL of USP Valsartan RS, and 0.025 µg/mL of USP Hydrochlorothiazide RS in *Diluent*
  Standard solution: 0.0005 mg/mL of USP Amlodipine Related Compound A RS, 0.0001 mg/mL of USP Benzothiadiazine Related Compound A RS, 0.0003 mg/mL of USP Amlodipine Besylate RS, 0.00015 mg/mL of USP Valsartan RS, and 0.00005 mg/mL of USP Hydrochlorothiazide RS in *Diluent*
  System suitability
  Samples: *System suitability solution, Sensitivity solution,* and *Standard solution*
  Suitability requirements
  Resolution: NLT 2.0 between any adjacent peaks of benzothiadiazine related compound A, hydrochlorothiazide, amlodipine related compound A, amlodipine, valsartan related compound B, and valsartan, *System suitability solution*
  Relative standard deviation: NMT 5.0% for amlodipine related compound A, benzothiadiazine related compound A, amlodipine, valsartan, and hydrochlorothiazide, *Standard solution*
  Signal-to-noise ratio: NLT 10 for amlodipine, valsartan, and hydrochlorothiazide, *Sensitivity solution*
  Analysis
  Samples: *Sample solution A, Sample solution B, Sample solution C,* and *Standard solution*
  Calculate the percentage of amlodipine related compound A in the portion of Tablets taken:

  $$Result = (r_U/r_S) \times (C_S/C_U) \times (M_{r1}/M_{r2}) \times 100$$

  r_U = peak response of amlodipine related compound A from *Sample solution A*
  r_S = peak response of amlodipine related compound A from the *Standard solution*
  C_S = concentration of USP Amlodipine Related Compound A RS in the *Standard solution* (mg/mL)
  C_U = nominal concentration of amlodipine in *Sample solution A* (mg/mL)

M_{r1} = molecular weight of amlodipine related compound A free base, 406.86
M_{r2} = molecular weight of amlodipine related compound A fumarate, 522.93

Calculate the percentage of any valsartan related degradation product in the portion of Tablets taken:

$$Result = (r_U/r_S) \times (C_S/C_U) \times 100$$

r_U = peak response of any valsartan related degradation product from *Sample solution B*
r_S = peak response of valsartan from the *Standard solution*
C_S = concentration of USP Valsartan RS in the *Standard solution* (mg/mL)
C_U = nominal concentration of valsartan in *Sample solution B* (mg/mL)

Calculate the percentage of benzothiadiazine related compound A in the portion of Tablets taken:

$$Result = (r_U/r_S) \times (C_S/C_U) \times 100$$

r_U = peak response of benzothiadiazine related compound A from *Sample solution C*
r_S = peak response of benzothiadiazine related compound A from the *Standard solution*
C_S = concentration of USP Benzothiadiazine Related Compound A RS in the *Standard solution* (mg/mL)
C_U = nominal concentration of hydrochlorothiazide in *Sample solution C* (mg/mL)

Calculate the percentage of chlorothiazide and hydrochlorothiazide dimer in the portion of Tablets taken:

$$Result = (r_U/r_S) \times (C_S/C_U) \times 100$$

r_U = peak response of chlorothiazide or hydrochlorothiazide dimer from *Sample solution C*
r_S = peak response of hydrochlorothiazide from the *Standard solution*
C_S = concentration of USP Hydrochlorothiazide RS in the *Standard solution* (mg/mL)
C_U = nominal concentration of hydrochlorothiazide in *Sample solution C* (mg/mL)

Calculate the percentage of each unspecified degradation product in the portion of Tablets taken:

$$Result = (r_U/r_S) \times (C_S/C_U) \times (M_{r1}/M_{r2}) \times 100$$

r_U = peak response of each unspecified degradation product from *Sample solution A*
r_S = peak response of amlodipine from the *Standard solution*
C_S = concentration of USP Amlodipine Besylate RS in the *Standard solution* (mg/mL)
C_U = nominal concentration of amlodipine in *Sample solution A* (mg/mL)
M_{r1} = molecular weight of amlodipine, 408.88
M_{r2} = molecular weight of amlodipine besylate, 567.05

Acceptance criteria: See *Table 6.* Disregard the amlodipine ethyl analog peak, the valsartan related compound B peak, and any peaks below 0.1%.

Table 6

Name	Relative Retention Time	Acceptance Criteria, NMT (%)
Benzothiadiazine related compound A[a]	0.60	1.0
Chlorothiazide[b]	0.62	0.50
Hydrochlorothiazide	0.64	—
Devaleryl valsartan[c]	0.71	0.2
Hydrochlorothiazide dimer[d]	0.89	0.50
Amlodipine related compound A[e]	0.96	0.5
Amlodipine	1.00	—
Valsartan related degradation product 1[f]	1.04	0.2
Amlodipine ethyl analog[g]	1.08	—
Valsartan related compound B[h]	1.22	—
Valsartan related degradation product 2[f]	1.27	0.2
Valsartan	1.36	—
Valsartan related degradation product 3[f]	1.51	0.2
Valsartan related degradation product 4[f]	1.62	0.2
Any other unspecified degradation product[i]	—	0.2
Total degradation products	—	2.0

[a] 4-Amino-6-chloro-1,3-benzenedisulfonamide.

[b] 6-Chloro-2H-1,2,4-benzothiadiazine-7-sulfonamide 1,1-dioxide.

[c] N-{[2'-(1H-Tetrazole-5-yl)biphenyl-4-yl]methyl}-L-valine.

[d] 6-Chloro-N-[(6-chloro-7-sulfamoyl-2,3-dihydro-4H-1,2,4-benzothiadiazine-4-yl 1,1-dioxide)methyl]3,4-dihydro-2H-1,2,4-benzothiadiazine-7-sulfonamide 1,1-dioxide.

[e] 3-Ethyl 5-methyl [2-(2-aminoethoxymethyl)-4-(2-chlorophenyl)-6-methyl-3,5-pyridinedicarboxylate].

[f] These are specified unidentified degradation products. No information is available about chemical structures or chemical names for these impurities.

[g] Diethyl 2-[(2-aminoethoxy)methyl]-4-(2-chlorophenyl)-6-methyl-1,4-dihydropyridine-3,5-dicarboxylate. Process related impurity given for information only.

[h] ● N-Butyryl-N-{[2'-(1H-tetrazole-5-yl)biphenyl-4-yl]-methyl}-L-valine. ● (IRA 1-Nov-2017) Process related impurity given for information only.

[i] Benzenesulfonic acid is the counter ion to the amlodipine, and peaks at RRT of 0.33 and 0.42 are not considered as degradation products.

Add the following:

●• LIMIT OF VALSARTAN RELATED COMPOUND A

[NOTE—Valsartan related compound A is a process impurity and a formulation specific degradation product.]

Mobile phase: n-Hexane, 2-propanol, and trifluoroacetic acid (850:150:1)

System suitability solution: 0.04 mg/mL each of USP Valsartan Related Compound A and USP Valsartan RS in *Mobile phase*

Standard solution: 0.001 mg/mL of USP Valsartan Related Compound A RS in *Mobile phase*

Sample solution: Nominally 0.5 mg/mL of valsartan in *Mobile phase* from a suitable amount of finely crushed powder from NLT 20 Tablets. Sonication may be necessary for complete dissolution. Pass through a suitable filter of 0.45-μm pore size.

Chromatographic system
(See *Chromatography* ⟨621⟩, *System Suitability*.)
Mode: LC
Detector: UV 230 nm
Column: 4.6-mm × 25-cm; 5-μm packing L40
Temperatures
  Autosampler: 10°
  Column: 30°
Flow rate: 0.8 mL/min
Injection volume: 20 μL
Run time: NLT 3.5 times the retention time of valsartan related compound A
System suitability
Samples: *System suitability solution* and *Standard solution*
[NOTE—The relative retention times of valsartan related compound A and valsartan are about 0.65 and 1.0, respectively.]
Suitability requirements
  Resolution: NLT 2.0 between valsartan and valsartan related compound A, *System suitability solution*
  Relative standard deviation: NMT 5.0% for valsartan related compound A, *Standard solution*
Analysis
Samples: *Standard solution* and *Sample solution*
Calculate the percentage of the valsartan related compound A in the portion of Tablets taken:

$$Result = (r_U/r_S) \times (C_S/C_U) \times 100$$

r_U = peak response of valsartan related compound A from the *Sample solution*
r_S = peak response of valsartan related compound A from the *Standard solution*
C_S = concentration of USP Valsartan Related Compound A RS in the *Standard solution* (mg/mL)
C_U = nominal concentration of valsartan in the *Sample solution* (mg/mL)
Acceptance criteria: NMT 1.0%● (IRA 1-Nov-2017)

ADDITIONAL REQUIREMENTS

- **PACKAGING AND STORAGE:** Store at controlled room temperature in tight containers in a dry place.
- **LABELING:** When more than one *Dissolution* test is given, the labeling states the *Dissolution* test used only if *Test 1* is not used.

Change to read:

- **USP REFERENCE STANDARDS** ⟨11⟩
  USP Amlodipine Besylate RS
  USP Amlodipine Related Compound A RS
    3-Ethyl 5-methyl [2-(2-aminoethoxymethyl)-4-(2-chlorophenyl)-6-methyl-3,5-pyridinedicarboxylate] fumarate.
    $C_{20}H_{23}ClN_2O_5 \cdot C_4H_4O_4$ 522.93
  USP Benzothiadiazine Related Compound A RS
    4-Amino-6-chloro-1,3-benzenedisulfonamide.
    $C_6H_8ClN_3O_4S_2$ 285.73
  USP Hydrochlorothiazide RS
  USP Valsartan RS
  ●USP Valsartan Related Compound A RS
    N-Valeryl-N-{[2'-(1H-tetrazole-5-yl)biphenyl-4-yl]methyl}-D-valine.
    $C_{24}H_{29}N_5O_3$ 435.52
  USP Valsartan Related Compound B RS
  ● (IRA 1-Nov-2017)

Amoxicillin

$C_{16}H_{19}N_3O_5S \cdot 3H_2O$ 419.45
4-Thia-1-azabicyclo[3.2.0]heptane-2-carboxylic acid,6-[[amino(4-hydroxyphenyl)acetyl]amino]-3,3-dimethyl-7-oxo-, trihydrate [2S-[2α,5α,6β(S*)]]-;
(2S,5R,6R)-6-[(R)-(–)-2-Amino-2-(p-hydroxyphenyl)acetamido]-3,3-dimethyl-7-oxo-4-thia-1-azabicyclo[3.2.0]heptane-2-carboxylic acid trihydrate [61336-70-7].
Anhydrous   365.41
    [26787-78-0].

DEFINITION
Amoxicillin contains NLT 900 µg/mg and NMT 1050 µg/mg of amoxicillin ($C_{16}H_{19}N_3O_5S$), calculated on the anhydrous basis.

IDENTIFICATION

Change to read:

- ■**A.**■1S (USP41) **INFRARED ABSORPTION** ⟨197K⟩

Add the following:

- ■• **B.** The retention time of the major peak of the *Sample solution* corresponds to that of the *Standard solution*, as obtained in the *Assay*.■1S (USP41)

ASSAY
- **PROCEDURE**
  Diluent: 6.8 g/L of monobasic potassium phosphate in water. Adjust with a 45% (w/w) solution of potassium hydroxide to a pH of 5.0 ± 0.1.
  Mobile phase: Acetonitrile and *Diluent* (1:24)
  Standard solution: 1.2 mg/mL of USP Amoxicillin RS in *Diluent*. [NOTE—Use this solution within 6 h.]
  Sample solution: 1.2 mg/mL of Amoxicillin in *Diluent*. [NOTE—Use this solution within 6 h.]
  Chromatographic system
  (See *Chromatography* ⟨621⟩, *System Suitability*.)
  Mode: LC
  Detector: UV 230 nm
  Column: 4-mm × 25-cm; packing L1
  Flow rate: 1.5 mL/min
  Injection volume: 10 µL
  System suitability
  Sample: *Standard solution*
  Suitability requirements
  Tailing factor: NMT 2.5
  Relative standard deviation: NMT 2.0%
  Analysis
  Samples: *Standard solution* and *Sample solution*
  Calculate the quantity, in µg/mg, of amoxicillin ($C_{16}H_{19}N_3O_5S$) in the portion of Amoxicillin taken:

$$Result = (r_U/r_S) \times (C_S/C_U) \times P$$

r_U = peak response from the *Sample solution*
r_S = peak response from the *Standard solution*
C_S = concentration of USP Amoxicillin RS in the *Standard solution* (mg/mL)
C_U = concentration of Amoxicillin in the *Sample solution* (mg/mL)

P = potency of amoxicillin in USP Amoxicillin RS (µg/mg)
Acceptance criteria: 900–1050 µg/mg of amoxicillin ($C_{16}H_{19}N_3O_5S$) on the anhydrous basis

IMPURITIES
- **ORGANIC IMPURITIES**
  Solution A: 2.72 g/L of monobasic potassium phosphate. Adjust with 1 N potassium hydroxide or 20% phosphoric acid to a pH of 5.0 ± 0.1.
  Solution B: Methanol
  Mobile phase: See *Table 1*.

Table 1

Time (min)	Solution A (%)	Solution B (%)
0	97	3
10	97	3
22	75	25
26	97	3

  System suitability solution: 12.5 µg/mL each of USP Amoxicillin Related Compound A RS and USP Amoxicillin Related Compound D RS in *Solution A*
  Standard solution: 12.5 µg/mL of USP Amoxicillin RS in *Solution A*
  Sample solution: 1.25 mg/mL of Amoxicillin in *Solution A*. [NOTE—Store this solution at 4° and use within 4 h.]
  Chromatographic system
  (See *Chromatography* ⟨621⟩, *System Suitability*.)
  Mode: LC
  Detector: UV 210 nm
  Column: 4.6-mm × 10-cm; 5-µm packing L1
  Temperatures
    Autosampler: 4°
    Column: 40°
  Flow rate: 1.5 mL/min
  Injection volume: 10 µL
  System suitability
  Samples: *System suitability solution* and *Standard solution*
  [NOTE—Identify peaks by the relative retention times in *Table 2*.]
  Suitability requirements
  Resolution: NLT 1.5 between amoxicillin related compound A and the second peak for amoxicillin related compound D, *System suitability solution*
  Relative standard deviation: NMT 10%, *Standard solution*
  Analysis
  Samples: *Standard solution* and *Sample solution*
  Calculate the percentage of each impurity in the portion of Amoxicillin taken:

$$Result = (r_U/r_S) \times (C_S/C_U) \times F \times 100$$

r_U = peak response of each impurity from the *Sample solution*
r_S = peak response of amoxicillin from the *Standard solution*
C_S = concentration of USP Amoxicillin RS in the *Standard solution* (µg/mL)
C_U = concentration of Amoxicillin in the *Sample solution* (mg/mL)
F = unit conversion factor, 0.001 mg/µg
Acceptance criteria: See *Table 2*. [NOTE—The reporting limit is 0.03 times the amoxicillin peak from the *Standard solution*.]

Table 2

Name	Relative Retention Time	Acceptance Criteria, NMT (%)
Amoxicillin related compound I[a] (D-hydroxyphenylglycine)	0.32	1.0
Amoxicillin related compound D[b,c] (amoxicillin open ring)	0.53	1.0
	0.68	1.0
Amoxicillin related compound A[d] (6-aminopenicillanic acid)	0.78	0.5
Amoxicillin related compound B[e,f] (L-amoxicillin)	0.87	—
Amoxicillin	1.0	—
Amoxicillin related compound G[g] (D-hydroxyphenyl glycylamoxicillin)	2.9	1.0
Amoxicillin related compound E[h,i] (amoxicillin penilloic derivative)	4.5	1.0
Amoxicillin related compound M[j] [N-(penicillan-6-yl) open ring amoxicillinamide]	6.0	1.0
Amoxicillin related compound F[e,k] (phenylpyrazinediol)	6.3	—
Amoxicillin related compound C[l] (amoxicillin rearrangement product)	6.4	1.0
Amoxicillin related compound E[h,i] (amoxicillin penilloic derivative)	6.7	1.0
Amoxicillin related compound J[m] (amoxicillin open ring dimer)	8.8	1.0
Amoxicillin related compound L[n] [N-(penicillan-6-yl) amoxicillinamide]	9.0	1.0
Any unspecified individual impurity	—	1.0
Total impurities	—	5.0

[a] (R)-2-Amino-2-(4-hydroxyphenyl)acetic acid.

[b] The chromatographic system resolves two penicilloic acids from each other.

[c] (4S)-2-{[(R)-2-Amino-2-(4-hydroxyphenyl)acetamido](carboxy)methyl}-5,5-dimethylthiazolidine-4-carboxylic acid.

[d] (2S,5R,6R)-6-Amino-3,3-dimethyl-7-oxo-4-thia-1-azabicyclo[3.2.0]heptane-2-carboxylic acid.

[e] These compounds are listed for information only and are not to be reported.

[f] (2S,5R,6R)-6-[(S)-2-Amino-2-(4-hydroxyphenyl)acetamido]-3,3-dimethyl-7-oxo-4-thia-1-azabicyclo[3.2.0]heptane-2-carboxylic acid.

[g] (2S,5R,6R)-6-{(R)-2-[(R)-2-Amino-2-(4-hydroxyphenyl)acetamido]-2-(4-hydroxyphenyl)acetamido}-3,3-dimethyl-7-oxo-4-thia-1-azabicyclo[3.2.0]heptane-2-carboxylic acid.

[h] The chromatographic system resolves two penilloic acids from each other.

[i] (4S)-2-{[(R)-2-Amino-2-(4-hydroxyphenyl)acetamido]methyl}-5,5-dimethylthiazolidine-4-carboxylic acid.

[j] (2S,5R,6R)-6-(2-[(R)-2-Amino-2-(4-hydroxyphenyl)acetamido]-2-((4S)-4-carboxy-5,5-dimethylthiazolidin-2-yl)acetamido)-3,3-dimethyl-7-oxo-4-thia-1-azabicyclo[3.2.0]heptane-2-carboxylic acid.

[k] 3-(4-Hydroxyphenyl)pyrazin-2-ol.

[l] (4S)-2-[5-(4-Hydroxyphenyl)-3,6-dioxopiperazin-2-yl]-5,5-dimethylthiazolidine-4-carboxylic acid.

[m] (2S,5R,6R)-6-((2R)-2-{2-[(R)-2-Amino-2-(4-hydroxyphenyl)acetamido]-2-[(4S)-4-carboxy-5,5-dimethylthiazolidin-2-yl]acetamido}-2-(4-hydroxyphenyl)acetamido)-3,3-dimethyl-7-oxo-4-thia-1-azabicyclo[3.2.0]heptane-2-carboxylic acid.

[n] (2S,5R,6R)-6-{(2S,5R,6R)-6-[(R)-2-Amino-2-(4-hydroxyphenyl)acetamido]-3,3-dimethyl-7-oxo-4-thia-1-azabicyclo[3.2.0]heptane-2-carboxamido}-3,3-dimethyl-7-oxo-4-thia-1-azabicyclo[3.2.0]heptane-2-carboxylic acid.

SPECIFIC TESTS
- **CRYSTALLINITY ⟨695⟩:** Meets the requirements
- **DIMETHYLANILINE ⟨223⟩:** Meets the requirements
- **PH ⟨791⟩**
  Sample solution: 2 mg/mL
  Acceptance criteria: 3.5–6.0
- **WATER DETERMINATION ⟨921⟩, Method I:** 11.5%–14.5%
- **STERILITY TESTS ⟨71⟩,** Test for Sterility of the Product to Be Examined, Direct Inoculation of the Culture Medium:
  Where the label states that Amoxicillin is sterile, it meets

the requirements, except to use Fluid Thioglycollate Medium containing polysorbate 80 solution (5 mg/mL) and an amount of sterile penicillinase sufficient to inactivate the amoxicillin in each tube, to use Soybean-Casein Digest Medium containing polysorbate 80 solution (5 mg/mL) and an amount of sterile penicillinase sufficient to inactivate the amoxicillin in each tube, and to shake the tubes once daily.
- **BACTERIAL ENDOTOXINS TEST ⟨85⟩:** Where the label states that Amoxicillin is sterile or Amoxicillin must be subjected to further processing during the preparation of injectable dosage forms, it contains NMT 0.25 USP Endotoxin Units/mg of amoxicillin.

ADDITIONAL REQUIREMENTS
- **PACKAGING AND STORAGE:** Preserve in tight containers, and store at controlled room temperature.
- **LABELING:** Where it is intended for use in preparing injectable dosage forms, the label states that it is intended for veterinary use only and that it is sterile or must be subjected to further processing during the preparation of injectable dosage forms. Label all other Amoxicillin to indicate that it is to be used in the manufacture of nonparenteral drugs only.

Change to read:

- **USP REFERENCE STANDARDS ⟨11⟩**
  USP Amoxicillin RS
  USP Amoxicillin Related Compound A RS
  (2S,5R,6R)-6-Amino-3,3-dimethyl-7-oxo-4-thia-1-azabicyclo[3.2.0]heptane-2-carboxylic acid;
  6-Aminopenicillanic acid.
  $C_8H_{12}N_2O_3S$ 216.26
  USP Amoxicillin Related Compound D RS
  (4S)-2-{[(R)-2-Amino-2-(4-hydroxyphenyl)acetamido](carboxy)methyl}-5,5-dimethylthiazolidine-4-carboxylic acid;
  Amoxicillin open ring.
  $C_{16}H_{21}N_3O_6S$ 383.42
  ● (CN 1-May-2018)

Delete the following:

■Anthrax Vaccine Adsorbed

DEFINITION
Anthrax Vaccine Adsorbed is a sterile, milky-white suspension made from cell-free filtrates of microaerophilic cultures of an avirulent, nonencapsulated strain of *Bacillus anthracis*. The final product contains no dead or live bacteria. The production cultures are grown in a chemically defined protein-free medium containing amino acids, vitamins, inorganic salts, and sugars. The sterile filtrate is adsorbed on sterile aluminum hydroxide, concentrated 10-fold, and resuspended in sterile physiological saline containing formaldehyde with benzethonium chloride as a preservative. Sublots may be combined to produce final lots. The product meets potency requirements when tested against the U.S. Reference Standard Anthrax Vaccine, in accordance with approved procedures (guinea pig intracutaneous challenge models).

IDENTIFICATION
- **A.**
  [NOTE—Perform analysis on the filtrate.]
  Trichloroacetic acid solution: Prepare a solution of trichloroacetic acid (see *Reagents, Indicators, and Solu-*

tions—*Reagent Specifications*) in water containing 100 g of trichloroacetic acid per 100 mL of the solution.

Sample buffer: Prepare a solution containing 141 mM tris(hydroxymethyl)aminomethane, 106 mM tris(hydroxymethyl)aminomethane hydrochloride, 0.51 mM edetate disodium, 2% (w/v) dodecyl lithium sulfate, 10% (v/v) glycerol, 0.22 mM Coomassie blue G-250, and 0.175 mM phenolsulfonphthalein. If necessary, adjust with hydrochloric acid or sodium hydroxide to a pH of 8.5.

Running buffer: Prepare a solution containing 25 mM tris(hydroxymethyl)aminomethane, 192 mM glycine, and 0.1% (w/v) dodecyl sodium sulfate (see *Reagents, Indicators, and Solutions—Reagent Specifications*) in water. If necessary, adjust with hydrochloric acid or sodium hydroxide to a pH of 8.5.

Transblotting buffer: Prepare a solution containing 12.5 mM tris(hydroxymethyl)aminomethane, 96 mM glycine, and 10% (v/v) methanol. If necessary, adjust with hydrochloric acid or sodium hydroxide to a pH of 8.0.

Blocking buffer: Prepare a solution containing 10 mM monobasic sodium phosphate, 150 mM sodium chloride, 5% (w/v) nonfat dry milk, and 0.05% (w/v) polysorbate 20. Adjust with sodium hydroxide to a pH of 7.4.

Primary antibody solutions: Prepare suitable monoclonal antibodies raised against the protective antigen (PA), the lethal factor (LF), and the edema factor (EF), respectively, of *Bacillus anthracis* in murine ascites cells, harvested, and used without further purification. Immediately before use, dilute each of the murine ascites fluids containing the monoclonal antibodies (1:1000) with the *Blocking buffer*.

Secondary antibody solution: Immediately before use, dissolve according to the manufacturer's instructions, if necessary, and dilute the stock horseradish peroxidase conjugated to goat anti-mouse IgG solution (1:1000) with *Blocking buffer*.

Chromogenic visualization solution: 150 mg/mL of 4-chloro-1-naphthol in water

Sample solution: Use anthrax vaccine filtrate as is.

Analysis: In a suitable centrifuge tube transfer (30/*c*) mL of the *Sample solution*, where *c* is the total protein concentration, in µg/mL, of the solution as determined in the test for *Total Protein*. Add 16.5/*c* mL of *Trichloroacetic acid solution*, and incubate for at least 10 min. Centrifuge at 9000 × *g* for about 10 min, decant off the supernatant, and hold the tube inverted to drain on a filter paper. Dissolve the pellet in 60 µL of *Sample buffer*, and transfer the solution to a polypropylene microfuge tube that has a lid. Close the lid tightly, secure with a lid-lock, and heat at 100° for 5 min. Allow the solution to cool to room temperature, and centrifuge at 10,000 × *g* for 15 s to collect the liquids. In a suitable device for polyacrylamide-gel electrophoresis (see *Biotechnology-Derived Articles—Polyacrylamide Gel Electrophoresis* ⟨1056⟩), add appropriate volumes of the *Running buffer* in the upper and the lower buffer chambers. Attach a 4%–20% gradient tris-glycine polyacrylamide slab gel sandwiched between two glass plates, such that the wells for sample application are exposed to the *Running buffer* in the upper buffer chamber. Apply about 20-µL aliquots of the treated *Sample solution* in three alternate lanes. [NOTE—Do not apply any solution in the outside lanes.] Connect the lower buffer chamber electrode to the positive terminal and the upper buffer chamber electrode to the negative terminal of a suitable power supply unit, and carry out the electrophoresis at a constant current of about 40 mA. When the dye-front is about 1 cm from the bottom of the gel (about 40 min), stop the current, and remove the gel from the gel assembly. [NOTE—Do not touch the gel with bare hands. Use gloves.]

Place three to four filter papers, cut to the size of the gel and soaked in the *Transblotting buffer*, on the anode plate of a suitable semidry electroblotter. Cut a nitrocellulose membrane to the same size as the gel plus 1–2 mm on each side, and "wet" the membrane by immersing it into the *Transblotting buffer* for about 15 s, such that there is no air bubble between the buffer and the membrane. Place the "wet" membrane immediately on the stack of filter papers, and remove all air bubbles between the membrane and filter paper by rolling a pipet, or equivalent, gently over the surface of the membrane. Place a few drops of the *Transblotting buffer* on the membrane, and then carefully place the gel on it. Gently roll a pipet, or equivalent, over the surface of the gel to ensure intimate contact between the gel and the membrane, making sure that there are no air bubbles in between. Place a filter paper cut to the size of the gel and soaked in the *Transblotting buffer*, such that there is no air bubble between the filter paper and the gel. Place two to three additional filter papers, prepared in a similar manner, on the top, and complete the transfer stack by placing the cathode plate on the top. Apply a current of about 250 mA, and continue transfer for 90 min.

Remove the membrane, and wash it quickly by immersing into water for 15 s. [NOTE—Do not touch the membrane with bare hands. Use gloves.] Cut the membrane into three strips such that each strip contains a lane containing the *Sample solution*, and mark the strips as PA, LF, and EF at the top. Place each strip in a heat-sealable bag, add 5 mL of *Blocking buffer*, and seal the bag. Incubate for 30 min with constant agitation. Open each bag, and pour out the *Blocking buffer*. Add 9 mL of the diluted *Primary antibody solution* against PA to the bag containing the strip marked PA. Similarly, add 9 mL of the diluted *Primary antibody solution* against LF and EF to the bags containing strips labeled LF and EF, respectively. Seal the bags, and incubate under agitation for 2 h at room temperature or overnight at 2°–8°. Remove the strips from the plastic bags, and place in separate plastic boxes. Add sufficient *Blocking buffer* so that each strip is completely immersed. Agitate for at least 30 min at room temperature with two changes of *Blocking buffer*. Remove the strips, and place each strip in a new heat-sealable plastic bag. Add 9 mL of the *Secondary antibody solution* to each plastic bag. Seal the bags, and incubate for 1 h at room temperature under agitation. Remove the strips from the plastic bags, and place in separate plastic boxes. Add sufficient *Blocking buffer* so that each strip is completely immersed. Agitate for at least 30 min at room temperature with two changes of the *Blocking buffer*. Transfer each strip into a new heat-sealable plastic bag, add 9 mL of *Chromogenic visualization solution* and 10 µL of 30% (v/v) hydrogen peroxide, and seal the bags. Incubate for 30 min under agitation. Transfer the strips into separate plastic boxes, and remove the excess 4-chloro-1-naphthol by incubating with water under agitation for 10 min.

Acceptance criteria: Visual observation indicates a strong positive band on the strip labeled PA, a faintly detectable band on the strip labeled LF, and no detectable band on the strip labeled EF.

ASSAY

- **RELATIVE POTENCY**

[NOTE—Perform analysis on the final product.]

Standard solutions: Dilute approved U.S. Reference Standard Anthrax Vaccine 1: 1.6, 1:4, 1:10, and 1:25 aseptically with a sterile 0.9% sodium chloride solution.

Sample solutions: Dilute Anthrax Vaccine Adsorbed, final product 1: 1.6, 1:4, 1:10, and 1:25 aseptically with a sterile 0.9% sodium chloride solution.

Analysis

Samples: *Standard solutions* and *Sample solutions*

Assign each dilution to a set of 12 randomly selected guinea pigs, strain Mdh:S(RA), 6 males and 6 females, each weighing 315–385 g on the day of vaccination. Inject the animals subcutaneously in the ventral abdomen with 0.5 mL of the assigned dilutions. On the 14th day post-vaccination, challenge the animals with approximately 1000 spores of *Bacillus anthracis* strain Vollum 1B, and record the deaths daily for a 10-day observation period. Record the numbers of surviving animals for each of the *Standard solutions* and the *Sample solutions* at the end of the test. Perform calculations by estimating best-fit lines for the *Standard solutions* and the *Sample solutions* using a logistic regression model that utilizes the number of animals that survived at the end of the test and the time to death for the animals that died. Evaluate statistically the lines corresponding to the *Standard solutions* and the *Sample solutions* for parallelism. Determine the common slope, and draw the parallel lines using the common slope. The relative potency of Anthrax Vaccine Adsorbed with respect to the corresponding U.S. Reference Standard Anthrax Vaccine is the antilog of the horizontal distance between the two parallel lines.

Acceptance criteria: The relative potency of Anthrax Vaccine Adsorbed is acceptable if it is between 0.53 and 1.79, both values inclusive.

OTHER COMPONENTS

- **ALUMINUM ⟨206⟩**

[NOTE—Perform analysis on the final product.]

Standard solutions: Prepare as directed for *Standard Preparations* in the chapter, except to prepare solutions containing 10, 20, 30, 40, and 50 μg/mL of aluminum.

Sample solution: Mix Anthrax Vaccine Adsorbed, final product well, and transfer 0.2 mL to a 10-mL volumetric flask. Add 0.5 mL of concentrated sulfuric acid and 0.5 mL of concentrated nitric acid, and mix gently. Incubate at room temperature for 30 min or until the solution becomes essentially clear. Dilute with water to volume.

Analysis: Proceed as directed for *Procedure* in the chapter. Plot the absorbances versus the content of aluminum, in μg/mL, for the *Standard solutions*, and draw a best-fit straight line through the points using a linear regression model. Calculate the amount of aluminum in Anthrax Vaccine Adsorbed, in mg/mL.

Acceptance criteria: The aluminum concentration is between 0.8 and 1.5 mg/mL.

- **FORMALDEHYDE**

[NOTE—Perform analysis on the final product.]

Potassium ferricyanide solution: Dissolve 2.5 g of potassium ferricyanide in about 100 mL of water, and mix.

Phenylhydrazine hydrochloride solution: Dissolve 4 g of phenylhydrazine hydrochloride in 100 mL of absolute alcohol, add 2 mL of water and mix.

Standard stock solution: Into a 100-mL volumetric flask containing 2.5 mL of water and 1 mL of sodium hydroxide TS 2, add 1.0 g of the formaldehyde solution to be examined, shake, and dilute with water to 100.0 mL. Determine the concentration of formaldehyde in percent (w/v) as follows. To 10.0 mL of the solution add 30.0 mL of 0.1 N iodine VS. Mix, and add 10 mL of sodium hydroxide TS 2. After 15 min, add 25 mL of diluted sulfuric acid and 4 mL of starch TS. Titrate with 0.1 N sodium thiosulphate VS. Each 1 mL of 0.05 M iodine is equivalent to 1.501 mg of formaldehyde (CH_2O).

Standard solutions: Dilute the *Standard stock solution* in water to obtain solutions having concentrations of 0.005%, 0.01%, and 0.02% (w/v).

Sample solution: Use Anthrax Vaccine Adsorbed, final product as is.

Analysis: To suitable glass centrifuge tubes transfer 1.0 mL each of water, the *Standard solutions*, and the *Sample solution*. To each tube, add 1.0 mL of *Potassium ferricyanide solution*, 4.0 mL of 18% (w/v) hydrochloric acid and 2.0 mL of *Phenylhydrazine hydrochloride solution*. Mix after each addition. Incubate for 50–60 min at room temperature. Centrifuge the solutions at 10,000 × *g* for at least 10 min, and measure absorbances of the supernatants at 540 nm using a suitable spectrophotometer (see *Ultraviolet-Visible Spectroscopy* ⟨857⟩). Plot the absorbances versus concentrations of formaldehyde, in mg/mL, in the *Standard solutions*, and draw the best-fit straight line through the points.

Calculate the percentage (w/v) of formaldehyde in the sample.

Acceptance criteria: The concentration of formaldehyde in Anthrax Vaccine Adsorbed is less than 0.02% (w/v).

- **BENZETHONIUM CHLORIDE**

[NOTE—Perform analysis on the final product.]

Citrate buffer: 25 g of citric acid monohydrate in about 60 mL of water, and adjust with a solution of sodium hydroxide to a pH of 4.5. Transfer the solution to a 100-mL volumetric flask. Dilute with water to volume and mix.

Dye solution: 50 mg of 2′,4′,5′,7′-tetrabromofluorescein in about 100 mL of water, and mix. Dilute 1 mL of this solution with water to 100 mL.

Docusate sodium solution: 50 μg/mL of docusate sodium

Standard solution A: 0.5 g of benzethonium chloride in a 100-mL volumetric flask, dissolve in 60 mL of water, dilute with water to volume, and mix.

Standard solutions B, C, D, and E: Dilute *Standard solution A* with water to obtain solutions having concentrations of 0.001%, 0.002%, 0.003%, and 0.004% (w/v), respectively.

Sample solution: Use Anthrax Vaccine Adsorbed, final product as is.

Titrimetric system

(See *Titrimetry* ⟨541⟩.)

Mode: Direct titration

Titrant: *Docusate sodium solution*

Endpoint detection: Visual

Analysis: Transfer 4.0 mL each of *Standard solutions B, C, D,* and *E* and the *Sample solution* to suitable glass centrifuge tubes. Add 1.0 mL of *Citrate buffer* and 0.4 mL of the *Dye solution* to each tube. Add 4.0 mL of 1,1,2,2-tetrachloroethane to each tube, and vigorously mix on a vortex mixer for 1 min. Centrifuge at about 1000 × *g* for at least 15 min to separate the organic layer from the aqueous layer. Transfer 2.0 mL of the organic layer from the tubes to another set of glass tubes. Add 4.0 mL of water and 0.5 mL of *Citrate buffer* to each tube, and mix on a vortex mixer for about 1 min. Titrate the benzethonium chloride-dye complex in each tube with the *Titrant* to the colorimetric endpoint indicated by the disappearance of the pink color of the organic layer. [NOTE—Vigorously mix the solution on a vortex mixer after each addition of the *Docusate sodium solution*.] Plot the volumes of *Docusate sodium solution* required versus the concentrations of benzethonium chloride in *Standard solutions B, C, D,* and *E*, and draw a best-fit straight line through the points. Determine the concentration of benzethonium chloride in the *Sample solution* from the volume of *Titrant* required to titrate the *Sample solution*.

Acceptance criteria: The concentration of benzethonium chloride in Anthrax Vaccine Adsorbed is between 0.0015% and 0.0030% (w/v).

SPECIFIC TESTS

• **83 KDA PROTEIN**

[NOTE—Perform tests on the filtrate.]

Trichloroacetic acid solution, Sample buffer, Running buffer, and **Sample solution:** Prepare as directed in *Identification* test *A.*

Staining solution: Prepare a solution of Coomassie blue G-250 having a concentration of 1.25 g/L in a mixture of methanol, acetic acid, and water (4:1:5, v/v).

Protein molecular weight standard solution: Reconstitute a vial of protein molecular weight standard mixture containing proteins of molecular weights at least in the range of 14–200 kDa, according to manufacturer's instruction. Dilute the solution with *Sample buffer* such that the concentration of each protein in the solution is about 0.5 µg/µL.

Analysis: In a suitable centrifuge tube transfer (10/*c*) mL of the *Sample solution*, where *c* is the total protein concentration, in µg/mL, of the solution as determined by the test for *Total Protein.* Add 5.5/*c* mL of *Trichloroacetic acid solution,* and incubate for at least 10 min. Centrifuge at 9000 × *g* for about 10 min, decant off the supernatant, and hold the tube inverted to drain on a filter paper. Dissolve the pellet in 20 µL of *Sample buffer,* and transfer the solution to a polypropylene microfuge tube with a lid. Transfer 20 µL of *Protein molecular weight standard solution* to another polypropylene microfuge tube with a lid. Close the lids tightly, secure with lid-locks, and heat both solutions at 100° for 5 min. Allow the solutions to cool to room temperature, and centrifuge at 10,000 × *g* for 15 s to collect the liquids. Apply the solutions to two consecutive lanes of a 4%–20% gradient tris-glycine polyacrylamide slab gel [NOTE—Do not apply any solution in the outside lanes.], and electrophorese as directed in *Identification* (see *Biotechnology-Derived Articles—Polyacrylamide Gel Electrophoresis* ⟨1056⟩). When the dye-front is about 1 cm from the bottom of the gel (about 40 min), stop the current, and remove the gel from the gel assembly. Soak the gel in a suitable volume of the *Staining solution* for at least 1 h, such that the gel is completely immersed in the *Staining solution* during staining. [NOTE—Do not touch the gel with bare hands. Use disposable gloves.] Destain the gel with a large volume of water under constant agitation with repeated changes of water until the background of the gel is completely color free. Using the molecular weights of the proteins in *Protein molecular weight standard solution,* identify the band corresponding to the PA (MW about 83 kDa) in the *Sample solution* lane. [NOTE—This band is also the predominant band in the lane of the *Sample solution.*] Scan the gel, and determine the relative amount (by peak area) of the 83 kDa band by densitometry in the lane of the *Sample solution.*

Acceptance criteria The content of 83 kDa band is NLT 35% of the total peak area.

• **TOTAL PROTEIN**

[NOTE—Perform tests on the filtrate.]

Standard solution A: Prepare a solution of albumin bovine serum (see *Reagents, Indicators, and Solutions—Reagent Specifications*) in water to obtain a known concentration of 2.0 mg/mL.

Standard solutions B, C, D, and **E:** Dilute *Standard solution A* with water to obtain solutions having protein concentrations of 4, 8, 16, and 24 µg/mL, respectively.

Sample solution: Use anthrax vaccine filtrate as is.

Analysis

(See *Biotechnology-Derived Articles—Total Protein Assay* ⟨1057⟩, *Method 3.*)

To a series of test tubes transfer 800 µL each of *Standard solutions B, C, D,* and *E* and the *Sample solution.* Also transfer 800 µL of water to be used as the blank. Add 200 µL of Coomassie blue G-250 dye solution (see *Reagents, Indicators, and Solutions—Reagent Specifications*) to each tube, and mix without foaming. Determine absorbances of the solutions at 595 nm using a suitable spectrophotometer (see *Ultraviolet-Visible Spectroscopy* ⟨857⟩), using the blank to set the instrument to zero.

[NOTE—Do not use quartz (silica) spectrophotometer cells; the dye binds to silica.]

Construct a standard curve by plotting the absorbances versus protein concentrations, in µg/mL, of *Standard solutions B, C, D,* and *E* and by drawing a best-fit straight line using the linear regression method. From the standard curve, determine the total protein concentration of the *Sample solution* using the absorbance value.

Acceptance criteria: The protein concentration is between 5 and 20 µg/mL.

• **SAFETY:** It meets the requirements when tested as directed in *Biological Reactivity Tests, In Vivo* ⟨88⟩, *Safety Tests—Biologicals.*

[NOTE—Perform tests on final product.]

• **STERILITY TESTS** ⟨71⟩: It meets the requirements when tested as directed for *Test for Sterility of the Product to Be Examined, Direct Inoculation of the Culture Medium.*

[NOTE—Perform tests on final product.]

• **PH** ⟨791⟩: 7.5–8.5

• **SODIUM CHLORIDE**

[NOTE—Perform tests on the final product.]

Standard solutions A and B: Prepare two solutions of sodium chloride in water having concentrations of 0.2 mM and 2.0 mM, respectively.

Sample solution: Transfer 0.5 mL of Anthrax Vaccine Adsorbed, final product to a 50-mL volumetric flask. Dilute with water to volume.

Analysis: Determine the voltage readings of *Standard solutions A* and *B* and the *Sample solution* using an ion-specific electrode specific for the chloride ion electrically coupled with a standard silver–silver chloride reference electrode. Plot the voltage readings versus concentration of chloride, in mg/mL, for *Standard solutions A* and *B,* and draw a straight line joining the points. Calculate the concentration of chloride ion in the *Sample solution* from the voltage reading. Assuming that the chloride ion comes entirely from sodium chloride, calculate the concentrations of sodium chloride in the *Sample solution.*

Acceptance criteria: The concentration of sodium chloride in Anthrax Vaccine Adsorbed is between 0.75% and 0.95% (w/v).

ADDITIONAL REQUIREMENTS

• **PACKAGING AND STORAGE:** Preserve in multiple-dose tight Type I glass containers. Store at a temperature between 2° and 8°. Do not freeze.

• **LABELING:** Label it to state that it is to be well shaken before use and that it is not to be frozen.

• **EXPIRATION DATE:** The expiration date is 18 months from the date of manufacture.■1S (USP41)

Aripiprazole Tablets

DEFINITION

Aripiprazole Tablets contain NLT 95.0% and NMT 105.0% of the labeled amount of aripiprazole ($C_{23}H_{27}Cl_2N_3O_2$).

IDENTIFICATION

• **A. INFRARED ABSORPTION** ⟨197K⟩

Standard: Add 30 mL of ethyl acetate to 30 mg of USP Aripiprazole RS. Shake for 10 min, centrifuge for NLT 5 min, and pass the supernatant through a suitable membrane filter. To the filtrate add 15 mL of water, shake for 5 min, and centrifuge for NLT 10 min. Transfer 20 mL of the upper layer to a container and add anhydrous magnesium sulfate, as needed. Shake well, pass through a suitable membrane filter, and evaporate the ethyl acetate on a water bath under reduced pressure. Use the residue. [NOTE—A centrifuge speed of 2000 rpm may be suitable.]

Sample: Grind a suitable number of Tablets and transfer a suitable portion of the ground Tablets, equivalent to 30 mg of aripiprazole, to an appropriate container. Add 30 mL of ethyl acetate, shake for 10 min, centrifuge for NLT 5 min, and pass the supernatant through a suitable membrane filter. To the filtrate add 15 mL of water, shake for 5 min, and centrifuge for NLT 10 min. Transfer 20 mL of the upper layer to a container and add a suitable amount of anhydrous magnesium sulfate. Shake well, pass through a suitable membrane filter, and evaporate the ethyl acetate on a water bath under reduced pressure. Use the residue. [NOTE—A centrifuge speed of 2000 rpm may be suitable.]

Analysis
Samples: *Standard* and *Sample*
Acceptance criteria: Meet the requirements
- **B.** The retention time of the aripiprazole peak of the *Sample solution* corresponds to that of the *Standard solution*, as obtained in the *Assay*.

ASSAY
- **PROCEDURE**
  Solution A: 2.8 g/L of anhydrous sodium sulfate in water
  Mobile phase: Acetonitrile, methanol, *Solution A*, and glacial acetic acid (33:11:56:1)
  Internal standard solution: 0.33 mg/mL of USP Propylparaben RS in *Mobile phase*
  Standard stock solution: 1 mg/mL of USP Aripiprazole RS in *Mobile phase*
  Standard solution: 0.2 mg/mL of USP Aripiprazole RS prepared as follows. Transfer 10.0 mL of *Standard stock solution* and 10.0 mL of *Internal standard solution* to a 50-mL volumetric flask, and dilute with *Mobile phase* to volume.
  Sample solution: Nominally 0.2 mg/mL of aripiprazole from Tablets prepared as follows. Powder NLT 20 Tablets and transfer a suitable portion of the powder to an appropriate volumetric flask. Add 40% of the final flask volume of *Mobile phase* and 20% of the final flask volume of *Internal standard solution*. Shake for 10 min, and dilute with *Mobile phase* to volume. Centrifuge, if necessary, and pass the supernatant through a suitable filter of NMT 0.5-μm pore size, discard the first 1 mL of filtrate, and use the subsequent filtrate.
  Chromatographic system
  (See *Chromatography* ⟨621⟩, *System Suitability*.)
  Mode: LC
  Detector: UV 254 nm
  Column: 4.6-mm × 25-cm; 5-μm packing L1
  Flow rate: 1 mL/min
  Injection volume: 10 μL
  Run time: NLT 2 times the retention time of aripiprazole
  System suitability
  Sample: *Standard solution*
  [NOTE—The relative retention times for aripiprazole and propylparaben are about 1.0 and 1.5, respectively.]
  Suitability requirements
  Resolution: NLT 8 between aripiprazole and propylparaben
  Tailing factor: NMT 1.7 for aripiprazole and for propylparaben
  Relative standard deviation: NMT 2.0% for the peak response ratio of aripiprazole to propylparaben

Analysis
Samples: *Standard solution* and *Sample solution*
Calculate the percentage of the labeled amount of aripiprazole ($C_{23}H_{27}Cl_2N_3O_2$) in the portion of Tablets taken:

$$Result = (R_U/R_S) \times (C_S/C_U) \times 100$$

R_U = peak response ratio of aripiprazole to propylparaben from the *Sample solution*
R_S = peak response ratio of aripiprazole to propylparaben from the *Standard solution*
C_S = concentration of USP Aripiprazole RS in the *Standard solution* (mg/mL)
C_U = nominal concentration of aripiprazole in the *Sample solution* (mg/mL)
Acceptance criteria: 95.0%–105.0%

PERFORMANCE TESTS

Change to read:

- **DISSOLUTION** ⟨711⟩
  •Test 1• (RB 1-Oct-2017)
  Medium: pH 1.2 hydrochloric acid buffer (Transfer 250 mL of 14.9 g/L of potassium chloride in water to a 1-L volumetric flask, add 425 mL of 0.2 N hydrochloric acid, and dilute with water to volume. Degas the resulting solution or pass the resulting solution through a filter under vacuum.), degassed; 900 mL
  Apparatus 2: 60 rpm
  Time: 30 min
  Procedure: Determine the percentage of the labeled amount of aripiprazole ($C_{23}H_{27}Cl_2N_3O_2$) dissolved by using either the *Spectrometric procedure* or the *Chromatographic procedure* described below.
  Spectrometric procedure
  Standard stock solution: 1 mg/mL of USP Aripiprazole RS in alcohol
  Standard solution: (L/900) mg/mL of USP Aripiprazole RS from *Standard stock solution* in *Medium*, where *L* is the label claim, in mg/Tablet
  Sample solution: Pass a portion of the solution under test through a suitable filter, discarding the first 5 mL of filtrate.
  Instrumental conditions
  Mode: UV
  Analytical wavelengths: 249 and 325 nm
  Cell length: 1 cm
  Blank: *Medium*
  Analysis
  Samples: *Standard solution* and *Sample solution*
  Calculate the percentage of the labeled amount of aripiprazole ($C_{23}H_{27}Cl_2N_3O_2$) dissolved:

  $$Result = (A_U/A_S) \times C_S \times V \times (1/L) \times 100$$

  A_U = absorbance at 249 nm minus the absorbance at 325 nm of the *Sample solution*
  A_S = absorbance at 249 nm minus the absorbance at 325 nm of the *Standard solution*
  C_S = concentration of USP Aripiprazole RS in the *Standard solution* (mg/mL)
  V = volume of *Medium*, 900 mL
  L = label claim (mg/Tablet)
  Chromatographic procedure
  Solution A: 2.8 g/L of anhydrous sodium sulfate
  Solution B: 13.9 g/L of glacial acetic acid and 23.9 g/L of sodium acetate in water
  Mobile phase: Acetonitrile, methanol, *Solution A*, and glacial acetic acid (40:10:50:1)
  Diluent: *Solution B* and methanol (50:50)
  Internal standard solution: 0.67 μg/mL of USP Propylparaben RS in *Diluent*

Standard stock solution A: 1 mg/mL of USP Aripiprazole RS in *Mobile phase*
Standard stock solution B: 0.002 mg/mL of USP Aripiprazole RS from *Standard stock solution A* in *Medium* passed through a suitable filter of NMT 0.5-μm pore size, discarding the first 6 mL of filtrate
Standard solution: 0.001 mg/mL of USP Aripiprazole RS from *Standard stock solution B* prepared by combining 5 mL of *Standard stock solution B* and 5 mL of *Internal standard solution*
Sample stock solution: Pass a portion of the solution under test through a suitable filter of NMT 0.5-μm pore size, discarding NLT the first 6 mL of filtrate.
Sample solution: Combine 2 mL of *Sample stock solution* with 2 mL of *Internal standard solution*.
Chromatographic system: Proceed as directed in the *Assay* except as follows.
Injection volume: 100 μL
● ● (RB 1-Oct-2017)
System suitability
Sample: *Standard solution*
[NOTE—The relative retention times for aripiprazole and propylparaben are about 1.0 and 1.8, respectively.]
Suitability requirements
Resolution: NLT 10 between aripiprazole and propylparaben
Relative standard deviation: NMT 1.5% for the peak response ratio of aripiprazole to propylparaben
Analysis
Samples: *Standard solution* and *Sample solution*
Calculate the percentage of the labeled amount of aripiprazole ($C_{23}H_{27}Cl_2N_3O_2$) dissolved:

$$Result = (R_U/R_S) \times C_S \times V \times (1/L) \times 100$$

R_U = peak response ratio of aripiprazole to propylparaben from the *Sample solution*
R_S = peak response ratio of aripiprazole to propylparaben from the *Standard solution*
C_S = concentration of USP Aripiprazole RS in the *Standard solution* (mg/mL)
V = volume of *Medium*, 900 mL
L = label claim (mg/Tablet)
Tolerances: NLT 75% (*Q*) of the labeled amount of aripiprazole ($C_{23}H_{27}Cl_2N_3O_2$) is dissolved.
● **Test 2:** If the product complies with this test, the labeling indicates that it meets USP *Dissolution Test 2*.
Medium: 0.1 N hydrochloric acid VS; 900 mL
Apparatus 2: 60 rpm
Time: 15 min
Buffer: 6.8 g/L of monobasic potassium phosphate in water. Adjust with 1 N phosphoric acid TS to a pH of 3.0.
Mobile phase: Acetonitrile and *Buffer* (40:60)
Standard stock solution: 0.11 mg/mL of USP Aripiprazole RS in solution prepared as follows. Transfer a suitable amount of USP Aripiprazole RS to an appropriate volumetric flask. Add 2% of the flask volume of acetonitrile and 70% of the flask volume of *Medium*. Sonication may be used to promote dissolution. Dilute with *Medium* to volume.
Standard solution: (*L*/900) mg/mL of USP Aripiprazole RS from *Standard stock solution* in *Medium*, where *L* is the label claim, in mg/Tablet
Sample solution: Pass a portion of the solution under test through a suitable filter, discarding NLT the first 5 mL of filtrate.
Chromatographic system
(See *Chromatography* ⟨621⟩, *System Suitability*.)

Mode: LC
Detector: UV 215 nm
Column: 4.6-mm × 15-cm; 5-μm packing L7
Column temperature: 40°
Flow rate: 1 mL/min
Injection volume: 5 μL
Run time: NLT 1.6 times the retention time of aripiprazole
System suitability
Sample: *Standard solution*
Suitability requirements
Tailing factor: NMT 1.5
Relative standard deviation: NMT 1.0%
Analysis
Samples: *Standard solution* and *Sample solution*
Calculate the percentage of the labeled amount of aripiprazole ($C_{23}H_{27}Cl_2N_3O_2$) dissolved:

$$Result = (r_U/r_S) \times C_S \times V \times (1/L) \times 100$$

r_U = peak response of aripiprazole from the *Sample solution*
r_S = peak response of aripiprazole from the *Standard solution*
C_S = concentration of USP Aripiprazole RS in the *Standard solution* (mg/mL)
V = volume of *Medium*, 900 mL
L = label claim (mg/Tablet)
Tolerances: NLT 80% (*Q*) of the labeled amount of aripiprazole ($C_{23}H_{27}Cl_2N_3O_2$) is dissolved.● (RB 1-Oct-2017)
● **UNIFORMITY OF DOSAGE UNITS ⟨905⟩:** Meet the requirements

IMPURITIES
● **ORGANIC IMPURITIES**
Protect solutions from light.
Buffer: 9.6 g/L of dibasic ammonium citrate, 1.6 g/L of citric acid, and 2.9 g/L of sodium dodecyl sulfate in water. Adjust with 11 g/L of dibasic ammonium citrate in water or 9.6 g/L of anhydrous citric acid in water to a pH of 4.7, if needed.
Mobile phase: Acetonitrile and *Buffer* (45:55)
Diluent: Acetonitrile, water, and glacial acetic acid (40:60:1)
System suitability solution: 0.5 mg/mL of USP Aripiprazole RS, and 0.0005 mg/mL each of USP Aripiprazole Related Compound F RS and USP Aripiprazole Related Compound G RS in *Diluent*
Sample solution: Nominally 0.5 mg/mL of aripiprazole from Tablets prepared as follows. Powder NLT 20 Tablets, transfer a suitable portion of the powder equivalent to NLT 4 mg of aripiprazole to an appropriate container, and add a suitable volume of *Diluent*. Shake for 10 min and centrifuge, if necessary. Pass the supernatant through a suitable filter of NMT 0.5-μm pore size, discard the first 1 mL of filtrate, and use the subsequent filtrate.
Chromatographic system
(See *Chromatography* ⟨621⟩, *System Suitability*.)
Mode: LC
Detector: UV 254 nm
Column: 4.6-mm × 15-cm; 5-μm packing L1
Flow rate: 1 mL/min
Injection volume: 20 μL
Run time: NLT 2 times the retention time of aripiprazole
System suitability
Sample: *System suitability solution*
[NOTE—See *Table 1* for the relative retention times.]
Suitability requirements
Resolution: NLT 3 between aripiprazole related compound G and aripiprazole
Signal-to-noise ratio: NLT 10 for aripiprazole related compound F and aripiprazole related compound G

Analysis
Sample: *Sample solution*
Calculate the percentage of each degradation product in the portion of Tablets taken:

$$Result = (r_U/r_T) \times 100$$

r_U = peak response of each degradation product from the *Sample solution*
r_T = sum of all the peak responses from the *Sample solution*

Acceptance criteria: See *Table 1.* Disregard peaks that are less than 0.1% of the aripiprazole peak.

Table 1

Name	Relative Retention Time	Acceptance Criteria, NMT (%)
Aripiprazole related compound F	0.54	0.3
Aripiprazole related compound G	0.81	0.3
Aripiprazole	1.0	—
Any individual unspecified degradation product	—	0.2
Total degradation products	—	1.0

ADDITIONAL REQUIREMENTS
- **PACKAGING AND STORAGE:** Preserve in tight containers. Store at controlled room temperature.

Add the following:

- **LABELING:** The labeling states the *Dissolution* test used only if *Test 1* is not used.● (RB 1-Oct-2017)
- **USP REFERENCE STANDARDS ⟨11⟩**
  USP Aripiprazole RS
  USP Aripiprazole Related Compound F RS
  4-(2,3-Dichlorophenyl)-1-[4-(2-oxo-1,2,3,4-tetrahydro-quinolin-7-yloxy)butyl]piperazine 1-oxide.
  $C_{23}H_{27}Cl_2N_3O_3$　　464.38
  USP Aripiprazole Related Compound G RS
  7-{4-[4-(2,3-Dichlorophenyl)piperazin-1-yl]butoxy}qui-nolin-2(1*H*)-one.
  $C_{23}H_{25}Cl_2N_3O_2$　　446.37
  USP Propylparaben RS

Azithromycin Tablets

DEFINITION
Azithromycin Tablets contain NLT 90.0% and NMT 110.0% of the labeled amount of azithromycin ($C_{38}H_{72}N_2O_{12}$).

IDENTIFICATION
- **A.** The retention time of the major peak of the *Sample solution* corresponds to that of the *Standard solution*, as obtained in the *Assay.*

ASSAY
- **PROCEDURE**
  Buffer: Dissolve 4.6 g of monobasic potassium phosphate anhydrous in 900 mL of water. Adjust with 1 N sodium hydroxide to a pH of 7.5, and dilute with water to 1 L.
  Mobile phase: Acetonitrile and *Buffer* (65:35)
  Standard solution: 1 mg/mL of USP Azithromycin RS in *Mobile phase.* Sonicate and shake as needed to dissolve.

Sample solution: Nominally 1 mg/mL of azithromycin in *Mobile phase* from NLT 20 Tablets, finely powdered. Sonicate and shake as needed to dissolve.
Chromatographic system
(See *Chromatography* ⟨621⟩, *System Suitability.*)
　Mode: LC
　Detector: UV 210 nm
　Column: 4.6-mm × 25-cm; 5-μm packing L1
　Column temperature: 50°
　Flow rate: 2 mL/min
　Injection volume: 100 μL
System suitability
　Sample: *Standard solution*
　Suitability requirements
　　Tailing factor: NMT 2.0
　　Relative standard deviation: NMT 2.0%
Analysis
　Samples: *Standard solution* and *Sample solution*
　Calculate the percentage of the labeled amount of azithromycin ($C_{38}H_{72}N_2O_{12}$) in the portion of Tablets taken:

$$Result = (r_U/r_S) \times (C_S/C_U) \times P \times F \times 100$$

r_U = peak response of azithromycin from the *Sample solution*
r_S = peak response of azithromycin from the *Standard solution*
C_S = concentration of USP Azithromycin RS in the *Standard solution* (mg/mL)
C_U = nominal concentration of azithromycin in the *Sample solution* (mg/mL)
P = potency of USP Azithromycin RS (μg/mg)
F = conversion factor, 0.001 mg/μg

Acceptance criteria: 90.0%–110.0%

PERFORMANCE TESTS
- **DISSOLUTION ⟨711⟩**
  Medium: pH 6.0 phosphate buffer; 900 mL
  Apparatus 2: 75 rpm
  Time: 30 min
  Solution A: 4.4 mg/mL of dibasic potassium phosphate and 0.5 mg/mL of sodium 1-octanesulfonate, adjusted with phosphoric acid to a pH of 8.20 ± 0.05
  Mobile phase: Acetonitrile, methanol, and *Solution A* (9:3:8)
  Diluent: 17.5 mg/mL of dibasic potassium phosphate. Adjust with phosphoric acid to a pH of 8.00 ± 0.05. Prepare a mixture of this solution and acetonitrile (80:20).
  Standard stock solution: Dissolve USP Azithromycin RS in *Medium* to obtain a solution having a known concentration of about (L/1000) mg/mL, where L is the label claim in mg/Tablet.
  Standard solution: Dilute the *Standard stock solution* with *Diluent* to obtain a solution having a known concentration of about (L/2000) mg/mL, where L is the label claim in mg/Tablet.
  Sample solution: Pass a portion of the solution under test through a suitable filter of 0.45-μm pore size. Dilute a portion of the filtrate with *Diluent* to obtain a solution having a theoretical concentration of about (L/2000) mg/mL, where L is the label claim in mg/Tablet, assuming complete dissolution.
  Chromatographic system
  (See *Chromatography* ⟨621⟩, *System Suitability.*)

Mode: LC
Detector: UV 210 nm
Column: 4.6-mm × 15-cm; 5-μm packing L1
Column temperature: 50°
Flow rate: 1.5 mL/min
Injection volume: 50 μL
System suitability
Sample: *Standard solution*
Suitability requirements
Tailing factor: NMT 2.0
Relative standard deviation: NMT 2.0%
Analysis
Samples: *Standard solution* and *Sample solution*
Calculate the percentage of the labeled amount of azithromycin ($C_{38}H_{72}N_2O_{12}$) dissolved:

$$Result = (r_U/r_S) \times (C_S/L) \times V \times 100$$

r_U = peak response of azithromycin from the *Sample solution*
r_S = peak response of azithromycin from the *Standard solution*
C_S = concentration of USP Azithromycin RS in the *Standard solution* (mg/mL)
L = label claim (mg/Tablet)
V = volume of *Medium*, 900 mL
Tolerances: NLT 80% (Q) of the labeled amount of azithromycin ($C_{38}H_{72}N_2O_{12}$) is dissolved.
- **UNIFORMITY OF DOSAGE UNITS ⟨905⟩:** Meet the requirements

IMPURITIES

Change to read:

- **ORGANIC IMPURITIES**
Protect all solutions containing azithromycin from light. Refrigerate the *Standard solution* and the *Sample solution* after preparation and during analysis, using a refrigerated autosampler set at 4°. The solutions must be analyzed within 24 h of preparation.
Solution A: Water and ammonium hydroxide (2000: 1.2). The pH of this solution is about 10.5.
Solution B: Acetonitrile, methanol, and ammonium hydroxide (1800: 200: 1.2)
Mobile phase: See *Table 1*.

Table 1

Time (min)	Solution A (%)	Solution B (%)
0	54	46
20	54	46
35	10	90
35.1	54	46
■50.1■1S (USP41)	54	46

Buffer: 1.7 g/L of monobasic ammonium phosphate in water. Adjust with ammonium hydroxide to a pH of 10.
Diluent A: Methanol, acetonitrile, and *Buffer* (350:300:350)
Diluent B: Methanol and *Buffer* (1:1)
System suitability stock solution: 0.1 mg/mL each of USP Desosaminylazithromycin RS and USP Azithromycin Related Compound F RS in acetonitrile
System suitability solution: 0.028 mg/mL each of USP Desosaminylazithromycin RS and USP Azithromycin Re-

lated Compound F RS from *System suitability stock solution* in *Diluent A*
Standard stock solution: 0.4 mg/mL of USP Azithromycin RS in acetonitrile. Sonicate and shake as needed to dissolve.
Standard solution: 0.02 mg/mL of azithromycin from the *Standard stock solution* in *Diluent A*
Sensitivity solution: 0.004 mg/mL of azithromycin from the *Standard solution* in *Diluent A*
Sample stock solution: Nominally 14.3 mg/mL of azithromycin prepared as follows. Weigh and finely powder NLT 20 Tablets. Transfer nominally 1430 mg of azithromycin to a 100-mL volumetric flask. Add 75 mL of acetonitrile, and sonicate for NLT 15 min. Shake by mechanical means for NLT 15 min. Allow the solution to equilibrate to room temperature, dilute with acetonitrile to volume, and mix.
Sample solution: Nominally 4 mg/mL of azithromycin prepared as follows. Centrifuge an aliquot of the *Sample stock solution* for NLT 15 min. Transfer 7.0 mL of the supernatant to a 25-mL volumetric flask, and dilute with *Diluent B* to volume.
Blank: *Diluent A*
Chromatographic system
(See *Chromatography* ⟨621⟩, *System Suitability*.)
Mode: LC
Detector: UV 210 nm
Column: 4.6-mm × 15-cm; 3.5-μm packing L1
Temperatures
Autosampler: 4°
Column: 50°
Flow rate: 1.2 mL/min
Injection volume: 100 μL
System suitability
Samples: *System suitability solution*, *Standard solution*, and *Sensitivity solution*
Suitability requirements
Resolution: NLT 1.0 between desosaminylazithromycin and azithromycin related compound F, *System suitability solution*
Relative standard deviation: NMT 2.0%, *Standard solution*
Signal-to-noise ratio: NLT 10, *Sensitivity solution*
Analysis
Samples: ■*Standard solution*,■1S (USP41) *Sample solution*, and *Blank*
Calculate the percentage of each impurity in the portion of Tablets taken:

$$Result = (r_U/r_S) \times (C_S/C_U) \times P \times F_1 \times (1/F_2) \times 100$$

r_U = peak response of each impurity from the *Sample solution*
r_S = peak response of azithromycin from the *Standard solution*
C_S = concentration of USP Azithromycin RS in the *Standard solution* (mg/mL)
C_U = nominal concentration of azithromycin in the *Sample solution* (mg/mL)
P = potency of USP Azithromycin RS (μg/mg)
F_1 = conversion factor, 0.001 mg/μg
F_2 = relative response factor (see *Table 2*)
Acceptance criteria: See *Table 2*. The reporting level for impurities is 0.1%. Disregard any peaks in the *Sample solution* that correspond to peaks in the *Blank*.

Table 2

Name	Relative Retention Time	Relative Response Factor	Acceptance Criteria, NMT (%)
Azithromycin N-oxide[a]	0.20	0.42	1.0
3'-(N,N-Didemethyl)-3'-N-formylazithromycin[b],■c (USP41)	0.29		
	0.30	1.7	1.0
3'-(N,N-Didemethyl)azithromycin (aminoazithromycin)[d]	0.34	0.49	0.5
Azithromycin related compound F[c],■1S (USP41)[e]	■0.40		
	0.46	5.5■1S (USP41)	1.0
Desosaminylazithromycin[f]	■0.47■1S (USP41)	1.1	0.5
N-Demethylazithromycin[g]	0.50	■0.47■1S (USP41)	0.7
3'-De(dimethylamino)-3'-oxoazithromycin[h]	0.87	■1.7■1S (USP41)	1.0
Azaerythromycin A[i,j]	0.94	—	—
Azithromycin	1.0	—	—
2-Desethyl-2-propylazithromycin[i,k]	1.10	—	—
3'-N-Demethyl-3'-N-[(4-methylphenyl)sulfonyl]azithromycin[i,l]	1.11	—	—
3-Deoxyazithromycin (azithromycin B)[i,m]	1.14	—	—

[a] (2R,3S,4R,5R,8R,10R,11R,12S,13S,14R)-13-[(2,6-Dideoxy-3-C-methyl-3-O-methyl-α-L-ribo-hexopyranosyl)oxy]-2-ethyl-3,4,10-trihydroxy-3,5,6,8,10,12,14-heptamethyl-11-[[3,4,6-trideoxy-3-(dimethylazinoyl)-β-D-xylo-hexopyranosyl]oxy]-1-oxa-6-azacyclopentadecan-15-one.

[b] (2R,3S,4R,5R,8R,10R,11R,12S,13S,14R)-13-[(2,6-Dideoxy-3-C-methyl-3-O-methyl-α-L-ribo-hexopyranosyl)oxy]-2-ethyl-3,4,10-trihydroxy-3,5,6,8,10,12,14-heptamethyl-11-[[3-formamido-3,4,6-trideoxy-β-D-xylo-hexopyranosyl]oxy]-1-oxa-6-azacyclopentadecan-15-one.

■c The system may resolve two rotamers. The limit is for the sum of the two rotamers.■1S (USP41)

[d] (2R,3S,4R,5R,8R,10R,11R,12S,13S,14R)-13-[(2,6-Dideoxy-3-C-methyl-3-O-methyl-α-L-ribo-hexopyranosyl)oxy]-2-ethyl-3,4,10-trihydroxy-3,5,6,8,10,12,14-heptamethyl-11-[[3-amino-3,4,6-trideoxy-β-D-xylo-hexopyranosyl]oxy]-1-oxa-6-azacyclopentadecan-15-one.

[e] 3'-(N-Demethyl)-3'-N-formylazithromycin; (2R,3S,4R,5R,8R,10R,11R,12S,13S,14R)-13-[(2,6-Dideoxy-3-C-methyl-3-O-methyl-α-L-ribo-hexopyranosyl)oxy]-2-ethyl-3,4,10-trihydroxy-3,5,6,8,10,12,14-heptamethyl-11-[[3-(N-methyl)formamido-3,4,6-trideoxy-β-D-xylo-hexopyranosyl]oxy]-1-oxa-6-azacyclopentadecan-15-one.

[f] (2R,3S,4R,5R,8R,10R,11R,12S,13S,14R)-2-Ethyl-3,4,10,13-tetrahydroxy-3,5,6,8,10,12,14-heptamethyl-11-[[3,4,6-trideoxy-3-dimethylamino-β-D-xylo-hexopyranosyl]oxy]-1-oxa-6-azacyclopentadecan-15-one.

[g] (2R,3S,4R,5R,8R,10R,11R,12S,13S,14R)-13-[(2,6-Dideoxy-3-C-methyl-3-O-methyl-α-L-ribo-hexopyranosyl)oxy]-2-ethyl-3,4,10-trihydroxy-3,5,6,8,10,12,14-heptamethyl-11-[[3,4,6-trideoxy-3-methylamino-β-D-xylo-hexopyranosyl]oxy]-1-oxa-6-azacyclopentadecan-15-one.

[h] (2R,3S,4R,5R,8R,10R,11R,12S,13S,14R)-13-[(2,6-Dideoxy-3,3-dimethyl-α-L-ribo-hexopyranosyl)oxy]-2-ethyl-3,4,10-trihydroxy-3,5,6,8,10,12,14-heptamethyl-11-[[3,4,6-trideoxy-3-oxo-β-D-xylo-hexopyranosyl]oxy]-1-oxa-6-azacyclopentadecan-15-one.

[i] Process impurities that are controlled in the drug substance are not to be reported. They are listed here for information only. The unspecified impurities and total impurities limits do not include these impurities.

[j] 9-Deoxo-9a-aza-9a-homoerythromycin A.

[k] (2R,3S,4R,5R,8R,10R,11R,12S,13S,14R)-13-[(2,6-Dideoxy-3-C-methyl-3-O-methyl-α-L-ribo-hexopyranosyl)oxy]-2-propyl-3,4,10-trihydroxy-3,5,6,8,10,12,14-heptamethyl-11-[[3,4,6-trideoxy-3-(dimethylamino)-β-D-xylo-hexopyranosyl]oxy]-1-oxa-6-azacyclopentadecan-15-one dihydrate.

[l] (2R,3S,4R,5R,8R,10R,11R,12S,13S,14R)-13-[(2,6-Dideoxy-3-C-methyl-3-O-methyl-α-L-ribo-hexopyranosyl)oxy]-2-ethyl-3,4,10-trihydroxy-3,5,6,8,10,12,14-heptamethyl-11-[[3-[N-(4-methylphenylsulfonyl)-N-methylamino]-3,4,6-trideoxy-β-D-xylo-hexopyranosyl]oxy]-1-oxa-6-azacyclopentadecan-15-one.

[m] (2R,3R,4S,5R,8R,10R,11R,12S,13S,14R)-13-[(2,6-Dideoxy-3-C-methyl-3-O-methyl-α-L-ribo-hexopyranosyl)oxy]-2-ethyl-4,10-dihydroxy-3,5,6,8,10,12,14-heptamethyl-11-[[3,4,6-trideoxy-3-(dimethylamino)-β-D-xylo-hexopyranosyl]oxy]-1-oxa-6-azacyclopentadecan-15-one.

Table 2 (Continued)

Name	Relative Retention Time	Relative Response Factor	Acceptance Criteria, NMT (%)
Any individual unspecified impurity[i]	—	1.0	0.2
Total impurities[i]	—	—	5.0

[a] (2R,3S,4R,5R,8R,10R,11R,12S,13S,14R)-13-[(2,6-Dideoxy-3-C-methyl-3-O-methyl-α-L-ribo-hexopyranosyl)oxy]-2-ethyl-3,4,10-trihydroxy-3,5,6,8,10,12,14-heptamethyl-11-[[3,4,6-trideoxy-3-(dimethylazinoyl)-β-D-xylo-hexopyranosyl]oxy]-1-oxa-6-azacyclopentadecan-15-one.

[b] (2R,3S,4R,5R,8R,10R,11R,12S,13S,14R)-13-[(2,6-Dideoxy-3-C-methyl-3-O-methyl-α-L-ribo-hexopyranosyl)oxy]-2-ethyl-3,4,10-trihydroxy-3,5,6,8,10,12,14-heptamethyl-11-[[3-formamido-3,4,6-trideoxy-β-D-xylo-hexopyranosyl]oxy]-1-oxa-6-azacyclopentadecan-15-one.

■c The system may resolve two rotamers. The limit is for the sum of the two rotamers.■1S (USP41)

[d] (2R,3S,4R,5R,8R,10R,11R,12S,13S,14R)-13-[(2,6-Dideoxy-3-C-methyl-3-O-methyl-α-L-ribo-hexopyranosyl)oxy]-2-ethyl-3,4,10-trihydroxy-3,5,6,8,10,12,14-heptamethyl-11-[[3-amino-3,4,6-trideoxy-β-D-xylo-hexopyranosyl]oxy]-1-oxa-6-azacyclopentadecan-15-one.

[e] 3'-(N-Demethyl)-3'-N-formylazithromycin; (2R,3S,4R,5R,8R,10R,11R,12S,13S,14R)-13-[(2,6-Dideoxy-3-C-methyl-3-O-methyl-α-L-ribo-hexopyranosyl)oxy]-2-ethyl-3,4,10-trihydroxy-3,5,6,8,10,12,14-heptamethyl-11-[[3-(N-methyl)formamido-3,4,6-trideoxy-β-D-xylo-hexopyranosyl]oxy]-1-oxa-6-azacyclopentadecan-15-one.

[f] (2R,3S,4R,5R,8R,10R,11R,12S,13S,14R)-2-Ethyl-3,4,10,13-tetrahydroxy-3,5,6,8,10,12,14-heptamethyl-11-[[3,4,6-trideoxy-3-dimethylamino-β-D-xylo-hexopyranosyl]oxy]-1-oxa-6-azacyclopentadecan-15-one.

[g] (2R,3S,4R,5R,8R,10R,11R,12S,13S,14R)-13-[(2,6-Dideoxy-3-C-methyl-3-O-methyl-α-L-ribo-hexopyranosyl)oxy]-2-ethyl-3,4,10-trihydroxy-3,5,6,8,10,12,14-heptamethyl-11-[[3,4,6-trideoxy-3-methylamino-β-D-xylo-hexopyranosyl]oxy]-1-oxa-6-azacyclopentadecan-15-one.

[h] (2R,3S,4R,5R,8R,10R,11R,12S,13S,14R)-13-[(2,6-Dideoxy-3,3-dimethyl-α-L-ribo-hexopyranosyl)oxy]-2-ethyl-3,4,10-trihydroxy-3,5,6,8,10,12,14-heptamethyl-11-[[3,4,6-trideoxy-3-oxo-β-D-xylo-hexopyranosyl]oxy]-1-oxa-6-azacyclopentadecan-15-one.

[i] Process impurities that are controlled in the drug substance are not to be reported. They are listed here for information only. The unspecified impurities and total impurities limits do not include these impurities.

[j] 9-Deoxo-9a-aza-9a-homoerythromycin A.

[k] (2R,3S,4R,5R,8R,10R,11R,12S,13S,14R)-13-[(2,6-Dideoxy-3-C-methyl-3-O-methyl-α-L-ribo-hexopyranosyl)oxy]-2-propyl-3,4,10-trihydroxy-3,5,6,8,10,12,14-heptamethyl-11-[[3,4,6-trideoxy-3-(dimethylamino)-β-D-xylo-hexopyranosyl]oxy]-1-oxa-6-azacyclopentadecan-15-one dihydrate.

[l] (2R,3S,4R,5R,8R,10R,11R,12S,13S,14R)-13-[(2,6-Dideoxy-3-C-methyl-3-O-methyl-α-L-ribo-hexopyranosyl)oxy]-2-ethyl-3,4,10-trihydroxy-3,5,6,8,10,12,14-heptamethyl-11-[[3-[N-(4-methylphenylsulfonyl)-N-methylamino]-3,4,6-trideoxy-β-D-xylo-hexopyranosyl]oxy]-1-oxa-6-azacyclopentadecan-15-one.

[m] (2R,3R,4S,5R,8R,10R,11R,12S,13S,14R)-13-[(2,6-Dideoxy-3-C-methyl-3-O-methyl-α-L-ribo-hexopyranosyl)oxy]-2-ethyl-4,10-dihydroxy-3,5,6,8,10,12,14-heptamethyl-11-[[3,4,6-trideoxy-3-(dimethylamino)-β-D-xylo-hexopyranosyl]oxy]-1-oxa-6-azacyclopentadecan-15-one.

ADDITIONAL REQUIREMENTS
- **PACKAGING AND STORAGE:** Preserve in tight containers. Store at controlled room temperature.
- **USP REFERENCE STANDARDS ⟨11⟩**
  USP Azithromycin RS
  USP Azithromycin Related Compound F RS
  3'-(N-Demethyl)-3'-N-formylazithromycin;
  (2R,3S,4R,5R,8R,10R,11R,12S,13S,14R)-13-[(2,6-Dideoxy-3-C-methyl-3-O-methyl-α-L-ribo-hexopyranosyl)oxy]-2-ethyl-3,4,10-trihydroxy-3,5,6,8,10,12,14-heptamethyl-11-[[3-(N-methyl)formamido-3,4,6-trideoxy-β-D-xylo-hexopyranosyl]oxy]-1-oxa-6-azacyclopentadecan-15-one.
  $C_{38}H_{70}N_2O_{13}$ 762.97
  USP Desosaminylazithromycin RS
  (2R,3S,4R,5R,8R,10R,11R,12S,13S,14R)-2-Ethyl-3,4,10,13-tetrahydroxy-3,5,6,8,10,12,14-heptamethyl-11-[[3,4,6-trideoxy-3-dimethylamino-β-D-xylo-hexopyranosyl]oxy]-1-oxa-6-azacyclopentadecan-15-one.
  $C_{30}H_{58}N_2O_9$ 590.79

Aztreonam

C$_{13}$H$_{17}$N$_5$O$_8$S$_2$ 435.43
Propanoic acid, 2-[[[1-(2-amino-4-thiazolyl)-2-[(2-methyl-4-oxo-1-sulfo-3-azetidinyl)amino]-2-oxoethylidene]amino]oxy]-2-methyl-, [2S-[2α,3β(Z)]]-;
(Z)-2-({[(2-Amino-4-thiazolyl){[(2S,3S)-2-methyl-4-oxo-1-sulfo-3-azetidinyl]carbamoyl}methylene]amino}oxy)-2-methylpropionic acid [78110-38-0].

DEFINITION
Aztreonam, which may be anhydrous or hydrated, contains NLT 92.0% and NMT 105.0% of aztreonam (C$_{13}$H$_{17}$N$_5$O$_8$S$_2$), calculated on the anhydrous and solvent-free basis.

IDENTIFICATION
- **A. INFRARED ABSORPTION ⟨197K⟩:** If a difference appears in the IR spectra of the analyte and the standard, dissolve equal portions of the test specimen and the Reference Standard in equal volumes of methanol. [NOTE—To achieve a complete dissolution, it is suggested to use about 25 mL of methanol for each 50 mg of material, and stir the mixture for 40 min at room temperature.] Evaporate the solutions to dryness under vacuum, and dry at 40° for 4 h under vacuum. Perform the test on the residues.

Add the following:

- **▪• B.** The retention time of the major peak of the *Sample solution* corresponds to that of the *Standard solution*, as obtained in the *Assay*.▪1S (USP41)

ASSAY
- **PROCEDURE**
  [NOTE—Store the *System suitability solution*, *Standard solution*, and *Sample solution* at 5°, and protect from light to prevent isomerization of aztreonam Z-isomer to aztreonam E-isomer.]
  Buffer: 6.8 mg/mL of monobasic potassium phosphate in water. Adjust with 1 M phosphoric acid to a pH of 3.0.
  Mobile phase: Methanol and *Buffer* (1:4)
  System suitability solution: 1 mg/mL of USP Aztreonam RS and 1 mg/mL of USP Aztreonam E-Isomer RS in *Mobile phase*
  Standard solution: 1 mg/mL of USP Aztreonam RS in *Mobile phase*
  Sample solution: 1 mg/mL of Aztreonam in *Mobile phase*
  Chromatographic system
  (See *Chromatography ⟨621⟩, System Suitability.*)
  Mode: LC
  Detector: UV 254 nm
  Column: 3.9-mm × 30-cm; 10-µm packing L1
  Flow rate: 1.5 mL/min
  Injection volume: 10 µL
  System suitability
  Samples: *System suitability solution* and *Standard solution*

[NOTE—The relative retention times for aztreonam and aztreonam E-isomer are 1.0 and 1.8, respectively.]
  Suitability requirements
  Resolution: NLT 2.0 between aztreonam and aztreonam E-isomer, *System suitability solution*
  Tailing factor: NMT 2 for aztreonam, *System suitability solution*
  Relative standard deviation: NMT 2.0%, *Standard solution*
  Analysis
  Samples: *Standard solution* and *Sample solution*
  Calculate the percentage of aztreonam (C$_{13}$H$_{17}$N$_5$O$_8$S$_2$) in the portion of Aztreonam taken:

$$Result = (r_U/r_S) \times (C_S/C_U) \times P \times F \times 100$$

  r_U = peak response from the *Sample solution*
  r_S = peak response from the *Standard solution*
  C_S = concentration of USP Aztreonam RS in the *Standard solution* (mg/mL)
  C_U = concentration of Aztreonam in the *Sample solution* (mg/mL)
  P = potency of USP Aztreonam RS (µg/mg)
  F = unit conversion factor, 0.001 mg/µg
  Acceptance criteria: 92.0%–105.0% on the anhydrous and solvent-free basis

IMPURITIES
- **RESIDUE ON IGNITION ⟨281⟩:** NMT 0.1%, the charred residue being moistened with 2 mL of nitric acid and 5 drops of sulfuric acid

Delete the following:

- **•• HEAVY METALS, *Method II* ⟨231⟩:** NMT 30 ppm• (Official 1-Jan-2018)
- **ORGANIC IMPURITIES**
  [NOTE—Store the *System suitability solution*, *Standard solution*, and *Sample solution* at 5°, and protect from light to prevent isomerization of aztreonam Z-isomer to aztreonam E-isomer.]
  Mobile phase, System suitability solution, Standard solution, Sample solution, Chromatographic system, and System suitability: Proceed as directed in the *Assay*.
  Analysis
  Samples: *Standard solution* and *Sample solution*
  Calculate the percentage of each impurity in the portion of Aztreonam taken:

$$Result = (r_U/r_S) \times (C_S/C_U) \times P \times F \times 100$$

  r_U = peak response of each impurity from the *Sample solution*
  r_S = peak response of aztreonam from the *Standard solution*
  C_S = concentration of USP Aztreonam RS in the *Standard solution* (mg/mL)
  C_U = concentration of Aztreonam in the *Sample solution* (mg/mL)
  P = potency of USP Aztreonam RS (µg/mg)
  F = unit conversion factor, 0.001 mg/µg
  Acceptance criteria: See *Table 1*.

Table 1

Name	Relative Retention Time	Acceptance Criteria, NMT (%)
Open-ring aztreonam[a] and open-ring desulfated aztreonam[b,c]	0.55	1.0
Aztreonam (Z-isomer)	1.0	—
Desulfated aztreonam[d]	1.6	1.5
Aztreonam E-isomer[e]	1.8	0.5
Aztreonam ethyl ester[f]	3.9	1.5
Any individual unspecified impurity	—	0.1
Total impurities	—	3.0

[a] (2S,3S)-2-{(Z)-2-[2-Aminothiazol-4-yl]-2-[2-carboxypropan-2-yloxyimino]acetamido}-3-(sulfoamino)butanoic acid.

[b] (2S,3S)-3-Amino-2-{(Z)-2-[2-aminothiazol-4-yl]-2-[2-carboxypropan-2-yloxyimino]acetamido}butanoic acid.

[c] Open-ring aztreonam and open-ring desulfated aztreonam coelute. The limit is for the sum of these two impurities.

[d] (Z)-2-({[(2-Amino-4-thiazolyl){[(2S,3S)-2-methyl-4-oxo-3-azetidinyl]carbamoyl}methylene]amino}oxy)-2-methylpropionic acid.

[e] (E)-2-({[(2-Amino-4-thiazolyl){[(2S,3S)-2-methyl-4-oxo-1-sulfo-3-azetidinyl]carbamoyl}methylene]amino}oxy)-2-methylpropionic acid.

[f] Ethyl (Z)-2-({[(2-amino-4-thiazolyl){[(2S,3S)-2-methyl-4-oxo-1-sulfo-3-azetidinyl]carbamoyl}methylene]amino}oxy)-2-methylpropionate.

SPECIFIC TESTS

- **STERILITY TESTS ⟨71⟩**, *Test for Sterility of the Product to Be Examined, Membrane Filtration*: Where the label states that Aztreonam is sterile, it meets the requirements using *Fluid A*, to which 23.4 g of sterile arginine has been added to each 1000 mL.
- **WATER DETERMINATION ⟨921⟩**, *Method I*: NMT 2.0%; if labeled as the hydrated form: 12.0%–18.0%. [NOTE—The term "hydrated form" refers to the α-form of Aztreonam, which is not a stoichiometric hydrate.]
- **BACTERIAL ENDOTOXINS TEST ⟨85⟩**: Where the label states that Aztreonam is sterile or must be subjected to further processing during the preparation of injectable dosage forms, it contains NMT 0.17 USP Endotoxin Units/mg of aztreonam.
- **LIMIT OF ALCOHOL**
  [NOTE—This test is to be performed if alcohol is used while manufacturing Aztreonam.]
  Standard solution: 0.004 mL/mL of alcohol from USP Alcohol Determination—Alcohol RS and 0.004 mL/mL of acetonitrile from USP Alcohol Determination—Acetonitrile RS in dimethylformamide. [NOTE—The *Standard solution* contains 0.4% alcohol and 0.4% acetonitrile.]
  Sample solution: 80 mg/mL of Aztreonam and 0.004 mL/mL of acetonitrile in dimethylformamide. [NOTE—Dissolve Aztreonam in dimethylformamide using 20% of the final volume. Add a suitable aliquot of USP Alcohol Determination—Acetonitrile RS, and dilute with dimethylformamide to volume. The concentration of acetonitrile in the *Sample solution* is 0.4%.]
  Chromatographic system
  (See *Chromatography ⟨621⟩, System Suitability*.)
  Mode: GC
  Detector: Flame ionization
  Column: 0.53-mm × 30-m; phase G43
  Film thickness: 3.0 µm
  Temperatures
  Injector: 210°
  Detector: 280°
  Column: See *Table 2*.

Table 2

Initial Temperature (°)	Temperature Ramp (°/min)	Final Temperature (°)	Hold Time at Final Temperature (min)
50	0	50	5

Table 2 (Continued)

Initial Temperature (°)	Temperature Ramp (°/min)	Final Temperature (°)	Hold Time at Final Temperature (min)
50	10	200	4

Carrier gas: Helium
Linear velocity: 35 cm/s
Injection mode: Split
Injection volume: 0.5 µL
Injection type: Split ratio, 5:1
System suitability
Sample: *Standard solution*
[NOTE—The relative retention times for alcohol and acetonitrile are 1.0 and 1.3, respectively.]
Suitability requirements
Resolution: NLT 2.0 between alcohol and acetonitrile
Tailing factor: NMT 1.5
Relative standard deviation: NMT 2.0%
Analysis
Samples: *Standard solution* and *Sample solution*
Calculate the percentage of alcohol in the portion of Aztreonam taken:

$$\text{Result} = (R_U/R_S) \times [C_S \times (D/C_U)] \times F \times 100$$

R_U = peak response ratio of alcohol to acetonitrile from the *Sample solution*
R_S = peak response ratio of alcohol to acetonitrile from the *Standard solution*
C_S = concentration of alcohol in the *Standard solution* (mL/mL)
D = density of alcohol (g/mL)
C_U = concentration of Aztreonam in the *Sample solution* (mg/mL)
F = unit conversion factor, 1000 mg/g
Acceptance criteria: NMT 4%

ADDITIONAL REQUIREMENTS
- **PACKAGING AND STORAGE:** Preserve in tight containers.
- **LABELING:** Where it is intended for use in preparing injectable dosage forms, the label states that it is sterile or must be subjected to further processing during the preparation of injectable dosage forms. Where it is the hydrated form, the label so indicates.

Change to read:

- **USP REFERENCE STANDARDS ⟨11⟩**
  USP Alcohol Determination—Acetonitrile RS
  C_2H_3N 41.05
  USP Alcohol Determination—Alcohol RS
  C_2H_5OH 46.07
  USP Aztreonam RS
  USP Aztreonam E-Isomer RS
  (E)-2-({[(2-Amino-4-thiazolyl){[(2S,3S)-2-methyl-4-oxo-1-sulfo-3-azetidinyl]carbamoyl}methylene]amino}oxy)-2-methylpropionic acid.
  $C_{13}H_{17}N_5O_8S_2$ 435.43
  ● ● (CN 1-May-2018)

Baclofen Tablets

DEFINITION
Baclofen Tablets contain NLT 90.0% and NMT 110.0% of the labeled amount of baclofen ($C_{10}H_{12}ClNO_2$).

IDENTIFICATION
- **A.** The retention time of the *Sample solution* corresponds to that of the *Standard solution*, as obtained in the *Assay*.

Add the following:

■• **B.** The UV spectrum of the major peak of the *Sample solution* corresponds to that of the *Standard solution*, as obtained in the *Assay*.■1S (USP41)

ASSAY

Change to read:

• **PROCEDURE**
  ■**Solution A:** 1.4 g/L of monobasic sodium phosphate and 1.7 g/L of sodium 1-pentanesulfonate in water. Adjust with 1.5 M phosphoric acid TS to a pH of 3.0.
  Solution B: Acetonitrile and methanol (50:50)
  Mobile phase: See *Table 1*.

Table 1

Time (min)	Solution A (%)	Solution B (%)
0	65	35
5	65	35
15	45	55
25	45	55
27	65	35
35	65	35

Diluent: *Solution A* and *Solution B* (65:35)
Standard solution: 200 µg/mL of USP Baclofen RS in *Diluent*
Sample solution: Nominally 200 µg/mL of baclofen prepared as follows. Finely powder NLT 20 Tablets and transfer a portion of the powder to an appropriate volumetric flask. Add *Diluent* to about 80% of the flask volume, sonicate for 10 min, and shake by mechanical means for 30 min. Dilute with *Diluent* to volume. Centrifuge a portion of this solution and use the supernatant.
Chromatographic system
  (See *Chromatography* ⟨621⟩, *System Suitability*.)
  Mode: LC
  Detector: UV 225 nm. For *Identification B*, use a diode array detector in the range of 200–400 nm.
  Column: 4.6-mm × 25-cm; 5-µm packing L1
  Column temperature: 35°
  Flow rate: 0.8 mL/min
  Injection volume: 10 µL
System suitability
  Sample: *Standard solution*
  Suitability requirements
    Tailing factor: NMT 2.0
    Relative standard deviation: NMT 1.0%
Analysis
  Samples: *Standard solution* and *Sample solution*
  Calculate the percentage of the labeled amount of baclofen ($C_{10}H_{12}ClNO_2$) in the portion of Tablets taken:

$$\text{Result} = (r_U/r_S) \times (C_S/C_U) \times 100$$

r_U = peak response from the *Sample solution*
r_S = peak response from the *Standard solution*
C_S = concentration of USP Baclofen RS in the *Standard solution* (µg/mL)
C_U = nominal concentration of baclofen in the *Sample solution* (µg/mL)■1S (USP41)

Acceptance criteria: 90.0%–110.0%

PERFORMANCE TESTS

Change to read:

• **DISSOLUTION** ⟨711⟩, *Procedure, Apparatus 1 and Apparatus 2, Immediate-Release Dosage Forms, Procedure for a pooled sample for immediate-release dosage forms*
  Medium: 0.01 N hydrochloric acid; 500 mL for Tablets containing NMT 10 mg of baclofen; 1000 mL for Tablets containing more than 10 mg of baclofen
  Apparatus 2: 50 rpm
  Time: 30 min
  ■**Solution A:** 62.7 g/L of sodium 1-pentanesulfonate in water■1S (USP41)
  Mobile phase: ■Methanol, 0.3 N acetic acid, and *Solution A* (44:55:2)■1S (USP41)
  Standard solution: USP Baclofen RS in *Medium*
  Sample solution: ■Use a portion of the solution under test.■1S (USP41)
  Chromatographic system
    (See *Chromatography* ⟨621⟩, *System Suitability*.)
    Mode: LC
    Detector: UV 265 nm
    Column: 3.9-mm × 30-cm; 10-µm packing L1
    Flow rate: 0.6 mL/min
    Injection volume: 190 µL
    ■**Run time:** NLT 2 times the retention time of the baclofen peak■1S (USP41)
  System suitability
    Sample: *Standard solution*
    Suitability requirements
      Relative standard deviation: NMT 2.0%
  Analysis
    Samples: *Standard solution* and *Sample solution*
    Calculate the percentage of the labeled amount of baclofen ($C_{10}H_{12}ClNO_2$) dissolved:

$$\text{Result} = (r_U/r_S) \times C_S \times V \times (1/L) \times 100$$

r_U = peak response from the *Sample solution*
r_S = peak response from the *Standard solution*
C_S = concentration of USP Baclofen RS in the *Standard solution* (mg/mL)
V = volume of *Medium*; 500 or 1000 mL
L = label claim (mg/Tablet)
  Tolerances: NLT 75% (Q) of the labeled amount of baclofen ($C_{10}H_{12}ClNO_2$) is dissolved.
• **UNIFORMITY OF DOSAGE UNITS** ⟨905⟩: Meet the requirements

IMPURITIES

Change to read:

• **ORGANIC IMPURITIES**
  ■**Solution A, Solution B, Mobile phase, Diluent, Sample solution,** and **Chromatographic system:** Proceed as directed in the *Assay*.
  Standard solution: 0.4 µg/mL of USP Baclofen RS and 8 µg/mL of USP Baclofen Related Compound A RS in *Diluent*
  System suitability
    Sample: *Standard solution*
    [NOTE—See *Table 2* for the relative retention times.]
    Suitability requirements
      Tailing factor: NMT 1.5 for baclofen
      Relative standard deviation: NMT 5.0% each for baclofen and baclofen related compound A

Analysis

Samples: *Standard solution* and *Sample solution*
Calculate the percentage of baclofen related compound A in the portion of Tablets taken:

$$Result = (r_U/r_S) \times (C_S/C_U) \times 100$$

r_U = peak response of baclofen related compound A from the *Sample solution*

r_S = peak response of baclofen related compound A from the *Standard solution*

C_S = concentration of USP Baclofen Related Compound A RS in the *Standard solution* (µg/mL)

C_U = nominal concentration of baclofen in the *Sample solution* (µg/mL)

Calculate the percentage of any individual degradation product in the portion of Tablets taken:

$$Result = (r_U/r_S) \times (C_S/C_U) \times 100$$

r_U = peak response of any individual degradation product from the *Sample solution*

r_S = peak response of baclofen from the *Standard solution*

C_S = concentration of USP Baclofen RS in the *Standard solution* (µg/mL)

C_U = nominal concentration of baclofen in the *Sample solution* (µg/mL)

Acceptance criteria: See *Table 2*.

Table 2

Name	Relative Retention Time	Acceptance Criteria, NMT (%)
Baclofen	1.0	—
Baclofen related compound A	3.0	4.0
Any individual degradation product	—	0.2
Total degradation products	—	1.0[a]

[a] Baclofen related compound A is not included in the total degradation products.

■1S *(USP41)*

ADDITIONAL REQUIREMENTS

- **PACKAGING AND STORAGE:** Preserve in well-closed containers. Store at controlled room temperature.
- **USP REFERENCE STANDARDS ⟨11⟩**
  USP Baclofen RS
  USP Baclofen Related Compound A RS
  4-(4-Chlorophenyl)-2-pyrrolidinone.
  $C_{10}H_{10}ClNO$ 195.65

Delete the following:

■BCG Vaccine

DEFINITION

BCG Vaccine conforms to the regulations of the FDA concerning biologics (see *Biologics* ⟨1041⟩). It is a dried, living culture of the bacillus Calmette-Guérin strain of *Mycobacterium tuberculosis* var. bovis, grown in a suitable medium from a seed strain of known history that has been maintained to preserve its capacity for conferring immunity. It contains an amount of viable bacteria such that inoculation, in the recommended dose, of tuberculin-negative persons results in an acceptable tuberculin conversion rate. It is free from other organisms, and contains a suitable stabilizer. It contains no antimicrobial agent.
[NOTE—Use the Vaccine immediately after its constitution, and discard any unused portion after 2 h.]

ADDITIONAL REQUIREMENTS

- **PACKAGING AND STORAGE:** Preserve in hermetic containers, preferably of Type I glass, at a temperature between 2° and 8°.
- **EXPIRATION DATE:** The expiration date is not later than 6 months after date of issue, or not later than 1 year after date of issue if stored at a temperature below 5°.■1S *(USP41)*

Benzethonium Chloride

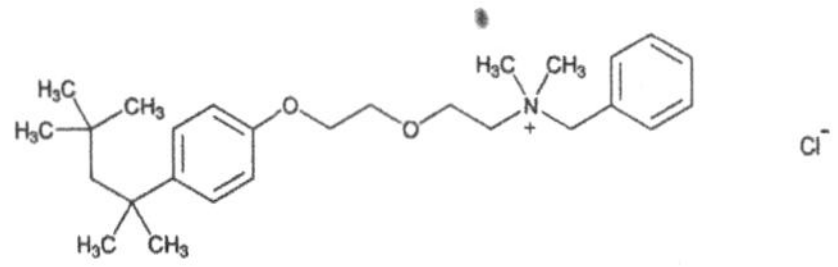

$C_{27}H_{42}ClNO_2$ 448.08
Benzenemethanaminium, N,N-dimethyl-N-[2-[2-[4-(1,1,3,3-tetramethylbutyl)phenoxy]ethoxy]ethyl]-, chloride;
Benzyldimethyl[2-[2-[p-(1,1,3,3-tetramethylbutyl)phenoxy]ethoxy]ethyl]ammonium chloride [121-54-0].

DEFINITION

Benzethonium Chloride contains NLT 97.0% and NMT 103.0% of benzethonium chloride ($C_{27}H_{42}ClNO_2$), calculated on the dried basis.

IDENTIFICATION

- **A.**
  Sample solution: 10 mg/mL
  Analysis: Add 2 mL of alcohol, 0.5 mL of 2 N nitric acid, and 1 mL of silver nitrate TS to 1 mL of the *Sample solution*.
  Acceptance criteria: A white precipitate, which is insoluble in 2 N nitric acid but soluble in 6 N ammonium hydroxide, is formed.

Change to read:

- **B.** ■**INFRARED ABSORPTION ⟨197⟩:** [NOTE—Methods described in ⟨197K⟩ or ⟨197A⟩ may be used.]■1S *(USP41)*
- **C.** The retention time of the major peak of the *Sample solution* corresponds to that of the *Standard solution*, as obtained in the *Assay*.

ASSAY

- **PROCEDURE**
  Buffer: Dilute 20 mL of triethylamine with water to 1000 mL, and adjust with phosphoric acid to a pH of 3.0.
  Mobile phase: Acetonitrile and *Buffer* (42:58)
  Diluent: Acetonitrile and water (42:58)
  System suitability solution: 0.15 mg/mL each of USP Benzethonium Chloride RS and USP Methylbenzethonium Chloride RS in *Diluent*
  Standard solution: 0.15 mg/mL of USP Benzethonium Chloride RS in *Diluent*
  Sample solution: 0.15 mg/mL of Benzethonium Chloride in *Diluent*
  Chromatographic system
  (See *Chromatography* ⟨621⟩, *System Suitability*.)

Mode: LC
Detector: UV 225 nm
Column: 4.6-mm × 15-cm; 5-µm packing L7
Column temperature: 40°
Flow rate: 1 mL/min
Injection volume: 10 µL
Run time: 1.5 times the retention time of the methylbenzethonium peak
System suitability
Sample: *System suitability solution*
[NOTE—The relative retention times for benzethonium and methylbenzethonium are 0.7 and 1.0, respectively.]
Suitability requirements
Resolution: NLT 7.0 between the benzethonium and methylbenzethonium peaks
Tailing factor: NMT 2.0 for the benzethonium peak
Relative standard deviation: NMT 1.0% for the benzethonium peak
Analysis
Samples: *Standard solution* and *Sample solution*
Calculate the percentage of benzethonium chloride ($C_{27}H_{42}ClNO_2$) in the portion of Benzethonium Chloride taken:

$$Result = (r_U/r_S) \times (C_S/C_U) \times 100$$

r_U = peak response of benzethonium from the *Sample solution*
r_S = peak response of benzethonium from the *Standard solution*
C_S = concentration of USP Benzethonium Chloride RS in the *Standard solution* (mg/mL)
C_U = concentration of Benzethonium Chloride in the *Sample solution* (mg/mL)
Acceptance criteria: 97.0%–103.0% on the dried basis

IMPURITIES
• **RESIDUE ON IGNITION** ⟨281⟩: NMT 0.1%

Add the following:

▪• **ORGANIC IMPURITIES**
Buffer, Mobile phase, Diluent, System suitability solution, and **Chromatographic system:** Proceed as directed in the *Assay*.
Standard solution: 1 µg/mL of USP Benzethonium Chloride RS in *Diluent*
Sample solution: 1 mg/mL of Benzethonium Chloride in *Diluent*
System suitability
Samples: *System suitability solution* and *Standard solution*
Suitability requirements: Proceed as directed in the *Assay*, except for *Relative standard deviation*
Relative standard deviation: NMT 5.0%, *Standard solution*
Analysis
Samples: *Standard solution* and *Sample solution*
Calculate the percentage of any individual unspecified impurity in the portion of Benzethonium Chloride taken:

$$Result = (r_U/r_S) \times (C_S/C_U) \times 100$$

r_U = peak response of any individual unspecified impurity from the *Sample solution*
r_S = peak response of benzethonium from the *Standard solution*
C_S = concentration of USP Benzethonium Chloride RS in the *Standard solution* (mg/mL)

C_U = concentration of Benzethonium Chloride in the *Sample solution* (mg/mL)
Acceptance criteria
Any individual unspecified impurity: 0.10%
Total impurities: 1.0%▪₁S (*USP41*)

SPECIFIC TESTS

Delete the following:

▪• **MELTING RANGE OR TEMPERATURE** ⟨741⟩: 158°–163°, the specimen having been dried previously▪₁S (*USP41*)
• **LOSS ON DRYING** ⟨731⟩
Analysis: Dry at 105° for 4 h.
Acceptance criteria: NMT 5.0%

ADDITIONAL REQUIREMENTS
• **PACKAGING AND STORAGE:** Preserve in tight, light-resistant containers.
• **USP REFERENCE STANDARDS** ⟨11⟩
USP Benzethonium Chloride RS
USP Methylbenzethonium Chloride RS

Add the following:

▪Brimonidine Tartrate

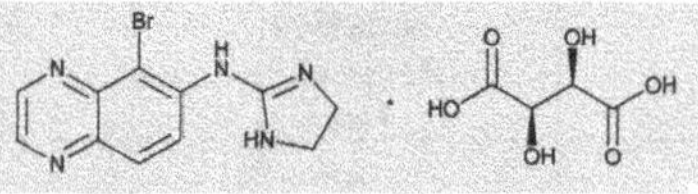

$C_{11}H_{10}BrN_5 \cdot C_4H_6O_6$　　　　　　442.22
6-Quinoxalinamine, 5-bromo-*N*-(4,5-dihydro-1*H*-imidazol-2-yl)-, [*R*-(*R**,*R**)]-2,3-dihydroxybutanedioate (1:1);
5-Bromo-6-(2-imidazolin-2-ylamino)quinoxaline L-tartrate (1:1). [70359-46-5].

DEFINITION
Brimonidine Tartrate contains NLT 98.0% and NMT 102.0% of brimonidine tartrate ($C_{11}H_{10}BrN_5 \cdot C_4H_6O_6$), calculated on the dried basis.

IDENTIFICATION
• **A. INFRARED ABSORPTION** ⟨197⟩: [NOTE—Methods described in ⟨197K⟩, ⟨197M⟩, or ⟨197A⟩ may be used.]
• **B.** The retention time of the major peak of the *Sample solution* corresponds to that of the *Standard solution*, as obtained in the *Assay*.

ASSAY
• **PROCEDURE**
Protect the solutions containing brimonidine tartrate from light.
Mobile phase: In a 1-L volumetric flask, dissolve 2.6 g of sodium 1-heptanesulfonate in 310 mL of methanol, add 2.5 mL of triethylamine and 7.5 mL of glacial acetic acid, and dilute with water to volume.
Standard solution: 1.3 mg/mL of USP Brimonidine Tartrate RS in water
Sample solution: 1.3 mg/mL of Brimonidine Tartrate in water
Chromatographic system
(See *Chromatography* ⟨621⟩, *System Suitability*.)

Mode: LC
Detector: UV 264 nm
Column: 4.6-mm × 25-cm; 5-μm packing L1
Column temperature: 30°
Flow rate: 1 mL/min
Injection volume: 20 μL
System suitability
  Sample: *Standard solution*
  Suitability requirements
    Tailing factor: NMT 1.5
    Relative standard deviation: NMT 0.73%
Analysis
  Samples: *Standard solution* and *Sample solution*
  Calculate the percentage of brimonidine tartrate
  ($C_{11}H_{10}BrN_5 \cdot C_4H_6O_6$) in the portion of Brimonidine
  Tartrate taken:

$$Result = (r_U/r_S) \times (C_S/C_U) \times 100$$

r_U = peak response from the *Sample solution*
r_S = peak response from the *Standard solution*
C_S = concentration of USP Brimonidine Tartrate RS
    in the *Standard solution* (mg/mL)
C_U = concentration of Brimonidine Tartrate in the
    Sample solution (mg/mL)
Acceptance criteria: 98.0%–102.0% on the dried basis

IMPURITIES
- **RESIDUE ON IGNITION ⟨281⟩:** NMT 0.3%
- **ORGANIC IMPURITIES**
  Protect the solutions containing brimonidine tartrate and
  related substances from light.
  Mobile phase: Proceed as directed in the *Assay*.
  System suitability solution: 1.3 mg/mL of USP
  Brimonidine Tartrate RS and 1.3 μg/mL of USP
  Brimonidine Related Compound E RS in water
  Sensitivity solution: 0.65 μg/mL of USP Brimonidine
  Tartrate RS in water
  Standard solution: 1.3 μg/mL of USP Brimonidine Tar-
  trate RS in water
  Sample solution: 1.3 mg/mL of USP Brimonidine Tar-
  trate RS in water
  Chromatographic system: Proceed as directed in the
  Assay, except for the *Run time*.
  Run time: NLT 3 times the retention time of
  brimonidine
  System suitability
    Samples: *System suitability solution* and *Sensitivity
    solution*
    [NOTE—The relative retention times for brimonidine re-
    lated compound E and brimonidine are about 0.93
    and 1.00, respectively.]
    Suitability requirements
      Resolution: NLT 1.5 between brimonidine related
      compound E and brimonidine, *System suitability
      solution*
      Signal-to-noise ratio: NLT 10, *Sensitivity solution*
  Analysis
    Samples: *Standard solution* and *Sample solution*
    Calculate the percentage of each impurity in the por-
    tion of Brimonidine Tartrate taken:

$$Result = (r_U/r_S) \times (C_S/C_U) \times 100$$

r_U = peak response of each individual impurity
    from the *Sample solution*
r_S = peak response of brimonidine from the
    Standard solution
C_S = concentration of USP Brimonidine Tartrate RS
    in the *Standard solution* (mg/mL)
C_U = concentration of Brimonidine Tartrate in the
    Sample solution (mg/mL)
Acceptance criteria: See *Table 1*. Disregard the tartrate
peak at a relative retention time of 0.09. The reporting
threshold is 0.05%.

Table 1

Name	Relative Retention Time	Acceptance Criteria, NMT (%)
Desbromobrimonidine[a]	0.86	0.1
Brimonidine	1.00	—
Any individual unspecified impurity	—	0.1
Total impurities	—	0.3

[a] *N*-(Quinoxalin-6-yl)imidazolidin-2-imine.

SPECIFIC TESTS
- **OPTICAL ROTATION ⟨781S⟩,** *Procedures, Specific Rotation*
  Sample solution: 10 mg/mL in water
  Acceptance criteria: +9.0° to +10.5°
- **LOSS ON DRYING ⟨731⟩**
  Analysis: Dry 1 g at 105° for 3 h.
  Acceptance criteria: NMT 0.5%

ADDITIONAL REQUIREMENTS
- **PACKAGING AND STORAGE:** Preserve in well-closed, light-
  resistant containers, and store at room temperature.
- **USP REFERENCE STANDARDS ⟨11⟩**
  USP Brimonidine Tartrate RS
  USP Brimonidine Related Compound E RS
  2-(5-Bromoquinoxalin-6-yl)guanidine.
  $C_9H_8BrN_5$ 266.10

■1S *(USP41)*

Add the following:

■Calcium Citrate Malate

$Ca_3(C_6H_5O_7)_2 \cdot 3CaC_4H_4O_5 \cdot 6H_2O$ 1122.97
1,2,3-Propanetricarboxylic acid, 2-hydroxy-, calcium salt
  mixture with 2-hydroxybutanedioic acid calcium salt
  (2:3:6), hexahydrate;
Calcium citrate malate (6:2:3), hexahydrate.

DEFINITION
Calcium Citrate Malate is a complex of calcium, citrate, and
malate. It contains NLT 23.0% and NMT 24.2% of calcium, calculated on the dried basis. The sum of citrate
and malate is NLT 73.0%, calculated on the dried basis.

IDENTIFICATION
- **A.**
  Sample: 0.5 g of Calcium Citrate Malate
  Analysis: Ignite completely the *Sample* at as low a temperature as possible, cool, and dissolve the residue in
  dilute glacial acetic acid (1:10). Filter, and add 10 mL of
  ammonium oxalate TS to the filtrate.
  Acceptance criteria: A voluminous white precipitate
  that is soluble in hydrochloric acid is formed.
- **B.** The retention times of the citric acid peak and the
  malic acid peak of the *Sample solution* correspond to
  those of the *System suitability solution*, as obtained in the
  test for *Content of Citrate, Malate, and Fumarate*.

ASSAY
- **PROCEDURE**
  Sample: 350 mg of Calcium Citrate Malate
  Titrimetric system
    (See *Titrimetry* ⟨541⟩.)

Mode: Direct titration
Titrant: 0.05 M edetate disodium VS
Endpoint detection: Visual
Analysis: Transfer the *Sample* into a 250-mL beaker, add 10 mL of water, 3 mL of 3 N hydrochloric acid, and swirl to dissolve. Add 90 mL of water and stir using a magnetic stirring bar. While stirring, add 30 mL of *Titrant* from the titration buret, and 25 mL of 1 N sodium hydroxide. Add 150 mg of hydroxy naphthol blue, and continue the titration to a blue endpoint. Perform a blank determination.
Calculate the percentage of calcium in the portion of Calcium Citrate Malate taken:

$$\text{Result} = \{[(V_S - V_B) \times M_A \times F]/W\} \times 100$$

V_S = *Titrant* volume consumed by the *Sample* (mL)
V_B = *Titrant* volume consumed by the blank (mL)
M_A = actual molarity of the *Titrant* (mmol/mL)
F = equivalency factor, 40.08 mg/mmol
W = *Sample* weight (mg)
Acceptance criteria: 23.0%–24.2% on the dried basis

IMPURITIES

- **LIMIT OF FLUORIDE**
  [NOTE—Prepare and store all solutions in plastic containers.]
  Buffer solution: 294 mg/mL of sodium citrate dihydrate in water
  Standard stock solution: 1.1052 mg/mL of USP Sodium Fluoride RS in water
  Standard solution: Transfer 1.0 mL of *Standard stock solution* to a 1000-mL volumetric flask, dilute with water to volume, and mix. Each milliliter of this solution contains 1 µg of fluoride ion.
  Sample solution: Transfer 1.0 g of Calcium Citrate Malate to a 100-mL beaker containing a plastic-coated stirring bar. Add 10 mL of water and place on a hot plate (medium heat). While stirring, add 10 mL of 1 N hydrochloric acid to dissolve. When dissolved, boil rapidly for 1 min, and transfer the solution to a 250-mL beaker. Cool rapidly to room temperature in an ice bath. Add 15 mL of *Buffer solution* and 10 mL of 0.2 M edetic acid, and mix. Adjust with 1 N hydrochloric acid or 1 N sodium hydroxide to a pH of 5.5 ± 0.1. Transfer the solution to a 100-mL volumetric flask, dilute with water to volume, and mix. Pour the solution back to the 250-mL beaker for performing the titration.
  Electrode system: Use a fluoride-specific ion-indicating electrode and a silver–silver chloride reference electrode connected to a pH meter capable of measuring potentials with a minimum reproducibility of ±0.2 mV (see *pH* ⟨791⟩).
  Analysis
  Samples: *Standard solution* and *Sample solution*
  Standard response line: Transfer 5.0, 25.0, and 50.0 mL of the *Standard solution* to three individual 250-mL beakers containing a plastic-coated stirring bar. Add 10 mL of 1 N hydrochloric acid, 15 mL of *Buffer solution*, and 0.2 M edetic acid to each beaker and mix. Adjust with 1 N hydrochloric acid or 1 N sodium hydroxide to a pH of 5.5 ± 0.1. Transfer the solutions to individual 100-mL volumetric flasks, dilute with water to volume, and mix. Pour the solutions back to the individual 250-mL beakers for performing the titration. Insert the electrodes into the solutions starting with the lowest concentration, stir for 15 min, and read the potential in millivolts. Between measurements, wash both reference and ion-selective electrodes with water and dry with cloth or paper towel. Plot the logarithms of the fluoride ion concentrations (0.05, 0.25, and 0.5 µg/mL) versus potential, in millivolts.
  Rinse and dry the electrodes, insert them into the *Sample solution*, stir for 5 min, and read the potential, in

millivolts. From the measured potential and the *Standard response line* determine the concentration (*C*), in µg/mL, of fluoride ion in the *Sample solution*.
Calculate the content of fluoride in the portion of Calcium Citrate Malate taken:

$$\text{Result} = (V \times C)/W$$

V = volume of the *Sample solution* (mL)
C = concentration of fluoride ion in the *Sample solution* determined from the *Standard response line* (µg/mL)
W = weight of Calcium Citrate Malate taken to prepare the *Sample solution* (g)
Acceptance criteria: NMT 30 µg/g
- **ELEMENTAL IMPURITIES—PROCEDURES ⟨233⟩**
  Acceptance criteria
  Arsenic: NMT 3.0 µg/g
  Lead: NMT 1.0 µg/g

SPECIFIC TESTS

- **CONTENT OF CITRATE, MALATE, AND FUMARATE**
  Diluent: 0.2 N hydrochloric acid
  Mobile phase: 50 mM of monobasic potassium phosphate in water. Adjust with phosphoric acid to a pH of 2.5.
  System suitability solution: 5 mg/mL of USP Calcium Citrate Malate RS in *Diluent*
  Citric acid standard solution: 1.8 mg/mL of USP Citric Acid RS in *Diluent*
  Malic acid standard solution: 1.8 mg/mL of USP Malic Acid RS in *Diluent*
  Fumaric acid standard solution: 20 µg/mL of USP Fumaric Acid RS in *Diluent*
  Sample solution: 5 mg/mL of Calcium Citrate Malate in *Diluent*
  Chromatographic system
  (See *Chromatography* ⟨621⟩, *System Suitability*.)
  Mode: LC
  Detector: UV 226 nm
  Column: 4.6-mm × 15-cm; 5-µm packing L1
  Column temperature: 35°
  Flow rate: 1.0 mL/min
  Injection volume: 10 µL
  System suitability
  Samples: *System suitability solution, Citric acid standard solution, Malic acid standard solution,* and *Fumaric acid standard solution*
  [NOTE—The relative retention times for malic acid, citric acid, and fumaric acid are 0.6, 1.0, and 1.4, respectively.]
  Suitability requirements
  Resolution: NLT 8.0 between malic acid and citric acid, *System suitability solution*
  Relative standard deviation: NMT 2.0% for each *Standard solution*
  Chromatogram similarity: The chromatogram of the *System suitability solution* is similar to the reference chromatogram provided with the lot of USP Calcium Citrate Malate RS being used.
  Analysis
  Samples: *Citric acid standard solution, Malic acid standard solution, Fumaric acid standard solution,* and *Sample solution*
  Separately calculate the percentage of citrate, malate, and fumarate in the portion of Calcium Citrate Malate taken:

$$\text{Result} = (r_U/r_S) \times (C_S/C_U) \times F \times 100$$

r_U = peak response of citric acid, malic acid, or fumaric acid from the *Sample solution*
r_S = peak response of citric acid, malic acid, or fumaric acid from the respective *Standard solutions*

C_S = concentration of USP Citric Acid RS, USP Malic Acid RS, or USP Fumaric Acid RS in the respective *Standard solutions* (mg/mL)

C_U = concentration of Calcium Citrate Malate in the *Sample solution* (mg/mL)

F = factor for converting molecular weight of the acid form to that of the salt form, 0.98

Acceptance criteria

Sum of citrate and malate: NLT 73.0% on the dried basis

Fumarate: NMT 0.1% on the dried basis

- **PH ⟨791⟩**
  Sample solution: 30 mg/mL in water. [NOTE—The solution is a slurry.]
  Acceptance criteria: 4.0–8.0
- **LOSS ON DRYING ⟨731⟩**
  Analysis: Dry at 150° for 4 h.
  Acceptance criteria: 8.0%–11.0%

ADDITIONAL REQUIREMENTS

- **PACKAGING AND STORAGE:** Preserve in tight containers.
- **USP REFERENCE STANDARDS ⟨11⟩**
  USP Calcium Citrate Malate RS
  USP Citric Acid RS
  USP Fumaric Acid RS
  USP Malic Acid RS
  USP Sodium Fluoride RS
  ■1S *(USP41)*

Carbidopa and Levodopa Extended-Release Tablets

DEFINITION

Carbidopa and Levodopa Extended-Release Tablets contain NLT 90.0% and NMT 110.0% of the labeled amount of carbidopa ($C_{10}H_{14}N_2O_4$) and levodopa ($C_9H_{11}NO_4$).

IDENTIFICATION

- **A.** The retention times of the major peaks of the *Sample solution* correspond to those of the *Standard solution*, as obtained in the *Assay.*

Add the following:

- **B.** The UV spectra of the major peaks of the *Sample solution* correspond to those of the *Standard solution*, as obtained in the *Assay.*■1S *(USP41)*

ASSAY

Change to read:

- **PROCEDURE**
  Protect the volumetric preparations from light.
  Solution A: 0.24 g/L of sodium 1-decanesulfonate in water
  Solution B: 11.6 g/L of monobasic sodium phosphate in water
  Mobile phase: *Solution A, Solution B,* and water (0.13: 95: 4.87), prepared as follows. Add 0.13% of the final volume of *Solution A* to 95% of the final volume of *Solution B.* Adjust with phosphoric acid to a pH of 2.8. Dilute with water to final volume.
  Standard solution: 0.1 mg/mL of USP Carbidopa RS and 0.4 mg/mL of USP Levodopa RS in solution, prepared as follows. Transfer accurately weighed portions of the Reference Standards into a suitable volumetric flask, and dissolve in 0.1 N phosphoric acid using 8% of the final volume. Sonication may be used to promote dissolution. Dilute with water to final volume.

Sample solution: Nominally 0.1 mg/mL of carbidopa and 0.4 mg/mL of levodopa from NLT 20 finely powdered Tablets, prepared as follows. Transfer an accurately weighed portion of the powder, equivalent to 1 Tablet weight, into a suitable volumetric flask, and dissolve in 0.1 N phosphoric acid, using 10% of the final volume. Sonicate for 10 min and then stir for 30 min. Dilute with water to volume and stir for another 20 min. Pass the solution through a suitable filter of 0.45-µm pore size.

Chromatographic system
(See *Chromatography* ⟨621⟩, *System Suitability.*)
Mode: LC
Detector: UV 280 nm. ■For *Identification B,* use a diode array detector in the range of 200–350 nm.
■1S *(USP41)*
Column: 4.6-mm × 10-cm; 5-µm packing L1
Flow rate: 2 mL/min
Injection volume: 20 µL
■**Run time:** NLT 4 times the retention time of levodopa■1S *(USP41)*

System suitability
Sample: *Standard solution*
[NOTE—The relative retention times for levodopa and carbidopa are 1.0 and 2.8, respectively.]
Suitability requirements
Tailing factor: NMT 1.5 for carbidopa; NMT 1.5 for levodopa
Resolution: NLT 6 between levodopa and carbidopa
Relative standard deviation: NMT 1.0% for carbidopa; NMT 1.0% for levodopa

Analysis
Samples: *Standard solution* and *Sample solution*
Calculate the percentage of the labeled amount of carbidopa ($C_{10}H_{14}N_2O_4$) or levodopa ($C_9H_{11}NO_4$) in the portion of Tablets taken:

$$\text{Result} = (r_U/r_S) \times (C_S/C_U) \times 100$$

r_U = peak response of carbidopa or levodopa from the *Sample solution*

r_S = peak response of carbidopa or levodopa from the *Standard solution*

C_S = concentration of USP Carbidopa RS or USP Levodopa RS in the *Standard solution* (mg/mL)

C_U = nominal concentration of carbidopa or levodopa in the *Sample solution* (mg/mL)

Acceptance criteria: 90.0%–110.0% each of the labeled amounts of carbidopa and levodopa

PERFORMANCE TESTS

Change to read:

- **DISSOLUTION ⟨711⟩**
  Test 1
  Medium: 0.1 N hydrochloric acid; 900 mL degassed with helium
  Apparatus 2: 50 rpm
  Times
  For Tablets that contain 25 mg of carbidopa and 100 mg of levodopa: 0.5, 1, and 4 h
  For Tablets that contain 50 mg of carbidopa and 200 mg of levodopa: 0.5, 1, 2.5, and 4 h
  Solution A: 0.24 g/L of sodium 1-decanesulfonate in water
  Solution B: 12.7 g/L of monobasic sodium phosphate in water
  Mobile phase: *Solution A, Solution B,* and water (0.13: 95: 4.87), prepared as follows. Add 0.13% of the final volume of *Solution A* to 95% of the final volume of *Solution B.* Adjust with phosphoric acid to a pH of 2.8. Dilute with water to final volume.

Standard solution: 0.03 mg/mL of USP Carbidopa RS and 0.1 mg/mL of USP Levodopa RS in *Medium.* Sonication may be used to aid in dissolution.

Sample solution

For Tablets that contain 25 mg of carbidopa and 100 mg of levodopa: Pass a portion of the solution under test through a suitable filter of 0.45-µm pore size and discard the first 1–3 mL.

For Tablets that contain 50 mg of carbidopa and 200 mg of levodopa: Pass a portion of the solution under test through a suitable filter of 0.45-µm pore size, discard the first 1–3 mL, and dilute with *Medium* (50:50).

Chromatographic system

(See *Chromatography* ⟨621⟩, *System Suitability.*)

Mode: LC

Detector: UV 280 nm

Column: 3.9-mm × 30-cm; 10-µm packing L1

Flow rate: 2 mL/min

Injection volume: 20 µL

■**Run time:** NLT 3 times the retention time of levodopa■₁ₛ (USP41)

System suitability

Sample: *Standard solution*

[NOTE—The relative retention times for levodopa and carbidopa are 0.4 and 1.0, respectively.]

Suitability requirements

Resolution: NLT 2.0 between levodopa and carbidopa

Relative standard deviation: NMT 2.0% for carbidopa and NMT 2.0% for levodopa for six replicate injections

Analysis

Samples: *Standard solution* and *Sample solution*

Calculate the concentration (C_i) of carbidopa ($C_{10}H_{14}N_2O_4$) or levodopa ($C_9H_{11}NO_4$) in the sample withdrawn from the vessel at each time point (i):

$$Result = (r_U/r_S) \times C_S \times D$$

r_U = peak response of carbidopa or levodopa from the *Sample solution*

r_S = peak response of carbidopa or levodopa from the *Standard solution*

C_S = concentration of USP Carbidopa RS or USP Levodopa RS in the *Standard solution* (mg/mL)

D = dilution factor for the *Sample solution*, if needed

Calculate the percentage of the labeled amount of carbidopa ($C_{10}H_{14}N_2O_4$) or levodopa ($C_9H_{11}NO_4$) dissolved at each time point (i):

$$Result_1 = C_1 \times V \times (1/L) \times 100$$

$$Result_2 = \{[C_2 \times (V - V_S)] + (C_1 \times V_S)\} \times (1/L) \times 100$$

$$Result_3 = (\{C_3 \times [V - (2 \times V_S)]\} + [(C_2 + C_1) \times V_S]) \times (1/L) \times 100$$

$$Result_4 = (\{C_4 \times [V - (3 \times V_S)]\} + [(C_3 + C_2 + C_1) \times V_S]) \times (1/L) \times 100$$

C_i = concentration of carbidopa or levodopa in the portion of sample withdrawn at time point i (mg/mL)

V = volume of the *Medium*, 900 mL

L = label claim of carbidopa or levodopa (mg/Tablet)

V_S = volume of the *Sample solution* withdrawn from the *Medium* (mL)

Tolerances

For Tablets that contain 25 mg of carbidopa and 100 mg of levodopa: See *Table 1.*

Table 1

Time Point (i)	Time (h)	Amount of Carbidopa Dissolved (%)	Amount of Levodopa Dissolved (%)
1	0.5	15–40	14–39
2	1	37–62	36–61
3	4	NLT 80	NLT 80

For Tablets that contain 50 mg of carbidopa and 200 mg of levodopa: See *Table 2.*

Table 2

Time Point (i)	Time (h)	Amount of Carbidopa Dissolved (%)	Amount of Levodopa Dissolved (%)
1	0.5	8–33	8–33
2	1	26–51	26–51
3	2.5	62–87	64–89
4	4	NLT 80	NLT 80

The percentages of the labeled amounts of carbidopa ($C_{10}H_{14}N_2O_4$) and levodopa ($C_9H_{11}NO_4$) dissolved at the times specified conform to *Dissolution* ⟨711⟩, *Acceptance Table 2.*

Test 2: If the product complies with this test, the labeling indicates that it meets USP *Dissolution Test 2.*

Medium: Simulated gastric fluid TS (prepared without enzymes); 900 mL

Apparatus 2: 50 rpm

Times: 0.5, 1, 2, and 3 h

Buffer: 6.8 g/L of monobasic potassium phosphate and 1.0 g/L of 1-hexanesulfonic acid in water. Adjust with phosphoric acid to a pH of 3.3.

Mobile phase: Filtered and degassed mixture of methanol and *Buffer* (20:80)

Standard solution: (L/900) mg/mL each of USP Carbidopa RS and USP Levodopa RS in *Medium*, where L is the label claim, in mg/Tablet

Sample solution: Pass a portion of the solution under test through a suitable filter of 0.45-µm pore size.

Chromatographic system

(See *Chromatography* ⟨621⟩, *System Suitability.*)

Mode: LC

Detector: UV 280 nm

Column: 4.6-mm × 15-cm; 5-µm packing L7

Flow rate: 1 mL/min

Injection volume: 20 µL

■**Run time:** NLT 2.5 times the retention time of levodopa■₁ₛ (USP41)

System suitability

Sample: *Standard solution*

[NOTE—The relative retention times for levodopa and carbidopa are 1.0 and 1.4, respectively.]

Suitability requirements

Resolution: NLT 2.0 between levodopa and carbidopa

Column efficiency: NLT 4000 theoretical plates for both carbidopa and levodopa

Tailing factor: NMT 2.0 for both carbidopa and levodopa

Relative standard deviation: NMT 1.0% for both carbidopa and levodopa

Analysis
  Samples: *Standard solution* and *Sample solution*
  Calculate the concentration (C_i) of carbidopa
  ($C_{10}H_{14}N_2O_4$) or levodopa ($C_9H_{11}NO_4$) in the sample
  withdrawn from the vessel at each time point (*i*):

$$\text{Result} = (r_U/r_S) \times C_S$$

r_U = peak response of carbidopa or levodopa from
         the *Sample solution*
r_S = peak response of carbidopa or levodopa from
         the *Standard solution*
C_S = concentration of USP Carbidopa RS or USP
         Levodopa RS in the *Standard solution*
         (mg/mL)
  Calculate the percentage of the labeled amount of
  carbidopa ($C_{10}H_{14}N_2O_4$) or levodopa ($C_9H_{11}NO_4$)
  dissolved at each time point (*i*):

$$\text{Result}_1 = C_1 \times V \times (1/L) \times 100$$

$$\text{Result}_2 = \{[C_2 \times (V - V_S)] + (C_1 \times V_S)\} \times (1/L) \times 100$$

$$\text{Result}_3 = (\{C_3 \times [V - (2 \times V_S)]\} + [(C_2 + C_1) \times V_S]) \times (1/L) \times 100$$

$$\text{Result}_4 = (\{C_4 \times [V - (3 \times V_S)]\} + [(C_3 + C_2 + C_1) \times V_S]) \times (1/L) \times 100$$

C_i = concentration of carbidopa or levodopa in the
         portion of sample withdrawn at time point *i*
         (mg/mL)
V = volume of the *Medium*, 900 mL
L = label claim of carbidopa or levodopa (mg/
         Tablet)
V_S = volume of the *Sample solution* withdrawn from
         the *Medium* (mL)
  Tolerances: See *Table 3*.

Table 3

Time Point (*i*)	Time (h)	Amount Dissolved (%)
1	0.5	20–35
2	1	35–60
3	2	65–95
4	3	NLT 80

  The percentages of the labeled amounts of carbidopa
  ($C_{10}H_{14}N_2O_4$) and levodopa ($C_9H_{11}NO_4$) dissolved at
  the times specified conform to *Dissolution* ⟨711⟩, *Acceptance Table 2*.
Test 3: If the product complies with this test, the labeling indicates that it meets USP *Dissolution Test 3*.
  Medium, Apparatus 2, Solution A, Solution B, Mobile phase, Standard solution, Chromatographic system, and **System suitability:** Proceed as directed in *Test 1*.
  Times: 0.5, 1, 2.5, and 4 h
  Sample solution: Pass a portion of the solution under test through a suitable filter.
  Analysis: Proceed as directed in *Test 1*.
  Tolerances: See *Table 4*.

Table 4

Time Point (*i*)	Time (h)	Amount Dissolved for Tablets That Contain 25 mg of Carbidopa and 100 mg of Levodopa (%)	Amount Dissolved for Tablets That Contain 50 mg of Carbidopa and 200 mg of Levodopa (%)
1	0.5	15–40	15–35
2	1	25–65	25–65
3	2.5	NLT 60	NLT 60
4	4	NLT 80	NLT 80

  The percentages of the labeled amounts of carbidopa
  ($C_{10}H_{14}N_2O_4$) and levodopa ($C_9H_{11}NO_4$) dissolved at
  the times specified conform to *Dissolution* ⟨711⟩, *Acceptance Table 2*.
Test 4: If the product complies with this test, the labeling indicates that it meets USP *Dissolution Test 4*.
  Medium: 0.1 N hydrochloric acid; 900 mL
  Apparatus 2: 50 rpm
  Times: 1, 3, and 6 h
  Solution A: 0.24 g/L of sodium 1-decanesulfonate in water
  Solution B: 11.6 g/L of monobasic sodium phosphate in water
  Mobile phase: *Solution A, Solution B,* and water
  (0.13: 95: 4.87), prepared as follows. Add 0.13% of the final volume of *Solution A* to 95% of the final volume of *Solution B*. Adjust with phosphoric acid to a pH of 2.8. Dilute with water to final volume.
  Standard solution: ($L/900$) mg/mL each of USP Carbidopa RS and USP Levodopa RS in *Medium*, where *L* is the label claim, in mg/Tablet
  Sample solution: Withdraw a 10.0-mL aliquot at each time point and pass a portion of the solution under test through a suitable filter. Replace the 10.0-mL aliquot withdrawn for analysis with a 10.0-mL aliquot of *Medium*.
  Chromatographic system
  (See *Chromatography* ⟨621⟩, *System Suitability*.)
  Mode: LC
  Detector: UV 280 nm
  Column: 3.9-mm × 30-cm; 10-µm packing L1
  Flow rate: 2 mL/min
  Injection volume: 50 µL
  Run time: NLT 3 times the retention time of levodopa
  System suitability
  Sample: *Standard solution*
  [NOTE—The relative retention times for levodopa and carbidopa are 1.0 and 2.5, respectively.]
  Suitability requirements
    Resolution: NLT 2.0 between levodopa and carbidopa
    Tailing factor: NMT 2.0 for both carbidopa and levodopa
    Relative standard deviation: NMT 2.0% for both carbidopa and levodopa
  Analysis
  Samples: *Standard solution* and *Sample solution*
  Calculate the concentration (C_i) of carbidopa
  ($C_{10}H_{14}N_2O_4$) or levodopa ($C_9H_{11}NO_4$) in the sample
  withdrawn from the vessel at each time point (*i*):

$$\text{Result} = (r_U/r_S) \times C_S$$

r_U = peak response of carbidopa or levodopa from
         the *Sample solution*
r_S = peak response of carbidopa or levodopa from
         the *Standard solution*

C_S = concentration of USP Carbidopa RS or USP Levodopa RS in the *Standard solution* (mg/mL)

Calculate the percentage of the labeled amount of carbidopa ($C_{10}H_{14}N_2O_4$) or levodopa ($C_9H_{11}NO_4$) dissolved at each time point (*i*):

$$Result_1 = C_1 \times V \times (1/L) \times 100$$

$$Result_2 = [(C_2 \times V) + (C_1 \times V_S)] \times (1/L) \times 100$$

$$Result_3 = [(C_3 \times V) + (C_2 + C_1) \times V_S] \times (1/L) \times 100$$

C_i = concentration of carbidopa or levodopa in the portion of sample withdrawn at time point *i* (mg/mL)
V = volume of the *Medium*, 900 mL
L = label claim of carbidopa or levodopa (mg/Tablet)
V_S = volume of the *Sample solution* withdrawn from the vessel and replaced with *Medium*, 10 mL

Tolerances: See *Table 5*.

Table 5

Time Point (*i*)	Time (h)	Amount Dissolved for Tablets That Contain 25 mg of Carbidopa and 100 mg of Levodopa (%)	Amount Dissolved for Tablets That Contain 50 mg of Carbidopa and 200 mg of Levodopa (%)
1	1	35–70	25–60
2	3	NLT 65	NLT 65
3	6	NLT 80	NLT 80

The percentages of the labeled amounts of carbidopa ($C_{10}H_{14}N_2O_4$) and levodopa ($C_9H_{11}NO_4$) dissolved at the times specified conform to *Dissolution* ⟨711⟩, *Acceptance Table 2*.

Test 5: If the product complies with this test, the labeling indicates that it meets USP *Dissolution Test 5*.
Medium: 0.1 N hydrochloric acid; 900 mL
Apparatus 2: 50 rpm
Times: 0.5, 1, 2.5, and 4 h
Mobile phase: 13.6 g/L of monobasic potassium phosphate adjusted with phosphoric acid to a pH of 3.0
Standard solution: (*L*/900) mg/mL each of USP Carbidopa RS and USP Levodopa RS in *Medium*, where *L* is the label claim, in mg/Tablet. [NOTE—This solution is stable for 1 day if stored at 23°–27°.]
Sample solution: Pass a portion of the solution under test through a suitable filter of 0.45-μm pore size, and discard the first 4–5 mL.
[NOTE—This solution is stable for 1 day if stored at 23°–27°.]
Chromatographic system
(See *Chromatography* ⟨621⟩, *System Suitability*.)
Mode: LC
Detector: UV 282 nm
Column: 4.6-mm × 15-cm; 5-μm packing L7
Flow rate: 1.5 mL/min
Injection volume: 20 μL
Run time: NLT 3 times the retention time of levodopa
System suitability
Sample: *Standard solution*
[NOTE—The relative retention times for levodopa and carbidopa are 1.0 and 1.6, respectively.]
Suitability requirements
Resolution: NLT 2.0 between levodopa and carbidopa

Tailing factor: NMT 2.0 for both carbidopa and levodopa
Relative standard deviation: NMT 2.0% for both carbidopa and levodopa
Analysis
Samples: *Standard solution* and *Sample solution*
Calculate the concentration (C_i) of carbidopa ($C_{10}H_{14}N_2O_4$) or levodopa ($C_9H_{11}NO_4$) in the sample withdrawn from the vessel at each time point (*i*):

$$Result = (r_U/r_S) \times C_S$$

r_U = peak response of carbidopa or levodopa from the *Sample solution*
r_S = peak response of carbidopa or levodopa from the *Standard solution*
C_S = concentration of USP Carbidopa RS or USP Levodopa RS in the *Standard solution* (mg/mL)

Calculate the percentage of the labeled amount of carbidopa ($C_{10}H_{14}N_2O_4$) or levodopa ($C_9H_{11}NO_4$) dissolved at each time point (*i*):

$$Result_1 = C_1 \times V \times (1/L) \times 100$$

$$Result_2 = \{[C_2 \times (V - V_S)] + (C_1 \times V_S)\} \times (1/L) \times 100$$

$$Result_3 = (\{C_3 \times [V - (2 \times V_S)]\} + [(C_2 + C_1) \times V_S]) \times (1/L) \times 100$$

$$Result_4 = (\{C_4 \times [V - (3 \times V_S)]\} + [(C_3 + C_2 + C_1) \times V_S]) \times (1/L) \times 100$$

C_i = concentration of carbidopa or levodopa in the portion of sample withdrawn at time point *i* (mg/mL)
V = volume of the *Medium*, 900 mL
L = label claim of carbidopa or levodopa (mg/Tablet)
V_S = volume of the *Sample solution* withdrawn from the *Medium* (mL)

Tolerances: See *Table 6*.

Table 6

Time Point (*i*)	Time (h)	Amount Dissolved for Tablets That Contain 25 mg of Carbidopa and 100 mg of Levodopa (%)	Amount Dissolved for Tablets That Contain 50 mg of Carbidopa and 200 mg of Levodopa (%)
1	0.5	25–45	20–40
2	1	40–65	30–60
3	2.5	NLT 65	NLT 55
4	4	NLT 80	NLT 75

The percentages of the labeled amounts of carbidopa ($C_{10}H_{14}N_2O_4$) and levodopa ($C_9H_{11}NO_4$) dissolved at the times specified conform to *Dissolution* ⟨711⟩, *Acceptance Table 2*.

Test 6: If the product complies with this test, the labeling indicates that it meets USP *Dissolution Test 6*.
Medium: 0.1 N hydrochloric acid; 900 mL degassed under vacuum
Apparatus 1: 75 rpm
Times: 0.5, 1, 2.5, and 3.5 h
Solution A: 0.24 g/L of sodium 1-decanesulfonate in water

Mobile phase: To each liter of 12.5 g/L of monobasic sodium phosphate dihydrate, add 1.3 mL of *Solution A* and adjust with phosphoric acid to a pH of 2.8.

Standard solution: 0.03 mg/mL of USP Carbidopa RS and 0.11 mg/mL of USP Levodopa RS in *Medium*

Sample solution

For Tablets that contain 25 mg of carbidopa and 100 mg of levodopa: Pass a portion of the solution under test through a suitable filter of 0.45-µm pore size, discard the first 2 mL, and use the remaining filtrate. Use within 24 h.

For Tablets that contain 50 mg of carbidopa and 200 mg of levodopa: Pass a portion of the solution under test through a suitable filter of 0.45-µm pore size, discard the first 2 mL, and dilute with *Medium* (50:50). Use within 24 h.

Chromatographic system

(See *Chromatography* ⟨621⟩, *System Suitability*.)

Mode: LC

Detector: UV 280 nm

Column: 3.9-mm × 30-cm; 10-µm packing L1

Flow rate: 2 mL/min

Injection volume: 20 µL

Run time: NLT 3 times the retention time of levodopa

System suitability

Sample: *Standard solution*

[NOTE—The relative retention times for levodopa and carbidopa are 1.0 and 2.8, respectively.]

Suitability requirements

Resolution: NLT 2.0 between levodopa and carbidopa

Tailing factor: NMT 2.0 for both levodopa and carbidopa

Relative standard deviation: NMT 2.0% for both levodopa and carbidopa

Analysis

Samples: *Standard solution* and *Sample solution*

Calculate the concentration (C_i) of carbidopa ($C_{10}H_{14}N_2O_4$) or levodopa ($C_9H_{11}NO_4$) in the sample withdrawn from the vessel at each time point (*i*):

$$\text{Result} = (r_U/r_S) \times C_S \times D$$

r_U = peak response of carbidopa or levodopa from the *Sample solution*

r_S = peak response of carbidopa or levodopa from the *Standard solution*

C_S = concentration of USP Carbidopa RS or USP Levodopa RS in the *Standard solution* (mg/mL)

D = dilution factor for the *Sample solution*, if needed

Calculate the percentage of the labeled amount of carbidopa ($C_{10}H_{14}N_2O_4$) or levodopa ($C_9H_{11}NO_4$) dissolved at each time point (*i*):

$$\text{Result}_1 = C_1 \times V \times (1/L) \times 100$$

$$\text{Result}_2 = \{[C_2 \times (V - V_S)] + (C_1 \times V_S)\} \times (1/L) \times 100$$

$$\text{Result}_3 = (\{C_3 \times [V - (2 \times V_S)]\} + [(C_2 + C_1) \times V_S]) \times (1/L) \times 100$$

$$\text{Result}_4 = (\{C_4 \times [V - (3 \times V_S)]\} + [(C_3 + C_2 + C_1) \times V_S]) \times (1/L) \times 100$$

C_i = concentration of carbidopa or levodopa in the portion of sample withdrawn at time point *i* (mg/mL)

V = volume of the *Medium*, 900 mL

L = label claim of carbidopa or levodopa (mg/Tablet)

V_S = volume of the *Sample solution* withdrawn from the *Medium* (mL)

Tolerances: See *Table 7*.

Table 7

Time Point (*i*)	Time (h)	Amount Dissolved for Tablets That Contain 25 mg of Carbidopa and 100 mg of Levodopa (%)	Amount Dissolved for Tablets That Contain 50 mg of Carbidopa and 200 mg of Levodopa (%)
1	0.5	15–40	10–30
2	1	35–60	25–50
3	2.5	NLT 70	NLT 65
4	3.5	NLT 85	NLT 80

The percentages of the labeled amounts of carbidopa ($C_{10}H_{14}N_2O_4$) and levodopa ($C_9H_{11}NO_4$) dissolved at the times specified conform to *Dissolution* ⟨711⟩, *Acceptance Table 2*.

- **UNIFORMITY OF DOSAGE UNITS** ⟨905⟩: Meet the requirements

IMPURITIES

- **ORGANIC IMPURITIES**

Protect all analytical solutions from light and maintain them at 2°–8° until they are injected.

Buffer: 6 g/L of anhydrous monobasic sodium phosphate in water. Adjust with phosphoric acid to a pH of 2.2.

Mobile phase: Alcohol and *Buffer* (5:95)

System suitability solution: 1 µg/mL of USP Levodopa Related Compound B RS and 125 µg/mL of USP Carbidopa RS in *Mobile phase*

Standard solution: 1.25 µg/mL of USP Carbidopa RS and 5 µg/mL of USP Levodopa RS in *Mobile phase*

Sensitivity solution: 0.125 µg/mL of USP Carbidopa RS and 0.5 µg/mL of USP Levodopa RS in *Mobile phase* from the *Standard solution*

Sample solution: Nominally 0.125 mg/mL of carbidopa and nominally 0.5 mg/mL of levodopa in *Mobile phase* from NLT 10 finely powdered Tablets, prepared as follows. Transfer an accurately weighed portion of the powder into a suitable volumetric flask, dissolve in *Mobile phase*, and pass through a suitable filter.

Chromatographic system

(See *Chromatography* ⟨621⟩, *System Suitability*.)

Mode: LC

Detector: UV 280 nm

Column: 4.6-mm × 15-cm; 5-µm packing L1

Autosampler temperature: 6°

Flow rate: 1 mL/min

Injection volume: 20 µL

Run time: ■NLT■1S (USP41) 6 times the retention time of carbidopa

System suitability

Samples: *System suitability solution*, *Standard solution*, and *Sensitivity solution*

[NOTE—For the relative retention times, see *Table 8*.]

Suitability requirements

Resolution: NLT 1.5 between carbidopa and levodopa related compound B, *System suitability solution*

Relative standard deviation: NMT 3.0% for both carbidopa and levodopa for five replicate injections, *Standard solution*

Signal-to-noise ratio: NLT 10 for carbidopa, *Sensitivity solution*

Analysis

Samples: *Standard solution* and *Sample solution*

Calculate the percentage of dihydroxybenzaldehyde, dihydroxyphenylacetone, and any unspecified carbidopa degradant based on the label claim of carbidopa in the portion of Tablets taken:

$$\text{Result} = (r_U/r_S) \times (C_S/C_U) \times (1/F) \times 100$$

r_U = peak response of dihydroxybenzaldehyde, dihydroxyphenylacetone, or any unspecified carbidopa degradant from the *Sample solution*

r_S = peak response of carbidopa from the *Standard solution*

C_S = concentration of USP Carbidopa RS in the *Standard solution* (mg/mL)

C_U = nominal concentration of carbidopa in the *Sample solution* (mg/mL)

F = relative response factor (see *Table 8*)

Calculate the percentage of levodopa related compound A and any unspecified levodopa degradant based on the label claim of levodopa in the portion of Tablets taken:

$$\text{Result} = (r_U/r_S) \times (C_S/C_U) \times (1/F) \times 100$$

r_U = peak response of levodopa related compound A or any unspecified levodopa degradant from the *Sample solution*

r_S = peak response of levodopa from the *Standard solution*

C_S = concentration of USP Levodopa RS in the *Standard solution* (mg/mL)

C_U = nominal concentration of levodopa in the *Sample solution* (mg/mL)

F = relative response factor (see *Table 8*)

Acceptance criteria: See *Table 8*. ■The reporting threshold is 0.05%, relative to the drug substance.

■1S (*USP41*)

Table 8

Name	Relative Retention Time	Relative Response Factor	Acceptance Criteria, NMT (%)
Levodopa related compound A[a,b]	0.9	0.8	0.1
Levodopa	1.0	—	—
Methyldopa[c,d]	1.9	—	—
Levodopa related compound B[a,d]	2.1	—	—
Carbidopa	2.3	—	—
Dihydrox-ybenzaldehyde[c,e]	5.7	5.9	0.2
Dihydroxypheny-lacetone[c,f]	6.3	1.0	1
3-O-Methyl-carbidopa[d,g]	6.9	—	—
Any unspecified carbidopa degradant	—	1.0	0.2

[a] Individual impurity based on label claim of levodopa.
[b] 3-(3,4,6-Trihydroxyphenyl)alanine.
[c] Individual impurity based on label claim of carbidopa.
[d] This impurity is listed for information only. It is monitored in the drug substance. This impurity is not to be reported and is not to be included in the total degradants.
[e] 3,4-Dihydroxybenzaldehyde.
[f] 3,4-Dihydroxyphenylacetone.
[g] (S)-2-Hydrazinyl-3-(4-hydroxy-3-methoxyphenyl)-2-methylpropanoic acid.

Table 8 (Continued)

Name	Relative Retention Time	Relative Response Factor	Acceptance Criteria, NMT (%)
Any unspecified levodopa degradant	—	1.0	0.1
Total degradants	—	—	4.0

[a] Individual impurity based on label claim of levodopa.
[b] 3-(3,4,6-Trihydroxyphenyl)alanine.
[c] Individual impurity based on label claim of carbidopa.
[d] This impurity is listed for information only. It is monitored in the drug substance. This impurity is not to be reported and is not to be included in the total degradants.
[e] 3,4-Dihydroxybenzaldehyde.
[f] 3,4-Dihydroxyphenylacetone.
[g] (S)-2-Hydrazinyl-3-(4-hydroxy-3-methoxyphenyl)-2-methylpropanoic acid.

ADDITIONAL REQUIREMENTS

- **PACKAGING AND S8TORAGE:** Preserve in well-closed, light-resistant containers, and store at controlled room temperature.
- **LABELING:** When more than one *Dissolution* test is given, the labeling states the *Dissolution* test used only if *Test 1* is not used.
- **USP REFERENCE STANDARDS ⟨11⟩**
  USP Carbidopa RS
  USP Levodopa RS
  USP Levodopa Related Compound B RS
  3-Methoxytyrosine.
  $C_{10}H_{13}NO_4$ 211.21

Carprofen

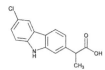

$C_{15}H_{12}ClNO_2$ 273.71
9H-Carbazole-2-acetic acid, 6-chloro-α-methyl-, (±)-; (±)-6-Chloro-α-methylcarbazole-2-acetic acid [53716-49-7].

DEFINITION
Carprofen contains NLT 98.0% and NMT 102.0% of carprofen ($C_{15}H_{12}ClNO_2$), calculated on the dried basis.

IDENTIFICATION

Change to read:

- **A. INFRARED ABSORPTION ■⟨197⟩:** [NOTE—Methods described in ⟨197K⟩ or ⟨197A⟩ may be used. If the spectra obtained in the solid state show differences, dissolve the substance to be examined and the reference substance separately in acetone, evaporate to dryness, and record new spectra using the residues.]■1S (*USP41*)
- **B.** The retention time of the major peak of the *Sample solution* corresponds to that of the *Standard solution*, as obtained in the *Assay*.

ASSAY

Change to read:

- **PROCEDURE**
  ■[NOTE—Protect all solutions containing carprofen from light.]■1S (*USP41*)

Mobile phase: Acetonitrile, methanol, glacial acetic acid, and water (40: 25: 0.2: 35)

System suitability stock solution: 16 µg/mL of USP Carprofen Related Compound A RS in *Mobile phase*. Sonicate if necessary. ■■1S (USP41)

Standard solution: 160 µg/mL of USP Carprofen RS in *Mobile phase*. Sonicate if necessary. ■■1S (USP41)

System suitability solution: 1.6 µg/mL of USP Carprofen Related Compound A RS and 16 µg/mL of USP Carprofen RS in *Mobile phase* prepared as follows. Mix 10 mL of *System suitability stock solution* and 10 mL of the *Standard solution* and dilute with *Mobile phase* to 100 mL. ■■1S (USP41)

Sample solution: 160 µg/mL of Carprofen in *Mobile phase* ■■1S (USP41)

Chromatographic system

(See *Chromatography* ⟨621⟩, *System Suitability*.)

Mode: LC

Detector: UV 239 nm

Column: 4.6-mm × 25-cm; 5-µm packing L1

Flow rate: 1 mL/min

Injection volume: 10 µL

System suitability

Sample: *System suitability solution*

Suitability requirements

Resolution: NLT 2.0 between carprofen and carprofen related compound A ■■1S (USP41)

Tailing factor: NMT 2.0 for the carprofen peak

Relative standard deviation: NMT 2.0% for the carprofen peak

Analysis

Samples: *Standard solution* and *Sample solution*

Calculate the percentage of carprofen ($C_{15}H_{12}ClNO_2$) in the portion of Carprofen taken:

$$Result = (r_U/r_S) \times (C_S/C_U) \times 100$$

r_U = peak response from the *Sample solution*

r_S = peak response from the *Standard solution*

C_S = concentration of USP Carprofen RS in the *Standard solution* (µg/mL)

C_U = concentration of Carprofen in the *Sample solution* (µg/mL)

Acceptance criteria: 98.0%–102.0% on the dried basis

IMPURITIES

• **RESIDUE ON IGNITION** ⟨281⟩: NMT 0.1%

■• **LIMIT OF ACETONE AND METHYLENE CHLORIDE**

Standard solution: 0.5 mg/mL of acetone and 0.06 mg/mL of methylene chloride in *N,N*-dimethylacetamide

Sample solution: 100 mg/mL of Carprofen in *N,N*-dimethylacetamide

Chromatographic system

Mode: GC

Detector: Flame ionization

Column: 0.53-mm × 30-m capillary column coated with 3.0-µm G43 stationary phase

Carrier gas: Nitrogen

Temperatures

Injector: 210°

Detector: 200°

Column: See *Table 1*.

Table 1

Initial Temperature (°)	Temperature Ramp (°/min)	Final Temperature (°)	Hold Time at Final Temperature (min)
80	0	80	4
80	30	190	3

Flow rate: 4.9 mL/min

Injection volume: 1 µL

Injection type: Split flow ratio, 10:1

System suitability

Sample: *Standard solution*

[NOTE—Acetone elutes before methylene chloride.]

Suitability requirements

Resolution: NLT 1.5 between acetone and methylene chloride

Relative standard deviation: NMT 10.0% for the acetone peak

Analysis

Samples: *Standard solution* and *Sample solution*

Calculate the percentage of each residual solvent in the portion of Carprofen taken:

$$Result = (r_U/r_S) \times (C_S/C_U) \times 100$$

r_U = peak response of the individual residual solvent in the *Sample solution*

r_S = peak response of the individual residual solvent in the *Standard solution*

C_S = concentration of individual residual solvent in the *Standard solution* (µg/mL)

C_U = concentration of carprofen in the *Sample solution* (µg/mL)

Acceptance criteria

Acetone: NMT 5000 ppm

Methylene chloride: NMT 600 ppm■1S (USP41)

• **ORGANIC IMPURITIES**

Mobile phase, System suitability solution, Sample solution, Chromatographic system, and **System suitability:** Proceed as directed in the *Assay*.

Analysis

Sample: *Sample solution*

Calculate the percentage of each impurity in the portion of Carprofen taken:

$$Result = (r_U/r_T) \times 100$$

r_U = peak response of each individual peak (other than the major peak of carprofen)

r_T = sum of all the peak responses

Acceptance criteria: See *Table 1*.

Table 1

Name	Relative Retention Time	Acceptance Criteria, NMT (%)
Carprofen related compound A (carbazole)	0.9	0.5
2-[1,1-Dimethoxy-2-hydroxypropyl]-6-chlorocarbazole	1.3	0.5
2-[2-Chloropro-pionyl]-6-chloro-9-acetylcarbazole	3.3	0.5

Table 1 *(Continued)*

Name	Relative Retention Time	Acceptance Criteria, NMT (%)
Any individual unspecified impurity	—	0.1
Total impurities	—	1.0

SPECIFIC TESTS
- **LOSS ON DRYING ⟨731⟩**
  Analysis: Dry at 105° for 2 h.
  Acceptance criteria: NMT 0.5%

ADDITIONAL REQUIREMENTS
- **PACKAGING AND STORAGE:** Preserve in tight, light-resistant containers. Store at 25°, excursions permitted between 15° and 30°.
- **LABELING:** Label it to indicate that it is intended for veterinary use only.
- **USP REFERENCE STANDARDS ⟨11⟩**
  USP Carprofen RS
  USP Carprofen Related Compound A RS
  Carbazole.
  $C_{12}H_9N$ 167.21

Cetylpyridinium Chloride

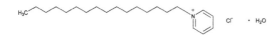

$C_{21}H_{38}ClN \cdot H_2O$	358.00
$C_{21}H_{38}ClN$	339.99

Pyridinium, 1-hexadecyl-, chloride, monohydrate;
1-Hexadecylpyridinium chloride monohydrate [6004-24-6].
Anhydrous [123-03-5].

DEFINITION
Cetylpyridinium Chloride contains NLT 98.0% and NMT 102.0% of cetylpyridinium chloride ($C_{21}H_{38}ClN$), calculated on the anhydrous basis.

IDENTIFICATION
- **A. INFRARED ABSORPTION ⟨197K⟩**
- **B.** The retention time of the major peak of the *Sample solution* corresponds to that of the *Standard solution*, as obtained in the *Assay.*

Change to read:

- **C. IDENTIFICATION TESTS—GENERAL ⟨191⟩,** *Chloride*
  Sample solution: 2 mg/mL in water
  Acceptance criteria: A 10-mL portion of the *Sample solution* meets the requirements •of test *A,*• (CN 1-May-2018) except that when silver nitrate TS is added, turbidity is produced rather than a curdy white precipitate.

ASSAY
- **PROCEDURE**
  Use 0.1% trifluoroacetic acid–rinsed glassware and silanized vials for all solutions containing cetylpyridinium chloride, as cetylpyridinium may react with the surface.
  Solution A: Trifluoroacetic acid and water (1:999)
  Solution B: Acetonitrile and trifluoroacetic acid (999:1)
  Mobile phase: *Solution A* and *Solution B* (62.5: 37.5)
  Standard solution: 0.25 mg/mL of USP Cetylpyridinium Chloride RS in *Solution A*

  Sample solution: 0.25 mg/mL of Cetylpyridinium Chloride in *Solution A*
  Chromatographic system
  (See *Chromatography* ⟨621⟩, *System Suitability.*)
  Mode: LC
  Detector: UV 258 nm
  Column: 2.1-mm × 10-cm; 5-µm packing L78
  Column temperature: 40°
  Flow rate: 0.6 mL/min
  Injection volume: 2 µL
  System suitability
  Sample: *Standard solution*
  Suitability requirements
  Tailing factor: NMT 1.5
  Relative standard deviation: NMT 0.73%
  Analysis
  Samples: *Standard solution* and *Sample solution*
  Calculate the percentage of cetylpyridinium chloride ($C_{21}H_{38}ClN$) in the portion of Cetylpyridinium Chloride taken:

$$Result = (r_U/r_S) \times (C_S/C_U) \times 100$$

r_U	= peak response from the *Sample solution*
r_S	= peak response from the *Standard solution*
C_S	= concentration of USP Cetylpyridinium Chloride RS in the *Standard solution* (mg/mL)
C_U	= concentration of Cetylpyridinium Chloride in the *Sample solution* (mg/mL)

Acceptance criteria: 98.0%–102.0% on the anhydrous basis

IMPURITIES
- **RESIDUE ON IGNITION ⟨281⟩:** NMT 0.2% on the anhydrous basis

Delete the following:

- •**HEAVY METALS,** *Method II* ⟨231⟩: NMT 20 ppm• (CN 1-Jan-2018)

Change to read:

- **ORGANIC IMPURITIES**
  Use 0.1% trifluoroacetic acid–rinsed glassware and silanized vials for all solutions containing cetylpyridinium chloride, as cetylpyridinium may react with the surface.
  Solution A, Solution B, Mobile phase, and **Chromatographic system:** Proceed as directed in the *Assay.*
  Standard solution: 2.5 µg/mL of USP Cetylpyridinium Chloride RS in *Solution A*
  Sample solution: 2.5 mg/mL of Cetylpyridinium Chloride in *Solution A*
  System suitability
  Sample: *Standard solution*
  Suitability requirements
  Relative standard deviation: NMT 2.0%
  Analysis
  Samples: *Standard solution* and *Sample solution*
  Calculate the percentage of each unspecified impurity in the portion of Cetylpyridinium Chloride taken:

$$Result = (r_U/r_S) \times (C_S/C_U) \times 100$$

r_U	= peak response of each unspecified impurity from the *Sample solution*
r_S	= peak response of cetylpyridinium from the *Standard solution*
C_S	= concentration of USP Cetylpyridinium Chloride RS in the *Standard solution* (mg/mL)
C_U	= concentration of Cetylpyridinium Chloride in the *Sample solution* (mg/mL)

Acceptance criteria: See *Table 1.* Disregard any impurity peaks less than 0.04%.

Table 1

Name	Relative Retention Time	Acceptance Criteria, NMT (%)
Cetylpyridinium chloride	1.0	—
Any unspecified impurity	—	0.1 (Postponed indefinitely) (RB 1-Aug-2017)
Total impurities	—	1.0

SPECIFIC TESTS

- **ACIDITY**
  Sample: 500 mg
  Analysis: Dissolve *Sample* in 50 mL of water, add phenolphthalein TS, and titrate with 0.020 N sodium hydroxide.
  Acceptance criteria: NMT 2.5 mL is required for neutralization.
- **WATER DETERMINATION ⟨921⟩**, *Method I:* 4.5%–5.5%

ADDITIONAL REQUIREMENTS

- **PACKAGING AND STORAGE:** Preserve in well-closed containers.
- **USP REFERENCE STANDARDS ⟨11⟩**
  USP Cetylpyridinium Chloride RS

Add the following:

▪Cholecalciferol Tablets

DEFINITION

Cholecalciferol Tablets contain NLT 90.0% and NMT 115.0% of the labeled amount of cholecalciferol ($C_{27}H_{44}O$).

IDENTIFICATION

- **A.** The retention time of the major peak of the *Sample solution* corresponds to that of the *Standard solution*, as obtained in the *Assay*.
- **B.** The UV spectrum of the major peak of the *Sample solution* corresponds to that of the *Standard solution*, as obtained in the *Assay*.

ASSAY

- **PROCEDURE**
  [NOTE—Use amber, low-actinic glassware.]
  Diluent: Water, dimethylformamide, and isopropyl alcohol (5:10:35, v/v)
  Mobile phase: Acetonitrile and water (70:30)
  Standard stock solution: 0.5 mg/mL of USP Cholecalciferol RS in isopropyl alcohol
  Ergocalciferol stock solution: 0.5 mg/mL of USP Ergocalciferol RS in isopropyl alcohol
  System suitability solution: Combine equal volumes of *Standard stock solution* and *Ergocalciferol stock solution* and dilute with *Diluent* to obtain a concentration of about 1 µg/mL each of cholecalciferol and ergocalciferol.
  Standard solution: 1 µg/mL of USP Cholecalciferol RS in *Diluent* from the *Standard stock solution*, prepared accurately
  Sample solution: Finely powder NLT 20 Tablets. Transfer a portion of the powder, nominally equivalent to 50 µg of cholecalciferol, into a 50-mL volumetric flask, add 5 mL of water and sonicate for 10 min with intermittent shaking. Add 10 mL of dimethylformamide, sonicate for 15 min with intermittent shaking, cool to room temperature, and dilute with isopropyl alcohol to

volume. Mix well and pass through a 0.45-µm nylon filter.
Chromatographic system
(See *Chromatography* ⟨621⟩, *System Suitability*.)
Mode: LC
Detector: UV 265 nm
Column: 4.6-mm × 15-cm; 2.7-µm packing L96
Column temperature: 40°
Flow rate: 1 mL/min
Injection volume: 20 µL
System suitability
Samples: *System suitability solution* and *Standard solution*
[NOTE—The relative retention times for cholecalciferol and ergocalciferol are 1.0 and 1.1, respectively.]
Suitability requirements
Resolution: NLT 1.5 between the cholecalciferol and ergocalciferol peaks, *System suitability solution*
Relative standard deviation: NMT 2.0%, *Standard solution*
Analysis
Samples: *Standard solution* and *Sample solution*
Calculate the percentage of the labeled amount of cholecalciferol ($C_{27}H_{44}O$) in the portion of Tablets taken:

$$\text{Result} = (r_U/r_S) \times (C_S/C_U) \times 100$$

r_U = peak area of cholecalciferol from the *Sample solution*
r_S = peak area of cholecalciferol from the *Standard solution*
C_S = concentration of cholecalciferol in the *Standard solution* (µg/mL)
C_U = nominal concentration of cholecalciferol in the *Sample solution* (µg/mL)

Acceptance criteria: 90.0%–115.0%

PERFORMANCE TESTS

- **DISSOLUTION ⟨711⟩**
  [NOTE—Perform this test under light conditions that minimize photodegradation.]
  Medium: 0.1% (w/v) octoxynol-9 in water; 500 mL
  Apparatus 2: 75 rpm
  Time: 30 min
  Mobile phase: Acetonitrile and water (70:30)
  Standard stock solution: 0.5 mg/mL of USP Cholecalciferol RS in isopropyl alcohol
  Standard solution: Dilute *Standard stock solution* with *Medium* to obtain the concentration equivalent to that expected in the *Sample solution*.
  Sample solution: Withdraw a portion of the solution under test, pass through a 0.45-µm PVDF filter, and use the pooled sample as the test specimen.
  Chromatographic system
  (See *Chromatography* ⟨621⟩, *System Suitability*.)
  Mode: LC
  Detector: UV 265 nm
  Column: 4.6-mm × 15-cm; 2.7-µm packing L96
  Column temperature: 40°
  Flow rate: 1 mL/min
  Injection volume: 100 µL
  System suitability
  Sample: *Standard solution*
  Suitability requirements
  Relative standard deviation: NMT 2.0%
  Analysis
  Samples: *Standard solution* and *Sample solution*
  Calculate the percentage of the labeled amount of cholecalciferol dissolved:

$$\text{Result} = (r_U/r_S) \times (C_S \times V/L) \times 100$$

r_U = peak area of cholecalciferol from the *Sample solution*

r_S = peak area of cholecalciferol from the *Standard solution*
C_S = concentration of cholecalciferol in the *Standard solution* (µg/mL)
V = volume of *Medium*, 500 mL
L = label claim of cholecalciferol (µg/Tablet)
Tolerances: NLT 75% (Q) of the labeled amount of cholecalciferol is dissolved.

- **UNIFORMITY OF DOSAGE UNITS ⟨905⟩:** Meet the requirements

ADDITIONAL REQUIREMENTS

- **PACKAGING AND STORAGE:** Preserve in tight, light-resistant containers.
- **LABELING:** Label the Tablets to indicate the content of cholecalciferol in µg.
- **USP REFERENCE STANDARDS ⟨11⟩**
  USP Cholecalciferol RS
  USP Ergocalciferol RS
  ■1S (USP41)

Chymotrypsin

Chymotrypsin [9004-07-3].

DEFINITION

Chymotrypsin is a proteolytic enzyme crystallized from an extract of the pancreas gland of the ox, *Bos taurus* L. (Fam. Bovidae). It contains NLT 1000 USP Chymotrypsin Units/mg, calculated on the dried basis, and NLT 90.0% and NMT 110.0% of the labeled potency, as determined by the *Assay*.

ASSAY

Change to read:

- **PROCEDURE**
  Monobasic potassium phosphate solution: 9.08 mg/mL of monobasic potassium phosphate in water
  Dibasic sodium phosphate solution: 9.46 mg/mL of anhydrous dibasic sodium phosphate in water
  Phosphate buffer: Mix 38.9 mL of *Monobasic potassium phosphate solution* and 61.1 mL of *Dibasic sodium phosphate solution*. If necessary, adjust by the dropwise addition of *Dibasic sodium phosphate solution* to a pH of 7.0.
  Substrate solution: Dissolve 23.7 mg of *N*-acetyl-L-tyrosine ethyl ester, suitable for use in assaying Chymotrypsin, in 50 mL of *Phosphate buffer*, with warming. When the solution is cool, dilute with additional *Phosphate buffer* to 100 mL. [NOTE—*Substrate solution* may be stored in the frozen state and used after thawing, but it is important to freeze it immediately after preparation.]
  Sample solution: Dissolve a quantity of Chymotrypsin in 0.0012 N hydrochloric acid to yield a solution containing 12–16 USP Chymotrypsin Units/mL. The dilution is correct if, during the conduct of the *Assay*, there is a change in absorbance of between 0.008 and 0.012 in each 30-s interval.
  ■**Blank solution:** Mix 0.2 mL of 0.0012 N hydrochloric acid and 3 mL of water.■1S (USP41)
  Analysis
    Samples: *Substrate solution, Sample solution,* ■and *Blank solution*■1S (USP41)
    [NOTE—Determine the suitability of the substrate and check the adjustment of the spectrophotometer by performing the *Analysis* using USP Chymotrypsin RS in place of the *Sample solution.*]
    Conduct the *Assay* in a suitable spectrophotometer equipped to maintain a temperature of 25 ± ■1.0°■1S (USP41) in the cell compartment. Determine the temperature in the reaction cell before and after the

absorbance measurement to ensure that the temperature does not change by more than ■1.0°. Pipet 3.0 mL of *Blank solution* into a 1-cm cell.■1S (USP41) Place the cell in the spectrophotometer, and adjust the instrument so that the absorbance will read ■0.00■1S (USP41) at 237 nm. Pipet 0.2 mL of *Sample solution* into another 1-cm cell, add 3 mL of *Substrate solution*, and place the cell in the spectrophotometer. [NOTE—Carefully follow this order of addition, and begin timing the reaction from the addition of the *Substrate solution.*] Read the absorbance at 30-s intervals for NLT 5 min. Repeat the procedure on the same dilution at least once. Absolute absorbance values are less important than a constant rate of absorbance change. If the rate of change fails to remain constant for NLT 3 min, repeat the test and, if necessary, use a lower concentration. The duplicate determination of the *Sample solution* matches the first determination, of the same dilution, in rate of absorbance change.
    Determine the average absorbance change per minute, using only the values within the 3-min portion of the curve where the rate of absorbance change is constant. Plot a curve of absorbance against time. One USP Chymotrypsin Unit is the activity causing a change in absorbance of 0.0075/min under the conditions specified in the *Assay*.
    Calculate the number of USP Chymotrypsin Units/mg in the portion of Chymotrypsin taken:

$$Result = (A_2 - A_1)/(T \times W \times F)$$

A_2 = absorbance straight-line initial reading
A_1 = absorbance straight-line final reading
T = time elapsed between the initial and final readings (min)
W = weight of Chymotrypsin in the volume of solution used in determining the absorbance (mg)
F = Chymotrypsin activity conversion factor, 0.0075/min

  Acceptance criteria: NLT 1000 USP Chymotrypsin Units/mg on the dried basis; 90.0%–110.0% of the labeled potency

IMPURITIES

- **RESIDUE ON IGNITION ⟨281⟩:** NMT 2.5%
- **LIMIT OF TRYPSIN**
  Tris buffer: Dissolve 294 mg of calcium chloride in 40 mL of 0.20 M tris(hydroxymethyl)aminomethane. Adjust with 1 N hydrochloric acid to a pH of 8.1, and dilute with water to 100 mL.
  Substrate solution: Transfer 98.5 mg of *p*-toluenesulfonyl-L-arginine methyl ester hydrochloride, suitable for use in assaying trypsin, to a 25-mL volumetric flask. Add 5 mL of *Tris buffer*, and swirl until the substrate dissolves. Add 0.25 mL of methyl red–methylene blue TS, and dilute with water to volume.
  Sample solution: 10 mg/mL of Chymotrypsin in water
  Analysis
    [NOTE—Determine the suitability of the substrate by performing the *Analysis* using the appropriate amount of USP Trypsin Crystallized RS in place of the *Sample solution.*]
    By means of a micropipet, transfer 50 µL of *Sample solution* to a depression on a white spot plate. Add 0.2 mL of *Substrate solution*.
  Acceptance criteria: No purple color develops within 3 min (NMT 1% of trypsin).

SPECIFIC TESTS

- **MICROBIAL ENUMERATION TESTS ⟨61⟩ and TESTS FOR SPECIFIED MICROORGANISMS ⟨62⟩:** It meets the requirements of the tests for absence of *Pseudomonas aeruginosa*, *Salmonella* species, and *Staphylococcus aureus*.

- **Loss on Drying ⟨731⟩**
  Analysis: Dry under vacuum at 60° for 4 h.
  Acceptance criteria: NMT 5.0%

ADDITIONAL REQUIREMENTS
- **Packaging and Storage:** Preserve in tight containers, and avoid exposure to excessive heat.
- **USP Reference Standards ⟨11⟩**
  USP Chymotrypsin RS
  USP Trypsin Crystallized RS

Chymotrypsin for Ophthalmic Solution

DEFINITION
Chymotrypsin for Ophthalmic Solution is sterile Chymotrypsin. When constituted as directed in the labeling, it yields a solution containing NLT 80.0% and NMT 120.0% of the labeled potency.

IDENTIFICATION
- **A.**
  Monobasic potassium phosphate solution: 9.08 mg/mL of monobasic potassium phosphate in water
  Dibasic sodium phosphate solution: 9.46 mg/mL of anhydrous dibasic sodium phosphate in water
  Phosphate buffer: Mix 38.9 mL of *Monobasic potassium phosphate solution* and 61.1 mL of *Dibasic sodium phosphate solution*. If necessary, adjust by the dropwise addition of *Dibasic sodium phosphate solution* to a pH of 7.0.
  Substrate solution: Transfer 237.0 mg of N-acetyl-L-tyrosine ethyl ester, suitable for use in assaying chymotrypsin, to a 100-mL volumetric flask, add 2 mL of alcohol, and swirl until solution is effected. Add 20 mL of *Phosphate buffer*, 1 mL of methyl red–methylene blue TS, and dilute with water to volume. If necessary, adjust by the dropwise addition of *Monobasic potassium phosphate solution* to a pH of 7.0.
  Sample solution: Dissolve the contents of 1 vial of Chymotrypsin for Ophthalmic Solution in 1 mL of saline TS.
  Analysis: Transfer 0.2 mL of the *Sample solution* to a suitable dish, and add 0.2 mL of the *Substrate solution*.
  Acceptance criteria: A purple color is produced within 3 min. [Note—This is distinct from trypsin, which produces no purple color within 3 min.]

ASSAY

Change to read:

- **Procedure**
  Monobasic potassium phosphate solution: 9.08 mg/mL of monobasic potassium phosphate in water
  Dibasic sodium phosphate solution: 9.46 mg/mL of anhydrous dibasic sodium phosphate in water
  Phosphate buffer: *Monobasic potassium phosphate solution* and *Dibasic sodium phosphate solution* (38.9: 61.1). If necessary, adjust by the dropwise addition of *Dibasic sodium phosphate solution* to a pH of 7.0.
  Substrate solution: Dissolve 23.7 mg of N-acetyl-L-tyrosine ethyl ester, suitable for use in assaying chymotrypsin, in 50 mL of *Phosphate buffer*, with warming. When the solution is cool, dilute with additional *Phosphate buffer* to 100 mL.
  [Note—*Substrate solution* may be stored in the frozen state and used after thawing, but it is important to freeze it immediately after preparation.]
  Sample stock solution: Dissolve the contents of 1 vial of Chymotrypsin for Ophthalmic Solution in 5.0 mL of 0.0012 N hydrochloric acid.

Sample solution: Dilute a volume (V_2, in mL) of the *Sample stock solution*, equivalent to 300 USP Chymotrypsin Units, with 0.0012 N hydrochloric acid to 25.0 mL. The dilution is correct if, during the conduct of the *Assay*, there is a change in absorbance of between 0.008 and 0.012 in each 30-s interval.
■**Blank solution:** Mix 0.2 mL of 0.0012 N hydrochloric acid and 3 mL of water.■₁S (USP41)

Analysis
Samples: *Substrate solution, Sample stock solution, Sample solution,* ■and *Blank solution*■₁S (USP41)
[Note—Determine the suitability of the substrate and check the adjustment of the spectrophotometer by performing the *Analysis* using USP Chymotrypsin RS in place of the *Sample solution*.]
Conduct the *Assay* in a suitable spectrophotometer equipped to maintain a temperature of 25 ± ■1.0°■₁S (USP41) in the cell compartment. Determine the temperature in the reaction cell before and after the absorbance measurement to ensure that the temperature does not change by more than ■1.0°. Pipet 3.0 mL of *Blank solution* into a 1-cm cell.■₁S (USP41) Place the cell in the spectrophotometer, and adjust the instrument so that the absorbance will read ■0.00■₁S (USP41) at 237 nm. Pipet 0.2 mL of *Sample solution* into another 1-cm cell, add 3 mL of *Substrate solution*, and place the cell in the spectrophotometer. [Note—Carefully follow this order of addition, and begin timing the reaction from the addition of the *Substrate solution*.] Read the absorbance at 30-s intervals for NLT 5 min. Repeat the procedure on the same dilution at least once. Absolute absorbance values are less important than a constant rate of absorbance change. If the rate of change fails to remain constant for NLT 3 min, repeat the test and, if necessary, use a lower concentration. The duplicate determination at the same dilution matches the first determination in rate of absorbance change.
Determine the average absorbance change per minute, using only the values within the 3-min portion of the curve where the rate of absorbance change is constant. Plot a curve of absorbance against time. One USP Chymotrypsin Unit is the activity causing a change in absorbance of 0.0075/min under the conditions specified in the *Assay*.
Calculate the percentage of the labeled potency of USP Chymotrypsin Units in a vial:

$$\text{Result} = [F_1 \times (V_1/V_2) \times (A_2 - A_1)]/(T \times F_2 \times F_3)$$

F_1 = total USP Chymotrypsin Units in the *Sample solution*, 300
V_1 = volume of the *Sample stock solution*, 5 mL
V_2 = volume as defined in the *Sample solution* (mL)
A_2 = absorbance straight-line initial reading
A_1 = absorbance straight-line final reading
T = time elapsed between the initial and final readings (min)
F_2 = number of USP Chymotrypsin Units in the solution on which the absorbance was determined, 2.4
F_3 = chymotrypsin activity conversion factor, 0.0075/min

Acceptance criteria: 80.0%–120.0% of the labeled potency

PERFORMANCE TESTS
- **Uniformity of Dosage Units ⟨905⟩**
  Analysis: Assay 10 individual units as directed in the *Assay*, and calculate the average of the 10 results.
  Acceptance criteria: Meets the requirements of the chapter and the average is 80.0%–120.0% of the labeled potency. The contents of NMT 2 vials deviate by more than 10% from the average content. The con-

tents of none of the vials deviate by more than 15% from the average.

IMPURITIES

- **LIMIT OF TRYPSIN**

    Tris buffer: Dissolve 294 mg of calcium chloride in 40 mL of 0.20 M tris(hydroxymethyl)aminomethane. Adjust with 1 N hydrochloric acid to a pH of 8.1, and dilute with water to 100 mL.

    Substrate solution: Transfer 98.5 mg of *p*-toluenesulfonyl-L-arginine methyl ester hydrochloride, suitable for use in assaying trypsin, to a 25-mL volumetric flask. Add 5 mL of *Tris buffer*, and swirl until the substrate dissolves. Add 0.25 mL of methyl red–methylene blue TS, and dilute with water to volume.

    Sample solution: 10 mg/mL of Chymotrypsin for Ophthalmic Solution

    Analysis

    [NOTE—Determine the suitability of the substrate by performing the *Analysis* using the appropriate amount of USP Trypsin Crystallized RS in place of the *Sample solution*.]

    By means of a micropipet, transfer 50 µL of the *Sample solution* to a depression on a white spot plate. Add 0.2 mL of the *Substrate solution*.

    Acceptance criteria: No purple color develops within 3 min (NMT 1% of trypsin).

SPECIFIC TESTS

- **PH ⟨791⟩:** 4.3–8.7, in the solution constituted as directed in the labeling
- **STERILITY TESTS ⟨71⟩:** Meets the requirements
- **COMPLETENESS OF SOLUTION ⟨641⟩:** It dissolves in the solvent and in the concentration recommended in the labeling to yield a clear solution.

ADDITIONAL REQUIREMENTS

- **PACKAGING AND STORAGE:** Preserve in single-dose containers, preferably of Type I glass, and avoid exposure to excessive heat.
- **USP REFERENCE STANDARDS ⟨11⟩**
    USP Chymotrypsin RS
    USP Trypsin Crystallized RS

Clarithromycin

$C_{38}H_{69}NO_{13}$ 747.95
Erythromycin, 6-O-methyl-;
6-O-Methylerythromycin [81103-11-9].

DEFINITION

Clarithromycin contains NLT 96.0% and NMT 102.0% of clarithromycin ($C_{38}H_{69}NO_{13}$), calculated on the anhydrous basis.

IDENTIFICATION

- **A. INFRARED ABSORPTION ⟨197K⟩**

Add the following:

- **B.** The retention time of the major peak of the *Sample solution* corresponds to that of *Standard solution 1*, as obtained in the *Assay*.■1S (USP41)

ASSAY

Change to read:

- **PROCEDURE**

    Solution A, Solution B, Mobile phase, Diluent, Standard solution 1, Standard solution 2, Standard solution 4, Sample solution, and Chromatographic system: Proceed as directed in *Organic Impurities*.

    System suitability

    Samples: *Standard solution 1, Standard solution 2,* and *Standard solution 4*

    [NOTE—See the relative retention times in *Table 2*. The typical retention time for clarithromycin is about 11 min.]

    Suitability requirements

    Peak-to-valley ratio: NLT 3.0, *Standard solution 4*
    The *Peak-to-valley ratio* is calculated as follows:

    $$Result = H_P/H_V$$

    H_P = height above the baseline of the clarithromycin impurity D peak, *Standard solution 4*
    H_V = height above the baseline of the lowest point of the curve separating the clarithromycin impurity D peak from the clarithromycin peak, *Standard solution 4*

    Tailing factor: NMT 1.7, *Standard solution 2*

    Relative standard deviation: NMT 1.5%, *Standard solution 1*

    Analysis

    Samples: *Standard solution 1* and *Sample solution*
    Calculate the percentage of clarithromycin ($C_{38}H_{69}NO_{13}$) in the portion of Clarithromycin taken:

    $$Result = (r_U/r_S) \times (C_S/C_U) \times 100$$

    r_U = peak ■1S (USP41) response from the *Sample solution*
    r_S = peak ■1S (USP41) response from *Standard solution 1*
    C_S = concentration of USP Clarithromycin RS in *Standard solution 1* (mg/mL)
    C_U = concentration of Clarithromycin in the *Sample solution* (mg/mL)

    Acceptance criteria: 96.0%–102.0% on the anhydrous basis

IMPURITIES

- **RESIDUE ON IGNITION ⟨281⟩**
    Sample: 0.5 g
    Acceptance criteria: NMT 0.2%

Delete the following:

- **HEAVY METALS**
    Diluent: 85% v/v dioxane in water
    Lead nitrate stock solution: Dissolve 159.8 mg of lead nitrate in 100 mL of water to which has been added 1 mL of nitric acid. Dilute with water to 1000 mL. Prepare and store this solution in glass containers free from soluble lead salts.
    Sample solution: 50 mg/mL in *Diluent*. Transfer 12 mL of this solution to a color-comparison tube.

Standard solution: 1 ppm of Pb, prepared by diluting *Lead nitrate stock solution* with *Diluent*. Add 10 mL of this solution and 2 mL of the *Sample solution* to a color-comparison tube.

Blank: Add 10 mL of *Diluent* and 2 mL of the *Sample solution* to a color-comparison tube.

Analysis
Samples: *Sample solution, Standard solution,* and *Blank*
To each of the three tubes add 2 mL of pH 3.5 acetate buffer, mix, then add 1.2 mL of thioacetamide–glycerin base TS, and mix.

Acceptance criteria: Compared to the *Blank*, the *Standard solution* shows a slight brown color. After 2 min, any brown color in the *Sample solution* is not more intense than that in the *Standard solution* (NMT 20 µg/g).

● (Official 1-Jan-2018)

Change to read:

● **ORGANIC IMPURITIES**
Solution A: 4.76 g/L of monobasic potassium phosphate. Adjust with dilute phosphoric acid (1 in 10) or potassium hydroxide (45% w/v) to a pH of 4.4. Pass this solution through a C18 filtration kit.
Solution B: Acetonitrile
Mobile phase: See *Table 1*.

Table 1

Time (min)	Solution A (%)	Solution B (%)
0	75	25
32	40	60
34	40	60
36	75	25
42	75	25

Diluent: Acetonitrile and water (1:1)
Standard solution 1: 1.5 mg/mL of USP Clarithromycin RS in acetonitrile and water (1:1). Dissolve first in acetonitrile, using 50% of the final volume, and dilute with water to volume.
Standard solution 2: 75 µg/mL of USP Clarithromycin RS from *Standard solution 1* in *Diluent*
Standard solution 3: 7.5 µg/mL of USP Clarithromycin RS from *Standard solution 2* in *Diluent*
Standard solution 4: 1.5 mg/mL of USP Clarithromycin Identity RS in acetonitrile and water (1:1). Dissolve first in acetonitrile, using 50% of the final volume, and dilute with water to volume.
Sample solution: 1.5 mg/mL of Clarithromycin in acetonitrile and water (1:1). Dissolve first in acetonitrile, using 50% of the final volume, and dilute with water to volume.
Chromatographic system
(See *Chromatography ⟨621⟩, System Suitability.*)
Mode: LC
Detector: UV 205 nm
Column: 4.6-mm × 10-cm; packing L1
Column temperature: 40°
Flow rate: 1.1 mL/min
Injection volume: 10 µL
System suitability
Samples: *Standard solution 2* and *Standard solution 4*
[NOTE—See the relative retention times in *Table 2*. The typical retention time for clarithromycin is about 11 min.]
Suitability requirements
Peak-to-valley ratio: NLT 3.0, *Standard solution 4*
The *Peak-to-valley ratio* is calculated as follows:

$$Result = H_P/H_V$$

H_P = height above the baseline of the clarithromycin impurity D peak, *Standard solution 4*
H_V = height above the baseline of the lowest point of the curve separating the clarithromycin impurity D peak from the clarithromycin peak, *Standard solution 4*
Tailing factor: NMT 1.7, *Standard solution 2*
Analysis
Samples: *Diluent, Standard solution 2, Standard solution 3, Standard solution 4,* and *Sample solution*
Calculate the percentage of each impurity in the portion of Clarithromycin taken:

$$Result = (r_U/r_S) \times (C_S/C_U) \times (1/F) \times 100$$

r_U = peak response of any individual impurity from the *Sample solution*
r_S = peak response of clarithromycin from *Standard solution 3*
C_S = concentration of USP Clarithromycin RS in *Standard solution 3* (mg/mL)
C_U = concentration of Clarithromycin in the *Sample solution* (mg/mL)
F = relative response factor (see *Table 2*)
Acceptance criteria: ■1S (USP41) The reporting threshold is 0.1%. Disregard the peaks eluting before impurity I and after impurity H.
Any individual impurity: NMT 1.0%. NMT four impurities exceed 0.4%.
Total impurities: NMT 3.5%

Table 2

Name	Relative Retention Time	Relative Response Factor
Clarithromycin impurity I[a]	0.38	1.0
Clarithromycin impurity A[b] (clarithromycin F)	0.42	1.0
Clarithromycin impurity J[c]	0.63	1.0
Clarithromycin impurity L[d]	0.74	1.0
Clarithromycin impurity B[e]	0.79	1.0
Clarithromycin impurity M[f]	0.81	1.0
Clarithromycin impurity C[g]	0.89	1.0
Clarithromycin impurity D[h]	0.96	1.0
Clarithromycin	1.0	—
Clarithromycin impurity N[i]	1.15	1.0
Clarithromycin related compound A[j]	1.27	1.0
Clarithromycin impurity F[k]	1.33	1.0
Clarithromycin impurity P[l]	1.35	1.0
Clarithromycin impurity O[m]	1.38	1.0

[a] 3-O-Decladinosyl-6-O-methylerythromycin A.
[b] 2-Demethyl-2-(hydroxymethyl)-6-O-methylerythromycin A.
[c] Erythromycin A (E)-9-oxime.
[d] 6-O-Methylerythromycin (Z)-9-oxime.
[e] 6-O-Methyl-15-norerythromycin A.
[f] 3''-N-Demethyl-6-O-methylerythromycin A (E)-9-oxime.
[g] 6-O-Methylerythromycin A (E)-9-oxime.
[h] 3''-N-Demethyl-6-O-methylerythromycin A.
[i] (10E)-10,11-Didehydro-11-deoxy-6-O-methylerythromycin A.
[j] 6,11-Di-O-methylerythromycin A.
[k] 6,12-Di-O-methylerythromycin A.
[l] 4',6-Di-O-methylerythromycin A.
[m] 6-O-Methylerythromycin A (Z)-9-(O-methyloxime).
[n] (1S,2R,5R,6S,7S,8R,9R,11Z)-2-Ethyl-6-hydroxy-9-methoxy-1,5,7,9,11,13-hexamethyl-8-[[3,4,6-trideoxy-3-(dimethylamino)-β-D-xylo-hexapyranosyl]oxy]-3,15-dioxabicyclo[10.2.1]pentadeca-11,13-dien-4-one (3-O-decladinosyl-8,9:10,11-dianhydro-6-O-methylerythromycin A)-9,12-hemiketal.
[o] 6-O-Methylerythromycin A (E)-9-(O-methyloxime).
[p] 3''-N-Demethyl-3'-N-formyl-6-O-methylerythromycin A.

Table 2 (Continued)

Name	Relative Retention Time	Relative Response Factor
Clarithromycin impurity K[n]	1.59	1.0
Clarithromycin impurity G[o]	1.72	3.7
Clarithromycin impurity H[p]	1.82	6.7

[a] 3-O-Decladinosyl-6-O-methylerythromycin A.
[b] 2-Demethyl-2-(hydroxymethyl)-6-O-methylerythromycin A.
[c] Erythromycin A (E)-9-oxime.
[d] 6-O-Methylerythromycin (Z)-9-oxime.
[e] 6-O-Methyl-15-norerythromycin A.
[f] 3″-N-Demethyl-6-O-methylerythromycin A (E)-9-oxime.
[g] 6-O-Methylerythromycin A (E)-9-oxime.
[h] 3″-N-Demethyl-6-O-methylerythromycin A.
[i] (10E)-10,11-Didehydro-11-deoxy-6-O-methylerythromycin A.
[j] 6,11-Di-O-methylerythromycin A.
[k] 6,12-Di-O-methylerythromycin A.
[l] 4′,6-Di-O-methylerythromycin A.
[m] 6-O-Methylerythromycin A (Z)-9-(O-methyloxime).
[n] (1S,2R,5R,6S,7S,8R,9R,11Z)-2-Ethyl-6-hydroxy-9-methoxy-1,5,7,9,11,13-hexamethyl-8-[[3,4,6-trideoxy-3-(dimethylamino)-β-D-xylo-hexapyranosyl]oxy]-3,15-dioxabicyclo[10.2.1]pentadeca-11,13-dien-4-one (3-O-decladinosyl-8,9:10,11-dianhydro-6-O-methylerythromycin A)-9,12-hemiketal.
[o] 6-O-Methylerythromycin A (E)-9-(O-methyloxime).
[p] 3″-N-Demethyl-3′-N-formyl-6-O-methylerythromycin A.

SPECIFIC TESTS
• **OPTICAL ROTATION ⟨781S⟩**, *Procedures, Specific Rotation*
  Sample solution: 10 mg/mL in methylene chloride
  Acceptance criteria: −94° to −102° (at 20°)
• **CRYSTALLINITY ⟨695⟩:** Meets the requirements
• **PH ⟨791⟩**
  Sample: 2-mg/mL suspension in methanol and water (1:19)
  Acceptance criteria: 8.0–10.0
• **WATER DETERMINATION ⟨921⟩**, *Method I:* NMT 2.0%

ADDITIONAL REQUIREMENTS
• **PACKAGING AND STORAGE:** Preserve in tight containers.
• **USP REFERENCE STANDARDS ⟨11⟩**
  USP Clarithromycin RS
  USP Clarithromycin Identity RS
  This is a mixture of clarithromycin, clarithromycin impurity D (3″-N-demethyl-6-O-methylerythromycin A; $C_{37}H_{67}NO_{13}$; 733.9), and other impurities.

Colchicine

$C_{22}H_{25}NO_6$ 399.44
Acetamide, N-(5,6,7,9-tetrahydro-1,2,3,10-tetramethoxy-9-oxobenzo[a]heptalen-7-yl)-, (S)-;
Colchicine [64-86-8].

DEFINITION
Colchicine is an alkaloid contained in various species of *Colchicum* and in other genera. It contains NLT 94.0% and

NMT 101.0% of colchicine ($C_{22}H_{25}NO_6$), calculated on the anhydrous, solvent-free basis.
[CAUTION—Colchicine is extremely poisonous.]

IDENTIFICATION
• **A. INFRARED ABSORPTION ⟨197K⟩**
  [NOTE—Disregard any peak occurring at 1735 cm⁻¹.]

ASSAY

Change to read:

• **PROCEDURE**
  [NOTE—Perform all dilutions in low-actinic glassware.]
  Mobile phase: Dilute 45 mL of 0.5 M monobasic potassium phosphate with water to 450 mL. Add 530 mL of methanol, cool to room temperature, and add methanol to bring the volume to 1000 mL. Adjust with 0.5 M phosphoric acid to a pH of 5.5 ± 0.05, and pass through a 0.45-μm membrane filter.
  Standard solution: 6 μg/mL of USP Colchicine RS in a mixture of methanol and water (1:1). This solution is stable for 4 months when stored tightly stoppered and in the dark.
  Sample solution: ■1S (USP41) 6 μg/mL of Colchicine in a mixture of methanol and water (1:1)
  Chromatographic system
  (See *Chromatography ⟨621⟩, System Suitability*.)
  Mode: LC
  Detector: UV 254 nm
  Column: 4.6-mm × 25-cm; packing L7
  Flow rate: 1.0 mL/min
  Injection volume: 20 μL
  System suitability
  Sample: *Standard solution*
  ■1S (USP41)
  Suitability requirements
  Column efficiency: NLT 4500 theoretical plates
  Relative standard deviation: NMT 2%
  Analysis
  Samples: *Standard solution* and *Sample solution*
  Measure the responses for all peaks recorded during 1.5 times the retention time for colchicine.
  Calculate the percentage of colchicine ($C_{22}H_{25}NO_6$) in the portion of Colchicine taken:

  $$Result = (r_U/r_S) \times (C_S/C_U) \times 100$$

  r_U = peak response from the *Sample solution*
  r_S = peak response from the *Standard solution*
  C_S = concentration of USP Colchicine RS in the *Standard solution* (μg/mL)
  C_U = concentration of Colchicine in the *Sample solution* (μg/mL)

  Acceptance criteria: 94.0%–101.0% on the anhydrous, solvent-free basis

IMPURITIES
• **LIMIT OF COLCHICEINE**
  Analysis: To 5 mL of a 10-mg/mL solution of colchicine, add 2 drops of ferric chloride TS.
  Acceptance criteria: No definite green color is produced.

Change to read:

• **LIMIT OF ETHYL ACETATE**
  ■**Internal standard solution:** Dilute 0.5 mL of n-propyl alcohol with water to 100 mL.
  Standard solution: Transfer 1.0 mL of ethyl acetate, 0.5 mL of diacetone alcohol, and 0.5 mL of n-propyl alcohol to a 1000-mL volumetric flask and dilute with water to volume. Mix well. This solution contains 0.9 mg/mL of ethyl acetate.

Sample solution: Add 250 mg of Colchicine, accurately weighed, to a 10-mL volumetric flask, and dissolve in about 8.0 mL of water. Add 1.0 mL of *Internal standard solution*, dilute with water to volume, and mix well.

Chromatographic system
(See *Chromatography* ⟨621⟩, *System Suitability*.)
Mode: GC
Detector: Flame ionization
Column: 0.53-mm × 30-m; coated with a 1-µm film of phase G16
Temperatures
Injection port: 180°
Detector: 220°
Column: See *Table 1*.

Table 1

Initial Temperature (°)	Temperature Ramp (°/min)	Final Temperature (°)	Hold Time at Final Temperature (min)
40	0	40	20
40	20	200	10

Carrier gas: Helium
Flow rate: 5.72 mL/min
Injection volume: 2 µL
Injection type: Split ratio, 15:1
System suitability
Sample: *Standard solution*
Suitability requirements
Tailing factor: NMT 2.0 for the menthol peak
Relative standard deviation: NMT 15.0% for the peak response ratios of ethyl acetate to the *n*-propyl alcohol peak, and of diacetone alcohol to the *n*-propyl alcohol peak, in replicate injections
Analysis
Samples: *Standard solution* and *Sample solution*
Calculate the percentage of ethyl acetate in the portion of Colchicine taken:

$$\text{Result} = (R_U/R_S) \times (C_S/C_U) \times 100$$

R_U = peak response ratio of ethyl acetate to *n*-propyl alcohol from the *Sample solution*
R_S = peak response ratio of ethyl acetate to *n*-propyl alcohol from the *Standard solution*
C_S = concentration of ethyl acetate in the *Standard solution* (mg/mL)
C_U = concentration of Colchicine in the *Sample solution* (mg/mL)■1S (USP41)
Acceptance criteria: NMT 8.0%
• CHROMATOGRAPHIC PURITY
Procedure: Proceed as directed in the *Assay*.
Acceptance criteria: NMT 5.0% other than that due to colchicine, eluting within 1.5 times the retention time for colchicine
• RESIDUAL SOLVENTS ⟨467⟩: Meets the requirements, except that the limit of chloroform is 100 ppm

SPECIFIC TESTS
• OPTICAL ROTATION ⟨781S⟩, *Procedures, Specific Rotation*
Sample solution: 10 mg/mL, in alcohol
Acceptance criteria: −240° to −250°, calculated on the anhydrous, solvent-free basis
• WATER DETERMINATION ⟨921⟩, *Method I*: NMT 2.0%

ADDITIONAL REQUIREMENTS
• PACKAGING AND STORAGE: Preserve in tight, light-resistant containers.
• USP REFERENCE STANDARDS ⟨11⟩
USP Colchicine RS

Delete the following:

■Cortisone Acetate Injectable Suspension

» Cortisone Acetate Injectable Suspension is a sterile suspension of Cortisone Acetate in a suitable aqueous medium. It contains not less than 90.0 percent and not more than 110.0 percent of the labeled amount of cortisone acetate ($C_{23}H_{30}O_6$).

Packaging and storage—Preserve in single-dose or multiple-dose containers, preferably of Type I glass.
USP Reference standards ⟨11⟩—
USP Cortisone Acetate RS
Identification—Mix 25 mL of water with a volume of Injectable Suspension equivalent to about 25 mg of cortisone acetate. Centrifuge, or allow the insoluble material to settle, then decant and discard the supernatant. Add 20 mL of methanol and, using agitation and warming as necessary, dissolve the residue. Evaporate the solvent on a steam bath with the aid of a current of air, then dry the residue at 105° for 30 minutes: the residue so obtained responds to *Identification* test A under *Cortisone Acetate*.
pH ⟨791⟩: between 5.0 and 7.0.
Other requirements—It meets the requirements under *Injections and Implanted Drug Products* ⟨1⟩.
Assay—
Mobile phase—Prepare as directed in the *Assay* under *Cortisone Acetate Tablets*.
Internal standard solution—Prepare a solution of prednisone in *Mobile phase* having a concentration of 0.5 mg per mL.
Standard preparation—Transfer about 12 mg of USP Cortisone Acetate RS, accurately weighed, to a stoppered, 50-mL conical flask. Add 20.0 mL of *Internal standard solution*, and sonicate for 5 minutes. Pass a portion through a polytef syringe filter, then combine 1 mL of the filtrate and 4 mL of *Mobile phase* to obtain the *Standard preparation*.
Resolution solution—Dissolve a quantity of hydrocortisone acetate in the *Standard preparation* to obtain a solution containing about 0.1 mg of hydrocortisone acetate per mL.
Assay preparation—Using a pipet calibrated "to contain," transfer 2.0 mL of freshly mixed Injectable Suspension to a volumetric flask of a size to give a cortisone acetate concentration of 2 mg per mL when diluted to volume. Rinse the suspension remaining in the pipet into the flask with isopropyl alcohol, dilute with isopropyl alcohol to volume, and sonicate for 3 minutes. Deliver a 3.0-mL aliquot of this solution to a stoppered, 25-mL conical flask, and evaporate on a steam bath with the aid of a current of air to dryness. Add 10.0 mL of *Internal standard solution*, insert the stopper, and sonicate for 5 minutes. Pass a portion through a polytef syringe filter, then combine approximately 1 mL of the filtrate and 4 mL of *Mobile phase* to obtain the *Assay preparation*.
Chromatographic system(see *Chromatography* ⟨621⟩)—Prepare as directed in the *Assay* under *Cortisone Acetate Tablets*. Chromatograph the *Resolution solution*, and record the peak responses as directed for *Procedure:* the resolution, *R*, between cortisone acetate and hydrocortisone acetate is not less than 2.2 (if necessary, add equal parts of *n*-butyl chloride and water-saturated *n*-butyl chloride to the *Mobile phase* to meet this requirement). Chromatograph the *Standard preparation*, and record the peak responses as directed for *Procedure:* the relative retention times are 0.6 for cortisone acetate and 1.0 for prednisone; and the relative stan-

dard deviation for replicate injections is not more than 2.0%.

Procedure—Proceed as directed in the *Assay* under *Cortisone Acetate Tablets*. Calculate the quantity, in mg, of cortisone acetate ($C_{23}H_{30}O_6$) in each mL of the Injectable Suspension taken by the formula:

$$W(V / 12)(R_U / R_S)$$

in which *V* is the capacity, in mL, of the volumetric flask used for the *Assay preparation*; and the other terms are as defined therein.
■1S (USP41)

Cyclopentolate Hydrochloride

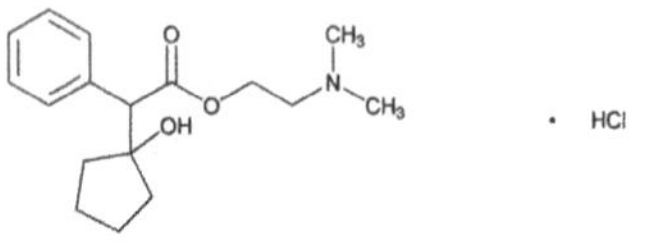

$C_{17}H_{25}NO_3 \cdot HCl$　　　　　　　　　327.85
Benzeneacetic acid, α-(1-hydroxycyclopentyl)-, 2-(dimethylamino)ethyl ester, hydrochloride, (±)-;
2-(Dimethylamino)ethyl (±)-1-hydroxy-α-phenylcyclopentaneacetate hydrochloride [5870-29-1].

DEFINITION
Cyclopentolate Hydrochloride contains NLT 98.0% and NMT 102.0% of cyclopentolate hydrochloride ($C_{17}H_{25}NO_3 \cdot HCl$), calculated on the dried basis.

IDENTIFICATION
• **A. INFRARED ABSORPTION ⟨197K⟩**

Add the following:

■• **B.** The retention time of the major peak of the *Sample solution* corresponds to that of the *Standard solution*, as obtained in the *Assay*.■1S (USP41)

Change to read:

• ■**C.**■1S (USP41) **IDENTIFICATION TESTS—GENERAL ⟨191⟩**, *Chemical Identification Tests, Chloride*
　Sample solution: 2 mg/mL
　Acceptance criteria: Meets the requirements

ASSAY

Change to read:

• **PROCEDURE**
　Buffer solution: Dissolve 660 mg of dibasic ammonium phosphate in 1000 mL of water. Adjust with phosphoric acid to a pH of 3.0 ± 0.1.
　Mobile phase: Acetonitrile and *Buffer solution* (7:3)
　Standard solution: 0.1 mg/mL of USP Cyclopentolate Hydrochloride RS in water
　Sample solution: 0.1 mg/mL of Cyclopentolate Hydrochloride in water
　Chromatographic system
　(See *Chromatography ⟨621⟩, System Suitability.*)

Mode: LC
Detector: UV 220 nm
Column: 4.6-mm × 15-cm; ■5-µm■1S (USP41) packing L15
Flow rate: 2 mL/min
Injection volume: 20 µL
System suitability
　Sample: *Standard solution*
　Suitability requirements
　■■1S (USP41)
　Tailing factor: NMT 2.0
　Relative standard deviation: NMT 2.0%
Analysis
　Samples: *Standard solution* and *Sample solution*
　Calculate the percentage of cyclopentolate hydrochloride ($C_{17}H_{25}NO_3 \cdot HCl$) in the portion of Cyclopentolate Hydrochloride taken:

$$Result = (r_U/r_S) \times (C_S/C_U) \times 100$$

r_U　= peak response from the *Sample solution*
r_S　= peak response from the *Standard solution*
C_S　= concentration of USP Cyclopentolate Hydrochloride RS in the *Standard solution* (mg/mL)
C_U　= concentration of Cyclopentolate Hydrochloride in the *Sample solution* (mg/mL)
Acceptance criteria: 98.0%–102.0% on the dried basis

IMPURITIES
• **RESIDUE ON IGNITION ⟨281⟩**: NMT 0.05%
• **ORGANIC IMPURITIES**
　Buffer solution, Mobile phase, Standard solution, Sample solution, Chromatographic system, and System suitability: Proceed as directed in the *Assay*, except for the *Run time*.
　Run time: NLT twice the retention time of cyclopentolate
　Analysis
　Sample: *Sample solution*
　Calculate the percentage of each impurity in the portion of Cyclopentolate Hydrochloride taken:

$$Result = (r_U/r_T) \times 100$$

r_U　= peak response of each impurity from the *Sample solution*
r_T　= sum of the responses of all of the peaks, excluding the solvent peak, from the *Sample solution*
　Acceptance criteria
　Individual impurity: NMT 1.0%
　Total impurities: NMT 2.0%

SPECIFIC TESTS
• **PH ⟨791⟩**
　Sample solution: 10 mg/mL
　Acceptance criteria: 4.5–5.5
• **LOSS ON DRYING ⟨731⟩**
　Sample: Dry at 105° for 4 h.
　Acceptance criteria: NMT 0.5%

ADDITIONAL REQUIREMENTS
• **PACKAGING AND STORAGE:** Preserve in tight containers, and store in a cold place.
• **USP REFERENCE STANDARDS ⟨11⟩**
　USP Cyclopentolate Hydrochloride RS

Delete the following:

■Dexamethasone Sodium Phosphate Inhalation Aerosol

» Dexamethasone Sodium Phosphate Inhalation Aerosol is a suspension, in suitable propellants and alcohol, in a pressurized container, of dexamethasone sodium phosphate ($C_{22}H_{28}FNa_2O_8P$) equivalent to not less than 90.0 percent and not more than 110.0 percent of the labeled amount of dexamethasone phosphate ($C_{22}H_{30}FO_8P$).

Packaging and storage—Preserve in tight, pressurized containers, and avoid exposure to excessive heat.

USP Reference standards ⟨11⟩—
USP Dexamethasone RS

Identification—Prepare a pH 9.0 buffer solution by dissolving 3.1 g of boric acid, 203 mg of magnesium chloride, and 860 mg of sodium hydroxide in water to make 1000 mL. Dissolve 50 mg of alkaline phosphatase enzyme in 50 mL of the pH 9.0 buffer solution, and transfer 5 mL of the resulting solution to a glass-stoppered, 50-mL tube containing 5 mL of the *Assay preparation* prepared as directed in the *Assay*. Incubate at 37° for 45 minutes, add 25 mL of methylene chloride, and shake for 2 minutes: the methylene chloride extract so obtained responds to the *Identification* test under *Dexamethasone Sodium Phosphate Injection*, beginning with "Evaporate 15 mL of the methylene chloride extract."

Alcohol Determination, *Method II* ⟨611⟩: between 1.7% and 2.3% of C_2H_5OH.

Delivered dose uniformity over the entire contents: meets the requirements for *Metered-Dose Inhalers* under *Aerosols, Nasal Sprays, Metered-Dose Inhalers, and Dry Powder Inhalers* ⟨601⟩.

PROCEDURE FOR DOSE UNIFORMITY—

Standard solution—Transfer about 10 mg of USP Dexamethasone RS, accurately weighed, to a 10-mL volumetric flask, dilute with alcohol to volume, and mix. Transfer 1.0 mL of this solution to a 100-mL volumetric flask, dilute with 0.1 N sulfuric acid to volume, and mix to obtain a solution having a known concentration of about 10 μg per mL.

Test solution—Discharge the minimum recommended dose into the sampling apparatus, and detach the inhaler as directed. Rinse the apparatus (filter and interior) with two 5.0-mL portions of 0.1 N sulfuric acid, and transfer the resulting solutions quantitatively to a 50-mL centrifuge tube containing 15 mL of methylene chloride that was previously chilled in a dry ice-acetone bath for a few minutes. Insert the stopper in the centrifuge tube, and shake cautiously, releasing the pressure occasionally. Allow the phases to separate, and equilibrate to room temperature. The aqueous phase is the *Test solution*.

Procedure—Transfer the *Test solution* and 10.0 mL of the *Standard solution* into separate flasks. Add 2.0 mL of 0.1 N sulfuric acid to each, and swirl to mix. Concomitantly determine the absorbances of both solutions in 1-cm cells at the wavelength of maximum absorbance at about 239 nm, with a suitable spectrophotometer, using 0.1 N sulfuric acid as the blank. Calculate the quantity, in μg, of dexamethasone phosphate ($C_{22}H_{30}FO_8P$) contained in the minimum dose by the formula:

$$10(472.45 / 392.47)(CN)(A_U / A_S)$$

in which 472.45 and 392.47 are the molecular weights of dexamethasone phosphate and dexamethasone, respectively; *C* is the concentration, in μg per mL, of USP Dexamethasone RS in the *Standard solution*; *N* is the number of sprays discharged to obtain the minimum recommended dose; and A_U and A_S are the absorbances of the solutions from the *Test solution* and the *Standard solution*, respectively.

Assay—

Standard preparation—Transfer about 40 mg of USP Dexamethasone RS, accurately weighed, to a 50-mL volumetric flask, dilute with alcohol to volume, and mix. Transfer 5.0 mL of this solution to a 500-mL volumetric flask, dilute with 0.1 N sulfuric acid to volume, and mix to obtain a solution having a known concentration of about 8 μg per mL.

Assay preparation—Weigh accurately a filled Inhalation Aerosol container, and record the weight (W_1). Place the container in a dry ice-acetone bath, and cool for 60 minutes. Remove the container from the bath, and carefully remove the valve with wire cutters, taking precautions to save all pieces of the valve and cap. With the aid of four 5-mL portions of 0.1 N sulfuric acid, transfer the contents of the container to a beaker previously chilled in the bath. Dry the rinsed empty container and all of its parts in an oven at 105° for 2 hours, cool, and weigh (W_2). Allow the contents of the beaker to warm to room temperature. After the bulk of the propellant has evaporated, quantitatively transfer the contents of the beaker, with the aid of several mL of 0.1 N sulfuric acid, to a 200-mL volumetric flask, dilute with 0.1 N sulfuric acid to volume, and mix. Transfer about 20 mL of this solution to a centrifuge tube, add 10 mL of methylene chloride, shake vigorously for 1 minute, and centrifuge. Pipet 10 mL of the clear supernatant into a 100-mL volumetric flask, dilute with 0.1 N sulfuric acid to volume, and mix.

Procedure—Concomitantly determine the absorbances of the *Assay preparation* and the *Standard preparation* in 1-cm cells at the wavelength of maximum absorbance at about 239 nm, with a suitable spectrophotometer, using 0.1 N sulfuric acid as the blank. Calculate the quantity, in mg, of dexamethasone phosphate ($C_{22}H_{30}FO_8P$) in each g of Inhalation Aerosol taken by the formula:

$$2(472.45 / 392.47)(A_U / A_S)[C / (W_1 - W_2)]$$

in which 472.45 and 392.47 are the molecular weights of dexamethasone phosphate and dexamethasone, respectively, A_U and A_S are the absorbances of the solutions from the *Assay preparation* and the *Standard preparation*, respectively, *C* is the concentration, in μg per mL, of USP Dexamethasone RS in the *Standard preparation*, and W_1 and W_2 are the weights, in g, as previously defined.
■1S (USP41)

Dorzolamide Hydrochloride and Timolol Maleate Ophthalmic Solution

DEFINITION

Dorzolamide Hydrochloride and Timolol Maleate Ophthalmic Solution is a sterile, isotonic, buffered, slightly viscous, aqueous solution of Dorzolamide Hydrochloride and Timolol Maleate. It contains an amount of dorzolamide hydrochloride ($C_{10}H_{16}N_2O_4S_3 \cdot$ HCl) equivalent to NLT 90.0% and NMT 110.0% of the labeled amount of dorzolamide ($C_{10}H_{16}N_2O_4S_3$), and also contains an amount of timolol maleate ($C_{13}H_{24}N_4O_3S \cdot C_4H_4O_4$) equivalent to NLT 90.0% and NMT 110.0% of the labeled amount of timolol ($C_{13}H_{24}N_4O_3S$). It may contain a suitable preservative.

IDENTIFICATION

- **A. THIN-LAYER CHROMATOGRAPHIC IDENTIFICATION TEST ⟨201⟩**

  Standard solution A: 1.5 mg/mL of USP Timolol Maleate RS in methanol

  Standard solution B: 5.0 mg/mL of USP Dorzolamide Hydrochloride RS in methanol

  Sample solution: Nominally equivalent to 5.0 mg/mL of dorzolamide from Ophthalmic Solution in methanol

  Chromatographic system

  Adsorbent: 0.25-mm layer of chromatographic silica gel mixture or equivalent

  Application volume: 20 µL

  Developing solvent system: Methylene chloride, methanol, and ammonium hydroxide (80:20:1)

  Analysis: Spot *Standard solution A*, *Standard solution B*, and the *Sample solution* approximately 2 cm from the bottom of the plate. Evaporate the solvent using a current of air. Saturate the developing tank with the *Developing solvent system*, and equilibrate for approximately 1 h prior to use. Develop the chromatogram in the *Developing solvent system* until the solvent front has moved about three-fourths of the length of the plate. Remove the plate from the developing tank, and allow the plate to air-dry in a fume hood. Examine the plate under short-wavelength UV light at 254 nm, or expose to iodine vapors.

  Acceptance criteria: The R_F values of the principal spots from the *Sample solution* correspond to the principal spots obtained from *Standard solution A* and *Standard solution B*.

- **B.** The retention time of the major peak of the *Sample solution* corresponds to that of the *Standard solution*, as obtained in the *Assay* for *Procedure 1: Dorzolamide*.

- **C.** The retention time of the major peak of the *Sample solution* corresponds to that of the *Standard solution*, as obtained in the *Assay* for *Procedure 2: Timolol*.

ASSAY

- **PROCEDURE 1: DORZOLAMIDE**

  Solution A: Acetonitrile

  Solution B: 0.2% (v/v) phosphoric acid in water

  Mobile phase: See *Table 1*.

Table 1

Time (min)	Solution A (%)	Solution B (%)
0	5	95
15.0	5	95
15.1	95	5
20.0	95	5
20.1	5	95
30.0	5	95

Diluent: Acetonitrile and *Solution B* (5:95)

Standard solution: 0.11 mg/mL of USP Dorzolamide Hydrochloride RS and 0.5 µg/mL each of USP Dorzolamide Related Compound B RS and USP Dorzolamide Related Compound D RS in *Diluent*

Sample solution: Nominally equivalent to 0.1 mg/mL of dorzolamide from Ophthalmic Solution in *Diluent*

Chromatographic system

(See *Chromatography* ⟨621⟩, *System Suitability*.)

Mode: LC

Detector: UV 253 nm

Column: 4.6-mm × 25-cm; 5-µm packing L7

Flow rate: 1.2 mL/min

Injection volume: 20 µL

System suitability

Sample: *Standard solution*

[NOTE—See *Table 2* for the relative retention times.]

Suitability requirements

Resolution: NLT 3.0 between dorzolamide and dorzolamide related compound D; NLT 3.0 between dorzolamide and dorzolamide related compound B

Relative standard deviation: NMT 2.0% for the dorzolamide peak

Analysis

Samples: *Standard solution* and *Sample solution*

Calculate the percentage of the labeled amount of dorzolamide ($C_{10}H_{16}N_2O_4S_3$) in the portion of Ophthalmic Solution taken:

$$Result = (r_U/r_S) \times (C_S/C_U) \times (M_{r1}/M_{r2}) \times 100$$

r_U = peak response of dorzolamide from the *Sample solution*

r_S = peak response of dorzolamide from the *Standard solution*

C_S = concentration of USP Dorzolamide Hydrochloride RS in the *Standard solution* (mg/mL)

C_U = nominal concentration of dorzolamide in the *Sample solution* (mg/mL)

M_{r1} = molecular weight of dorzolamide, 324.44

M_{r2} = molecular weight of dorzolamide hydrochloride, 360.90

Acceptance criteria: 90.0%–110.0%

Change to read:

- **PROCEDURE 2: TIMOLOL**

  Buffer: Transfer 22 g of monobasic sodium phosphate into a 2000-mL volumetric flask. Dissolve in 1995 mL of water, and adjust with phosphoric acid to a pH of 2.8. Dilute with water to volume.

  Mobile phase: Methanol and *Buffer* (40:60)

  System suitability solution: Transfer 88 mg of USP Timolol Maleate RS into a 50-mL volumetric flask. Transfer 8 mL of 0.1 M sodium hydroxide into the flask, mix, and heat at 70° for 15 h. Dilute with *Mobile phase* to volume, and mix well. Transfer 5 mL of this solution into a 25-mL volumetric flask, and add 28 mg of USP Dorzolamide Hydrochloride RS into the same flask. Dilute with *Mobile phase* to volume. [NOTE—The preparation generates timolol impurity G and timolol ■related compound■$_{1S\ (USP41)}$ B.]

  Standard solution: 0.35 mg/mL of USP Timolol Maleate RS in *Mobile phase*

  Sample solution: Nominally equivalent to 0.25 mg/mL of timolol from Ophthalmic Solution in *Mobile phase*

  Chromatographic system

  (See *Chromatography* ⟨621⟩, *System Suitability*.)

  Mode: LC

  Detector: UV 295 nm

  Column: 4.6-mm × 25-cm; 5-µm packing L1

  Column temperature: 40°

  Flow rate: 1 mL/min

  Injection volume: 20 µL

  System suitability

  Sample: *System suitability solution*

  [NOTE—See *Table 3* for the relative retention times.]

  Suitability requirements

  Resolution: NLT 1.5 between timolol impurity G and timolol ■related compound■$_{1S\ (USP41)}$ B

  Relative standard deviation: NMT 2.5% for timolol for five replicate injections

Analysis

Samples: *Standard solution* and *Sample solution*

Calculate the percentage of the labeled amount of timolol ($C_{13}H_{24}N_4O_3S$) in the portion of Ophthalmic Solution taken:

$$Result = (r_U/r_S) \times (C_S/C_U) \times (M_{r1}/M_{r2}) \times 100$$

r_U = peak response from the *Sample solution*
r_S = peak response from the *Standard solution*
C_S = concentration of USP Timolol Maleate RS in the *Standard solution* (mg/mL)
C_U = nominal concentration of timolol in the *Sample solution* (mg/mL)
M_{r1} = molecular weight of timolol, 316.42
M_{r2} = molecular weight of timolol maleate, 432.49

Acceptance criteria: 90.0%–110.0%

IMPURITIES

Change to read:

- **ORGANIC IMPURITIES: DORZOLAMIDE HYDROCHLORIDE**
  Mobile phase, Standard solution, Sample solution, and Chromatographic system: Proceed as directed in the *Assay* for *Procedure 1: Dorzolamide.*
  System suitability
  Sample: *Standard solution*
  Suitability requirements
  Resolution: NLT 3.0 between dorzolamide and dorzolamide related compound D; NLT 3.0 between dorzolamide and dorzolamide related compound B
  Relative standard deviation: NMT 2.0% for dorzolamide
  Analysis
  Samples: *Standard solution* and *Sample solution*
  Calculate the percentage of dorzolamide related compound D in the portion of Ophthalmic Solution taken:

  $$Result = (r_U/r_S) \times (C_S/C_U) \times (M_{r1}/M_{r2}) \times 100$$

  r_U = peak area of dorzolamide related compound D from the *Sample solution*
  r_S = peak area of dorzolamide related compound D from the *Standard solution*
  C_S = concentration of USP Dorzolamide Related Compound D RS in the *Standard solution* (mg/mL)
  C_U = nominal concentration of dorzolamide in the *Sample solution* (mg/mL)
  M_{r1} = molecular weight of dorzolamide, 324.44
  M_{r2} = molecular weight of dorzolamide related compound D, 332.85

  Calculate the percentage of dorzolamide related compound B in the portion of Ophthalmic Solution taken:

  $$Result = (r_U/r_S) \times (C_S/C_U) \times (M_{r1}/M_{r2}) \times 100$$

  r_U = peak area of dorzolamide related compound B from the *Sample solution*
  r_S = peak area of dorzolamide related compound B from the *Standard solution*
  C_S = concentration of USP Dorzolamide Related Compound B RS in the *Standard solution* (mg/mL)
  C_U = nominal concentration of dorzolamide in the *Sample solution* (mg/mL)
  M_{r1} = molecular weight of dorzolamide, 324.44
  M_{r2} = molecular weight of dorzolamide related compound B, 360.90

  Calculate the percentage of any individual unspecified impurity in the portion of Ophthalmic Solution taken:

  $$Result = (r_U/r_T) \times 100$$

r_U = peak area of any individual unspecified impurity from the *Sample solution*
r_T = sum of all the peak areas from the *Sample solution*

Acceptance criteria: See *Table 2.* ■The reporting threshold is 0.10%.■₁S (USP41)

Table 2

Name	Relative Retention Time	Acceptance Criteria, NMT (%)
Maleic acid	0.33	Disregard
Dorzolamide related compound D■₁S (USP41)	0.83	0.5
Dorzolamide	1.00	—
Dorzolamide related compound B■₁S (USP41)	1.17	2.0
Any individual unspecified impurity	—	0.5
Total impurities■ₐ₁S (USP41)	—	3.0

ₐ ■It is the sum of all impurities in *Table 2* and dorzolamide maleic acid adducts in *Table 5.*■₁S (USP41)

Change to read:

- **ORGANIC IMPURITIES: TIMOLOL MALEATE**
  Mobile phase, System suitability solution, and Sample solution: Prepare as directed in the *Assay* for *Procedure 2: Timolol.*
  Standard stock solution: Use the *Standard solution* as prepared in the *Assay* for *Procedure 2: Timolol.*
  Standard solution: 3.5 µg/mL of USP Timolol Maleate RS from the *Standard stock solution* in *Mobile phase*
  Chromatographic system: Proceed as directed in the *Assay* for *Procedure 2: Timolol* except for the *Run time.*
  Run time: NLT 2 times the retention time of timolol
  System suitability
  Sample: *System suitability solution*
  Suitability requirements
  Resolution: NLT 1.5 between timolol impurity G and timolol ■related compound■₁S (USP41) B
  Relative standard deviation: NMT 2.5% for timolol for five replicate injections
  Analysis
  Samples: *Sample solution* and *Standard solution*
  Calculate the percentage of each impurity in the portion of Ophthalmic Solution taken:

  $$Result = (r_U/r_S) \times (C_S/C_U) \times (M_{r1}/M_{r2}) \times 100$$

  r_U = peak area of each impurity from the *Sample solution*
  r_S = peak area of timolol from the *Standard solution*
  C_S = concentration of USP Timolol Maleate RS in the *Standard solution* (mg/mL)
  C_U = nominal concentration of timolol in the *Sample solution* (mg/mL)
  M_{r1} = molecular weight of timolol, 316.42
  M_{r2} = molecular weight of timolol maleate, 432.49

  Acceptance criteria: See *Table 3.* ■The reporting threshold is 0.10%.■₁S (USP41)

Table 3

Name	Relative Retention Time	Acceptance Criteria, NMT (%)
Dorzolamide and maleic acid	0.49	Disregard
Timolol impurity G[a]	0.58	0.5
Timolol ■related compound■1S (USP41) B[b]	0.70	1.0
Timolol	1.00	—
Timolol ■related compound■1S (USP41) D[c]	1.51	0.5
Any individual unspecified impurity	—	0.6
Total impurities	—	2.0

[a] 4-Morpholino-1,2,5-thiadiazol-3-ol 1-oxide.
[b] 3-(*tert*-Butylamino)-2-(4-morpholino-1,2,5-thiadiazol-3-yloxy)propan-1-ol.
[c] 4-Morpholino-1,2,5-thiadiazol-3-ol.

Add the following:

■• LIMIT OF DORZOLAMIDE MALEIC ACID ADDUCTS
   Solution A, Solution B, Standard solution, Sample solution, Chromatographic system, and **System suitability:** Proceed as directed in the *Assay* for *Procedure 1: Dorzolamide.*
   Mobile phase: See *Table 4.* Return to original conditions and re-equilibrate the system for 6 min.

Table 4

Time (min)	Solution A (%)	Solution B (%)
0	5	95
15.0	5	95
15.1	13	87
20.0	13	87
25.0	95	5
29.0	95	5

Analysis
   Samples: *Standard solution* and *Sample solution*
   Calculate the percentage of dorzolamide maleic acid adduct in the portion of Ophthalmic Solution taken:

$$\text{Result} = (r_U/r_S) \times (C_S/C_U) \times (M_{r1}/M_{r2}) \times 100$$

r_U = peak area of dorzolamide maleic acid adduct from the *Sample solution*
r_S = peak area of dorzolamide from the *Standard solution*
C_S = concentration of USP Dorzolamide Hydrochloride RS in the *Standard solution* (mg/mL)
C_U = nominal concentration of dorzolamide in the *Sample solution* (mg/mL)
M_{r1} = molecular weight of dorzolamide, 324.44
M_{r2} = molecular weight of dorzolamide hydrochloride, 360.90
   Acceptance criteria: See *Table 5.*

Table 5

Name	Relative Retention Time	Acceptance Criteria, NMT (%)
Dorzolamide	1.00	—

[a] The chromatographic system resolves the two epimers from each other.
[b] N-Ethyl-N-[(4S,6S)-6-methyl-7,7-dioxido-2-sulfamoyl-5,6-dihydro-4H-thieno[2,3-b]thiopyran-4-yl]aspartic acid.

Table 5 *(Continued)*

Name	Relative Retention Time	Acceptance Criteria, NMT (%)
Dorzolamide maleic acid adducts[a],[b]	1.71	0.5
	1.78	0.5

[a] The chromatographic system resolves the two epimers from each other.
[b] N-Ethyl-N-[(4S,6S)-6-methyl-7,7-dioxido-2-sulfamoyl-5,6-dihydro-4H-thieno[2,3-b]thiopyran-4-yl]aspartic acid.

■1S (USP41)

SPECIFIC TESTS
• **STERILITY TESTS ⟨71⟩:** Meets the requirements
• **PH ⟨791⟩:** 5.4–5.9 at 22°

ADDITIONAL REQUIREMENTS
• **PACKAGING AND STORAGE:** Preserve in tight containers protected from light, at controlled room temperature.

Change to read:

• **USP REFERENCE STANDARDS ⟨11⟩**
   USP Dorzolamide Hydrochloride RS
   USP Dorzolamide Related Compound B RS
   ■(4RS,6SR)-4-(Ethylamino)-6-methyl-5,6-dihydro-4H-thieno[2,3-b]thiopyran-2-sulfonamide 7,7-dioxide hydrochloride.■1S (USP41)
   $C_{10}H_{16}N_2O_4S_3 \cdot HCl$ 360.90
   USP Dorzolamide Related Compound D RS
   (4S,6S)-4-Amino-6-methyl-5,6-dihydro-4H-thieno[2,3-b]thiopyran-2-sulfonamide 7,7-dioxide hydrochloride.
   $C_8H_{12}N_2O_4S_3 \cdot HCl$ 332.85
   USP Timolol Maleate RS

Doxycycline Hyclate Capsules

DEFINITION
Doxycycline Hyclate Capsules contain the equivalent of NLT 90.0% and NMT 120.0% of the labeled amount of doxycycline ($C_{22}H_{24}N_2O_8$).

IDENTIFICATION
• **A.** The retention time of the major peak of the *Sample solution* corresponds to that of the *Standard solution*, as obtained in the *Assay.*

Add the following:

■• B. INFRARED ABSORPTION ⟨197A⟩
   Standard solution: Transfer about 25 mg of USP Doxycycline Hyclate RS to a suitable flask. Add 25 mL of acetonitrile and mix for approximately 5 min with a magnetic stir bar. Pass the solution through a suitable filter, and remove the solvent by natural evaporation or by using a rotary evaporator under vacuum.
   Sample solution: Transfer the contents of NLT 10 Capsules, equivalent to 25 mg of doxycycline hyclate, to a suitable flask. Add 25 mL of acetonitrile and mix for approximately 5 min with a magnetic stir bar. Pass the solution through a suitable filter, and remove the solvent by natural evaporation or by using a rotary evaporator under vacuum.
   Analysis: Examine the spectra of the *Standard solution* and the *Sample solution* in the range between 2000 and 650 cm⁻¹.
   Acceptance criteria: The *Sample solution* exhibits bands at about 1663, 1611, 1576, 1453, 1213, 1037, 1002, 935, and 659 cm⁻¹, similar to the *Standard solution.*
   ■1S (USP41)

ASSAY
- ### PROCEDURE
  Protect solutions containing doxycycline from light.
  Solution A: Transfer 3.1 g of monobasic potassium phosphate, 0.5 g of edetate disodium, and 0.5 mL of triethylamine to a 1000-mL volumetric flask. Add about 850 mL of water and mix. Dilute with water to volume and adjust with 1 N sodium hydroxide VS to a pH of 8.5 ± 0.2.
  Solution B: Methanol
  Mobile phase: See *Table 1*.

Table 1

Time (min)	Solution A (%)	Solution B (%)
0.0	90	10
2.0	90	10
4.0	60	40
6.0	90	10
9.0	90	10

Diluent: 0.01 N hydrochloric acid
System suitability stock solution 1: 1 mg/mL each of USP Doxycycline Related Compound A RS and USP Methacycline Hydrochloride RS in *Diluent*
System suitability stock solution 2: 1.2 mg/mL of USP Doxycycline Hyclate RS in *Diluent*
System suitability solution: Transfer 5 mL of *System suitability stock solution 2* to a 25-mL volumetric flask, heat on a steam bath for 60 min, and evaporate to dryness on a hot plate, taking care not to char the residue. Dissolve the residue in *Diluent*, add 0.5 mL of *System suitability stock solution 1*, and dilute with *Diluent* to volume. Pass the solution through a suitable filter and use the filtrate.
This solution contains a mixture of 4-epidoxycycline, doxycycline related compound A, methacycline, and doxycycline. When stored in a refrigerator, this solution may be used for 14 days.
Standard solution: 0.3 mg/mL of USP Doxycycline Hyclate RS in *Diluent*. Sonicate as needed to dissolve.
Sample solution: Nominally 0.25 mg/mL of doxycycline in *Diluent*, prepared as follows. Empty as completely as possible the contents of NLT 20 Capsules. Mix the combined contents and transfer a suitable portion of the powder to a suitable volumetric flask. Add 75% of the final volume of *Diluent*, sonicate for about 5 min, shake for about 15 min, and dilute with *Diluent* to volume. Pass a portion of this solution through a suitable filter of 0.2-μm pore size.
Chromatographic system
(See *Chromatography ⟨621⟩, System Suitability*.)
Mode: LC
Detector: UV 350 nm
Column: 2.1-mm × 5-cm; 1.7-μm packing L7. [NOTE— A 1.7-μm guard column with packing L7 was used during method validation.]
Column temperature: 60°
Flow rate: 0.6 mL/min
Injection volume: 5 μL
System suitability
Samples: *System suitability solution* and *Standard solution*
[NOTE—See *Table 2* for relative retention times.]
Suitability requirements
Resolution: NLT 1.5 between methacycline and 4-epidoxycycline; NLT 1.5 between 4-epidoxycycline and doxycycline related compound A; NLT 1.5 be-
tween doxycycline related compound A and doxycycline, *System suitability solution*
Tailing factor: NMT 1.5, *Standard solution*
Relative standard deviation: NMT 2.0%, *Standard solution*
Analysis
Samples: *Standard solution* and *Sample solution*
Calculate the percentage of the labeled amount of doxycycline ($C_{22}H_{24}N_2O_8$) in the portion of Capsules taken:

$$\text{Result} = (r_U/r_S) \times (C_S/C_U) \times P \times F \times 100$$

r_U = peak response from the *Sample solution*
r_S = peak response from the *Standard solution*
C_S = concentration of USP Doxycycline Hyclate RS in the *Standard solution* (mg/mL)
C_U = nominal concentration of doxycycline in the *Sample solution* (mg/mL)
P = potency of doxycycline in USP Doxycycline Hyclate RS (μg/mg)
F = conversion factor, 0.001 mg/μg
Acceptance criteria: 90.0%–120.0%

PERFORMANCE TESTS
- ### DISSOLUTION ⟨711⟩
  Medium: Water; 900 mL
  Apparatus 2: 75 rpm, the distance between the blade and the inside bottom of the vessel being maintained at 4.5 ± 0.5 cm during the test
  Time: 30 min
  Standard solution: USP Doxycycline Hyclate RS in *Medium*
  Sample solution: Dilute with *Medium* to a concentration that is similar to the *Standard solution*.
  Instrumental conditions
  Mode: UV
  Analytical wavelength: 276 nm
  Analysis
  Samples: *Standard solution* and *Sample solution*
  Calculate the percentage (Q) of the labeled amount of doxycycline ($C_{22}H_{24}N_2O_8$) dissolved:

$$\text{Result} = (A_U/A_S) \times (C_S/L) \times V \times 100$$

A_U = absorbance of the *Sample solution*
A_S = absorbance of the *Standard solution*
C_S = concentration of doxycycline in the *Standard solution* (mg/mL)
L = label claim (mg/Capsule)
V = volume of *Medium*, 900 mL
Tolerances: NLT 80% (Q) of the labeled amount of doxycycline ($C_{22}H_{24}N_2O_8$) is dissolved.
- ### UNIFORMITY OF DOSAGE UNITS ⟨905⟩: Meet the requirements

IMPURITIES

Change to read:

- ### ORGANIC IMPURITIES
  Mobile phase, Diluent, System suitability solution, Sample solution, and **Chromatographic system:** Proceed as directed in the *Assay*.
  Standard solution: 1.5 μg/mL of USP Doxycycline Hyclate RS in *Diluent*
  System suitability
  Samples: *System suitability solution* and *Standard solution*

Suitability requirements
Resolution: NLT 1.5 between methacycline and 4-epidoxycycline; NLT 1.5 between 4-epidoxycycline and doxycycline related compound A; NLT 1.5 between doxycycline related compound A and doxycycline, *System suitability solution*
Relative standard deviation: NMT 5.0% for the doxycycline peak, *Standard solution*
Analysis
Samples: *Sample solution* and *Standard solution*
Calculate the percentage of each impurity in the portion of Capsules taken:

$$Result = (r_U/r_S) \times (C_S/C_U) \times P \times F \times 100$$

r_U = peak response of each impurity from the *Sample solution*
r_S = peak response of doxycycline from the *Standard solution*
C_S = concentration of USP Doxycycline Hyclate RS in the *Standard solution* (mg/mL)
C_U = nominal concentration of doxycycline in the *Sample solution* (mg/mL)
P = potency of doxycycline in USP Doxycycline Hyclate RS (µg/mg)
F = conversion factor, 0.001 mg/µg
Acceptance criteria: See *Table 2*. Disregard any impurity peaks less than 0.2%.

Table 2

Name	Relative Retention Time	Acceptance Criteria, NMT (%)
Methacycline[a,b]	0.64	—
4-Epidoxycycline[c]	0.79	●1.0● (RB 1-May-2017)
Doxycycline related compound A (6-epidoxycycline)[a,d]	0.88	—
Doxycycline	1.0	—
Any individual unspecified impurity	—	0.5
Total impurities	—	2.0

[a] Process impurities are controlled in the drug substance and are not to be reported here. They are not included in total impurities.
[b] (4S,4aR,5S,5aR,12aS)-4-(Dimethylamino)-1,4,4a,5,5a,6,11,12a-octahydro-3,5,10,12,12a-pentahydroxy-6-methylene-1,11-dioxo-2-naphthacene-carboxamide.
[c] (4R,4aR,5S,5aR,6R,12aS)-4-(Dimethylamino)-1,4,4a,5,5a,6,11,12a-octahydro-3,5,10,12,12a-pentahydroxy-6-methyl-1,11-dioxo-2-naphthacenecarboxamide.
[d] (4S,4aR,5S,5aR,6S,12aS)-4-(Dimethylamino)-1,4,4a,5,5a,6,11,12a-octahydro-3,5,10,12,12a-pentahydroxy-6-methyl-1,11-dioxo-2-naphthacenecarboxamide.

ADDITIONAL REQUIREMENTS

• **PACKAGING AND STORAGE:** Preserve in tight, light-resistant containers. Store at controlled room temperature.
• **USP REFERENCE STANDARDS ⟨11⟩**
USP Doxycycline Hyclate RS
USP Doxycycline Related Compound A RS
[NOTE—May be available as a free base or a hydrochloride salt.]
(4S,4aR,5S,5aR,6S,12aS)-4-(Dimethylamino)-1,4,4a,5,5a,6,11,12a-octahydro-3,5,10,12,12a-pentahydroxy-6-methyl-1,11-dioxo-2-naphthacenecarboxamide.

$C_{22}H_{24}N_2O_8$ 444.43
(4S,4aR,5S,5aR,6S,12aS)-4-(Dimethylamino)-1,4,4a,5,5a,6,11,12a-octahydro-3,5,10,12,12a-pentahydroxy-6-methyl-1,11-dioxo-2-naphthacenecarboxamide, monohydrochloride.
$C_{22}H_{24}N_2O_8 \cdot HCl$ 480.13
USP Methacycline Hydrochloride RS

Doxycycline Hyclate Tablets

DEFINITION
Doxycycline Hyclate Tablets contain the equivalent of NLT 90.0% and NMT 120.0% of the labeled amount of doxycycline ($C_{22}H_{24}N_2O_8$).

IDENTIFICATION
• **A.** The retention time of the major peak of the *Sample solution* corresponds to that of the *Standard solution*, as obtained in the *Assay*.

Add the following:

■• **B. INFRARED ABSORPTION ⟨197A⟩**
Standard solution: Transfer about 25 mg of USP Doxycycline Hyclate RS to a suitable flask. Add 25 mL of acetonitrile and mix for approximately 5 min with a magnetic stir bar. Pass the solution through a suitable filter, and remove the solvent by natural evaporation or by using a rotary evaporator under vacuum.
Sample solution: Transfer powdered Tablets (NLT 25), equivalent to 25 mg of doxycycline hyclate, to a suitable flask. Add 25 mL of acetonitrile and mix for approximately 5 min with a magnetic stir bar. Pass the solution through a suitable filter, and remove the solvent by natural evaporation or by using a rotary evaporator under vacuum.
Analysis: Examine the spectra of the *Standard solution* and the *Sample solution* in the range between 2000 and 650 cm⁻¹.
Acceptance criteria: The *Sample solution* exhibits bands at about 1663, 1611, 1576, 1453, 1213, 1037, 1002, 935, and 659 cm⁻¹, similar to the *Standard solution*.
■1S (USP41)

ASSAY
• **PROCEDURE**
Protect solutions containing doxycycline from light.
Solution A: Transfer 3.1 g of monobasic potassium phosphate, 0.5 g of edetate disodium, and 0.5 mL of triethylamine to a 1000-mL volumetric flask. Add about 850 mL of water and mix. Dilute with water to volume and adjust with 1 N sodium hydroxide to a pH of 8.5 ± 0.2.
Solution B: Methanol
Mobile phase: See *Table 1*.

Table 1

Time (min)	Solution A (%)	Solution B (%)
0.0	90	10
2.0	90	10
4.0	60	40
6.0	90	10
9.0	90	10

Diluent: 0.01 N hydrochloric acid
System suitability stock solution 1: 1 mg/mL each of USP Doxycycline Related Compound A RS and USP Methacycline Hydrochloride RS in *Diluent*

System suitability stock solution 2: 1.2 mg/mL of USP Doxycycline Hyclate RS in *Diluent*

System suitability solution: Transfer 5 mL of *System suitability stock solution 2* to a 25-mL volumetric flask, heat on a steam bath for 60 min, and evaporate to dryness on a hot plate, taking care not to char the residue. Dissolve the residue in *Diluent*, add 0.5 mL of *System suitability stock solution 1*, and dilute with *Diluent* to volume. Pass the solution through a suitable filter and use the filtrate.

This solution contains a mixture of 4-epidoxycycline, doxycycline related compound A, methacycline, and doxycycline. When stored in a refrigerator, this solution may be used for 14 days.

Standard solution: 0.3 mg/mL of USP Doxycycline Hyclate RS in *Diluent*. Sonicate as needed to dissolve.

Sample solution: Nominally 0.25 mg/mL of doxycycline in *Diluent*, prepared as follows. Transfer a suitable portion of NLT 20 finely powdered Tablets to a suitable volumetric flask. Add 50% of the final volume of *Diluent*, sonicate for about 5 min, shake for about 15 min, and dilute with *Diluent* to volume. Pass a portion of this solution through a suitable filter of 0.2-µm pore size.

Chromatographic system
(See *Chromatography* ⟨621⟩, *System Suitability*.)
  Mode: LC
  Detector: UV 350 nm
  Column: 2.1-mm × 5-cm; 1.7-µm packing L7. [NOTE—A 1.7-µm guard column with packing L7 was used during method validation.]
  Column temperature: 60°
  Flow rate: 0.6 mL/min
  Injection volume: 5 µL

System suitability
  Samples: *System suitability solution* and *Standard solution*
  [NOTE—See *Table 2* for relative retention times.]
  Suitability requirements
    Resolution: NLT 1.5 between methacycline and 4-epidoxycycline; NLT 1.5 between 4-epidoxycycline and doxycycline related compound A; NLT 1.5 between doxycycline related compound A and doxycycline, *System suitability solution*
    Tailing factor: NMT 1.5, *Standard solution*
    Relative standard deviation: NMT 2.0%, *Standard solution*

Analysis
  Samples: *Standard solution* and *Sample solution*
  Calculate the percentage of the labeled amount of doxycycline ($C_{22}H_{24}N_2O_8$) in the portion of Tablets taken:

$$Result = (r_U/r_S) \times (C_S/C_U) \times P \times F \times 100$$

r_U = peak response from the *Sample solution*
r_S = peak response from the *Standard solution*
C_S = concentration of USP Doxycycline Hyclate RS in the *Standard solution* (mg/mL)
C_U = nominal concentration of doxycycline in the *Sample solution* (mg/mL)
P = potency of doxycycline in USP Doxycycline Hyclate RS (µg/mg)
F = conversion factor, 0.001 mg/µg

Acceptance criteria: 90.0%–120.0%

PERFORMANCE TESTS

- **DISSOLUTION ⟨711⟩**
  Protect solutions containing doxycycline from light.
  Test 1
    Medium: Water; 900 mL
    Apparatus 2: 75 rpm, the distance between the blade and the inside bottom of the vessel being maintained at 4.5 ± 0.5 cm during the test

  Time: 90 min
  Standard solution: USP Doxycycline Hyclate RS in *Medium*
  Sample solution: Dilute with *Medium*, if necessary, to a concentration that is similar to the *Standard solution*.
  Instrumental conditions
    (See *Ultraviolet-Visible Spectroscopy* ⟨857⟩.)
    Mode: UV-Vis
    Analytical wavelength: 276 nm
  Analysis
    Samples: *Standard solution* and *Sample solution*
    Calculate the percentage of the labeled amount of doxycycline ($C_{22}H_{24}N_2O_8$) dissolved:

$$Result = (A_U/A_S) \times (C_S/L) \times V \times 100$$

A_U = absorbance of the *Sample solution*
A_S = absorbance of the *Standard solution*
C_S = concentration of doxycycline in the *Standard solution* (mg/mL)
L = label claim (mg/Tablet)
V = volume of *Medium*, 900 mL

  Tolerances: NLT 85% (*Q*) of the labeled amount of doxycycline ($C_{22}H_{24}N_2O_8$) is dissolved.

Test 2: If the product complies with this test, the labeling indicates that it meets USP *Dissolution Test 2*.
  Medium: Water; 900 mL
  Apparatus 2: 50 rpm, the distance between the blade and the inside bottom of the vessel being maintained at 4.5 ± 0.5 cm during the test
  Time: 30 min
  Standard solution: 22 µg/mL of doxycycline from USP Doxycycline Hyclate RS, in *Medium*
  Sample solution: Pass a portion of the solution under test through a suitable filter.
  Blank: *Medium*
  Instrumental conditions
    (See *Ultraviolet-Visible Spectroscopy* ⟨857⟩.)
    Mode: UV-Vis
    Analytical wavelength: 276 nm
    Cell: 0.5 cm
  Analysis
    Samples: *Standard solution* and *Sample solution*
    Calculate the percentage of the labeled amount of doxycycline ($C_{22}H_{24}N_2O_8$) dissolved:

$$Result = (A_U/A_S) \times (C_S/L) \times V \times 100$$

A_U = absorbance of the *Sample solution*
A_S = absorbance of the *Standard solution*
C_S = concentration of doxycycline in the *Standard solution* (mg/mL)
L = label claim (mg/Tablet)
V = volume of *Medium*, 900 mL

  Tolerances: NLT 85% (*Q*) of the labeled amount of doxycycline is dissolved.

- **UNIFORMITY OF DOSAGE UNITS ⟨905⟩:** Meet the requirements

IMPURITIES

Change to read:

- **ORGANIC IMPURITIES**
  Mobile phase, Diluent, System suitability solution, Sample solution, and Chromatographic system: Proceed as directed in the *Assay*.

Standard solution: 1.5 µg/mL of USP Doxycycline Hyclate RS in *Diluent*
System suitability
  Samples: *System suitability solution* and *Standard solution*
  Suitability requirements
    Resolution: NLT 1.5 between methacycline and 4-epidoxycycline; NLT 1.5 between 4-epidoxycycline and doxycycline related compound A; NLT 1.5 between doxycycline related compound A and doxycycline, *System suitability solution*
    Relative standard deviation: NMT 5.0% for the doxycycline peak, *Standard solution*
Analysis
  Samples: *Sample solution* and *Standard solution*
  Calculate the percentage of each impurity in the portion of Tablets taken:

$$Result = (r_U/r_S) \times (C_S/C_U) \times P \times F \times 100$$

r_U = peak response of each impurity from the *Sample solution*
r_S = peak response of doxycycline from the *Standard solution*
C_S = concentration of USP Doxycycline Hyclate RS in the *Standard solution* (mg/mL)
C_U = nominal concentration of doxycycline in the *Sample solution* (mg/mL)
P = potency of doxycycline in USP Doxycycline Hyclate RS (µg/mg)
F = conversion factor, 0.001 mg/µg
Acceptance criteria: See *Table 2*. Disregard any impurity peaks less than 0.2%.

Table 2

Name	Relative Retention Time	Acceptance Criteria, NMT (%)
Methacycline[a,b]	0.64	—
4-Epidoxycycline[c]	0.79	●1.5● (RB 1-Aug-2017)
Doxycycline related compound A (6-epidoxycycline)[a,d]	0.88	—
Doxycycline	1.0	—
Any individual unspecified impurity	—	0.5
Total impurities	—	2.0

[a] Process impurities are controlled in the drug substance and are not to be reported here. They are not included in total impurities.

[b] (4S,4aR,5S,5aR,12aS)-4-(Dimethylamino)-1,4,4a,5,5a,6,11,12a-octahydro-3,5,10,12,12a-pentahydroxy-6-methylene-1,11-dioxo-2-naphthacenecarboxamide.

[c] (4R,4aR,5S,5aR,6R,12aS)-4-(Dimethylamino)-1,4,4a,5,5a,6,11,12a-octahydro-3,5,10,12,12a-pentahydroxy-6-methyl-1,11-dioxo-2-naphthacenecarboxamide.

[d] (4S,4aR,5S,5aR,6S,12aS)-4-(Dimethylamino)-1,4,4a,5,5a,6,11,12a-octahydro-3,5,10,12,12a-pentahydroxy-6-methyl-1,11-dioxo-2-naphthacenecarboxamide.

ADDITIONAL REQUIREMENTS

• **PACKAGING AND STORAGE:** Preserve in tight, light-resistant containers. Store at controlled room temperature.
• **LABELING:** When more than one *Dissolution* test is given, the labeling states the *Dissolution* test used only if *Test 1* is not used.
• **USP REFERENCE STANDARDS ⟨11⟩**
  USP Doxycycline Hyclate RS
  USP Doxycycline Related Compound A RS. [NOTE—May be available as a free base or a hydrochloride salt.]
  (4S,4aR,5S,5aR,6S,12aS)-4-(Dimethylamino)-1,4,4a,5,5a,6,11,12a-octahydro-3,5,10,12,12a-pentahydroxy-6-methyl-1,11-dioxo-2-naphthacenecarboxamide.
  $C_{22}H_{24}N_2O_8$ 444.43

(4S,4aR,5S,5aR,6S,12aS)-4-(Dimethylamino)-1,4,4a,5,5a,6,11,12a-octahydro-3,5,10,12,12a-pentahydroxy-6-methyl-1,11-dioxo-2-naphthacenecarboxamide, monohydrochloride.
$C_{22}H_{24}N_2O_8 \cdot HCl$ 480.13
USP Methacycline Hydrochloride RS

Doxycycline Hyclate Delayed-Release Tablets

DEFINITION
Doxycycline Hyclate Delayed-Release Tablets contain an amount of Doxycycline Hyclate equivalent to NLT 90.0% and NMT 120.0% of the labeled amount of doxycycline ($C_{22}H_{24}N_2O_8$).

IDENTIFICATION
• **A.** The retention time of the major peak of the *Sample solution* corresponds to that of the *Standard solution*, as obtained in the *Assay*.

ASSAY
• **PROCEDURE**
  Mobile phase: Transfer 0.77 g of ammonium acetate, 0.75 g of sodium hydroxide, 0.50 g of tetrabutylammonium hydrogen sulfate, and 0.40 g of edetate disodium to a 1000-mL volumetric flask. Add 850 mL of water, and dissolve. Add 70 g of tertiary butyl alcohol with the aid of water, dilute with water to volume, and adjust with acetic acid or ammonium hydroxide to a pH of 9.00 ± 0.05.
  Standard solution: 1.16 mg/mL of doxycycline hyclate in methanol and water (1:9). Transfer USP Doxycycline Hyclate RS to a suitable volumetric flask, and add methanol to 10% of the final volume. Sonicate for 5 min or until dissolved. Dilute with water to volume. Protect the *Standard solution* from light. Calculate the concentration, C_S, in mg/mL of doxycycline, using the designated potency, in µg/mg of doxycycline in USP Doxycycline Hyclate RS.
  Sample solution: Equivalent to 1 mg/mL of doxycycline in a mixture of methanol and water (1:9) from NLT 10 Tablets, crushed. Prepare the solution as follows. Weigh and crush NMT 2 Tablets at a time in a suitable mortar. Transfer a weighed portion of the powder to a suitable volumetric flask, add methanol to 10% of the final volume, and sonicate. Dilute with water to volume, sonicating as necessary. Pass through a suitable filter. Protect the *Sample solution* from light.
  Chromatographic system
  (See *Chromatography ⟨621⟩, System Suitability*.)
  Mode: LC
  Detector: UV 270 nm
  Column: 4.6-mm × 25-cm; packing L21
  Column temperature: 52 ± 2°
  Flow rate: 1 mL/min
  Injection volume: 15 µL
  Run time: 1.7 times the retention time of the doxycycline peak
  System suitability
  Sample: *Standard solution*
  Suitability requirements
    Tailing factor: NMT 2.0
    Relative standard deviation: NMT 2.0% from six replicate injections
  Analysis
  Samples: *Standard solution* and *Sample solution*
  Calculate the percentage of the labeled amount of doxycycline ($C_{22}H_{24}N_2O_8$) in the portion of Tablets taken:

$$Result = (r_U/r_S) \times (C_S/C_U) \times 100$$

r_U = peak response from the *Sample solution*
r_S = peak response from the *Standard solution*
C_S = concentration of doxycycline in the *Standard solution* (mg/mL)
C_U = nominal concentration of doxycycline in the *Sample solution* (mg/mL)
Acceptance criteria: 90.0%–120.0%

PERFORMANCE TESTS

Change to read:

• **DISSOLUTION ⟨711⟩**
  Test 1: Proceed as directed for *Dissolution* ⟨711⟩, *Procedure, Apparatus 1 and Apparatus 2, Delayed-Release Dosage Forms, Method B Procedure.*
  Acid stage
    Medium: 0.06 N hydrochloric acid; 900 mL, degassed with helium
    Apparatus 1: 50 rpm
    Time: 20 min
    Standard solution: 0.128 mg/mL of USP Doxycycline Hyclate RS in *Medium.* Calculate the concentration, C_S, in mg/mL of doxycycline, using the designated potency, in μg/mg of doxycycline in USP Doxycycline Hyclate RS. [NOTE—Sonicate if necessary to dissolve.]
    Sample solution: Pass portions of the solution under test through a suitable PVDF filter of 0.45-μm pore size.
    Detector: UV 346 nm
    Cell: 0.1-cm quartz
    Blank: *Medium*
    Analysis
      Samples: *Standard solution* and *Sample solution*
      Calculate the percentage of the labeled amount of doxycycline ($C_{22}H_{24}N_2O_8$) dissolved:

$$\text{Result} = (A_U/A_S) \times (C_S/L) \times V \times 100$$

A_U = absorbance of the *Sample solution*
A_S = absorbance of the *Standard solution*
C_S = concentration of doxycycline in the *Standard solution* (mg/mL)
L = label claim (mg/Tablet)
V = volume of *Medium*, 900 mL
    Tolerances
      Level 1 (6 Tablets tested): No individual value is more than 30% of the labeled amount of doxycycline ($C_{22}H_{24}N_2O_8$) dissolved in 20 min.
      Level 2 (6 Tablets tested): NMT 2 individual values of the 12 tested are greater than 30% of the labeled amount of doxycycline ($C_{22}H_{24}N_2O_8$) in 20 min.
  Buffer stage
    Conduct this stage of testing on separate Tablets, selecting those that were not previously subjected to the *Acid stage* testing.
    Medium: pH 5.5 neutralized phthalate buffer (see *Reagents, Indicators, and Solutions—Buffers*); 900 mL, degassed
    Apparatus 1: 50 rpm
    Time: 30 min
    Standard solution: 0.128 mg/mL of USP Doxycycline Hyclate RS in *Medium.* Calculate the concentration, C_S, in mg/mL of doxycycline, using the designated potency, in μg/mg of doxycycline in USP Doxycycline Hyclate RS. [NOTE—Sonicate if necessary to dissolve.]
    Sample solution: Pass portions of the solution under test through a suitable PVDF filter of 0.45-μm pore size.
    Analysis: Determine the percentage of doxycycline ($C_{22}H_{24}N_2O_8$) dissolved by the procedure described for the *Acid stage.*
    Tolerances: NLT 85% (Q) of the labeled amount of doxycycline ($C_{22}H_{24}N_2O_8$) is dissolved.

  Test 2: If the product complies with this test, the labeling indicates that the product meets USP *Dissolution Test 2.* Proceed as directed for *Dissolution* ⟨711⟩, *Procedure, Apparatus 1 and Apparatus 2, Delayed-Release Dosage Forms, Method B Procedure.*
  Acid stage
    Medium, Apparatus 1, Time, Blank, and **Analysis:** Proceed as directed for *Acid stage* in *Test 1.*
    Standard solution: (L/900) mg/mL of USP Doxycycline Hyclate RS in *Medium.* Calculate the concentration, C_S, in mg/mL of doxycycline, using the designated potency, in μg/mg of doxycycline in USP Doxycycline Hyclate RS. Sonicate if necessary to dissolve.
    Sample solution: Pass portions of the solution under test through a suitable filter.
    Detector: UV 345 nm
    Cell: See *Table 1.*

Table 1

Tablet Strength (mg/Tablet)	Cell Size (cm)
75	0.5
100	0.5
150	0.2

    Tolerances
      Level 1 (6 Tablets tested): No individual value is more than 50% of the labeled amount of doxycycline ($C_{22}H_{24}N_2O_8$) dissolved in 20 min.
      Level 2 (6 Tablets tested): NMT 2 individual values of the 12 tested are greater than 50% of the labeled amount of doxycycline ($C_{22}H_{24}N_2O_8$) in 20 min.
  Buffer stage
    Conduct this stage of testing on separate Tablets, selecting those that were not previously subjected to the *Acid stage* testing.
    Medium: pH 5.5 neutralized phthalate buffer (see *Reagents, Indicators, and Solutions—Buffers*); 1000 mL, degassed
    Apparatus 1 and **Analysis:** Proceed as directed for *Buffer stage* in *Test 1.*
    Time: 45 min
    Standard solution: (L/1000) mg/mL of USP Doxycycline Hyclate RS in *Medium.* Calculate the concentration, C_S, in mg/mL of doxycycline, using the designated potency, in μg/mg of doxycycline in USP Doxycycline Hyclate RS. Sonicate if necessary to dissolve.
    Sample solution: Pass portions of the solution under test through a suitable filter.
    Detector and **Cell:** Proceed as directed for *Acid stage* in *Test 2.*
    Tolerances: NLT 70% (Q) of the labeled amount of doxycycline ($C_{22}H_{24}N_2O_8$) is dissolved.
  Test 3: If the product complies with this test, the labeling indicates that the product meets USP *Dissolution Test 3.* Proceed as directed for *Dissolution* ⟨711⟩, *Procedure, Apparatus 1 and Apparatus 2, Delayed-Release Dosage Forms, Method B Procedure.*
  Acid stage
    Apparatus 1 and **Time:** Proceed as directed for *Acid stage* in *Test 1.*
    Medium: 0.06 N hydrochloric acid; 900 mL
    Standard solution: Prepare the solutions as directed in *Table 2* from USP Doxycycline Hyclate RS in *Medium.* Calculate the concentration, C_S, in mg/mL of doxycycline, using the designated potency, in μg/mg of doxycycline in USP Doxycycline Hyclate RS.

Table 2

Tablet Strength (mg/Tablet)	Concentration of Doxycycline (mg/mL)
75	0.1
100	0.1
150	0.17

Sample solution: Pass portions of the solution under test through a suitable filter.
Detector: UV 345 nm
Cell: 0.2 cm
Blank: *Medium*
Analysis
  Samples: *Standard solution* and *Sample solution*
  Calculate the percentage of the labeled amount of doxycycline ($C_{22}H_{24}N_2O_8$) dissolved:

$$Result = (A_U/A_S) \times (C_S/L) \times V \times 100$$

A_U = absorbance of the *Sample solution*
A_S = absorbance of the *Standard solution*
C_S = concentration of doxycycline in the *Standard solution* (mg/mL)
L = label claim (mg/Tablet)
V = volume of *Medium*, 900 mL
  Tolerances: See *Table 3*.

Table 3

Level	Number of Tablets Tested	Tolerances	
		Tablets Labeled to Contain 75 or 100 mg of Doxycycline	Tablets Labeled to Contain 150 mg of Doxycycline
A_1	6	No individual value exceeds 50% at 20 min.	No individual value exceeds 30% at 20 min.
A_2	6	Average of 12 units ($A_1 + A_2$) is NMT 50% at 20 min, and no individual unit is greater than 65% dissolved.	Average of 12 units ($A_1 + A_2$) is NMT 30% at 20 min, and no individual unit is greater than 45% dissolved.
A_3	12	Average of 24 units ($A_1 + A_2 + A_3$) is NMT 50% at 20 min, and no individual unit is greater than 65% dissolved.	Average of 24 units ($A_1 + A_2 + A_3$) is NMT 30% at 20 min, and no individual unit is greater than 45% dissolved.

Buffer stage
Conduct this stage of testing on separate Tablets, selecting those that were not previously subjected to the *Acid stage* testing.
Medium: pH 5.5 neutralized phthalate buffer (see *Reagents, Indicators, and Solutions—Buffers*); 1000 mL
Apparatus 1: 50 rpm
Time: 60 min
Standard solution: Prepare the solutions as directed in *Table 4* from USP Doxycycline Hyclate RS in *Medium*. Calculate the concentration, C_S, in mg/mL of doxycycline, using the designated potency, in μg/mg of doxycycline in USP Doxycycline Hyclate RS.

Table 4

Tablet Strength (mg/Tablet)	Concentration of Doxycycline (mg/mL)
75	0.1
100	0.1
150	0.15

Sample solution: Pass portions of the solution under test through a suitable filter.
Detector: UV 345 nm
Cell: 0.2 cm
Blank: *Medium*
Analysis
  Samples: *Standard solution* and *Sample solution*
  Calculate the percentage of the labeled amount of doxycycline ($C_{22}H_{24}N_2O_8$) dissolved:

$$Result = (A_U/A_S) \times (C_S/L) \times V \times 100$$

A_U = absorbance of the *Sample solution*
A_S = absorbance of the *Standard solution*
C_S = concentration of doxycycline in the *Standard solution* (mg/mL)
L = label claim (mg/Tablet)
V = volume of *Medium*, 1000 mL
  Tolerances: See *Table 5*.

Table 5

Tablets Labeled to Contain 75 or 100 mg of Doxycycline	Tablets Labeled to Contain 150 mg of Doxycycline
NLT 80% (*Q*) of the labeled amount of doxycycline ($C_{22}H_{24}N_2O_8$) is dissolved.	NLT 70% (*Q*) of the labeled amount of doxycycline ($C_{22}H_{24}N_2O_8$) is dissolved.

Test 4: If the product complies with this test, the labeling indicates that the product meets USP *Dissolution Test 4*. Proceed as directed for *Dissolution ⟨711⟩, Procedure, Apparatus 1 and Apparatus 2, Delayed-Release Dosage Forms, Method B Procedure*.
Acid stage
  Medium: 0.06 N hydrochloric acid; 900 mL, degassed
  Apparatus 1: 50 rpm
  Time: 20 min
  Standard solution: 0.1 mg/mL of doxycycline from USP Doxycycline Hyclate RS in *Medium*. Calculate the concentration, C_S, in mg/mL of doxycycline, using the designated potency, in μg/mg of doxycycline in USP Doxycycline Hyclate RS.
  Sample solution: Pass portions of the solution under test through a suitable filter.
  Detector: UV 345 nm
  Cell: 0.2-cm quartz
  Blank: *Medium*
  Analysis
    Samples: *Standard solution* and *Sample solution*
    Calculate the percentage of the labeled amount of doxycycline ($C_{22}H_{24}N_2O_8$) dissolved:

$$Result = (A_U/A_S) \times (C_S/L) \times V \times 100$$

A_U = absorbance of the *Sample solution*
A_S = absorbance of the *Standard solution*
C_S = concentration of doxycycline in the *Standard solution* (mg/mL)
L = label claim (mg/Tablet)
V = volume of *Medium*, 900 mL
  Tolerances
    Level 1 (6 Tablets tested): No individual value is more than 30% of the labeled amount of doxycycline ($C_{22}H_{24}N_2O_8$) dissolved in 20 min.

Level 2 (6 Tablets tested): NMT 2 individual values of the 12 tested are greater than 30% of the labeled amount of doxycycline ($C_{22}H_{24}N_2O_8$) in 20 min.

Buffer stage

Conduct this stage of testing on separate Tablets, selecting those that were not previously subjected to the *Acid stage* testing.

Medium: pH 5.5 neutralized phthalate buffer (see *Reagents, Indicators, and Solutions—Buffers*); 1000 mL, degassed

Apparatus 1: 50 rpm

Time: 30 min

Standard solution: 0.1 mg/mL of doxycycline from USP Doxycycline Hyclate RS in *Medium*

Sample solution: Pass portions of the solution under test through a suitable filter. Calculate the concentration, C_s, in mg/mL of doxycycline, using the designated potency, in µg/mg of doxycycline in USP Doxycycline Hyclate RS.

Blank: *Medium*

Analysis

Samples: *Standard solution* and *Sample solution*

Calculate the percentage of the labeled amount of doxycycline ($C_{22}H_{24}N_2O_8$) dissolved:

$$Result = (A_U/A_S) \times (C_S/L) \times V \times 100$$

A_U = absorbance of the *Sample solution*
A_S = absorbance of the *Standard solution*
C_S = concentration of doxycycline in the *Standard solution* (mg/mL)
L = label claim (mg/Tablet)
V = volume of *Medium*, 1000 mL

Tolerances: NLT 75% (*Q*) of the labeled amount of doxycycline ($C_{22}H_{24}N_2O_8$) is dissolved.

•**Test 5:** If the product complies with this test, the labeling indicates that the product meets USP *Dissolution Test 5*. Proceed as directed for *Dissolution ⟨711⟩, Procedure, Apparatus 1 and Apparatus 2, Delayed-Release Dosage Forms, Method B Procedure.*

Acid stage

Medium: 0.06 N hydrochloric acid; 900 mL

Apparatus 1: 100 rpm

Time: 20 min

Standard solution: 0.06 mg/mL of doxycycline from USP Doxycycline Hyclate RS in *Medium*. Calculate the concentration, C_s, in mg/mL of doxycycline, using the designated potency, in µg/mg of doxycycline in USP Doxycycline Hyclate RS.

Sample solution: Pass portions of the solution under test through a suitable filter.

Detector: UV 345 nm

Cell: 1.0 cm

Blank: *Medium*

Analysis

Samples: *Standard solution* and *Sample solution*

Calculate the percentage of the labeled amount of doxycycline ($C_{22}H_{24}N_2O_8$) dissolved:

$$Result = (A_U/A_S) \times (C_S/L) \times V \times 100$$

A_U = absorbance of the *Sample solution*
A_S = absorbance of the *Standard solution*
C_S = concentration of doxycycline in the *Standard solution* (mg/mL)
L = label claim (mg/Tablet)
V = volume of *Medium*, 900 mL

Tolerances: See *Table 6*.

Table 6

Level	Number of Tablets Tested	Tolerances
A_1	6	No individual value exceeds 50% at 20 min.
A_2	6	Average of 12 units ($A_1 + A_2$) is NMT 50% at 20 min, and no individual unit is greater than 65% dissolved.
A_3	12	Average of 24 units ($A_1 + A_2 + A_3$) is NMT 50% at 20 min, and no individual unit is greater than 65% dissolved.

Buffer stage

Conduct this stage of testing on separate Tablets, selecting those that were not previously subjected to the *Acid stage* testing.

Medium: pH 5.5 neutralized phthalate buffer (see *Reagents, Indicators, and Solutions—Buffers*); 900 mL

Apparatus 1: 100 rpm

Time: 30 min

Standard solution: 0.06 mg/mL of doxycycline from USP Doxycycline Hyclate RS in *Medium*. Calculate the concentration, C_s, in mg/mL of doxycycline, using the designated potency, in µg/mg of doxycycline in USP Doxycycline Hyclate RS.

Sample solution: Pass portions of the solution under test through a suitable filter.

Blank: *Medium*

Analysis

Samples: *Standard solution* and *Sample solution*

Calculate the percentage of the labeled amount of doxycycline ($C_{22}H_{24}N_2O_8$) dissolved:

$$Result = (A_U/A_S) \times (C_S/L) \times V \times 100$$

A_U = absorbance of the *Sample solution*
A_S = absorbance of the *Standard solution*
C_S = concentration of doxycycline in the *Standard solution* (mg/mL)
L = label claim (mg/Tablet)
V = volume of *Medium*, 900 mL

Tolerances: NLT 80% (*Q*) of the labeled amount of doxycycline ($C_{22}H_{24}N_2O_8$) is dissolved.• (RB 1-Aug-2017)

• **UNIFORMITY OF DOSAGE UNITS ⟨905⟩:** Meet the requirements

IMPURITIES

Change to read:

• **ORGANIC IMPURITIES**

Mobile phase, Sample solution, and **Chromatographic system:** Proceed as directed in the *Assay*.

Standard stock solution: 1.16 mg/mL of doxycycline hyclate in methanol and water (1:9). Transfer USP Doxycycline Hyclate RS to a suitable volumetric flask, and add methanol to 10% of the final volume. Sonicate for 5 min or until dissolved. Dilute with water to volume. Protect the solution from light. Calculate the concentration, in mg/mL of doxycycline, using the designated potency, in µg/mg of doxycycline in USP Doxycycline Hyclate RS.

Standard solution: 0.02 mg/mL of doxycycline from the *Standard stock solution*. Protect the solution from light.

Sensitivity solution: 1 µg/mL of doxycycline from the *Standard solution*. Protect the solution from light.

System suitability stock solution: 0.04 mg/mL each of USP Oxytetracycline Hydrochloride RS, USP Methacycline Hydrochloride RS, and USP Doxycycline Related Compound A RS. Protect the solution from light.

System suitability solution: Transfer 5 mL of the *Standard stock solution* into a 25-mL volumetric flask. Heat on a steam bath for 60 min, and gently evaporate to dryness on a hot plate (partial degradation of doxycycline to 4-epidoxycycline). Add 3 mL of the *System suitability stock solution* to the flask, and dilute with water to volume. Pass through a suitable filter. Protect the solution from light.

System suitability
Samples: *Standard solution, Sensitivity solution,* and *System suitability solution*
Suitability requirements
Signal-to-noise ratio: NLT 10 for doxycycline, *Sensitivity solution*
Resolution: NLT 1.5 between doxycycline and 6-epidoxycycline, *System suitability solution*
Tailing factor: NMT 2.0, *Standard solution*
Relative standard deviation: NMT 5.0%, *Standard solution*
Analysis
Samples: *Sample solution* and *Standard solution*
Calculate the percentage of each impurity in the portion of Tablets taken:

$$Result = (r_U/r_S) \times (C_S/C_U) \times (1/F) \times 100$$

r_U = peak response of each impurity from the *Sample solution*
r_S = peak response of doxycycline from the *Standard solution*
C_S = concentration of doxycycline in the *Standard solution* (mg/mL)
C_U = nominal concentration of doxycycline in the *Sample solution* (mg/mL)
F = relative response factor (see *Table •7)•* (RB 1-Aug-2017)

Acceptance criteria: See *Table •7.•* (RB 1-Aug-2017)

Table •7• (RB 1-Aug-2017)

Name	Relative Retention Time	Relative Response Factor	Acceptance Criteria, NMT (%)
Oxytetracycline	0.3	1.0	0.5
4-Epidoxycycline[a]	0.4	1.0	1.0
Methacycline	0.6	1.0	2.0
6-Epidoxycycline (doxycycline related compound A)[b]	0.7	0.86	2.0
Doxycycline	1.0	—	—

[a] (4R,4aR,5S,5aR,6R,12aS)-4-(Dimethylamino)-1,4,4a,5,5a,6,11,12a-octahydro-3,5,10,12,12a-pentahydroxy-6-methyl-1,11-dioxo-2-naphthacenecarboxamide monohydrate.
[b] (4S,4aR,5S,5aR,6S,12aS)-4-(Dimethylamino)-1,4,4a,5,5a,6,11,12a-octahydro-3,5,10,12,12a-pentahydroxy-6-methyl-1,11-dioxo-2-naphthacenecarboxamide monohydrate.

ADDITIONAL REQUIREMENTS
- **PACKAGING AND STORAGE:** Preserve in tight, light-resistant containers. Store at controlled room temperature.
- **LABELING:** When more than one *Dissolution* test is given, the labeling states the test used only if *Test 1* is not used.
- **USP REFERENCE STANDARDS ⟨11⟩**
  USP Doxycycline Hyclate RS
  USP Doxycycline Related Compound A RS
  6-Epidoxycycline, or (4S,4aR,5S,5aR,6S,12aS)-4-(dimethylamino)-3,5,10,12,12a-pentahydroxy-6-methyl-1,11-dioxo-1,4,4a,5,5a,6,11,12a-octahydrotetracene-2-carboxamide.

$C_{22}H_{24}N_2O_8$ 444.43
USP Methacycline Hydrochloride RS
USP Oxytetracycline Hydrochloride RS

Duloxetine Delayed-Release Capsules

DEFINITION
Duloxetine Delayed-Release Capsules contain an amount of Duloxetine Hydrochloride equivalent to NLT 90.0% and NMT 110.0% of the labeled amount of duloxetine ($C_{18}H_{19}NOS$).

IDENTIFICATION
- **A. INFRARED ABSORPTION ⟨197F⟩**
  Buffer: 6.9 g/L of monobasic sodium phosphate in water adjusted with 5 N sodium hydroxide to a pH of 7.5
  Spectral range: 1650 cm⁻¹ to 900 cm⁻¹
  Standard: 1 mg/mL of USP Duloxetine Hydrochloride RS in methylene chloride. Shake the contents, and sonicate for 1 min. Transfer 15 mL of filtrate into a separatory funnel, and add 15 mL of *Buffer*. Collect the organic layer, and evaporate to dryness. Redissolve the residue with a few drops of methylene chloride, and transfer to a potassium bromide or sodium chloride plate. Allow it to dry.
  Sample: 1 mg/mL of duloxetine, from the contents of NLT 10 Capsules in methylene chloride. Proceed as directed in the *Standard*.
  Acceptance criteria: Meet the requirements
- **B.** The retention time of the major peak of the *Sample solution* corresponds to that of the *Standard solution*, as obtained in the *Assay*.

ASSAY

Change to read:

- **PROCEDURE**
  Protect solutions of duloxetine from light.
  Buffer A: 3.4 g/L of monobasic potassium phosphate in water. To 1 L of this solution add 15 mL of triethylamine, and adjust with phosphoric acid to a pH of 5.5.
  Buffer B: 0.2 g/L of monobasic ammonium phosphate and 4.5 g/L of dibasic potassium phosphate in water. Adjust with phosphoric acid to a pH of 8.0.
  Mobile phase: Methanol, tetrahydrofuran, and *Buffer A* (323:90:587)
  Diluent: Methanol and *Buffer B* (50:50)
  System suitability solution: 0.1 mg/mL of USP Duloxetine Hydrochloride RS, 0.05 mg/mL of •α-naphthol,• (RB 1-Aug-2017) 0.01 mg/mL of USP Duloxetine Related Compound F RS, and 0.025 mg/mL of USP Duloxetine Related Compound H RS in *Diluent*. [NOTE—Add 1 mL of methanol before diluting to volume to assist with dissolving contents. Duloxetine related compound H is used for peak identification purposes in this solution.]
  Standard solution: 0.1 mg/mL of USP Duloxetine Hydrochloride RS in *Diluent*
  Sample solution: Nominally 0.1 mg/mL of duloxetine from the contents of NLT 5 Capsules, in *Diluent*
  Chromatographic system
  (See *Chromatography ⟨621⟩, System Suitability*.)
  [NOTE—It is recommended to preheat the *Mobile phase* to 45°.]

Mode: LC
Detector: UV 230 nm
Column: 4.6-mm × 7.5-cm; 3- or 3.5-μm packing L7
Column temperature: 45°
Flow rate: 1.5 mL/min
Injection volume: 10 μL
Run time: 6 times the retention time of duloxetine
System suitability
  Samples: *System suitability solution* and *Standard solution*
  [NOTE—See •*Table 2*• (RB 1-Aug-2017) in *Organic Impurities* for relative retention times.]
  Suitability requirements
    Resolution: NLT 1.6 between duloxetine and duloxetine related compound F; NLT 2 between •α-naphthol• (RB 1-Aug-2017) and duloxetine related compound H, *System suitability solution*
    Relative standard deviation: NMT 1.5%, *Standard solution*
Analysis
  Samples: *Standard solution* and *Sample solution*
  Calculate the percentage of the labeled amount of duloxetine ($C_{18}H_{19}NOS$) in the portion of Capsules taken:

$$Result = (r_U/r_S) \times (C_S/C_U) \times (M_{r1}/M_{r2}) \times 100$$

r_U = peak response from the *Sample solution*
r_S = peak response from the *Standard solution*
C_S = concentration of USP Duloxetine Hydrochloride RS in the *Standard solution* (mg/mL)
C_U = nominal concentration of duloxetine in the *Sample solution* (mg/mL)
M_{r1} = molecular weight of duloxetine free base, 297.42
M_{r2} = molecular weight of duloxetine hydrochloride, 333.88
Acceptance criteria: 90.0%–110.0%

PERFORMANCE TESTS

Change to read:

- **DISSOLUTION ⟨711⟩**
  Test 1
    Acid stage
      Acid stage medium: •0.1 N hydrochloric acid VS;• (RB 1-Aug-2017) 1000 mL
      Apparatus 1: 100 rpm
      Time: 2 h
    Buffer stage
      Buffer stage medium: pH 6.8 phosphate buffer; 1000 mL
      Apparatus 1: 100 rpm
      Time: 60 min for Capsules containing 20% w/w pellets; 90 min for Capsules containing 32% w/w pellets
    Buffer A and **Mobile phase:** Proceed as directed in the *Assay*.
    Standard stock solution: 0.28 mg/mL of USP Duloxetine Hydrochloride RS, •equivalent to 0.25 mg/mL of duloxetine,• (RB 1-Aug-2017) in *Buffer stage medium*. Use a small amount of methanol, not exceeding 2% of the final volume, to dissolve duloxetine.
    Acid stage standard solution: •0.0023 mg/mL of USP Duloxetine Hydrochloride RS, equivalent to 0.002 mg/mL of duloxetine,• (RB 1-Aug-2017) from the *Standard stock solution* diluted with *Buffer stage medium*
    Buffer stage standard solution: •0.023 mg/mL of USP Duloxetine Hydrochloride RS, equivalent to 0.02 mg/mL of duloxetine,• (RB 1-Aug-2017) from the *Standard stock solution* diluted with *Buffer stage medium*
    Sample solution: After 2 h in the *Acid stage medium*, pass a portion of the solution under test through a

suitable filter. Transfer the basket containing the pellets to the vessel containing the *Buffer stage medium*. After the appropriate time in the *Buffer stage medium*, pass a portion of the solution under test through a suitable filter.
    Chromatographic system
    (See *Chromatography* ⟨621⟩, *System Suitability*.)
      Mode: LC
      Detector: UV 230 nm
      Column: 4.6-mm × 7.5-cm; 3- or 3.5-μm packing L7
      Column temperature: 45°
      Flow rate: 1.5 mL/min
      Injection volume: 10 μL
    System suitability
      Sample: *Acid stage standard solution*
      [NOTE—The relative retention times for duloxetine and •α-naphthol• (RB 1-Aug-2017) are 1.0 and 1.4, respectively.]
      Suitability requirements
        Tailing factor: NMT 1.5
        Relative standard deviation: NMT 2.0%
    Analysis
      Samples: *Acid stage standard solution, Buffer stage standard solution,* and *Sample solution*
      Calculate the concentration of duloxetine in the *Acid stage medium* (C_1):

$$Result = (r_U/r_S) \times C_S \times (M_{r1}/M_{r2})$$

r_U = peak response of duloxetine from the *Sample solution*
r_S = peak response of duloxetine from the *Acid stage standard solution*
C_S = concentration of USP Duloxetine Hydrochloride RS in the *Acid stage standard solution* (mg/mL)
M_{r1} = molecular weight of duloxetine free base, 297.42
M_{r2} = molecular weight of duloxetine hydrochloride, 333.88
      Calculate the equivalent concentration of duloxetine from •α-naphthol• (RB 1-Aug-2017) in the *Acid stage medium* (C_2):

$$Result = (r_U/r_S) \times C_S \times (M_{r1}/M_{r2}) \times (M_{r1}/M_{r3})$$

r_U = peak response of •α-naphthol• (RB 1-Aug-2017) from the *Sample solution*
r_S = peak response of duloxetine from the *Acid stage standard solution*
C_S = concentration of USP Duloxetine Hydrochloride RS in the *Acid stage standard solution* (mg/mL)
M_{r1} = molecular weight of duloxetine free base, 297.42
M_{r2} = molecular weight of duloxetine hydrochloride, 333.88
M_{r3} = molecular weight of •α-naphthol,• (RB 1-Aug-2017) 144.17
      Calculate the percentage of the labeled amount of duloxetine •dissolved• (RB 1-Aug-2017) in the *Acid stage medium* (Q_A):

$$Result = (C_1 + C_2) \times V \times (1/L) \times 100$$

C_1 = concentration of duloxetine in the *Acid stage medium* (mg/mL)
C_2 = equivalent concentration of duloxetine from •α-naphthol• (RB 1-Aug-2017) in the *Acid stage medium* (mg/mL)
V = volume of *Medium*, 1000 mL
L = label claim of duloxetine (mg/Capsule)

Calculate the percentage of the labeled amount of duloxetine •dissolved• (RB 1-Aug-2017) in the *Buffer stage medium*:

$$Result = [(r_U/r_S) \times (C_S/L) \times V \times (M_{r1}/M_{r2}) \times 100] + Q_A$$

r_U = peak response of duloxetine from the *Sample solution*
r_S = peak response of duloxetine from the *Buffer stage standard solution*
C_S = concentration of USP Duloxetine Hydrochloride RS in the *Buffer stage standard solution* (mg/mL)
L = label claim (mg/Capsule)
V = volume of *Medium*, 1000 mL
M_{r1} = molecular weight of duloxetine free base, 297.42
M_{r2} = molecular weight of duloxetine hydrochloride, 333.88
Q_A = percentage of the labeled amount of duloxetine •dissolved• (RB 1-Aug-2017) in the *Acid stage medium*

Tolerances
Acid stage: No individual unit releases more than 10% of the labeled amount of duloxetine in 2 h.
Buffer stage
For Capsules containing 20% w/w pellets: NLT 75% (*Q*) of the labeled amount of duloxetine is dissolved in 60 min.
For Capsules labeled to contain 32% w/w pellets: NLT 75% (*Q*) of the labeled amount of duloxetine is dissolved in 90 min.
Test 2: If the product complies with this test, the labeling indicates that it meets USP *Dissolution Test 2*. Protect solutions of duloxetine from light.
Acid stage
Acid stage medium: •0.1 N hydrochloric acid VS;• (RB 1-Aug-2017) 750 mL
Apparatus 2: 100 rpm
Time: 2 h in *Acid stage medium*
Buffer stage
Buffer stage medium: pH 6.8 phosphate buffer (after 2 h, add 250 mL of •76 g/L of tribasic sodium phosphate,• (RB 1-Aug-2017) previously heated to 37 ± 0.5°, to the *Acid stage medium*); 1000 mL
Apparatus 2: 100 rpm
Time: 3 h in *Buffer stage medium*. The time in *Buffer stage medium* includes the time in *Acid stage medium*.
Solution A: A mixture of triethylamine and water prepared as follows. Add 15 mL of triethylamine to 1 L of water and adjust with phosphoric acid to a pH of 2.5 ± 0.05.
Mobile phase: Acetonitrile and *Solution A* (40:60)
Diluent: •0.1 N hydrochloric acid VS• (RB 1-Aug-2017) and •76 g/L of tribasic sodium phosphate,• (RB 1-Aug-2017) (75:25)
Standard stock solution: 0.46 mg/mL of USP Duloxetine Hydrochloride RS, equivalent to 0.4 mg/mL of duloxetine, prepared as follows. Transfer a suitable amount of USP Duloxetine Hydrochloride RS to an appropriate volumetric flask and dissolve in 50% of the final flask volume of *Mobile phase*. Dilute with *Mobile phase* to volume.
Standard solution: 0.046 mg/mL of USP Duloxetine Hydrochloride RS, equivalent to 0.04 mg/mL of duloxetine, from the *Standard stock solution* in *Diluent*
Acid stage sample solution and **Buffer stage sample solution:** Pass a portion of the solution under test through a suitable filter, and use the filtrate. [NOTE—A cannula-style filter with a 20-μm pore size may be suitable.]
Chromatographic system
(See *Chromatography* ⟨621⟩, *System Suitability*.)

Mode: LC
Detector: UV 290 nm
Column: 4.6-mm × 15.0-cm; 3-μm packing L1
Column temperature: 40°
Flow rate: 1.3 mL/min
Injection volume: 10 μL
System suitability
Sample: *Standard solution*
Suitability requirements
Tailing factor: NMT 2.5
Relative standard deviation: NMT 2.0%
Analysis
Samples: *Standard solution*, *Acid stage sample solution*, and *Buffer stage sample solution*
Calculate the percentage of the labeled amount of duloxetine ($C_{18}H_{19}NOS$) dissolved in *Acid stage medium*:

$$Result = (r_U/r_S) \times C_S \times (M_{r1}/M_{r2}) \times V \times (1/L) \times 100$$

r_U = peak response of duloxetine from the *Acid stage sample solution*
r_S = peak response of duloxetine from the *Standard solution*
C_S = concentration of USP Duloxetine Hydrochloride RS in the *Standard solution* (mg/mL)
M_{r1} = molecular weight of duloxetine free base, 297.42
M_{r2} = molecular weight of duloxetine hydrochloride, 333.88
V = volume of *Acid stage medium*, 750 mL
L = label claim of duloxetine (mg/Capsule)
Calculate the percentage of the labeled amount of duloxetine ($C_{18}H_{19}NOS$) dissolved in *Buffer stage medium*:

$$Result = (r_U/r_S) \times C_S \times (M_{r1}/M_{r2}) \times V \times (1/L) \times 100$$

r_U = peak response of duloxetine from the *Buffer stage sample solution*
r_S = peak response of duloxetine from the *Standard solution*
C_S = concentration of USP Duloxetine Hydrochloride RS in the *Standard solution* (mg/mL)
M_{r1} = molecular weight of duloxetine free base, 297.42
M_{r2} = molecular weight of duloxetine hydrochloride, 333.88
V = volume of *Buffer stage medium*, 1000 mL
L = label claim of duloxetine (mg/Capsule)
Tolerances
Acid stage: For each individual value, NMT 10% of the labeled amount of duloxetine ($C_{18}H_{19}NOS$). The percentage of the labeled amount of duloxetine dissolved at the time specified conforms to *Dissolution* ⟨711⟩, •• (RB 1-Aug-2017) *Acceptance Table 3*.
Buffer stage: NLT 80% (*Q*) of the labeled amount of duloxetine ($C_{18}H_{19}NOS$). The percentage of the labeled amount of duloxetine dissolved at the time specified conforms to *Dissolution* ⟨711⟩, •• (RB 1-Aug-2017) *Acceptance Table 4*.
•**Test 3:** If the product complies with this test, the labeling indicates that it meets USP *Dissolution Test 3*. Protect solutions of duloxetine from light.
Acid stage
Acid stage medium: 0.1 N hydrochloric acid VS with pepsin (mix 8.5 mL of hydrochloric acid and 3.2 g of pepsin in 1 L of water); 1000 mL
Apparatus 1: 100 rpm
Time: 2 h in *Acid stage medium*
Buffer stage
Buffer stage medium: pH 6.8 phosphate buffer (6.8 g/L of monobasic potassium phosphate and

0.9 g/L of sodium hydroxide in water, adjusted with phosphoric acid or 1 N sodium hydroxide VS to a pH of 6.80); 1000 mL

Apparatus 1: 100 rpm

Time: 3 h in *Buffer stage medium*. The time in *Buffer stage medium* includes the time in *Acid stage medium*.

Procedure: After 2 h in the *Acid stage medium*, withdraw a sample from the solution and immediately filter. Remove and rinse each basket with NMT 25 mL of 0.1 N hydrochloric acid VS. Then transfer the baskets to the *Buffer stage medium*.

Solution A: 2.7 g/L of monobasic potassium phosphate in water. Add 2.0 mL of triethylamine per liter of solution and adjust with phosphoric acid to a pH of 6.0.

Mobile phase: Acetonitrile and *Solution A* (38:62)

Standard stock solution: 1.1 mg/mL of USP Duloxetine Hydrochloride RS, equivalent to 1.0 mg/mL of duloxetine, prepared as follows. Transfer a suitable amount of USP Duloxetine Hydrochloride RS to an appropriate volumetric flask and dissolve in 60% of the flask volume of water. Sonication may be used to promote dissolution. Dilute with water to volume.

System suitability stock solution: 0.011 mg/mL of USP Duloxetine Hydrochloride RS from the *Standard stock solution* in 0.1 N hydrochloric acid VS. Store this solution in a 37° water bath for 30 min.

System suitability solution: 0.002 mg/mL of USP Duloxetine Hydrochloride RS from the *System suitability stock solution* in *Mobile phase*. Pass the resulting solution through a suitable filter and use the filtrate.

Acid stage standard stock solution: 0.11 mg/mL of USP Duloxetine Hydrochloride RS, equivalent to 0.10 mg/mL of duloxetine, from the *Standard stock solution* in water

Acid stage standard solution: $(L/50,000)$ mg/mL of duloxetine from the *Standard stock solution* in *Mobile phase*, where L is the label claim, in mg/Capsule

Buffer stage standard solution: $(L/1,000)$ mg/mL of duloxetine from the *Standard stock solution* in *Buffer stage medium*, where L is the label claim, in mg/Capsule

Acid stage sample solution: Transfer 2 mL of the solution under test to a suitable container and dilute with *Mobile phase* to 10 mL. Pass a portion of the resulting solution through a suitable filter, discard NLT 3 mL, and use the filtrate.

Buffer stage sample solution: Pass a portion of the solution under test through a suitable filter, discard NLT 1 mL, and use the filtrate.

Chromatographic system
(See *Chromatography ⟨621⟩, System Suitability.*)
Mode: LC
Detector: UV 230 nm
Column: 4.6-mm × 15.0-cm; 3.5-μm packing L1
Column temperature: 50°
Flow rate: 1.1 mL/min
Injection volume: 10 μL
Run time: NLT 2 times the retention time of duloxetine

System suitability
Samples: *System suitability solution* and *Buffer stage standard solution*
[NOTE—The relative retention times for duloxetine and α-naphthol are 1.0 and 1.7, respectively.]
Suitability requirements
Resolution: NLT 5 between duloxetine and α-naphthol, *System suitability solution*
Tailing factor: NMT 2.0, *Buffer stage standard solution*
Relative standard deviation: NMT 2.0%, *Buffer stage standard solution*

Analysis
Samples: *Acid stage standard solution, Buffer stage standard solution, Acid stage sample solution,* and *Buffer stage sample solution*
Calculate the concentration of duloxetine ($C_{18}H_{19}NOS$) dissolved in the *Acid stage medium* (C_1):

$$Result = (r_U/r_S) \times C_S \times D \times (M_{r1}/M_{r2})$$

r_U = peak response of duloxetine from the *Acid stage sample solution*
r_S = peak response of duloxetine from the *Acid stage standard solution*
C_S = concentration of USP Duloxetine Hydrochloride RS in the *Acid stage standard solution* (mg/mL)
D = dilution factor of the *Acid stage sample solution,* 5
M_{r1} = molecular weight of duloxetine free base, 297.42
M_{r2} = molecular weight of duloxetine hydrochloride, 333.88

Calculate the equivalent concentration of duloxetine from α-naphthol in the *Acid stage medium* (C_2):

$$Result = (r_U/r_S) \times C_S \times D \times (1/F) \times (M_{r1}/M_{r2})$$

r_U = peak response of α-naphthol from the *Acid stage sample solution*
r_S = peak response of duloxetine from the *Acid stage standard solution*
C_S = concentration of USP Duloxetine Hydrochloride RS in the *Acid stage standard solution* (mg/mL)
D = dilution factor of the *Acid stage sample solution,* 5
F = relative response factor of α-naphthol, 1.7
M_{r1} = molecular weight of duloxetine free base, 297.42
M_{r2} = molecular weight of duloxetine hydrochloride, 333.88

Calculate the equivalent concentration of duloxetine from all of the unspecified degradation products in the *Acid stage medium* (C_3):

$$Result = (r_i/r_S) \times C_S \times D \times (M_{r1}/M_{r2})$$

r_i = sum of the peak responses from all of the unspecified degradation products in the *Acid stage sample solution*
r_S = peak response of duloxetine from the *Acid stage standard solution*
C_S = concentration of USP Duloxetine Hydrochloride RS in the *Acid stage standard solution* (mg/mL)
D = dilution factor of the *Acid stage sample solution,* 5
M_{r1} = molecular weight of duloxetine free base, 297.42
M_{r2} = molecular weight of duloxetine hydrochloride, 333.88

Calculate the percentage of the labeled amount of duloxetine dissolved in the *Acid stage medium* (Q_A):

$$Result = (\Sigma C_i) \times V \times (1/L) \times 100$$

C_i = concentration or equivalent concentration of duloxetine in the *Acid stage medium* (mg/mL)
V = volume of *Acid stage medium,* 1000 mL
L = label claim of duloxetine (mg/Capsule)

Calculate the percentage of the labeled amount of duloxetine dissolved in both the *Acid stage medium* and the *Buffer stage medium*:

$$Result = [(r_U/r_S) \times C_S \times (M_{r1}/M_{r2}) \times V \times (1/L) \times 100] + Q_A$$

r_U = peak response of duloxetine from the *Buffer stage sample solution*

r_S = peak response of duloxetine from the *Buffer stage standard solution*

C_S = concentration of USP Duloxetine Hydrochloride RS in the *Buffer stage standard solution* (mg/mL)

M_{r1} = molecular weight of duloxetine free base, 297.42

M_{r2} = molecular weight of duloxetine hydrochloride, 333.88

V = volume of *Buffer stage medium*, 1000 mL

L = label claim (mg/Capsule)

Q_A = percentage of the labeled amount of duloxetine dissolved in the *Acid stage medium*

Tolerances

Acid stage: For each individual value, NMT 10% of the labeled amount of duloxetine ($C_{18}H_{19}NOS$). The percentage of the labeled amount of duloxetine dissolved at the time specified conforms to *Dissolution* ⟨711⟩, *Acceptance Table 3*.

Buffer stage: NLT 75% (Q) of the labeled amount of duloxetine ($C_{18}H_{19}NOS$). The percentage of the labeled amount of duloxetine dissolved at the time specified conforms to *Dissolution* ⟨711⟩, *Acceptance Table 4*.

Test 4: If the product complies with this test, the labeling indicates that it meets USP *Dissolution Test 4*. Protect solutions of duloxetine from light.

Acid stage

Acid stage medium: 0.1 N hydrochloric acid VS; 1000 mL

Apparatus 1: 100 rpm

Time: 2 h in *Acid stage medium*

Buffer stage

Buffer stage medium: pH 6.8 phosphate buffer (6.8 g/L of monobasic potassium phosphate and 0.9 g/L of sodium hydroxide in water, adjusted with phosphoric acid or 1 N sodium hydroxide VS to a pH of 6.80); 1000 mL

Apparatus 1: 100 rpm

Time: 3 h in *Buffer stage medium*. The time in *Buffer stage medium* includes the time in *Acid stage medium*.

Procedure: After 2 h in the *Acid stage medium*, withdraw a sample from the solution under test and immediately filter. Remove the *Acid stage medium* and add the *Buffer stage medium*.

Solution A: Acetonitrile and water (20:80). To each liter add 1.0 mL of phosphoric acid.

Solution B: Acetonitrile

Mobile phase: See *Table 1*.

Table 1

Time (min)	Solution A (%)	Solution B (%)
0	100	0
10	35	65
11	100	0
15	100	0

Acid stage standard stock solution: 0.011 mg/mL of USP Duloxetine Hydrochloride RS, equivalent to 0.010 mg/mL of duloxetine, in methanol. Use this solution within 10 h.

Acid stage standard solution: (L/20,000) mg/mL of duloxetine from the *Standard stock solution* in solution prepared as follows, where *L* is the label claim, in mg/Capsule. Transfer a suitable volume of *Acid stage standard stock solution* to an appropriate volumetric flask. Add 45% of the flask volume of 0.1 N hydrochloric acid VS and dilute with 0.1 N sodium hydroxide VS to volume. Use this solution within 10 h.

Buffer stage standard stock solution: 0.67 mg/mL of USP Duloxetine Hydrochloride RS, equivalent to 0.6 mg/mL of duloxetine, in acetonitrile

Buffer stage standard solution: (L/1,000) mg/mL of duloxetine from *Buffer stage standard stock solution* in *Buffer stage medium*

Acid stage sample stock solution: Pass a portion of the solution under test through a suitable filter, discard NLT 1 mL, and use the filtrate. Use this solution within 4 h.

Acid stage sample solution: Dilute 5.0 mL of the *Acid stage sample stock solution* with 0.1 N sodium hydroxide to 10 mL. Use this solution within 4 h.

Buffer stage sample solution: Pass a portion of the solution under test through a suitable filter, discard NLT 2 mL, and use the filtrate. Further dilute with *Buffer stage medium*, if needed.

Chromatographic system
(See *Chromatography* ⟨621⟩, *System Suitability*.)

Mode: LC

Detector: UV 230 nm

Column: 4.6-mm × 10.0-cm; 5-μm packing L1

Flow rate: 1 mL/min

Injection volume: 10 μL

System suitability

Sample: *Acid stage standard solution*

[NOTE—The relative retention times for duloxetine 4-naphthyl isomer, duloxetine, and α-naphthol are 0.8, 1.0, and 1.5, respectively.]

Suitability requirements

Tailing factor: NMT 2.0

Relative standard deviation: NMT 2.0%

Instrumental conditions
(See *Ultraviolet-Visible Spectroscopy* ⟨857⟩.)

Mode: UV

Analytical wavelength: 291 nm

Blank: *Buffer stage medium*

System suitability

Sample: *Buffer stage standard solution*

Suitability requirements

Relative standard deviation: NMT 2.0%

Analysis

Samples: *Acid stage standard solution, Buffer stage standard solution, Acid stage sample solution,* and *Buffer stage sample solution*

Calculate the concentration of duloxetine ($C_{18}H_{19}NOS$) dissolved in the *Acid stage medium* (C_1):

$$Result = (r_U/r_S) \times C_S \times D \times (M_{r1}/M_{r2})$$

r_U = peak response of duloxetine from the *Acid stage sample solution*

r_S = peak response of duloxetine from the *Acid stage standard solution*

C_S = concentration of USP Duloxetine Hydrochloride RS in the *Acid stage standard solution* (mg/mL)

D = dilution factor of the *Acid stage sample solution*, 2

M_{r1} = molecular weight of duloxetine free base, 297.42

M_{r2} = molecular weight of duloxetine hydrochloride, 333.88

Calculate the equivalent concentration of duloxetine from α-naphthol in the *Acid stage medium* (C_2):

$$Result = (r_U/r_S) \times C_S \times D \times (1/F) \times (M_{r1}/M_{r2})$$

r_U = peak response of α-naphthol from the *Acid stage sample solution*

r_S = peak response of duloxetine from the *Acid stage standard solution*

C_S = concentration of USP Duloxetine Hydrochloride RS in the *Acid stage standard solution* (mg/mL)

D = dilution factor of the *Acid stage sample solution*, 2

F = relative response factor of α-naphthol, 2.0

M_{r1} = molecular weight of duloxetine free base, 297.42

M_{r2} = molecular weight of α-naphthol, 144.17

Calculate the equivalent concentration of duloxetine from duloxetine 4-naphthyl isomer (4-[3-(Methylamino)-1-(thiophen-2-yl)propyl]naphthalen-1-ol) in the *Acid stage medium* (C_3):

$$Result = (r_U/r_S) \times C_2 \times D \times (1/F) \times (M_{r1}/M_{r2})$$

r_U = peak response of duloxetine 4-naphthyl isomer from the *Acid stage sample solution*

r_S = peak response of duloxetine from the *Acid stage standard solution*

C_2 = equivalent concentration of duloxetine from α-naphthol in the *Acid stage medium* (mg/mL)

D = dilution factor of the *Acid stage sample solution*, 2

F = relative response factor of duloxetine 4-naphthyl isomer, 0.70

M_{r1} = molecular weight of duloxetine free base, 297.42

M_{r2} = molecular weight of duloxetine 4-naphthyl isomer, 297.42

Calculate the percentage of the labeled amount of duloxetine dissolved in *Acid stage medium* (Q_A):

$$Result = \Sigma(C_i) \times V \times (1/L) \times 100$$

C_i = concentration or equivalent concentration of duloxetine in the *Acid stage medium* (mg/mL) associated with duloxetine, α-naphthol, and duloxetine 4-naphthyl isomer

V = volume of *Acid stage medium*, 1000 mL

L = label claim of duloxetine (mg/Capsule)

Calculate the percentage of the labeled amount of duloxetine dissolved in the *Buffer stage medium*:

$$Result = (A_U/A_S) \times [C_S \times (M_{r1}/M_{r2})] \times V \times D \times (1/L) \times 100$$

A_U = absorbance of duloxetine from the *Buffer stage sample solution*

A_S = absorbance of duloxetine from the *Buffer stage standard solution*

C_S = concentration of USP Duloxetine Hydrochloride RS in the *Buffer stage standard solution* (mg/mL)

M_{r1} = molecular weight of duloxetine free base, 297.42

M_{r2} = molecular weight of duloxetine hydrochloride, 333.88

V = volume of *Buffer stage medium*, 1000 mL

D = dilution factor of the *Buffer stage sample solution*, if needed

L = label claim (mg/Capsule)

Tolerances

Acid stage: NMT 10% of the labeled amount of duloxetine ($C_{18}H_{19}NOS$). The percentage of the labeled amount of duloxetine dissolved at the time specified conforms to *Dissolution* ⟨711⟩, *Acceptance Table 3*.

Buffer stage: NLT 75% (Q) of the labeled amount of duloxetine ($C_{18}H_{19}NOS$). The percentage of the labeled amount of duloxetine dissolved at the time specified conforms to *Dissolution* ⟨711⟩, *Acceptance Table 4*.● (RB 1-Aug-2017)

• **UNIFORMITY OF DOSAGE UNITS** ⟨905⟩: Meet the requirements

IMPURITIES

Change to read:

• **ORGANIC IMPURITIES**

Protect solutions of duloxetine from light.

Buffer A, Buffer B, Mobile phase, Diluent, System suitability solution, Standard solution, Sample solution, Chromatographic system, and **System suitability:** Proceed as directed in the *Assay*.

Analysis

Sample: *Sample solution*

Calculate the percentage of each impurity in the portion of Capsules taken:

$$Result = (r_U/r_T) \times 100$$

r_U = peak response for each impurity

r_T = sum of all the peak responses

Acceptance criteria: See ●*Table 2.*

Table 2● (RB 1-Aug-2017)

Name	Relative Retention Time	Acceptance Criteria, NMT (%)
Duloxetine	1.0	—
Duloxetine related compound F[a]	1.1	—
●α-Naphthol● (RB 1-Aug-2017)[b]	1.5	0.2
Duloxetine related compound H[c]	2.2	0.2
Any individual unspecified degradation product	—	0.2
Total impurities	—	0.4

[a] This is a process impurity that is included in *Table 1* for identification purposes only. It is controlled in the drug substance and is not to be reported or included in total impurities.

[b] ●Naphthalen-1-ol.● (RB 1-Aug-2017)

[c] ●May not be present in all formulations.● (RB 1-Aug-2017)

ADDITIONAL REQUIREMENTS

• **PACKAGING AND STORAGE:** Preserve in tight containers. Store at controlled room temperature.

• **LABELING:** The labeling states with which *Dissolution* test the article complies, if other than *Test 1*.

• **USP REFERENCE STANDARDS** ⟨11⟩

USP Duloxetine Hydrochloride RS

USP Duloxetine Related Compound F RS

(*S*)-*N*-Methyl-3-(naphthalen-1-yloxy)-3-(thiophen-3-yl)propan-1-amine hydrochloride.

$C_{18}H_{19}NOS \cdot HCl$ 333.88

USP Duloxetine Related Compound H RS

(*S*)-4-{Methyl[3-(naphthalen-1-yloxy)-3-(thiophen-2-yl)propyl]amino}-4-oxobutanoic acid.

$C_{22}H_{23}NO_4S$ 397.49

Estradiol Benzoate

C$_{25}$H$_{28}$O$_3$ 376.49
Estra-1,3,5(10)-triene-3,17-diol, (17β)-, 3-benzoate;
Estradiol 3-benzoate [50-50-0].

DEFINITION
Estradiol Benzoate contains NLT 97.0% and NMT 103.0% of
estradiol benzoate (C$_{25}$H$_{28}$O$_3$), calculated on the dried
basis.

IDENTIFICATION

Change to read:

- **A. INFRARED ABSORPTION ■⟨197⟩:** [NOTE—Methods described in ⟨197K⟩ or ⟨197A⟩ may be used. If the spectra
  obtained in the solid state show differences, dissolve the
  substance to be examined and the reference substance
  separately in acetone, evaporate to dryness, and record
  new spectra using the residues.]■1S (USP41)
- **B.** The retention time of the major peak of the *Sample
  solution* corresponds to that of the *Standard solution*, as
  obtained in the *Assay*.

ASSAY

Change to read:

- **PROCEDURE**
  Mobile phase: Acetonitrile and water (7:3)
  System suitability solution: Transfer 20.0 mg each of
  USP Estradiol Benzoate RS and estradiol 17-acetate to a
  100-mL volumetric flask. Add 70 mL of acetonitrile, and
  sonicate until dissolved. Add 25 mL of water, mix well,
  and allow to equilibrate to ambient temperature. Dilute
  with water to volume.
  Standard solution: Transfer 20.0 mg of USP Estradiol
  Benzoate RS to a 100-mL volumetric flask. Add 70 mL
  of acetonitrile, and sonicate until dissolved. Add 25 mL
  of water, mix well, and allow to equilibrate to ambient
  temperature. Dilute with water to volume.
  Sample solution: Transfer 20.0 mg of Estradiol Benzo-
  ate to a 100-mL volumetric flask. Add 70 mL of acetoni-
  trile, and sonicate until dissolved. Add 25 mL of water,
  mix well, and allow to equilibrate to ambient tempera-
  ture. Dilute with water to volume.
  Chromatographic system
  (See *Chromatography* ⟨621⟩, *System Suitability*.)
  Mode: LC
  Detector: UV 230 nm
  Columns
   Guard: 4.6-mm × 4.5-cm; packing L1
   Analytical: 4.6-mm × 25-cm; 5-μm packing L1
  Flow rate: 1.5 mL/min
  Injection volume: 20 μL
  System suitability
  Samples: *System suitability solution* and *Standard
  solution*
  [NOTE—The relative retention times for estradiol 17-ace-
  tate and estradiol benzoate are about 0.5 and 1.0,
  respectively.]

Suitability requirements
 Resolution: NLT 6.0 between estradiol 17-acetate
 and estradiol benzoate, *System suitability solution*
 ■1S (USP41)
 Tailing factor: NMT 2.0, *System suitability solution*
 Relative standard deviation: NMT 1.5%, *Standard
 solution*
Analysis
 Samples: *Standard solution* and *Sample solution*
 Calculate the percentage of estradiol benzoate
 (C$_{25}$H$_{28}$O$_3$) in the portion of Estradiol Benzoate taken:

$$\text{Result} = (r_U/r_S) \times (C_S/C_U) \times 100$$

r_U = peak response from the *Sample solution*
r_S = peak response from the *Standard solution*
C_S = concentration of USP Estradiol Benzoate RS in
        the *Standard solution* (mg/mL)
C_U = concentration of Estradiol Benzoate in the
        Sample solution (mg/mL)
Acceptance criteria: 97.0%–103.0% on the dried basis

IMPURITIES
- **RESIDUE ON IGNITION ⟨281⟩**
  Sample: 250 mg
  Acceptance criteria: NMT 0.2%

Change to read:

- **LIMIT OF METHANOL AND DICHLOROMETHANE:** ■Proceed as
  directed in *Residual Solvents* ⟨467⟩.■1S (USP41)
  Acceptance criteria: The sum of methanol and methyl-
  ene chloride is NMT 0.20%.
- **ORGANIC IMPURITIES**
  Diluent: Methylene chloride and alcohol (2:1)
  Standard solution: 5 mg/mL of USP Estradiol Benzoate
  RS in *Diluent*
  Sample solution A: 5 mg/mL of Estradiol Benzoate in
  Diluent
  Sample solution B: 0.1 mg/mL of Estradiol Benzoate in
  Diluent from *Sample solution A*
  Chromatographic system
  (See *Chromatography* ⟨621⟩, *General Procedures, Thin-
  Layer Chromatography.*)
  Mode: TLC
  Adsorbent: 0.25-mm layer of chromatographic silica
  gel mixture
  Developing solvent system: Toluene and ethyl ace-
  tate (70:30)
  Spray reagent: 50 mg/mL of ammonium molybdate
  in 10% sulfuric acid
  Analysis
  Samples: *Standard solution, Sample solution A*, and
  Sample solution B
  To the plate apply 20-μL aliquots of the *Standard solution* and *Sample solution A* and 20-, 15-, 10-, 5-, and
  2-μL aliquots of *Sample solution B*. The volumetric series of *Sample solution B* represents 2.0%, 1.5%,
  1.0%, 0.5%, and 0.2% of the concentration of Estradiol Benzoate within the *Sample solution A* spot.
  Allow the spots to dry, and develop the chromatogram until the solvent front has moved about three-
  fourths of the length of the plate. Spray the plate
  thoroughly with *Spray reagent*, and dry. Heat the
  plate in a drying oven for 10 min at about 115°.
  Calculate the relative retardation factor (relative to estradiol benzoate) of all spots within the lanes for
  Sample solution A and *Sample solution B*.
  Determine the percentages of each impurity by comparing the intensity of the impurity spots within *Sample solution A* to those of the main spots obtained
  from the series of *Sample solution B*, ignoring any impurity peak less intense than the main spots found in

the *Sample solution B* lane containing 0.2% of the amount of estradiol benzoate of *Sample solution A*.
Acceptance criteria: See *Table 1*.

Table 1

Name	Relative Retardation Factor	Acceptance Criteria, NMT (%)
Estradiol[a]	0.84	1.0
Estradiol benzoate	1.00	—
17a-Estradiol benzoate[b]	1.15	1.0
Estrone[c]	1.21	1.0
Any individual unspecified impurity	—	1.0
Total impurities	—	2.0

[a] Estra-1,3,5(10)-triene-3,17b-diol.
[b] Estra-1,3,5(10)-triene-3,17a-diol 3-benzoate.
[c] Estra-1,3,5(10)-triene-17-one, 3-hydroxy.

SPECIFIC TESTS
- **OPTICAL ROTATION ⟨781S⟩,** *Procedures, Specific Rotation*
  Sample solution: 10 mg/mL, previously dried in dioxane
  Acceptance criteria: +57.0° to +63.0°
- **LOSS ON DRYING ⟨731⟩**
  Analysis: Dry at 100°–105° for 3 h.
  Acceptance criteria: NMT 0.5%
- **PARTICLE SIZE DISTRIBUTION ESTIMATION BY ANALYTICAL SIEVING ⟨786⟩**
  Suspension fluid: To a mixture of glycerin and water (60:40, w/w) add a sufficient quantity of polysorbate 20 to obtain a solution having a concentration of 125 µL of polysorbate 20 per 100 g of solution.
  Sample suspension: Saturate the *Suspension fluid* by adding 100 mg of fine Estradiol Benzoate per 100 g of *Suspension fluid*, and sonicate for 10 min. Pass the resulting suspension through a nylon filter of 0.45-µm pore size. To the filtrate, add 50 mg of Estradiol Benzoate per mL of the filtered, saturated *Suspension fluid*, and mix on a vortex mixer until dispersed (about 1 min).
  Analysis: Using a suitable multi-wavelength particle size analyzer,[1] determine the particle size distribution within the *Sample suspension*, analyzing the results in the range of 5–600 µm.
  Acceptance criteria: NMT 50% of the particles are less than 30 µm, and NLT 90% of the particles are less than 450 µm. The mean diameter of fine grade Estradiol Benzoate is NMT 100 µm, and the mean diameter of coarse grade Estradiol Benzoate is 100–200 µm.

ADDITIONAL REQUIREMENTS
- **PACKAGING AND STORAGE:** Preserve in tight, light-resistant containers.
- **LABELING:** Label it to indicate that it is for veterinary use only. Label it to indicate whether it is coarse grade or fine grade.
- **USP REFERENCE STANDARDS ⟨11⟩**
  USP Estradiol Benzoate RS

Eszopiclone Tablets

DEFINITION
Eszopiclone Tablets contain NLT 90.0% and NMT 110.0% of the labeled amount of eszopiclone ($C_{17}H_{17}ClN_6O_3$).

[1] A suitable multi-wavelength particle size analyzer is model LS 13 320, obtained from Beckman Coulter, Inc., Fullerton, CA, or equivalent.

IDENTIFICATION
- **A. INFRARED ABSORPTION ⟨197K⟩**
  Standard: USP Eszopiclone RS
  Sample: Nominally 37.5 mg of eszopiclone from Tablets prepared as follows. Powder a number of Tablets, and mix the resulting powder. Transfer a portion of powder, equivalent to 37.5 mg of eszopiclone, to a suitable container, add 30 mL of acetone, and shake. Dilute with acetone to 50 mL and pass the resulting solution through a suitable filter. Evaporate the filtrate to dryness on a water bath and dry the residue in an oven at 60° for 2 h.
  Acceptance criteria: Meets the requirements
- **B.** The retention time of the major peak of the *Sample solution* corresponds to that of the *Standard solution*, as obtained in the *Assay*.

ASSAY
- **PROCEDURE**
  Solution A: 1.4 g/L of anhydrous dibasic sodium phosphate in water
  Mobile phase: Acetonitrile and *Solution A* (25:75) adjusted with dilute phosphoric acid to a pH of 6.5 ± 0.05
  Standard stock solution: 0.5 mg/mL of USP Eszopiclone RS prepared as follows. Transfer a suitable quantity of USP Eszopiclone RS to an appropriate volumetric flask and add 50% of the final flask volume of acetonitrile. Sonication may be used to promote dissolution. Dilute with acetonitrile to volume.
  Standard solution: 0.03 mg/mL of USP Eszopiclone RS from *Standard stock solution* in *Mobile phase* passed through a suitable filter of 0.45-µm pore size. Use the filtrate.
  Sample stock solution: Nominally 0.2 mg/mL of eszopiclone from Tablets prepared as follows. Transfer NLT 5 intact Tablets to a suitable volumetric flask. Add 5% of the final flask volume of *Solution A* and sonicate in cool water for 5 min with constant shaking. Add 30% of the final flask volume of acetonitrile and sonicate for 15 min. Dilute with acetonitrile to volume. Centrifuge the resulting solution and use the supernatant.
  Sample solution: Nominally 0.03 mg/mL of eszopiclone from *Sample stock solution* in *Mobile phase* passed through a suitable filter of 0.45-µm pore size. Use the filtrate.
  Chromatographic system
  (See *Chromatography ⟨621⟩, System Suitability*.)
  Mode: LC
  Detector: UV 303 nm
  Column: 4.6-mm × 15.0-cm; 5-µm packing L1
  Column temperature: 30°
  Flow rate: 1.5 mL/min
  Injection volume: 50 µL
  Run time: NLT 1.9 times the retention time of eszopiclone
  System suitability
  Sample: *Standard solution*
  Suitability requirements
  Tailing factor: NMT 2.0
  Relative standard deviation: NMT 2.0%
  Analysis
  Samples: *Standard solution* and *Sample solution*
  Calculate the percentage of the labeled amount of eszopiclone ($C_{17}H_{17}ClN_6O_3$) in the portion of Tablets taken:

  $$Result = (r_U/r_S) \times (C_S/C_U) \times 100$$

  r_U = peak response from the *Sample solution*
  r_S = peak response from the *Standard solution*
  C_S = concentration of USP Eszopiclone RS in the *Standard solution* (mg/mL)
  C_U = nominal concentration of eszopiclone in the *Sample solution* (mg/mL)

Acceptance criteria: 90.0%–110.0%

PERFORMANCE TESTS

Change to read:

- **DISSOLUTION ⟨711⟩**
  Test 1● (RB 1-Aug-2017)
  Medium: 0.1 N hydrochloric acid; 500 mL
  Apparatus 2:   50 rpm
  Time: 30 min
  Solution A: 1.4 g/L of anhydrous dibasic sodium phosphate in water
  Mobile phase: Acetonitrile and *Solution A* (30:70) adjusted with dilute phosphoric acid (1 in 10) to a pH of 6.5 ± 0.05
  Standard stock solution: 0.1 mg/mL of USP Eszopiclone RS in acetonitrile. Sonication may be used to promote dissolution.
  Standard solution: (*L*/500) mg/mL of USP Eszopiclone RS from *Standard stock solution* in *Medium*, where *L* is the Tablet label claim in mg. Pass the resulting solution through a suitable filter of 0.45-μm pore size and use the filtrate.
  Sample solution: Pass a portion of the solution under test through a suitable filter of 0.45-μm pore size and use the filtrate.
  Chromatographic system
  (See *Chromatography* ⟨621⟩, *System Suitability*.)
  Mode: LC
  Detector: UV 303 nm
  Column: 4.6-mm × 15.0-cm; 5-μm packing L1
  Column temperature: 30°
  Flow rate: 1.2 mL/min
  Injection volume: 100 μL
  Run time: NLT 1.5 times the retention time of eszopiclone
  System suitability
  Sample: *Standard solution*
  Suitability requirements
  Tailing factor: NMT 2.0
  Relative standard deviation: NMT 2.0%
  Analysis
  Samples: *Standard solution* and *Sample solution*
  Calculate the percentage of the labeled amount of eszopiclone ($C_{17}H_{17}ClN_6O_3$) dissolved:

  $$Result = (r_U/r_S) \times C_S \times V \times (1/L) \times 100$$

  r_U = peak response from the *Sample solution*
  r_S = peak response from the *Standard solution*
  C_S = concentration of USP Eszopiclone RS in the *Standard solution* (mg/mL)
  V = volume of *Medium*, 500 mL
  L = label claim (mg/Tablet)
  Acceptance criteria: NLT 80% (*Q*) of the labeled amount of eszopiclone ($C_{17}H_{17}ClN_6O_3$) is dissolved.
  Test 2
  Medium: 0.1 N hydrochloric acid VS; 500 mL
  Apparatus 2:   50 rpm
  Time: 20 min
  Buffer: To each liter of water add 1.0 mL of phosphoric acid and adjust with 2 N sodium hydroxide TS to a pH of 4.0.
  Mobile phase: Acetonitrile and *Buffer* (20:80)
  Standard stock solution: 0.1 mg/mL of USP Eszopiclone RS in *Medium*. Sonication may be used to promote dissolution.
  Standard solution: (*L*/500) mg/mL of USP Eszopiclone RS from *Standard stock solution* in *Medium*, where *L* is the label claim in mg/Tablet. Pass the resulting solution through a suitable filter of 0.45-μm pore size and use the filtrate.

Sample solution: Pass a portion of the solution under test through a suitable filter of 0.45-μm pore size and use the filtrate.
Chromatographic system
(See *Chromatography* ⟨621⟩, *System Suitability*.)
Mode: LC
Detector: UV 303 nm
Column: 4.6-mm × 15.0-cm; 5-μm packing L1
Column temperature: 45°
Flow rate: 1 mL/min
Injection volume: 80 μL
Run time: NLT 1.5 times the retention time of eszopiclone
System suitability
Sample: *Standard solution*
Suitability requirements
Tailing factor: NMT 2.0
Relative standard deviation: NMT 2.0%
Analysis
Samples: *Standard solution* and *Sample solution*
Calculate the percentage of the labeled amount of eszopiclone ($C_{17}H_{17}ClN_6O_3$) dissolved:

$$Result = (r_U/r_S) \times C_S \times V \times (1/L) \times 100$$

r_U = peak response from the *Sample solution*
r_S = peak response from the *Standard solution*
C_S = concentration of USP Eszopiclone RS in the *Standard solution* (mg/mL)
V = volume of *Medium*, 500 mL
L = label claim (mg/Tablet)
Tolerances: NLT 80% (*Q*) of the labeled amount of eszopiclone ($C_{17}H_{17}ClN_6O_3$) is dissolved.● (RB 1-Aug-2017)
- **UNIFORMITY OF DOSAGE UNITS ⟨905⟩:**   Meets the requirements

IMPURITIES

Change to read:

- **ORGANIC IMPURITIES**
  Protect all solutions from light.
  Solution A: 8.1 g/L of ●sodium dodecyl sulfate● (RB 1-Aug-2017) and 6.9 g/L of monobasic sodium phosphate in water. Sonicate for NLT 15 min and do not let the temperature of the water bath exceed 25°. Pass the resulting solution through a suitable filter of 0.45-μm pore size. Foam may form during filtration.
  Mobile phase: Acetonitrile and *Solution A* (37:63) adjusted with dilute phosphoric acid (1 in 100) to a pH of 4.8 ± 0.05
  Diluent: Acetonitrile and *Solution A* (37:63) adjusted with dilute phosphoric acid (1 in 100) to a pH of 2.5 ± 0.05
  System suitability solution: 0.008 mg/mL each of USP Eszopiclone Related Compound A RS and USP Eszopiclone RS in *Diluent*. Sonication may be used to promote dissolution.
  Standard solution: 0.008 mg/mL of USP Eszopiclone RS in *Diluent* passed through a suitable membrane filter of 0.45-μm pore size. Use the filtrate. Sonication may be used to promote dissolution.
  Sample solution: Nominally 0.8 mg/mL of eszopiclone in *Diluent* prepared as follows. Crush NLT 20 Tablets to a fine powder and transfer a suitable portion to an appropriate volumetric flask. Add 60% of the final flask volume of *Diluent*, sonicate for 15 min in cold water with periodic shaking, and dilute with *Diluent* to volume. Pass the resulting solution through a suitable membrane filter of 0.45-μm pore size, and use the filtrate.
  Chromatographic system
  (See *Chromatography* ⟨621⟩, *System Suitability*.)

Mode: LC
Detector: UV 303 nm
Column: 4.6-mm × 25-cm; 5-µm packing L1
Column temperature: 30°
Flow rate: 1.5 mL/min
Injection volume: 50 µL
Run time: NLT 2 times the retention time of eszopiclone
System suitability
Samples: *System suitability solution* and *Standard solution*
Suitability requirements
Resolution: NLT 10 between eszopiclone related compound A and eszopiclone, *System suitability solution*
Tailing factor: NMT 2.0 for eszopiclone, *Standard solution*
Relative standard deviation: NMT 5.0%, *Standard solution*
Analysis
Samples: *Standard solution* and *Sample solution*
Calculate the percentage of each degradation product in the portion of Tablets taken:

$$Result = (r_U/r_S) \times (C_S/C_U) \times (1/F) \times 100$$

r_U = peak response of each degradation product from the *Sample solution*
r_S = peak response of eszopiclone from the *Standard solution*
C_S = concentration of USP Eszopiclone RS in the *Standard solution* (mg/mL)
C_U = nominal concentration of eszopiclone in the *Sample solution* (mg/mL)
F = relative response factor (see *Table 1*)
Acceptance criteria: See *Table 1*. Disregard peaks less than 0.04%.

Table 1

Name	Relative Retention Time	Relative Response Factor	Acceptance Criteria, NMT (%)
Zopiclone alcohol[a]	0.11	1.7	1.0
2-Amino-5-chloropyridine	0.21	0.76	1.0
Eszopiclone related compound A	0.44	0.86	1.0
Eszopiclone	1.0	—	—
Any individual unspecified degradation product	—	1.0	0.50
Total degradation products	—	—	2.0

[a] 6-(5-Chloropyridin-2-yl)-7-hydroxy-6,7-dihydro-5*H*-pyrrolo[3,4-*b*]pyrazin-5-one.

ADDITIONAL REQUIREMENTS
• **PACKAGING AND STORAGE:** Preserve in tight containers. Store at controlled room temperature.

Add the following:

•• **LABELING:** The labeling states the *Dissolution* test used only if *Test 1* is not used.• (RB 1-Aug-2017)

Glycine

$C_2H_5NO_2$ 75.07
Glycine [56-40-6].

DEFINITION
Glycine contains NLT 98.5% and NMT 101.5% of glycine ($C_2H_5NO_2$), calculated on the dried basis.

IDENTIFICATION
• **A. INFRARED ABSORPTION ⟨197M⟩**

ASSAY
• **PROCEDURE**
Sample: 150 mg of Glycine
Blank: 100 mL of glacial acetic acid
Titrimetric system
(See *Titrimetry ⟨541⟩*.)
Mode: Direct titration
Titrant: 0.1 N perchloric acid VS
Endpoint detection: Visual
Analysis: Dissolve the *Sample* in 100 mL of glacial acetic acid, and add 1 drop of crystal violet TS. Titrate with the *Titrant* to a green endpoint. Perform the *Blank* determination.
Calculate the percentage of glycine ($C_2H_5NO_2$) in the *Sample* taken:

$$Result = \{[(V_S - V_B) \times N \times F]/W\} \times 100$$

V_S = *Titrant* volume consumed by the *Sample* (mL)
V_B = *Titrant* volume consumed by the *Blank* (mL)
N = actual normality of the *Titrant* (mEq/mL)
F = equivalency factor, 75.07 mg/mEq
W = *Sample* weight (mg)
Acceptance criteria: 98.5%–101.5% on the dried basis

IMPURITIES
• **RESIDUE ON IGNITION ⟨281⟩:** NMT 0.1%
• **CHLORIDE AND SULFATE ⟨221⟩,** *Chloride*
Standard solution: 0.10 mL of 0.020 N hydrochloric acid
Sample: 1 g of Glycine
Acceptance criteria: NMT 0.007%
• **CHLORIDE AND SULFATE ⟨221⟩,** *Sulfate*
Standard solution: 0.20 mL of 0.020 N sulfuric acid
Sample: 3 g of Glycine
Acceptance criteria: NMT 0.0065%

Delete the following:

•• **HEAVY METALS,** *Method I* ⟨231⟩: NMT 20 ppm• (Official 1-Jan-2018)
• **HYDROLYZABLE SUBSTANCES**
Sample solution: 100 mg/mL of Glycine
Analysis: Boil 10 mL of the *Sample solution* for 1 min, and set aside for 2 h.
Acceptance criteria: The solution appears as clear and as mobile as 10 mL of the same solution that has not been boiled.

Add the following:

■• **RELATED COMPOUNDS**
Solution A: Transfer 2.16 g of octanesulfonic acid sodium salt to a 1000-mL volumetric flask, add 900 mL of HPLC grade water and 2.0 mL of perchloric acid, and mix to dissolve. Adjust with 5 N sodium hydroxide solution to a pH of 2.2. Dilute with HPLC grade water to volume. Pass the solution through a membrane filter of 0.2-μm pore size.
Solution B: Acetonitrile
Mobile phase: Gradient elution. See *Table 1.*

Table 1

Time (min)	Solution A (%)	Solution B (%)
0	100	0
7	100	0
13	90	10
18	90	10
35	100	0
45	100	0

Standard solution: A mixture of 0.005 mg/mL each of USP Glycine RS, USP Diglycine RS, USP Triglycine RS, and glycine anhydride,[1] and 0.0025 mg/mL of monochloroacetic acid[2] in HPLC grade water. [NOTE—Monochloroacetic acid may be omitted from the *Standard solution* if the article being tested does not contain this substance.]
Sample solution: Transfer 125 mg of Glycine into a 25-mL volumetric flask, dissolve in and dilute with HPLC grade water to volume.
Blank: HPLC grade water
Chromatographic system
(See *Chromatography ⟨621⟩, System Suitability.*)
Mode: LC
Detector: UV 200 nm
Column: 4.6-mm × 15-cm; 3-μm packing L1
Column temperature: 25°
Flow rate: 1 mL/min
Injection volume: 20 μL
System suitability
Samples: *Standard solution* and *Blank*
[NOTE—See *Table 2* for the relative retention times.]
Suitability requirements
  Interference peaks: Compare the chromatogram obtained from the *Standard solution* with that obtained from the *Blank.* Any peak area from the *Blank* that overlaps or co-elutes with the amino acid peak from the *Standard solution* is NMT 2.0% of that amino acid peak area.
  Resolution: NLT 2.0 between the diglycine and triglycine peaks, *Standard solution*
  Relative standard deviation: NMT 5.0% each for the specified peaks, *Standard solution*
Analysis
Samples: *Standard solution, Sample solution,* and *Blank*
Separately inject the *Blank, Standard solution,* and *Sample solution* into the chromatograph. Compare the chromatogram from the *Sample solution* with that from the *Blank.* Disregard any peak observed in both the *Sample solution* and the *Blank.* Identify the amino acid impurities in the *Sample solution* by comparing with those specified in the *Standard solution.*
Separately calculate the percentage of each specified impurity in the portion of Glycine taken:

$$\text{Result} = (r_U/r_S) \times (C_S/C_U) \times 100$$

[1] Analytical grade with purity NLT 99.0%.
[2] Analytical grade with purity NLT 99.0%.

r_U = peak response of glycine anhydride, monochloroacetic acid, diglycine, or triglycine from the *Sample solution*
r_S = peak response of glycine anhydride, monochloroacetic acid, diglycine, or triglycine from the *Standard solution*
C_S = concentration of glycine anhydride, monochloroacetic acid, USP Diglycine RS, or USP Triglycine RS in the *Standard solution* (mg/mL)
C_U = concentration of Glycine in the *Sample solution* (mg/mL)
Separately calculate the percentage of iminodiacetic acid, hexamethylenetetramine, and any unspecified impurity in the portion of Glycine taken:

$$\text{Result} = (r_U/r_S) \times (C_S/C_U) \times 100$$

r_U = peak response of iminodiacetic acid, hexamethylenetetramine, or any unspecified impurity from the *Sample solution*
r_S = peak response of glycine from the *Standard solution*
C_S = concentration of USP Glycine RS in the *Standard solution* (mg/mL)
C_U = concentration of Glycine in the *Sample solution* (mg/mL)
Acceptance criteria: See *Table 2.* [NOTE—Disregard any impurity peak less than 0.05%.]

Table 2

Name	Relative Retention Time	Acceptance Criteria, NMT (%)
Glycine anhydride	0.25	0.1
Monochloroacetic acid	0.44	a
Iminodiacetic acid	0.60	0.1
Glycine	1.00	—
Diglycine	1.70	0.1
Triglycine	1.80	0.1
Hexamethylenetetramine	2.47	0.1
Any unspecified impurity	—	b
Total impurities	—	1.0

a The limit should be controlled as per International Council for Harmonisation (ICH) M7.

b The limit should be based on the maximum daily dose (MDD) of the drug products.

■1S (USP41)

SPECIFIC TESTS
• **LOSS ON DRYING ⟨731⟩**
  Analysis: Dry at 105° for 2 h.
  Acceptance criteria: NMT 0.2%

ADDITIONAL REQUIREMENTS

Change to read:

• **PACKAGING AND STORAGE:** Preserve in well-closed containers ■at room temperature.■1S (USP41)

Change to read:

• **USP REFERENCE STANDARDS ⟨11⟩**
  ■USP Diglycine RS■1S (USP41)
  USP Glycine RS
  ■USP Triglycine RS■1S (USP41)

Delete the following:

∎Hydrocortisone Acetate Ophthalmic Ointment

DEFINITION
Hydrocortisone Acetate Ophthalmic Ointment is Hydrocortisone Acetate in a suitable ophthalmic ointment base. It contains NLT 90.0% and NMT 110.0% of the labeled amount of total steroids, calculated as $C_{23}H_{32}O_6$. It is sterile.

IDENTIFICATION
• A. THIN-LAYER CHROMATOGRAPHIC IDENTIFICATION TEST ⟨201⟩
  Sample solution: Transfer a quantity of Ophthalmic Ointment equivalent to 5 mg of hydrocortisone acetate to a flask, add 5 mL of methanol, and heat on a steam bath for 5 min with frequent mixing. Cool to solidify the Ophthalmic Ointment base, and filter. Use the filtrate.
  Spray reagent: 70% Methanolic sulfuric acid solution
  Analysis: Proceed as directed in the chapter. Locate the spots by spraying the dried plate with *Spray reagent*. Heat the plate for 20–30 min at 90°, allow to cool, and view under long-wavelength UV light.
  Acceptance criteria: The R_F value and fluorescence of the principal spot of the *Sample solution* correspond to those of the *Standard solution*.

ASSAY
• ASSAY FOR STEROIDS ⟨351⟩
  Standard solution: Proceed as directed in the chapter for *Standard Preparation* using USP Hydrocortisone Acetate RS.
  Sample solution: Transfer a portion of Ophthalmic Ointment equivalent to 10 mg of hydrocortisone acetate to a flask, and add 30 mL of alcohol. Heat on a steam bath to melt the Ophthalmic Ointment base. Cool to solidify the Ophthalmic Ointment base, and filter the alcohol solution into a 100-mL volumetric flask. Repeat the extraction with three 20-mL portions of alcohol, and add alcohol to volume. Pipet 10 mL of this solution into a 100-mL volumetric flask, and add alcohol to volume. Pipet 20 mL of the resulting solution into a glass-stoppered, 50-mL conical flask.
  Analysis: Proceed as directed in the chapter. Calculate the percentage of the total amount of steroids, as $C_{23}H_{32}O_6$, in the portion of Ophthalmic Ointment taken:

$$Result = (A_U/A_S) \times (C_S/C_U) \times 100$$

  A_U = absorbance of the *Sample solution*
  A_S = absorbance of the *Standard solution*
  C_S = concentration of the *Standard solution* (mg/mL)
  C_U = nominal concentration of hydrocortisone acetate in the *Sample solution* (mg/mL)
  Acceptance criteria: 90.0%–110.0%

SPECIFIC TESTS
• STERILITY TESTS ⟨71⟩: Meets the requirements
• OTHER REQUIREMENTS: It meets the requirements for *Particulate and Foreign Matter* and *Container Contents* in *Ophthalmic Products—Quality Tests* ⟨771⟩, *Drug Product Quality, Universal Tests, Particulate and Foreign Matter* and *Container Contents*.

ADDITIONAL REQUIREMENTS
• PACKAGING AND STORAGE: Preserve in collapsible ophthalmic ointment tubes.

• USP REFERENCE STANDARDS ⟨11⟩
  USP Hydrocortisone Acetate RS
  ∎1S *(USP41)*

Delete the following:

∎Hydroxyzine Pamoate Oral Suspension

DEFINITION
Hydroxyzine Pamoate Oral Suspension contains hydroxyzine pamoate ($C_{21}H_{27}ClN_2O_2 \cdot C_{23}H_{16}O_6$) equivalent to NLT 90.0% and NMT 110.0% of the labeled amount of hydroxyzine hydrochloride ($C_{21}H_{27}ClN_2O_2 \cdot 2HCl$).

IDENTIFICATION
• A. The retention time of the major peak of the *Sample solution* corresponds to that of the *Standard solution*, as obtained in the *Assay*.

ASSAY
• PROCEDURE
  Buffer: 7.0 g/L of monobasic sodium phosphate in water adjusted with phosphoric acid to a pH of 4.4 and filtered through a polytef membrane filter of 5-μm pore size
  Mobile phase: Methanol and *Buffer* (50:50)
  Standard solution: 0.18 mg/mL of USP Hydroxyzine Pamoate RS in methanol (equivalent to 0.1 mg/mL of hydroxyzine hydrochloride)
  Sample solution: Nominally equivalent to 0.1 mg/mL of hydroxyzine hydrochloride from Oral Suspension prepared as follows. Transfer a suitable volume of Oral Suspension, freshly mixed and free from air bubbles, to an appropriate volumetric flask. Dissolve in and dilute with methanol to volume. Pass this solution through a polytef membrane filter of 1-μm or finer pore size.
  Chromatographic system
  (See *Chromatography* ⟨621⟩, *System Suitability*.)
  Mode: LC
  Detector: UV 232 nm
  Column: 4.6-mm × 25-cm; packing L9
  Flow rate: 2.5 mL/min
  Injection volume: 25 μL
  System suitability
  Sample: *Standard solution*
  Suitability requirements
    Relative standard deviation: NMT 2.0% for 4 replicate injections
  Analysis
  Samples: *Standard solution* and *Sample solution*
  Calculate the percentage of hydroxyzine pamoate ($C_{21}H_{27}ClN_2O_2 \cdot C_{23}H_{16}O_6$) equivalent to the labeled amount of hydroxyzine hydrochloride ($C_{21}H_{27}ClN_2O_2 \cdot 2HCl$) in the portion of Oral Suspension taken:

$$Result = (r_U/r_S) \times (C_S/C_U) \times (M_{r1}/M_{r2}) \times 100$$

  r_U = peak response from the *Sample solution*
  r_S = peak response from the *Standard solution*
  C_S = concentration of USP Hydroxyzine Pamoate RS in the *Standard solution* (mg/mL)
  C_U = nominal equivalent concentration of hydroxyzine hydrochloride in the *Sample solution* (mg/mL)
  M_{r1} = molecular weight of hydroxyzine hydrochloride, 447.83
  M_{r2} = molecular weight of hydroxyzine pamoate, 763.27

Acceptance criteria: 90.0%–110.0%

PERFORMANCE TESTS
• **UNIFORMITY OF DOSAGE UNITS ⟨905⟩:** Meets the requirements for oral suspension packaged in single-unit containers
• **DELIVERABLE VOLUME ⟨698⟩:** Meets the requirements for oral suspension packaged in multiple-unit containers

SPECIFIC TESTS
• **PH ⟨791⟩:** 4.5–7.0

ADDITIONAL REQUIREMENTS
• **PACKAGING AND STORAGE:** Preserve in tight, light-resistant containers.
• **USP REFERENCE STANDARDS ⟨11⟩**
  USP Hydroxyzine Pamoate RS
  ■15 *(USP41)*

Isoleucine

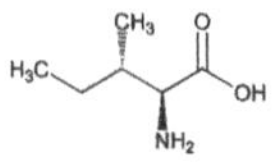

C₆H₁₃NO₂   131.17
L-Isoleucine [73-32-5].

DEFINITION
Isoleucine contains NLT 98.5% and NMT 101.5% of L-isoleucine ($C_6H_{13}NO_2$), calculated on the dried basis.

IDENTIFICATION
• **A. INFRARED ABSORPTION ⟨197K⟩**

ASSAY
• **PROCEDURE**
  Sample: 130 mg of Isoleucine
  Blank: Mix 3 mL of formic acid and 50 mL of glacial acetic acid.
  Titrimetric system
  (See *Titrimetry* ⟨541⟩.)
  Mode: Direct titration
  Titrant: 0.1 N perchloric acid VS
  Endpoint detection: Potentiometric
  Analysis: Dissolve the *Sample* in 3 mL of formic acid and 50 mL of glacial acetic acid. Titrate with the *Titrant*. Perform the blank determination.
  Calculate the percentage of L-isoleucine ($C_6H_{13}NO_2$) in the *Sample* taken:

$$Result = \{[(V_S - V_B) \times N_A \times F]/W\} \times 100$$

V_S = *Titrant* volume consumed by the *Sample* (mL)
V_B = *Titrant* volume consumed by the *Blank* (mL)
N_A = actual normality of the *Titrant* (mEq/mL)
F = equivalency factor, 131.2 mg/mEq
W = *Sample* weight (mg)
  Acceptance criteria: 98.5%–101.5% on the dried basis

IMPURITIES
• **RESIDUE ON IGNITION ⟨281⟩:** NMT 0.3%
• **CHLORIDE AND SULFATE ⟨221⟩,** *Chloride*
  Standard solution: 0.50 mL of 0.020 N hydrochloric acid

Sample: 0.73 g of Isoleucine
Acceptance criteria: NMT 0.05%
• **CHLORIDE AND SULFATE ⟨221⟩,** *Sulfate*
  Standard solution: 0.10 mL of 0.020 N sulfuric acid
  Sample: 0.33 g of Isoleucine
  Acceptance criteria: NMT 0.03%
• **IRON ⟨241⟩:** NMT 30 ppm

Delete the following:

•**HEAVY METALS,** *Method I* ⟨231⟩**:** NMT 15 ppm• (Official 1-Jan-2018)

Change to read:

• **RELATED COMPOUNDS**
  • (RB 1-Aug-2017)
  System suitability solution: 0.4 mg/mL each of USP L-Isoleucine RS and USP L-Valine RS in 0.1 N hydrochloric acid
  Standard solution: 0.05 mg/mL of USP L-Isoleucine RS in 0.1 N hydrochloric acid. [NOTE—This solution has a concentration equivalent to 0.5% of that of the *Sample solution*.]
  Sample solution: 10 mg/mL of Isoleucine in 0.1 N hydrochloric acid
  Chromatographic system
  (See *Chromatography* ⟨621⟩, *General Procedures, Thin-Layer Chromatography*.)
  Mode: TLC
  Adsorbent: 0.25-mm layer of chromatographic silica gel mixture
  Application volume: 5 µL
  Developing solvent system: Butyl alcohol, glacial acetic acid, and water (3:1:1)
  Spray reagent: 2 mg/mL of ninhydrin in a mixture of butyl alcohol and 2 N acetic acid (95:5)
  System suitability
  Sample: *System suitability solution*
  Suitability requirements: The chromatogram of the *System suitability solution* exhibits two clearly separated spots.
  Analysis
  Samples: *System suitability solution, Standard solution,* and *Sample solution*
  After air-drying the plate, spray with *Spray reagent*, and heat between 100° and 105° for 15 min. Examine the plate under white light.
  Acceptance criteria: Any secondary spot of the *Sample solution* is not larger or more intense than the principal spot of the *Standard solution*.
  Individual impurities: NMT 0.5%
  Total impurities: NMT 2.0%

SPECIFIC TESTS
• **OPTICAL ROTATION ⟨781S⟩,** *Procedures, Specific Rotation*
  Sample solution: 40 mg/mL in 6 N hydrochloric acid
  Acceptance criteria: +38.9° to +41.8°
• **PH ⟨791⟩**
  Sample solution: 10 mg/mL in water
  Acceptance criteria: 5.5–7.0
• **LOSS ON DRYING ⟨731⟩**
  Analysis: Dry at 105° for 3 h.
  Acceptance criteria: NMT 0.3%

ADDITIONAL REQUIREMENTS
• **PACKAGING AND STORAGE:** Preserve in well-closed containers.

Change to read:

- **USP Reference Standards ⟨11⟩**
  USP L-Isoleucine RS
  ● (RB 1-Aug-2017)
  USP L-Valine RS

Levocarnitine

C$_7$H$_{15}$NO$_3$ 161.20
(*R*)-3-Carboxy-2-hydroxy-*N,N,N*-trimethyl-1-propanaminium, inner salt;
(*R*)-(3-Carboxy-2-hydroxypropyl)trimethylammonium, inner salt [541-15-1].

DEFINITION
Levocarnitine contains NLT 97.0% and NMT 103.0% of levocarnitine (C$_7$H$_{15}$NO$_3$), calculated on the anhydrous basis.

IDENTIFICATION
- **A. Infrared Absorption ⟨197K⟩**
  Analysis: Dry the sample and USP Levocarnitine RS under vacuum at 50° for 5 h.
  Acceptance criteria: Meets the requirements

Add the following:

■**• B.** The retention time of the major peak of the derivatized *Sample solution* corresponds to that of the levocarnitine peak of the derivatized *System suitability solution*, as obtained in the test for *Enantiomeric Purity*.■1S (USP41)

ASSAY
- **Procedure**
  Sample: 100 mg of Levocarnitine
  Blank: A mixture of 3 mL of formic acid and 50 mL of glacial acetic acid
  Titrimetric system
  (See *Titrimetry* ⟨541⟩.)
  Mode: Direct titration
  Titrant: 0.1 N perchloric acid VS
  Endpoint detection: Visual
  Analysis: Dissolve the *Sample* in a mixture of 3 mL of formic acid and 50 mL of glacial acetic acid. Add 2 drops of crystal violet TS, and titrate with the *Titrant* to an emerald green endpoint. Perform the blank determination.
  Calculate the percentage of levocarnitine (C$_7$H$_{15}$NO$_3$) in the portion of Levocarnitine taken:

$$Result = \{[(V_S - V_B) \times N \times F]/W\} \times 100$$

  V_S = *Titrant* volume consumed by the *Sample* (mL)
  V_B = *Titrant* volume consumed by the *Blank* (mL)
  N = actual normality of the *Titrant* (mEq/mL)
  F = equivalency factor, 161.2 mg/mEq
  W = *Sample* weight (mg)
  Acceptance criteria: 97.0%–103.0% on the anhydrous basis

IMPURITIES
- **Residue on Ignition ⟨281⟩:** NMT 0.5%
- **Chloride and Sulfate ⟨221⟩,** *Chloride*
  Standard solution: 0.50 mL of 0.020 N hydrochloric acid

Sample: 0.090 g of Levocarnitine
Acceptance criteria: NMT 0.4%

Delete the following:

●**• Heavy Metals ⟨231⟩:** NMT 20 ppm● (Official 1-Jan-2018)

Add the following:

■**• Enantiomeric Purity**
  Buffer solution: Mix thoroughly 2000 mL of water with 5 mL of phosphoric acid and add accurately 13.6 mL of triethylamine dropwise while stirring.
  Solution A: Mix 1500 mL of *Buffer solution* and 500 mL of acetonitrile. Adjust the solution with phosphoric acid to a pH of 2.6.
  Solution B: Acetonitrile
  Carbonate buffer solution: Transfer 338 mg of sodium carbonate and 152 mg of sodium bicarbonate to a 100-mL volumetric flask, and dissolve in and dilute with water to volume.
  Sodium hydroxide solution: 30% solution of sodium hydroxide in water
  Acetate buffer solution: Transfer 0.3 mL of glacial acetic acid to a 100-mL volumetric flask, add 90 mL of water to dissolve, adjust with *Sodium hydroxide solution* to a pH of 4.2, and dilute with water to volume.
  Derivatization reagent: (+)-1-(9-Fluorenyl)ethyl chloroformate solution [(+)-FLEC]
  System suitability solution: 1.25 mg/mL of USP Levocarnitine RS in water
  Sample solution: 1.25 mg/mL of Levocarnitine in water
  Blank: Water
  Chromatographic system
  (See *Chromatography* ⟨621⟩, *System Suitability*.)
  Mode: LC
  Detector: Fluorescence
   Excitation wavelength: 260 nm
   Emission wavelength: 315 nm
  Column: 4.6-mm × 7.5-cm; 2.7-µm packing L1
  Column temperature: 30°
  Flow rate: 1.5 mL/min
  Injection volume: 20.0 µL
  Mobile phase: See *Table 1.*

Table 1

Time (min)	Solution A (%)	Solution B (%)
0.0	100	0
7.4	100	0
7.5	2	98
9.1	2	98
9.3	100	0
11.0	100	0

  After each sequence of samples, rinse the column with water for 10 min and then with acetonitrile and water (98:2) for another 10 min.
  System suitability
  [NOTE—Proceed with preparation and analysis of the derivatized *System suitability solution* as directed in *Analysis*. Relative retention times are about 0.87 and 1.0 for the (+)-FLEC derivatives of D-carnitine and L-carnitine, respectively.]
  Sample: Derivatized *System suitability solution*
  Suitability requirements
   Resolution: NLT 2.0 between (+)-FLEC derivatives of D-carnitine and L-carnitine
  Analysis: Transfer 30.0 µL of the *Blank, System suitability solution,* and *Sample solution* to separate 10-mL test tubes. Add 30 µL of *Carbonate buffer solution* and 80 µL of *Derivatization reagent* to each test tube and mix by

vortex mixer. Allow the solutions to react for 1 h at 45° over a water bath. Cool the test tubes to room temperature, add 5.0 mL of *Acetate buffer solution* to each test tube, mix by vortex mixer, and transfer to vials for chromatographic analyses.

Separately inject equal volumes of derivatized *Blank*, derivatized *System suitability solution*, and derivatized *Sample solution* into the chromatograph and record the chromatograms. Identify the two diastereomer peaks due to (+)-FLEC derivatives of D-carnitine and L-carnitine in the chromatograms of the derivatized *System suitability solution* and derivatized *Sample solution*. Depending on the purity of the derivatizing reagent, these two peaks may contain co-eluting enantiomers of (−)-FLEC derivatives with D- and L-carnitines, which are accounted in the percentage calculations below. There should be no peaks observed at the retention times of D- and L-carnitine derivatives in the chromatogram of the derivatized *Blank*.

Calculate the percentage of L-carnitine derivative (R_L) from the derivatized *Sample solution*:

$$\text{Result} = r_L/(r_L + r_D) \times 100$$

r_L = peak response of the L-carnitine derivative from the derivatized *Sample solution*
r_D = peak response of the D-carnitine derivative from the derivatized *Sample solution*

Calculate the corrected percentage of L-carnitine ($C_7H_{15}NO_3$) (C_L) in the portion of Levocarnitine taken:

$$\text{Result} = (R_L - P_B)/(P_A - P_B)$$

R_L = percentage of L-carnitine derivative, calculated previously
P_B = percentage of (−)-FLEC as determined for (+)-1-(9-Fluorenyl)ethyl chloroformate solution (see *Reagents, Indicators, and Solutions—Reagent Specifications*)
P_A = percentage of (+)-FLEC as determined for (+)-1-(9-Fluorenyl)ethyl chloroformate solution (see *Reagents, Indicators, and Solutions—Reagent Specifications*)

Calculate the corrected percentage of D-carnitine in the portion of Levocarnitine taken:

$$\text{Result} = 100 - C_L$$

C_L = corrected percentage of L-carnitine, calculated previously

Acceptance criteria: NMT 0.2% of D-carnitine■1S (USP41)

• **LIMIT OF POTASSIUM**
[NOTE—The *Standard solution* and the *Sample solutions* may be modified, if necessary, to obtain solutions of suitable concentrations adaptable to the linear or working range of the instrument.]

Standard solution: 31.25 µg/mL of potassium in water, prepared from potassium chloride, previously dried at 105° for 2 h

Sample stock solution: 0.625 mg/mL of Levocarnitine in water

Sample solution A: Transfer 20.0 mL of the *Sample stock solution* to a 25-mL volumetric flask, and dilute with water to volume. This solution contains 500 µg/mL of Levocarnitine and 0 µg/mL of added potassium from the *Standard solution*.

Sample solution B: Transfer 20.0 mL of the *Sample stock solution* to a 25-mL volumetric flask, add 2.0 mL of the *Standard solution*, and dilute with water to volume. This solution contains 500 µg/mL of Levocarnitine and 2.5 µg/mL of added potassium from the *Standard solution*.

Sample solution C: Transfer 20.0 mL of the *Sample stock solution* to a 25-mL volumetric flask, add 4.0 mL of the *Standard solution*, and dilute with water to vol-

ume. This solution contains 500 µg/mL of Levocarnitine and 5.0 µg/mL of added potassium from the *Standard solution*.

Blank: Water

Instrumental conditions
(See *Atomic Absorption Spectroscopy* ⟨852⟩.)
Mode: Atomic absorption spectrophotometry
Analytical wavelength: 766.7 nm
Lamp: Potassium hollow-cathode
Flame: Air–acetylene

Analysis
Samples: *Sample solution A, Sample solution B, Sample solution C*, and *Blank*

Determine the absorbances of the solutions against the *Blank*. Plot the absorbances of the three *Sample solutions* versus their added potassium concentrations, in µg/mL. Draw the straight line best fitting the three points, and extrapolate the line until it intercepts the concentration axis. From the intercept determine the concentration, in µg/mL, of potassium in *Sample solution A*.

Calculate the percentage of potassium in the portion of Levocarnitine taken:

$$\text{Result} = (C_K/C_U) \times 100$$

C_K = concentration of potassium in *Sample solution A* (µg/mL), determined from the intercept of the linear regression line
C_U = concentration of Levocarnitine in *Sample solution A* (µg/mL)

Acceptance criteria: NMT 0.2%

• **LIMIT OF SODIUM**
[NOTE—The *Standard solution* and the *Sample solutions* may be modified, if necessary, to obtain solutions of suitable concentrations adaptable to the linear or working range of the instrument.]

Standard solution: 250 µg/mL of sodium in water, prepared from sodium chloride, previously dried at 105° for 2 h

Sample stock solution: 40.0 mg/mL of Levocarnitine in water

Sample solution A: Transfer 20.0 mL of the *Sample stock solution* to a 25-mL volumetric flask, and dilute with water to volume. This solution contains 32 mg/mL of Levocarnitine and 0 µg/mL of added sodium from the *Standard solution*.

Sample solution B: Transfer 20.0 mL of the *Sample stock solution* to a 25-mL volumetric flask, add 2.0 mL of the *Standard solution*, and dilute with water to volume. This solution contains 32 mg/mL of Levocarnitine and 20 µg/mL of added sodium from the *Standard solution*.

Sample solution C: Transfer 20.0 mL of the *Sample stock solution* to a 25-mL volumetric flask, add 4.0 mL of the *Standard solution*, and dilute with water to volume. This solution contains 32 mg/mL of Levocarnitine and 40 µg/mL of added sodium from the *Standard solution*.

Blank: Water

Instrumental conditions
(See *Atomic Absorption Spectroscopy* ⟨852⟩.)
Mode: Atomic absorption spectrophotometry
Analytical wavelength: 589.0 nm
Lamp: Sodium hollow-cathode
Flame: Air–acetylene

Analysis
Samples: *Sample solution A, Sample solution B, Sample solution C*, and *Blank*

Determine the absorbances of the solutions against the *Blank*. Plot the absorbances of the three *Sample solutions* versus their added sodium concentrations, in µg/mL. Draw the straight line best fitting the three points, and extrapolate the line until it intercepts the concentration axis. From the intercept determine the concentration, in µg/mL, of sodium in *Sample solution A*.

Calculate the percentage of sodium in the portion of Levocarnitine taken:

$$Result = (C_{Na}/C_U) \times 100$$

C_{Na} = concentration of sodium in *Sample solution A* (µg/mL), determined from the intercept of the linear regression line

C_U = concentration of Levocarnitine in *Sample solution A* (µg/mL)

Acceptance criteria: NMT 0.1%

SPECIFIC TESTS

■• **OPTICAL ROTATION ⟨781S⟩,** *Specific Rotation*
Sample solution: 100 mg/mL in water
Acceptance criteria: −29° to −32°■1S (USP41)
• **PH ⟨791⟩**
Sample solution: 50 mg/mL
Acceptance criteria: 5.5–9.5
• **WATER DETERMINATION ⟨921⟩:** NMT 4.0%

ADDITIONAL REQUIREMENTS

• **PACKAGING AND STORAGE:** Preserve in tight containers ■at temperatures between −15° and 35°. Protect from light.
■1S (USP41)
• **USP REFERENCE STANDARDS ⟨11⟩**
USP Levocarnitine RS

Lidocaine

C₁₄H₂₂N₂O   234.34

$C_{14}H_{22}N_2O$ 234.34
Acetamide, 2-(diethylamino)-*N*-(2,6-dimethylphenyl)-;
2-(Diethylamino)-2′,6′-acetoxylidide [137-58-6].

DEFINITION
Lidocaine contains NLT 97.5% and NMT 102.5% of lidocaine ($C_{14}H_{22}N_2O$).

IDENTIFICATION

• **A. INFRARED ABSORPTION ■⟨197⟩:** [NOTE—Methods described under ⟨197K⟩ or ⟨197A⟩ may be used.]■1S (USP41)
Sample: Previously dried under vacuum over silica gel for 24 h
■**Acceptance criteria:** Meets the requirements■1S (USP41)
• **B.** The retention time of the major peak of the *Sample solution* corresponds to that of the *Standard solution*, as obtained in the *Assay*.

ASSAY

• **PROCEDURE**
Solution A: Water and glacial acetic acid (930:50). Adjust with 1 N sodium hydroxide to a pH of 3.4.
Mobile phase: Acetonitrile and *Solution A* (20:80)
■■1S (USP41)
Standard solution: 1.7 mg/mL of USP Lidocaine RS in *Mobile phase*, prepared as follows. Dissolve 85 mg of USP Lidocaine RS with 0.5 mL of 1 N hydrochloric acid, warming if necessary, in a 50-mL flask. Dilute with *Mobile phase* to volume.
System suitability stock solution: 220 µg/mL of methylparaben in *Mobile phase*
System suitability solution: Mix 2 mL of *System suitability stock solution* and 20 mL of *Standard solution*.
Sample solution: 1.7 mg/mL of Lidocaine in *Mobile phase*, prepared as follows. Dissolve 85 mg of Lidocaine with 0.5 mL of 1 N hydrochloric acid, warming if necessary, in a 50-mL flask. Dilute with *Mobile phase* to volume.
Chromatographic system
(See *Chromatography* ⟨621⟩, *System Suitability*.)
Mode: LC
Detector: UV 254 nm
Column: 3.9-mm × 30-cm; ■4-µm■1S (USP41) packing L1
Flow rate: 1.5 mL/min
Injection volume: 20 µL
System suitability
Samples: *Standard solution* and *System suitability solution*
Suitability requirements
Resolution: NLT 3.0 between lidocaine and methylparaben, *System suitability solution*
Relative standard deviation: NMT 1.5%, *Standard solution*
Analysis
Samples: *Standard solution* and *Sample solution*
Calculate the percentage of lidocaine ($C_{14}H_{22}N_2O$) in the portion of Lidocaine taken:

$$Result = (r_U/r_S) \times (C_S/C_U) \times 100$$

r_U = peak response of lidocaine from the *Sample solution*

r_S = peak response of lidocaine from the *Standard solution*

C_S = concentration of USP Lidocaine RS in the *Standard solution* (mg/mL)

C_U = concentration of Lidocaine in the *Sample solution* (mg/mL)

Acceptance criteria: 97.5%–102.5%

IMPURITIES
• **RESIDUE ON IGNITION ⟨281⟩:** NMT 0.1%
• **CHLORIDE AND SULFATE ⟨221⟩,** *Chloride*
Sample: 1.0 g
Analysis: Dissolve the *Sample* in a mixture of 3 mL of 2 N nitric acid and 12 mL of water, and add 1 mL of silver nitrate TS.
Acceptance criteria: The turbidity does not exceed that produced by 50 µL of 0.020 N hydrochloric acid (NMT 0.0035%).
• **CHLORIDE AND SULFATE ⟨221⟩,** *Sulfate*
Sample: 100 mg
Analysis: Dissolve the *Sample* in a mixture of 1 mL of 2 N nitric acid and 10 mL of water. Filter if necessary, and add 1 mL of barium chloride TS.
Acceptance criteria: The turbidity does not exceed that produced by 0.10 mL of 0.020 N sulfuric acid (NMT 0.1%).

Delete the following:

•• HEAVY METALS, Method I ⟨231⟩
Sample: 1.0 g
Analysis: Dissolve the *Sample* in a mixture of 2 mL of
3 N hydrochloric acid and 10 mL of water. Evaporate
on a steam bath to dryness, and dissolve the residue in
25 mL of water.
Acceptance criteria: NMT 20 ppm• (Official 1-Jan-2018)

Add the following:

■• ORGANIC IMPURITIES
Solution A: 4.85 g/L of monobasic potassium phos-
phate in water. Adjust with sodium hydroxide solution
to a pH of 8.0.
Mobile phase: Acetonitrile and *Solution A* (30:70)
Standard solution: 0.5 µg/mL of USP Ropivacaine Re-
lated Compound A RS and 5 µg/mL each of USP Lido-
caine Related Compound H RS and USP Lidocaine RS in
Mobile phase
Sample solution: 5 mg/mL of Lidocaine in *Mobile phase*
Chromatographic system
(See *Chromatography ⟨621⟩, System Suitability.*)
Mode: LC
Detector: UV 230 nm
Column: 3.9-mm × 15-cm; 5-µm packing L1
Column temperature: 30°
Flow rate: 1 mL/min
Injection volume: 20 µL
System suitability
Sample: *Standard solution*
[NOTE—See *Table 1* for relative retention times.]
Suitability requirements
Resolution: NLT 1.5 between the lidocaine related
compound H and 2,6-dimethylaniline (ropivacaine re-
lated compound A free base) peaks
Relative standard deviation: NMT 10.0% for 2,6-
dimethylaniline
Analysis
Samples: *Standard solution* and *Sample solution*
Calculate the percentage of lidocaine related compound
H in the portion of Lidocaine taken:

$$\text{Result} = (r_U/r_S) \times (C_S/C_U) \times 100$$

r_U = peak response of lidocaine related compound
H from the *Sample solution*
r_S = peak response of lidocaine related compound
H from the *Standard solution*
C_S = concentration of USP Lidocaine Related
Compound H RS in the *Standard solution*
(µg/mL)
C_U = concentration of Lidocaine in the *Sample
solution* (µg/mL)

Calculate the percentage of 2,6-dimethylaniline
(ropivacaine related compound A free base) in the
portion of Lidocaine taken:

$$\text{Result} = (r_U/r_S) \times (C_S/C_U) \times (M_{r1}/M_{r2}) \times 100$$

r_U = peak response of 2,6-dimethylaniline from the
Sample solution
r_S = peak response of 2,6-dimethylaniline from the
Standard solution
C_S = concentration of USP Ropivacaine Related
Compound A RS in the *Standard solution*
(µg/mL)
C_U = concentration of Lidocaine in the *Sample
solution* (µg/mL)
M_{r1} = molecular weight of 2,6-dimethylaniline,
121.18
M_{r2} = molecular weight of ropivacaine related
compound A, 157.64

Calculate the percentage of any unspecified impurity in
the portion of Lidocaine taken:

$$\text{Result} = (r_U/r_S) \times (C_S/C_U) \times 100$$

r_U = peak response of each unspecified impurity
from the *Sample solution*
r_S = peak response of lidocaine from the *Standard
solution*
C_S = concentration of USP Lidocaine RS in the
Standard solution (µg/mL)
C_U = concentration of Lidocaine in the *Sample
solution* (µg/mL)
Acceptance criteria: See *Table 1.*

Table 1

Name	Relative Retention Time	Acceptance Criteria, NMT (%)
Lidocaine related compound H	0.38	0.10
2,6-Dimethylaniline	0.42	0.01
Lidocaine	1.0	—
Any unspecified impurity	—	0.10
Total impurities	—	0.5

■1S *(USP41)*

SPECIFIC TESTS

Delete the following:

■• MELTING RANGE OR TEMPERATURE ⟨741⟩: 66°–69°■1S *(USP41)*

ADDITIONAL REQUIREMENTS
• **PACKAGING AND STORAGE:** Preserve in well-closed containers. Store at room temperature.

Change to read:

• **USP REFERENCE STANDARDS ⟨11⟩**
USP Lidocaine RS
■USP Lidocaine Related Compound H RS
2-Chloro-*N*-(2,6-dimethylphenyl)acetamide.
$C_{10}H_{12}ClNO$ 197.66
USP Ropivacaine Related Compound A RS
2,6-Dimethylaniline hydrochloride.
$C_8H_{11}N \cdot HCl$ 157.64■1S *(USP41)*

Lidocaine Hydrochloride Oral Topical Solution

DEFINITION
Lidocaine Hydrochloride Oral Topical Solution contains NLT
95.0% and NMT 105.0% of the labeled amount of lido-
caine hydrochloride ($C_{14}H_{22}N_2O \cdot HCl$). It contains a suitable flavor and/or sweetening agent.

IDENTIFICATION

Change to read:

• **A. INFRARED ABSORPTION ⟨197K⟩**
Sample: Place in a separator a volume of Oral Topical
Solution, nominally equivalent to 300 mg of lidocaine
hydrochloride, and extract with four 15-mL portions of
chloroform, discarding the chloroform extracts. Add

2 mL of 2 N sodium hydroxide to the aqueous solution remaining in the separator, and extract with four 15-mL portions of chloroform. Combine the chloroform extracts, and evaporate ■₁₅ (USP41) to dryness. Dissolve the crystals in solvent hexane, evaporate ■the solvent, ■₁₅ (USP41) and dry the residue under vacuum over silica gel for 24 h. ■[NOTE—A rotary evaporator may be used.]■₁₅ (USP41)
Acceptance criteria: Residue obtained from the *Sample* meets the requirements.
- **B.** The retention time of the major peak of the *Sample solution* corresponds to that of the *Standard solution*, as obtained in the *Assay*.

ASSAY

Change to read:

- **PROCEDURE**
  Solution A: 4.85 g/L of monobasic potassium phosphate. Adjust with 10 N sodium hydroxide solution to a pH of 8.0.
  Mobile phase: Acetonitrile and *Solution A* (30:70) ■■₁₅ (USP41)
  Standard solution: 0.85 mg/mL of USP Lidocaine RS (equivalent to 1 mg/mL of lidocaine hydrochloride) in *Mobile phase*
  Sample solution: Nominally 1 mg/mL of lidocaine hydrochloride from Oral Topical Solution in *Mobile phase*
  Chromatographic system
  (See *Chromatography* ⟨621⟩, *System Suitability*.)
  Mode: LC
  Detector: UV 230 nm
  Column: 4.6-mm × 15-cm; 3.5-μm packing L1
  Column temperature: 45°
  Flow rate: 1 mL/min
  Injection volume: 20 μL
  System suitability
    Sample: ■■₁₅ (USP41) *Standard solution*
    ■■₁₅ (USP41)
    Suitability requirements
    ■■₁₅ (USP41)
      Tailing factor: NMT 2.0
      Relative standard deviation: NMT 2.0%
  Analysis
    Samples: *Standard solution* and *Sample solution*
    Calculate the percentage of the labeled amount of lidocaine hydrochloride ($C_{14}H_{22}N_2O \cdot HCl$) in the portion of Oral Topical Solution taken:

$$Result = (r_U/r_S) \times (C_S/C_U) \times (M_{r1}/M_{r2}) \times 100$$

r_U = peak response of lidocaine from the *Sample solution*
r_S = peak response of lidocaine from the *Standard solution*
C_S = concentration of USP Lidocaine RS in the *Standard solution* (mg/mL)
C_U = nominal concentration of lidocaine hydrochloride in the *Sample solution* (mg/mL)
M_{r1} = molecular weight of lidocaine hydrochloride, 270.80
M_{r2} = molecular weight of lidocaine, 234.34
Acceptance criteria: 95.0%–105.0%

IMPURITIES

Change to read:

- **ORGANIC IMPURITIES**
  Solution A, Mobile phase, ■■₁₅ (USP41) and **Chromatographic system:** Proceed as directed in the *Assay*.

Standard solution: 0.0043 mg/mL of USP Lidocaine RS, 0.005 mg/mL of USP Lidocaine Related Compound H RS, and 0.00065 mg/mL of USP Ropivacaine Related Compound A RS (equivalent to 0.0005 mg/mL of 2,6-dimethylaniline) in *Mobile phase*
Sample solution: Nominally 5 mg/mL of lidocaine hydrochloride from Oral Topical Solution in *Mobile phase*
System suitability
  Sample: ■■₁₅ (USP41) *Standard solution*
  Suitability requirements
    Resolution: NLT 1.5 between the lidocaine related compound H and ■2,6-dimethylaniline (ropivacaine related compound A free base) peaks■₁₅ (USP41)
    Relative standard deviation: NMT 2.0% for lidocaine, ■lidocaine related compound H, and 2,6-dimethylaniline■₁₅ (USP41)
Analysis
  Samples: *Standard solution* and *Sample solution*
  Calculate the percentage of lidocaine related compound H in the portion of Oral Topical Solution taken:

$$Result = (r_U/r_S) \times (C_S/C_U) \times 100$$

r_U = peak response of lidocaine related compound H from the *Sample solution*
r_S = peak response of lidocaine related compound H from the *Standard solution*
C_S = concentration of USP Lidocaine Related Compound H RS in the *Standard solution* (mg/mL)
C_U = nominal concentration of lidocaine hydrochloride in the *Sample solution* (mg/mL)

Calculate the percentage of ■2,6-■₁₅ (USP41)dimethylaniline in the portion of Oral Topical Solution taken:

$$Result = (r_U/r_S) \times (C_S/C_U) \times (M_{r1}/M_{r2}) \times 100$$

r_U = peak response of ■2,6-■₁₅ (USP41)dimethylaniline from the *Sample solution*
r_S = peak response of ■2,6-■₁₅ (USP41)dimethylaniline from the *Standard solution*
C_S = concentration of USP Ropivacaine Related Compound A RS in the *Standard solution* (mg/mL)
C_U = nominal concentration of lidocaine hydrochloride in the *Sample solution* (mg/mL)
M_{r1} = molecular weight of ■2,6-dimethylaniline, 121.18■₁₅ (USP41)
M_{r2} = molecular weight of ■ropivacaine related compound A, 157.64■₁₅ (USP41)

Calculate the percentage of any ■unspecified degradation product■₁₅ (USP41) in the portion of Oral Topical Solution taken:

$$Result = (r_U/r_S) \times (C_S/C_U) \times (M_{r1}/M_{r2}) \times 100$$

r_U = peak response of ■any unspecified degradation product■₁₅ (USP41) from the *Sample solution*
r_S = peak response of lidocaine from the *Standard solution*
C_S = concentration of USP Lidocaine RS in the *Standard solution* (mg/mL)
C_U = nominal concentration of lidocaine hydrochloride in the *Sample solution* (mg/mL)
M_{r1} = molecular weight of lidocaine hydrochloride, 270.80
M_{r2} = molecular weight of lidocaine, 234.34
Acceptance criteria: See *Table 1*. ■■₁₅ (USP41)

Table 1

Name	Relative Retention Time	Acceptance Criteria, NMT (%)
Lidocaine related compound H	0.33	■0.5■₁ₛ (USP41)
■2,6-■₁ₛ (USP41)Dimethylaniline	0.37	■0.5■₁ₛ (USP41)
Lidocaine	1.0	—
Any ■unspecified degradation product■₁ₛ (USP41)	—	■0.5■₁ₛ (USP41)
Total ■degradation products■₁ₛ (USP41)	—	■2.0■₁ₛ (USP41)

SPECIFIC TESTS
• **PH ⟨791⟩:** 5.0–7.0

ADDITIONAL REQUIREMENTS
• **PACKAGING AND STORAGE:** Preserve in tight containers. Store at controlled room temperature.

Change to read:

• **USP REFERENCE STANDARDS ⟨11⟩**
USP Lidocaine RS
USP Lidocaine Related Compound H RS
■2-Chloro-*N*-(2,6-dimethylphenyl)acetamide.■₁ₛ (USP41)
$C_{10}H_{12}ClNO$ 197.66
USP Ropivacaine Related Compound A RS
2,6-Dimethylaniline hydrochloride.
$C_8H_{11}N \cdot HCl$ 157.64

Lidocaine Hydrochloride Topical Solution

DEFINITION
Lidocaine Hydrochloride Topical Solution contains NLT 95.0% and NMT 105.0% of the labeled amount of lidocaine hydrochloride ($C_{14}H_{22}N_2O \cdot HCl$).

IDENTIFICATION

Change to read:

• **A. INFRARED ABSORPTION ⟨197K⟩**
Sample: Place in a separator a volume of Topical Solution, nominally equivalent to 200 mg of lidocaine hydrochloride, and extract with four 15-mL portions of chloroform, discarding the chloroform extracts. Add 2 mL of 2 N sodium hydroxide to the aqueous solution remaining in the separator, and extract with four 15-mL portions of chloroform. Combine the chloroform extracts, and evaporate ■■₁ₛ (USP41) to dryness. Dissolve the crystals in solvent hexane, evaporate ■the solvent, ■₁ₛ (USP41) and dry the residue under vacuum over silica gel for 24 h. ■[NOTE—A rotary evaporator may be used.]■₁ₛ (USP41)
Acceptance criteria: The residue obtained from the *Sample* meets the requirements.
• **B.** The retention time of the major peak of the *Sample solution* corresponds to that of the *Standard solution*, as obtained in the *Assay*.

ASSAY
• **PROCEDURE**
Solution A: Water and glacial acetic acid (930:50). Adjust with 1 N sodium hydroxide to a pH of 3.4.

Mobile phase: Acetonitrile and *Solution A* (20:80)
Standard solution: 1.7 mg/mL of USP Lidocaine RS (equivalent to 2 mg/mL of lidocaine hydrochloride) in *Mobile phase*, prepared as follows. Transfer a weighed quantity of USP Lidocaine RS to a suitable volumetric flask, and add 1 N hydrochloric acid to fill 1% of the final volume. Warm if necessary, and dilute with *Mobile phase* to volume.
System suitability stock solution: 220 µg/mL of USP Methylparaben RS in *Mobile phase*
System suitability solution: Mix 2 mL of *System suitability stock solution* with 20 mL of the *Standard solution*.
Sample solution: Nominally 2 mg/mL of lidocaine hydrochloride from Topical Solution in *Mobile phase*
Chromatographic system
(See *Chromatography* ⟨621⟩, *System Suitability*.)
Mode: LC
Detector: UV 254 nm
Column: 3.9-mm × 30-cm; 10-µm packing L1
Flow rate: 1.5 mL/min
Injection volume: 20 µL
System suitability
Samples: *Standard solution* and *System suitability solution*
Suitability requirements
Resolution: NLT 3.0 between lidocaine and methylparaben, *System suitability solution*
Relative standard deviation: NMT 1.5%, *Standard solution*
Analysis
Samples: *Standard solution* and *Sample solution*
Calculate the percentage of the labeled amount of lidocaine hydrochloride ($C_{14}H_{22}N_2O \cdot HCl$) in the portion of Topical Solution taken:

$$Result = (r_U/r_S) \times (C_S/C_U) \times (M_{r1}/M_{r2}) \times 100$$

r_U = peak response of lidocaine from the *Sample solution*
r_S = peak response of lidocaine from the *Standard solution*
C_S = concentration of USP Lidocaine RS in the *Standard solution* (mg/mL)
C_U = nominal concentration of lidocaine hydrochloride in the *Sample solution* (mg/mL)
M_{r1} = molecular weight of lidocaine hydrochloride, 270.80
M_{r2} = molecular weight of lidocaine, 234.34
Acceptance criteria: 95.0%–105.0%

IMPURITIES

Change to read:

• **ORGANIC IMPURITIES**
Solution A, Mobile phase, and ■Sample solution:■₁ₛ (USP41) Prepare as directed in the *Assay*.
■■₁ₛ (USP41)
Standard solution: 0.0017 mg/mL of USP Lidocaine RS ■(equivalent to 0.002 mg/mL of lidocaine hydrochloride),■₁ₛ (USP41) 0.0026 mg/mL of USP Ropivacaine Related Compound A RS (equivalent to 0.002 mg/mL of 2,6-dimethylaniline), and 0.002 mg/mL of USP Lidocaine Related Compound H RS in *Mobile phase*
■■₁ₛ (USP41)
Chromatographic system
(See *Chromatography* ⟨621⟩, *System Suitability*.)

Mode: LC
Detector: UV 254 nm
Column: 4.6-mm × 25-cm; 5-μm packing L1
Flow rate: 1.5 mL/min
Injection volume: 50 μL
System suitability
Sample: ■1S (USP41) *Standard solution*
[NOTE—See *Table 1* for the relative retention times.]
Suitability requirements
Resolution: NLT 2.0 between the lidocaine related compound H and ■2,6-dimethylaniline (ropivacaine related compound A free base) peaks■1S (USP41)
Relative standard deviation: NMT 2.0% for lidocaine, ■lidocaine related compound H, and 2,6-dimethylaniline■1S (USP41)
Analysis
Samples: *Sample solution* and *Standard solution*
Calculate the percentage of lidocaine related compound H in the portion of Topical Solution taken:

$$Result = (r_U/r_S) \times (C_S/C_U) \times 100$$

r_U = peak response of lidocaine related compound H from the *Sample solution*
r_S = peak response of lidocaine related compound H from the *Standard solution*
C_S = concentration of USP Lidocaine Related Compound H RS in the *Standard solution* (mg/mL)
C_U = nominal concentration of lidocaine hydrochloride in the *Sample solution* (mg/mL)

Calculate the percentage of ■2,6-■1S (USP41) dimethylaniline in the portion of Topical Solution taken:

$$Result = (r_U/r_S) \times (C_S/C_U) \times (M_{r1}/M_{r2}) \times 100$$

r_U = peak response of ■2,6-■1S (USP41) dimethylaniline from the *Sample solution*
r_S = peak response of ■2,6-■1S (USP41) dimethylaniline from the *Standard solution*
C_S = concentration of USP Ropivacaine Related Compound A RS in the *Standard solution* (mg/mL)
C_U = nominal concentration of lidocaine hydrochloride in the *Sample solution* (mg/mL)
M_{r1} = molecular weight of ■2,6-dimethylaniline, 121.18■1S (USP41)
M_{r2} = molecular weight of ■ropivacaine related compound A, 157.64■1S (USP41)

Calculate the percentage of any ■unspecified degradation product■1S (USP41) in the portion of Topical Solution taken:

$$Result = (r_U/r_S) \times (C_S/C_U) \times (M_{r1}/M_{r2}) \times 100$$

r_U = peak response of ■any unspecified degradation product■1S (USP41) from the *Sample solution*
r_S = peak response of lidocaine from the *Standard solution*
C_S = concentration of USP Lidocaine RS in the *Standard solution* (mg/mL)
C_U = nominal concentration of lidocaine hydrochloride in the *Sample solution* (mg/mL)
M_{r1} = molecular weight of lidocaine hydrochloride, 270.80
M_{r2} = molecular weight of lidocaine, 234.34
Acceptance criteria: See *Table 1*. ■1S (USP41)

Table 1

Name	Relative Retention Time	Acceptance Criteria, NMT (%)
Lidocaine	1.0	—
■2,6-■1S (USP41)Dimethylaniline	3.2	■0.5■1S (USP41)
Lidocaine related compound H	3.8	■0.5■1S (USP41)
Any unspecified ■degradation product■1S (USP41)	—	■0.5■1S (USP41)
Total ■degradation products■1S (USP41)	—	2.0

SPECIFIC TESTS
• **PH** ⟨791⟩: 5.0–7.0

ADDITIONAL REQUIREMENTS
• **PACKAGING AND STORAGE:** Preserve in tight containers. Store at controlled room temperature.

Change to read:

• **USP REFERENCE STANDARDS** ⟨11⟩
USP Lidocaine RS
USP Lidocaine Related Compound H RS
■2-Chloro-*N*-(2,6-dimethylphenyl)acetamide.■1S (USP41)
$C_{10}H_{12}ClNO$ 197.66
USP Methylparaben RS
USP Ropivacaine Related Compound A RS
2,6-Dimethylaniline hydrochloride.
$C_8H_{11}N \cdot HCl$ 157.64

Mebendazole Tablets

DEFINITION
Mebendazole Tablets contain NLT 90.0% and NMT 110.0% of the labeled amount of mebendazole ($C_{16}H_{13}N_3O_3$).

IDENTIFICATION

Change to read:

• **A.** ■The UV spectrum of the major peak of the *Sample solution* corresponds to that of the *Standard solution*, as obtained in the *Assay*.■1S (USP41)

Add the following:

■• **B.** The retention time of the major peak of the *Sample solution* corresponds to that of the *Standard solution*, as obtained in the *Assay*.■1S (USP41)

ASSAY

Change to read:

• **PROCEDURE**
■**Solution A:** 7.5 g/L of ammonium acetate in water
Solution B: Acetonitrile
Mobile phase: See *Table 1*.

Table 1

Time (min)	Solution A (%)	Solution B (%)
0	80	20
15	70	30

Table 1 *(Continued)*

Time (min)	Solution A (%)	Solution B (%)
20	10	90
25	10	90
26	80	20
30	80	20

Diluent: *N,N*-Dimethyl formamide
Standard solution: 0.05 mg/mL of USP Mebendazole RS in *Diluent*. Sonicate, if necessary, to dissolve.
Sample solution: Nominally 0.05 mg/mL of mebendazole in *Diluent*, prepared as follows. Transfer a suitable quantity of mebendazole from NLT 20 finely powdered Tablets into a suitable volumetric flask. Add *Diluent* to about 80% of the flask volume and sonicate for 30 min. Dilute with *Diluent* to volume and pass through a suitable filter of 0.45-μm pore size.
Chromatographic system
(See *Chromatography* ⟨621⟩, *System Suitability*.)
Mode: LC
Detector: UV 250 nm. For *Identification A*, use a diode array detector in the range of 200–400 nm.
Column: 4.6-mm × 10-cm; 3-μm packing L1
Column temperature: 40°
Flow rate: 1.2 mL/min
Injection volume: 10 μL
System suitability
Sample: *Standard solution*
Suitability requirements
Tailing factor: NMT 2.0
Relative standard deviation: NMT 2.0%■1S (USP41)
Analysis
Samples: *Standard solution* and *Sample solution*
Calculate the percentage of the labeled amount of mebendazole ($C_{16}H_{13}N_3O_3$) in the portion of Tablets taken:

$$\text{Result} = (r_U/r_S) \times (C_S/C_U) \times 100$$

r_U = peak response of mebendazole from the *Sample solution*
r_S = peak response of mebendazole from the *Standard solution*
C_S = concentration of USP Mebendazole RS in the *Standard solution* (mg/mL)
C_U = nominal concentration of mebendazole in the *Sample solution* (mg/mL)
Acceptance criteria: 90.0%–110.0%

PERFORMANCE TESTS
• **DISSOLUTION** ⟨711⟩
Medium: 0.1 N hydrochloric acid containing 1.0% sodium lauryl sulfate; 900 mL
Apparatus 2: 75 rpm
Time: 120 min
Solution A: Dissolve 8.0 g of sodium hydroxide in 2 L of water. Add 3.0 g of sodium lauryl sulfate, and mix. Add 20 mL of phosphoric acid, and adjust with phosphoric acid to a pH of 2.5.
Mobile phase: Acetonitrile and *Solution A* (3:7)
Standard solution: 0.5 mg/mL of USP Mebendazole RS prepared as follows. Transfer the appropriate amount of USP Mebendazole RS to a volumetric flask. Add 20% of the final volume of formic acid, and dissolve. Dilute with methanol to volume. Dilute a portion of this solution with *Medium* to obtain a solution having a known concentration similar to the expected concentration in the solution under test.
Chromatographic system
(See *Chromatography* ⟨621⟩, *System Suitability*.)

Mode: LC
Detector: UV 254 nm
Column: 4.6-mm × 3-cm; packing L7
Flow rate: 1 mL/min
Injection volume: 10 μL
System suitability
Sample: *Standard solution*
Suitability requirements
Relative standard deviation: NMT 2.0%
Analysis: Determine the percentage of mebendazole ($C_{16}H_{13}N_3O_3$) dissolved.
Tolerances: NLT 75% (*Q*) of the labeled amount of mebendazole ($C_{16}H_{13}N_3O_3$) is dissolved.

Change to read:

• **UNIFORMITY OF DOSAGE UNITS** ⟨905⟩: Meet the requirements
■■1S (USP41)

IMPURITIES

Add the following:

■• **ORGANIC IMPURITIES**
Solution A, Solution B, Mobile phase, Diluent, and **Chromatographic system:** Proceed as directed in the *Assay*.
System suitability solution: 0.1 mg/mL of USP Mebendazole RS and 0.002 mg/mL of USP Mebendazole Related Compound D RS in *Diluent*. Sonicate, if necessary, to dissolve.
Standard solution: 0.002 mg/mL of USP Mebendazole RS in *Diluent*. Sonicate, if necessary, to dissolve.
Sample solution: Nominally 1 mg/mL of mebendazole in *Diluent*, prepared as follows. Transfer a suitable quantity of mebendazole from NLT 20 powdered Tablets into a suitable volumetric flask. Add *Diluent* to about 40% of the flask volume and sonicate for about 30 min. Dilute with *Diluent* to volume and pass through a suitable filter of 0.45-μm pore size.
System suitability
Samples: *System suitability solution* and *Standard solution*
Suitability requirements
Resolution: NLT 1.5 between mebendazole and mebendazole related compound D, *System suitability solution*
Relative standard deviation: NMT 5.0%, *Standard solution*
Analysis
Samples: *Standard solution* and *Sample solution*
Calculate the percentage of each impurity in the portion of Tablets taken:

$$\text{Result} = (r_U/r_S) \times (C_S/C_U) \times 100$$

r_U = peak response of each impurity from the *Sample solution*
r_S = peak response of mebendazole from the *Standard solution*
C_S = concentration of USP Mebendazole RS in the *Standard solution* (mg/mL)
C_U = nominal concentration of mebendazole in the *Sample solution* (mg/mL)
Acceptance criteria: See *Table 2*. Disregard any peak below 0.05%.

Table 2

Name	Relative Retention Time	Acceptance Criteria, NMT (%)
Mebendazole	1.0	—
Mebendazole related compound D[a]	1.1	—
Any individual unspecified impurity	—	0.2
Total impurities	—	1.0

[a] This is a process-related impurity and not included in the total impurities.

■1S (*USP41*)

ADDITIONAL REQUIREMENTS
• **PACKAGING AND STORAGE:** Preserve in well-closed containers.

Change to read:

• **USP REFERENCE STANDARDS ⟨11⟩**
USP Mebendazole RS
■USP Mebendazole Related Compound D RS
Methyl 5-benzoyl-1-methylbenzimidazol-2-yl carbamate.
$C_{17}H_{15}N_3O_3$ 309.32■1S (*USP41*)

Meloxicam Oral Suspension

DEFINITION
Meloxicam Oral Suspension contains NLT 90.0% and NMT 110.0% of the labeled amount of meloxicam ($C_{14}H_{13}N_3O_4S_2$).

IDENTIFICATION

Delete the following:

■• **A. THIN-LAYER CHROMATOGRAPHIC IDENTIFICATION TEST ⟨201⟩**
Standard solution: 0.25 mg/mL, prepared by dissolving USP Meloxicam RS in 1 mL of water and diluting with acetone to volume
Sample solution: Nominally 0.25 mg/mL of meloxicam prepared as follows. Transfer a quantity of meloxicam nominally equivalent to 2.5 mg, to a 10 mL volumetric flask. Dilute with acetone to volume. Mix for 10 min. If necessary, pass through fluted filter paper
Developing solvent system: Chloroform, methanol, and ammonium hydroxide (80:20:1)
Analysis
Samples: *Standard solution* and *Sample solution*
Proceed as directed in the chapter. After removing the plate from the chamber and drying, examine the chromatograms under UV light at 254 nm.
Acceptance criteria: The R_F value (approximately 0.45) of the principal dark spot obtained from the *Sample solution* corresponds to that obtained from the *Standard solution*.■1S (*USP41*)

Add the following:

■• **A.** The UV absorption spectrum of the meloxicam peak of the *Sample solution* exhibits maxima and minima at the same wavelengths as those of the *Standard solution*, as obtained in the *Assay*.■1S (*USP41*)
• **B.** The retention time of the major peak of the *Sample solution* corresponds to that of the *Standard solution*, as obtained in the *Assay*.

ASSAY

Change to read:

• **PROCEDURE**
Buffer: Dissolve 2 g of monohydrate citric acid and 2 g of boric acid in 1000 mL of water, and adjust with dihydrate trisodium citrate to a pH of 2.9.
Solution A: Acetonitrile, methanol, and *Buffer* (200:260:565)
Mobile phase: Dissolve 200 mg of sodium dodecyl sulfate in 1000 mL of *Solution A*.
Diluent: Dissolve 3 g of boric acid and 1.5 g of dihydrate trisodium citrate in 1000 mL of water, and adjust with 2 M sodium hydroxide to a pH of 8.3. Mix 420 mL of the resulting buffer with 420 mL of methanol and 160 mL of acetonitrile.
Related compound standard stock solution: 8.4 µg/mL of USP Meloxicam Related Compound B RS prepared as follows. Transfer 21 mg of USP Meloxicam Related Compound B RS into a 100-mL volumetric flask. Add 3.0 mL of dimethylformamide, 15 mL of methanol, and about 60 mL of *Diluent*. Sonicate, and mix until dissolved. Cool to room temperature. Dilute with *Diluent* to volume. Dilute further with *Diluent* to a concentration of 8.4 µg/mL.
System suitability solution: Transfer a volume of Oral Suspension, nominally equivalent to 15 mg of meloxicam, to a 50-mL volumetric flask. Add 3.0 mL of *Related compound standard stock solution*. Add 3.0 mL of dimethylformamide. Swirl the flask, and allow to stand for 5 min. Add 15 mL of methanol. Dilute with *Diluent* to just below volume. Sonicate for 30 min, mixing the flask vigorously about every 5 min. Cool to room temperature. Dilute with *Diluent* to volume. Mix, and allow particulates to settle. Pass through a 0.45-µm membrane filter with a fiberglass prefilter.
Standard stock solution: Transfer about 67 mg of USP Meloxicam RS into a 100-mL volumetric flask. Add 3.0 mL of dimethylformamide. Swirl the flask, and allow to stand for 5 min. Add 15 mL of methanol. Dilute with *Diluent* to just below volume. Sonicate for 30 min, and mix until dissolved. Cool to room temperature. Dilute with *Diluent* to volume.
Standard solution: ■0.3■1S (*USP41*) mg/mL of USP Meloxicam RS in *Diluent* from *Standard stock solution*
Sample solution: Nominally 0.3 mg/mL of meloxicam prepared as follows. Transfer a volume of Oral Suspension, nominally equivalent to 15 mg of meloxicam, to a 50-mL volumetric flask. Add 3.0 mL of dimethylformamide. Swirl the flask, and allow to stand for about 5 min. Add 15 mL of methanol. Dilute with *Diluent* to just below volume. Sonicate for 30 min, mixing the flask vigorously about every 5 min. Cool to room temperature. Dilute with *Diluent* to volume. Mix, and allow particulates to settle. Pass through a 0.45-µm membrane filter with a fiberglass prefilter.
Chromatographic system
(See *Chromatography* ⟨621⟩, *System Suitability*.)
Mode: LC
Detector: UV 360 nm. For *Identification A*, use a diode array detector in the range of 200–400 nm.
■■1S (*USP41*)
Column: 4-mm × 12.5-cm; 5-µm packing L1
Column temperature: 40°
Flow rate: 1.0 mL/min
Run time: ■NLT 2 times the retention time of meloxicam■1S (*USP41*)
Injection volume: 10 µL
System suitability
Samples: *System suitability solution* and *Standard solution*
■■1S (*USP41*)

Suitability requirements
Resolution: NLT 1.5 between meloxicam and any other adjacent peak, ■₁ₛ (USP41) *System suitability solution*
Tailing factor: NMT 2.0 for the meloxicam peak, ■₁ₛ (USP41) *System suitability solution*
Relative standard deviation: NMT 1.5%, ■₁ₛ (USP41) *Standard solution*
Analysis
Samples: *Standard solution* and *Sample solution* ■₁ₛ (USP41)
Calculate the percentage of the labeled amount of meloxicam ($C_{14}H_{13}N_3O_4S_2$) in the portion of Oral Suspension taken:

$$Result = (r_U/r_S) \times (C_S/C_U) \times 100$$

r_U = peak area of meloxicam from the *Sample solution* ■₁ₛ (USP41)
r_S = peak area of meloxicam from the *Standard solution* ■₁ₛ (USP41)
C_S = concentration of USP Meloxicam RS in the *Standard solution* (mg/mL)
C_U = nominal concentration of meloxicam in the *Sample solution* (mg/mL)
Acceptance criteria: 90.0%–110.0%

PERFORMANCE TESTS
* **DISSOLUTION ⟨711⟩**
Medium: pH 7.5 phosphate buffer; 900 mL
Apparatus 2: 25 rpm
Time: 15 min
Standard solution: Transfer about 20.83 mg of USP Meloxicam RS into a 100-mL volumetric flask. Dissolve in 5 mL of methanol and 1 mL of 0.1 M sodium hydroxide, and dilute with *Medium* to volume. Dilute with *Medium* to a final concentration of 8.3 µg/mL of meloxicam.
Sample solution: Shake each sample for 15 min. Weigh six portions, equivalent to 7.5 mg of the Oral Suspension, into separate tared 10-mL beakers, and record each weight. Introduce each of the samples to the middle of the dissolution vessels, and rinse each beaker with 20 mL of the *Medium* withdrawn from the vessel. Carefully lower the paddle to the appropriate height and start the rotation. After completion of the dissolution, pass a 20-mL aliquot through a nylon filter having 0.45-µm porosity, discarding the first 3 mL of the filtrate.
Instrumental conditions
Mode: UV-Vis
Analytical wavelength: At about 362 nm (wavelength of maximum absorbance)
Blank: *Medium*
Analysis
Samples: *Standard solution* and *Sample solution*
Calculate the percentage of the labeled amount of meloxicam ($C_{14}H_{13}N_3O_4S_2$) dissolved:

$$Result = (A_U/A_S) \times C_S \times (1/W_U) \times (1/L) \times d \times V \times 100$$

A_U = absorbance of the *Sample solution*
A_S = absorbance of the *Standard solution*
C_S = concentration of USP Meloxicam RS in the *Standard solution* (mg/mL)
W_U = weight of the Oral Suspension taken (mg)
L = label claim (mg/mL)
d = density of the Oral Suspension (g/mL)
V = volume of *Medium*, 900 mL
Tolerances: NLT 75% (Q) of the labeled amount of meloxicam ($C_{14}H_{13}N_3O_4S_2$) is dissolved.

IMPURITIES

Change to read:

* **ORGANIC IMPURITIES**
Buffer, Solution A, Mobile phase, Diluent, Related compound standard stock solution, and **Sample solution:** Proceed as directed in the *Assay.*
Sensitivity solution: 0.08 µg/mL of USP Meloxicam Related Compound B RS in *Diluent* from *Related compound standard stock solution*
■**Standard solution:**₁ₛ (USP41) 0.5 µg/mL of USP Meloxicam Related Compound B RS in *Diluent* from *Related compound standard stock solution*
Chromatographic system: Proceed as directed in the *Assay,* ■except for the *Detector.*
Detector: UV 260 and 360 nm■₁ₛ (USP41)
System suitability
Samples: *Sensitivity solution* and ■*Standard solution*₁ₛ (USP41)
Suitability requirements
Tailing factor: NMT 2.0 for the meloxicam related compound B peak at 260 nm, ■*Standard solution*₁ₛ (USP41)
Relative standard deviation: NMT 10% for meloxicam related compound B at 260 nm, ■₁ₛ (USP41) *Sensitivity solution*
Analysis
Samples: ■*Standard solution*₁ₛ (USP41) and *Sample solution* ■₁ₛ (USP41)
Calculate the percentage of meloxicam related compound B in the portion of Oral Suspension taken:

$$Result = (r_U/r_S) \times (C_S/C_U) \times 100$$

r_U = peak area of meloxicam related compound B in the *Sample solution* at 260 nm
r_S = peak area of meloxicam related compound B in the ■*Standard solution*₁ₛ (USP41) at 260 nm
C_S = concentration of USP Meloxicam Related Compound B RS in the ■*Standard solution*₁ₛ (USP41) (mg/mL)
C_U = nominal concentration of meloxicam in the *Sample solution* (mg/mL)
Calculate the percentage of each unknown degradation product in the portion of Oral Suspension taken:

$$Result = (r_U/r_T) \times 100$$

r_U = peak area of any unknown degradation product in the *Sample solution* at 360 nm
r_T = sum of peak areas of meloxicam and all impurities in the *Sample solution* at 360 nm
Acceptance criteria
Meloxicam related compound B: NMT 0.15%
Any individual unknown degradation product: NMT 0.2%
Total degradation products: NMT 0.5%

SPECIFIC TESTS
* **MICROBIAL ENUMERATION TESTS ⟨61⟩** and **TESTS FOR SPECIFIED MICROORGANISMS ⟨62⟩:** The total aerobic microbial count does not exceed 10^2 cfu/g or 10^2 cfu/mL. The total yeasts and molds count does not exceed 5×10^1 cfu/g or 5×10^1 cfu/mL. It meets the requirements of the test for the absence of *Escherichia coli.*
* **PH ⟨791⟩:** 3.5–4.5
* **VISCOSITY—ROTATIONAL METHODS ⟨912⟩**
Analysis: Determine at 20° by using a shear rate programmable rotational viscometer.

Acceptance criteria: 40–100 centipoises

ADDITIONAL REQUIREMENTS
• **PACKAGING AND STORAGE:** Preserve in well-closed containers. Store at 25°, excursions permitted between 15° and 30°.

Change to read:

• **USP REFERENCE STANDARDS ⟨11⟩**
USP Meloxicam RS
USP Meloxicam Related Compound B RS
■5-Methylthiazol-2-amine.
$C_4H_6N_2S$ 114.175■₁ₛ (USP4T)

Delete the following:

■Metaproterenol Sulfate Inhalation Aerosol

» Metaproterenol Sulfate Inhalation Aerosol is a suspension of microfine Metaproterenol Sulfate in fluorochlorohydrocarbon propellants in a pressurized container. It contains not less than 90.0 percent and not more than 110.0 percent of the labeled amount of metaproterenol sulfate [$(C_{11}H_{17}NO_3)_2 \cdot H_2SO_4$].

Packaging and storage—Preserve in small, nonreactive, light-resistant aerosol containers equipped with metered-dose valves and provided with oral inhalation actuators.

USP Reference standards ⟨11⟩—
USP Metaproterenol Sulfate RS

Identification—The UV absorption spectrum of the solution from the *Assay preparation*, obtained as directed in the *Assay*, exhibits maxima and minima at the same wavelengths as that of the *Standard preparation* prepared as directed in the *Assay*.

Delivered dose uniformity over the entire contents: meets the requirements for *Metered-Dose Inhalers* under *Aerosols, Nasal Sprays, Metered-Dose Inhalers, and Dry Powder Inhalers* ⟨601⟩.

PROCEDURE FOR DOSE UNIFORMITY—

Standard preparation—Using a suitable quantity of USP Metaproterenol Sulfate RS, accurately weighed, prepare a solution in 0.01 N hydrochloric acid to obtain a solution having a known concentration of 0.05 mg per mL.

Test preparation—Discharge the minimum recommended dose into the sampling apparatus and detach the inhaler as directed. Rinse the apparatus (filter and interior) with four 5.0-mL portions of 0.01 N hydrochloric acid, and quantitatively transfer the rinsings to a 25-mL volumetric flask. Dilute with 0.01 N hydrochloric acid to volume, and mix.

Procedure—Transfer 20.0 mL portions of the *Standard preparation*, the *Test preparation*, and 0.01 N hydrochloric acid to serve as a blank to separate centrifuge tubes. Add 10.0 mL of chloroform to each, shake by mechanical means for 5 minutes, and separate the layers by centrifuging for 5 minutes. Determine the absorbances of the respective aqueous layers in 1-cm cells, at the wavelength of maximum absorbance at about 276 nm, with a suitable spectrophotometer, against the blank. Calculate the quantity, in

mg, of metaproterenol sulfate [$(C_{11}H_{17}NO_3)_2 \cdot H_2SO_4$] contained in the minimum dose taken by the formula:

$$12.5CN(A_U / A_S)$$

in which C is the concentration, in mg per mL, of USP Metaproterenol Sulfate RS in the *Standard preparation*; N is the number of sprays discharged to obtain the minimum dose; and A_U and A_S are the absorbances of the solutions from the *Test preparation* and the *Standard preparation*, respectively.

Particle size—Prime the valve of an Inhalation Aerosol container by alternately shaking and firing it several times, and then actuate one measured spray onto a clean, dry microscope slide held 5 cm from the end of the oral inhalation actuator, perpendicular to the direction of the spray. Carefully rinse the slide with about 2 mL of chloroform, and allow to dry. Examine the slide under a microscope equipped with a calibrated ocular micrometer, using 450× magnification. Focus on the particles of 25 fields of view near the center of the test specimen pattern, and note the size of the great majority of individual particles: they are less than 5 μm along the longest axis. Record the number and size of all individual crystalline particles (not agglomerates) more than 10 μm in length measured along the longest axis: not more than 10 such particles are observed.

Water—Transfer the contents of a weighed container to the titration vessel by attaching the valve stem to an inlet tube. Weigh the empty container and determine the weight of the specimen taken. The water content, determined by *Method I* under *Water Determination* ⟨921⟩, is not more than 0.075%.

Assay—Cool an accurately weighed Inhalation Aerosol container for 10 minutes in a bath consisting of a mixture of acetone and solid carbon dioxide. Cut the valve from the aerosol container and allow the container to warm to room temperature. When most of the propellants have evaporated, transfer the residue in the container to a 250-mL separator with the aid of 30 mL of chloroform and 50 mL of 0.01 N hydrochloric acid. Reserve the valve and the empty container. Shake the separator for 1 minute and allow the phases to separate. Transfer the chloroform phase to a second 250-mL separator and the aqueous phase to a 250-mL volumetric flask. Wash the chloroform phase with two 50-mL portions of 0.01 N hydrochloric acid, add the washings to the 250-mL volumetric flask, dilute with 0.01 N hydrochloric acid to volume, and mix. Transfer an accurately measured volume of this stock solution, equivalent to about 10 mg of metaproterenol sulfate, to a 100-mL volumetric flask, dilute with 0.01 N hydrochloric acid to volume, and mix. Dissolve an accurately weighed quantity of USP Metaproterenol Sulfate RS in 0.01 N hydrochloric acid, and dilute quantitatively and stepwise with the same solvent to obtain a Standard solution having a known concentration of about 100 μg per mL. Concomitantly determine the absorbances of both solutions at the wavelength of maximum absorbance at about 276 nm, with a suitable spectrophotometer, using 0.01 N hydrochloric acid as the blank. Rinse the empty aerosol container and the valve with water and dry them at 105° for 10 minutes, allow to cool, and weigh. Subtract the weight thus obtained from the original weight of the Inhalation Aerosol container to obtain the weight of the Inhalation Aerosol taken. Calculate the quantity, in mg, of metaproterenol sulfate [$(C_{11}H_{17}NO_3)_2 \cdot H_2SO_4$] in each mL of the Inhalation Aerosol taken by the formula:

$$25(C / V)(d / W)(A_U / A_S)$$

in which C is the concentration, in μg per mL, of USP Metaproterenol Sulfate RS in the Standard solution, V is the volume, in mL, of stock solution taken, W is the weight, in g, of the Inhalation Aerosol taken, and A_U and A_S are the absorbances of the solution from the Inhalation Aerosol and the Standard solution, respectively. [The density, d, is determined as follows: Weigh a known volume (*v*) of the Inhalation Aerosol in a suitable 5-mL gas-tight syringe equipped with a linear valve. Calibrate the volume of the syringe by filling to the 5-mL mark with dichlorotetrafluoroethane withdrawn from a plastic-coated glass vial sealed with a neoprene multiple-dose rubber stopper and an aluminum seal, using 1.456 g per mL as the density of the calibrating liquid. Maintain the dichlorotetrafluoroethane, the Inhalation Aerosol sample, and the syringe (protected from becoming wet) at 25° in a water bath. Obtain the sample, equivalent to the same volume as that obtained during the sampling procedure, from the Inhalation Aerosol by means of a sampling device consisting of a replaceable rubber septum engaged in the plate threads at one end of a threaded fitting, the opposite end of which contains a sharpened tube capable of puncturing the aerosol container, and a rubber gasket around the tube to prevent leakage of the container contents after puncture.* Calculate the density taken by the formula:

$$w / v$$

in which *w* is the weight of the volume, *v*, of the Inhalation Aerosol taken.]∎1S (*USP41*)

Methotrexate Injection

DEFINITION

Methotrexate Injection is a sterile solution of Methotrexate in Water for Injection prepared with the aid of Sodium Hydroxide. It contains NLT 90.0% and NMT 110.0% of the labeled amount of methotrexate ($C_{20}H_{22}N_8O_5$).

IDENTIFICATION

• **A. INFRARED ABSORPTION ⟨197K⟩**
  Sample: Dilute, if necessary, a volume of Injection, equivalent to about 25 mg of methotrexate, with water to obtain a solution with a concentration of about 2.5 mg/mL. Adjust with 0.1 N hydrochloric acid to a pH of 4.0. Place the slurry in a 50-mL centrifuge tube, and centrifuge. Decant the supernatant, add 25 mL of acetone, shake, and pass through a solvent-resistant membrane filter of 0.45-µm pore size. Air-dry the filtered precipitate.
  Acceptance criteria: Meets the requirements

Add the following:

∎• **B.** The retention time of the major peak of the *Sample solution* corresponds to that of the *Standard solution*, as obtained in the *Assay*.∎1S (*USP41*)

ASSAY

Change to read:

• **PROCEDURE**
  ∎**Buffer:** 3.4 mg/mL of anhydrous monobasic sodium phosphate in water. Adjust with 1 N sodium hydroxide to a pH of 6.0.
  Solution A: Acetonitrile and *Buffer* (5:95)
  Solution B: Acetonitrile and *Buffer* (50:50)
  Mobile phase: See *Table 1*.

Table 1

Time (min)	Solution A (%)	Solution B (%)
0.0	100	0
30	50	50
34	50	50
35	100	0
40	100	0

Standard solution: 0.2 mg/mL of USP Methotrexate RS in *Solution A* prepared as follows. Add a sufficient amount of USP Methotrexate RS to a suitable volumetric flask and add dimethyl sulfoxide equivalent to 5% of the flask volume. Sonicate to achieve dissolution, then dilute with *Solution A* to volume.
Sample solution: Nominally 0.2 mg/mL of methotrexate from Injection prepared as follows. Transfer a sufficient amount of Injection to an appropriate volumetric flask. Add about 5% of the flask volume of dimethyl sulfoxide and sonicate for 2 min at ambient temperature, then add 30% of the flask volume of *Solution A* and sonicate. Dilute with *Solution A* to volume.
Chromatographic system
(See *Chromatography* ⟨621⟩, *System Suitability*.)
  Mode: LC
  Detector: UV 280 nm
  Column: 4.6-mm × 25-cm; 5-µm packing L1
  Flow rate: 1 mL/min
  Injection volume: 20 µL
System suitability
  Sample: *Standard solution*
  Suitability requirements
    Tailing factor: NMT 2.0
    Relative standard deviation: NMT 2.0%∎1S (*USP41*)
Analysis
  Samples: *Standard solution* and *Sample solution*
  Calculate the percentage of the labeled amount of methotrexate ($C_{20}H_{22}N_8O_5$) in the portion of Injection taken:

$$Result = (r_U/r_S) \times (C_S/C_U) \times 100$$

r_U = peak response from the *Sample solution*
r_S = peak response from the *Standard solution*
C_S = concentration of USP Methotrexate RS in the *Standard solution* (µg/mL)
C_U = nominal concentration of methotrexate in the *Sample solution* (µg/mL)
Acceptance criteria: 90.0%–110.0%

IMPURITIES

Add the following:

∎• **ORGANIC IMPURITIES**
  Solution A, Solution B, Mobile phase, Sample solution, and Chromatographic system: Proceed as directed in the *Assay*.
  Standard solution: 0.2 µg/mL each of USP Methotrexate RS, USP Methotrexate Related Compound B RS, USP Methotrexate Related Compound C RS, and USP Methotrexate Related Compound E RS in *Solution A* prepared as follows. Add a sufficient amount of each Reference Standard to a suitable volumetric flask and add dimethyl sulfoxide equivalent to 5% of the flask volume. Sonicate to achieve dissolution, then dilute with *Solution A* to volume. Sonicate if necessary to aid dissolution.
  Sample solution: Nominally 0.2 mg/mL of methotrexate from Injection prepared as directed in the *Assay*

---

* A suitable sampling system is available from Alltek Associates, P. O. Box 498, Arlington Heights, IL 60006.

System suitability

Sample: *Standard solution*

[NOTE—See *Table 2* for relative retention times.]

Suitability requirements

Resolution: NLT 1.5 between methotrexate related compound B and methotrexate related compound C

Relative standard deviation: NMT 5.0% each for methotrexate, methotrexate related compound B, methotrexate related compound C, and methotrexate related compound E

Analysis

Samples: *Standard solution* and *Sample solution*

Calculate the percentage of methotrexate related compound B and methotrexate related compound C in the portion of Injection taken:

$$Result = (r_U/r_S) \times (C_S/C_U) \times 100$$

r_U = peak response of each corresponding impurity from the *Sample solution*

r_S = peak response of each corresponding Reference Standard from the *Standard solution*

C_S = concentration of each corresponding Reference Standard in the *Standard solution* (µg/mL)

C_U = nominal concentration of methotrexate in the *Sample solution* (µg/mL)

Calculate the percentage of methotrexate related compound E free acid in the portion of Injection taken:

$$Result = (r_U/r_S) \times (C_S/C_U) \times (M_{r1}/M_{r2}) \times 100$$

r_U = peak response from the *Sample solution*

r_S = peak response from the *Standard solution*

C_S = concentration of USP Methotrexate Related Compound E RS in the *Standard solution* (µg/mL)

C_U = nominal concentration of methotrexate in the *Sample solution* (µg/mL)

M_{r1} = molecular weight of methotrexate related compound E free acid, 325.33

M_{r2} = molecular weight of USP Methotrexate Related Compound E RS, 343.56

[NOTE—USP Methotrexate Related Compound E RS is 4-{[(2,4-Diaminopteridin-6-yl)methyl](methyl)amino}benzoic acid, hemihydrochloride.]

Calculate the percentage of any individual unspecified degradation product in the portion of Injection taken:

$$Result = (r_U/r_S) \times (C_S/C_U) \times 100$$

r_U = peak response of each unspecified degradation product from the *Sample solution*

r_S = peak response of methotrexate from the *Standard solution*

C_S = concentration of USP Methotrexate RS in the *Standard solution* (µg/mL)

C_U = nominal concentration of methotrexate in the *Sample solution* (µg/mL)

Acceptance criteria: See *Table 2*. The reporting threshold is 0.1%.

Table 2

Name	Relative Retention Time	Acceptance Criteria, NMT (%)
Methotrexate related compound B	0.67	0.3
Methotrexate related compound C	0.73	3.0

[a] 4-{[(2,4-Diaminopteridin-6-yl)methyl](methyl)amino}benzoic acid.

Table 2 *(Continued)*

Name	Relative Retention Time	Acceptance Criteria, NMT (%)
Methotrexate	1.0	—
Methotrexate related compound E free acid[a]	1.41	0.3
Any individual unspecified degradation product	—	0.2
Total unspecified degradation products	—	1.0

[a] 4-{[(2,4-Diaminopteridin-6-yl)methyl](methyl)amino}benzoic acid.

■1S (USP41)

SPECIFIC TESTS
- **PH ⟨791⟩:** 7.0–9.0
- **BACTERIAL ENDOTOXINS TEST ⟨85⟩:** NMT 0.4 USP Endotoxin Units/mg of methotrexate sodium
- **OTHER REQUIREMENTS:** Meets the requirements in *Injections and Implanted Drug Products* ⟨1⟩

ADDITIONAL REQUIREMENTS

Change to read:

- **PACKAGING AND STORAGE:** Preserve in single-dose or in multiple-dose containers, preferably of Type I glass, protected from light. ■Store at controlled room temperature. ■1S (USP41)

Change to read:

- **USP REFERENCE STANDARDS ⟨11⟩**
  - ● (CN 1-May-2018)
  USP Methotrexate RS
  ■USP Methotrexate Related Compound B RS
  (*S*)-2-{4-[(2,4-Diaminopteridin-6-yl)methylamino]benzamido}pentanedioic acid.
  $C_{19}H_{20}N_8O_5$ 440.41
  USP Methotrexate Related Compound C RS
  (*S*)-2-(4-{[(2-Amino-4-oxo-1,4-dihydropteridin-6-yl)methyl](methyl)amino}benzamido)pentanedioic acid.
  $C_{20}H_{21}N_7O_6$ 455.42
  USP Methotrexate Related Compound E RS
  4-{[(2,4-Diaminopteridin-6-yl)methyl](methyl)amino}benzoic acid, hemihydrochloride.
  $C_{15}H_{15}N_7O_2 \cdot \frac{1}{2}HCl$ 343.56 (anhydrous)
  $C_{15}H_{15}N_7O_2$ 325.33 (free acid)■1S (USP41)

Miconazole Nitrate

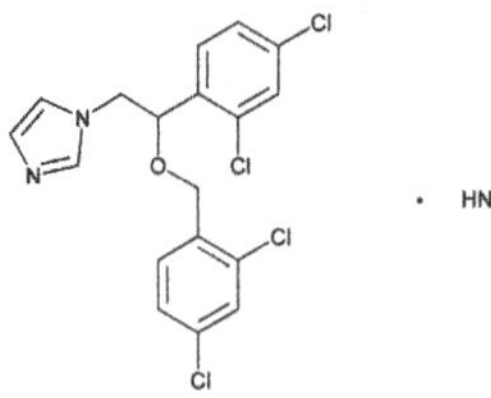

$C_{18}H_{14}Cl_4N_2O \cdot HNO_3$ 479.14

1*H*-Imidazole, 1-[2-(2,4-dichlorophenyl)-2-[(2,4-dichlorophenyl)methoxy]ethyl]-, mononitrate;

1-[2,4-Dichloro-β-[(2,4-dichlorobenzyl)oxy]phenethyl]imidazole mononitrate [22832-87-7].

DEFINITION

Miconazole Nitrate contains NLT 98.0% and NMT 102.0% of miconazole nitrate ($C_{18}H_{14}Cl_4N_2O \cdot HNO_3$), calculated on the dried basis.

IDENTIFICATION

Change to read:

- **A.** **INFRARED ABSORPTION** ■⟨197⟩: [NOTE—Methods described in ⟨197K⟩ or ⟨197A⟩ may be used.]■₁S *(USP41)*

Delete the following:

■● **B.** **ULTRAVIOLET ABSORPTION** ⟨197U⟩
  Diluent: 0.1 N hydrochloric acid in isopropyl alcohol (1 in 10)
  Sample solution: 400 µg/mL sample in *Diluent*
  Acceptance criteria: Meets the requirements■₁S *(USP41)*

Add the following:

■● **B.** The retention time of the major peak of the *Sample solution* corresponds to that of the *Standard solution*, as obtained in the *Assay.*■₁S *(USP41)*

ASSAY

Change to read:

- **PROCEDURE**
  ■**Solution A:** Methanol, water, and 1 M triethylammonium acetate (30:70:1)
  Solution B: Acetonitrile, methanol, and 1 M triethylammonium acetate (25: 75: 0.2)
  Mobile phase: See *Table 1*.

Table 1

Time (min)	Solution A (%)	Solution B (%)
0	70	30
5	70	30
10	44	56
27	44	56
30	25	75
35	25	75
36	70	30
40	70	30

  Diluent: Methanol and water (70:30)
  System suitability solution: 0.1 mg/mL of USP Miconazole Nitrate RS and 6 µg/mL of USP Miconazole Related Compound F RS in *Diluent*. Sonication may be needed to aid dissolution.
  Standard solution: 0.1 mg/mL of USP Miconazole Nitrate RS in *Diluent*. Sonication may be needed to aid dissolution.
  Sample solution: 0.1 mg/mL of Miconazole Nitrate in *Diluent*. Sonication may be needed to aid dissolution.
  Chromatographic system
  (See *Chromatography* ⟨621⟩, *System Suitability*.)
  Mode: LC
  Detector: UV 215 nm
  Column: 4.6-mm × 10-cm; 2.6-µm packing L11
  Column temperature: 40°
  Flow rate: 0.8 mL/min
  Injection volume: 10 µL
  System suitability
  Samples: *System suitability solution* and *Standard solution*

[NOTE—The relative retention times for miconazole related compound F and miconazole are 0.96 and 1.0, respectively.]
  Suitability requirements
  Resolution: NLT 1.5 between miconazole related compound F and miconazole, *System suitability solution*
  Tailing factor: NMT 2.0, *Standard solution*
  Relative standard deviation: NMT 0.73%, *Standard solution*
  Analysis
  Samples: *Standard solution* and *Sample solution*
  Calculate the percentage of miconazole nitrate ($C_{18}H_{14}Cl_4N_2O \cdot HNO_3$) in the portion of Miconazole Nitrate taken:

$$\text{Result} = (r_U/r_S) \times (C_S/C_U) \times 100$$

r_U = peak response of miconazole from the *Sample solution*
r_S = peak response of miconazole from the *Standard solution*
C_S = concentration of USP Miconazole Nitrate RS in the *Standard solution* (mg/mL)
C_U = concentration of Miconazole Nitrate in the *Sample solution* (mg/mL)■₁S *(USP41)*
  Acceptance criteria: 98.0%–102.0% on the dried basis

IMPURITIES

- **RESIDUE ON IGNITION** ⟨281⟩: NMT 0.2%

Change to read:

- **ORGANIC IMPURITIES**
  ■**Solution A, Solution B, Mobile phase, Diluent,** and **Chromatographic system:** Proceed as directed in the *Assay*.
  Standard solution: 1.2 µg/mL each of USP Miconazole Nitrate RS, USP Econazole Nitrate RS, USP Miconazole Related Compound C RS, USP Miconazole Related Compound F RS, and USP Miconazole Related Compound I RS in *Diluent*
  Sample solution: 600 µg/mL of Miconazole Nitrate in *Diluent*. Sonication may be needed to aid dissolution.
  System suitability
  Sample: *Standard solution*
  [NOTE—See *Table 2* for relative retention times.]
  Suitability requirements
  Resolution: NLT 1.5 between miconazole related compound C and miconazole related compound I; NLT 1.5 between miconazole related compound I and econazole; and NLT 1.5 between miconazole related compound F and miconazole
  Relative standard deviation: NMT 3.0% for miconazole
  Analysis
  Samples: *Standard solution* and *Sample solution*
  Calculate the percentage of miconazole related compound C, miconazole related compound F, miconazole related compound I, or econazole nitrate in the portion of Miconazole Nitrate taken:

$$\text{Result} = (r_U/r_S) \times (C_S/C_U) \times 100$$

r_U = peak response of miconazole related compound C, miconazole related compound F, miconazole related compound I, or econazole nitrate from the *Sample solution*
r_S = peak response of miconazole related compound C, miconazole related compound F, miconazole related compound I, or econazole nitrate from the *Standard solution*

C_S = concentration of USP Miconazole Related Compound C RS, USP Miconazole Related Compound F RS, USP Miconazole Related Compound I RS, or USP Econazole Nitrate RS in the *Standard solution* (µg/mL)

C_U = concentration of Miconazole Nitrate in the *Sample solution* (µg/mL)

Calculate the percentage of each specified and any individual unspecified impurity in the portion of Miconazole Nitrate taken:

$$Result = (r_U/r_S) \times (C_S/C_U) \times 100$$

r_U = peak response of each specified and any individual unspecified impurity from the *Sample solution*

r_S = peak response of miconazole from the *Standard solution*

C_S = concentration of USP Miconazole Nitrate RS in the *Standard solution* (µg/mL)

C_U = concentration of Miconazole Nitrate in the *Sample solution* (µg/mL)

Acceptance criteria: See *Table 2*.

Table 2

Name	Relative Retention Time	Acceptance Criteria, NMT (%)
Deschlorobenzyl econazole[a]	0.22	0.25
Miconazole quarternary salt[b]	0.57	0.25
Miconazole benzyl analog[c]	0.65	0.25
Miconazole related compound C	0.74	0.25
Miconazole related compound I	0.76	0.25
Econazole nitrate	0.78	0.25
Miconazole 2,6-isomer[d]	0.87	0.25
Miconazole 2,5-isomer[e]	0.94	0.25
Miconazole related compound F	0.96	0.25
Miconazole	1.0	—
Any individual unspecified impurity	—	0.10
Total impurities	—	0.5

[a] 1-(2,4-Dichlorophenyl)-2-(1H-imidazol-1-yl)ethanol.
[b] 2-(3-{2-[(2,4-Dichlorobenzyl)oxy]-2-(2,4-dichlorophenyl)ethyl}-1H-imidazol-3-ium-1-yl)-2-methylpropanoate.
[c] 1-[2-(Benzyloxy)-2-(2,4-dichlorophenyl)ethyl]-1H-imidazole.
[d] 1-{2-[(2,6-Dichlorobenzyl)oxy]-2-(2,4-dichlorophenyl)ethyl}-1H-imidazole.
[e] 1-{2-[(2,5-Dichlorobenzyl)oxy]-2-(2,4-dichlorophenyl)ethyl}-1H-imidazole.

■1S (USP41)

SPECIFIC TESTS

Add the following:

■• **OPTICAL ROTATION** ⟨781S⟩, *Procedures, Specific Rotation*
Sample solution: 10 mg/mL of Miconazole Nitrate in methanol

Acceptance criteria: −0.10° to +0.10°■1S (USP41)
• **LOSS ON DRYING** ⟨731⟩
Analysis: Dry at 105° for 2 h.
Acceptance criteria: NMT 0.5%

ADDITIONAL REQUIREMENTS

Change to read:

• **PACKAGING AND STORAGE:** Preserve in well-closed containers, protected from light. ■Store at controlled room temperature.■1S (USP41)

Change to read:

• **USP REFERENCE STANDARDS** ⟨11⟩
USP Econazole Nitrate RS
USP Miconazole Nitrate RS
■USP Miconazole Related Compound C RS
2-[(2,4-Dichlorobenzyl)oxy]-2-(2,4-dichlorophenyl)ethan-1-amine hydrochloride.
$C_{15}H_{13}Cl_4NO \cdot HCl$ 401.53
USP Miconazole Related Compound F RS
1-{2-[(3,4-Dichlorobenzyl)oxy]-2-(2,4-dichlorophenyl)ethyl}-1H-imidazole.
$C_{18}H_{14}Cl_4N_2O$ 416.13
USP Miconazole Related Compound I RS
1-{2-[(2-Chlorobenzyl)oxy]-2-(2,4-dichlorophenyl)ethyl}-1H-imidazole mononitrate.
$C_{18}H_{15}Cl_3N_2O \cdot HNO_3$ 444.69■1S (USP41)

Miconazole Nitrate Topical Powder

DEFINITION
Miconazole Nitrate Topical Powder contains NLT 90.0% and NMT 110.0% of the labeled amount of miconazole nitrate ($C_{18}H_{14}Cl_4N_2O \cdot HNO_3$).

IDENTIFICATION

Change to read:

• **A.**
Sample: Transfer nominally 100 mg of miconazole nitrate from Topical Powder to a 50-mL beaker, disperse in 40 mL of methanol, and mix for a minimum of 5 min. Allow to settle for 5–10 min and filter into a 100-mL beaker. Evaporate on a steam bath ■or by a rotary evaporator■1S (USP41) to dryness. Dry the residue at 105° for 10 min.
Acceptance criteria: The IR absorption spectrum of a potassium bromide dispersion of the residue obtained from the *Sample* exhibits maxima only at the same wavelengths as that of a similar preparation of USP Miconazole Nitrate RS.

Add the following:

■• **B.** The retention time of the major peak of the *Sample solution* corresponds to that of the *Standard solution*, as obtained in the *Assay*.■1S (USP41)

ASSAY

Change to read:

- **PROCEDURE**
  ■**Buffer:** 4.6 g/L of dibasic potassium phosphate trihydrate in water. Adjust with phosphoric acid to a pH of 7.5.
  Solution A: Acetonitrile and *Buffer* (65:35)
  Solution B: Acetonitrile
  Solution C: Acetonitrile, water, and phosphoric acid (50: 50: 0.05)
  Mobile phase: See *Table 1*.

Table 1

Time (min)	Solution A (%)	Solution B (%)	Solution C (%)	Flow rate (mL/min)
0	100	0	0	1.0
17.0	86	14	0	1.0
17.1	0	0	100	3.0
28.0	0	0	100	3.0
28.1	100	0	0	2.0
38.0	100	0	0	2.0
38.1	100	0	0	1.0
40	100	0	0	1.0

Diluent: Acetonitrile and water (50:50)
Standard stock solution: 2 mg/mL of USP Miconazole Nitrate RS in *Diluent*. Sonication may be needed to aid dissolution.
Standard solution: 0.2 mg/mL of USP Miconazole Nitrate RS in *Diluent* from the *Standard stock solution*
Sample solution: Nominally 0.2 mg/mL of miconazole nitrate in *Diluent* prepared as follows. Transfer an appropriate amount of miconazole nitrate from a portion of the Topical Powder to a suitable volumetric flask. Add *Diluent* equivalent to 50% of the flask volume, shake for 30 min, and sonicate for 10 min. Dilute with *Diluent* to volume. Pass a portion of the solution through a suitable filter of 0.45-μm pore size.
Chromatographic system
  (See *Chromatography* ⟨621⟩, *System Suitability*.)
  Mode: LC
  Detector: UV 220 nm
  Column: 4.6-mm × 25-cm; 5-μm packing L7
  Column temperature: 32°
  Flow rate: See *Table 1*.
  Injection volume: 5 μL
System suitability
  Sample: *Standard solution*
  Suitability requirements
    Tailing factor: NMT 2.0
    Relative standard deviation: NMT 2.0%
Analysis
  Samples: *Standard solution* and *Sample solution*
  Calculate the percentage of the labeled amount of miconazole nitrate ($C_{18}H_{14}Cl_4N_2O \cdot HNO_3$) in the portion of Topical Powder taken:

$$Result = (r_U/r_S) \times (C_S/C_U) \times 100$$

r_U = peak response of miconazole from the *Sample solution*
r_S = peak response of miconazole from the *Standard solution*
C_S = concentration of USP Miconazole Nitrate RS in the *Standard solution* (mg/mL)
C_U = nominal concentration of miconazole nitrate in the *Sample solution* (mg/mL)■15 *(USP41)*

Acceptance criteria: 90.0%–110.0%

IMPURITIES

Add the following:

- ■• **ORGANIC IMPURITIES**
  Buffer, Solution B, Solution C, Diluent, Standard stock solution, and **Sample solution:** Prepare as directed in the *Assay*.
  Solution A: Acetonitrile and *Buffer* (35:65)
  Mobile phase: See *Table 2*.

Table 2

Time (min)	Solution A (%)	Solution B (%)	Solution C (%)	Flow rate (mL/min)
0	100	0	0	1.0
55.0	30.8	69.2	0	1.0
55.1	0	0	100	3.0
68.0	0	0	100	3.0
68.1	100	0	0	2.0
83.0	100	0	0	2.0
83.1	100	0	0	1.0
85.0	100	0	0	1.0

System suitability solution: 0.2 mg/mL of USP Miconazole Nitrate RS from the *Standard stock solution* and 0.2 μg/mL of USP Miconazole Related Compound C RS in *Diluent*
Standard solution: 2 μg/mL of USP Miconazole Nitrate RS in *Diluent* from the *Standard stock solution*
Sensitivity solution: 0.1 μg/mL of USP Miconazole Nitrate RS in *Diluent* from the *Standard solution*
Chromatographic system
  (See *Chromatography* ⟨621⟩, *System Suitability*.)
  Mode: LC
  Detector: UV 220 nm
  Column: 4.6-mm × 25-cm; 5-μm packing L7
  Column temperature: 32°
  Flow rate: See *Table 2*.
  Injection volume: 15 μL
System suitability
  Samples: *System suitability solution*, *Standard solution*, and *Sensitivity solution*
  Suitability requirements
    Resolution: NLT 1.5 between miconazole related compound C and miconazole, *System suitability solution*
    Relative standard deviation: NMT 10.0%, *Standard solution*
    Signal-to-noise ratio: NLT 10, *Sensitivity solution*
Analysis
  Samples: *Standard solution* and *Sample solution*
  Calculate the percentage of miconazole related compound C and any individual unspecified degradation product in the portion of Topical Powder taken:

$$Result = (r_U/r_S) \times (C_S/C_U) \times 100$$

r_U = peak response of miconazole related compound C or any individual unspecified degradation product from the *Sample solution*
r_S = peak response of miconazole from the *Standard solution*
C_S = concentration of USP Miconazole Nitrate RS in the *Standard solution* (μg/mL)
C_U = nominal concentration of miconazole nitrate in the *Sample solution* (μg/mL)
Acceptance criteria: See *Table 3*.

Table 3

Name	Relative Retention Time	Acceptance Criteria, NMT (%)
Miconazole	1.0	—
Miconazole related compound C	1.06	0.25
Any individual unspecified degradation product	—	0.10
Total impurities	—	1.0

■1S (USP41)

PERFORMANCE TESTS
• **MINIMUM FILL ⟨755⟩:** Meets the requirements

SPECIFIC TESTS
• **MICROBIAL ENUMERATION TESTS ⟨61⟩ and TESTS FOR SPECIFIED MICROORGANISMS ⟨62⟩:** The total count does not exceed 10² cfu/g. It meets the requirements of the tests for the absence of *Staphylococcus aureus* and *Pseudomonas aeruginosa*.

ADDITIONAL REQUIREMENTS

Change to read:

• **PACKAGING AND STORAGE:** Preserve in well-closed containers. ■Store at controlled room temperature.■1S (USP41)

Change to read:

• **USP REFERENCE STANDARDS ⟨11⟩**
USP Miconazole Nitrate RS
■USP Miconazole Related Compound C RS
2-[(2,4-Dichlorobenzyl)oxy]-2-(2,4-dichlorophenyl)ethan-1-amine.
$C_{15}H_{13}Cl_4NO$ 365.08■1S (USP41)

Minocycline Hydrochloride

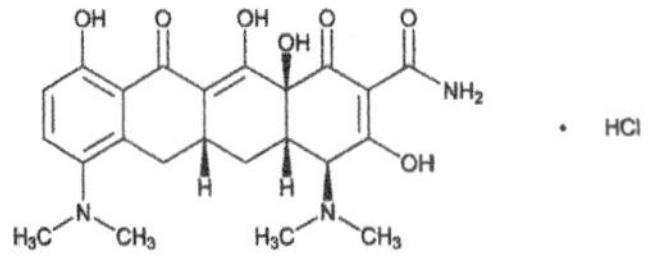

$C_{23}H_{27}N_3O_7 \cdot HCl$ 493.94
2-Naphthacenecarboxamide, 4,7-bis(dimethylamino)-1,4,4a, 5,5a,6,11,12a-octahydro-3,10,12,12a-tetrahydroxy-1,11dioxo-, monohydrochloride, [4S-(4α,4aα,5aα,12aα)]-;
4,7-Bis(dimethylamino)-1,4,4a,5,5a,6,11,12a-octahydro-3,10,12,12a-tetrahydroxy-1,11-dioxo-2-naphthacene-carboxamide monohydrochloride [13614-98-7].

DEFINITION
Minocycline Hydrochloride contains the equivalent of NLT 890 µg and NMT 950 µg of minocycline ($C_{23}H_{27}N_3O_7$) per mg, calculated on the anhydrous basis.

IDENTIFICATION

Change to read:

• ■**A.**■1S (USP41) **INFRARED ABSORPTION ⟨197K⟩:** Dry the Standard and Sample at 100° for 2 h before use.

Add the following:

■• **B.** The retention time of the major peak of the *Sample solution* corresponds to that of the *Standard solution*, as obtained in the *Assay*.■1S (USP41)

ASSAY
• **PROCEDURE**
[NOTE—Protect the *Standard solution* and *Sample solution* from light, store in a refrigerator, and use within 3 h.]
Mobile phase: Dimethylformamide, tetrahydrofuran, 0.2 M ammonium oxalate, and 0.01 M edetate disodium TS (120:80:600:180). Adjust with ammonium hydroxide to a pH of 7.2.
System suitability solution: Dissolve 10 mg of USP Minocycline Hydrochloride RS in 20 mL of 0.2 M ammonium oxalate. Heat on a water bath at 60° for 3 h, allow to cool, and dilute with water to 25.0 mL.
Standard solution: Equivalent to 500 µg/mL of minocycline ($C_{23}H_{27}N_3O_7$) from USP Minocycline Hydrochloride RS in water
Sample solution: Equivalent to 500 µg/mL of minocycline ($C_{23}H_{27}N_3O_7$) from Minocycline Hydrochloride in water
Chromatographic system
(See *Chromatography* ⟨621⟩, *System Suitability*.)
Mode: LC
Detector: UV 280 nm
Column: 4.6-mm × 25-cm; 5-µm packing L1
Column temperature: 40°
Flow rate: 1.5 mL/min
Injection volume: 20 µL
System suitability
Samples: *System suitability solution* and *Standard solution*
[NOTE—The relative retention times for epiminocycline and minocycline are 0.7 and 1.0, respectively.]
Suitability requirements
Resolution: NLT 4.6 between epiminocycline and minocycline, *System suitability solution*
Tailing factor: 0.9–2.0, *Standard solution*
Relative standard deviation: NMT 2.0%, *Standard solution*
Analysis
Samples: *Standard solution* and *Sample solution*
Calculate the quantity, in µg/mg, of minocycline ($C_{23}H_{27}N_3O_7$) in the portion of Minocycline Hydrochloride taken:

$$Result = (r_U/r_S) \times (C_S/C_U) \times P$$

r_U = peak response from the *Sample solution*
r_S = peak response from the *Standard solution*
C_S = concentration of minocycline in the *Standard solution* (µg/mL)
C_U = concentration of minocycline in the *Sample solution* (µg/mL)
P = potency of USP Minocycline Hydrochloride RS (µg/mg)
Acceptance criteria: 890–950 µg/mg on the anhydrous basis

IMPURITIES
• **RESIDUE ON IGNITION ⟨281⟩:** NMT 0.15%

Delete the following:

■• **HEAVY METALS,** *Method II* ⟨231⟩: NMT 50 ppm• (Official 1-Jan-2018)

Change to read:

- **ORGANIC IMPURITIES**

  Mobile phase, System suitability solution, Standard solution, Chromatographic system, and System suitability: Proceed as directed in the *Assay*.
  [NOTE—Protect the *Standard solution* and the *Sample solutions* from light, store in a refrigerator, and use within 3 h.]
  Sample solution 1: 0.25 mg/mL of Minocycline Hydrochloride ■in water■1S (USP41)
  Sample solution 2: 5 µg/mL of Minocycline Hydrochloride in water
  Sample solution 3: 3 µg/mL of Minocycline Hydrochloride in water
  Run time: 2.6 times the retention time of minocycline, *Sample solution 1*
  Analysis
    Samples: *Sample solution 1*, *Sample solution 2*, and *Sample solution 3*
    Calculate the percentage of epiminocycline in the portion of Minocycline Hydrochloride taken:

$$Result = (r_{E1}/r_{M3}) \times D_1 \times 100$$

r_{E1} = peak response of epiminocycline from *Sample solution 1*
r_{M3} = peak response of minocycline from *Sample solution 3*
D_1 = dilution factor for *Sample solution 3*

Calculate the total percentage of impurities other than epiminocycline in the portion of Minocycline Hydrochloride taken:

$$Result = (r_T/r_{M2}) \times D_2 \times 100$$

r_T = sum of the peak responses of all impurities other than epiminocycline from *Sample solution 1*
r_{M2} = peak response of minocycline from *Sample solution 2*
D_2 = dilution factor for *Sample solution 2*

Acceptance criteria
  Individual impurities: NMT 1.2% epiminocycline
  Total impurities (excluding epiminocycline): NMT 2.0%

SPECIFIC TESTS
- **CRYSTALLINITY ⟨695⟩:** Meets the requirements
- **PH ⟨791⟩**
  Sample: 10 mg/mL of minocycline in solution
  Acceptance criteria: 3.5–4.5
- **WATER DETERMINATION ⟨921⟩, *Method I*:** 4.3%–8.0%
- **STERILITY TESTS ⟨71⟩:** Where the label states that Minocycline Hydrochloride is sterile, it meets the requirements.
- **BACTERIAL ENDOTOXINS TEST ⟨85⟩:** Where the label states that Minocycline Hydrochloride is sterile or must be subjected to further processing during the preparation of injectable dosage forms, it contains NMT 1.25 USP Endotoxin Units/mg of minocycline.

ADDITIONAL REQUIREMENTS
- **PACKAGING AND STORAGE:** Preserve in tight containers, protected from light.
- **LABELING:** Where it is intended for use in preparing injectable dosage forms, the label states that it is sterile or must be subjected to further processing during the preparation of injectable dosage forms.

Change to read:

- **USP REFERENCE STANDARDS ⟨11⟩**
  ● (CN 1-May-2018)
  USP Minocycline Hydrochloride RS

Montelukast Sodium Oral Granules

DEFINITION
Montelukast Sodium Oral Granules contain Montelukast Sodium equivalent to NLT 90.0% and NMT 108.0% of the labeled amount of montelukast ($C_{35}H_{36}ClNO_3S$).
[NOTE—Avoid exposure of samples containing montelukast to light.]

IDENTIFICATION
- **A. ULTRAVIOLET ABSORPTION ⟨197U⟩**
  Diluent: Methanol and water (3:1)
  Standard solution: 3.3 µg/mL of USP Montelukast Dicyclohexylamine RS in *Diluent*
  Sample stock solution: Nominally 0.02 mg/mL of montelukast prepared as follows. Transfer the contents of one packet to a suitable volumetric flask, add 66% of the flask volume of *Diluent*, shake well, and sonicate for 15 min with occasional shaking. Cool to room temperature, dilute with *Diluent* to volume, and mix well.
  Sample solution: Nominally 2 µg/mL of montelukast in *Diluent* from the *Sample stock solution*. Pass a portion of the resulting solution through a suitable filter of 0.45-µm pore size or centrifuge to obtain a clear solution.
  Wavelength range: 210–400 nm
  Acceptance criteria: The *Sample solution* exhibits maxima only at the same wavelengths as the *Standard solution*.
- **B.** The retention time of the major peak of the *Sample solution* corresponds to that of the *Standard solution*, as obtained in the *Assay*.

ASSAY
- **PROCEDURE**
  Diluent: Methanol and water (3:1)
  Solution A: 0.2% (v/v) trifluoroacetic acid in water
  Solution B: Methanol and acetonitrile (3:2)
  Mobile phase: See *Table 1*.

Table 1

Time (min)	Solution A (%)	Solution B (%)
0	48	52
5	45	55
12	45	55
22	25	75
23	25	75
25	48	52
30	48	52

Standard solution: 0.33 mg/mL of USP Montelukast Dicyclohexylamine RS in *Diluent*
System suitability solution: Transfer 10 mL of the *Standard solution* to a clear 10-mL volumetric flask, add 4 µL of hydrogen peroxide, and mix well. Expose the flask for at least 4 h to ambient light or 10 min to a 4 klx cool white light. [NOTE—Montelukast is partially converted to the *cis*-isomer under these conditions.]
Sensitivity solution: 0.33 µg/mL of USP Montelukast Dicyclohexylamine RS in *Diluent* from the *Standard solution*
Sample solution: Nominally 0.24 mg/mL of montelukast prepared as follows. Transfer the equivalent of 60 mg of montelukast from the contents of the pack-

ets (NLT 15) to a 500-mL volumetric flask, and add 250 mL of *Diluent*. Shake well and sonicate for 30 min, with occasional shaking. Pass a portion of the resulting solution through a suitable filter of 0.45-µm pore size or centrifuge to obtain a clear solution.

Chromatographic system
(See *Chromatography* ⟨621⟩, *System Suitability*.)
Mode: LC
Detector: UV 255 nm
Columns
  Guard: 3.0-mm × 4-mm; packing L11
  Analytical: 4.6-mm × 10-cm; 3-µm packing L11
Column temperature: 50°
Flow rate: 1.5 mL/min
Injection volume: 20 µL
Run time: 2 times the retention time of montelukast
System suitability
Samples: *Standard solution, System suitability solution,* and *Sensitivity solution*
[NOTE—The relative retention times for the *cis*-isomer and montelukast are about 0.92 and 1.0, respectively.]
Suitability requirements
  Resolution: NLT 1.5 between the *cis*-isomer and montelukast, *System suitability solution*
  Relative standard deviation: NMT 2.0% for five injections, *Standard solution*
  Signal-to-noise ratio: NLT 10, *Sensitivity solution*
Analysis
Samples: *Standard solution* and *Sample solution*
Calculate the percentage of the labeled amount of montelukast ($C_{35}H_{36}ClNO_3S$) in the portion of Oral Granules taken:

$$Result = (r_U/r_S) \times (C_S/C_U) \times (M_{r1}/M_{r2}) \times 100$$

r_U = peak response from the *Sample solution*
r_S = peak response from the *Standard solution*
C_S = concentration of USP Montelukast Dicyclohexylamine RS in the *Standard solution* (mg/mL)
C_U = nominal concentration of montelukast in the *Sample solution* (mg/mL)
M_{r1} = molecular weight of montelukast, 586.18
M_{r2} = molecular weight of montelukast dicyclohexylamine, 767.50
Acceptance criteria: 90.0%–108.0%

PERFORMANCE TESTS

Change to read:

- **DISSOLUTION ⟨711⟩**
Test 1
  Medium: 0.5% (w/v) sodium dodecyl sulfate in water; 900 mL. Do not deaerate.
  Apparatus 1: 100 mesh; 50 rpm
  Time: 15 min
  Solution A: 0.2% (v/v) trifluoroacetic acid in water
  Solution B: 0.2% (v/v) trifluoroacetic acid in acetonitrile
  Mobile phase: *Solution A* and *Solution B* (1:1)
  Standard stock solution: 0.33 mg/mL of USP Montelukast Dicyclohexylamine RS in methanol (equivalent to 0.25 mg/mL of montelukast)
  Standard solution: (*L*/900) mg/mL of montelukast in *Medium* from the *Standard stock solution*, where *L* is the label claim in mg/packet of montelukast
  Sample solution: Place the entire contents of one packet in the basket. At the appropriate time point, pass a portion of the solution under test through a suitable filter to obtain a clear solution. Discard the first 10 mL of the filtrate.
  Chromatographic system
  (See *Chromatography* ⟨621⟩, *System Suitability*.)

Mode: LC
Detector: UV 389 nm
Column: 3.0-mm × 10-cm; 5-µm packing L11
Column temperature: 50°
Flow rate: 0.9 mL/min
Injection volume: 25 µL
Run time: 1.5 times the retention time of montelukast
System suitability
Sample: *Standard solution*
Suitability requirements
  Tailing factor: NMT 1.5
  Relative standard deviation: NMT 2.0%
Analysis
Samples: *Standard solution* and *Sample solution*
Calculate the percentage of the labeled amount of montelukast ($C_{35}H_{36}ClNO_3S$) dissolved:

$$Result = (r_U/r_S) \times C_S \times V \times (1/L) \times 100$$

r_U = peak response of montelukast from the *Sample solution*
r_S = peak response of montelukast from the *Standard solution*
C_S = concentration of montelukast in the *Standard solution* (mg/mL)
V = volume of *Medium*, 900 mL
L = label claim (mg/packet)
Tolerances: NLT 85% (*Q*) of the labeled amount of montelukast ($C_{35}H_{36}ClNO_3S$) is dissolved.
Test 2: If the product complies with this test, the labeling indicates that it meets USP *Dissolution Test 2*.
Medium: 0.5% (w/v) sodium dodecyl sulfate in water; 900 mL
Apparatus 1: 100 mesh; 50 rpm
Time: 15 min
Solution A: 0.07 g/L of monobasic sodium phosphate
Solution B: Acetonitrile
Mobile phase: *Solution A* and *Solution B* (45:55). Add 1.33 mL/L of triethylamine and adjust with phosphoric acid to a pH of 6.7.
Standard stock solution: 0.1 mg/mL of montelukast from montelukast sodium hydrate prepared as follows. Transfer a suitable amount of montelukast sodium hydrate to an appropriate volumetric flask. Dissolve in 4% of the flask volume of methanol and dilute with *Medium* to volume. Determine the water content of montelukast sodium hydrate at the time of use.
Standard solution: 0.004 mg/mL of montelukast in *Medium* from the *Standard stock solution*
Sample solution: Place the entire contents of one packet in the basket. At the appropriate time point, centrifuge a portion of the solution under test.
Chromatographic system
(See *Chromatography* ⟨621⟩, *System Suitability*.)
Mode: LC
Detector: UV 225 nm
Column: 4.6-mm × 5-cm; 1.8-µm packing L1
Column temperature: 35°
Flow rate: 1 mL/min
Injection volume: 100 µL
Run time: 1.5 times the retention time of montelukast
System suitability
Sample: *Standard solution*
Suitability requirements
  Relative standard deviation: NMT 2.0%
Analysis
Samples: *Standard solution* and *Sample solution*
Calculate the percentage of the labeled amount of montelukast ($C_{35}H_{36}ClNO_3S$) dissolved:

$$Result = (r_U/r_S) \times C_S \times V \times (1/L) \times 100$$

r_U = peak response from the *Sample solution*

r_S = peak response from the *Standard solution*
C_S = concentration of montelukast in the *Standard solution* (mg/mL)
V = volume of *Medium*, 900 mL
L = label claim (mg/packet)

Tolerances: NLT 80% (Q) of the labeled amount of montelukast ($C_{35}H_{36}ClNO_3S$) is dissolved.

Test 3: If the product complies with this test, the labeling indicates that it meets USP *Dissolution Test 3*.
Medium: 0.5% (w/v) sodium dodecyl sulfate in water; 900 mL
Apparatus 2: 50 rpm
Time: 10 min
Solution A: 2.72 g/L of monobasic potassium phosphate in water
Mobile phase: Acetonitrile and *Solution A* (70:30)
Diluent: Acetonitrile and water (50:50)
System suitability solution: Expose a portion of *Standard solution* in a clear glass vial to direct room light for about 30 min.
Standard stock solution: 0.524 mg/mL of USP Montelukast Dicyclohexylamine RS in *Diluent* (equivalent to 0.4 mg/mL of montelukast)
Standard solution: 0.0065 mg/mL of USP Montelukast Dicyclohexylamine RS in *Medium* from the *Standard stock solution* (equivalent to 0.005 mg/mL of montelukast)
Sample solution: Transfer the entire contents of one packet to the dissolution vessel. At the specified time point, withdraw 10 mL of sample from the dissolution vessel. Pass a portion of the solution under test through a suitable filter. Discard the first 5 mL of the filtrate.
Chromatographic system
(See *Chromatography* ⟨621⟩, *System Suitability*.)
Mode: LC
Detector: UV 281 nm
Column: 4.6-mm × 3-cm; 3-µm packing L1
Column temperature: 40°
Flow rate: 0.8 mL/min
Injection volume: 25 µL
Run time: About 1.5 times the retention time of montelukast
System suitability
Samples: *System suitability solution* and *Standard solution*
[NOTE—The relative retention times for *Z*-isomer and montelukast are 0.8 and 1.0, respectively.]
Suitability requirements
Resolution: NLT 2.0 between the *Z*-isomer and montelukast, *System suitability solution*
Tailing factor: NMT 2.0 for montelukast, *System suitability solution*
Relative standard deviation: NMT 2.0%, *Standard solution*
Analysis
Samples: *Standard solution* and *Sample solution*
Calculate the percentage of the labeled amount of montelukast ($C_{35}H_{36}ClNO_3S$) dissolved:

$$\text{Result} = (r_U/r_S) \times C_S \times V \times (1/L) \times (M_{r1}/M_{r2}) \times 100$$

r_U = peak response from the *Sample solution*
r_S = peak response from the *Standard solution*
C_S = concentration of USP Montelukast Dicyclohexylamine RS in the *Standard solution* (mg/mL)
V = volume of *Medium*, 900 mL
L = label claim (mg/packet)
M_{r1} = molecular weight of montelukast, 586.18
M_{r2} = molecular weight of montelukast dicyclohexylamine, 767.50

Tolerances: NLT 80% (Q) of the labeled amount of montelukast ($C_{35}H_{36}ClNO_3S$) is dissolved.

•**Test 4:** If the product complies with this test, the labeling indicates that it meets USP *Dissolution Test 4*.
Medium: 0.5% (w/v) sodium dodecyl sulfate in water; 900 mL
Apparatus 1: 100 mesh; 50 rpm
Time: 20 min
Solution A: 3.9 g/L of sodium phosphate monobasic dihydrate in water. Adjust with dilute phosphoric acid to a pH of 3.7.
Mobile phase: Acetonitrile and *Solution A* (80:20)
Diluent: *Medium*
Standard solution: 0.005 mg/mL of montelukast in *Diluent* from montelukast sodium hydrate. Determine the water content of montelukast sodium hydrate at the time of use.
Sample solution: Place the entire contents of one packet in the basket. At the specified time point, withdraw 10 mL of sample from the dissolution vessel. Pass a portion of the solution under test through a suitable filter paper. Discard the first 3 mL of the filtrate.
Chromatographic system
(See *Chromatography* ⟨621⟩, *System Suitability*.)
Mode: LC
Detector: UV 254 nm
Column: 4.6-mm × 15-cm; 5-µm packing L1
Temperatures
Autosampler: 20°
Column: 28°
Flow rate: 1.5 mL/min
Injection volume: 50 µL
Run time: NLT 1.5 times the retention time of montelukast
System suitability
Sample: *Standard solution*
Suitability requirements
Tailing factor: NMT 2.0 for montelukast
Relative standard deviation: NMT 2.0%
Analysis
Samples: *Standard solution* and *Sample solution*
Calculate the percentage of the labeled amount of montelukast ($C_{35}H_{36}ClNO_3S$) dissolved:

$$\text{Result} = (r_U/r_S) \times C_S \times V \times (1/L) \times 100$$

r_U = peak response from the *Sample solution*
r_S = peak response from the *Standard solution*
C_S = concentration of montelukast in the *Standard solution* (mg/mL)
V = volume of *Medium*, 900 mL
L = label claim (mg/packet)
Tolerances: NLT 80% (Q) of the labeled amount of montelukast ($C_{35}H_{36}ClNO_3S$) is dissolved.• (RB 1-Oct-2017)

• **UNIFORMITY OF DOSAGE UNITS** ⟨905⟩
Procedure for content uniformity
Solution A, Solution B, Mobile phase, and **System suitability:** Proceed as directed in *Dissolution Test 1*.
Standard solution: 26.4 µg/mL of USP Montelukast Dicyclohexylamine RS in methanol
Sample solution: Nominally 0.02 mg/mL of montelukast prepared as follows. Transfer the contents of one packet to a suitable volumetric flask, add 66% of the flask volume of methanol, shake well, and sonicate for 15 min with occasional shaking. Cool to room temperature, dilute with methanol to volume, and mix well. Pass a portion of the resulting solution through a suitable filter of 0.45-µm pore size or centrifuge to obtain a clear solution.
Chromatographic system: Proceed as directed in *Dissolution Test 1*, except use an *Injection volume* of 5 µL.
Analysis
Samples: *Standard solution* and *Sample solution*
Calculate the percentage of the labeled amount of montelukast ($C_{35}H_{36}ClNO_3S$) in the packet taken:

$$\text{Result} = (r_U/r_S) \times (C_S/C_U) \times (M_{r1}/M_{r2}) \times 100$$

r_U = peak response from the *Sample solution*
r_S = peak response from the *Standard solution*
C_S = concentration of USP Montelukast Dicyclohexylamine RS in the *Standard solution* (mg/mL)
C_U = nominal concentration of montelukast in the *Sample solution* (mg/mL)
M_{r1} = molecular weight of montelukast, 586.18
M_{r2} = molecular weight of montelukast dicyclohexylamine, 767.50

Acceptance criteria: Meet the requirements

IMPURITIES

Change to read:

- **ORGANIC IMPURITIES**
  Diluent, Solution A, Solution B, Mobile phase, Standard solution, System suitability solution, Sensitivity solution, Sample solution, Chromatographic system, and **System suitability:** Proceed as directed in the *Assay.*
  Analysis
  Samples: *Standard solution* and *Sample solution*
  Calculate the percentage of any individual degradation product in the portion of Oral Granules taken:

  $$Result = (r_U/r_S) \times (C_S/C_U) \times (M_{r1}/M_{r2}) \times (1/F) \times 100$$

  r_U = peak response of any individual degradation product from the *Sample solution*
  r_S = peak response of montelukast from the *Standard solution*
  C_S = concentration of USP Montelukast Dicyclohexylamine RS in the *Standard solution* (mg/mL)
  C_U = nominal concentration of montelukast in the *Sample solution* (mg/mL)
  M_{r1} = molecular weight of montelukast, 586.18
  M_{r2} = molecular weight of montelukast dicyclohexylamine, 767.50
  F = relative response factor (see *Table 2*)

  Acceptance criteria: See *Table 2*. Disregard any peak with an area less than that of the *Sensitivity solution*.

Table 2

Name	Relative Retention Time	Relative Response Factor	Acceptance Criteria, NMT (%)
Sulfoxide impurity[a,b]	0.45	1.0	●1.0● (RB 1-Oct-2017)
Montelukast ketone impurity[c]	0.71	1.7	0.2

[a] These two impurities are not resolved by the method and need to be integrated together to determine conformance.
[b] [1-[[[1-[3-[(*E*)-2-(7-Chloroquinolin-2-yl)ethenyl]phenyl]-3-[2-(1-hydroxy-1-methylethyl)phenyl]propyl]sulfinyl]methyl]cyclopropyl]acetic acid.
[c] (*E*)-1-{3-[2-(7-Chloroquinolin-2-yl)vinyl]phenyl}-3-[2-(2-hydroxypropan-2-yl)phenyl]propan-1-one.
[d] [1-[[[(1*R*)-1-[3-[(*Z*)-2-(7-Chloroquinolin-2-yl)ethenyl]phenyl]-3-[2-(1-hydroxy-1-methylethyl)phenyl]propyl]sulfanyl]methyl]cyclopropyl]acetic acid.
[e] This is a process impurity and is included in the table for identification only. This impurity is controlled in the drug substance. It is not to be reported for the drug product and should not be included in the total impurities.
[f] [1-[[[(1*R*)-3-(2-Acetylphenyl)-1-[3-[(*E*)-2-(7-chloroquinolin-2-yl)ethenyl]phenyl]propyl]sulfanyl]methyl]cyclopropyl]acetic acid.
[g] (1-{[(*R*)-1-(3-[(*R*)-1-{[1-(Carboxymethyl)cyclopropyl]methylthio}-2-(7-chloroquinolin-2-yl)ethyl]phenyl}-3-[2-(2-hydroxypropan-2-yl)phenyl]propylthio]methyl}cyclopropyl)acetic acid.
[h] (1-{[(*R*)-1-(3-[(*S*)-1-{[1-(Carboxymethyl)cyclopropyl]methylthio}-2-(7-chloroquinolin-2-yl)ethyl]phenyl)-3-[2-(2-hydroxypropan-2-yl)phenyl]propylthio]methyl}cyclopropyl)acetic acid.
[i] [1-[[[(1*R*)-1-[3-[(*E*)-2-(7-Chloroquinolin-2-yl)ethenyl]phenyl]propyl]sulfanyl]methyl]cyclopropyl]acetic acid.

Table 2 *(Continued)*

Name	Relative Retention Time	Relative Response Factor	Acceptance Criteria, NMT (%)
cis-Isomer[d]	0.92	1.0	0.2
Montelukast	1.0	—	—
Methylketone impurity[e,f]	1.04	—	—
Michael adduct 1[g,e]	1.16	—	—
Michael adduct 2[h,e]	1.18	—	—
Methylstyrene impurity[i,e]	1.55	—	—
Any other individual degradation product	—	1.0	0.2
Total impurities	—	—	●1.5● (RB 1-Oct-2017)

[a] These two impurities are not resolved by the method and need to be integrated together to determine conformance.
[b] [1-[[[1-[3-[(*E*)-2-(7-Chloroquinolin-2-yl)ethenyl]phenyl]-3-[2-(1-hydroxy-1-methylethyl)phenyl]propyl]sulfinyl]methyl]cyclopropyl]acetic acid.
[c] (*E*)-1-{3-[2-(7-Chloroquinolin-2-yl)vinyl]phenyl}-3-[2-(2-hydroxypropan-2-yl)phenyl]propan-1-one.
[d] [1-[[[(1*R*)-1-[3-[(*Z*)-2-(7-Chloroquinolin-2-yl)ethenyl]phenyl]-3-[2-(1-hydroxy-1-methylethyl)phenyl]propyl]sulfanyl]methyl]cyclopropyl]acetic acid.
[e] This is a process impurity and is included in the table for identification only. This impurity is controlled in the drug substance. It is not to be reported for the drug product and should not be included in the total impurities.
[f] [1-[[[(1*R*)-3-(2-Acetylphenyl)-1-[3-[(*E*)-2-(7-chloroquinolin-2-yl)ethenyl]phenyl]propyl]sulfanyl]methyl]cyclopropyl]acetic acid.
[g] (1-{[(*R*)-1-(3-[(*R*)-1-{[1-(Carboxymethyl)cyclopropyl]methylthio}-2-(7-chloroquinolin-2-yl)ethyl]phenyl}-3-[2-(2-hydroxypropan-2-yl)phenyl]propylthio]methyl}cyclopropyl)acetic acid.
[h] (1-{[(*R*)-1-(3-[(*S*)-1-{[1-(Carboxymethyl)cyclopropyl]methylthio}-2-(7-chloroquinolin-2-yl)ethyl]phenyl)-3-[2-(2-hydroxypropan-2-yl)phenyl]propylthio]methyl}cyclopropyl)acetic acid.
[i] [1-[[[(1*R*)-1-[3-[(*E*)-2-(7-Chloroquinolin-2-yl)ethenyl]phenyl]propyl]sulfanyl]methyl]cyclopropyl]acetic acid.

ADDITIONAL REQUIREMENTS
- **PACKAGING AND STORAGE:** Preserve in tight containers, protected from light. Store at controlled room temperature.
- **LABELING:** When more than one *Dissolution* test is given, the labeling states the test used only if *Test 1* is not used.
- **USP REFERENCE STANDARDS ⟨11⟩**
  USP Montelukast Dicyclohexylamine RS
  $C_{35}H_{36}ClNO_3S \cdot C_{12}H_{23}N$ 767.50

Moxifloxacin Hydrochloride

$C_{21}H_{24}FN_3O_4 \cdot HCl$ 437.89
(4a*S*-*cis*)-1-Cyclopropyl-6-fluoro-1,4-dihydro-8-methoxy-7-(octahydro-6*H*-pyrrolo[3,4-*b*]pyridin-6-yl)-4-oxo-3-quinolinecarboxylic acid, monohydrochloride;
1-Cyclopropyl-6-fluoro-1,4-dihydro-8-methoxy-7-[(4a*S*,7a*S*)-octahydro-6*H*-pyrrolo[3,4-*b*]pyridin-6-yl]-4-oxo-3-quinolinecarboxylic acid, monohydrochloride [186826-86-8].

DEFINITION

Moxifloxacin Hydrochloride contains NLT 98.0% and NMT 102.0% of moxifloxacin hydrochloride ($C_{21}H_{24}FN_3O_4 \cdot HCl$), calculated on the anhydrous basis.

IDENTIFICATION

- **A. INFRARED ABSORPTION** ⟨197K⟩
- **B.** The retention time of the major peak of the *Sample solution* corresponds to that of the *Standard solution*, as obtained in the *Assay*.
- **C. IDENTIFICATION TESTS—GENERAL** ⟨191⟩, *Chloride*
  Sample solution: To a solution (1 in 160) add diluted nitric acid, and filter.
  Acceptance criteria: Meets the requirements

ASSAY

- **PROCEDURE**
  Buffer: Dissolve 0.5 g of tetrabutylammonium hydrogen sulfate and 1.0 g of monobasic potassium phosphate in water, add 2 mL of phosphoric acid, dilute with water to 1000 mL, mix, and pass through a filter of 0.45-μm pore size.
  Mobile phase: Methanol and *Buffer* (28:72)
  Diluent: Add 20 mg of anhydrous sodium sulfite to 1000 mL of *Buffer*, mix gently, and pass through a filter of 0.45-μm pore size.
  System suitability solution: 0.1 mg/mL of USP Moxifloxacin Hydrochloride RS and 1 μg/mL of USP Moxifloxacin Related Compound A RS, in *Diluent*
  Standard solution: 0.1 mg/mL of USP Moxifloxacin Hydrochloride RS in *Diluent*
  Sample solution: 0.1 mg/mL of Moxifloxacin Hydrochloride in *Diluent*
  Chromatographic system
  (See *Chromatography* ⟨621⟩, *System Suitability*.)
  Mode: LC
  Detector: UV 293 nm
  Column: 4.0-mm × 25-cm; 5-μm packing L11
  Column temperature: 45°
  Flow rate: 0.9 mL/min
  Injection volume: 25 μL
  System suitability
  Samples: *System suitability solution* and *Standard solution*
  [NOTE—The relative retention times for moxifloxacin and moxifloxacin related compound A are about 1.0 and 1.2, respectively.]
  Suitability requirements
  Resolution: NLT 1.5 between moxifloxacin and moxifloxacin related compound A, *System suitability solution*
  Tailing factor: NMT 2.0, *Standard solution*
  Relative standard deviation: NMT 0.73%, *Standard solution*
  Analysis
  Samples: *Standard solution* and *Sample solution*
  Calculate the percentage of moxifloxacin hydrochloride ($C_{21}H_{24}FN_3O_4 \cdot HCl$) in the portion of Moxifloxacin Hydrochloride taken:

$$\text{Result} = (r_U/r_S) \times (C_S/C_U) \times 100$$

r_U = peak response from the *Sample solution*
r_S = peak response from the *Standard solution*
C_S = concentration of USP Moxifloxacin Hydrochloride RS in the *Standard solution* (mg/mL)
C_U = concentration of Moxifloxacin Hydrochloride in the *Sample solution* (mg/mL)

Acceptance criteria: 98.0%–102.0% on the anhydrous basis

IMPURITIES

- **RESIDUE ON IGNITION** ⟨281⟩: NMT 0.1%
- **CHLORIDE AND SULFATE** ⟨221⟩, *Sulfate*
  Sample: 0.6 g
  Acceptance criteria: 0.04%; the *Sample* shows no more sulfate than corresponds to 0.25 mL of 0.020 N sulfuric acid.
- **ORGANIC IMPURITIES**
  Protect all solutions containing moxifloxacin from light.
  Mobile phase, Diluent, System suitability solution, and **Sample solution:** Prepare as directed in the *Assay*.
  Standard solution: 2 μg/mL of USP Moxifloxacin Hydrochloride RS in *Diluent*
  Sensitivity solution: 0.05 μg/mL of USP Moxifloxacin Hydrochloride RS from the *Standard solution* in *Diluent*. Store the *Sensitivity solution* under refrigeration and protected from light.
  Chromatographic system: Proceed as directed in the *Assay* with a run time of two times the retention time of moxifloxacin.
  System suitability
  Samples: *System suitability solution, Standard solution,* and *Sensitivity solution*
  Suitability requirements
  Resolution: NLT 1.5 between moxifloxacin and moxifloxacin related compound A, *System suitability solution*
  Tailing factor: NMT 2.0, *Standard solution*
  Relative standard deviation: NMT 2.0%, *Standard solution*
  Signal-to-noise ratio: NLT 10, *Sensitivity solution*
  Analysis
  Samples: *Sample solution* and *Standard solution*
  Calculate the percentage of each impurity in the portion of Moxifloxacin Hydrochloride taken:

$$\text{Result} = (r_U/r_S) \times (C_S/C_U) \times (1/F) \times 100$$

r_U = peak response of each impurity from the *Sample solution*
r_S = peak response of moxifloxacin from the *Standard solution*
C_S = concentration of USP Moxifloxacin Hydrochloride RS in the *Standard solution* (mg/mL)
C_U = concentration of Moxifloxacin Hydrochloride in the *Sample solution* (mg/mL)
F = relative response factor (see *Table 1*)

Acceptance criteria: See *Table 1*.

Table 1

Name	Relative Retention Time	Relative Response Factor	Acceptance Criteria, NMT (%)
Moxifloxacin	1.0	—	—
Moxifloxacin related compound A[a]	1.15	1.0	0.1
Moxifloxacin related compound B[b]	1.32	0.71	0.1
Moxifloxacin related compound C[c]	1.48	1.0	0.1
Moxifloxacin related compound D[d]	1.71	1.0	0.1

[a] 1-Cyclopropyl-6,8-difluoro-1,4-dihydro-7-[(4aS,7aS)-octahydro-6H-pyrrolo[3,4-b]pyridin-6-yl]-4-oxo-3-quinolinecarboxylic acid.
[b] 1-Cyclopropyl-6,8-dimethoxy-1,4-dihydro-7-[(4aS,7aS)-octahydro-6H-pyrrolo[3,4-b]pyridin-6-yl]-4-oxo-3-quinolinecarboxylic acid.
[c] 1-Cyclopropyl-8-ethoxy-6-fluoro-1,4-dihydro-7-[(4aS,7aS)-octahydro-6H-pyrrolo[3,4-b]pyridin-6-yl]-4-oxo-3-quinolinecarboxylic acid.
[d] 1-Cyclopropyl-8-fluoro-6-methoxy-1,4-dihydro-7-[(4aS,7aS)-octahydro-6H-pyrrolo[3,4-b]pyridin-6-yl]-4-oxo-3-quinolinecarboxylic acid.
[e] 1-Cyclopropyl-6-fluoro-8-hydroxy-1,4-dihydro-7-[(4aS,7aS)-octahydro-6H-pyrrolo[3,4-b]pyridin-6-yl]-4-oxo-3-quinolinecarboxylic acid.

Table 1 (Continued)

Name	Relative Retention Time	Relative Response Factor	Acceptance Criteria, NMT (%)
Moxifloxacin related compound E[e]	1.83	0.29	0.1
Other individual impurity	—	1.0	0.1
Total impurities	—	—	0.5

[a] 1-Cyclopropyl-6,8-difluoro-1,4-dihydro-7-[(4a*S*,7a*S*)-octahydro-6*H*-pyrrolo[3,4-*b*]pyridin-6-yl]-4-oxo-3-quinolinecarboxylic acid.
[b] 1-Cyclopropyl-6,8-dimethoxy-1,4-dihydro-7-[(4a*S*,7a*S*)-octahydro-6*H*-pyrrolo[3,4-*b*]pyridin-6-yl]-4-oxo-3-quinolinecarboxylic acid.
[c] 1-Cyclopropyl-8-ethoxy-6-fluoro-1,4-dihydro-7-[(4a*S*,7a*S*)-octahydro-6*H*-pyrrolo[3,4-*b*]pyridin-6-yl]-4-oxo-3-quinolinecarboxylic acid.
[d] 1-Cyclopropyl-8-fluoro-6-methoxy-1,4-dihydro-7-[(4a*S*,7a*S*)-octahydro-6*H*-pyrrolo[3,4-*b*]pyridin-6-yl]-4-oxo-3-quinolinecarboxylic acid.
[e] 1-Cyclopropyl-6-fluoro-8-hydroxy-1,4-dihydro-7-[(4a*S*,7a*S*)-octahydro-6*H*-pyrrolo[3,4-*b*]pyridin-6-yl]-4-oxo-3-quinolinecarboxylic acid.

Change to read:

- **ENANTIOMERIC PURITY**
  Protect all solutions containing moxifloxacin from light.
  Buffer: 0.47 g/L of anhydrous cupric sulfate and 1.31 g/L of L-isoleucine in water. Adjust with 0.1 N sodium hydroxide to a pH of 4.50.
  Solution A: Methanol and *Buffer* (500:1500)
  Solution B: Methanol and *Buffer* (225:450)
  Mobile phase: See *Table 2.*

Table 2

Time (min)	Solution A (%)	Solution B (%)
0	100	0
50	100	0
51	0	100
61	0	100
62	100	0
85	100	0

  System suitability solution: 8 mg/mL of USP Moxifloxacin Hydrochloride RS and 8 µg/mL of USP Moxifloxacin Related Compound G RS in *Solution A*
  Sensitivity solution: 0.8 µg/mL of USP Moxifloxacin Related Compound G RS in *Solution A*
  Sample solution: 8 mg/mL of Moxifloxacin Hydrochloride in *Solution A*
  Chromatographic system
  (See *Chromatography* ⟨621⟩, *System Suitability*.)
  Mode: LC
  Detector: UV 295 nm
  Column: 3.0-mm × 15-cm; 3-µm packing L1
  Flow rate: 0.42 mL/min
  Injection volume: 1.5 µL
  System suitability
  Samples: *System suitability solution* and *Sensitivity solution*
  [NOTE—The relative retention times for moxifloxacin related compound G and moxifloxacin are 0.78 and 1.0, respectively.]
  Suitability requirements
  Resolution: NLT 2.0 between moxifloxacin related compound G and moxifloxacin, *System suitability solution*

  Signal-to-noise ratio: NLT 5, *Sensitivity solution*
  Analysis
  Sample: *Sample solution*
  Calculate the percentage of moxifloxacin related compound G in the portion of Moxifloxacin Hydrochloride taken:

  $$Result = [r_U/(r_S + r_U)] \times 100$$

  r_U = peak response of moxifloxacin related compound G from the *Sample solution*
  r_S = peak response of moxifloxacin from the *Sample solution*
  Acceptance criteria: ●NMT 0.15%● (RB 1-Aug-2017)

SPECIFIC TESTS
- **MICROBIAL ENUMERATION TESTS** ⟨61⟩ and **TESTS FOR SPECIFIED MICROORGANISMS** ⟨62⟩
  Total aerobic microbial count: NMT 10^3 cfu/g
  Total combined molds and yeasts count: NMT 10^2 cfu/g
- **PH** ⟨791⟩
  Sample solution: 2 mg/mL
  Acceptance criteria: 3.9–4.6
- **WATER DETERMINATION** ⟨921⟩, *Method I, Method Ia*: NMT 4.5%

ADDITIONAL REQUIREMENTS
- **PACKAGING AND STORAGE:** Preserve in tight, light-resistant containers. Store at room temperature.
- **USP REFERENCE STANDARDS** ⟨11⟩
  USP Moxifloxacin Hydrochloride RS
  USP Moxifloxacin Related Compound A RS
    1-Cyclopropyl-6,8-difluoro-1,4-dihydro-7-[(4a*S*,7a*S*)-octahydro-6*H*-pyrrolo[3,4-*b*]pyridin-6-yl]-4-oxo-3-quinolinecarboxylic acid.
    $C_{20}H_{21}F_2N_3O_3$ 389.40
  USP Moxifloxacin Related Compound G RS
    1-Cyclopropyl-6-fluoro-1,4-dihydro-8-methoxy-7-[(4a*R*,7a*R*)-octahydro-6*H*-pyrrolo[3,4-*b*]pyridin-6-yl]-4-oxo-3-quinolinecarboxylic acid, monohydrochloride.
    $C_{21}H_{24}FN_3O_4 \cdot HCl$ 437.89

Naproxen Sodium Tablets

DEFINITION
Naproxen Sodium Tablets contain NLT 90.0% and NMT 110.0% of the labeled amount of naproxen sodium ($C_{14}H_{13}NaO_3$).

IDENTIFICATION
- **A. IDENTIFICATION TESTS—GENERAL** ⟨191⟩, *Chemical Identification Tests, Sodium*
  Sample: Transfer an amount nominally equivalent to about 250 mg of naproxen sodium from finely powdered Tablets to a centrifuge tube. Add 12 mL of water and 1 mL of hydrochloric acid. A dense white precipitate is formed. Centrifuge the mixture. Use the clear supernatant for the test.
  Acceptance criteria: Meets the requirements
- **B.** The retention time of the major peak of the *Sample solution* corresponds to that of the *Standard solution*, as obtained in the *Assay*.
- **C.** The UV absorption spectra of the major peak of the *Sample solution* and that of the *Standard solution* exhibit maxima and minima at the same wavelengths, as obtained in the *Assay*.

ASSAY

Change to read:

- **PROCEDURE**
  Mobile phase: Acetonitrile, water, and glacial acetic acid (450:540:10)
  Standard solution: 0.1 mg/mL of USP Naproxen Sodium RS in *Mobile phase*
  •**Sample stock solution:** Nominally 1.0 mg/mL of naproxen sodium from Tablets prepared as follows. Transfer an appropriate amount of naproxen sodium from NLT 20 Tablets, finely powdered, to a suitable volumetric flask. Add 15% of the volume of water and sonicate for 5 min. Add 50% of the volume of *Mobile phase* and sonicate for an additional 30 min, shaking intermittently. Allow the solution to cool to room temperature and then dilute with *Mobile phase* to volume. Centrifuge or pass a portion of this solution through a suitable filter.• (IRA 1-May-2018)
  Sample solution: Nominally equivalent to 0.1 mg/mL of naproxen sodium in *Mobile phase* from *Sample stock solution*
  Chromatographic system
  (See *Chromatography* ⟨621⟩, *System Suitability*.)
  Mode: LC
  Detector: UV 254 nm, diode array
  Column: 4.6-mm × 15-cm; 5-μm packing L7
  Flow rate: 1.2 mL/min
  Injection volume: 20 μL
  Run time: NLT 2 times the retention time of naproxen
  System suitability
  Sample: *Standard solution*
  Suitability requirements
  Tailing factor: NMT 2.0
  Relative standard deviation: NMT 2.0%
  Analysis
  Samples: *Standard solution* and *Sample solution*
  Calculate the percentage of the labeled amount of naproxen sodium ($C_{14}H_{13}NaO_3$) in the portion of Tablets taken:

$$Result = (r_U/r_S) \times (C_S/C_U) \times 100$$

  r_U = peak response of naproxen from the *Sample solution*
  r_S = peak response of naproxen from the *Standard solution*
  C_S = concentration of USP Naproxen Sodium RS in the *Standard solution* (mg/mL)
  C_U = nominal concentration of naproxen sodium in the *Sample solution* (mg/mL)
  Acceptance criteria: 90.0%–110.0%

PERFORMANCE TESTS
- **DISSOLUTION ⟨711⟩**
  Buffer: 0.1 M of a phosphate buffer with a pH of 7.4, containing 2.62 g/L of monobasic sodium phosphate and 11.50 g/L of anhydrous dibasic sodium phosphate in water
  Medium: *Buffer*, 900 mL
  Apparatus 2: 50 rpm
  Time: 45 min
  Standard solution: 50 μg/mL of USP Naproxen Sodium RS in *Medium*
  Sample solution: Dilute a filtered portion of the solution under test with *Medium* as necessary to obtain a nominal concentration of 50 μg/mL of naproxen sodium ($C_{14}H_{13}NaO_3$).
  Instrumental conditions
  Mode: UV
  Analytical wavelength: About 332 nm (maximum absorbance)

Analysis
Samples: *Standard solution* and *Sample solution*
Calculate the percentage of the labeled amount of naproxen sodium ($C_{14}H_{13}NaO_3$) dissolved.
Tolerances: NLT 80% (*Q*) of the labeled amount of naproxen sodium ($C_{14}H_{13}NaO_3$) is dissolved.
- **UNIFORMITY OF DOSAGE UNITS ⟨905⟩:** Meet the requirements

IMPURITIES

Change to read:

- **ORGANIC IMPURITIES**
  Solution A: Dissolve 1.36 g of monobasic potassium phosphate in 1 L of water. Adjust with triethylamine to a pH of 6.5. Pass through a suitable filter of 0.45-μm pore size.
  Solution B: Acetonitrile
  Diluent: Acetonitrile and *Solution A* (50:50)
  Mobile phase: See *Table 1.*

Table 1

Time (min)	Solution A (%)	Solution B (%)
0	85	15
5	85	15
25	60	40
45	50	50
50	85	15
60	85	15

  Standard stock solution 1: •0.05 mg/mL• (IRA 1-May-2018) of USP Naproxen Sodium RS in *Diluent* •• (IRA 1-May-2018)
  Standard stock solution 2: 0.01 mg/mL of USP Naproxen Related Compound A RS in methanol
  Standard stock solution 3: 0.01 mg/mL of USP Naproxen Related Compound L RS in methanol
  System suitability solution: 0.5 mg/mL of USP Naproxen Sodium RS and 0.5 μg/mL of USP Naproxen Related Compound A RS in *Diluent*, from *Standard stock solution 1* and *Standard stock solution 2*, respectively
  Standard solution: 1.0 μg/mL of USP Naproxen Sodium RS, and 0.5 μg/mL each of USP Naproxen Related Compound A RS and USP Naproxen Related Compound L RS in *Diluent*, from *Standard stock solution 1*, *Standard stock solution 2*, and *Standard stock solution 3*, respectively
  •**Sample stock solution:** Nominally 1.0 mg/mL of naproxen sodium from Tablets prepared as follows. Transfer an appropriate amount of naproxen sodium from NLT 20 Tablets, finely powdered, to a suitable volumetric flask. Add 15% of the volume of water and sonicate for 5 min. Add 50% of the volume of *Mobile phase* described in the *Assay* and sonicate for an additional 30 min, shaking intermittently. Allow the solution to cool to room temperature and then dilute with *Mobile phase* described in the *Assay* to volume. Centrifuge or pass a portion of this solution through a suitable filter.• (IRA 1-May-2018)
  Sample solution: Nominally equivalent to 0.55 mg/mL of naproxen sodium in *Diluent* from the *Sample stock solution*
  Chromatographic system
  (See *Chromatography* ⟨621⟩, *System Suitability*.)

Mode: LC
Detector: UV 236 nm
Column: 4.6-mm × 15-cm; 5-µm packing L7
Column temperature: 40°
Flow rate: 1.0 mL/min
Injection volume: 10 µL
System suitability
Samples: *System suitability solution* and *Standard solution*
Suitability requirements
Resolution: NLT 6.0 between naproxen related compound A and naproxen, *System suitability solution*
Relative standard deviation: NMT 5.0% for naproxen, naproxen related compound A, and naproxen related compound L, *Standard solution*
Analysis
Samples: *Standard solution* and *Sample solution*
Calculate the percentage of naproxen related compound A and naproxen related compound L in the portion of Tablets taken:

$$Result = (r_U/r_S) \times (C_S/C_U) \times 100$$

r_U = peak response of naproxen related compound A or naproxen related compound L from the *Sample solution*
r_S = peak response of naproxen related compound A or naproxen related compound L from the *Standard solution*
C_S = concentration of USP Naproxen Related Compound A RS or USP Naproxen Related Compound L RS in the *Standard solution* (mg/mL)
C_U = nominal concentration of naproxen sodium in the *Sample solution* (mg/mL)

Calculate the percentage of naproxen methyl ester and any individual unspecified degradation product in the portion of Tablets taken:

$$•Result = (r_U/r_S) \times (C_S/C_U) \times 100• \text{ (IRA 1-May-2018)}$$

r_U = peak response of naproxen methyl ester or any individual unspecified degradation product from the *Sample solution*
r_S = peak response of naproxen from the *Standard solution*
C_S = concentration of USP Naproxen Sodium RS in the *Standard solution* (mg/mL)
C_U = nominal concentration of naproxen sodium in the *Sample solution* (mg/mL)
● (IRA 1-May-2018)

Acceptance criteria: See *Table 2*. Disregard any peaks below LOQ (0.004% for naproxen methyl ester and any individual unspecified degradation product, 0.002% for naproxen related compound A, and 0.006% for naproxen related compound L).

Table 2

Name	Relative Retention Time	●● (IRA 1-May-2018)	Acceptance Criteria, NMT (%)
Naproxen related compound A[a]	0.63	●● (IRA 1-May-2018)	0.2
Naproxen	1.00	●● (IRA 1-May-2018)	—
Naproxen related compound L[b]	2.32	●● (IRA 1-May-2018)	0.2
Naproxen methyl ester[c]	3.19	●● (IRA 1-May-2018)	0.2

[a] 6-Methoxy-2-naphthoic acid.
[b] 1-(6-Methoxynaphthalen-2-yl)ethanone.
[c] (S)-Methyl 2-(6-methoxynaphthalen-2-yl)propanoate.

Table 2 (Continued)

Name	Relative Retention Time	●● (IRA 1-May-2018)	Acceptance Criteria, NMT (%)
Any individual unspecified degradation product	—	●● (IRA 1-May-2018)	0.2
Total impurities	—	●● (IRA 1-May-2018)	1.5

[a] 6-Methoxy-2-naphthoic acid.
[b] 1-(6-Methoxynaphthalen-2-yl)ethanone.
[c] (S)-Methyl 2-(6-methoxynaphthalen-2-yl)propanoate.

ADDITIONAL REQUIREMENTS
• **PACKAGING AND STORAGE:** Preserve in well-closed containers.
• **USP REFERENCE STANDARDS ⟨11⟩**
USP Naproxen Sodium RS
USP Naproxen Related Compound A RS
6-Methoxy-2-naphthoic acid.
$C_{12}H_{10}O_3$ 202.21
USP Naproxen Related Compound L RS
1-(6-Methoxynaphthalen-2-yl)ethanone.
$C_{13}H_{12}O_2$ 200.23

Nicotine Transdermal System

DEFINITION

Change to read:

Nicotine Transdermal System contains NLT ■85%■1S (USP41) and NMT ■115%■1S (USP41) of the labeled amount of nicotine ($C_{10}H_{14}N_2$).

IDENTIFICATION
• **A.** The retention time of the major peak of the *Sample solution* corresponds to that of the *Standard solution*, as obtained in the *Assay*.

Add the following:

■• **B.** The UV spectrum of the major peak of the *Sample solution* corresponds to that of the *Standard solution*, as obtained in the *Assay*.■1S (USP41)

ASSAY

Change to read:

• **PROCEDURE**
■**Solution A:** Dissolve 1.1 g of monobasic potassium phosphate and 7.3 g of dibasic potassium phosphate in 1 L of water. [NOTE—The pH of this solution is between 7.5 and 7.6.]
Solution B: Methanol
Mobile phase: See *Table 1*.

Table 1

Time (min)	Solution A (%)	Solution B (%)
0	95	5
20	52.5	47.5
20.1	95	5
25	95	5

Extraction solvent: Methanol and tetrahydrofuran (90:10)

Standard stock solution: 3.0 mg/mL of USP Nicotine Bitartrate Dihydrate RS on the anhydrous basis (equivalent to about 1 mg/mL of nicotine) in *Extraction solvent*

Standard solution: 0.15 mg/mL of USP Nicotine Bitartrate Dihydrate RS on the anhydrous basis (equivalent to about 0.05 mg/mL of nicotine) in *Solution A* from the *Standard stock solution*

System suitability stock solution: 1 mg/mL each of USP Nicotine Related Compound E RS and USP Nicotine Related Compound D RS in *Extraction solvent*

System suitability solution: 0.15 mg/mL of Nicotine Bitartrate Dihydrate RS on the anhydrous basis and 0.1 mg/mL each of USP Nicotine Related Compound D RS and USP Nicotine Related Compound E RS in *Solution A* from the *Standard stock solution* and the *System suitability stock solution*

Sample stock solution: Nominally 1 mg/mL of nicotine from NLT 10 Transdermal System units prepared as follows. Transfer the required number of units to a suitable flask carefully ensuring that no adhesive contacts the walls. Add a suitable volume of *Extraction solvent*. Stopper the flask and seal to minimize the loss of the *Extraction solvent*. Shake the flask using a suitable ■ shaker for 2 h.

Sample solution: Nominally 0.05 mg/mL of nicotine in *Solution A* from the *Sample stock solution*. Pass the solution through a suitable filter of 0.45-μm pore size.

Alternative sample preparation: If necessary, the *Sample stock solution* and the *Sample solution* may be prepared using the following alternative procedure.

Sample stock solution: Transfer one Transdermal System without the liner to a suitable 100-mL centrifuge tube with stopper. [NOTE—Cut Transdermal Systems larger than 2.5 cm² into 3–5-mm strips.] Add 10 mL of methylene chloride and a stirrer bar. Stopper the flask and stir the contents for NLT 4 h at room temperature. [NOTE—500 rpm for stirring speed is suitable.] Add 50 mL of 0.5% (v/v) phosphoric acid solution and continue extraction for another 1 h. Centrifuge at about 1000 rpm for NLT 5 min. Prepare separately the required number of extracts from the required number of Transdermal Systems following the same procedure described above. Combine equal volumes of the aqueous layer from each extract to obtain the *Sample stock solution*.

Sample solution: Nominally 0.03–0.05 mg/mL of nicotine from a suitable volume of the *Sample stock solution* and water

Chromatographic system
(See *Chromatography ⟨621⟩, System Suitability*.)
Mode: LC
Detector: UV 260 nm
Column: 4.6-mm × 15-cm; 3.5-μm packing L1
Column temperature: 45 ± 2°
Flow rate: 1.0 mL/min
Injection volume: 80 μL
System suitability
Samples: *System suitability solution* and *Standard solution*
Suitability requirements
Resolution: NLT 1.5 between nicotine related compound D and nicotine, *System suitability solution*
Relative standard deviation: NMT 2.0%, *Standard solution*
Analysis
Samples: *Standard solution* and *Sample solution*
Calculate the percentage of the labeled amount of nicotine ($C_{10}H_{14}N_2$) in the portion of Transdermal System taken:

$$Result = (r_U/r_S) \times (C_S/C_U) \times (M_{r1}/M_{r2}) \times 100$$

r_U = peak response of nicotine from the *Sample solution*
r_S = peak response of nicotine from the *Standard solution*
C_S = concentration of USP Nicotine Bitartrate Dihydrate RS on the anhydrous basis in the *Standard solution* (mg/mL)
C_U = nominal concentration of nicotine in the *Sample solution* (mg/mL)
M_{r1} = molecular weight of nicotine, 162.23
M_{r2} = molecular weight of anhydrous nicotine bitartrate, 462.41

Acceptance criteria: 85%–115%■₁ₛ (USP41)

PERFORMANCE TESTS

Change to read:

• **DRUG RELEASE ⟨724⟩**
Test 1: If the product complies with this test, the labeling indicates that it meets USP *Drug Release Test 1*.
Medium: Phosphoric acid solution (1 in 1000); 250 mL, in a tall-form beaker
Apparatus 7: Proceed as directed in the chapter, using the transdermal system holder–cylinder (see ■*Drug Release ⟨724⟩, Figure 5b*).
Sample solution: Center the Transdermal System onto a dry, unused 10-cm × 10-cm piece of Cuprophan dialysis membrane with the adhesive side against the membrane, taking care to eliminate air bubbles between the membrane and the release surface. Attach the membrane to the cylinder using two Parker O-rings, such that one of the borders of the Transdermal System is aligned to the groove and it is wrapped around the cylinder. The filled beakers are weighed and pre-equilibrated to 32.0 ± 0.3°, before immersing the test sample. Reciprocate at a frequency of about 30 cycles/min with an amplitude of 2.0 ± 0.1 cm. At the end of each time interval, transfer the test sample to a fresh beaker containing the appropriate volume of *Medium*, weighed and pre-equilibrated to 32.0 ± 0.3°. At the end of each release interval, allow the beakers to cool to room temperature, make up for evaporative losses by adding water to obtain the original weight, and mix.■₁ₛ (USP41)
Times: 2, 12, and 24 h
Mobile phase: Transfer 0.2 mL of *N,N*-dimethyloctylamine to a 1-L volumetric flask, add 220 mL of acetonitrile, and mix. Add 300 mL of water, 0.2 mL of glacial acetic acid, 0.20 g of anhydrous sodium acetate, and 0.55 g of sodium 1-dodecanesulfonate, and dilute with water to volume. Mix for 1 h until clear. [NOTE—Equilibration of the column may take as long as 3 h.]
Standard solution: ■0.15 mg/mL of USP Nicotine Bitartrate Dihydrate RS on the anhydrous basis (or 0.05 mg/mL of nicotine as free base)■₁ₛ (USP41) in *Medium* ■■₁ₛ (USP41)
System suitability solution: ■Transfer an amount of USP Nicotine Bitartrate Dihydrate RS equivalent to about 8 mg of nicotine■₁ₛ (USP41) to a 100-mL volumetric flask, and dissolve in 10 mL of acetonitrile. Add 5 mL of 30% hydrogen peroxide, and allow 15 min to react. Dilute with *Medium* to volume, and mix. Transfer 20 mL of this solution to a 100-mL volumetric flask, and dilute with *Standard solution* to volume.
Chromatographic system
(See *Chromatography ⟨621⟩, System Suitability*.)

Mode: LC
Detector: UV 254 nm
Column: 4.6-mm × 15-cm; packing L1
Flow rate: 1 mL/min
Injection volume: 50 µL
System suitability
  Sample: *System suitability solution*
  Suitability requirements
   Resolution: NLT 1.1 between nicotine and any degradation peaks
   Tailing factor: NMT 2.0
   Relative standard deviation: NMT 1.5%
Analysis
  Samples: *Standard solution* and *Sample solution*
Tolerances: See *Table 2*.

Table 2

Time (h)	Amount Released (%)
0–2	31–87
2–12	62–191
12–24	85–261

■The percentages of the labeled amount of nicotine ($C_{10}H_{14}N_2$) released■₁ₛ ₍USP41₎ at the times specified, conform to *Dissolution* ⟨711⟩, *Acceptance Table 1*.
Test 2: If the product complies with this test, the labeling indicates that it meets USP *Drug Release Test 2*.
Buffer: 8 g/L of sodium chloride, 0.2 g/L of potassium chloride, 1.7 g/L of dibasic sodium phosphate, and 0.2 g/L of monobasic potassium phosphate in water
Medium: *Buffer*; 500 mL
Apparatus 6: 50 rpm, double-sided tape being used to attach the Transdermal System to the cylinder
Times: 6 and 24 h
Mobile phase: ■Acetonitrile, triethylamine, and water (300:1:700)■₁ₛ ₍USP41₎
Standard solution: ■0.6 mg/mL of USP Nicotine Bitartrate Dihydrate RS on the anhydrous basis (equivalent to about 0.2 mg/mL of nicotine) in *Medium*■₁ₛ ₍USP41₎
Sample solution: At each of the test times, withdraw a 2-mL aliquot of the solution under test. Replace the aliquots withdrawn for analysis with fresh portions of *Medium*.
Chromatographic system
  (See *Chromatography* ⟨621⟩, *System Suitability*.)
  Mode: LC
  Detector: UV 260 nm
  Column: 4.6-mm × 12.5-cm; packing L1
  Flow rate: 1 mL/min
  Injection volume: 100 µL
System suitability
  Sample: *Standard solution* ■₁ₛ ₍USP41₎
  Suitability requirements
   ■₁ₛ ₍USP41₎
   Tailing factor: NMT 2.0
   Relative standard deviation: NMT 2.0%
Analysis
  Samples: *Standard solution* and *Sample solution*
Tolerances: See *Table 3*.

Table 3

Time (h)	Amount Released (%)
6	71–157
24	156–224

■The percentages of the labeled amount of nicotine ($C_{10}H_{14}N_2$) released■₁ₛ ₍USP41₎ at the times specified, conform to *Dissolution* ⟨711⟩, *Acceptance Table 1*.

Test 3: If the product complies with this test, the labeling indicates that it meets USP *Drug Release Test 3*.
Medium: Water; 900 mL
Apparatus 5: 50 rpm, the stainless steel disk assembly being replaced with a 5-cm watch glass for an 11-mg Transdermal System and an 8-cm watch glass for a 22-mg Transdermal System
Times: 1, 2, and 4 h
Standard solution: USP Nicotine Bitartrate Dihydrate RS in water having a known concentration of nicotine similar to that of the *Sample solution*.
■**Sample solution:** At the specified times, withdraw a suitable volume of the solution under test.■₁ₛ ₍USP41₎
Instrumental conditions
  Mode: UV
  Analytical wavelength: 259 nm
  Blank: Water
Analysis
  Samples: *Standard solution* and *Sample solution*
Tolerances: See *Table 4*.

Table 4

Time (h)	Amount Released (%)
1	35–75
2	55–95
4	NLT 73

■The percentages of the labeled amount of nicotine ($C_{10}H_{14}N_2$) released■₁ₛ ₍USP41₎ at the times specified, conform to *Table 5*.

Table 5

Level	Tested	Criteria
L_1	6	No individual value lies outside each of the stated ranges and no individual value is less than the stated amount at the final test time.
L_2	6	The average value of the 12 units (L_1 + L_2) lies within each of the stated ranges and is NLT the stated amount at the final test time; none is more than 5% of the labeled content outside each of the stated ranges; and none is more than 5% of the labeled content below the stated amount at the final test time.
L_3	12	The average value of the 24 units (L_1 + L_2 + L_3) lies within each of the stated ranges and is NLT the stated amount at the final test time; NMT 2 of the 24 units are more than 5% of labeled content outside each of the stated ranges; NMT 2 of the 24 units are more than 5% of the labeled content below the stated amount at the final test time; and none of the units is more than 10% of the labeled content outside each of the stated ranges or more than 10% of the labeled content below the stated amount at the final test time.

Test 4: If the product complies with this test, the labeling indicates that it meets USP *Drug Release Test 4*.
Medium: 0.025 N hydrochloric acid; 600 mL
Apparatus 5: 50 rpm, a convex screen being used to hold the Transdermal System in position during testing

Times: 4 and 16 h
Standard solution: USP Nicotine Bitartrate Dihydrate RS in water having a known concentration of nicotine similar to that of the *Sample solution*
■**Sample solution:** At the specified times, withdraw a suitable volume of the solution under test.■1S (USP41)
Instrumental conditions
  Mode: UV
  Analytical wavelength: 259 nm
  Blank: Water
Analysis
  Samples: *Standard solution* and *Sample solution*
  Tolerances: See *Table 6*.

Table 6

Time (h)	Amount Released (%)
4	36–66
16	72–112

■The percentages of the labeled amount of nicotine ($C_{10}H_{14}N_2$) released■1S (USP41) at the times specified, conform to *Dissolution ⟨711⟩, Acceptance Table 1*.
Test 5: If the product complies with this test, the labeling indicates that it meets USP *Drug Release Test 5*.
Buffer, Medium, and **Apparatus 6:** Proceed as directed in *Test 2*.
Times: 3, 6, and 24 h
■**Mobile phase,**■1S (USP41) **Standard solution, Sample solution, Chromatographic system, System suitability,** and **Analysis:** Proceed as directed in *Test 2*, except to use an *Injection volume* of 30 µL.
Tolerances: See *Table 7*.

Table 7

Time (h)	Amount Released (%)
3	79–112
6	108–141
24	156–202

■The percentages of the labeled amount of nicotine ($C_{10}H_{14}N_2$) released■1S (USP41) at the times specified, conform to *Dissolution ⟨711⟩, Acceptance Table 1*.
- **UNIFORMITY OF DOSAGE UNITS ⟨905⟩:** Meets the requirements

IMPURITIES

Add the following:

■• **ORGANIC IMPURITIES**
  Solution A, Solution B, Mobile phase, Standard solution, System suitability solution, Sample solution, and **Chromatographic system:** Proceed as directed in the *Assay*.
  Diluent: Tetrahydrofuran, methanol, and *Solution A* (0.5: 4.5: 95)
  Sensitivity solution: 0.15 µg/mL of USP Nicotine Bitartrate Dihydrate RS (equivalent to about 0.05 µg/mL of nicotine) in *Diluent* from the *Standard solution*
  System suitability
    Samples: *System suitability solution* and *Sensitivity solution*
    [NOTE—See *Table 8* for the relative retention times. The 1R,2S isomer of nicotine related compound E is a small peak that precedes the 1S,2S isomer, which is the major peak.]
  Suitability requirements
    Resolution: NLT 3 between nicotine related compound D and nicotine, *System suitability solution*; NLT 1.2 between the (1R,2S) and (1S,2S) isomers of nicotine related compound E, *System suitability solution*
    Signal-to-noise ratio: NLT 10 for nicotine, *Sensitivity solution*

Table 8

Name	Relative Retention Time	Relative Response Factor	Acceptance Criteria, NMT (%)		
			7 mg/24 h	14 mg/24 h	21 mg/24 h
Nicotinic acid[a]	0.15	1.3	0.5	0.5	0.5
Nicotine related compound E (1R,2S isomer)	0.25	0.76	0.5	0.5	0.5
Nicotine related compound E (1S,2S isomer)	0.27	0.76	0.5	0.5	0.5
Nicotine related compound F[b,c]	0.38	—	—	—	—
Nicotine related compound C[d]	0.54	1.0	2.8	2.6	1.8
Nicotine related compound G[b,e]	0.64	—	—	—	—
Nicotine related compound A[b,f]	0.74	—	—	—	—
Nicotine related compound D	0.85	1.6	5.6	3.2	2.6
Nicotine	1.00	—	—	—	—
Nicotine related compound B[g]	1.19	1.9	0.5	0.5	0.5

[a] 3-Pyridine carboxylic acid.
[b] Process impurity; controlled in drug substance and not to be included in total impurities.
[c] (S)-3-(Pyrrolidin-2-yl)pyridine; also known as nornicotine.
[d] (S)-1-Methyl-5-(pyridin-3-yl)pyrrolidin-2-one; also known as cotinine.
[e] (S)-3-(Piperidin-2-yl)pyridine; also known as anabasine.
[f] (S)-1,2,3,6-Tetrahydro-2,3′-bipyridine; also known as anatabine.
[g] 3-(1-Methyl-1H-pyrrol-2-yl)pyridine; also known as nicotyrine.

Table 8 (Continued)

Name	Relative Retention Time	Relative Response Factor	Acceptance Criteria, NMT (%)		
			7 mg/24 h	14 mg/24 h	21 mg/24 h
Any other unspecified impurity	—	1.0	0.6	0.5	0.5
Total impurities	—	—	8.3	5.8	4.4

ᵃ 3-Pyridine carboxylic acid.
ᵇ Process impurity; controlled in drug substance and not to be included in total impurities.
ᶜ (S)-3-(Pyrrolidin-2-yl)pyridine; also known as nornicotine.
ᵈ (S)-1-Methyl-5-(pyridin-3-yl)pyrrolidin-2-one; also known as cotinine.
ᵉ (S)-3-(Piperidin-2-yl)pyridine; also known as anabasine.
ᶠ (S)-1,2,3,6-Tetrahydro-2,3'-bipyridine; also known as anatabine.
ᵍ 3-(1-Methyl-1H-pyrrol-2-yl)pyridine; also known as nicotyrine.

Analysis
Sample: *Sample solution*
Calculate the percentage of each impurity in the portion of Transdermal System taken:

$$Result = (r_U/r_T) \times (1/F) \times 100$$

r_U = peak response of each impurity from the *Sample solution*
r_T = sum of all the peak responses from the *Sample solution*
F = relative response factor (see *Table 8*)
Acceptance criteria: See *Table 8*. Disregard peaks that are less than 0.05% of the nicotine peak. ∎1S (USP41)

ADDITIONAL REQUIREMENTS
- **PACKAGING AND STORAGE:** Preserve in the hermetic, light-resistant, unit-dose pouch.
- **LABELING:** The labeling indicates the *Drug Release Test* with which the product complies.

Change to read:

- **USP REFERENCE STANDARDS ⟨11⟩**
  USP Nicotine Bitartrate Dihydrate RS
  ∎$C_{10}H_{14}N_2 \cdot (C_4H_6O_6)_2 \cdot 2H_2O$ 498.44
  USP Nicotine Related Compound D RS
  3-(4,5-Dihydro-3H-pyrrol-2-yl)pyridine fumarate;
  Also known as Myosmine.
  $C_9H_{10}N_2 \cdot C_4H_4O_4$ 262.26
  USP Nicotine Related Compound E RS
  (1RS,2S)-1-Methyl-2-(pyridin-3-yl)pyrrolidine 1-oxide oxalate;
  Also known as Nicotine N-oxide.
  [NOTE—This may be a mixture of (1R,2S) and (1S,2S) isomers.]
  $C_{10}H_{14}N_2O \cdot C_2H_2O_4$ 268.27∎1S (USP41)

Nifedipine Extended-Release Tablets

DEFINITION
Nifedipine Extended-Release Tablets contain NLT 90.0% and NMT 110.0% of the labeled amount of nifedipine ($C_{17}H_{18}N_2O_6$). [NOTE—Nifedipine, when exposed to daylight and certain wavelengths of artificial light, readily converts to a nitrosophenylpyridine derivative. Exposure to UV light leads to the formation of a nitrophenylpyridine derivative. Perform assays and tests in the dark or under golden fluorescent or other low-actinic light. Use low-actinic glassware.]

IDENTIFICATION
- **A.** The retention time of the *Sample solution* corresponds to that of the *Standard solution*, as obtained in the *Assay*.

- **B. ULTRAVIOLET ABSORPTION ⟨197U⟩**
  Standard stock solution and **Sample stock solution:** Prepare as directed in the *Assay*.
  Standard solution: 0.02 mg/mL of USP Nifedipine RS in *Mobile phase* from the *Standard stock solution*
  Sample solution: Nominally 0.02 mg/mL of nifedipine in *Mobile phase* from the *Sample stock solution*

ASSAY
- **PROCEDURE**
  [NOTE—Conduct the *Assay* promptly after preparation of the *Standard solution* and the *Sample solution*.]
  Mobile phase: Acetonitrile, methanol, and water (25:25:50)
  Standard stock solution: 1 mg/mL of USP Nifedipine RS in methanol
  Standard solution: 0.1 mg/mL of USP Nifedipine RS from the *Standard stock solution* in *Mobile phase*
  Sample stock solution: Dissolve an amount equivalent to 420 mg of nifedipine from powdered Tablets in 130 mL of water in a 250-mL volumetric flask; or transfer the intact Tablets to a 400-mL, high-speed blender cup containing 130 mL of water. Homogenize until a uniform suspension is achieved (about 2 min), and transfer the suspension with the aid of a mixture of acetonitrile and methanol (1:1) to a 250-mL volumetric flask. Dilute with a mixture of acetonitrile and methanol (1:1) to volume, and stir for 30 min. Centrifuge the resulting suspension to obtain a clear supernatant.
  Sample solution: Nominally 0.1 mg/mL of nifedipine prepared as follows. Transfer 3.0 mL of the *Sample stock solution* to a 50-mL volumetric flask, dilute with *Mobile phase* to volume, and filter. [NOTE—Reserve a portion of this solution for use as the *Sample solution* in the test for *Organic Impurities*.]
  Chromatographic system
  (See *Chromatography ⟨621⟩, System Suitability*.)
  Mode: LC
  Detector: UV 265 nm
  Columns
    Guard: 2.1-mm × 3-cm; packing L1
    Analytical: 4.6-mm × 25-cm; 5-μm packing L1
  Flow rate: 1 mL/min
  Injection volume: 25 μL
  System suitability
  Sample: *Standard solution*
  Suitability requirements
    Column efficiency: NLT 4000 theoretical plates
    Tailing factor: NMT 1.5
    Relative standard deviation: NMT 1.0%
  Analysis
  Samples: *Standard solution* and *Sample solution*
  Calculate the percentage of the labeled amount of nifedipine ($C_{17}H_{18}N_2O_6$) in the portion of Tablets taken:

$$Result = (r_U/r_S) \times (C_S/C_U) \times 100$$

r_U = peak response from the *Sample solution*
r_S = peak response from the *Standard solution*

C_S = concentration of USP Nifedipine RS in the *Standard solution* (mg/mL)

C_U = nominal concentration of nifedipine in the *Sample solution* (mg/mL)

Acceptance criteria: 90.0%–110.0%

PERFORMANCE TESTS

Change to read:

- **DISSOLUTION ⟨711⟩**
  Test 1: If the product complies with this test, the labeling indicates that it meets USP *Dissolution Test 1*.
  Medium: Water; 50 mL
  Apparatus 7: (See *Drug Release* ⟨724⟩.) 15–30 cycles/min. Do not use the reciprocating disk; use a 25-cm Plexiglas rod, the perimeter of the Tablets being affixed to the rod with a water-insoluble glue. The solution containers are 25-mm test tubes, 150–200 mm in length, and the water bath is maintained at 37 ± 0.5°. At the end of each specified test interval, the systems are transferred to the next row of new test tubes containing 50 mL of fresh *Medium*.
  Times: 4, 8, 12, 16, 20, and 24 h
  Diluent: Methanol and water (1:1)
  Standard solution: Transfer 50 mg of USP Nifedipine RS to a 100-mL volumetric flask. Dissolve in 50 mL of methanol, and dilute with water to volume. Quantitatively dilute this solution with *Diluent* to obtain solutions having suitable known concentrations.
  Sample solution: Use portions of the solution under test, passed through a suitable filter of 0.4-μm pore size, suitably diluted with methanol, and stepwise if necessary, with *Diluent* to obtain a final mixture consisting of equal parts of methanol and water.
  Instrumental conditions
  (See *Ultraviolet-Visible Spectroscopy* ⟨857⟩.)
  Mode: UV
  Analytical wavelength: 338 nm
  Cell: 0.5 cm
  Analysis: Determine the amount of nifedipine ($C_{17}H_{18}N_2O_6$) released in the *Sample solution* at each 4-h interval from UV absorbances. [NOTE—For the 4-h time period, determine the absorbance at 456 nm, and use this determination to correct for excipient interference.]
  Tolerances: See *Table 1*.

Table 1

Time (h)	Amount Dissolved[a] (%)
4	5–17
8	—
12	43–80
16	—
20	—
24	NLT 80

[a] The amount dissolved is expressed in terms of the labeled Tablet strength rather than in terms of the labeled total contents.

The cumulative percentages of the labeled amount of nifedipine ($C_{17}H_{18}N_2O_6$), released at the times specified, conform to *Dissolution* ⟨711⟩, *Acceptance Table 2*.

Test 2: If the product complies with this test, the labeling indicates that it meets USP *Dissolution Test 2*.
Solution A: Dissolve 330.9 g of dibasic sodium phosphate and 38 g of citric acid in water in a 1-L volumetric flask. Add 10 mL of phosphoric acid, and dilute with water to volume.
Medium: Mix 125.0 mL of *Solution A* and 1 L of 10% sodium lauryl sulfate solution, and dilute to 10 L. Adjust, if necessary, to a pH of 6.8; 900 mL.

Apparatus 2: 50 rpm, with sinkers (see *Dissolution* ⟨711⟩, *Figure 2a*)
Times: 3, 6, and 12 h
Mobile phase: Acetonitrile and water (7:3)
Standard stock solution: 1.11 mg/mL of USP Nifedipine RS in methanol
Standard solution: 0.1 mg/mL of USP Nifedipine RS from the *Standard stock solution* in *Medium*
Sample solution: Pass a portion of the solution under test through a suitable filter.
Chromatographic system
(See *Chromatography* ⟨621⟩, *System Suitability*.)
Mode: LC
Detector: UV 350 nm
Column: 4.0-mm × 125-mm; 3-μm packing L1
Temperature: 40°
Flow rate: 1.5 mL/min
Injection volume: 20 μL
System suitability
Sample: *Standard solution*
Suitability requirements
Column efficiency: NLT 2000 theoretical plates
Tailing factor: NMT 1.5
Relative standard deviation: NMT 2.0%
Analysis
Samples: *Standard solution* and *Sample solution*
Determine the amount of nifedipine ($C_{17}H_{18}N_2O_6$) dissolved.
Tolerances: See *Table 2*.

Table 2

Time (h)	Amount Dissolved (%)
3	10–30
6	40–65
12	NLT 80

The percentages of the labeled amount of nifedipine ($C_{17}H_{18}N_2O_6$), • (RB 1-Aug-2017) dissolved at the times specified, conform to *Dissolution* ⟨711⟩, *Acceptance Table 2*.

Test 3: If the product complies with this test, the labeling indicates that it meets USP *Dissolution Test 3*.
For Tablets labeled to contain 30 mg of nifedipine: Phase 1
Medium: 0.05 M phosphate buffer, pH 7.5; 900 mL
Apparatus 2: 100 rpm
Time: 1 h
Standard solution: 0.034 mg/mL of USP Nifedipine RS in *Medium*. [NOTE—If necessary, a volume of methanol, not exceeding 10% of the final volume, can be used to help solubilize nifedipine.]
Sample solution: Pass a portion of the solution under test through a suitable filter.
Instrumental conditions
(See *Ultraviolet-Visible Spectroscopy* ⟨857⟩.)
Mode: UV
Analytical wavelength: 238 nm
Cell: 0.5 cm
Analysis: [NOTE—After the run, take the Tablet out of the dissolution vessel, adapt a sinker to it, and transfer the Tablet with the sinker to the dissolution vessel containing the *Medium* for *Phase 2*.] Determine the amount of nifedipine ($C_{17}H_{18}N_2O_6$) released in *Phase 1*, using filtered portions of the *Sample solution*, in comparison with the *Standard solution*, using the *Medium* as the blank.
For Tablets labeled to contain 30 mg of nifedipine: Phase 2
Medium: 0.5% sodium lauryl sulfate in simulated gastric fluid without enzyme, pH 1.2; 900 mL

Apparatus 2: 100 rpm
Times: 1, 4, 8, and 12 h
Standard solution: 0.034 mg/mL of USP Nifedipine RS in *Medium*. [NOTE—If necessary, a volume of methanol, not exceeding 10% of the final volume, can be used to help solubilize nifedipine.]
Sample solution: Pass a portion of the solution under test through a suitable filter.
Instrumental conditions
(See *Ultraviolet-Visible Spectroscopy* ⟨857⟩.)
Mode: UV
Analytical wavelength: 238 nm
Analysis: Determine the amount of nifedipine ($C_{17}H_{18}N_2O_6$) released in *Phase 2*, using filtered portions of the *Sample solution*, in comparison with the *Standard solution*, using *Medium* as the blank.
Tolerances: See *Table 3*.

Table 3

Time (h)	Amount Dissolved[a] (%)
1	NMT 30
4	30–55
8	NLT 60
12	NLT 80

[a] For each dosage unit, add the amount dissolved in phosphate buffer, pH 7.5 from *Phase 1* to the amount dissolved at each time point in *Phase 2*.

The cumulative percentages of the labeled amount of nifedipine ($C_{17}H_{18}N_2O_6$), • ● (RB 1-Aug-2017) dissolved at the times specified, conform to *Dissolution* ⟨711⟩, *Acceptance Table 2*.
For Tablets labeled to contain 60 mg of nifedipine:
Phase 1
Medium: 0.05 M phosphate buffer, pH 7.5; 900 mL
Apparatus 2: 100 rpm
Time: 25 min
Standard solution: 0.067 mg/mL of USP Nifedipine RS in *Medium*. [NOTE—If necessary, a volume of methanol, not exceeding 10% of the final volume, can be used to help solubilize nifedipine.]
Sample solution: Pass a portion of the solution under test through a suitable filter.
Instrumental conditions
(See *Ultraviolet-Visible Spectroscopy* ⟨857⟩.)
Mode: UV
Analytical wavelength: 238 nm
Analysis: [NOTE—After the run, take the Tablet out of the dissolution vessel, adapt a sinker to it, and transfer the Tablet with the sinker to the dissolution vessel containing the *Medium* for *Phase 2*.] Determine the amount of nifedipine ($C_{17}H_{18}N_2O_6$) released in *Phase 1*, using filtered portions of the *Sample solution*, in comparison with the *Standard solution*, using the *Medium* as the blank.
For Tablets labeled to contain 60 mg of nifedipine:
Phase 2
Medium: 0.5% sodium lauryl sulfate in simulated gastric fluid without enzyme, pH 1.2; 900 mL
Apparatus 2: 100 rpm
Times: 1, 4, 8, and 12 h
Standard solution: 0.067 mg/mL of USP Nifedipine RS in *Medium*. [NOTE—If necessary, a volume of methanol, not exceeding 10% of the final volume, can be used to help solubilize nifedipine.]
Sample solution: Pass a portion of the solution under test through a suitable filter.
Instrumental conditions
(See *Ultraviolet-Visible Spectroscopy* ⟨857⟩.)
Mode: UV
Analytical wavelength: 238 nm
Analysis: Determine the amount of nifedipine ($C_{17}H_{18}N_2O_6$) released in *Phase 2*, using filtered por-

tions of the *Sample solution*, in comparison with the *Standard solution*, using the *Medium* as the blank.
Tolerances: See *Table 4*.

Table 4

Time (h)	Amount Dissolved[a] (%)
1	NMT 30
4	40–70
8	NLT 70
12	NLT 80

[a] For each dosage unit, add the amount dissolved in phosphate buffer, pH 7.5 from *Phase 1* to the amount dissolved at each time point in *Phase 2*.

The cumulative percentages of the labeled amount of nifedipine ($C_{17}H_{18}N_2O_6$), released in vivo and dissolved at the times specified, conform to *Dissolution* ⟨711⟩, *Acceptance Table 2*.
Test 4: If the product complies with this test, the labeling indicates that the product meets USP *Dissolution Test 4*.
Medium: 0.5% sodium lauryl sulfate in simulated gastric fluid without enzyme, pH 1.2; 900 mL
Apparatus 2: 100 rpm
Times: 1, 4, and 12 h
Standard solution: 0.067 mg/mL of USP Nifedipine RS for Tablets labeled to contain 60 mg, and 0.034 mg/mL of USP Nifedipine RS for Tablets labeled to contain 30 mg, in *Medium*. [NOTE—If necessary, a volume of methanol, not exceeding 10% of the final volume, can be used to help solubilize nifedipine.]
Sample solution: Pass a portion of the solution under test through a suitable filter.
Instrumental conditions
(See *Ultraviolet-Visible Spectroscopy* ⟨857⟩.)
Mode: UV
Analytical wavelength: UV 238 nm
Cell: 1 cm
Analysis: Determine the amount of nifedipine ($C_{17}H_{18}N_2O_6$) released, using filtered portions of the *Sample solution*, in comparison with the *Standard solution*, using the *Medium* as the blank.
Tolerances: See *Table 5* and *Table 6*.

Table 5

For Tablets Labeled to Contain 30 mg of Nifedipine	
Time (h)	Amount Dissolved (%)
1	12–35
4	44–67
12	NLT 80

Table 6

For Tablets Labeled to Contain 60 mg of Nifedipine	
Time (h)	Amount Dissolved (%)
1	10–30
4	40–63
12	NLT 80

The cumulative percentages of the labeled amount of nifedipine ($C_{17}H_{18}N_2O_6$), released at the times specified, conform to *Dissolution* ⟨711⟩, *Acceptance Table 2*.
Test 5: If the product complies with this test, the labeling indicates that the product meets USP *Dissolution Test 5*.
Medium: Water; 50 mL
Apparatus 7: (See *Drug Release* ⟨724⟩.) Use a 25-cm Plexiglas rod, the perimeter of the Tablets being af-

fixed to the rod with a water-insoluble glue; 30 dips/min. The solution containers are 25-mm test tubes, 150–200 mm in length, and the water bath is maintained at 37 ± 0.5°.

Times: 4, 12, and 24 h
Diluent A: Methanol and acetonitrile (1:1)
Diluent B: *Diluent A* and water (1:1)
Standard stock solution: 50 mg of USP Nifedipine RS in *Diluent A* and water (50:50)
Standard solutions: 0.01, 0.05, and 0.20 mg/mL solutions, from the *Standard stock solution* in *Diluent B*, that are used at 4-, 12-, and 24-h samplings
Sample solution: Pass a portion of the solution under test through a suitable filter.
Instrumental conditions
(See *Ultraviolet-Visible Spectroscopy ⟨857⟩*.)
Mode: UV
Analytical wavelength: 238 nm
Cell: 0.5 cm
Analysis: [NOTE—For the 4-h time period, filter the solution under test, and determine the absorbance at 456 nm. Use this absorbance value to correct for excipient interference at the other time points.] Determine the amount of nifedipine released at each interval on portions of the *Sample solution* passed through a suitable filter of 0.45-μm pore size, suitably diluted, if necessary, with *Diluent A* and water to obtain a final mixture of water, methanol, and acetonitrile (2:1:1), in comparison with the appropriate *Standard solution*, using *Diluent B* as the blank.
Tolerances: See *Table 7*.

Table 7

Time (h)	Amount Dissolved (%)
4	NMT 14
12	39–75
24	NLT 75

The cumulative percentages of the labeled amount of nifedipine, • • (RB 1-Aug-2017) dissolved at the times specified, conform to *Dissolution ⟨711⟩, Acceptance Table 2*.
Test 6: If the product complies with this test, the labeling indicates that it meets USP *Dissolution Test 6*.
Medium: Simulated gastric fluid without enzyme containing 0.5% of sodium lauryl sulfate, pH 1.2; 900 mL, deaerated
Apparatus 1: 100 rpm
Times: 1, 4, and 12 h
Standard stock solution: 0.33 mg/mL of USP Nifedipine RS in methanol
Standard solution: Quantitatively dilute the *Standard stock solution* with *Medium* to obtain a solution having a concentration of about 0.033 mg/mL.
Sample solution: Pass a portion of the solution under test through a suitable filter of 0.45-μm pore size.
Instrumental conditions
(See *Ultraviolet-Visible Spectroscopy ⟨857⟩*.)
Mode: UV
Analytical wavelength: 329 nm
Cell: 0.5 cm
Blank: *Medium*
Tolerances: See *Table 8*.

Table 8

Time (h)	Amount Dissolved (%)
1	NMT 15
4	20 • (RB 1-Aug-2017)–40
12	NLT 80

The cumulative percentages of the labeled amount of nifedipine ($C_{17}H_{18}N_2O_6$) dissolved at the times specified conform to *Dissolution ⟨711⟩, Acceptance Table 2*.
Test 7: If the product complies with this test, the labeling indicates that it meets USP *Dissolution Test 7*.
Medium: Simulated gastric fluid without enzyme containing 0.5% sodium lauryl sulfate, pH 1.2; 900 mL
Apparatus 2: 100 rpm, with three-prong sinker
Times: 1, 4, and 12 h
Standard solution: (L/900) mg/mL of USP Nifedipine RS in *Medium*, where L is the label claim, in mg/Tablet, of nifedipine. A small amount of methanol, not exceeding 6%–7% of the final volume of the first dilution, can be used to solubilize nifedipine.
Sample solution: Pass a portion of the solution under test through a suitable filter.
Instrumental conditions
(See *Ultraviolet-Visible Spectroscopy ⟨857⟩*.)
Mode: UV
Analytical wavelength: 238 nm
Cell: 1 mm, flow cell
Blank: *Medium*
Tolerances: See *Table 9*.

Table 9

Time (h)	Amount Dissolved (%)
1	NMT 15
4	25–50
12	NLT 80

The cumulative percentages of the labeled amount of nifedipine ($C_{17}H_{18}N_2O_6$) dissolved at the times specified conform to *Dissolution ⟨711⟩, Acceptance Table 2*.
Test 8: If the product complies with this test, the labeling indicates that it meets USP *Dissolution Test 8*.
Acid stage medium: Simulated gastric fluid without enzyme containing 3% polysorbate 80, pH 1.2; 250 mL
Apparatus 3: 20 dpm, 20-mesh polypropylene screen on the bottom; 1 min drip time. The Tablet is automatically transferred by the apparatus to the next set of vessels for each time point.
Time: 1 h
Buffer stage medium: 0.01 M sodium phosphate buffer, pH 6.8, containing 3% polysorbate 80 (dissolve 8.3 g of monobasic sodium phosphate and 1 g of sodium hydroxide in 6 L of water, adjust with either diluted sodium hydroxide or phosphoric acid to a pH of 6.8 ± 0.05, and add 180 g of polysorbate 80); 250 mL
Times: 2, 8, 12, and 24 h
Mobile phase: Acetonitrile, methanol, and water (35:35:30)
Standard stock solution: 1 mg/mL of USP Nifedipine RS in *Buffer stage medium*. An amount of methanol, about 40% of the final volume, can be used to dissolve nifedipine.
Standard solution: (L/1000) mg/mL in *Buffer stage medium*, from the *Standard stock solution*, where L is the label claim in mg/Tablet
Sample solution: Pass a portion of the solution under test through a suitable filter.
Chromatographic system
(See *Chromatography ⟨621⟩, System Suitability*.)

Mode: LC
Detector: UV 338 nm
Column: 4.6-mm × 25-cm; packing L1
Temperature: 30°
Flow rate: 1.5 mL/min
Injection volume: 10 µL
System suitability
Sample: *Standard solution*
Suitability requirements
Column efficiency: NLT 4000 theoretical plates
Tailing factor: NMT 1.7
Relative standard deviation: NMT 2.0%
Analysis: Calculate the percentage of the labeled amount of nifedipine dissolved at each time point.
At 1 h:

$$D_1 = (r_U/r_S) \times (C_S/L) \times V \times 100$$

At 2 h:

$$D = (r_U/r_S) \times (C_S/L) \times V \times 100$$

$$D_2 = D_1 + D$$

At 8 h:

$$D = (r_U/r_S) \times (C_S/L) \times V \times 100$$

$$D_8 = D_2 + D$$

At 12 h:

$$D = (r_U/r_S) \times (C_S/L) \times V \times 100$$

$$D_{12} = D_8 + D$$

At 24 h:

$$D = (r_U/r_S) \times (C_S/L) \times V \times 100$$

$$D_{24} = D_{12} + D$$

r_U = peak response from the *Sample solution*
r_S = peak response from the *Standard solution*
C_S = concentration of the *Standard solution* (mg/mL)
L = label claim (mg/Tablet)
V = volume of *Medium*, 250 mL
Tolerances
Acid stage: NMT 5% of the labeled amount of nifedipine is dissolved in 1 h.
Buffer stage: See *Table 10*.

Table 10

Time (h)	Amount Dissolved (%)
1	NMT 5
2	0–10
8	25–60
12	45–85
24	NLT 80

The cumulative percentages of the labeled amount of nifedipine ($C_{17}H_{18}N_2O_6$) dissolved at the times specified conform to *Dissolution* ⟨711⟩, *Acceptance Table 2*.
Test 9: If the product complies with this test, the labeling indicates that it meets USP *Dissolution Test 9*.
Medium: 0.03 M phosphate/citrate buffer, pH 6.8 with 1% sodium lauryl sulfate (to a solution of 4.1 g/L of dibasic sodium phosphate and 0.475 g/L of citric

acid monohydrate in water, add 10 g/L of sodium lauryl sulfate. Adjust if necessary, with phosphoric acid to a pH of 6.8); 900 mL
Apparatus 2: 50 rpm, with a suitable sinker
Times: 3, 6, and 12 h
Standard stock solution: 0.33 mg/mL of USP Nifedipine RS in methanol
Standard solution: Prepare the corresponding USP Nifedipine RS solutions in *Medium* as directed in *Table 11*.

Table 11

Tablet Strength (mg)	Concentration (mg/mL)
30	0.033
60	0.066
90	0.099

Sample solution: Pass a portion of the solution under test at each time point through a suitable filter.
Instrumental conditions
(See *Ultraviolet-Visible Spectroscopy* ⟨857⟩.)
Mode: UV
Analytical wavelength: 346 nm
Cell: 1 cm
Blank: *Medium*
Analysis
Samples: *Standard solutions* and *Sample solution*
Calculate the concentration (C_i) of nifedipine ($C_{17}H_{18}N_2O_6$) in the sample withdrawn from the vessel at each time point (i):

$$\text{Result}_i = (A_U/A_S) \times C_S$$

A_U = absorbance of the *Sample solution* at each time point
A_S = absorbance of the *Standard solution*
C_S = concentration of USP Nifedipine RS in the *Standard solution* (mg/mL)
Calculate the percentage of the labeled amount of nifedipine ($C_{17}H_{18}N_2O_6$) dissolved at each time point (i):

$$\text{Result}_1 = C_1 \times V \times (1/L) \times 100$$

$$\text{Result}_2 = \{[C_2 \times (V - V_S)] + (C_1 \times V_S)\} \times (1/L) \times 100$$

$$\text{Result}_3 = (\{C_3 \times [V - (2 \times V_S)]\} + [(C_2 + C_1) \times V_S]) \times (1/L) \times 100$$

C_i = concentration of nifedipine in the *Sample solution* at the specified time point (i) (mg/mL)
V = volume of the *Medium*, 900 mL
L = label claim (mg/Tablet)
V_S = volume of the *Sample solution* withdrawn at each time point (i) (mL)
Tolerances: See *Table 12*.

Table 12

Time Point (*i*)	Time (h)	Amount Dissolved (%)	
		Tablets Labeled to Contain 30 mg and 60 mg of Nifedipine	Tablets Labeled to Contain 90 mg of Nifedipine
1	3	15–40	10–35
2	6	43–73	40–65
3	12	NLT 80	NLT 80

The percentages of the labeled amount of Nifedipine ($C_{17}H_{18}N_2O_6$) dissolved at the times specified conform to *Dissolution* ⟨711⟩, *Acceptance Table 2*.

•**Test 10:** If the product complies with this test, the labeling indicates that the product meets USP *Dissolution Test 10*.

Medium: pH 6.8 phosphate buffer with 0.5% sodium lauryl sulfate (transfer 442.1 g of dibasic sodium phosphate and 38 g of citric acid in a 1-L volumetric flask. Add water to dissolve, add 10 mL of phosphoric acid, and dilute with water to volume. Transfer 60 g of sodium lauryl sulfate to a suitable container. Add 150 mL of the phosphate solution above and 11,850 mL of water. Mix well and adjust with phosphoric acid or sodium hydroxide to a pH of 6.8); 900 mL

Apparatus 2: 50 rpm, with sinkers (see *Dissolution* ⟨711⟩, *Figure 2a*)

Times: 2, 8, and 16 h

Mobile phase: Methanol and water (60:40)

Standard solution: 0.06 mg/mL of USP Nifedipine RS prepared as follows. Transfer 12 mg of USP Nifedipine RS into a 200-mL volumetric flask. Add 20 mL of methanol, and dilute with *Medium* to volume. [NOTE—Sonication may be needed to aid dissolution.]

Sample solution: Withdraw a 10-mL aliquot at each time point. Pass a portion of the solution under test through a suitable filter.

Chromatographic system
(See *Chromatography* ⟨621⟩, *System Suitability*.)
Mode: LC
Detector: UV 380 nm
Column: 4.6-mm × 7.5-mm; 3.5-μm packing L60
Temperature: 45°
Flow rate: 1 mL/min
Injection volume: 20 μL

System suitability
Sample: *Standard solution*
Suitability requirements
Column efficiency: NLT 3000 theoretical plates
Tailing factor: NMT 1.5
Relative standard deviation: NMT 3.0%

Analysis
Samples: *Standard solution* and *Sample solution*
Calculate the concentration (C_i) of nifedipine ($C_{17}H_{18}N_2O_6$) in the sample withdrawn from the vessel at each time point (*i*):

$$Result_i = (r_U/r_S) \times C_S$$

r_U = peak response of nifedipine in the *Sample solution* at each time point
r_S = peak response of nifedipine in the *Standard solution*
C_S = concentration of USP Nifedipine RS in the *Standard solution* (mg/mL)

Calculate the percentage of the labeled amount of nifedipine ($C_{17}H_{18}N_2O_6$) dissolved at each time point (*i*):

$$Result_1 = C_1 \times V \times (1/L) \times 100$$

$$Result_2 = \{[C_2 \times (V - V_S)] + (C_1 \times V_S)\} \times (1/L) \times 100$$

$$Result_3 = (\{C_3 \times [V - (2 \times V_S)]\} + [(C_2 + C_1) \times V_S]) \times (1/L) \times 100$$

C_i = concentration of nifedipine in the *Sample solution* at the specified time point (*i*) (mg/mL)
V = volume of the *Medium*, 900 mL
L = label claim (mg/Tablet)
V_S = volume of the *Sample solution* withdrawn at each time point (*i*) (mL)

Tolerances: See *Table 13*.

Table 13

Time Point (*i*)	Time (h)	Amount Dissolved (%)	
		Tablets Labeled to Contain 30 and 60 mg of Nifedipine	Tablets Labeled to Contain 90 mg of Nifedipine
1	2	NMT 30	NMT 15
2	8	53–83	35–58
3	16	NLT 80	NLT 75

The percentages of the labeled amount of nifedipine ($C_{17}H_{18}N_2O_6$) dissolved at the times specified, conform to *Dissolution* ⟨711⟩, *Acceptance Table 2*.• (RB 1-Aug-2017)

•**Test 11:** If the product complies with this test, the labeling indicates that the product meets USP *Dissolution Test 11*.

Medium: 1.25% sodium lauryl sulfate in water (transfer 12.5 g of sodium lauryl sulfate to 1 L of water); 900 mL

Apparatus 2: 100 rpm

Times: 1, 2, 4 and 10 h

Standard solution: 0.033 mg/mL of USP Nifedipine RS for Tablets labeled to contain 30 mg prepared as follows. Transfer an appropriate amount of USP Nifedipine RS into a suitable volumetric flask. Add methanol to 1% volume of the flask, and dilute with *Medium* to volume. [NOTE—Sonication may be needed to aid the dissolution.]

Sample solution: A portion of the solution under test at the time points specified

Instrumental conditions
(See *Ultraviolet-Visible Spectroscopy* ⟨857⟩.)
Mode: UV
Analytical wavelengths: 230–246 nm, from the difference between first derivative values at the wavelengths of maximum and minimum in the wavelength range from 230 to 246 nm
Cell: 1 mm
Blank: *Medium*

Analysis: Use an automatic dissolution system with an appropriate dissolution software. Determine the amount of nifedipine ($C_{17}H_{18}N_2O_6$) dissolved, using portions of the *Sample solution*, in comparison with the *Standard solution*.

Tolerances: See *Table 14*.

Table 14

For Tablets Labeled to Contain 30 mg of Nifedipine	
Time (h)	Amount Dissolved (%)
1	NMT 25
2	15–40
4	35–70
10	NLT 85

The cumulative percentages of the labeled amount of nifedipine ($C_{17}H_{18}N_2O_6$), dissolved at the times specified, conform to *Dissolution* ⟨711⟩, *Acceptance Table 2*.

Test 12: If the product complies with this test, the labeling indicates that the product meets USP *Dissolution Test 12*.

Medium: pH 6.8 phosphate buffer with 1.25% sodium lauryl sulfate (transfer 6 g of monobasic sodium phosphate and 112 mL of 0.2 N sodium hydroxide in a 1-L volumetric flask containing 800 mL of water. Mix to dissolve, and dilute with water to volume. Adjust with phosphoric acid or sodium hydroxide to a pH of 6.8. Transfer 12.5 g of sodium lauryl sulfate in 1 L of the phosphate solution); 900 mL

Apparatus 2: 50 rpm

Times: 2, 6, 8 and 16 h

Standard solution: 0.067 mg/mL of USP Nifedipine RS for Tablets labeled to contain 60 mg prepared as follows. Transfer an appropriate amount of USP Nifedipine RS into a suitable volumetric flask. Add methanol to 1% volume of the flask, and dilute with *Medium* to volume.

[NOTE—Sonication may be needed to aid the dissolution.]

Sample solution: A portion of the solution under test at the time points specified

Instrumental conditions

(See *Ultraviolet-Visible Spectroscopy* ⟨857⟩.)

Mode: UV

Analytical wavelengths: 230–246 nm, from the difference between first derivative values at the wavelengths of maximum and minimum in the wavelength range from 230 to 246 nm

Cell: 1 mm

Blank: *Medium*

Analysis: Use an automatic dissolution system with an appropriate dissolution software. Determine the amount of nifedipine ($C_{17}H_{18}N_2O_6$) dissolved, using portions of the *Sample solution*, in comparison with the *Standard solution*.

Tolerances: See *Table 15*.

Table 15

For Tablets Labeled to Contain 60 mg of Nifedipine	
Time (h)	Amount Dissolved (%)
2	NMT 20
6	28–53
8	43–68
16	NLT 80

The cumulative percentages of the labeled amount of nifedipine ($C_{17}H_{18}N_2O_6$), dissolved at the times specified, conform to *Dissolution* ⟨711⟩, *Acceptance Table 2*.

● (RB 1-Oct-2017)

- **UNIFORMITY OF DOSAGE UNITS** ⟨905⟩: Meet the requirements

IMPURITIES

- **ORGANIC IMPURITIES**

[NOTE—Conduct this test promptly after preparation of the *Standard nifedipine solution* and the *Sample solution*.]

Mobile phase: Acetonitrile, methanol, and water (25:25:50)

Quantitative limit stock solution A: 1 mg/mL of USP Nifedipine Nitrophenylpyridine Analog RS in methanol

Quantitative limit solution A: 6 µg/mL of USP Nifedipine Nitrophenylpyridine Analog RS from *Quantitative limit stock solution A* in *Mobile phase*

Quantitative limit stock solution B: 1 mg/mL of USP Nifedipine Nitrosophenylpyridine Analog RS in methanol

Quantitative limit solution B: 1.5 µg/mL of USP Nifedipine Nitrosophenylpyridine Analog RS from *Quantitative limit stock solution B* in *Mobile phase*

Standard nifedipine stock solution: 1 mg/mL of USP Nifedipine RS in methanol

Standard nifedipine solution: 0.3 mg/mL of USP Nifedipine RS from *Standard nifedipine stock solution* in *Mobile phase*

System suitability solution: *Quantitative limit solution A*, *Quantitative limit solution B*, and *Standard nifedipine solution* (1:1:1)

Standard solution: *Mobile phase*, *Quantitative limit solution A*, and *Quantitative limit solution B* (1:1:1)

[NOTE—Each mL of this solution contains about 2 µg of USP Nifedipine Nitrophenylpyridine Analog RS and 0.5 µg of USP Nifedipine Nitrosophenylpyridine Analog RS.]

Sample solution: Use a portion of the *Sample solution* prepared as directed in the *Assay*.

Chromatographic system

(See *Chromatography* ⟨621⟩, *System Suitability*.)

Mode: LC

Detector: UV 265 nm

Columns

Guard: 2.1-mm × 3-cm; packing L1

Analytical: 4.6-mm × 25-cm; packing L1

Flow rate: 1 mL/min

Injection volume: 25 µL

System suitability

Sample: *System suitability solution*

Suitability requirements

Resolution: NLT 1.5 between the nitrophenylpyridine analog and nitrosophenylpyridine analog peaks; NLT 1.0 between the nitrosophenylpyridine analog and nifedipine peaks

Relative standard deviation: NMT 10% for each analog

Analysis

Samples: *Standard solution* and *Sample solution*

Calculate the percentage of each analog in the portion of Tablets taken:

$$Result = (r_U/r_S) \times (C_S/C_U) \times 100$$

r_U = peak response of each analog from the *Sample solution*

r_S = peak response of each analog from the *Standard solution*

C_S = concentration of the appropriate analog USP Reference Standard in the *Standard solution* (µg/mL)

C_U = nominal concentration of nifedipine in the *Sample solution* (µg/mL)

Acceptance criteria: NMT 2.0% of nifedipine nitrophenylpyridine analog and NMT 0.5% of nifedipine nitrosophenylpyridine analog, both relative to the nifedipine content

ADDITIONAL REQUIREMENTS

- **PACKAGING AND STORAGE:** Preserve in tight, light-resistant containers, and store at controlled room temperature.
- **LABELING:** The labeling indicates the *Dissolution* test with which the product complies.
- **USP REFERENCE STANDARDS** ⟨11⟩

USP Nifedipine RS

USP Nifedipine Nitrophenylpyridine Analog RS

Dimethyl 4-(2-nitrophenyl)-2,6-dimethylpyridine-3,5-dicarboxylate.

$C_{17}H_{16}N_2O_6$ 344.33

USP Nifedipine Nitrosophenylpyridine Analog RS

Dimethyl 4-(2-nitrosophenyl)-2,6-dimethylpyridine-3,5-dicarboxylate.

$C_{17}H_{16}N_2O_5$ 328.33

Norelgestromin

C$_{21}$H$_{29}$NO$_2$ 327.46
18,19-Dinorpregn-4-en-20-yn-3-one, 13-ethyl-17-hydroxy-,
oxime, (17α)-;
13-Ethyl-17-hydroxy-18,19-dinor-17α-pregn-4-en-20-yn-
3-one oxime [53016-31-2].

DEFINITION
Norelgestromin is a mixture of (E)- and (Z)-isomers having a
ratio of (E)- to (Z)-isomer between 1.3 and 1.6, and the
sum of both isomers is NLT 98.0% and NMT 102.0% of
norelgestromin (C$_{21}$H$_{29}$NO$_2$), calculated on the anhydrous
basis.

IDENTIFICATION
- **A. INFRARED ABSORPTION ⟨197K⟩**
- **B.** The retention time of the major peak of the *Sample
  solution* corresponds to that of the *Standard solution*, as
  obtained in the *Assay*.

ASSAY

Change to read:

- **PROCEDURE**
  Mobile phase: Cyclohexane and absolute alcohol
  (100:2)
  Diluent: Cyclohexane and absolute alcohol (90:10)
  System suitability solution: 1.5 mg/mL of USP
  Norelgestromin RS and 8 µg/mL of USP Norelgestromin
  Related Compound A RS in *Diluent*
  Standard solution: 1.5 mg/mL of USP Norelgestromin
  RS in *Diluent*
  Sample solution: 1.5 mg/mL of Norelgestromin in
  Diluent
  Chromatographic system
  (See *Chromatography ⟨621⟩, System Suitability.*)
  Mode: LC
  Detector: UV 210 nm
  Column: 4.6-mm × 25-cm; 5-µm packing L20
  Column temperature: 50°
  Flow rate: 1.2 mL/min
  Injection volume: 25 µL
  Run time: ■NLT■$_{1S \ (USP41)}$ 1.6 times the retention time
  of (Z)-norelgestromin
  System suitability
  Samples: *System suitability solution* and *Standard
  solution*
  [NOTE—The relative retention times for the (Z)-isomer of
  norelgestromin related compound A, (E)-norelges-
  tromin, and (Z)-norelgestromin are about 0.77, 0.85,
  and 1.0, respectively.]
  Suitability requirements
  Resolution: NLT 1.4 between the (Z)-isomer of
  norelgestromin related compound A and (E)-norelges-
  tromin, *System suitability solution*
  Tailing factor: 0.8–1.2 for both (E)- and (Z)-norelges-
  tromin, ■■$_{1S \ (USP41)}$ *Standard solution*
  Relative standard deviation: NMT 0.73% for both
  (E)- and (Z)-norelgestromin, ■■$_{1S \ (USP41)}$ *Standard
  solution*

Analysis
Samples: *Standard solution* and *Sample solution*
Calculate the percentage of norelgestromin (C$_{21}$H$_{29}$NO$_2$)
in the portion of Norelgestromin taken:

$$\text{Result} = \{[(r_{UE} \times F) + r_{UZ}]/[(r_{SE} \times F) + r_{SZ}]\} \times (C_S/C_U) \times 100$$

r_{UE}	= peak response of (E)-norelgestromin from the *Sample solution*
F	= response factor for (E)-norelgestromin, 1.04
r_{UZ}	= peak response of (Z)-norelgestromin from the *Sample solution*
r_{SE}	= peak response of (E)-norelgestromin from the *Standard solution*
r_{SZ}	= peak response of (Z)-norelgestromin from the *Standard solution*
C_S	= concentration of USP Norelgestromin RS in the *Standard solution* (mg/mL)
C_U	= concentration of Norelgestromin in the *Sample solution* (mg/mL)

Calculate the ratio of (E)- to (Z)-norelgestromin:

$$\text{Result} = (r_{UE} \times F)/r_{UZ}$$

r_{UE}	= peak response of (E)-norelgestromin from the *Sample solution*
F	= response factor for (E)-norelgestromin, 1.04
r_{UZ}	= peak response of (Z)-norelgestromin from the *Sample solution*

Acceptance criteria
Both isomers: 98.0%–102.0% on the anhydrous basis
Ratio of (E)- to (Z)-isomer: 1.3–1.6

IMPURITIES
- **RESIDUE ON IGNITION ⟨281⟩:** NMT 0.2%

Change to read:

- **ORGANIC IMPURITIES**
  **Mobile phase, Diluent, System suitability solution,
  Standard solution, Sample solution,** and **Chromato-
  graphic system:** Proceed as directed in the *Assay*.
  Sensitivity solution: 1.5 µg/mL of USP Norelgestromin
  RS in *Diluent* from the *Standard solution*
  System suitability
  Samples: *System suitability solution, Standard solution,*
  and *Sensitivity solution*
  Suitability requirements
  Resolution: NLT 1.4 between the (Z)-isomer of
  norelgestromin related compound A and (E)-norelges-
  tromin, *System suitability solution*
  Tailing factor: 0.8–1.2 for both (E)- and (Z)-norelges-
  tromin, ■■$_{1S \ (USP41)}$ *Standard solution*
  Relative standard deviation: NMT 0.73% for both
  (E)- and (Z)-norelgestromin, ■■$_{1S \ (USP41)}$ *Standard
  solution*
  Signal-to-noise ratio: NLT 3 for both (E)- and (Z)-
  norelgestromin, *Sensitivity solution*
  Analysis
  Samples: *Standard solution* and *Sample solution*
  Calculate the percentage of each impurity in the por-
  tion of Norelgestromin taken:

$$\text{Result} = \{r_U/[(r_{SE} \times F) + r_{SZ}]\} \times (C_S/C_U) \times 100$$

r_U	= peak response of each impurity from the *Sample solution*
r_{SE}	= peak response of (E)-norelgestromin from the *Standard solution*
F	= response factor for (E)-norelgestromin, 1.04
r_{SZ}	= peak response of (Z)-norelgestromin from the *Standard solution*
C_S	= concentration of USP Norelgestromin RS in the *Standard solution* (mg/mL)

C_U = concentration of Norelgestromin in the *Sample solution* (mg/mL)

Acceptance criteria: See *Table 1*. Disregard peaks that are less than 0.05% of the total peak areas of (*E*)- and (*Z*)-norelgestromin.

Table 1

Name	Relative Retention Time	Acceptance Criteria, NMT (%)
Norgestrel[a]	0.37	0.5
(*E*)- and (*Z*)-Norgestimate[b]	0.43[c], 0.47[d]	0.5[e]
Norelgestromin 5(10)-ene[f,g]	0.68	—
Norelgestromin related compound A[g]	0.73[h], 0.77[i]	—
(*E*)-Norelgestromin	0.85	—
(*Z*)-Norelgestromin	1.0	—
Any other individual impurity	—	0.10
Total impurities	—	1.0

[a] (±)-13-Ethyl-17-hydroxy-18,19-dinor-17α-pregn-4-en-20-yn-3-one.

[b] 18,19-Dinor-17-pregn-4-en-20-yn-3-one, 17-(acetyloxy)-13-ethyl-,oxime, (17α)-(+)-; (+)-13-Ethyl-17-hydroxy-18,19-dinor-17α-pregn-4-en-20-yn-3-one oxime acetate (ester).

[c] (*E*)-Norgestimate.

[d] (*Z*)-Norgestimate.

[e] The combined limits for (*E*)- and (*Z*)-norgestimate are NMT 0.5%.

[f] 13-Ethyl-17-hydroxy-18,19-dinor-17α-pregn-5(10)-en-20-yn-3-one oxime.

[g] This is not a specified impurity and is included in this table for identification only. It is not to be reported or included in the total impurities.

[h] (*E*)-Isomer of norelgestromin related compound A.

[i] (*Z*)-Isomer of norelgestromin related compound A.

SPECIFIC TESTS

- **OPTICAL ROTATION ⟨781S⟩,** *Procedures, Specific Rotation*
  Sample solution: 5 mg/mL in alcohol and water (75:25)
  Acceptance criteria: +35° to +41°
- **WATER DETERMINATION ⟨921⟩,** *Method I, Method Ic*: NMT 1.0%

ADDITIONAL REQUIREMENTS

- **PACKAGING AND STORAGE:** Preserve in well-closed containers, and store at controlled room temperature.
- **USP REFERENCE STANDARDS ⟨11⟩**
  USP Norelgestromin RS
  USP Norelgestromin Related Compound A RS
  Mixture of (*E*)- and (*Z*)-isomers.
  13-Ethyl-17-hydroxy-18,19-dinor-17α-pregn-5(6)-en-20-yn-3-one oxime.
  $C_{21}H_{29}NO_2$ 327.46

Octinoxate

$C_{18}H_{26}O_3$ 290.40

2-Propenoic acid, 3-(4-methoxyphenyl)-, 2-ethylhexyl ester;
2-Ethylhexyl *p*-methoxycinnamate [5466-77-3].

DEFINITION

Octinoxate contains NLT 95.0% and NMT 105.0% of octinoxate ($C_{18}H_{26}O_3$), calculated on the as-is basis.

IDENTIFICATION

Change to read:

- **A. INFRARED ABSORPTION** ■⟨197⟩: [NOTE—Methods described in ⟨197F⟩ or ⟨197A⟩ may be used.]■1S (USP41)

Change to read:

- **B.** ■The retention time of the octinoxate peak of the *Sample solution* corresponds to that of the *Standard solution*, as obtained in the *Assay*.■1S (USP41)

ASSAY

Change to read:

- **PROCEDURE**
  ■**System suitability stock solution:**■1S (USP41) 5% (v/v) ■USP Benzyl Benzoate RS■1S (USP41) in acetone
  ■**System suitability solution:** 50 mg/mL of USP Octinoxate RS in *System suitability stock solution*■1S (USP41)
  Standard solution: 50 mg/mL of USP Octinoxate RS in ■acetone■1S (USP41)
  Sample solution: Transfer 5 mL of Octinoxate to a 100-mL volumetric flask, and dilute with ■acetone■1S (USP41) to volume.
  Chromatographic system
  (See *Chromatography* ⟨621⟩, *System Suitability*.)
  Mode: GC
  Detector: Flame ionization
  Column: 0.32-mm × 25-m; 0.25-µm thickness of phase G1
  Carrier gas: Helium
  Temperatures
  Injection port: 250°
  Detector: 300°
  Column: See *Table 1*.

Table 1

Initial Temperature (°)	Temperature Ramp (°/min)	Final Temperature (°)	Hold Time at Final Temperature (min)
80	22	300	10

Flow rate: 2 mL/min
Injection volume: 1 µL
Injection type: Split ratio, 85:1
System suitability
  Samples: ■ *System suitability solution* and■1S (USP41) *Standard solution*
  [NOTE—The relative retention times for benzyl benzoate and octinoxate are about 0.68 and 1.0, respectively.]
  Suitability requirements
  Resolution: NLT 20 between benzyl benzoate and octinoxate, ■*System suitability solution*■1S (USP41)
  Relative standard deviation: NMT 2.0%, ■*Standard solution*■1S (USP41)
Analysis
  Samples: *Standard solution* and *Sample solution*
  Calculate the percentage of octinoxate ($C_{18}H_{26}O_3$) in the portion of Octinoxate taken:

$$\blacksquare Result = (r_U/r_S) \times (C_S/C_U) \times 100 \blacksquare 1S\ (USP41)$$

r_{U}■1S (USP41) = peak response ■of octinoxate■1S (USP41) from the *Sample solution*

r_{S}■1S (USP41) = peak response ■of octinoxate■1S (USP41) from the *Standard solution*

C_S = concentration of USP Octinoxate RS in the *Standard solution* (mg/mL)

C_U　　= concentration of Octinoxate in the *Sample solution* (mg/mL)
　Acceptance criteria:　95.0%–105.0% on the as-is basis

IMPURITIES

Change to read:

- ● ORGANIC IMPURITIES
　■System suitability stock solution, System suitability solution,■1S (USP41) Standard solution, Chromatographic system, and System suitability:　Proceed as directed in the *Assay*.
　Sample solution:　Transfer 5 mL of Octinoxate to a 100-mL volumetric flask, and dilute with acetone to volume.
　Analysis
　Sample:　*Sample solution*
　Calculate the percentage of each impurity in the portion of Octinoxate taken:

$$Result = (r_U/r_T) \times 100$$

r_U　　= peak response of each impurity from the *Sample solution*
r_T　　= sum of all the peak responses from the *Sample solution*
　Acceptance criteria
　Any individual impurity:　NMT 0.5%
　Total impurities:　NMT 2.0%

SPECIFIC TESTS

- ● SPECIFIC GRAVITY ⟨841⟩:　1.005–1.013
- ● REFRACTIVE INDEX ⟨831⟩:　1.542–1.548 at 20°
- ● ACIDITY
　Sample:　5 mL of Octinoxate
　Analysis:　Add 50 mL of alcohol to the *Sample*, and mix. Add 4 drops of phenolphthalein TS, and titrate with 0.1 N sodium hydroxide.
　Acceptance criteria:　NMT 0.8 mL of 0.1 N sodium hydroxide is required.

ADDITIONAL REQUIREMENTS

- ● PACKAGING AND STORAGE:　Preserve in tight containers, and store in a cool place.

Change to read:

- ● USP REFERENCE STANDARDS ⟨11⟩
　■USP Benzyl Benzoate RS
　Benzoic acid, phenylmethyl ester.
　$C_{14}H_{12}O_2$　212.24■1S (USP41)
　USP Octinoxate RS

Octisalate

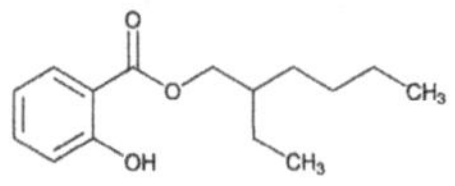

$C_{15}H_{22}O_3$　　　　　　　　　　　　　　　250.33
Benzoic acid, 2-hydroxy-, 2-ethylhexyl ester;
2-Ethylhexyl salicylate [118-60-5].

DEFINITION

Change to read:

Octisalate contains NLT 95.0% and NMT 105.0% of octisalate ($C_{15}H_{22}O_3$), ■calculated on the as-is basis.■1S (USP41)

IDENTIFICATION

Change to read:

- ● A.　■INFRARED ABSORPTION ⟨197⟩:　[NOTE—Methods described in ⟨197F⟩ or ⟨197A⟩ may be used.]■1S (USP41)

Change to read:

- ● B.　■The retention time of the major peak of the *Sample solution* corresponds to that of the *Standard solution*, as obtained in the *Assay*.■1S (USP41)

ASSAY

- ● PROCEDURE
　Standard solution:　20 mg/mL of USP Octisalate RS in *tert*-butyl methyl ether
　Sample solution:　20 mg/mL of Octisalate in *tert*-butyl methyl ether
　Chromatographic system
　(See *Chromatography* ⟨621⟩, *System Suitability*.)
　Mode:　GC
　Detector:　Flame ionization
　Column:　0.32-mm × 25-m; coated with a 0.1-μm film of phase G1
　Temperatures
　Injector:　240°
　Detector:　260°
　Column:　See *Table 1*.

Table 1

Initial Temperature (°)	Temperature Ramp (°/min)	Final Temperature (°)	Hold Time at Final Temperature (min)
60	8	240	10

　Carrier gas:　Helium
　Flow rate:　6 mL/min
　Injection volume:　1 μL
　Injection type:　Split; split ratio 50:1. [NOTE—Split ratio can be modified to optimize the performance.]
　System suitability
　Sample:　*Standard solution*
　Suitability requirements
　Resolution:　NLT 1.0 between octisalate and any other peak
　Relative standard deviation:　NMT 2.0%
　Analysis
　Samples:　*Standard solution* and *Sample solution*
　Calculate the percentage of octisalate ($C_{15}H_{22}O_3$) in the portion of Octisalate taken:

$$Result = (r_U/r_S) \times (C_S/C_U) \times 100$$

r_U　　= peak response from the *Sample solution*
r_S　　= peak response from the *Standard solution*
C_S　　= concentration of USP Octisalate RS in the *Standard solution* (mg/mL)
C_U　　= concentration of Octisalate in the *Sample solution* (mg/mL)

Acceptance criteria: 95.0%–105.0% on the as-is basis

IMPURITIES
- **ORGANIC IMPURITIES**
  Standard solution, Sample solution, Chromatographic system, and **System suitability:**   Proceed as directed in the *Assay*.
  Analysis
  Sample: *Sample solution*
  Calculate the percentage of each impurity in the portion of Octisalate taken:

$$Result = (r_U/r_T) \times 100$$

r_U = peak response of each impurity from the *Sample solution*
r_T = sum of all the peak responses from the *Sample solution*
  Acceptance criteria
  Individual impurities: NMT 0.5%
  Total impurities: NMT 2.0%

SPECIFIC TESTS
- **SPECIFIC GRAVITY ⟨841⟩:**   1.011–1.016
- **REFRACTIVE INDEX ⟨831⟩:**   1.500–1.503 at 20°
- **ACIDITY**
  Sample solution: 5.0 mL of measured Octisalate
  Titrimetric system
  Mode: Direct titration
  Titrant: 0.1 N sodium hydroxide
  Endpoint detection: Visual
  Analysis: Transfer 50 mL of alcohol to a suitable container, add 1 mL of phenol red TS, and add sufficient *Titrant* to obtain a persistent pink color. Transfer 50 mL of this solution to a suitable container, add the *Sample solution*, mix, and titrate with *Titrant*.
  Acceptance criteria: NMT 0.2 mL of 0.1 N sodium hydroxide per milliliter of Octisalate is required for neutralization.

ADDITIONAL REQUIREMENTS
- **PACKAGING AND STORAGE:**   Preserve in tight containers.
- **USP REFERENCE STANDARDS ⟨11⟩**
  USP Octisalate RS

Octocrylene

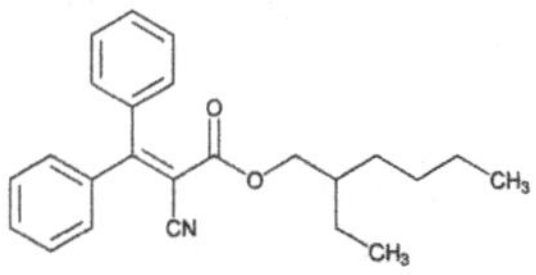

$C_{24}H_{27}NO_2$ 361.48
2-Propenoic acid, 2-cyano-3,3-diphenyl-, 2-ethylhexyl ester;
2-Ethylhexyl 2-cyano-3,3-diphenylacrylate [6197-30-4].

DEFINITION
Octocrylene contains NLT 95.0% and NMT 105.0% of octocrylene ($C_{24}H_{27}NO_2$).

IDENTIFICATION

Change to read:

- ■**A.** ■1S *(USP41)* **ULTRAVIOLET ABSORPTION ⟨197U⟩**
  Sample solution: 25 µg/mL in methanol
  Analytical wavelength: 303 nm
  Acceptance criteria: NMT 3.0%, calculated on the as-is basis

Add the following:

- ■● **B.**   The retention time of major peak of the *Sample solution* corresponds to that of the *Standard solution*, as obtained in the *Assay*.■1S *(USP41)*

ASSAY
- **PROCEDURE**
  Standard solution: 21 mg/mL of USP Octocrylene RS in acetone
  Sample solution: 21 mg/mL of Octocrylene in acetone
  Chromatographic system
  (See *Chromatography* ⟨621⟩, *System Suitability*.)
  Mode: GC
  Detector: Flame ionization
  Column: 0.32-mm × 60-m; coated with a 0.25-µm film of phase G1
  Temperatures
  Injection port: 300°
  Detector: 300°
  Column: See *Table 1*.

Table 1

Initial Temperature (°)	Temperature Ramp (°/min)	Final Temperature (°)	Hold Time at Final Temperature (min)
80	4	280	10

  Carrier gas: Helium
  Flow rate: 6 mL/min
  Injection volume: 1 µL
  Injection type: Split ratio, 30:1
  System suitability
  Sample: *Standard solution*
  Suitability requirements
  Resolution: NLT 1.0 between octocrylene and any other adjacent peak
  Relative standard deviation: NMT 2.0%
  Analysis
  Samples: *Standard solution* and *Sample solution*
  Calculate the percentage of octocrylene ($C_{24}H_{27}NO_2$) in the portion of Octocrylene taken:

$$Result = (r_U/r_S) \times (C_S/C_U) \times 100$$

r_U = peak response from the *Sample solution*
r_S = peak response from the *Standard solution*
C_S = concentration of USP Octocrylene RS in the *Standard solution* (mg/mL)
C_U = concentration of Octocrylene in the *Sample solution* (mg/mL)
  Acceptance criteria: 95.0%–105.0%

IMPURITIES
- **ORGANIC IMPURITIES**
  Standard solution, Sample solution, Chromatographic system, and **System suitability:**   Proceed as directed in the *Assay*.
  Analysis
  Sample: *Sample solution*
  Calculate the percentage of each impurity in the portion of Octocrylene taken:

$$Result = (r_U/r_T) \times 100$$

r_U = peak response of each impurity from the *Sample solution*
r_T = sum of all the peak responses from the *Sample solution*

Acceptance criteria
  Individual impurities: NMT 0.5%
  Total impurities: NMT 2.0%

SPECIFIC TESTS
- **SPECIFIC GRAVITY ⟨841⟩:** 1.045–1.055
- **REFRACTIVE INDEX ⟨831⟩:** 1.561–1.571 at 20°
- **ACIDITY**
  Sample: 6 g of Octocrylene
  Titrimetric system
    (See *Titrimetry* ⟨541⟩.)
    Mode: Direct titration
    Titrant: 0.1 N sodium hydroxide
    Endpoint detection: Visual
  Analysis: To 60 mL of alcohol, add 1 mL of phenol-phthalein TS and sufficient *Titrant* to obtain a persistent pink color. Transfer 60 mL of this solution to a suitable container, add the *Sample*, mix, and titrate with *Titrant* until a persistent pink color is obtained.
  Acceptance criteria: NMT 0.18 mL of *Titrant* is required

ADDITIONAL REQUIREMENTS
- **PACKAGING AND STORAGE:** Preserve in tight containers.
- **USP REFERENCE STANDARDS ⟨11⟩**
  USP Octocrylene RS

Olmesartan Medoxomil Tablets

DEFINITION
Olmesartan Medoxomil Tablets contain NLT 93.0% and NMT 105.0% of the labeled amount of olmesartan medoxomil ($C_{29}H_{30}N_6O_6$).

IDENTIFICATION
- **A.** The UV absorption spectra of the major peak of the *Sample solution* exhibit maxima and minima at the same wavelengths as those of the corresponding peak of the *Standard solution*, as obtained in the *Assay*.
- **B.** The retention time of the major peak of the *Sample solution* corresponds to that of the *Standard solution*, as obtained in the *Assay*.

ASSAY

Change to read:

- **PROCEDURE**
  Solution A: 3.1 g/L of formic acid
  Solution B: Acetonitrile and *Solution A* (10:90)
  Solution C: Acetonitrile and *Solution A* (90:10)
  Mobile phase: See *Table 1*.

Table 1

Time (min)	Solution B (%)	Solution C (%)
0	68.8	31.2
1.5	37.5	62.5
1.6	68.8	31.2
3.0	68.8	31.2

Diluent: Acetonitrile and water (60:40)
Standard solution: 40 µg/mL of USP Olmesartan Medoxomil RS in *Diluent*
Sample stock solution: Prepare solutions of nominal concentrations of olmesartan medoxomil in *Diluent* as follows. To NLT 10 Tablets for 5- •● (RB 1-Aug-2017) and 20-mg Tablet strengths and NLT 5 Tablets for 40-mg Tablet strength in a 200-mL volumetric flask, add *Diluent* to volume. Sonicate with occasional shaking to dis-

integrate the Tablets completely, centrifuge the suspension, and use the supernatant.
Sample solution: Nominally 40 µg/mL of olmesartan medoxomil in *Diluent* from *Sample stock solution*
Chromatographic system
  (See *Chromatography* ⟨621⟩, *System Suitability*.)
  Mode: LC
  Detector: UV 249 nm. For *Identification B*, use a diode array detector in the range of 200–400 nm.
  Column: 2.1-mm × 5-cm; 1.7-µm packing L1
  Column temperature: 35°
  Flow rate: 0.6 mL/min
  Injection volume: 1 µL
System suitability
  Sample: *Standard solution*
  Suitability requirements
    Tailing factor: NMT 2.0
    Relative standard deviation: NMT 1.0%
Analysis
  Samples: *Standard solution* and *Sample solution*
  Calculate the percentage of the labeled amount of olmesartan medoxomil ($C_{29}H_{30}N_6O_6$) in the portion of Tablets taken:

$$Result = (r_U/r_S) \times (C_S/C_U) \times 100$$

r_U = peak response of olmesartan medoxomil from the *Sample solution*
r_S = peak response of olmesartan medoxomil from the *Standard solution*
C_S = concentration of USP Olmesartan Medoxomil RS in the *Standard solution* (µg/mL)
C_U = nominal concentration of olmesartan medoxomil in the *Sample solution* (µg/mL)
Acceptance criteria: 93.0%–105.0%

PERFORMANCE TESTS

Change to read:

- **DISSOLUTION ⟨711⟩**
  •Test 1● (RB 1-Aug-2017)
    Medium: pH 6.8 phosphate buffer (see *Reagents, Indicators, and Solutions—Buffer Solutions*)
    For Tablets labeled to contain 5 mg: 500 mL
    For Tablets labeled to contain 20 and 40 mg: 1000 mL
    Apparatus 2: 50 rpm
    Time: 30 min
    Diluent: Acetonitrile and water (60:40)
    Standard stock solution: 2 mg/mL of USP Olmesartan Medoxomil RS in *Diluent*
    Standard solution: (L/V) mg/mL of USP Olmesartan Medoxomil RS in *Medium*, where L is the label claim in mg/Tablet and V is the volume of the *Medium* in mL from the *Standard stock solution*
    Sample solution: Pass a portion of the solution under test through a glass fiber filter of 1.2-µm pore size.
    Instrumental conditions
      (See *Ultraviolet-Visible Spectroscopy* ⟨857⟩.)
      Mode: UV
      Analytical wavelength: 258 nm
      Cells
        For Tablets labeled to contain 5 and 20 mg: 1 cm
        For Tablets labeled to contain 40 mg: 0.5 cm
      Blank: *Medium*
    Analysis
      Samples: *Standard solution* and *Sample solution*
      Calculate the percentage of the labeled amount of olmesartan medoxomil ($C_{29}H_{30}N_6O_6$) dissolved:

$$Result = (A_U/A_S) \times C_S \times V \times (1/L) \times 100$$

A_U = absorbance of the *Sample solution*
A_S = absorbance of the *Standard solution*

C_S = concentration of the *Standard solution* (mg/mL)
V = volume of *Medium* (see *Medium*)
L = label claim (mg/Tablet)
Tolerances: NLT 75% (*Q*) of the labeled amount of olmesartan medoxomil ($C_{29}H_{30}N_6O_6$) is dissolved.
•Test 2: If the product complies with this test, the labeling indicates that it meets USP *Dissolution Test 2*.
Medium: pH 7.2 phosphate buffer (see *Reagents, Indicators, and Solutions—Buffer Solutions*); 900 mL
Apparatus 2: 75 rpm
Time: 30 min
Standard stock solution: 0.2 mg/mL of USP Olmesartan Medoxomil RS prepared as follows. Transfer an appropriate amount of USP Olmesartan Medoxomil RS into a suitable volumetric flask. Dissolve in 30% of the flask volume of acetonitrile. Dilute with *Medium* to volume and mix.
Standard solution: (*L*/1000) mg/mL of USP Olmesartan Medoxomil RS in *Medium*, from the *Standard stock solution*, where *L* is the label claim in mg/Tablet
Sample solution: Pass a portion of the solution under test through a suitable filter of 0.45-μm pore size and discard the first few milliliters of the filtrate.
Instrumental conditions
  Mode: UV
  Analytical wavelength: 257 nm
  Cell: 1 cm
  Blank: *Medium*
Analysis
  Samples: *Standard solution* and *Sample solution*
  Calculate the percentage of the labeled amount of olmesartan medoxomil ($C_{29}H_{30}N_6O_6$) dissolved:

$$Result = (A_U/A_S) \times C_S \times V \times (1/L) \times 100$$

A_U = absorbance of the *Sample solution*
A_S = absorbance of the *Standard solution*
C_S = concentration of the *Standard solution* (mg/mL)
V = volume of *Medium*, 900 mL
L = label claim (mg/Tablet)
Tolerances: NLT 80% (*Q*) of the labeled amount of olmesartan medoxomil ($C_{29}H_{30}N_6O_6$) is dissolved.• (RB 1-Aug-2017)

• **UNIFORMITY OF DOSAGE UNITS ⟨905⟩:** Meet the requirements

IMPURITIES
• **ORGANIC IMPURITIES**
  Buffer: 0.015 M monobasic potassium phosphate. Adjust with phosphoric acid to a pH of 3.5.
  Solution A: Acetonitrile and *Buffer* (20:80)
  Solution B: Acetonitrile and *Buffer* (79:21)
  Mobile phase: See *Table 2*.

Table 2

Time (min)	Solution A (%)	Solution B (%)
0	75	25
10	75	25
35	0	100
45	0	100

Diluent: Acetonitrile and water (90:10)
System suitability solution: 0.01 mg/mL each of USP Olmesartan Medoxomil RS and USP Olmesartan Medoxomil Related Compound A RS in *Diluent*
Standard solution: 0.01 mg/mL of USP Olmesartan Medoxomil RS in *Diluent*

Sensitivity solution: 0.002 mg/mL of USP Olmesartan Medoxomil RS in *Diluent* from the *Standard solution*
Sample solution: Nominally 1 mg/mL of olmesartan medoxomil in *Diluent* prepared as follows. Dissolve a suitable number of Tablets in *Diluent*. Sonicate and/or shake occasionally to disintegrate the Tablets completely. Centrifuge and pass the supernatant through a suitable filter of 0.45-μm pore size.
Chromatographic system
(See *Chromatography ⟨621⟩, System Suitability*.)
  Mode: LC
  Detector: UV 250 nm
  Column: 4.6-mm × 10-cm; 3.5-μm packing L7
  Column temperature: 40°
  Flow rate: 1 mL/min
  Injection volume: 10 μL
System suitability
  Samples: *System suitability solution* and *Sensitivity solution*
  Suitability requirements
    Resolution: NLT 5 between olmesartan medoxomil and olmesartan medoxomil related compound A, *System suitability solution*
    Relative standard deviation: NMT 2.0% for both peaks, *System suitability solution*
    Signal-to-noise ratio: NLT 30, *Sensitivity solution*
Analysis
  Samples: *Standard solution* and *Sample solution*
  Calculate the percentage of each degradation product in the portion of Tablets taken:

$$Result = (r_U/r_S) \times (C_S/C_U) \times (1/F) \times 100$$

r_U = peak response of each degradation product from the *Sample solution*
r_S = peak response of olmesartan medoxomil from the *Standard solution*
C_S = concentration of USP Olmesartan Medoxomil RS in the *Standard solution* (mg/mL)
C_U = nominal concentration of olmesartan medoxomil in the *Sample solution* (mg/mL)
F = relative response factor (see *Table 3*)
Acceptance criteria: See *Table 3*. Disregard peaks below 0.1%.

Table 3

Name	Relative Retention Time	Relative Response Factor	Acceptance Criteria, NMT (%)
Olmesartan[a]	0.2	1.0	2.5
Olmesartan medoxomil related compound A[b]	0.7	1.6	—
Olmesartan medoxomil	1.0	—	—
Olmesartan dimer[c]	1.2	0.8	0.5
Olefinic impurity[d]	1.5	1.0	0.6

[a] 1-{[2′-(1*H*-Tetrazol-5-yl)biphenyl-4-yl]methyl}-4-(2-hydroxypropan-2-yl)-2-propyl-1*H*-imidazole-5-carboxylic acid.
[b] This is a process-related impurity that is controlled in the drug substance.
[c] 1-({2′-(1*H*-Tetrazol-5-yl)-[1,1′-biphenyl]-4-yl}methyl)-4-(2-{[1-({2′-(1*H*-tetrazol-5-yl)-[1,1′-biphenyl]-4-yl}methyl)-4-(2-hydroxypropan-2-yl)-2-propyl-1*H*-imidazole-5-carbonyl]oxy}propan-2-yl)-2-propyl-1*H*-imidazole-5-carboxylic acid.
[d] (5-Methyl-2-oxo-1,3-dioxol-4-yl)methyl 1-((2′-(1*H*-tetrazol-5-yl)biphenyl-4-yl)methyl)-4-(prop-1-en-2-yl)-2-propyl-1*H*-imidazole-5-carboxylate.

Table 3 *(Continued)*

Name	Relative Retention Time	Relative Response Factor	Acceptance Criteria, NMT (%)
Any unspecified degradation product	—	1.0	0.2
Total degradation products	—	—	4.1

[a] 1-{[2'-(1*H*-Tetrazol-5-yl)biphenyl-4-yl]methyl}-4-(2-hydroxypropan-2-yl)-2-propyl-1*H*-imidazole-5-carboxylic acid.

[b] This is a process-related impurity that is controlled in the drug substance.

[c] 1-({2'-(1*H*-Tetrazol-5-yl)-[1,1'-biphenyl]-4-yl}methyl)-4-(2-{[1-({2'-(1*H*-tetrazol-5-yl)-[1,1'-biphenyl]-4-yl}methyl)-4-(2-hydroxypropan-2-yl)-2-propyl-1*H*-imidazole-5-carbonyl]oxy}propan-2-yl)-2-propyl-1*H*-imidazole-5-carboxylic acid.

[d] (5-Methyl-2-oxo-1,3-dioxol-4-yl)methyl 1-((2'-(1*H*-tetrazol-5-yl)biphenyl-4-yl)methyl)-4-(prop-1-en-2-yl)-2-propyl-1*H*-imidazole-5-carboxylate.

ADDITIONAL REQUIREMENTS
- **PACKAGING AND STORAGE:** Preserve in well-closed containers. Store at controlled room temperature.

Add the following:

- **• LABELING:** When more than one *Dissolution* test is given, the labeling states the *Dissolution* test used only if *Test 1* is not used.• (RB 1-Aug-2017)
- **USP REFERENCE STANDARDS ⟨11⟩**
  USP Olmesartan Medoxomil RS
  USP Olmesartan Medoxomil Related Compound A RS
  1-{[2'-(1*H*-Tetrazol-5-yl)biphenyl-4-yl]methyl}-4,4-dimethyl-2-propyl-1*H*-furo[3,4-*d*]imidazol-6(4*H*)-one.
  $C_{24}H_{24}N_6O_2$ 428.49

Omega-3-Acid Ethyl Esters

DEFINITION
Omega-3-Acid Ethyl Esters is a mixture of ethyl esters, principally the ethyl esters of eicosapentaenoic acid (EPAee) (C20:5 n–3, EE) and docosahexaenoic acid (DHAee) (C22:6 n–3, EE). It may also contain ethyl esters of alpha-linolenic acid (C18:3 n–3, EE), moroctic acid (C18:4 n–3, EE), eicosatetraenoic acid (C20:4 n–3, EE), heneicosapentaenoic acid (C21:5 n–3, EE), and docosapentaenoic acid (C22:5 n–3, EE). Tocopherol may be added as an antioxidant.

IDENTIFICATION
- **A.** The retention times of the principal peaks in *Test solution 4* correspond to those of eicosapentaenoic acid ethyl ester and docosahexaenoic acid ethyl ester in *Standard solution 1b* and *Standard solution 1a*, as obtained in the *Assay*.
- **B.** It meets the acceptance criteria in *Table 1* of the *Assay*.

ASSAY
- **CONTENT OF EPAEE, DHAEE, AND TOTAL OMEGA-3-ACID ETHYL ESTERS**
  (See *Fats and Fixed Oils* ⟨401⟩, *Procedures, Omega-3 Fatty Acids Determination and Profile.*)
  Test solution 3, Test solution 4, Standard solution 1a, Standard solution 1b, System suitability solution 1, Chromatographic system, and **System suitability:** Proceed as directed in *Fats and Fixed Oils* ⟨401⟩, *Procedures, Omega-3 Fatty Acids Determination and Profile.*

Analysis
  Samples: *Test solution 3, Test solution 4, Standard solution 1a,* and *Standard solution 1b*
  Calculate the content of EPAee and DHAee in the portion of Omega-3-Acid Ethyl Esters taken:

$$Result = (R_U/R_S) \times (C_S/C_U)$$

R_U = peak area ratio of the EPAee or DHAee peak to the internal standard peak from *Test solution 3*

R_S = peak area ratio of the EPAee peak to the internal standard peak from *Standard solution 1b* or DHAee peak to the internal standard peak from *Standard solution 1a*

C_S = concentration of USP Eicosapentaenoic Acid Ethyl Ester RS in *Standard solution 1b* or USP Docosahexaenoic Acid Ethyl Ester RS in *Standard solution 1a* (mg/mL)

C_U = concentration of Omega-3-Acid Ethyl Esters in *Test solution 3* (g/mL)

Calculate the content of total omega-3-acid ethyl esters in the portion of Omega-3-Acid Ethyl Esters taken:

$$Result = r_{FAn-3ee}[(EPAee + DHAee)/(r_{EPAee} + r_{DHAee})] + EPAee + DHAee$$

$r_{FAn-3ee}$ = sum of the peak areas of alpha-linolenic acid ethyl ester (C18:3 n–3, EE), moroctic acid ethyl ester (C18:4 n–3, EE), eicosatetraenoic acid ethyl ester (C20:4 n–3, EE), heneicosapentaenoic acid ethyl ester (C21:5 n–3, EE), and docosapentaenoic acid ethyl ester (C22:5 n–3, EE) in *Test solution 4*

$EPAee$ = content of EPAee (mg/g)
$DHAee$ = content of DHAee (mg/g)
r_{EPAee} = peak area of EPAee in *Test solution 4*
r_{DHAee} = peak area of DHAee in *Test solution 4*

  Acceptance criteria: It conforms to the acceptance criteria in *Table 1*. Articles labeled as Omega-3-Acid Ethyl Esters type A meet *Acceptance Criteria II*.

Table 1

Name	Relative Retention Time	Acceptance Criteria I		Acceptance Criteria II (for articles labeled as Omega-3-Acid Ethyl Esters type A)	
		NLT	NMT	NLT	NMT
C18:3 n–3, EE[a]	0.585	—	—	—	—
C18:4 n–3, EE[b]	0.608	—	—	—	—
C20:4 n–3, EE[c]	0.777	—	—	—	—
C20:5 n–3, EE (EPAee)[d]	0.796	430 mg/g	495 mg/g	365 mg/g	435 mg/g
C21:5 n–3, EE[e]	0.889	—	—	—	—

[a] Alpha-linolenic acid ethyl ester.
[b] Moroctic acid ethyl ester.
[c] Eicosatetraenoic acid ethyl ester.
[d] Eicosapentaenoic acid ethyl ester.
[e] Heneicosapentaenoic acid ethyl ester.
[f] Docosapentaenoic acid ethyl ester (clupanodonic acid ethyl ester).
[g] Docosahexaenoic acid ethyl ester.

Table 1 (Continued)

Name	Relative Retention Time	Acceptance Criteria I		Acceptance Criteria II (for articles labeled as Omega-3-Acid Ethyl Esters type A)	
		NLT	NMT	NLT	NMT
C22:5 n–3, EE[f]	0.977	—	—	—	—
C22:6 n–3, EE (DHAee)[g]	1.000	347 mg/g	403 mg/g	290 mg/g	360 mg/g
EPAee + DHAee	—	800 mg/g	880 mg/g	700 mg/g	749 mg/g
Total omega-3-acid ethyl esters	—	90% (w/w)	—	78% (w/w)	—

[a] Alpha-linolenic acid ethyl ester.
[b] Moroctic acid ethyl ester.
[c] Eicosatetraenoic acid ethyl ester.
[d] Eicosapentaenoic acid ethyl ester.
[e] Heneicosapentaenoic acid ethyl ester.
[f] Docosapentaenoic acid ethyl ester (clupanodonic acid ethyl ester).
[g] Docosahexaenoic acid ethyl ester.

IMPURITIES
- **FATS AND FIXED OILS ⟨401⟩:** NMT 0.1 ppm each of lead (Pb), cadmium (Cd), arsenic (As), and mercury (Hg)
- **CHOLESTEROL**
  Internal standard stock solution: 3 mg/mL of 5α-cholestane in *n*-heptane. [NOTE—Prepare fresh before use.]
  Internal standard solution: 0.3 mg/mL of 5α-cholestane in *n*-heptane. [NOTE—Prepare fresh before use.]
  Standard stock solution: 3.0 mg/mL of cholesterol in *n*-heptane. [NOTE—This solution is stable for 6 months stored in a freezer.] Transfer 1.0 mL of this solution to a 10.0-mL volumetric flask. Dilute with *n*-heptane to volume. [NOTE—Prepare this solution fresh daily.]
  Standard solution: Transfer 1.0 mL each of the *Standard stock solution* and the *Internal standard solution* to a 15-mL centrifuge tube. Prepare as directed in the *Sample solution* beginning with "Evaporate to dryness".
  Alpha tocopherol stock solution: 1.5–2.0 mg/mL of USP Alpha Tocopherol RS in *n*-heptane. [NOTE—This solution is stable for 12 months stored in a freezer.]
  System suitability solution: Mix 1.0 mL of the *Standard stock solution*, 1.0 mL of the *Internal standard stock solution*, and 2.0 mL of the *Alpha tocopherol stock solution* in a 50-mL volumetric flask. Evaporate to dryness with the aid of heat, and dilute with ethyl acetate to volume. Dilute 1.0 mL of this solution with ethyl acetate to 10.0 mL. [NOTE—This solution is stable for 6 months stored in a freezer.]
  Sample solution: Transfer 100 mg of Omega-3-Acid Ethyl Esters to a 15-mL centrifuge tube. Add 1.0 mL of the *Internal standard solution*. Evaporate to dryness at about 50° with a gentle stream of nitrogen. Add 0.5 mL of 50% potassium hydroxide and 3 mL of alcohol, fill the tube with nitrogen, and cap. Heat the sample at 100° for 60 min, using a heating block. Cool for about 10 min. Add 6 mL of water to the tube, and shake for 1 min. Extract the solution four times with 2.5-mL portions of ethyl ether, using a vortex mixer or suitable shaker for 1 min for each extraction. Transfer and combine the extracts into a large centrifuge tube, and wash

with 5 mL of water, mixing completely with gentle inversion. Remove the water phase, and add 5 mL of 0.5 M potassium hydroxide to the ether phase, mixing carefully to avoid an emulsion. Remove the potassium hydroxide, and add another 5 mL of water, mixing carefully. Transfer the ether phase to a small centrifuge tube. [NOTE—If an emulsion has occurred, a small amount of sodium chloride may be added to obtain a separation of the phases.] Evaporate the ether phase to dryness under a stream of nitrogen with careful heating. Dissolve the sample in 600 μL of ethyl acetate, and mix well. Transfer 200 μL of this solution to a sample vial, and dilute with ethyl acetate to about 2 mL.
  Chromatographic system
  (See *Chromatography* ⟨621⟩, *System Suitability*.)
  Mode: GC
  Detector: Flame ionization
  Column: 0.25-mm × 30-m capillary; coated with a G27 phase of 0.25-μm thickness
  Temperatures
  Injection port: 320°
  Detector: 300°
  Column: See *Table 2.*

Table 2

Initial Temperature (°)	Temperature Ramp (°/min)	Final Temperature (°)	Hold Time at Final Temperature (min)
170	0	170	1
170	4	320	1.5

  Carrier gas: Helium
  Flow rate: 1.3 mL/min
  Injection volume: 1 μL
  Injection type: Splitless injection system
  System suitability
  Sample: *System suitability solution*
  Suitability requirements
  Resolution: NLT 1.2 between alpha tocopherol and cholesterol
  Analysis
  Samples: *Standard solution* and *Sample solution*
  Calculate the content of total cholesterol in the portion of Omega-3-Acid Ethyl Esters taken:

$$Result = (R_U/R_S) \times (W_S/W_U)$$

  R_U = peak area ratio of the cholesterol peak to the internal standard from the *Sample solution*
  R_S = peak area ratio of the cholesterol peak to the internal standard from the *Standard solution*
  W_S = weight of cholesterol in the *Standard solution* (mg)
  W_U = weight of Omega-3-Acid Ethyl Esters in the *Sample solution* (g)
  Acceptance criteria: NMT 3.0 mg/g
- **OLIGOMERS**
  Mobile phase: Tetrahydrofuran
  System suitability solution: Monodocosahexaenoin, didocosahexaenoin, and tridocosahexaenoin[1] in *Mobile phase*, with concentrations of about 0.5, 0.3, and 0.2 mg/mL, respectively.
  Sample solution 1: 5.0 mg/mL of Omega-3-Acid Ethyl Esters in tetrahydrofuran
  Sample solution 2: [NOTE—Use *Sample solution 2* where the results of this test using *Sample solution 1* exceed the *Acceptance criteria* due to the presence of monoglycerides.] Weigh 50 mg of Omega-3-Acid Ethyl Esters into a quartz tube, add 1.5 mL of a 20-g/L solution of sodium hydroxide in methanol, cover with nitrogen, cap tightly with a polytef-lined cap, mix, and heat

---
[1] Suitable grades of monodocosahexaenoin, didocosahexaenoin, and tridocosahexaenoin may be obtained from Nu-Chek Prep.

on a water bath for 7 min. Allow to cool. Add 2.0 mL of boron trichloride–methanol solution, cover with nitrogen, cap tightly, mix, and heat on a water bath for 30 min. Cool to 40°–50°, add 1 mL of isooctane, cap, and shake vigorously for NLT 30 s. Immediately add 5 mL of saturated sodium chloride solution, cover with nitrogen, cap, and shake thoroughly for NLT 15 s. Transfer the upper layer to a separate tube. Shake the methanol layer with 1 mL of isooctane. Wash the combined isooctane extracts with two quantities, each of 1 mL of water. Carefully evaporate the solvent under a stream of nitrogen, then add 10.0 mL of tetrahydrofuran to the residue. Add a small amount of anhydrous sodium sulfate, and filter.

Chromatographic system
(See *Chromatography ⟨621⟩, System Suitability*.)
Mode: LC
Detector: Differential refractometer
Columns: Three concatenated, 7.8-mm × 30-cm; 7-μm packing L21, with pore sizes in the range of 5–50 nm, arranged with decreasing pore size from the injector to the detector to fulfill the system suitability requirements
Flow rate: 0.8 mL/min
Injection volume: 40 μL
System suitability
Sample: *System suitability solution*
Suitability requirements
  Elution order: Tridocosahexaenoin, didocosahexaenoin, and monodocosahexaenoin
  Resolution: NLT 2.0 between monodocosahexaenoin and didocosahexaenoin; NLT 1.0 between didocosahexaenoin and tridocosahexaenoin
Analysis
Samples: *Sample solution 1* and *Sample solution 2*
Measure the areas of the major peaks.
Calculate the percentage of oligomers in the portion of Omega-3-Acid Ethyl Esters taken to prepare *Sample solution 1*:

$$Result = (r_i/r_T) \times 100$$

r_i = sum of the areas of the peaks with a retention time less than that of the ethyl esters peaks
r_T = sum of the areas of all peaks
Calculate the percentage of oligomers in the portion of Omega-3-Acid Ethyl Esters taken to prepare *Sample solution 2*:

$$Result = (r_i/r_T) \times 100$$

r_i = sum of the areas of all peaks with a retention time less than that of the methyl esters peaks
r_T = sum of the areas of all peaks
Acceptance criteria: NMT 1.0% of oligomers

• **LIMIT OF DIOXINS, FURANS, AND POLYCHLORINATED BIPHENYLS (PCBs):** Determine the content of polychlorinated dibenzo-para-dioxins (PCDDs) and polychlorinated dibenzofurans (PCDFs) by method No. 1613 revision B of the Environmental Protection Agency. Determine the content of polychlorinated biphenyls (PCBs) by method No. 1668 revision A of the Environmental Protection Agency.
Acceptance criteria: The sum of PCDDs and PCDFs is NMT 1 pg/g of WHO toxic equivalents. The sum of PCBs (polychlorinated biphenyls, IUPAC congeners PCB-28, PCB-52, PCB-101, PCB-118, PCB-138, PCB-153, and PCB-180) is NMT 0.5 ppm.

• **LIMIT OF TOTAL UNIDENTIFIED FATTY ACID ETHYL ESTERS**
[NOTE—This test is not required for articles labeled as Omega-3-Acid Ethyl Esters type A.]
From the chromatogram obtained with *Test solution 4* in the *Assay* for *Content of EPAee, DHAee, and Total Omega-3-Acid Ethyl Esters*, determine the peak area of the larg-

est single unidentified peak with a relative retention time different from those in *Table 3*.

Table 3

Identified Ethyl Ester	Relative Retention Time
Phytanic acid	0.416
C16:3 n–4	0.431
C16:4 n–1	0.468
C18:3 n–6	0.557
C18:3 n–4	0.574
C18:3 n–3	0.585
C18:4 n–3	0.608
C18:4 n–1	0.618
Furan acid 5	0.691
C19:5	0.710
C20:3 n–6	0.720
C20:4 n–6	0.736
Furan acid 7	0.744
C20:4 n–3	0.777
Furan acid 8	0.783
EPA	0.796
Furan acid 9	0.867
C21:5 n–3	0.889
C22:4	0.917
Furan acid 10	0.922
C22:5 n–6	0.939
Furan acid 11	0.963
C22:5 n–3	0.977
DHA	1.000

Calculate the content of unidentified fatty acid esters in area percentage:

$$Result = 100 - (100 \times \Sigma \, Aiee/r_T)$$

$Aiee$ = peak area of each identified ethyl ester in *Table 3*
r_T = sum of the areas of all peaks except solvents and BHT
Acceptance criteria: The area of the largest single unidentified peak is NMT 0.5% of the total area. The total area of unidentified peaks as calculated above is NMT 2%.

• **LIMIT OF NON-OMEGA-3-ACID ETHYL ESTERS**
[NOTE—This test is only required for articles labeled as Omega-3-Acid Ethyl Esters type A.]
From the chromatogram obtained with *Test solution 4* in the *Assay* for *Content of EPAee, DHAee, and Total Omega-3-Acid Ethyl Esters*, calculate the amounts of C18:1 n–9 ethyl ester and C20:4 n–6 ethyl ester in the portion of Omega-3-Acid Ethyl Esters taken:

$$Result = (Aiee/r_T) \times 100$$

$Aiee$ = peak area of C18:1 n–9 ethyl ester or C20:4 n–6 ethyl ester
r_T = sum of the areas of all peaks except solvents and BHT
Acceptance criteria
  C18:1 n–9 ethyl ester: NMT 6.0%
  C20:4 n–6 ethyl ester: NMT 4.0%

SPECIFIC TESTS
• **FATS AND FIXED OILS ⟨401⟩**, *Procedures, Acid Value*: NMT 2.0
• **FATS AND FIXED OILS ⟨401⟩**, *Procedures, Anisidine Value*: NMT 15
• **FATS AND FIXED OILS ⟨401⟩**, *Procedures, Peroxide Value*: NMT 10.0

- **ABSORBANCE**
  Sample solution: Transfer 300 mg, accurately weighed, to a 50-mL volumetric flask. Dissolve in and dilute immediately with isooctane to volume. Pipet 2.0 mL into a 50-mL volumetric flask, and dilute with isooctane to volume.
  Acceptance criteria: NMT 0.55, determined at 233 nm, with isooctane being used as the blank

ADDITIONAL REQUIREMENTS
- **PACKAGING AND STORAGE:** Preserve in tight, light-resistant containers under a nitrogen atmosphere. Store at controlled room temperature.

Change to read:

- **LABELING:** The label states the content of DHA ethyl ester and EPA ethyl ester in mg/g, the sum of the EPA and DHA ethyl esters contents in mg/g, and the content of the total omega-3-acid ethyl esters in weight percentage (w/w). It also states the name of any added antioxidant. Articles ▪which▪1S (USP41) meet *Acceptance Criteria II* of the *Assay* and the *Limit of Non-Omega-3-Acid Ethyl Esters* are labeled as Omega-3-Acid Ethyl Esters type A.

Change to read:

- **USP REFERENCE STANDARDS ⟨11⟩**
  ▪● (CN 1-May-2018)
  USP Alpha Tocopherol RS

Omega-3-Acid Ethyl Esters Capsules

DEFINITION
Omega-3-Acid Ethyl Esters Capsules contain Omega-3-Acid Ethyl Esters, with NLT 95.0% and NMT 105.0% of the labeled sum of eicosapentaenoic acid ethyl ester (EPAee) and docosahexaenoic acid ethyl ester (DHAee) and NLT 95% of the labeled amount of total omega-3-acid ethyl esters, as the sum of alpha-linolenic acid ethyl ester (C18:3 n–3, EE), moroctic acid ethyl ester (C18:4 n–3, EE), eicosatetraenoic acid ethyl ester (C20:4 n–3, EE), eicosapentaenoic acid ethyl ester (EPAee) (C20:5 n–3, EE), heneicosapentaenoic acid ethyl ester (C21:5 n–3, EE), docosapentaenoic acid ethyl ester (C22:5 n–3, EE), and docosahexaenoic acid ethyl ester (DHAee) (C22:6 n–3, EE). Tocopherol may be added as an antioxidant.

IDENTIFICATION
- **A.** The retention times of the peaks for eicosapentaenoic acid ethyl ester and docosahexaenoic acid ethyl ester of the *Sample solution* correspond to those of the *Standard solution*, as obtained in the *Assay* for *Content of EPAee, DHAee, and Total Omega-3-Acid Ethyl Esters*.
- **B.** It complies with the *Acceptance criteria* in the test for *Concentration of Omega-3-Acid Ethyl Esters* in *Specific Tests*.

ASSAY
- **CONTENT OF EPAEE, DHAEE, AND TOTAL OMEGA-3-ACID ETHYL ESTERS**
  [NOTE—Carry out the procedure as rapidly as possible, avoiding exposure to actinic light, oxidizing agents, oxidation catalysts (e.g., copper and iron), and air.]
  Antioxidant solution: 50 mg/L of butylated hydroxytoluene in isooctane
  Retention time identification solution: Prepare a mixture containing suitable concentrations of alpha-linolenic acid ethyl ester (C18:3 n–3, EE), moroctic acid ethyl ester (C18:4 n–3, EE), eicosatetraenoic acid ethyl ester (C20:4 n–3, EE), heneicosapentaenoic acid ethyl

ester (C21:5 n–3, EE), and docosapentaenoic acid ethyl ester (C22:5 n–3, EE) in *Antioxidant solution*.[1]
Internal standard solution: 7.0 mg/mL of USP Methyl Tricosanoate RS in *Antioxidant solution*
System suitability solution: 5.5 mg/mL of docosahexaenoic acid methyl ester and 0.5 mg/mL of tetracos-15-enoic acid methyl ester in *Antioxidant solution*
Standard solution: Dissolve 60.0 mg of USP Docosahexaenoic Acid Ethyl Ester RS and 90.0 mg of USP Eicosapentaenoic Acid Ethyl Ester RS in 10.0 mL of *Internal standard solution*.
Sample solution: Weigh NLT 10 Capsules in a tared weighing bottle. With a sharp blade, carefully open the Capsules, without loss of shell material, and transfer the combined Capsule contents to a 100-mL beaker. Remove any adhering substance from the emptied Capsules by washing with several small portions of diethyl ether. Discard the washings, and allow the empty Capsules to air-dry over a period of NMT 30 min, taking precautions to avoid uptake or loss of moisture. Weigh the empty Capsules in the original tared weighing bottle, and calculate the average fill weight per Capsule (W_{AF}). Transfer an amount of the combined Capsule contents equivalent to 225 mg of the labeled amount of total omega-3-acid ethyl esters to a suitable flask, and dissolve with 10.0 mL of *Internal standard solution*.
Chromatographic system
(See *Chromatography* ⟨621⟩, *System Suitability*.)
Mode: GC
Detector: Flame ionization
Column: 0.25-mm × 25–50-m fused silica capillary; coated with a 0.25-μm film of phase G16
Temperatures
Injection port: 250°
Detector: 270°
Column: See *Table 1*.

Table 1

Initial Temperature (°)	Temperature Ramp (°/min)	Final Temperature (°)	Hold Time at Final Temperature (min)
170	0	170	2
170	3.5	255	9

Carrier gas: Hydrogen or helium
Linear velocity: Adjust to obtain a retention time for docosahexaenoic acid ethyl ester of 26 ± 3 min.
Injection volume: 1 μL
Injection type: Split; split ratio, 1:220
System suitability
Samples: *System suitability solution* and *Standard solution*
Suitability requirements
Resolution: NLT 1.2 between the docosahexaenoic acid methyl ester and tetracos-15-enoic acid methyl ester peaks, *System suitability solution*
Relative standard deviation: NMT 2.0% for the ratios of the peak responses of DHAee and EPAee relative to the internal standard, *Standard solution*
Analysis
Samples: *Retention time identification solution*, *Standard solution*, and *Sample solution*
Identify the retention times of the relevant fatty acid ethyl esters by comparing the peaks from the *Sample solution* with those from the *Retention time identification solution*.
Calculate the content, in mg/g, of EPAee and DHAee in the portion of Capsules taken:

$$Result = (R_U/R_S) \times (C_S/C_U)$$

[1] The relevant fatty acid ethyl esters are available from Nu-Chek Prep, Inc. (www.nu-chekprep.com); Cayman Chemical (www.caymanchem.com); and Carbosynth (www.carbosynth.com).

R_U = peak area ratio of the EPAee or DHAee peak to the internal standard peak from the *Sample solution*

R_S = peak area ratio of the EPAee or DHAee peak to the internal standard peak from the *Standard solution*

C_S = concentration of USP Eicosapentaenoic Acid Ethyl Ester RS or USP Docosahexaenoic Acid Ethyl Ester RS in the *Standard solution* (mg/mL)

C_U = Capsule fill content of the *Sample solution* (g/mL)

Calculate the percentage of the labeled sum of EPAee and DHAee in the portion of Capsules taken:

$$Result = (EPAee + DHAee) \times W_{AF} \times (100/L)$$

$EPAee$ = content of EPAee in the portion of Capsules taken (mg/g)

$DHAee$ = content of DHAee in the portion of Capsules taken (mg/g)

W_{AF} = average fill weight of the Capsules taken (g)

L = sum of the labeled content of EPAee and DHAee (mg/Capsule)

Calculate the percentage of the labeled amount of total omega-3-acid ethyl esters in the portion of Capsules taken:

$$Result = \{r_{FAn-3ee} \times [(EPAee + DHAee)/(r_{EPAee} + r_{DHAee})] + EPAee + DHAee\} \times W_{AF} \times (100/L)$$

$r_{FAn-3ee}$ = sum of the peak areas of alpha-linolenic acid ethyl ester (C18:3 n–3, EE), moroctic acid ethyl ester (C18:4 n–3, EE), eicosatetraenoic acid ethyl ester (C20:4 n–3, EE), heneicosapentaenoic acid ethyl ester (C21:5 n–3, EE), and docosapentaenoic acid ethyl ester (C22:5 n–3, EE) from the *Sample solution*

$EPAee$ = content of EPAee (mg/g)

$DHAee$ = content of DHAee (mg/g)

r_{EPAee} = peak area of EPAee from the *Sample solution*

r_{DHAee} = peak area of DHAee from the *Sample solution*

W_{AF} = average fill weight of the Capsules taken (g)

L = label claim of total omega-3-acids ethyl esters (mg/Capsule)

Acceptance criteria: 95.0%–105.0% of the labeled sum of EPAee and DHAee and NLT 95.0% of the labeled amount of total omega-3-acid ethyl esters per Capsule

PERFORMANCE TESTS

- **UNIFORMITY OF DOSAGE UNITS** ⟨905⟩, *Weight Variation*: Meet the requirements
- **DISINTEGRATION** ⟨701⟩
  Medium, tier 1: Water
  Medium, tier 2: Simulated gastric fluid TS
  Time: 30 min
  Analysis: Perform the test with water as *Medium, tier 1*. Repeat the test with simulated gastric fluid TS as *Medium, tier 2*, if the disintegration time is more than 30 min in *Medium, tier 1*.
  Acceptance criteria: Meet the requirements

IMPURITIES

- **OLIGOMERS**
  Mobile phase: Tetrahydrofuran
  System suitability solution: Monodocosahexaenoin, didocosahexaenoin, and tridocosahexaenoin in *Mobile phase*, with concentrations of about 0.5, 0.3, and 0.2 mg/mL, respectively. [NOTE—Suitable grades of monodocosahexaenoin, didocosahexaenoin, and tridocosahexaenoin may be obtained from Nu-Chek Prep.]
  Sample solution 1: 5.0 mg/mL of the Capsule contents in tetrahydrofuran

Sample solution 2: [NOTE—Use *Sample solution 2* where the results of this test using *Sample solution 1* exceed the *Acceptance criteria* due to the presence of monoglycerides.] Weigh 50 mg of the Capsule contents into a quartz tube, add 1.5 mL of a 20-g/L solution of sodium hydroxide in methanol, cover with nitrogen, cap tightly with a polytef-lined cap, mix, and heat on a water bath for 7 min. Allow to cool. Add 2.0 mL of boron trichloride–methanol solution, cover with nitrogen, cap tightly, mix, and heat on a water bath for 30 min. Cool to 40°–50°, add 1 mL of isooctane, cap, and shake vigorously for NLT 30 s. Immediately add 5 mL of saturated sodium chloride solution, cover with nitrogen, cap, and shake thoroughly for NLT 15 s. Transfer the upper layer to a separate tube. Shake the methanol layer with 1 mL of isooctane. Wash the combined isooctane extracts with 2 quantities, each of 1 mL of water. Carefully evaporate the solvent under a stream of nitrogen, then add 10.0 mL of tetrahydrofuran to the residue. Add a small amount of anhydrous sodium sulfate, and filter.

Chromatographic system
(See *Chromatography* ⟨621⟩, *System Suitability*.)
Mode: LC
Detector: Differential refractometer
Columns: Three concatenated, 7.8-mm × 30-cm; 7-μm packing L21, with pore sizes in the range of 5–50 nm, arranged with decreasing pore size from the injector to the detector to fulfill the system suitability requirements
Flow rate: 0.8 mL/min
Injection volume: 40 μL
System suitability
Sample: *System suitability solution*
Suitability requirements
Elution order: Tridocosahexaenoin, didocosahexaenoin, and monodocosahexaenoin
Resolution: NLT 2.0 between monodocosahexaenoin and didocosahexaenoin; NLT 1.0 between didocosahexaenoin and tridocosahexaenoin
Analysis
Samples: *Sample solution 1* and *Sample solution 2*
Measure the areas of the major peaks.
Calculate the percentage of oligomers in the portion of omega-3-acid ethyl esters taken to prepare *Sample solution 1*:

$$Result = (r_I/r_T) \times 100$$

r_I = sum of the peak areas with retention times less than that of the ethyl esters peak from *Sample solution 1*

r_T = sum of the areas of all peaks from *Sample solution 1*

Calculate the percentage of oligomers in the portion of the Capsules contents taken to prepare *Sample solution 2*:

$$Result = (r_I/r_T) \times 100$$

r_I = sum of the peak areas with retention times less than that of the methyl esters peak from *Sample solution 2*

r_T = sum of the areas of all peaks from *Sample solution 2*

Acceptance criteria: NMT 2% of oligomers

SPECIFIC TESTS

- **CONCENTRATION OF OMEGA-3-ACID ETHYL ESTERS**
  Antioxidant solution, Retention time identification solution, Internal standard solution, System suitability solution, Standard solution, Sample solution, Chromatographic system, System suitability, and Analysis: Proceed as directed in the *Assay* for *Content of EPAee, DHAee, and Total Omega-3-Acid Ethyl Esters*.

Calculate the concentration, in mg/g, of EPAee and DHAee in the portion of Capsules taken:

$$Result = (R_U/R_S) \times (C_S/C_U)$$

R_U = peak area ratio of the EPAee or DHAee peak to the internal standard peak from the *Sample solution*

R_S = peak area ratio of the EPAee or DHAee peak to the internal standard peak from the *Standard solution*

C_S = concentration of USP Eicosapentaenoic Acid Ethyl Ester RS or USP Docosahexaenoic Acid Ethyl Ester RS in the *Standard solution* (mg/mL)

C_U = Capsule fill content of the *Sample solution* (g/mL)

Calculate the concentration, in mg/g, of total omega-3-acids ethyl esters in the portion of Capsules taken:

$$Result = r_{FAn-3ee} \times [(EPAee + DHAee)/(r_{EPAee} + r_{DHAee})] + EPAee + DHAee$$

$r_{FAn-3ee}$ = sum of the peak areas of alpha-linolenic acid ethyl ester (C18:3 n–3, EE), moroctic acid ethyl ester (C18:4 n–3, EE), eicosatetraenoic acid ethyl ester (C20:4 n–3, EE), heneicosapentaenoic acid ethyl ester (C21:5 n–3, EE), and docosapentaenoic acid ethyl ester (C22:5 n–3, EE) from the *Sample solution*

$EPAee$ = content of EPAee (mg/g)

$DHAee$ = content of DHAee (mg/g)

r_{EPAee} = peak area of EPAee from the *Sample solution*

r_{DHAee} = peak area of DHAee from the *Sample solution*

Acceptance criteria: It meets the requirements in *Table 2*. Capsules labeled as containing Omega-3-Acid Ethyl Esters type A meet *Acceptance Criteria II*.

Table 2

Name	Acceptance Criteria I		Acceptance Criteria II (for Capsules labeled as containing Omega-3-Acid Ethyl Esters type A)	
	NLT	NMT	NLT	NMT
EPAee	430 mg/g	495 mg/g	365 mg/g	435 mg/g
DHAee	347 mg/g	403 mg/g	290 mg/g	360 mg/g
EPAee + DHAee	800 mg/g	880 mg/g	700 mg/g	749 mg/g
Total omega-3-acid ethyl esters[a]	90% (w/w)	—	78% (w/w)	—

[a] Sum of alpha-linolenic acid ethyl ester (C18:3 n–3, EE), moroctic acid ethyl ester (C18:4 n–3, EE), eicosatetraenoic acid ethyl ester (C20:4 n–3, EE), heneicosapentaenoic acid ethyl ester (EPAee) (C20:5 n–3, EE), heneicosapentaenoic acid ethyl ester (C21:5 n–3, EE), docosapentaenoic acid ethyl ester (C22:5 n–3, EE), and docosahexaenoic acid ethyl ester (DHAee) (C22:6 n–3, EE).

• **FATS AND FIXED OILS ⟨401⟩,** *Procedures, Acid Value*
Sample solution: Dissolve about 5.0 g of the oil, accurately weighed, in 100 mL of a mixture of equal volumes of alcohol and ether (which has been neutralized to phenolphthalein with 0.1 M potassium hydroxide) contained in a flask.
Acceptance criteria: NMT 2.0
• **FATS AND FIXED OILS ⟨401⟩,** *Procedures, Anisidine Value*:
NMT 25
• **FATS AND FIXED OILS ⟨401⟩,** *Procedures, Peroxide Value*:
NMT 10 mEq/kg

• **ABSORBANCE**
Sample solution: Transfer 300 mg, accurately weighed, to a 50-mL volumetric flask. Dissolve in and dilute immediately with isooctane to volume. Pipet 2.0 mL into a 50-mL volumetric flask, and dilute with isooctane to volume.
Acceptance criteria: NMT 0.60, determined at 233 nm in a 1-cm cell, with isooctane being used as the blank
• **MICROBIAL ENUMERATION TESTS ⟨61⟩:** NMT 10^3 cfu/g for the total aerobic microbial count, and NMT 10^2 cfu/g for the total combined yeasts and molds count.
• **TESTS FOR SPECIFIED MICROORGANISMS ⟨62⟩:** Meet the requirements for absence of *Escherichia coli* in 1 g and for absence of *Salmonella* species in 10 g

ADDITIONAL REQUIREMENTS
• **PACKAGING AND STORAGE:** Preserve in tight containers, and store at controlled room temperature. Do not freeze. Protect from light.

Change to read:

• **LABELING:** The label states the amount of docosahexaenoic acid (DHA) ethyl ester and eicosapentaenoic acid (EPA) ethyl ester, and the minimum amount of total content of omega-3-acid ethyl esters in mg/Capsule. Capsules ■which■₁S (USP41) meet *Acceptance Criteria II* of the test for *Concentration of Omega-3-Acid Ethyl Esters* are labeled as containing Omega-3-Acid Ethyl Esters type A. It also states the name and content of any added antioxidant.
• **USP REFERENCE STANDARDS ⟨11⟩**
USP Docosahexaenoic Acid Ethyl Ester RS
All *cis*-4,7,10,13,16,19-docosahexaenoic ethyl ester.
$C_{24}H_{36}O_2$ 356.55
USP Eicosapentaenoic Acid Ethyl Ester RS
All *cis*-5,8,11,14,17-eicosapentaenoic ethyl ester.
$C_{22}H_{34}O_2$ 330.51
USP Methyl Tricosanoate RS
Tricosanoic acid methyl ester.
$C_{24}H_{48}O_2$ 368.64

Oxybutynin Chloride Extended-Release Tablets

DEFINITION
Oxybutynin Chloride Extended-Release Tablets contain NLT 90.0% and NMT 110.0% of the labeled amount of oxybutynin chloride ($C_{22}H_{31}NO_3 \cdot HCl$).

IDENTIFICATION
• **A. INFRARED ABSORPTION ⟨197⟩**
Standard: Dissolve 15 mg of USP Oxybutynin Chloride RS in 5 mL of water. Adjust with 0.1 N sodium hydroxide to a pH of between 7 and 8. Extract the solution twice with 10 mL of ether. Combine the extracts, evaporate the ether, and dry under vacuum over silica gel for at least 30 min. Redissolve the dried residue in a small amount of acetone, transfer the solution to an IR salt plate, and evaporate to cast a thin film.
Sample: Add a quantity of finely powdered Tablets, equivalent to about 15 mg of oxybutynin chloride, to 5 mL of water per Tablet. Mix for 1 min. Adjust with 0.1 N sodium hydroxide to a pH between 7 and 8. Extract the solution twice with 10 mL of ether. Combine the extracts, evaporate the ether, and dry under vacuum over silica gel for at least 30 min. Redissolve the dried residue in a small amount of acetone, transfer the solution to an IR salt plate, and evaporate to cast a thin film.

- **B.** The retention time of the major peak of the *Sample solution* corresponds to that of the *Standard solution*, as obtained in the *Assay*.

ASSAY
- **PROCEDURE**
  Diluent: Use water adjusted with phosphoric acid to a pH of 3.5.
  Solution A: Methanol and acetonitrile (1:1)
  Mobile phase: Acetonitrile, triethylamine, and water (700:3:1300). Adjust with phosphoric acid to a pH of 3.9.
  Impurity stock solution: 0.11 mg/mL of USP Oxybutynin Related Compound A RS in acetonitrile
  Standard stock solution: 0.37 mg/mL of USP Oxybutynin Chloride RS in acetonitrile
  System suitability solution: Transfer 10 mL of the *Standard stock solution* and 1 mL of the *Impurity stock solution* to a 100-mL volumetric flask, and dilute with *Diluent* to volume.
  Standard solution: 0.1 mg/mL of USP Oxybutynin Chloride RS in *Diluent* from the *Standard stock solution*
  Sample solution
    For Tablets that contain 5 mg of oxybutynin chloride: Place 10 Tablets in a 500-mL volumetric flask, add 150 mL of *Solution A*, and stir for at least 4 h or until dissolved. Dilute with *Diluent* to volume. Mix thoroughly, centrifuge, and use the clear supernatant.
    For Tablets that contain 10 mg or more of oxybutynin chloride: Place 10 Tablets in a 1000-mL volumetric flask, add 300 mL of *Solution A*, and stir for at least 4 h or until dissolved. Dilute with *Diluent* to volume. If necessary, make a further dilution with *Diluent* to obtain a solution having a final concentration equivalent to 0.1 mg/mL of oxybutynin chloride. Mix thoroughly, centrifuge, and use the clear supernatant.
  Chromatographic system
  (See *Chromatography* ⟨621⟩, *System Suitability*.)
    Mode: LC
    Detector: UV 220 nm
    Column: 4.6-mm × 15-cm; packing L11
    Flow rate: 1.5 mL/min
    Injection volume: 50 µL
  System suitability
    Sample: *System suitability solution*
    [NOTE—The relative retention times for oxybutynin and oxybutynin related compound A are about 1.0 and 1.6, respectively.]
    Suitability requirements
      Resolution: NLT 1.5 between oxybutynin and oxybutynin related compound A
      Tailing factor: Greater than 0.75 and NMT 2.5 for each peak
      Relative standard deviation: NMT 3% for each compound for six replicate injections
  Analysis
    Samples: *Standard solution* and *Sample solution*
    Calculate the percentage of the labeled amount of oxybutynin chloride ($C_{22}H_{31}NO_3 \cdot HCl$) in the portion of Tablets taken:

$$Result = (r_U/r_S) \times (C_S/C_U) \times 100$$

r_U = peak response from the *Sample solution*
r_S = peak response from the *Standard solution*
C_S = concentration of USP Oxybutynin Chloride RS in the *Standard solution* (mg/mL)
C_U = nominal concentration of oxybutynin chloride in the *Sample solution* (mg/mL)

Acceptance criteria: 90.0%–110.0%

PERFORMANCE TESTS

Change to read:

- **DISSOLUTION ⟨711⟩**
  Test 1
    Medium: Simulated gastric fluid without enzyme; 50 mL
    Apparatus 7: See *Drug Release* ⟨724⟩, 30 cycles/min; 2–3-cm amplitude, at 37.0 ± 0.5°
    Times: 4, 10, and 24 h
    Solution A: 4.83 g/L of monobasic sodium phosphate in water. Add 2.3 mL/L of triethylamine, and adjust with phosphoric acid to a pH of 2.2 ± 0.2.
    Mobile phase: Acetonitrile and *Solution A* (7:13)
    Solution B: To 1 L of water add phosphoric acid dropwise to a pH of 3.5, and mix well.
    Standard stock solutions: 250, 300, and 350 µg/mL of USP Oxybutynin Chloride RS in acetonitrile
    Standard solutions: Prepare a series of dilutions of the *Standard stock solutions* in *Solution B* having final concentrations similar to those expected in the *Sample solution*.
    System suitability solution: Use a medium range *Standard solution* of USP Oxybutynin Chloride RS.
    Sample solution: Use portions of the solution under test. If the solution is cloudy, centrifuge at 2000 rpm for 10 min, and use the supernatant.
  Chromatographic system
  (See *Chromatography* ⟨621⟩, *System Suitability*.)
    Mode: LC
    Detector: UV 230 nm
    Column: 4.6-mm × 5-cm; packing L11
    Column temperature: 35°
    Flow rate: 1.5 mL/min
    Injection volume: 50 µL
  System suitability
    Sample: *System suitability solution*
    Suitability requirements
      Tailing factor: Greater than 0.5 and less than 2.5
      Relative standard deviation: NMT 2.0%
  Analysis
    Samples: *Standard solutions* and *Sample solution*
    Construct a calibration curve by plotting the peak response versus concentration of the *Standard solutions*. A weighing factor, $1/x$, is applied to the regression line of the calibration curve to enhance the accuracy of the low standard concentrations. Determine the percentage of oxybutynin chloride ($C_{22}H_{31}NO_3 \cdot HCl$) dissolved in each interval from a linear regression analysis of the calibration curve.
    Tolerances: See *Tables 1* and *2*.

Table 1. For Tablets Labeled to Contain 5 or 10 mg of Oxybutynin Chloride

Time (h)	Amount Dissolved
4	NMT 20%
10	34.5%–59.5%
24	NLT 80%

Table 2. For Tablets Labeled to Contain 15 mg of Oxybutynin Chloride

Time (h)	Amount Dissolved
4	NMT 20%
10	34.5%–59.5%
24	NLT 75%

The percentages of the labeled amount of oxybutynin chloride ($C_{22}H_{31}NO_3 \cdot HCl$) dissolved at the times specified conform to *Dissolution* ⟨711⟩, *Acceptance Table 2*.

Test 2: If the product complies with this test, the labeling indicates that the product meets USP *Dissolution Test 2*.

Acid stage medium: Simulated gastric fluid, without enzymes, pH 1.2 ± 0.05; 250 mL (first row)

Buffer stage medium: Simulated intestinal fluid, without enzymes, pH 6.8 ± 0.1; 250 mL (rows 2–4)

Apparatus 3: 25 dips/min; 20-mesh polypropylene screen on top and bottom; 30 s drip time

Times: 2 h in the *Acid stage medium* (first row); 4, 8, and 16 h (corresponding to 2, 6, and 14 h after changing the medium) in the *Buffer stage medium* (rows 2–4)

Solution A: Transfer 1 mL of triethylamine to 1000 mL of water. Adjust with phosphoric acid to a pH of 3.50 ± 0.05.

Mobile phase: Acetonitrile and *Solution A* (4:1)

Standard stock solution: 0.2 mg/mL of USP Oxybutynin Chloride RS in *Acid stage medium*

Working standard solution: Transfer 5.0 mL of the *Standard stock solution* for Tablets labeled to contain 5 mg, transfer 10 mL for Tablets labeled to contain 10 mg, or transfer 15 mL for Tablets labeled to contain 15 mg to a 100-mL volumetric flask. Dilute with *Buffer stage medium* to volume.

Sample solution: Centrifuge a portion of the solution under test at approximately 3000 rpm for 10 min. Use the supernatant.

Chromatographic system
(See *Chromatography* ⟨621⟩, *System Suitability*.)
Mode: LC
Detector: UV 203 nm
Column: 4.6-mm × 25-cm; packing L7
Flow rate: 1.5 mL/min
Injection volume: 25 µL
System suitability
Sample: *Working standard solution*
Suitability requirements
Tailing factor: NMT 2.0
Relative standard deviation: NMT 3.0%
Analysis
Samples: *Working standard solution* and *Sample solution*
Calculate the percentage of the labeled amount of oxybutynin chloride ($C_{22}H_{31}NO_3 \cdot HCl$) dissolved at each time point (C_{T2}, C_{T4}, C_{T8}, C_{T16}):

$$C_i = (r_U/r_S) \times (C_S/L) \times V \times 100$$

r_U = peak response from the *Sample solution*
r_S = peak response from the *Working standard solution*
C_S = concentration of the *Working standard solution* (mg/mL)
L = label claim (mg/Tablet)
V = volume of *Medium*, 250 mL
C_{T2} = percentage dissolved at 2 h, C_2
C_{T4} = percentage dissolved at 4 h, $C_2 + C_4$
C_{T8} = percentage dissolved at 8 h, $C_2 + C_4 + C_8$
C_{T16} = percentage dissolved at 16 h, $C_2 + C_4 + C_8 + C_{16}$

Tolerances: See *Tables 3* and *4*.

Table 3. For Tablets Labeled to Contain 5 or 10 mg of Oxybutynin Chloride

Time (h)	Amount Dissolved
2	0%–10%
4	10%–30%

Table 3. For Tablets Labeled to Contain 5 or 10 mg of Oxybutynin Chloride (Continued)

Time (h)	Amount Dissolved
8	40%–65%
16	NLT 80%

Table 4. For Tablets Labeled to Contain 15 mg of Oxybutynin Chloride

Time (h)	Amount Dissolved
2	0%–10%
4	10%–30%
8	35%–65%
16	NLT 75%

The percentages of the labeled amount of oxybutynin chloride ($C_{22}H_{31}NO_3 \cdot HCl$) dissolved at the times specified conform to *Dissolution* ⟨711⟩, *Acceptance Table 2*.

Test 3: If the product complies with this test, the labeling indicates that the product meets USP *Dissolution Test 3*.

Medium: Simulated gastric fluid without enzyme; 50 mL

Apparatus 7: See *Drug Release* ⟨724⟩. Use acrylic rods. 30 dips/min, 37.0 ± 0.5°, 10 s drip time. Dip time interval: row 1, 1 h; row 2, 3 h; row 3, 6 h; row 4, 5 h; row 5, 9 h.

Times: 4, 10, and 24 h

pH 2.3 phosphate buffer: 3.4 g/L of monobasic potassium phosphate in water. Adjust with phosphoric acid or 2 N potassium hydroxide to a pH of 2.30 ± 0.05.

Standard solution: ($L/200$) mg/mL of USP Oxybutynin Chloride RS in *Medium*, where L is the label claim, in mg/Tablet

Sample solution: Pass a portion of the solution under test through a suitable nylon filter of 0.45-µm pore size, discarding the first few mL.

Mobile phase: *pH 2.3 phosphate buffer* and acetonitrile (7:3)

Chromatographic system
(See *Chromatography* ⟨621⟩, *System Suitability*.)
Mode: LC
Detector: UV 220 nm
Column: 4.6-mm × 15-cm; packing L10
Flow rate: 1.0 mL/min
Injection volume: 10 µL
System suitability
Sample: *Standard solution*
Suitability requirements
Tailing factor: NMT 2.0
Relative standard deviation: NMT 2.0%
Analysis
Samples: *Standard solution* and *Sample solution*
Calculate the amount, in mg, of oxybutynin chloride ($C_{22}H_{31}NO_3 \cdot HCl$) dissolved at each time interval:

$$Result = (r_U/r_S) \times (C_S/L) \times V$$

r_U = peak response from the *Sample solution*
r_S = peak response from the *Standard solution*
C_S = concentration of the *Standard solution* (mg/mL)
L = label claim (mg/Tablet)
V = volume of *Medium*, 50 mL

Calculate the percentage of the labeled amount of oxybutynin dissolved:

$$Result = \Sigma(\text{amount dissolved at current time interval} + \text{amount dissolved at previous time intervals}) \times 100/L$$

Tolerances: See *Table 5.*

Table 5

Time (h)	Amount Dissolved
4	NMT 25%
10	40%–65%
24	NLT 75%

The percentages of the labeled amount of oxybutynin chloride ($C_{22}H_{31}NO_3 \cdot HCl$) dissolved at the times specified conform to *Dissolution* ⟨711⟩, *Acceptance Table 2.*

Test 4: If the product complies with this test, the labeling indicates that the product meets USP *Dissolution Test 4.*

Acid stage medium: 0.1 N hydrochloric acid; 900 mL

Buffer stage medium: pH 6.0 sodium phosphate buffer with 0.2% of sodium lauryl sulfate; 900 mL

Apparatus 2: 50 rpm, with sinkers. [NOTE—A suitable sinker is available as catalog number CAPWHT-2S from www.QLA-LLC.com.]

Times: 2 h in the *Acid stage medium*; 4, 6, and 14 h (corresponding to 2, 4, 12 h after changing the medium) in the *Buffer stage medium*

Standard solution: (L/1000) mg/mL of USP Oxybutynin Chloride RS in *Buffer stage medium*, where L is the label claim, in mg/Tablet

Sample solution: Pass a portion of the solution under test through a suitable PVDF filter of 0.45-μm pore size.

pH 3.5 phosphate buffer: 6.94 g/L of monobasic potassium phosphate in water. Adjust with diluted phosphoric acid to a pH of 3.50 ± 0.05.

Mobile phase: *pH 3.5 phosphate buffer* and acetonitrile (1:1)

Chromatographic system
(See *Chromatography* ⟨621⟩, *System Suitability*.)
Mode: LC
Detector: UV 210 nm
Column: 4.6-mm × 15-cm; packing L7
Flow rate: 1.0 mL/min
Injection volume: 20 μL
System suitability
Sample: *Standard solution*
Suitability requirements
 Column efficiency: NLT 2000 theoretical plates
 Tailing factor: NMT 2.0
 Relative standard deviation: NMT 2.0%
Analysis
Samples: *Standard solution* and *Sample solution*
Calculate the concentration (C_i) in mg/mL of oxybutynin chloride ($C_{22}H_{31}NO_3 \cdot HCl$) at each time point ($i$):

$$C_i = (r_U/r_S) \times C_S$$

r_U = peak response from the *Sample solution*
r_S = peak response from the *Standard solution*
C_S = concentration of the *Standard solution* (mg/mL)

Calculate the cumulative percentage of the labeled amount of oxybutynin chloride ($C_{22}H_{31}NO_3 \cdot HCl$) dissolved ($Q_i$) at each time point ($i$):
At i = 1

$$Q_1 = (C_1 \times V/L) \times 100$$

At i = 2 to n

$$\frac{(C_1 \times 900) + \sum\limits_{j=2}^{n-1} C_j V_s + C_n \times [900 - (n-2)V_s] \times 100}{L}$$

i = 1, 2, ..., n
j = 2, 3, ..., n–1
C_i = concentration of oxybutynin chloride in the *Sample solution* at time point i (mg/mL)
C_j = concentration of oxybutynin chloride in the *Sample solution* at time point 2 through n–1 (mg/mL)
V_s = sampling volume (mL)
L = label claim (mg/Tablet)
Tolerances: See *Table 6.*

Table 6

Time (h)	Amount Dissolved
2	NMT 10%
4	10%–40%
6	40%–75%
14	NLT 85%

The percentages of the labeled amount of oxybutynin chloride ($C_{22}H_{31}NO_3 \cdot HCl$) dissolved at the times specified conform to *Dissolution* ⟨711⟩, *Acceptance Table 2.*

Test 5: If the product complies with this test, the labeling indicates that the product meets USP *Dissolution Test 5.*

Medium: Acetate buffer pH 4.5, prepared as follows. Transfer 2.99 g of sodium acetate to a 1000-mL volumetric flask, dissolve in 700 mL of water, adjust with glacial acetic acid to a pH of 4.5, and dilute with water to volume; 900 mL.

Apparatus 2: 75 rpm
Times: 2, 8, 12, and 24 h
Standard stock solution: 0.28 mg/mL of USP Oxybutynin Chloride RS in acetonitrile. Use sonication, if necessary.

Standard solution: (L/900) mg/mL of USP Oxybutynin Chloride RS in *Medium*, where L is the label claim, in mg/Tablet, from the *Standard stock solution*

Sample solution: Pass a portion of the solution under test through a suitable PVDF filter of 0.45-μm pore size, discarding the first few mL of the filtrate. Replace the portion of solution withdrawn with an equal volume of *Medium*.

pH 3.5 phosphate buffer: 6.94 g/L of monobasic potassium phosphate in water. Adjust with phosphoric acid to a pH of 3.50 ± 0.05.

Mobile phase: *pH 3.5 phosphate buffer* and acetonitrile (1:1)

Chromatographic system
(See *Chromatography* ⟨621⟩, *System Suitability*.)
Mode: LC
Detector: UV 210 nm
Column: 4.6-mm × 15-cm; 5-μm packing L7
Flow rate: 1.0 mL/min
Injection volume: 20 μL
System suitability
Sample: *Standard solution*
Suitability requirements
 Column efficiency: NLT 2000 theoretical plates
 Tailing factor: NMT 2.0
 Relative standard deviation: NMT 2.0% for six replicate injections
Analysis
Samples: *Standard solution* and *Sample solution*
Calculate the concentration (C_i), in mg/mL, of oxybutynin chloride ($C_{22}H_{31}NO_3 \cdot HCl$) in the sample withdrawn from the vessel at each point (i):

$$Result_i = (r_U/r_S) \times C_S$$

r_U = peak response from the *Sample solution*
r_S = peak response from the *Standard solution*

C_S = concentration of the *Standard solution* (mg/mL)

Calculate the percentage of the labeled amount of oxybutynin chloride ($C_{22}H_{31}NO_3 \cdot HCl$) dissolved at each time point (*i*):

$$Result_1 = C_1 \times V \times (1/L) \times 100$$

$$Result_2 = [(C_2 \times V) + (C_1 \times V_S)] \times (1/L) \times 100$$

$$Result_3 = \{(C_3 \times V) + [(C_2 + C_1) \times V_S]\} \times (1/L) \times 100$$

$$Result_4 = \{(C_4 \times V) + [(C_3 + C_2 + C_1) \times V_S]\} \times (1/L) \times 100$$

C_i = concentration of oxybutynin chloride in the portion of the sample withdrawn at the specified time point (mg/mL)
V = volume of *Medium*, 900 mL
L = label claim (mg/Tablet)
V_S = volume of the *Sample solution* withdrawn at each time point and replaced with *Medium* (mL)

Tolerances: See *Table 7*.

Table 7

Time (h)	Amount Dissolved
2	NMT 10%
8	30%–50%
12	55%–75%
24	NLT 85%

The percentages of the labeled amount of oxybutynin chloride ($C_{22}H_{31}NO_3 \cdot HCl$) dissolved at the times specified conform to *Dissolution ⟨711⟩, Acceptance Table 2*.

•**Test 6:** If the product complies with this test, the labeling indicates that the product meets USP *Dissolution Test 6*.

Medium: Simulated gastric fluid without enzyme; 50 mL

Apparatus 7: See *Drug Release ⟨724⟩*; Tablets glued to stainless steel rods with water insoluble glue. At the end of each specified test interval, the systems are transferred to the next row of new tubes containing 50 mL of fresh *Medium*, 30 cycles/min; 2–3 cm amplitude.

Times: 4, 10, and 24 h

Calculate the percentage of the labeled amount of oxybutynin chloride ($C_{22}H_{31}NO_3 \cdot HCl$) dissolved by using the following method.

Buffer: 4.83 g/L of monobasic sodium phosphate in water. Add 2.3 mL/L of triethylamine, and adjust with phosphoric acid to a pH of 2.2 ± 0.2.

Mobile phase: Acetonitrile and *Buffer* (25:75)

Diluent: To 1 L of water add phosphoric acid dropwise to a pH of 3.5, and mix well.

Standard stock solution: 0.5 mg/mL of USP Oxybutynin Chloride RS in acetonitrile

Standard solution: 0.05 mg/mL of USP Oxybutynin Chloride RS in *Diluent* from *Standard stock solution*

Sample solution: Pass a portion of the solution under test through a suitable PVDF filter of 0.45-µm pore size, discarding the first few milliliters of the filtrate. Dilute with *Diluent*, if necessary, to obtain a solution with a concentration similar to that of the *Standard solution*.

Chromatographic system
(See *Chromatography ⟨621⟩, System Suitability*.)

Mode: LC
Detector: UV 230 nm
Column: 4.6-mm × 5-cm; 5-µm packing L11
Column temperature: 35°
Flow rate: 1.5 mL/min
Injection volume: 50 µL
System suitability
Sample: *Standard solution*
Suitability requirements
Tailing factor: 0.5–2.5
Relative standard deviation: NMT 2.0%
Analysis
Samples: *Standard solution* and *Sample solution*
Calculate the concentration (C_i), in mg/mL, of oxybutynin chloride ($C_{22}H_{31}NO_3 \cdot HCl$) in the sample withdrawn from the vessel at each time point (*i*) shown in *Table 8*:

$$C_i = (r_U/r_S) \times C_S$$

r_U = peak response of oxybutynin from the *Sample solution*
r_S = peak response of oxybutynin from the *Standard solution*
C_S = concentration of USP Oxybutynin Chloride RS in the *Standard solution* (mg/mL)

Calculate the percentage of the labeled amount of oxybutynin chloride ($C_{22}H_{31}NO_3 \cdot HCl$) dissolved at each time point shown in *Table 8*:

$$Result_1 = C_1 \times V \times D \times (1/L) \times 100$$

$$Result_2 = (C_2 + C_1) \times V \times D \times (1/L) \times 100$$

$$Result_3 = (C_1 + C_2 + C_3) \times V \times D \times (1/L) \times 100$$

C_i = concentration of oxybutynin chloride in the portion of sample withdrawn at time point *i* (mg/mL)
V = volume of *Medium*, 50 mL
D = dilution factor for the *Sample solution*
L = label claim (mg/Tablet)

Tolerances: See *Table 8*.

Table 8

Time (h)	Amount Dissolved (%)
4	NMT 20
10	35–60
24	NLT 80

The percentages of the labeled amount of oxybutynin chloride ($C_{22}H_{31}NO_3 \cdot HCl$) dissolved at the times specified conform to *Dissolution ⟨711⟩, Acceptance Table 2*.• (RB 1-Aug-2017)

• **UNIFORMITY OF DOSAGE UNITS ⟨905⟩:** Meet the requirements

IMPURITIES
• **ORGANIC IMPURITIES**
Diluent, Solution A, Mobile phase, Impurity stock solution, System suitability solution, Sample solution, Chromatographic system, and **System suitability:** Proceed as directed in the *Assay*.
Impurity standard solution: 1 µg/mL of USP Oxybutynin Related Compound A RS in *Diluent* from the *Impurity stock solution*
Analysis
Samples: *Impurity standard solution* and *Sample solution*

Calculate the percentage of each impurity in the portion of Tablets taken:

$$Result = (r_U/r_S) \times (C_S/C_U) \times 100$$

r_U = peak response of each impurity from the *Sample solution*
r_S = peak response from the *Impurity standard solution*
C_S = concentration of USP Oxybutynin Related Compound A RS in the *Standard solution* (mg/mL)
C_U = nominal concentration of the *Sample solution* (mg/mL)

[NOTE—Disregard any peak less than 0.1%.]

Acceptance criteria
Individual impurities: NMT 1% of oxybutynin related compound A is found.
Total impurities: NMT 2%

ADDITIONAL REQUIREMENTS
- **PACKAGING AND STORAGE:** Preserve in tight containers. Store at controlled room temperature.
- **LABELING:** When more than one *Dissolution* test is given, the labeling states the *Dissolution* test used only if *Test 1* is not used.
- **USP REFERENCE STANDARDS ⟨11⟩**
  USP Oxybutynin Chloride RS
  USP Oxybutynin Related Compound A RS
  Phenylcyclohexylglycolic acid.
  $C_{14}H_{18}O_3$ 234.30

Pantoprazole Sodium

$C_{16}H_{14}F_2N_3NaO_4S \cdot 1.5H_2O$ 432.37
1*H*-Benzimidazole, 5-(difluoromethoxy)-2-[[(3,4-dimethoxy-2-pyridyl)methyl]sulfinyl]-, sodium salt, hydrate (2:3);
5-(Difluoromethoxy)-2-[[(3,4-dimethoxy-2-pyridyl)methyl]sulfinyl]benzimidazole, sodium salt, sesquihydrate [164579-32-2].

DEFINITION
Pantoprazole Sodium contains NLT 98.0% and NMT 102.0% of pantoprazole sodium ($C_{16}H_{14}F_2N_3NaO_4S$), calculated on the anhydrous basis.

IDENTIFICATION

Change to read:

- **A. INFRARED ABSORPTION ■⟨197⟩:** [NOTE—Methods described in ⟨197K⟩ or ⟨197A⟩ may be used.]■1S (USP41)
- **B.** The retention time of the major peak of the *Sample solution* corresponds to that of the *Standard solution*, as obtained in the *Assay*.

Change to read:

- **C. ●IDENTIFICATION TESTS—GENERAL ⟨191⟩,** *Chemical Identification Tests, Sodium:●* (CN 1-May-2018) Meets the requirements of ●test A.● (CN 1-May-2018)

ASSAY

Change to read:

- **PROCEDURE**
  ■[NOTE—Protect solutions containing pantoprazole sodium from light.]■1S (USP41)
  Ammonium phosphate buffer: 1.32 g/L of dibasic ammonium phosphate in water, adjusted with phosphoric acid to a pH of 7.5
  Acetonitrile–methanol mixture: Acetonitrile and methanol (7:3)
  Solution A: *Acetonitrile–methanol mixture* and *Ammonium phosphate buffer* (15:85)
  Solution B: *Acetonitrile–methanol mixture*
  Mobile phase: See *Table 1*. Return to original conditions and re-equilibrate the system for 10 min.

Table 1

Time (min)	Solution A (%)	Solution B (%)
0	86	14
10	86	14
35	42	58

Diluent: Dilute 25 mL of ammonium hydroxide with water to 500 mL.
System suitability stock solution: 0.5 mg/mL each of USP Pantoprazole Sodium RS, USP Pantoprazole Related Compound A RS, and USP Pantoprazole Related Compound B RS in a mixture of acetonitrile and water (1:1)
System suitability solution: 0.005 mg/mL each of USP Pantoprazole Sodium RS, USP Pantoprazole Related Compound A RS, and USP Pantoprazole Related Compound B RS in *Diluent*, from *System suitability stock solution*
Standard stock solution: 0.4 mg/mL of USP Pantoprazole Sodium RS, dissolved first in a mixture of acetonitrile and water (1:1) using 10%–20% of the final volume, and then diluted with *Diluent* to volume
Standard solution: 0.06 mg/mL of USP Pantoprazole Sodium RS in *Diluent*, from *Standard stock solution*
Sample stock solution: Transfer about 20 mg of Pantoprazole Sodium to a 50-mL volumetric flask. Dissolve in 5–10 mL of a mixture of acetonitrile and water (1:1), and dilute with *Diluent* to volume.
Sample solution: 0.06 mg/mL of Pantoprazole Sodium in *Diluent*, from *Sample stock solution*
Chromatographic system
(See *Chromatography* ⟨621⟩, *System Suitability*.)
Mode: LC
Detector: UV 285 nm
Column: 3.9-mm × 15-cm; 4-μm packing L1
Temperatures
Autosampler: 4°
Column: 30°
Flow rate: 1 mL/min
Injection volume: 20 μL
System suitability
Samples: *System suitability solution* and *Standard solution*
[NOTE—Identify the components based on their relative retention times (see *Table 2*).]
Suitability requirements
Resolution: NLT 10.0 between pantoprazole related compound A and pantoprazole, *System suitability solution*
Relative standard deviation: ■NMT 0.73%,■1S (USP41) *Standard solution*

Analysis

Samples: *Standard solution* and *Sample solution*

Calculate the percentage of pantoprazole sodium ($C_{16}H_{14}F_2N_3NaO_4S$) in the portion of Pantoprazole Sodium taken:

$$Result = (r_U/r_S) \times (C_S/C_U) \times 100$$

r_U = peak response from the *Sample solution*
r_S = peak response from the *Standard solution*
C_S = concentration of USP Pantoprazole Sodium RS in the *Standard solution* (mg/mL)
C_U = concentration of Pantoprazole Sodium in the *Sample solution* (mg/mL)

Acceptance criteria: 98.0%–102.0% on the anhydrous basis

IMPURITIES

Delete the following:

•• **HEAVY METALS,** *Method II* ⟨231⟩: NMT 20 ppm• (Official 1-Jan-2018)

Change to read:

• **ORGANIC IMPURITIES**

[NOTE—On the basis of the synthetic route, perform either *Test 1* or *Test 2*. *Test 2* is recommended when impurities C, D, E, and F are potential related compounds.]

■[NOTE—Protect solutions containing pantoprazole sodium from light.]■1S (USP41)

Test 1

■1S (USP41)

Ammonium phosphate buffer, Mobile phase, Diluent, System suitability solution, Standard stock solution, Sample stock solution, and **Chromatographic system:** Proceed as directed in the *Assay*.

Standard solution: 0.0004 mg/mL of USP Pantoprazole Sodium RS in *Diluent*, from *Standard stock solution*

Sample solution: *Sample stock solution*

System suitability

Samples: *System suitability solution* ■and *Standard solution*■1S (USP41)

[NOTE—See *Table 2* for relative retention times.]

Suitability requirements

Resolution: NLT 10.0 between pantoprazole related compound A and pantoprazole, *System suitability solution*

■**Relative standard deviation:** NMT 10.0%, *Standard solution*■1S (USP41)

Analysis

Samples: *Standard solution* and *Sample solution*

Calculate the percentage of each impurity in the portion of Pantoprazole Sodium taken:

$$Result = (r_U/r_S) \times (C_S/C_U) \times 100$$

r_U = peak response of each impurity from the *Sample solution*
r_S = peak response of pantoprazole from the *Standard solution*
C_S = concentration of USP Pantoprazole Sodium RS in the *Standard solution* (mg/mL)
C_U = concentration of Pantoprazole Sodium in the *Sample solution* (mg/mL)

Acceptance criteria: See *Table 2*. The reporting level for impurities is 0.05%.

Table 2

Name	Relative Retention Time	Acceptance Criteria, NMT (%)
■Pantoprazole sulfone■1S (USP41) (pantoprazole related compound A)	0.52	0.20
Pantoprazole	1.0	—
■Pantoprazole sulfide■1S (USP41) (pantoprazole related compound B)	1.7	0.15
Any other individual impurity	—	0.10
Total impurities	—	0.5

Test 2

Solution A: 1.74 g/L of dibasic potassium phosphate adjusted with a solution of phosphoric acid (330 g/L) to a pH of 7.00 ± 0.05

Solution B: Acetonitrile

Mobile phase: See *Table 3*. Return to original conditions and re-equilibrate the system for 15 min.

Table 3

Time (min)	Solution A (%)	Solution B (%)
0	80	20
40	20	80

Diluent: Acetonitrile and 0.001 N sodium hydroxide (1:1)

System suitability solution: About 0.46 mg/mL of USP Pantoprazole Sodium RS, and about 1.3 µg/mL each of USP Pantoprazole Related Compound A RS, USP Pantoprazole Related Compound B RS, USP Pantoprazole Related Compound C RS, USP Pantoprazole Related Compound D and F Mixture RS, and USP Pantoprazole Related Compound E RS in *Diluent*

Standard solution: 0.03 mg/mL of USP Pantoprazole Sodium RS in *Diluent*

Sample solution: 0.46 mg/mL of Pantoprazole Sodium in *Diluent*

Chromatographic system

(See *Chromatography* ⟨621⟩, *System Suitability*.)

Mode: LC

Detector: UV 290 and 305 nm

Column: 4.6-mm × 12.5-cm; 5-µm packing L1

Column temperature: 40°

Flow rate: 1 mL/min

Injection volume: 20 µL

System suitability

Samples: *System suitability solution* and *Standard solution* at 290 nm

[NOTE—See *Table 4* for relative retention times.]

Suitability requirements

Resolution: NLT 1.5 between pantoprazole related compound E and pantoprazole related compound D and F, *System suitability solution*

Tailing factor: NMT 2.0, *Standard solution*

Relative standard deviation: NMT 5.0%, *Standard solution*

Analysis

[NOTE—Pantoprazole related compound C is monitored at 305 nm, and all other compounds are monitored at 290 nm.]

Samples: *Standard solution* and *Sample solution*

Calculate the percentage of each impurity in the portion of Pantoprazole Sodium taken:

$$Result = (r_U/r_S) \times (C_S/C_U) \times (1/F) \times 100$$

r_U = peak response of each impurity from the *Sample solution*
r_S = peak response of pantoprazole sodium from the *Standard solution*

C_S = concentration of USP Pantoprazole Sodium RS in the *Standard solution* (mg/mL)

C_U = concentration of Pantoprazole Sodium in the *Sample solution* (mg/mL)

F = relative response factor (see *Table 4*)

Acceptance criteria: See *Table 4* for individual impurities. The reporting level for impurities is 0.05%.

■**Table 4**

Name	Relative Retention Time	Relative Response Factor	Acceptance Criteria, NMT (%)
Benzimidazolethiol derivative (pantoprazole related compound C)	0.6	3.3	0.10[a]
Pantoprazole sulfone (pantoprazole related compound A)	0.9	1.0	0.20
Pantoprazole	1.0	—	—
N^1-Methyl pantoprazole (pantoprazole related compound D) and N^3-Methyl pantoprazole (pantoprazole related compound F)	1.2	1.0	0.20[b]
Pantoprazole dimer (pantoprazole related compound E)	1.3	1.0	0.10
Pantoprazole sulfide (pantoprazole related compound B)	1.5	1.0	0.15
Any other individual impurity	—	—	0.10
Total impurities	—	—	0.5

[a] At 305 nm.

[b] Impurities D and F are not fully resolved and should be integrated together.

■1S (USP41)

SPECIFIC TESTS

Change to read:

• **WATER DETERMINATION ⟨921⟩,** *Method I:* ■4.5%■1S (USP41)–8.0%

ADDITIONAL REQUIREMENTS
• **PACKAGING AND STORAGE:** Preserve in well-closed, light-resistant containers. Store at room temperature.
• **LABELING:** If a test for *Organic Impurities* other than *Test 1* is used, then the labeling states the test with which the article complies.
• **USP REFERENCE STANDARDS ⟨11⟩**
USP Pantoprazole Sodium RS
USP Pantoprazole Related Compound A RS
5-(Difluoromethoxy)-2-[[(3,4-dimethoxy-2-pyridyl)methyl]sulfonyl]-1*H*-benzimidazole.
$C_{16}H_{15}F_2N_3O_5S$ 399.37
USP Pantoprazole Related Compound B RS
5-(Difluoromethoxy)-2-[[(3,4-dimethoxy-2-pyridyl)methyl]thio]-1*H*-benzimidazole.
$C_{16}H_{15}F_2N_3O_3S$ 367.37
USP Pantoprazole Related Compound C RS
5-(Difluoromethoxy)-1*H*-benzimidazole-2-thiol.
$C_8H_6F_2N_2OS$ 216.21
USP Pantoprazole Related Compound D and F Mixture RS
A mixture of 5-(difluoromethoxy)-2-[(*RS*)-[(3,4-dimethoxypyridin-2-yl)methyl]sulfinyl]-1-methyl-1*H*-benzimidazole and 6-(difluoromethoxy)-2-[(*RS*)-[(3,4-dimethoxypyridin-2-yl)methyl]sulfinyl]-1-methyl-1*H*-benzimidazole.
$C_{17}H_{17}F_2N_3O_4S$ 397.40
USP Pantoprazole Related Compound E RS
A mixture of the stereoisomers of 6,6'-bis(difluoromethoxy)-2,2'-bis[[(3,4-dimethoxypyridin-2-yl)methyl]sulfinyl]-1*H*,1'*H*-5,5'-bibenzimidazolyl.
$C_{34}H_{28}F_4N_6O_8S_2$ 764.74

Pentazocine

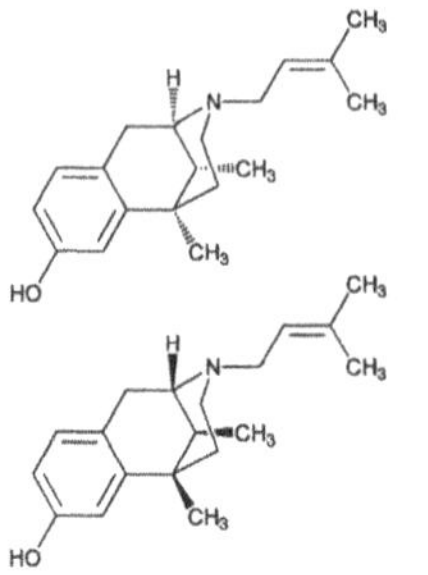

$C_{19}H_{27}NO$ 285.42
2,6-Methano-3-benzazocin-8-ol, 1,2,3,4,5,6-hexahydro-6,11-dimethyl-3-(3-methyl-2-butenyl)-, (2α,6α,11*R**)-;
(2*R**,6*R**,11*R**)-1,2,3,4,5,6-Hexahydro-6,11-dimethyl-3-(3-methyl-2-butenyl)-2,6-methano-3-benzazocin-8-ol
[359-83-1].

DEFINITION

Change to read:

Pentazocine contains NLT 98.0% and NMT ■102.0%■1S (USP41) of pentazocine ($C_{19}H_{27}NO$), calculated on the dried basis.

IDENTIFICATION

Change to read:

• **A. ■INFRARED ABSORPTION ⟨197⟩:** [NOTE—Methods described in ⟨197K⟩ or ⟨197A⟩ may be used.]■1S (USP41)

Delete the following:

■• **B. ULTRAVIOLET ABSORPTION ⟨197U⟩**
Sample solution: 80 µg/mL in 0.01 N hydrochloric acid
Analytical wavelength: 278 nm
Acceptance criteria: Absorptivities do not differ by more than 3.0%, calculated on the dried basis.■1S (USP41)

Add the following:

■• **B.** The retention time of the pentazocine peak of the *Sample solution* corresponds to that of the *Standard solution*, as obtained in the *Assay.*■1S (USP41)

ASSAY

Change to read:

• **PROCEDURE**
■**Solution A:** 15 mM sodium borate in water. Adjust with 10 N sodium hydroxide to a pH of 10.0.

Solution B: Methanol
Mobile phase: See *Table 1*.

Table 1

Time (min)	Solution A (%)	Solution B (%)
0	85	15
15	15	85
20	15	85
21	85	15
25	85	15

Diluent: Methanol, phosphoric acid, and water (500:1:500)
Standard solution: 0.025 mg/mL of USP Pentazocine RS in *Diluent*
Sample solution: 0.025 mg/mL of Pentazocine in *Diluent*
Chromatographic system
(See *Chromatography* ⟨621⟩, *System Suitability*.)
Mode: LC
Detector: UV 225 nm
Column: 4.6-mm × 10-cm; 2.6-μm packing L1
Column temperature: 40°
Flow rate: 0.5 mL/min
Injection volume: 20 μL
System suitability
Sample: *Standard solution*
Suitability requirements
Tailing factor: NMT 2.0
Relative standard deviation: NMT 0.73%
Analysis
Samples: *Standard solution* and *Sample solution*
Calculate the percentage of pentazocine ($C_{19}H_{27}NO$) in the portion of Pentazocine taken:

$$Result = (r_U/r_S) \times (C_S/C_U) \times 100$$

r_U = peak response of pentazocine from the *Sample solution*
r_S = peak response of pentazocine from the *Standard solution*
C_S = concentration of USP Pentazocine RS in the *Standard solution* (mg/mL)
C_U = concentration of Pentazocine in the *Sample solution* (mg/mL)■1S (USP41)
Acceptance criteria: 98.0%–■102.0%■1S (USP41) on the dried basis

IMPURITIES
• **RESIDUE ON IGNITION** ⟨281⟩: NMT 0.2%

Delete the following:

■• **ORDINARY IMPURITIES** ⟨466⟩
Standard solution: Methanol
Test solution: Methanol
Eluant: Chloroform, methanol, and isopropylamine (94:3:3)
Visualization: Heat the plate in an oven at 105° for 15 min. Cool, follow with visualization technique 17, and view under short-wavelength UV light.
Acceptance criteria: Meets the requirements■1S (USP41)

Add the following:

■• **ORGANIC IMPURITIES**
Solution A, Solution B, Mobile phase, Diluent, and Chromatographic system: Proceed as directed in the *Assay*.
Sensitivity solution: 0.0006 mg/mL of USP Pentazocine RS in *Diluent*

Standard solution: 0.002 mg/mL of USP Pentazocine RS in *Diluent*
Sample solution: 2 mg/mL of Pentazocine in *Diluent*. Sonicate to dissolve, if necessary.
System suitability
Samples: *Sensitivity solution* and *Standard solution*
Suitability requirements
Relative standard deviation: NMT 5.0%, *Standard solution*
Signal-to-noise ratio: NLT 10, *Sensitivity solution*
Analysis
Samples: *Standard solution* and *Sample solution*
Calculate the percentage of each impurity in the portion of Pentazocine taken:

$$Result = (r_U/r_S) \times (C_S/C_U) \times 100$$

r_U = peak response of each impurity from the *Sample solution*
r_S = peak response of pentazocine from the *Standard solution*
C_S = concentration of USP Pentazocine RS in the *Standard solution* (mg/mL)
C_U = concentration of Pentazocine in the *Sample solution* (mg/mL)
Acceptance criteria: See *Table 2*. The reporting threshold is 0.03%.

Table 2

Name	Relative Retention Time	Acceptance Criteria, NMT (%)
Norpentazocine[a]	0.6	0.15
Pentazocine hydration product[b]	0.9	0.15
Pentazocine	1.0	—
Any unspecified impurity	—	0.10
Total impurities	—	1.0

[a] (2R,6R,11R)-1,2,3,4,5,6-Hexahydro-6,11-dimethyl-2,6-methano-3-benzazocin-8-ol.
[b] (2R,6R,11R)-3-(3-Hydroxy-3-methylbutyl)-6,11-dimethyl-1,2,3,4,5,6-hexahydro-2,6-methanobenzo[d]azocin-8-ol.

■1S (USP41)

SPECIFIC TESTS

Delete the following:

■• **MELTING RANGE OR TEMPERATURE** ⟨741⟩: 147°–158°, with slight darkening■1S (USP41)

Add the following:

■• **BACTERIAL ENDOTOXINS TEST** ⟨85⟩: The level of bacterial endotoxins is such that the requirement in the relevant dosage form monograph(s) in which Pentazocine is used can be met. Where the label states that Pentazocine must be subjected to further processing during the preparation of injectable dosage forms, the level of bacterial endotoxins is such that the requirement in the relevant dosage form monograph(s) in which Pentazocine is used can be met.■1S (USP41)
• **LOSS ON DRYING** ⟨731⟩
Analysis: Dry at a pressure of NMT 5 mm of mercury at 60° to constant weight.
Acceptance criteria: NMT 1.0%

ADDITIONAL REQUIREMENTS
• **PACKAGING AND STORAGE:** Preserve in tight, light-resistant containers.

Add the following:

■● LABELING: Where Pentazocine must be subjected to further processing during the preparation of injectable dosage forms to ensure acceptable levels of bacterial endotoxins, it is so labeled.■1S (USP41)

● **USP REFERENCE STANDARDS ⟨11⟩**
USP Pentazocine RS

Delete the following:

■Perphenazine Injection

» Perphenazine Injection is a sterile solution of Perphenazine in Water for Injection, prepared with the aid of Citric Acid. It contains not less than 90.0 percent and not more than 110.0 percent of the labeled amount of $C_{21}H_{26}ClN_3OS$, as the citrate.

Packaging and storage—Preserve in single-dose or multiple-dose containers, preferably of Type I glass, protected from light.

Change to read:

USP Reference standards ⟨11⟩—
● ● (CN 1-May-2018)
USP Perphenazine RS
[NOTE—Throughout the following procedures, protect test or assay specimens, the USP Reference Standard, and solutions containing them, by conducting the procedures without delay, under subdued light, or using low-actinic glassware.]
Identification—Dilute 1 mL with methanol to 5 mL. Apply 5 µL each of this solution and a solution of *USP Perphenazine RS* in methanol containing 1 mg per mL to a suitable thin-layer chromatographic plate, coated with a 0.25-mm layer of chromatographic silica gel. Develop the chromatogram in a solvent system consisting of a mixture of acetone and ammonium hydroxide (200:1) until the solvent front has moved about 15 cm. Air-dry the plate, and spray lightly with a solution of iodoplatinic acid prepared by dissolving 100 mg of chloroplatinic acid in 1 mL of 1 N hydrochloric acid, adding 25 mL of potassium iodide solution (4 in 100), diluting with water to 100 mL, and adding 0.50 mL of formic acid: the R_F value of the principal spot obtained from the Injection corresponds to that obtained from the Standard solution.
Bacterial Endotoxins Test ⟨85⟩—It contains not more than 35.7 USP Endotoxin Units per mg of perphenazine.
pH ⟨791⟩: between 4.2 and 5.6.
Other requirements—It meets the requirements under *Injections and Implanted Drug Products ⟨1⟩*.
Assay—
Acid-alcohol solution—Transfer 10 mL of hydrochloric acid to a 1000-mL flask containing 500 mL of alcohol and 300 mL of water. Dilute with water to volume.
Palladium chloride solution—Dissolve 100 mg of palladium chloride in a mixture of 1 mL of hydrochloric acid and 50 mL of water in a 100-mL volumetric flask, heating on a steam bath to effect solution. Cool, dilute with water to volume, and mix. Store in an amber bottle and use within 30 days. On the day of use, transfer 50 mL to a 500-mL

volumetric flask, add 4 mL of hydrochloric acid and 4.1 g of anhydrous sodium acetate, dilute with water to volume, and mix.
Standard preparation—Dissolve an accurately weighed quantity of *USP Perphenazine RS* in *Acid-alcohol solution* to obtain a solution having a known concentration of about 150 µg per mL.
Assay preparation—Dilute 3.0 mL of Injection with *Acid-alcohol solution* to 100 mL in a volumetric flask.
Procedure—Mix 10.0 mL each of the *Assay preparation* and the *Standard preparation* with 15.0 mL of *Palladium chloride solution*, filter, if necessary, and concomitantly determine the absorbances of these solutions, against a reagent blank, in 1-cm cells at the wavelength of maximum absorbance at about 480 nm, with a suitable spectrophotometer. Calculate the quantity, in mg, of $C_{21}H_{26}ClN_3OS$ in the volume of Injection taken by the formula:

$$0.1C(A_U / A_S)$$

in which C is the concentration, in µg per mL, of *USP Perphenazine RS* in the *Standard preparation*, and A_U and A_S are the absorbances of the solutions from the *Assay preparation* and the *Standard preparation*, respectively.
■1S (USP41)

Delete the following:

■Perphenazine Oral Solution

» Perphenazine Oral Solution contains not less than 90.0 percent and not more than 110.0 percent of the labeled amount of perphenazine ($C_{21}H_{26}ClN_3OS$).

Packaging and storage—Preserve in well-closed, light-resistant containers.
USP Reference standards ⟨11⟩—
USP Perphenazine RS
[NOTE—Throughout the following procedures, protect test or assay specimens, the USP Reference Standard, and solutions containing them, by conducting the procedures without delay, under subdued light, or using low-actinic glassware.]
Identification—It meets the requirements for the *Identification* test under *Perphenazine Injection*.
Uniformity of dosage units ⟨905⟩—
FOR ORAL SOLUTION PACKAGED IN SINGLE-UNIT CONTAINERS: meets the requirements.
Deliverable volume ⟨698⟩—
FOR ORAL SOLUTION PACKAGED IN MULTIPLE-UNIT CONTAINERS: meets the requirements.
Limit of perphenazine sulfoxide—
Mobile phase, Resolution solution, Standard preparation, and*Chromatographic system*—Proceed as directed in the *Assay*.
Test preparation—Transfer an accurately measured portion of Oral Solution, equivalent to about 16 mg of perphenazine, to a 200-mL volumetric flask, dissolve in and dilute with methanol to volume, mix, and filter.
Procedure—Inject a volume (about 10 µL) of the *Test preparation* into the chromatograph, record the chromatogram, and measure the peak responses. Calculate the per-

centage of perphenazine sulfoxide in the portion of Oral Solution taken by the formula:

$$100(r_i / r_s)$$

in which r_i is the peak response of perphenazine sulfoxide (relative retention time of about 0.72); and r_s is the sum of the responses of all the peaks: not more than 5.0% of perphenazine sulfoxide is found.

Assay—

Mobile phase—Prepare a filtered and degassed mixture of 0.01 M ammonium acetate, acetonitrile, and methanol (48:39:13). Adjust with glacial acetic acid to a pH of 4.5. Make adjustments if necessary (see *System Suitability* under *Chromatography* ⟨621⟩).

Resolution solution—Dissolve suitable quantities of brompheniramine maleate and USP Perphenazine RS in methanol to obtain a solution having known concentrations of about 40 µg per mL and 8 µg per mL, respectively.

Standard preparation—Dissolve an accurately weighed quantity of USP Perphenazine RS in methanol, dilute quantitatively, and stepwise if necessary, with methanol to obtain a solution having a known concentration of about 8.0 µg per mL, and filter.

Assay preparation—Transfer an accurately measured portion of Oral Solution, equivalent to about 16 mg of perphenazine, to a 200-mL volumetric flask, dissolve in and dilute with methanol to volume, and mix. Dilute quantitatively, and stepwise if necessary, with methanol to obtain a solution having a concentration of about 8.0 µg per mL, and filter.

Chromatographic system (see *Chromatography* ⟨621⟩)—The liquid chromatograph is equipped with a 254-nm detector and a 3.9-mm × 30-cm column that contains packing L11. The flow rate is about 1.5 mL per minute. Chromatograph the *Resolution solution,* and record the peak responses as directed for *Procedure:* the relative retention times are about 0.6 for brompheniramine and 1.0 for perphenazine; and the resolution, *R,* between brompheniramine and perphenazine is not less than 3.0. Chromatograph the *Standard preparation,* and record the peak responses as directed for *Procedure:* the tailing factor is not more than 3.0; and the relative standard deviation for replicate injections is not more than 2.0%.

Procedure—Separately inject equal volumes (about 10 µL) of the *Standard preparation* and the *Assay preparation* into the chromatograph, record the chromatograms, and measure the responses for the major peaks. Calculate the quantity, in mg, of perphenazine ($C_{21}H_{26}ClN_3OS$) in the portion of Oral Solution taken by the formula:

$$2000C(r_U / r_S)$$

in which *C* is the concentration, in mg per mL, of USP Perphenazine RS in the *Standard preparation;* and r_U and r_S are the peak responses obtained from the *Assay preparation* and the *Standard preparation,* respectively.

▪1S (USP41)

Delete the following:

▪Perphenazine Syrup

» Perphenazine Syrup contains not less than 90.0 percent and not more than 110.0 percent of the labeled amount of perphenazine ($C_{21}H_{26}ClN_3OS$).

USP Reference standards ⟨11⟩—
USP Perphenazine RS
[NOTE—Throughout the following procedures, protect test or assay specimens, the USP Reference Standard, and solutions containing them, by conducting the procedures without delay, under subdued light, or using low-actinic glassware.]

Identification—Add 10 mL of water to a volume of Syrup, equivalent to about 4 mg of perphenazine, render alkaline by dropwise addition of sodium hydroxide to a pH of 11 to 12, and extract with four 5-mL portions of chloroform, combining the extracts through a bed of anhydrous sodium sulfate in a funnel into a beaker. Evaporate the extracts on a steam bath nearly to dryness, and dissolve the residue in 4 mL of methanol: the solution so obtained responds to the *Identification* test under *Perphenazine Injection.*

Uniformity of dosage units ⟨905⟩—

FOR SYRUP PACKAGED IN SINGLE-UNIT CONTAINERS: meets the requirements.

Deliverable volume ⟨698⟩—

FOR SYRUP PACKAGED IN MULTIPLE-UNIT CONTAINERS: meets the requirements.

Assay—

Acid-alcohol solution and *Palladium chloride solution*—Prepare as directed in the *Assay* under *Perphenazine Injection.*

Standard preparation—Dissolve an accurately weighed quantity of *USP Perphenazine RS* in *Acid-alcohol solution* to obtain a solution having a known concentration of about 160 µg per mL.

Assay preparation—Transfer an accurately measured volume of Syrup, equivalent to about 6 mg of perphenazine, to a 25-mL volumetric flask, dilute with water to volume, and mix. Transfer 10 mL to a 125-mL separator, add 25 mL of water, adjust with ammonium hydroxide to a pH of 10 to 11, and extract with four 20-mL portions of chloroform, filtering the extracts through anhydrous sodium sulfate. Evaporate the combined extracts on a steam bath with the aid of a stream of nitrogen to about 5 mL. Complete the evaporation without application of heat, and dissolve the residue in 15.0 mL of *Acid-alcohol solution,* filtering if necessary.

Procedure—Mix 10.0 mL each of the *Assay preparation* and the *Standard preparation* with 15.0 mL of *Palladium chloride solution,* filter if necessary, and concomitantly determine the absorbances of these solutions, against a reagent blank, in 1-cm cells at the wavelength of maximum absorbance at about 480 nm, with a suitable spectrophotometer. Calculate the quantity, in mg, of perphenazine ($C_{21}H_{26}ClN_3OS$) in each mL of the Syrup taken by the formula:

$$0.0375(C/V)(A_U / A_S)$$

in which *C* is the concentration, in µg per mL, of *USP Perphenazine RS* in the *Standard preparation;* *V* is the volume, in mL, of Syrup taken; and A_U and A_S are the absorbances of the solutions from the *Assay preparation* and the *Standard preparation,* respectively.

▪1S (USP41)

Phenoxybenzamine Hydrochloride Capsules

DEFINITION

Phenoxybenzamine Hydrochloride Capsules contain NLT 90.0% and NMT 110.0% of the labeled amount of phenoxybenzamine hydrochloride ($C_{18}H_{22}ClNO \cdot HCl$).

IDENTIFICATION

- **A.** The UV absorption spectra of the phenoxybenzamine peak of the *Sample solution* exhibit maxima and minima at the same wavelengths as those of the corresponding peak from the *Standard solution*, as obtained in the *Assay*.
- **B.** The retention time of the major peak of the *Sample solution* corresponds to that of the *Standard solution*, as obtained in the *Assay*.

ASSAY

Change to read:

- **PROCEDURE**
  Solution A: 2.2 mg/mL of anhydrous monobasic sodium phosphate in water. Adjust with phosphoric acid to a pH of 3.0.
  Mobile phase: Filtered and degassed mixture of *Solution A* and acetonitrile (45:55)
  Standard solution: 0.2 mg/mL of USP Phenoxybenzamine Hydrochloride RS in acetonitrile. [NOTE—Sonicate if necessary.]
  System suitability solution: 10 mL of the *Standard solution* and 0.5 mL of 0.1 N sodium hydroxide taken in a vial. [NOTE—Basic solutions of phenoxybenzamine hydrochloride will produce the known degradant, tertiary amine phenoxybenzamine—the second major peak that elutes before the phenoxybenzamine peak and has a relative retention time of about 0.3 and an unknown related substance. Severe degradation of the drug substance will be observed if the solution is allowed to stand for more than 1 h.]
  Sample solution: Nominally 0.2 mg/mL of phenoxybenzamine hydrochloride in acetonitrile prepared as follows. Remove, as completely as possible, the contents of NLT 20 Capsules. Transfer a portion of the mixed powder, equivalent to about 10 mg of phenoxybenzamine hydrochloride, to a 50-mL volumetric flask. Add about 40 mL of acetonitrile, and sonicate for 15 min with occasional swirling. Cool, and dilute with acetonitrile to volume to obtain the concentration, based on the label claim. Allow the sample to stand undisturbed for 30 min such that the undissolved material settles to the bottom. Transfer the top clear solution into HPLC vials, and use as the *Sample solution*.
  Chromatographic system
  (See *Chromatography ⟨621⟩, System Suitability.*)
  Mode: LC
  Detector
   Assay: UV 268 nm
   Identification A: Diode array, UV 240–340 nm
  Column: 4.6-mm × 150-cm; •5 µm• (RB 1-Oct-2017) packing L7
  Flow rate: 1 mL/min
  Injection volume: 10 µL
  System suitability
  Samples: *Standard solution* and *System suitability solution*
  • (RB 1-Oct-2017)
  Suitability requirements
   Resolution: NLT 4 between phenoxybenzamine and the unknown peak eluting after the phenoxybenzamine peak (at about 9.4 min), *System suitability solution*
   Relative standard deviation: NMT 2%, *Standard solution*
  Analysis
  Samples: *Standard solution* and *Sample solution*
  Calculate the percentage of the labeled amount of phenoxybenzamine hydrochloride ($C_{18}H_{22}ClNO \cdot HCl$) in the portion of Capsules taken:

$$Result = (r_U/r_S) \times (C_S/C_U) \times 100$$

r_U = peak response •of phenoxybenzamine• (RB 1-Oct-2017) from the *Sample solution*
r_S = peak response •of phenoxybenzamine• (RB 1-Oct-2017) from the *Standard solution*
C_S = concentration of USP Phenoxybenzamine Hydrochloride RS in the *Standard solution* (mg/mL)
C_U = nominal concentration of phenoxybenzamine hydrochloride in the *Sample solution* (mg/mL)
Acceptance criteria: 90.0%–110.0%

PERFORMANCE TESTS

Change to read:

- **DISSOLUTION ⟨711⟩**
  Medium: 0.1 N hydrochloric acid; 500 mL
  Apparatus 1: 100 rpm
  Time: 45 min
  Buffer: 2.2 g/L of monobasic sodium phosphate in water. Adjust with phosphoric acid to a pH of 3.00 ± 0.05.
  Mobile phase: *Buffer* and acetonitrile (9:11)
  Standard solution: 0.02 mg/mL of USP Phenoxybenzamine Hydrochloride RS in *Medium*
  Sample solution: Pass a portion of the solution under test through a suitable filter of 0.45-µm pore size.
  Chromatographic system
  (See *Chromatography ⟨621⟩, System Suitability.*)
  Mode: LC
  Detector: UV 268 nm
  Column: 4.6-mm × 150-cm; packing L7
  Flow rate: 1 mL/min
  Injection volume: 10 µL
  System suitability
  Sample: *Standard solution*
  Suitability requirements
   Relative standard deviation: NMT 2%
  Calculate the percentage of the labeled amount of phenoxybenzamine hydrochloride ($C_{18}H_{22}ClNO \cdot HCl$) dissolved:

$$Result = (r_U/r_S) \times (C_S/L) \times V \times 100$$

r_U = peak response •of phenoxybenzamine• (RB 1-Oct-2017) from the *Sample solution*
r_S = peak response •of phenoxybenzamine• (RB 1-Oct-2017) from the *Standard solution*
C_S = concentration of USP Phenoxybenzamine Hydrochloride RS from the *Standard solution* (mg/mL)
L = label claim (mg/Capsule)
V = volume of *Medium*, 500 mL
Tolerances: NLT 75% (*Q*) of the labeled amount of phenoxybenzamine hydrochloride ($C_{18}H_{22}ClNO \cdot HCl$) is dissolved.

- **UNIFORMITY OF DOSAGE UNITS ⟨905⟩:** Meet the requirements

IMPURITIES

Change to read:

- **ORGANIC IMPURITIES**
  Solution A, Mobile phase, •• (RB 1-Aug-2017) System suitability solution, Sample solution, Chromatographic system, and System suitability: Proceed as directed in the *Assay*.

Analysis
Sample: • (RB 1-Aug-2017) *Sample solution*
Calculate the percentage of each •degradation product• (RB 1-Aug-2017) in the portion of Capsules taken:

$$Result = (r_U/r_T) \times (1/F) \times 100$$

r_U = peak response of •each degradation product• (RB 1-Aug-2017) from the *Sample solution*
r_T = sum of all the peak responses from the *Sample solution*
F = relative response factor •(see *Table 1*)• (RB 1-Aug-2017)

Acceptance criteria: •See *Table 1*.

Table 1

Name	Relative Retention Time	Relative Response Factor	Acceptance Criteria (NMT %)
Phenoxybenzamine tertiary amine[a]	0.3	1.1	•1.5• (RB 1-Oct-2017)
Phenoxybenzamine	1.0	—	—
Any unspecified degradation product	—	1.0	0.2
Total degradation products[b]	—	—	•2.0• (RB 1-Oct-2017)

[a] 2-[Benzyl(1-phenoxypropan-2-yl)amino]ethan-1-ol.
[b] Includes specified and unspecified degradation products.

• (RB 1-Aug-2017)

ADDITIONAL REQUIREMENTS
• **PACKAGING AND STORAGE:** Preserve in well-closed containers.
• **USP REFERENCE STANDARDS ⟨11⟩**
   USP Phenoxybenzamine Hydrochloride RS

Pilocarpine Hydrochloride Tablets

DEFINITION
Pilocarpine Hydrochloride Tablets contain NLT 90.0% and NMT 110.0% of the labeled amount of pilocarpine hydrochloride ($C_{11}H_{16}N_2O_2 \cdot HCl$).

IDENTIFICATION

Change to read:

• ■A.■1S (USP41) The retention time of the major peak of the *Sample solution* corresponds to the major peak of the *Standard solution*, as obtained in the *Assay*.

Add the following:

■• B. The UV spectrum of the major peak of the *Sample solution* corresponds to that of the *Standard solution*, as obtained in the *Assay*.■1S (USP41)

ASSAY

Change to read:

• **PROCEDURE**
   Solution A: 10 N sodium hydroxide, 85% phosphoric acid, triethylamine, and water (7:6:1:500). Adjust with 10 N sodium hydroxide to a pH of 3.0.

Mobile phase: Methanol and *Solution A* (3:100)
Standard solution: 50 µg/mL of USP Pilocarpine Hydrochloride RS
System suitability solution: Transfer 10 mL of the *Standard solution* to a test tube. Add 100 µL of 2 N sodium hydroxide, mix well, and allow it to stand for 5 min. Add 100 µL of 2 N hydrochloric acid and mix well. [NOTE—This preparation contains pilocarpine, isopilocarpine, and two unidentified compounds.]
Sample stock solution: ■Nominally 0.1 mg/mL of pilocarpine hydrochloride in water prepared as follows.
■1S (USP41) Place Tablets, equivalent to 50 mg of pilocarpine hydrochloride, in a 500-mL volumetric flask. Fill the flask 75% full with water. Stir for at least 30 min or more if necessary, until the Tablets are completely disintegrated and the powder is finely dispersed. Dilute with water to volume.
Sample solution: ■Nominally 50 µg/mL of pilocarpine hydrochloride in water from *Sample stock solution*.
■1S (USP41) Pass a suitable amount of solution through a PVDF filter of 0.45-µm pore size, and discard the first 5 mL ■of the filtrate.■1S (USP41)
Chromatographic system
(See *Chromatography* ⟨621⟩, *System Suitability*.)
Mode: LC
Detector: UV 215 nm. ■For *Identification B*, use a diode array detector in the range of 190–400 nm.
■1S (USP41)
Column: 4.6-mm × 15-cm; 5-µm packing L1
Flow rate: 1.5 mL/min
Injection volume: 20 µL
System suitability
Samples: *Standard solution* and *System suitability solution*
[NOTE—The relative retention times for isopilocarpine, pilocarpine, and two unidentified peaks are 0.9, 1.0, 1.2, and 1.5, respectively.]
Suitability requirements
Resolution: NLT 1.2 between isopilocarpine and pilocarpine; NLT 1.2 between pilocarpine and the peak at a relative retention time of 1.2; NLT 1.2 between the peaks at relative retention times of 1.2 and 1.5, *System suitability solution*
■1S (USP41)
Tailing factor: NMT 1.5, *Standard solution*
Relative standard deviation: NMT 2.0%, *Standard solution*
Analysis
Samples: *Standard solution* and *Sample solution*
Calculate the percentage ■of the labeled amount■1S (USP41) of pilocarpine hydrochloride ($C_{11}H_{16}N_2O_2 \cdot HCl$) in the portion of Tablets taken:

$$Result = (r_U/r_S) \times (C_S/C_U) \times 100$$

r_U = peak response of pilocarpine hydrochloride from the *Sample solution*
r_S = peak response of pilocarpine hydrochloride from the *Standard solution*
C_S = concentration of USP Pilocarpine Hydrochloride RS in the *Standard solution* (mg/mL)
C_U = nominal concentration of pilocarpine hydrochloride in the *Sample solution* (mg/mL)

Acceptance criteria: 90.0%–110.0%

PERFORMANCE TESTS

Change to read:

- **DISSOLUTION ⟨711⟩**
  Medium: 0.1 N hydrochloric acid; 500 mL
  Apparatus 2: 50 rpm
  Time: 45 min
  Buffer solution: 13.5 mL of phosphoric acid and 3.0 mL of triethylamine in 1000 mL of water. Adjust with phosphoric acid or 10 N sodium hydroxide to a pH of 3.
  Mobile phase: Methanol and *Buffer solution* (3:17)
  Standard stock solution: 0.1 mg/mL of USP Pilocarpine Hydrochloride RS in *Medium*
  Standard solution
    For Tablets labeled to contain 7.5 mg: Transfer 15.0 mL of the *Standard stock solution* to a 100-mL volumetric flask, and dilute with *Medium* to volume.
    For Tablets labeled to contain 5 mg: Transfer 5.0 mL of the *Standard stock solution* to a 50-mL volumetric flask, and dilute with *Medium* to volume.
  Sample solution: Pass the solution under test through a suitable polyethylene filter of 45-μm pore size.
  Chromatographic system
    (See *Chromatography ⟨621⟩, System Suitability.*)
    Mode: LC
    Detector: UV 215 nm
    Column: 4.6-mm × 15-cm; packing L1
    Flow rate: 1 mL/min
    Injection volume: 20 μL
  System suitability
    Sample: *Standard solution*
    Suitability requirements
      ■1S (USP41)
      Tailing factor: NMT 2.0
      Relative standard deviation: NMT 2.0%
  Analysis
    Samples: *Standard solution* and *Sample solution*
    Calculate the percentage of pilocarpine hydrochloride ($C_{11}H_{16}N_2O_2 \cdot HCl$) dissolved:

$$Result = (r_U/r_S) \times (C_S/L) \times V \times 100$$

r_U = peak response from the *Sample solution*
r_S = peak response from the *Standard solution*
C_S = concentration of the *Standard solution* (mg/mL)
L = label claim (mg/Tablet)
V = volume of *Medium*, 500 mL

Tolerances: NLT 75% (Q) of the labeled amount of pilocarpine hydrochloride ($C_{11}H_{16}N_2O_2 \cdot HCl$) is dissolved.

Change to read:

- **UNIFORMITY OF DOSAGE UNITS ⟨905⟩**
  Procedure for content uniformity
    Mobile phase, Standard solution, System suitability solution, Chromatographic system, and **System suitability:** Proceed as directed in the *Assay.*
    Sample solution: Place 1 Tablet in a suitable volumetric flask, fill the flask about 75% full with water, and vigorously stir for NLT 30 min to ensure complete disintegration. Dilute with water to volume to obtain a final concentration of 0.05 mg/mL of pilocarpine hydrochloride. Pass the solution through a PVDF filter of 0.45-μm pore size.

Analysis
  Samples: *Standard solution* and *Sample solution*
  Calculate the percentage ■of the labeled amount■1S (USP41) of pilocarpine hydrochloride ($C_{11}H_{16}N_2O_2 \cdot HCl$) in the portion of Tablets taken:

$$Result = (r_U/r_S) \times (C_S/C_U) \times 100$$

r_U = peak response of pilocarpine hydrochloride from the *Sample solution*
r_S = peak response of pilocarpine hydrochloride from the *Standard solution*
C_S = concentration of USP Pilocarpine Hydrochloride RS in the *Standard solution* (mg/mL)
C_U = nominal concentration of pilocarpine hydrochloride in the *Sample solution* (mg/mL)

Acceptance criteria: Meet the requirements

IMPURITIES

Change to read:

- **ORGANIC IMPURITIES**
  Procedure
    Mobile phase, System suitability solution, Sample stock solution, and **System suitability:** Proceed as directed in the *Assay.*
    Standard solution: 0.5 μg/mL of USP Pilocarpine Hydrochloride RS
    Sample solution: ■Nominally 100 μg/mL of pilocarpine hydrochloride in water from *Sample stock solution.* Pass a suitable amount of solution through a PVDF filter of 0.45-μm pore size, and discard the first 5 mL of the filtrate.■1S (USP41)
  Chromatographic system
    (See *Chromatography ⟨621⟩, System Suitability.*)
    Mode: LC
    Detector: UV 215 nm
    Column: 4.6-mm × 15-cm; 5-μm packing L1
    Flow rate: 1.5 mL/min
    Injection volume: 100 μL
  Analysis
    Samples: *Standard solution* and *Sample solution*
    Calculate the percentage of each impurity in the portion of Tablets taken:

$$Result = (r_U/r_S) \times (C_S/C_U) \times (1/F) \times 100$$

r_U = peak response of each impurity from the *Sample solution*
r_S = peak response of pilocarpine hydrochloride from the *Standard solution*
C_S = concentration of USP Pilocarpine Hydrochloride RS in the *Standard solution* (mg/mL)
C_U = nominal concentration of pilocarpine hydrochloride in the *Sample solution* (mg/mL)
F = relative response factor for each impurity (see *Table 1*)

Acceptance criteria: See *Table 1.*

Table 1

Name	Relative Retention Time	Relative Response Factor	Acceptance Criteria, NMT (%)
Isopilocarpine	0.9	0.79	1.0
Pilocarpine	1.0	1.0	—
Pilocarpic acid	1.2	1.0	0.5

Table 1 (Continued)

Name	Relative Retention Time	Relative Response Factor	Acceptance Criteria, NMT (%)
■Any individual un-specified impurity■1S (USP41)	—	1.0	0.2
Total impurities	—	—	1.2

ADDITIONAL REQUIREMENTS

- **PACKAGING AND STORAGE:** Preserve in tight containers, and store at controlled room temperature.
- **USP REFERENCE STANDARDS ⟨11⟩**
  USP Pilocarpine Hydrochloride RS

Pralidoxime Chloride

Change to read:

C₇H₉ClN₂O   172.61

Pyridinium, 2-[(hydroxyimino)methyl]-1-methyl-, chloride
■(*E*)-;■1S (USP41)
■(*E*)-■1S (USP41)2-Formyl-1-methylpyridinium chloride oxime
■[14018-50-9].
Unspecified isomer■1S (USP41) [51-15-0].

DEFINITION

Pralidoxime Chloride contains NLT 97.0% and NMT 102.0% of pralidoxime chloride (C₇H₉ClN₂O), calculated on the dried basis.

IDENTIFICATION

Change to read:

- **A. ■INFRARED ABSORPTION ⟨197⟩:** [NOTE—Methods described in ⟨197K⟩, ⟨197M⟩, or ⟨197A⟩ may be used.]■1S (USP41)
- **B. IDENTIFICATION TESTS—GENERAL ⟨191⟩,** *Chemical Identification Tests, Chloride:* A solution (1 in 10) meets the requirements.
- **C.** The retention time of the major peak of the *Sample solution* corresponds to that of the *Standard solution*, as obtained in the *Assay.*

ASSAY

Change to read:

- **PROCEDURE**
  ■Solution A: Prepare a solution containing 8 mM sodium octanesulfonate and 2 mM tetraethylammonium chloride as follows. Transfer 1.87 g of sodium octanesulfonate monohydrate and 330 mg of tetraethylammonium chloride to a 1-L volumetric flask, add water to dissolve the mixture, and dilute with water to volume. Adjust with 0.01 N hydrochloric acid to a pH of 4.3.
  Mobile phase: Acetonitrile and *Solution A* (17:83)
  Diluent: Acetonitrile and water (17:83)
  Standard stock solution: 1.25 mg/mL of USP Pralidoxime Chloride RS in water. Use sonication to dissolve, if necessary.
  Standard solution: 0.125 mg/mL of USP Pralidoxime Chloride RS in *Diluent* from the *Standard stock solution*

Sample stock solution: 1.25 mg/mL of Pralidoxime Chloride in water. Use sonication to dissolve if necessary.
Sample solution: 0.125 mg/mL of Pralidoxime Chloride in *Diluent* from the *Sample stock solution.* [NOTE—This solution is stable for up to 6 h when stored at room temperature protected from light.]
Chromatographic system
(See *Chromatography* ⟨621⟩, *System Suitability.*)
  Mode: LC
  Detector: UV 270 nm
  Column: 4.6-mm × 15-cm; 3- or 3.5-μm packing L1
  Flow rate: 0.5 mL/min
  Injection volume: 10 μL
System suitability
  Sample: *Standard solution*
  [NOTE—USP Pralidoxime Chloride RS contains pralidoxime *anti*-isomer as a minor component. The relative retention times for pralidoxime *anti*-isomer and pralidoxime are 0.9 and 1.0, respectively.]
  Suitability requirements
    Resolution: NLT 2.0 between the pralidoxime *anti*-isomer and pralidoxime peaks
    Tailing factor: NMT 1.5 for the pralidoxime chloride peak
    Relative standard deviation: NMT 0.73% for the pralidoxime chloride peak
Analysis
  Samples: *Standard solution* and *Sample solution*
  Calculate the percentage of pralidoxime chloride (C₇H₉ClN₂O) in the portion of Pralidoxime Chloride taken:

$$Result = (r_U/r_S) \times (C_S/C_U) \times 100$$

r_U	= peak response of pralidoxime from the *Sample solution*
r_S	= peak response of pralidoxime from the *Standard solution*
C_S	= concentration of USP Pralidoxime Chloride RS in the *Standard solution* (μg/mL)
C_U	= concentration of Pralidoxime Chloride in the *Sample solution* (μg/mL)■1S (USP41)

Acceptance criteria: 97.0%–102.0% on the dried basis

OTHER COMPONENTS

- **CONTENT OF CHLORIDE**
  Sample solution: Dissolve 300 mg of Pralidoxime Chloride in 150 mL of water.
  Analysis: Add 20 mL of glacial acetic acid and 10 drops of (*p-tert*-octylphenoxy)nonaethoxyethanol to the *Sample solution*, and titrate with 0.1 N silver nitrate VS, determining the endpoint potentiometrically. Perform a blank determination, and make any necessary corrections. Each milliliter of 0.1 N silver nitrate is equivalent to 3.545 mg of chloride.
  Acceptance criteria: 20.2%–20.8% on the dried basis

IMPURITIES

- **RESIDUE ON IGNITION ⟨281⟩:** NMT 0.5%

Delete the following:

- ●**HEAVY METALS ⟨231⟩,** *Method I:* 0.002%● (Official 1-Jan-2018)

Add the following:

- ■● **ORGANIC IMPURITIES**
  Solution A, Mobile phase, Diluent, Sample solution, and Chromatographic system: Proceed as directed in the *Assay.*
  Standard stock solution: Use the *Standard solution* prepared as directed in the *Assay.*

Standard solution: 0.125 µg/mL of USP Pralidoxime Chloride RS in *Diluent* from the *Standard stock solution*

Sensitivity solution: 0.0625 µg/mL of USP Pralidoxime Chloride RS in *Diluent* from the *Standard solution*

System suitability

Samples: *Standard stock solution, Standard solution, and Sensitivity solution*

Suitability requirements

Resolution: NLT 2.0 between the pralidoxime *anti*-isomer and pralidoxime peaks, *Standard stock solution*

Relative standard deviation: NMT 5.0% for the pralidoxime chloride peak, *Standard solution*

Signal-to-noise ratio: NLT 10, *Sensitivity solution*

Analysis

Samples: *Sample solution* and *Standard solution*

Calculate the percentage of each impurity in the portion of Pralidoxime Chloride taken:

$$Result = (r_U/r_S) \times (C_S/C_U) \times 100$$

r_U = peak response of each impurity from the *Sample solution*

r_S = peak response of pralidoxime from the *Standard solution*

C_S = concentration of USP Pralidoxime Chloride RS in the *Standard solution* (µg/mL)

C_U = concentration of Pralidoxime Chloride in the *Sample solution* (µg/mL)

Acceptance criteria: See *Table 1*. The reporting level for impurities is 0.05%.

Table 1

Name	Relative Retention Time	Acceptance Criteria, NMT (%)
Pyridine-2-aldoxime	0.7	0.5
Pralidoxime *anti*-isomer[a]	0.9	2
Pralidoxime	1.0	—
Any other individual impurity	—	0.10
Total impurities	—	3

[a] (Z)-2-[(Hydroxyimino)methyl]-1-methylpyridin-1-ium chloride.

■1S (USP41)

SPECIFIC TESTS

Delete the following:

■• **MELTING RANGE OR TEMPERATURE** ⟨741⟩: 215°– 225°, with decomposition■1S (USP41)

• **LOSS ON DRYING** ⟨731⟩

Analysis: Dry at 105° for 3 h.

Acceptance criteria: NMT 2.0%

• **STERILITY TESTS** ⟨71⟩: Where the label states that Pralidoxime Chloride is sterile, it meets the requirements.

• **BACTERIAL ENDOTOXINS TEST** ⟨85⟩: Where the label states that Pralidoxime Chloride is sterile or must be subjected to further processing during the preparation of injectable dosage forms, it contains NMT 0.10 USP Endotoxin Units/mg of pralidoxime chloride.

ADDITIONAL REQUIREMENTS

• **PACKAGING AND STORAGE:** Preserve in well-closed containers.

• **LABELING:** Where it is intended for use in preparing injectable dosage forms, the label states that it is sterile or must be subjected to further processing during the preparation of injectable dosage forms.

Change to read:

• **USP REFERENCE STANDARDS** ⟨11⟩

■• (CN 1-May-2018)

USP Pralidoxime Chloride RS

Pralidoxime Chloride for Injection

DEFINITION

Pralidoxime Chloride for Injection contains NLT 90.0% and NMT 110.0% of the labeled amount of pralidoxime chloride ($C_7H_9ClN_2O$).

IDENTIFICATION

Change to read:

• **A.** ■**INFRARED ABSORPTION** ⟨197⟩: [NOTE—Methods described in ⟨197K⟩, ⟨197M⟩, or ⟨197A⟩ may be used.]■1S (USP41)

• **B. IDENTIFICATION TESTS—GENERAL** ⟨191⟩, *Chemical Identification Tests, Chloride*: A solution (1 in 10) meets the requirements.

• **C.** The retention time of the major peak of the *Sample solution* corresponds to that of the *Standard solution*, as obtained in the *Assay*.

ASSAY

Change to read:

• **PROCEDURE**

■**Solution A:** Prepare a solution containing 8 mM sodium octanesulfonate and 2 mM tetraethylammonium chloride as follows. Transfer 1.87 g of sodium octanesulfonate monohydrate and 330 mg of tetraethylammonium chloride to a 1-L volumetric flask, add water to dissolve the mixture, and dilute with water to volume. Adjust with 0.01 N hydrochloric acid to a pH of 4.3.

Mobile phase: Acetonitrile and *Solution A* (17:83)

Diluent: Acetonitrile and water (17:83)

Standard stock solution: 1.25 mg/mL of USP Pralidoxime Chloride RS in water. Use sonication to dissolve, if necessary.

Standard solution: 0.125 mg/mL of USP Pralidoxime Chloride RS in *Diluent* from the *Standard stock solution*

Sample stock solution: Nominally 1.25 mg/mL of pralidoxime chloride prepared as follows. Select a number of containers of Pralidoxime Chloride for Injection, the combined contents of which are equivalent to about 10 g of pralidoxime chloride. Dissolve the contents of each container in water and combine all of the solutions in a 1000-mL volumetric flask. Rinse each container with water and add the rinsings to the volumetric flask. Dilute with water to volume and mix. Transfer 25.0 mL of the resulting solution to a 200-mL volumetric flask and dilute with water to volume.

Sample solution: Nominally 0.125 mg/mL of pralidoxime chloride in *Diluent* from the *Sample stock solution*. [NOTE—This solution is stable for up to 6 h when stored at room temperature protected from light.]

Chromatographic system

(See *Chromatography* ⟨621⟩, *System Suitability*.)

Mode: LC
Detector: UV 270 nm
Column: 4.6-mm × 15-cm; 3- or 3.5-µm packing L1
Flow rate: 0.5 mL/min
Injection volume: 10 µL
System suitability
Sample: *Standard solution*
[NOTE—USP Pralidoxime Chloride RS contains pralidoxime *anti*-isomer as a minor component. The relative retention times for pralidoxime *anti*-isomer and pralidoxime are 0.9 and 1.0, respectively.]
Suitability requirements
 Resolution: NLT 2.0 between the pralidoxime *anti*-isomer and pralidoxime peaks
 Tailing factor: NMT 1.5 for the pralidoxime chloride peak
 Relative standard deviation: NMT 1.0% for the pralidoxime chloride peak
Analysis
Samples: *Standard solution* and *Sample solution*
Calculate the percentage of the labeled amount of pralidoxime chloride ($C_7H_9ClN_2O$) in the portion of Pralidoxime Chloride for Injection taken:

$$Result = (r_U/r_S) \times (C_S/C_U) \times 100$$

r_U = peak response of pralidoxime from the *Sample solution*
r_S = peak response of pralidoxime from the *Standard solution*
C_S = concentration of USP Pralidoxime Chloride RS in the *Standard solution* (µg/mL)
C_U = nominal concentration of pralidoxime chloride in the *Sample solution* (µg/mL)■1S (USP41)
Acceptance criteria: 90.0%–110.0%

PERFORMANCE TESTS
• **UNIFORMITY OF DOSAGE UNITS ⟨905⟩:** Meets the requirements

IMPURITIES

Delete the following:

•• **HEAVY METALS ⟨231⟩,** *Method I:* NMT 0.002%• (Official 1-Jan-2018)

Add the following:

■• **ORGANIC IMPURITIES**
 Solution A, Mobile phase, Diluent, Sample solution, and **Chromatographic system:** Proceed as directed in the *Assay.*
 Standard stock solution: Use the *Standard solution* prepared as directed in the *Assay.*
 Standard solution: 0.125 µg/mL of USP Pralidoxime Chloride RS in *Diluent* from the *Standard stock solution*
 System suitability
 Samples: *Standard stock solution* and *Standard solution*
 Suitability requirements
  Resolution: NLT 2.0 between the pralidoxime *anti*-isomer and pralidoxime peaks, *Standard stock solution*
  Relative standard deviation: NMT 5.0% for the pralidoxime chloride peak, *Standard solution*
 Analysis
 Samples: *Sample solution* and *Standard solution*
 Calculate the percentage of each impurity in the portion of Pralidoxime Chloride for Injection taken:

$$Result = (r_U/r_S) \times (C_S/C_U) \times 100$$

r_U = peak response of each impurity from the *Sample solution*

r_S = peak response of pralidoxime from the *Standard solution*
C_S = concentration of USP Pralidoxime Chloride RS in the *Standard solution* (µg/mL)
C_U = nominal concentration of pralidoxime chloride in the *Sample solution* (µg/mL)
Acceptance criteria: See *Table 1.*

Table 1

Name	Relative Retention Time	Acceptance Criteria, NMT (%)
Pyridine-2-aldoxime	0.7	0.5
Pralidoxime *anti*-isomer[a]	0.9	2
Pralidoxime	1.0	—
Any other individual impurity	—	0.2
Total impurities	—	3

[a] (Z)-2-[(Hydroxyimino)methyl]-1-methylpyridin-1-ium chloride.

■1S (USP41)

SPECIFIC TESTS

Delete the following:

■• **COMPLETENESS OF SOLUTION ⟨641⟩**
 Sample solution: Dissolve the contents of 1 container in 10 mL of water.
 Acceptance criteria: It yields a clear solution.■1S (USP41)
• **CONSTITUTED SOLUTION:** At the time of use, it meets the requirements for *Injections and Implanted Drug Products ⟨1⟩, Product Quality Tests Common to Parenteral Dosage Forms, Specific Tests, Completeness and clarity of solutions*
• **BACTERIAL ENDOTOXINS TEST ⟨85⟩:** It contains NMT 0.10 USP Endotoxin Units/mg of pralidoxime chloride.
• **PH ⟨791⟩:** 3.5–4.5, in a solution (1 in 20)
• **LOSS ON DRYING ⟨731⟩**
 Analysis: Dry at 105° for 3 h.
 Acceptance criteria: NMT 2.0%
• **STERILITY TESTS ⟨71⟩:** Meets the requirements
• **OTHER REQUIREMENTS:** It meets the requirements for *Labeling ⟨7⟩, Labels and Labeling for Injectable Products.*

ADDITIONAL REQUIREMENTS
• **PACKAGING AND STORAGE:** Preserve as described in *Packaging and Storage Requirements ⟨659⟩, Injection Packaging.*

Change to read:

• **USP REFERENCE STANDARDS ⟨11⟩**
 • (CN 1-May-2018)
 USP Pralidoxime Chloride RS

Add the following:

■Prasugrel Hydrochloride

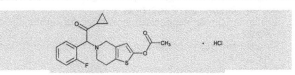

$C_{20}H_{20}FNO_3S \cdot HCl$ 409.90

Ethanone, 2-[2-(acetyloxy)-6,7-dihydrothieno[3,2-*c*]pyridin-5(4*H*)-yl]-1-cyclopropyl-2-(2-fluorophenyl)-, hydrochloride; 5-[2-Cyclopropyl-1-(2-fluorophenyl)-2-oxoethyl]-4,5,6,7-tetrahydrothieno[3,2-*c*]pyridin-2-yl acetate hydrochloride [389574-19-0].

DEFINITION
Prasugrel Hydrochloride contains NLT 97.0% and NMT 102.0% of prasugrel hydrochloride ($C_{20}H_{20}FNO_3S \cdot HCl$), calculated on the anhydrous and solvent-free basis.

IDENTIFICATION
- **A. INFRARED ABSORPTION ⟨197⟩:** [NOTE—Methods described in ⟨197K⟩ or ⟨197A⟩ may be used.]
- **B.** The retention time of the prasugrel peak of the *Sample solution* corresponds to that of the *Standard solution*, as obtained in the *Assay*.
- **C. IDENTIFICATION TESTS—GENERAL ⟨191⟩,** *Chemical Identification Tests, Chloride*: Meets the requirements

ASSAY
- **PROCEDURE**
  Buffer: 10 mM monobasic potassium phosphate in water. Adjust with phosphoric acid to a pH of 2.8.
  Mobile phase: Acetonitrile and *Buffer* (35:65)
  Diluent: Acetonitrile and water (70:30)
  Standard solution: 0.1 mg/mL of USP Prasugrel Hydrochloride RS in *Diluent*
  Sample solution: 0.1 mg/mL of Prasugrel Hydrochloride in *Diluent*
  Chromatographic system
  (See *Chromatography* ⟨621⟩, *System Suitability*.)
    Mode: LC
    Detector: UV 260 nm
    Column: 4.6-mm × 15-cm; 5-µm packing L1
    Column temperature: 40°
    Flow rate: 1 mL/min
    Injection volume: 10 µL
    Run time: NLT 2.5 times the retention time of prasugrel
  System suitability
    Sample: *Standard solution*
    Suitability requirements
      Tailing factor: NMT 2.0%
      Relative standard deviation: NMT 1.0%
  Analysis
    Samples: *Standard solution* and *Sample solution*
    Calculate the percentage of prasugrel hydrochloride ($C_{20}H_{20}FNO_3S \cdot HCl$) in the portion of Prasugrel Hydrochloride taken:

$$Result = (r_U/r_S) \times (C_S/C_U) \times 100$$

r_U = peak response of prasugrel from the *Sample solution*
r_S = peak response of prasugrel from the *Standard solution*
C_S = concentration of USP Prasugrel Hydrochloride RS in the *Standard solution* (mg/mL)
C_U = concentration of Prasugrel Hydrochloride in the *Sample solution* (mg/mL)
Acceptance criteria: 97.0%–102.0% on the anhydrous and solvent-free basis

IMPURITIES
- **RESIDUE ON IGNITION ⟨281⟩:** NMT 0.2%
- **ORGANIC IMPURITIES, PROCEDURE 1**
  Buffer: 10 mM monobasic potassium phosphate in water
  Mobile phase: Acetonitrile, tetrahydrofuran, and *Buffer* (10:25:65)
  Diluent: Acetonitrile and water (70:30)
  Solution A: 150 µL of piperidine in 50 mL of acetonitrile
  System suitability stock solution: 0.1 mg/mL of USP Prasugrel Hydrochloride RS in *Diluent* prepared as follows. Transfer 5 mg of USP Prasugrel Hydrochloride RS to a 50-mL volumetric flask. Add 20 mL of *Diluent* and mix to dissolve. Add 1 mL of *Solution A* and dilute with *Diluent* to the volume. Heat the solution at 50° for 1 h and cool to room temperature.
  System suitability solution: 0.02 mg/mL of USP Prasugrel Hydrochloride RS from the *System suitability stock solution* in *Diluent*
  Standard solution: 0.015 mg/mL of USP Prasugrel Hydrochloride RS in *Diluent*
  Sensitivity solution: 0.3 µg/mL of USP Prasugrel Hydrochloride RS from the *Standard solution* in *Diluent*
  Sample solution: 1.5 mg/mL of Prasugrel Hydrochloride in *Diluent*
  Chromatographic system
  (See *Chromatography* ⟨621⟩, *System Suitability*.)
    Mode: LC
    Detector: UV 240 nm
    Column: 4.6-mm × 15-cm; 3-µm packing L1
    Temperatures
      Autosampler: 10°
      Column: 40°
    Flow rate: 0.9 mL/min
    Injection volume: 10 µL
    Run time: NLT 2 times the retention time of prasugrel
  System suitability
    Samples: *System suitability solution, Standard solution,* and *Sensitivity solution*
    [NOTE—See *Table 1* for the relative retention times.]
    Suitability requirements
      Resolution: NLT 1.5 between desacetyl prasugrel diastereomer 1 and desacetyl prasugrel diastereomer 2 peaks, *System suitability solution*
      Relative standard deviation: NMT 2.0%, *Standard solution*
      Signal-to-noise ratio: NLT 10, *Sensitivity solution*
  Analysis
    Samples: *Standard solution* and *Sample solution*
    Calculate the percentage of each specified process impurity in the portion of Prasugrel Hydrochloride taken:

$$Result = (r_U/r_S) \times (C_S/C_U) \times 100$$

r_U = peak response of each specified impurity from the *Sample solution*
r_S = peak response of prasugrel from the *Standard solution*
C_S = concentration of USP Prasugrel Hydrochloride RS in the *Standard solution* (mg/mL)
C_U = concentration of Prasugrel Hydrochloride in the *Sample solution* (mg/mL)
Acceptance criteria: See *Table 1*.

Table 1

Name	Relative Retention Time	Acceptance Criteria, NMT (%)
Desacetyl prasugrel diastereomer 1[a]	0.43	—
Desacetyl prasugrel diastereomer 2[a]	0.45	—
Desfluoro prasugrel[b]	0.9	0.20
Prasugrel	1.0	—

[a] 5-[2-Cyclopropyl-1-(2-fluorophenyl)-2-oxoethyl]-5,6,7,7a-tetrahydrothieno[3,2-*c*]pyridin-2(4*H*)-one. Desacetyl prasugrel diastereomer 1 and desacetyl prasugrel diastereomer 2 are a pair of diastereomers. They are used for resolution measurement only.
[b] 5-(2-Cyclopropyl-2-oxo-1-phenylethyl)-4,5,6,7-tetrahydrothieno[3,2-*c*]pyridin-2-yl acetate.
[c] 5-[2-Cyclopropyl-1-(4-fluorophenyl)-2-oxoethyl]-4,5,6,7-tetrahydrothieno[3,2-*c*]pyridin-2-yl acetate.
[d] 5-[2-Cyclopropyl-1-(3-fluorophenyl)-2-oxoethyl]-4,5,6,7-tetrahydrothieno[3,2-*c*]pyridin-2-yl acetate.

Table 1 *(Continued)*

Name	Relative Retention Time	Acceptance Criteria, NMT (%)
4-Fluoro prasugrel[c]	1.2	0.15
3-Fluoro prasugrel[d]	1.3	0.30

[a] 5-[2-Cyclopropyl-1-(2-fluorophenyl)-2-oxoethyl]-5,6,7,7a-tetrahydrothieno[3,2-c]pyridin-2(4H)-one. Desacetyl prasugrel diastereomer 1 and desacetyl prasugrel diastereomer 2 are a pair of diastereomers. They are used for resolution measurement only.

[b] 5-(2-Cyclopropyl-2-oxo-1-phenylethyl)-4,5,6,7-tetrahydrothieno[3,2-c]pyridin-2-yl acetate.

[c] 5-[2-Cyclopropyl-1-(4-fluorophenyl)-2-oxoethyl]-4,5,6,7-tetrahydrothieno[3,2-c]pyridin-2-yl acetate.

[d] 5-[2-Cyclopropyl-1-(3-fluorophenyl)-2-oxoethyl]-4,5,6,7-tetrahydrothieno[3,2-c]pyridin-2-yl acetate.

- **ORGANIC IMPURITIES, PROCEDURE 2**
  Buffer: 25 mM monobasic potassium phosphate in water. Adjust with phosphoric acid to a pH of 4.0.
  Solution A: Acetonitrile and *Buffer* (10:90)
  Solution B: Acetonitrile and water (90:10)
  Solution C: 150 µL of piperidine in 50 mL of acetonitrile
  Mobile phase: See *Table 2*.

Table 2

Time (min)	Solution A (%)	Solution B (%)
0	100	0
2	100	0
30	0	100
37	0	100
38	100	0
45	100	0

  Diluent: Acetonitrile and water (70:30)
  System suitability solution: 0.1 mg/mL of USP Prasugrel Hydrochloride RS in *Diluent* prepared as follows. Transfer 5 mg of USP Prasugrel Hydrochloride RS to a 50-mL volumetric flask. Add 20 mL of *Diluent* and mix to dissolve. Add 1 mL of *Solution C* and dilute with *Diluent* to volume. Heat the solution at 50° for 1 h and cool to room temperature.
  Standard solution: 0.1 mg/mL of USP Prasugrel Hydrochloride RS in *Diluent*
  Sensitivity solution: 2 µg/mL of USP Prasugrel Hydrochloride RS from the *Standard solution* in *Diluent*
  Sample solution: 10 mg/mL of Prasugrel Hydrochloride in *Diluent*
  Chromatographic system
  (See *Chromatography* ⟨621⟩, *System Suitability*.)
  Mode: LC
  Detector: UV 210 nm
  Column: 4.6-mm × 15-cm; 4-µm packing L87
  Column temperature: 45°
  Flow rate: 1.5 mL/min
  Injection volume: 5 µL
  System suitability
  Samples: *System suitability solution, Standard solution,* and *Sensitivity solution*
  [NOTE—See *Table 3* for the relative retention times.]
  Suitability requirements
  Resolution: NLT 0.9 between the desacetyl prasugrel diastereomer 1 and desacetyl prasugrel diastereomer 2 peaks, *System suitability solution*
  Relative standard deviation: NMT 2.0%, *Standard solution*

Signal-to-noise ratio: NLT 10, *Sensitivity solution*
Analysis
  Samples: *Standard solution* and *Sample solution*
  Calculate the percentage of each specified and unspecified degradation product in the portion of Prasugrel Hydrochloride taken:

$$Result = (r_U/r_S) \times (C_S/C_U) \times (1/F) \times 100$$

r_U = peak response of each degradation product from the *Sample solution*
r_S = peak response of prasugrel from the *Standard solution*
C_S = concentration of USP Prasugrel Hydrochloride RS in the *Standard solution* (mg/mL)
C_U = concentration of Prasugrel Hydrochloride in the *Sample solution* (mg/mL)
F = relative response factor
Acceptance criteria: See *Table 3*.

Table 3

Name	Relative Retention Time	Relative Response Factor	Acceptance Criteria, NMT (%)
Desacetyl hydroxyprasugrel[a]	0.74	1.0	0.15
Prasugrel diketone[b]	0.78	1.0	0.20
Desacetyl prasugrel diastereomer 1[c]	0.86	1.0	0.20
Desacetyl prasugrel diastereomer 2[c]	0.87	1.0	0.50
Prasugrel	1.0	—	—
Prasugrel chlorobutyryl analog[d]	1.06	0.73	0.30
Any individual unspecified degradation product	—	1.0	0.10
Total degradation products	—	—	1.0

[a] 5-[2-Cyclopropyl-1-(2-fluorophenyl)-2-oxoethyl]-7a-hydroxy-5,6,7,7a-tetrahydrothieno[3,2-c]pyridin-2(4H)-one.

[b] 1-Cyclopropyl-2-(2-fluorophenyl)ethane-1,2-dione.

[c] 5-[2-Cyclopropyl-1-(2-fluorophenyl)-2-oxoethyl]-5,6,7,7a-tetrahydrothieno[3,2-c]pyridin-2(4H)-one. Desacetyl prasugrel diastereomer 1 and desacetyl prasugrel diastereomer 2 are a pair of diastereomers.

[d] 5-[5-Chloro-1-(2-fluorophenyl)-2-oxopentyl]-4,5,6,7-tetrahydrothieno[3,2-c]pyridin-2-yl acetate.

SPECIFIC TESTS
- **WATER DETERMINATION** ⟨921⟩, *Method I, Method Ic:* NMT 0.2%

ADDITIONAL REQUIREMENTS
- **PACKAGING AND STORAGE:** Preserve in well-closed containers. Store at room temperature.
- **USP REFERENCE STANDARDS** ⟨11⟩
  USP Prasugrel Hydrochloride RS
  ■1S *(USP41)*

Pravastatin Sodium

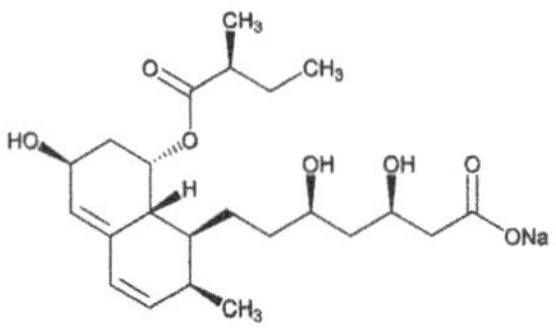

$C_{23}H_{35}NaO_7$ 446.52

1-Naphthaleneheptanoic acid, 1,2,6,7,8,8a-hexahydro-β,δ,
6-trihydroxy-2-methyl-8-(2-methyl-1-oxobutoxy)-,
monosodium salt, [1S-[1α(βS*,δS*),2α,6α,8β(R*),8aα]]-;
Sodium (βR,δR,1S,2S,6S,8S,8aR)-1,2,6,7,8,8a-hexahydro-β,δ,
6,8-tetrahydroxy-2-methyl-1-naphthaleneheptanoate, 8-
[(2S)-2-methylbutyrate] [81131-70-6].

DEFINITION
Pravastatin Sodium contains NLT 97.5% and NMT 102.0%
of pravastatin sodium ($C_{23}H_{35}NaO_7$), calculated on the anhydrous and solvent-free basis.

IDENTIFICATION
- **A. INFRARED ABSORPTION ⟨197K⟩**

Change to read:

- **B. IDENTIFICATION TESTS—GENERAL ⟨191⟩**, *Chemical Identification Tests, Sodium:* Meets the requirements ■of test
A● (CN 1-May-2018)

Add the following:

- ■● **C.** The retention time of the major peak of the *Sample
solution* corresponds to that of the *Standard solution*, as
obtained in the *Assay*.■1S (USP41)

ASSAY

Change to read:

- **PROCEDURE**
  Solution A: 0.08 M phosphoric acid solution. Adjust
  with a 25% sodium hydroxide solution to a pH of 5.5.
  Solution B: Acetonitrile and *Solution A* (20:80)
  Solution C: Acetonitrile
  Mobile phase: See *Table 1.*

Table 1

Time (min)	Solution B (%)	Solution C (%)
0	100	0
7.0	90	10
10.0	62.5	37.5
17.0	62.5	37.5
17.1	100	0
20.0	100	0

System suitability solution: 0.25 mg/mL of USP Pravastatin 1,1,3,3-Tetramethylbutylamine RS and 0.001 mg/
mL of USP Pravastatin Related Compound A RS in
methanol
Standard solution: 0.25 mg/mL of USP Pravastatin 1,1,
3,3-Tetramethylbutylamine RS in methanol
Sample solution: 0.2 mg/mL of Pravastatin Sodium in
methanol
Chromatographic system
(See *Chromatography ⟨621⟩, System Suitability.*)

Mode: LC
Detector: UV 238 nm
Column: 4.0-mm × 10-cm; 3-μm packing L1
Flow rate: 1 mL/min
Injection volume: 10 μL
System suitability
Sample: *System suitability solution*
[NOTE—The relative retention times for pravastatin and
pravastatin related compound A are about 1.0 and
1.2, respectively.]
Suitability requirements
Resolution: NLT 1.2 between pravastatin and pravas-
tatin related compound A
Relative standard deviation: NMT 2.0% for the
pravastatin peak
Analysis
Samples: *Standard solution* and *Sample solution*
■1S (USP41) Calculate the percentage of pravastatin so-
dium ($C_{23}H_{35}NaO_7$) in the portion of Pravastatin Sodium taken:

$$Result = (r_U/r_S) \times (C_S/C_U) \times (M_{r1}/M_{r2}) \times 100$$

r_U = peak response of pravastatin from the *Sample
solution*
r_S = peak response of pravastatin from the
Standard solution
C_S = concentration of ■USP Pravastatin 1,1,3,3-
Tetramethylbutylamine RS■1S (USP41) in the
Standard solution (mg/mL)
C_U = concentration of Pravastatin Sodium in the
Sample solution (mg/mL)
M_{r1} = molecular weight of pravastatin sodium,
446.52
M_{r2} = molecular weight of pravastatin 1,1,3,3-
tetramethylbutylamine, 553.78
Acceptance criteria: 97.5%–102.0% on the anhydrous
and solvent-free basis

IMPURITIES

Delete the following:

- ■● **HEAVY METALS ⟨231⟩**, *Method II:* NMT 20 ppm● (Official 1-
Jan-2018)

Change to read:

- **ORGANIC IMPURITIES**
  [NOTE—The *Standard solution* and the *Sample solution* are
  maintained at 15° until injected into the
  chromatograph.]
  Diluent: Methanol and water (50:50)
  Solution A: 0.08 M phosphoric acid solution. Adjust
  with triethylamine to a pH of 7.0.
  Solution B: Acetonitrile, *Solution A*, and water
  (18:30:52)
  Solution C: Acetonitrile, *Solution A*, and water
  (60:30:10)
  Mobile phase: See *Table 2.*

Table 2

Time (min)	Solution B (%)	Solution C (%)
0	100	0
3.0	100	0
26.5	0	100
26.6	100	0
30.0	100	0

System suitability solution: 0.6 mg/mL of USP Pravastatin 1,1,3,3-Tetramethylbutylamine RS and 0.001 mg/

mL of USP Pravastatin Related Compound A RS in *Diluent*. [NOTE—USP Pravastatin Related Compound A RS is a sodium salt of 3α-hydroxyisocompactin acid.]
Standard solution: 1.25 µg/mL of USP Pravastatin 1,1, 3,3-Tetramethylbutylamine RS in *Diluent*
Sample solution: 0.5 mg/mL of Pravastatin Sodium in *Diluent*
Chromatographic system
  (See *Chromatography ⟨621⟩, System Suitability.*)
  Mode: LC
  Detector: UV 238 nm
  Column: 4.6-mm × 7.5-cm; 3.5-µm packing L1.
    [NOTE—Alternatively, a 4.0-mm × 10-cm; 3-µm packing L1 can be used.]
  Flow rate: 1 mL/min
  Injection volume: 10 µL
System suitability
  Samples: *System suitability solution* and *Standard solution*
  [NOTE—The relative retention times for pravastatin and pravastatin related compound A are about 1.0 and 1.1, respectively. ■■1S (USP41)]
  Suitability requirements
    Resolution: NLT 2.0 between pravastatin and pravastatin related compound A, *System suitability solution*
    Relative standard deviation: NMT 10.0%, *Standard solution*
  Analysis
    Samples: *Standard solution* and *Sample solution*
    ■■1S (USP41) Calculate the percentage of each ■specified or any unspecified■1S (USP41) impurity in the portion of Pravastatin Sodium taken:

$$Result = (r_U/r_S) \times (C_S/C_U) \times (M_{r1}/M_{r2}) \times 100$$

r_U = peak response of each impurity from the *Sample solution*
r_S = peak response of pravastatin from the *Standard solution*
C_S = concentration of ■USP Pravastatin 1,1,3,3-Tetramethylbutylamine RS■1S (USP41) in the *Standard solution* (mg/mL)
C_U = concentration of Pravastatin Sodium in the *Sample solution* (mg/mL)
M_{r1} = molecular weight of pravastatin sodium, 446.52
M_{r2} = molecular weight of pravastatin 1,1,3,3-tetramethylbutylamine, 553.78

Acceptance criteria: See *Table 3*. The reporting level for impurities is 0.05%. ■■1S (USP41)

Table 3

Name	Relative Retention Time	Acceptance Criteria, NMT (%)
3″-Hydroxypravastatin	0.33	0.2
6′-Epi-pravastatin	0.92	0.3
■Pravastatin	1.0	—■1S (USP41)
■Pravastatin related compound A■1S (USP41)	1.1	0.2
Pentanoyl impurity■■1S (USP41)	1.2	0.2
Pravastatin lactone	1.8	0.2
Compactin	3.1	0.2

■a ■1S (USP41) (3R,5R)-3,5-Dihydroxy-7-[(1S,2S,6S,8S,8aR)-6-hydroxy-2-methyl-8-[[(2S)-2-methylpentanoyl]oxy]-1,2,6,7,8,8a-hexahydronaphthalen-1-yl]heptanoic acid.

Table 3 (*Continued*)

Name	Relative Retention Time	Acceptance Criteria, NMT (%)
Any ■unspecified■1S (USP41) impurity	—	■0.10■1S (USP41)
Total impurities	—	0.6

■a ■1S (USP41) (3R,5R)-3,5-Dihydroxy-7-[(1S,2S,6S,8S,8aR)-6-hydroxy-2-methyl-8-[[(2S)-2-methylpentanoyl]oxy]-1,2,6,7,8,8a-hexahydronaphthalen-1-yl]heptanoic acid.

SPECIFIC TESTS

Change to read:

- **LIMIT OF ALCOHOL** (if present)
  Standard stock solution 1: Pipet 2 mL of dehydrated alcohol into a 100-mL volumetric flask, and dilute with water to volume.
  Standard stock solution 2: Pipet 10 mL of *Standard stock solution 1* into a 100-mL volumetric flask, and dilute with water to volume.
  Sample stock solution: Transfer 0.2 g of Pravastatin Sodium to a 20-mL volumetric flask, and dilute with water to volume.
  Sample solution: Pipet 5 mL of the *Sample stock solution* into a vial fitted with a septum and a crimp cap, add 1 mL of water, seal the vial, and mix. Heat the sealed vial at 80° for 60 min.
  Standard solution: Pipet 1 mL of *Standard stock solution 2* into a vial fitted with a septum and a crimp cap, and calculate the amount of alcohol (W_A) added in grams (the specific gravity of dehydrated alcohol is 0.79 g/mL). Add 5 mL of the *Sample solution* to the same vial, and seal the vial. Heat the sealed vial at 80° for 60 min.
  Blank solution: Pipet 6 mL of water into a vial fitted with a septum and a crimp cap, and seal the vial. Heat the sealed vial at 80° for 60 min.
  Chromatographic system
    (See *Chromatography ⟨621⟩, System Suitability.*)
    Mode: GC
    Detector: Flame ionization
    Column: 0.53-mm × 30-m fused silica capillary; coated with a 3-µm film of stationary phase G43
    Temperatures
      Transfer line: 85°
      Injection port: 140°
      Detector: 250°
      Column: See *Table 4.*

Table 4

Initial Temperature (°)	Temperature Ramp (°/min)	Final Temperature (°)	Hold Time at Final Temperature (min)
40	0	40	20
40	10	240	—
240	0	240	20

Carrier gas: Helium
Flow rate: Linear velocity of 35 cm/s
Injection volume: 1 mL
Injection type: Split ratio, 1:5
System suitability
  Sample: *Blank solution*
  Suitability requirement: No interfering peaks are observed.

Analysis
Samples: *Sample solution* and *Standard solution*
Calculate the percentage of alcohol in the portion of Pravastatin Sodium taken:

$$\text{Result} = [r_U/(r_S - r_U)] \times (W_A/W) \times D \times 100 \text{ ■}_{1S} \text{ (USP41)}$$

r_U = peak response of alcohol from the *Sample solution*
r_S = peak response of alcohol from the *Standard solution*
W_A = amount of alcohol added (g)
W = weight of Pravastatin Sodium taken to prepare the *Sample solution* (g)
■D = dilution factor for the *Sample solution*, 4 ■$_{1S}$ (USP41)

Acceptance criteria: NMT 3.0%
- **OPTICAL ROTATION ⟨781S⟩**, *Procedures, Specific Rotation*
  Sample solution: 5 mg/mL in water
  Acceptance criteria: +150° to +160° (at 20°), calculated on the anhydrous and solvent-free basis
- **pH ⟨791⟩:** 7.2–9.0, in a solution (1 in 20)
- **WATER DETERMINATION ⟨921⟩**, *Method I:* NMT 4.0%

ADDITIONAL REQUIREMENTS
- **PACKAGING AND STORAGE:** Preserve in tight containers. Store as per labeling instructions. Possible storage conditions could include the following, in the presence of stability data supporting the condition: Store under nitrogen in a cold place. Store at room temperature.

Change to read:

- **USP REFERENCE STANDARDS ⟨11⟩**
  USP Pravastatin 1,1,3,3-Tetramethylbutylamine RS
  ■2,4,4-Trimethylpentan-2-amine (3R,5R)-3,5-dihydroxy-7-[(1S,2S,6S,8S,8aR)-6-hydroxy-2-methyl-8-{[(S)-2-methylbutanoyl]oxy}-1,2,6,7,8,8a-hexahydronaphthalen-1-yl]heptanoate.
  $C_{23}H_{36}O_7 \cdot C_8H_{19}N$ 553.78 ■$_{1S}$ (USP41)
  USP Pravastatin Sodium RS
  USP Pravastatin Related Compound A RS
  ■Sodium (3R,5R)-3,5-dihydroxy-7-[(1S,2R,3S,8S,8aR)-3-hydroxy-2-methyl-8-[[(2S)-2-methylbutanoyl]oxy]-1,2,3,7,8,8a-hexahydronaphthalen-1-yl]heptanoate.
  $C_{23}H_{35}NaO_7$ 446.51 ■$_{1S}$ (USP41)

Pyridostigmine Bromide Tablets

DEFINITION
Pyridostigmine Bromide Tablets contain NLT 95.0% and NMT 105.0% of the labeled amount of pyridostigmine bromide ($C_9H_{13}BrN_2O_2$).

IDENTIFICATION
- **A.** The retention time of the major peak of the *Sample solution* corresponds to that of the *Standard solution*, as obtained in the *Assay.*
- **B. IDENTIFICATION TESTS—GENERAL ⟨191⟩**, *Chemical Identification Tests, Bromide*
  Sample solution: Shake a quantity of finely powdered Tablets, equivalent to 100 mg of pyridostigmine bromide, with 20 mL of water for 5 min, and filter the mixture. Use the filtrate.
  Acceptance criteria: Meet the requirements

ASSAY
- **PROCEDURE**
  Mobile phase: Dissolve 1 g of sodium 1-heptanesulfonate in 500 mL of water in a 1000-mL volumetric flask, and add 5.0 mL of triethylamine and 100 mL of aceto-

nitrile. Dilute with water to volume, and mix. Adjust with phosphoric acid to a pH of 3.0.
Diluent: Mix 11.2 g of phosphoric acid with 500 mL of water, and adjust with a 50% sodium hydroxide solution to a pH of 7.0. Dilute with water to 1000 mL.
Standard solution: 0.25 mg/mL of USP Pyridostigmine Bromide RS in *Diluent*
Sample solution: Nominally 0.25 mg/mL of pyridostigmine bromide prepared as follows. Finely powder NLT 20 Tablets and transfer a portion of the powder, equivalent to about 50 mg of pyridostigmine bromide, to a suitable volumetric flask. Add about 50% of the flask volume of *Diluent,* and shake for 30 min. Dilute with *Diluent* to volume, mix, and centrifuge. Use the supernatant.
Chromatographic system
(See *Chromatography ⟨621⟩, System Suitability.*)
  Mode: LC
  Detector: UV 270 nm
  Column: 4-mm × 30-cm; packing L1
  Flow rate: 2 mL/min
  Injection volume: 20 µL
System suitability
  Sample: *Standard solution*
  Suitability requirements
    Tailing factor: NMT 1.5
    Relative standard deviation: NMT 1.0%
Analysis
  Samples: *Standard solution* and *Sample solution*
  Calculate the percentage of the labeled amount of pyridostigmine bromide ($C_9H_{13}BrN_2O_2$) in the portion of Tablets taken:

$$\text{Result} = (r_U/r_S) \times (C_S/C_U) \times 100$$

r_U = peak response from the *Sample solution*
r_S = peak response from the *Standard solution*
C_S = concentration of USP Pyridostigmine Bromide RS in the *Standard solution* (mg/mL)
C_U = nominal concentration of pyridostigmine bromide in the *Sample solution* (mg/mL)

Acceptance criteria: 95.0%–105.0%

PERFORMANCE TESTS
- **DISSOLUTION ⟨711⟩**
  Medium: Water; 900 mL
  Apparatus 2: 50 rpm
  Time: 60 min
  Standard solution: USP Pyridostigmine Bromide RS in *Medium* at a known concentration approximately the same as that of the *Sample solution*
  Sample solution: Dilute with *Medium* and filter to obtain a concentration that is similar to that of the *Standard solution.*
  Instrumental conditions
    Mode: UV
    Analytical wavelength: 270 nm
  Analysis
    Samples: *Standard solution* and *Sample solution*
    Calculate the percentage of the labeled amount of pyridostigmine bromide ($C_9H_{13}BrN_2O_2$) dissolved:

$$\text{Result} = (A_U/A_S) \times C_S \times V \times (1/L) \times 100$$

A_U = absorbance of the *Sample solution*
A_S = absorbance of the *Standard solution*
C_S = concentration of USP Pyridostigmine Bromide RS in the *Standard solution* (mg/mL)
V = volume of *Medium*, 900 mL
L = label claim of pyridostigmine bromide (mg/Tablet)

Tolerances: NLT 80% (Q) of the labeled amount of pyridostigmine bromide ($C_9H_{13}BrN_2O_2$) is dissolved.
- **UNIFORMITY OF DOSAGE UNITS ⟨905⟩:** Meet the requirements

IMPURITIES

Change to read:

- **ORGANIC IMPURITIES**
  Solution A: 4.3 g/L of sodium dodecyl sulfate in water. Adjust with phosphoric acid to a pH of 2.0.
  Mobile phase: Acetonitrile and *Solution A* (30:70)
  System suitability solution: 5 µg/mL each of USP Pyridostigmine Bromide RS and USP Pyridostigmine Related Compound A RS in *Mobile phase*
  Sensitivity solution: 0.4 µg/mL of USP Pyridostigmine Bromide RS in *Mobile phase*
  Standard solution 1: 0.005 mg/mL of USP Pyridostigmine Bromide RS in *Mobile phase*
  Standard solution 2: 0.06 mg/mL of USP Pyridostigmine Bromide RS in *Mobile phase*
  Sample solution: Nominally 1 mg/mL of pyridostigmine bromide prepared as follows. Transfer a portion of powdered Tablets equivalent to 100 mg of pyridostigmine bromide to a suitable volumetric flask with 100 mL of *Mobile phase*. Shake for 30 min, and pass a portion of the solution through a glass fiber filter.
  Chromatographic system
  (See *Chromatography* ⟨621⟩, *System Suitability*.)
  Mode: LC
  Detector: UV 220 nm
  Column: 4.6-mm × 25-cm; 5-µm packing L1
  Flow rate: 1.1 mL/min
  Injection volume: 20 µL
  Run time: •NLT• (IRA 1-Nov-2017) 2 times the retention time of pyridostigmine
  System suitability
  Samples: *System suitability solution, Sensitivity solution,* and *Standard solution 1*
  [NOTE—See *Table 1* for the relative retention times.]
  System suitability requirements
  Resolution: NLT 1.5 between pyridostigmine and pyridostigmine related compound A, *System suitability solution*
  Relative standard deviation: NMT 5.0%, *Standard solution 1*
  Signal-to-noise ratio: NLT 10, *Sensitivity solution*
  Analysis
  Samples: *Standard solution 1, Standard solution 2,* and *Sample solution*
  Calculate the percentage of pyridostigmine related compound A and any individual unspecified degradation product in the portion of Tablets taken:

$$\text{Result} = (r_U/r_S) \times (C_S/C_U) \times 100$$

r_U = peak response of •pyridostigmine related compound A or any individual unspecified degradation product• (IRA 1-Nov-2017) from the *Sample solution*
r_S = peak response of pyridostigmine from *Standard solution 1*
C_S = concentration of USP Pyridostigmine Bromide RS in *Standard solution 1* (mg/mL)
C_U = nominal concentration of pyridostigmine in the *Sample solution* (mg/mL)

Calculate the percentage of pyridostigmine related compound B in the portion of Tablets taken:

$$\text{Result} = (r_U/r_S) \times (C_S/C_U) \times 100$$

r_U = peak response of pyridostigmine related compound B from the *Sample solution*
r_S = peak response of pyridostigmine from *Standard solution 2*
C_S = concentration of USP Pyridostigmine Bromide RS in *Standard solution 2* (mg/mL)

C_U = nominal concentration of pyridostigmine in the *Sample solution* (mg/mL)
Acceptance criteria: See *Table 1*. Disregard any peak below 0.04%.

Table 1

Name	Relative Retention Time	Acceptance Criteria, NMT (%)
Pyridostigmine related compound B[a]	0.75	•0.2• (IRA 1-Nov-2017)
Pyridostigmine related compound A	0.92	•0.2• (IRA 1-Nov-2017)
Pyridostigmine	1.0	—
Any individual unspecified degradation product	—	0.2
Total •• (IRA 1-Nov-2017) degradation products	—	•0.5• (IRA 1-Nov-2017)

[a] 3-Hydroxy-1-methylpyridin-1-ium bromide.

ADDITIONAL REQUIREMENTS
- **PACKAGING AND STORAGE:** Preserve in tight, light-resistant containers. Store at controlled room temperature.
- **USP REFERENCE STANDARDS** ⟨11⟩
  USP Pyridostigmine Bromide RS
  USP Pyridostigmine Related Compound A RS
  Pyridin-3-yl dimethylcarbamate.
  $C_8H_{10}N_2O_2$ 166.18

Add the following:

•Raltegravir Tablets

DEFINITION
Raltegravir Tablets contain an amount of Raltegravir Potassium equivalent to NLT 95.0% and NMT 105.0% of the labeled amount of raltegravir ($C_{20}H_{20}FN_6O_5$).

IDENTIFICATION
- **A. INFRARED ABSORPTION** ⟨197K⟩ or ⟨197A⟩
  Sample: Grind a Tablet, and use a suitable amount of the powdered Tablet to prepare a specimen.
  Acceptance criteria: The spectrum obtained from the *Sample* shows bands at approximately 1633, 1515, 1188, 810, and 728 cm⁻¹, similar to the spectrum from the Standard similarly obtained. [NOTE—Peak positions may vary slightly between instruments (within ±10 cm⁻¹). Other peaks may be present in the spectra that do not appear in this list.]
- **B.** The retention time of the major peak of the *Sample solution* corresponds to that of the *Standard solution*, as obtained in the *Assay*.

ASSAY
- **PROCEDURE**
  Buffer: 1.36 g/L of monobasic potassium phosphate in water. Adjust with phosphoric acid to a pH of 2.5.
  Mobile phase: Acetonitrile and *Buffer* (29:71)
  Solution A: Acetonitrile and water (50:50)
  Diluent: Acetonitrile and water (30:70)
  Standard solution: 0.22 mg/mL of USP Raltegravir Potassium RS in *Diluent*
  Sample stock solution: Nominally equivalent to 8 mg/mL of raltegravir from Tablets prepared as follows. Transfer NLT 10 Tablets to a suitable volumetric flask and dilute with *Solution A* to volume. Stir the flask vig-

orously for 1 h. Centrifuge a portion of the solution and use the supernatant for *Sample solution* preparation.

Sample solution: Nominally 0.2 mg/mL of raltegravir in *Diluent* from *Sample stock solution*

Chromatographic system
(See *Chromatography* ⟨621⟩, *System Suitability*.)
Mode: LC
Detector: UV 210 nm
Column: 4.6-mm × 15-cm; 5-μm packing L1
Column temperature: 40°
Flow rate: 2 mL/min
Injection volume: 30 μL
Run time: NLT 1.5 times the retention time of raltegravir

System suitability
Sample: *Standard solution*
Suitability requirements
Tailing factor: NMT 1.5
Relative standard deviation: NMT 2.0%

Analysis
Samples: *Standard solution* and *Sample solution*
Calculate the percentage of the labeled amount of raltegravir ($C_{20}H_{20}FN_6O_5$) in the portion of Tablets taken:

$$Result = (r_U/r_S) \times (C_S/C_U) \times (M_{r1}/M_{r2}) \times 100$$

r_U = peak response of raltegravir from the *Sample solution*
r_S = peak response of raltegravir from the *Standard solution*
C_S = concentration of USP Raltegravir Potassium RS in the *Standard solution* (mg/mL)
C_U = nominal concentration of raltegravir in the *Sample solution* (mg/mL)
M_{r1} = molecular weight of raltegravir, 444.44
M_{r2} = molecular weight of raltegravir potassium, 482.51

Acceptance criteria: 95.0%–105.0%

PERFORMANCE TESTS
* **DISSOLUTION ⟨711⟩**
Medium: Water; 900 mL, deaerated
Apparatus 2: 100 rpm with sinker
Times: 15 and 60 min
Buffer: 1.36 g/L of monobasic potassium phosphate in water. Adjust with phosphoric acid to a pH of 3.0.
Mobile phase: Acetonitrile and *Buffer* (38:62)
Diluent: Acetonitrile and water (20:80)
Standard solution: 0.48 mg/mL of USP Raltegravir Potassium RS in *Diluent*. Sonicate, if necessary, to dissolve prior to final dilution.
Sample solution: Pass a portion of the solution under test through a suitable filter.
Chromatographic system
(See *Chromatography* ⟨621⟩, *System Suitability*.)
Mode: LC
Detector: UV 303 nm
Column: 4.6-mm × 10-cm; packing L1
Column temperature: 40°
Flow rate: 5 mL/min
Injection volume: 10 μL
Run time: 1 min
System suitability
Sample: *Standard solution*
Suitability requirements
Tailing factor: NMT 2.0
Relative standard deviation: NMT 3.0%
Analysis
Samples: *Standard solution* and *Sample solution*
Calculate the percentage of the labeled amount of raltegravir ($C_{20}H_{20}FN_6O_5$) dissolved:

$$Result = (r_U/r_S) \times C_S \times (1/L) \times V \times D \times (M_{r1}/M_{r2}) \times 100$$

r_U = peak response from the *Sample solution*
r_S = peak response from the *Standard solution*
C_S = concentration of the USP Raltegravir Potassium RS in the *Standard solution* (mg/mL)
L = label claim (mg/Tablet)
V = volume of *Medium*, 900 mL
D = dilution factor for the *Sample solution*, if needed
M_{r1} = molecular weight of raltegravir, 444.44
M_{r2} = molecular weight of raltegravir potassium, 482.51

Tolerances: 15%–45% of the labeled amount of raltegravir is dissolved in 15 min, and NLT 70% (Q) of the labeled amount of raltegravir is dissolved in 60 min.

* **UNIFORMITY OF DOSAGE UNITS ⟨905⟩:** Meet the requirements

IMPURITIES
* **ORGANIC IMPURITIES**
Buffer, Mobile phase, Solution A, Diluent, Sample solution, and **Chromatographic system:** Proceed as directed in the *Assay*.
Peak identification solution: Prepare a solution containing 2 mg/mL of USP Raltegravir Potassium RS in 1 N sodium hydroxide solution. Stir the solution for 2 h at room temperature. Transfer 5 mL of this solution to a 50-mL volumetric flask and add 5 mL of 1 N hydrochloric acid. Dilute with *Diluent* to volume. [NOTE—In situ degradation generates the raltegravir amine and raltegravir oxalylacetohydrazide analog peaks along with a small peak for raltegravir oxalyl analog impurity.]
System suitability solution: 0.1 mg/mL of USP Raltegravir Potassium RS and 0.2 μg/mL of USP Raltegravir Related Compound E RS in *Diluent*
Standard stock solution: Use the *Standard solution* prepared in the *Assay*.
Standard solution: 0.44 μg/mL of USP Raltegravir Potassium RS in *Diluent* from *Standard stock solution*
System suitability
Samples: *System suitability solution* and *Standard solution*
[NOTE—See *Table 1* for relative retention times.]
Suitability requirements
Resolution: NLT 1.5 between raltegravir related compound E and raltegravir, *System suitability solution*
Relative standard deviation: NMT 10.0%, *Standard solution*
Analysis
Samples: *Sample solution, Peak identification solution,* and *Standard solution*
Calculate the percentage of any individual impurity in the portion of Tablets taken:

$$Result = (r_U/r_S) \times (C_S/C_U) \times (M_{r1}/M_{r2}) \times (1/F) \times 100$$

r_U = peak response of any individual impurity from the *Sample solution*
r_S = peak response of raltegravir from the *Standard solution*
C_S = concentration of USP Raltegravir Potassium RS in the *Standard solution* (mg/mL)
C_U = nominal concentration of raltegravir in the *Sample solution* (mg/mL)
M_{r1} = molecular weight of raltegravir, 444.44
M_{r2} = molecular weight of raltegravir potassium, 482.51
F = relative response factor (see *Table 1*)

Acceptance criteria: See *Table 1*. Reporting threshold is 0.1%.

Table 1

Name	Relative Retention Time	Relative Response Factor	Acceptance Criteria, NMT (%)
Raltegravir amine[a]	0.14	1.0	—[b]
Raltegravir formididyl analog[c]	0.29	1.0	—[b]
Raltegravir oxalyl analog[d]	0.33	1.0	0.3
Raltegravir oxalylacetohydrazide analog[e]	0.48	0.75	0.5
Raltegravir related compound E	0.83	1.0	—[b]
Raltegravir	1.0	—	—
Any individual unspecified impurity	—	1.0	0.2
Total impurities	—	—	0.8

[a] 2-(2-Aminopropan-2-yl)-N-(4-fluorobenzyl)-5-hydroxy-1-methyl-6-oxo-1,6-dihydropyrimidine-4-carboxamide.

[b] This is a process impurity controlled in the drug substance and not monitored in the drug product.

[c] (E)-2-(2-(2-{[(Dimethylamino)methylidene]amino}propan-2-yl)-N-(4-fluorobenzyl)-5-hydroxy-1-methyl-6-oxo-1,6-dihydropyrimidine-4-carboxamide.

[d] 2-[(2-{4-[(4-Fluorobenzyl)carbamoyl]-5-hydroxy-1-methyl-6-oxo-1,6-dihydropyrimidin-2-yl}propan-2-yl)amino]-2-oxoacetic acid.

[e] 2-[2-[2-(2-Acetylhydrazinyl)-2-oxoacetamido]propan-2-yl]-N-(4-fluorobenzyl)-5-hydroxy-1-methyl-6-oxo-1,6-dihydropyrimidine-4-carboxamide.

ADDITIONAL REQUIREMENTS
- **PACKAGING AND STORAGE:** Preserve in tight containers. Store at controlled room temperature.
- **USP REFERENCE STANDARDS ⟨11⟩**
  USP Raltegravir Potassium RS
  USP Raltegravir Related Compound E RS
  N-{2-[4-(Benzylcarbamoyl)-5-hydroxy-1-methyl-6-oxo-1,6-dihydropyrimidin-2-yl]propan-2-yl}-5-methyl-1,3,4-oxadiazole-2-carboxamide.
  $C_{20}H_{22}N_6O_5$ 426.43

∎1S (USP41)

Add the following:

∎Raltegravir Chewable Tablets

DEFINITION
Raltegravir Chewable Tablets contain an amount of Raltegravir Potassium equivalent to NLT 95.0% and NMT 105.0% of the labeled amount of raltegravir ($C_{20}H_{21}FN_6O_5$).

IDENTIFICATION
- **A. INFRARED ABSORPTION ⟨197K⟩ or ⟨197A⟩**
  Sample: Grind a Tablet, and use a suitable amount of the powdered Chewable Tablet to prepare a specimen.
  Acceptance criteria: The spectrum obtained from the *Sample* shows bands at approximately 1633, 1515, 1188, 810, and 728 cm⁻¹, similar to the spectrum from the Standard similarly obtained. [NOTE—Peak positions may vary slightly between instruments (within ±10 cm⁻¹). Other peaks may be present in the spectra that do not appear in this list.]
- **B.** The retention time of the major peak of the *Sample solution* corresponds to that of the *Standard solution*, as obtained in the *Assay*.

ASSAY
- **PROCEDURE**
  Buffer: 1.36 g/L of monobasic potassium phosphate in water. Adjust with phosphoric acid to a pH of 3.0.
  Solution A: Acetonitrile and *Buffer* (20:80)
  Solution B: Acetonitrile
  Mobile phase: See *Table 1.*

Table 1

Time (min)	Solution A (%)	Solution B (%)
0	100	0
25	50	50
25.1	100	0
30	100	0

Diluent: Acetonitrile and water (30:70)
Standard solution: 0.11 mg/mL of USP Raltegravir Potassium RS in *Diluent*
Sample stock solution: Nominally equivalent to 1 mg/mL of raltegravir from Chewable Tablets prepared as follows. Transfer NLT 10 Chewable Tablets to a suitable volumetric flask and dilute with *Diluent* to 20% of the flask volume. Stir the contents of the flask for about 10 min to break apart the Chewable Tablets. Dilute with *Diluent* to volume and stir the contents of the flask for about 1 h. Centrifuge a portion of the solution and use the supernatant for *Sample solution* preparation.
Sample solution: Nominally 0.1 mg/mL of raltegravir from the *Sample stock solution* in *Diluent*
Chromatographic system
(See *Chromatography* ⟨621⟩, *System Suitability*.)
Mode: LC
Detector: UV 220 nm
Column: 4.6-mm × 25-cm; 5-µm packing L1
Column temperature: 40°
Flow rate: 1 mL/min
Injection volume: 15 µL
System suitability
Sample: *Standard solution*
Suitability requirements
Tailing factor: NMT 1.5
Relative standard deviation: NMT 2.0%
Analysis
Samples: *Standard solution* and *Sample solution*
Calculate the percentage of the labeled amount of raltegravir ($C_{20}H_{21}FN_6O_5$) in the portion of Chewable Tablets taken:

$$\text{Result} = (r_U/r_S) \times (C_S/C_U) \times (M_{r1}/M_{r2}) \times 100$$

r_U	= peak response of raltegravir from the *Sample solution*
r_S	= peak response of raltegravir from the *Standard solution*
C_S	= concentration of USP Raltegravir Potassium RS in the *Standard solution* (mg/mL)
C_U	= nominal concentration of raltegravir in the *Sample solution* (mg/mL)
M_{r1}	= molecular weight of raltegravir, 444.44
M_{r2}	= molecular weight of raltegravir potassium, 482.51

Acceptance criteria: 95.0%–105.0%

PERFORMANCE TESTS
- **DISSOLUTION ⟨711⟩**
  Medium: Water; 900 mL, deaerated
  Apparatus 2: 50 rpm
  Time: 15 min
  Buffer: 1.36 g/L of monobasic potassium phosphate in water. Adjust with phosphoric acid to a pH of 3.0.

Mobile phase: Acetonitrile and *Buffer* (38:62)
Diluent: Acetonitrile and water (30:70)
Standard solution: (*L*/900) mg/mL of raltegravir from USP Raltegravir Potassium RS in *Diluent*, where *L* is the label claim in mg/Chewable Tablet
Sample solution: Pass a portion of the solution under test through a suitable filter.
Chromatographic system
(See *Chromatography* ⟨621⟩, *System Suitability*.)
Mode: LC
Detector: UV 303 nm
Column: 4.6-mm × 10-cm; packing L1
Column temperature: 40°
Flow rate: 5 mL/min
Injection volume: 30 µL
Run time: 1 min
System suitability
Sample: *Standard solution*
Suitability requirements
Relative standard deviation: NMT 2.0%
Analysis
Samples: *Standard solution* and *Sample solution*
Calculate the percentage of the labeled amount of raltegravir ($C_{20}H_{21}FN_6O_5$) dissolved:

$$Result = (r_U/r_S) \times C_S \times (1/L) \times V \times D \times (M_{r1}/M_{r2}) \times 100$$

r_U = peak response of raltegravir from the *Sample solution*
r_S = peak response of raltegravir from the *Standard solution*
C_S = concentration of the USP Raltegravir Potassium RS in the *Standard solution* (mg/mL)
L = label claim (mg/Chewable Tablet)
V = volume of *Medium*, 900 mL
D = dilution factor for the *Sample solution*, if applicable
M_{r1} = molecular weight of raltegravir, 444.44
M_{r2} = molecular weight of raltegravir potassium, 482.51
Tolerances: NLT 85% (*Q*) of the labeled amount of raltegravir is dissolved.
• **UNIFORMITY OF DOSAGE UNITS ⟨905⟩:** Meet the requirements

IMPURITIES
• **ORGANIC IMPURITIES**
Solution A, Mobile phase, Diluent, Sample solution, and Chromatographic system: Proceed as directed in the *Assay*.
Peak identification solution: Prepare a solution containing 2 mg/mL of USP Raltegravir Potassium RS in 1 N sodium hydroxide solution. Stir the solution for 2 h at room temperature. Transfer 5 mL of this solution to a 50-mL volumetric flask and add 5 mL of 1 N hydrochloric acid. Dilute with *Diluent* to volume. [NOTE—In situ degradation generates the raltegravir amine and raltegravir oxalylacetohydrazide analog peaks along with a small peak for raltegravir oxalyl analog impurity.]
System suitability solution: 0.1 mg/mL of USP Raltegravir Potassium RS and 0.2 µg/mL of USP Raltegravir Related Compound E RS in *Diluent*
Standard stock solution: Use the *Standard solution* prepared in the *Assay*.
Standard solution: 0.22 µg/mL of USP Raltegravir Potassium RS in *Diluent* from *Standard stock solution*
System suitability
Samples: *System suitability solution* and *Standard solution*
[NOTE—See *Table 2* for relative retention times.]
Suitability requirements
Resolution: NLT 1.5 between raltegravir related compound E and raltegravir, *System suitability solution*
Relative standard deviation: NMT 10.0%, *Standard solution*

Analysis
Samples: *Sample solution, Peak identification solution,* and *Standard solution*
Calculate the percentage of any individual impurity in the portion of Chewable Tablets taken:

$$Result = (r_U/r_S) \times (C_S/C_U) \times (M_{r1}/M_{r2}) \times (1/F) \times 100$$

r_U = peak response of any individual impurity from the *Sample solution*
r_S = peak response of raltegravir from the *Standard solution*
C_S = concentration of USP Raltegravir Potassium RS in the *Standard solution* (mg/mL)
C_U = nominal concentration of raltegravir in the *Sample solution* (mg/mL)
M_{r1} = molecular weight of raltegravir, 444.44
M_{r2} = molecular weight of raltegravir potassium, 482.51
F = relative response factor (see *Table 2*)
Acceptance criteria: See *Table 2*. Reporting threshold is 0.1%.

Table 2

Name	Relative Retention Time	Relative Response Factor	Acceptance Criteria, NMT (%)
Raltegravir amine[a]	0.42	1.0	—[b]
Raltegravir formididyl analog[c]	0.53	1.0	—[b]
Raltegravir oxalyl analog[d]	0.69	0.70	0.2
Raltegravir oxaly-lacetohydra-zide analog[e]	0.81	0.63	0.3
Raltegravir related compound E	0.96	1.0	—[b]
Raltegravir	1.0	—	—
Any individual unspecified impurity	—	1.0	0.2
Total impurities	—	—	0.8

[a] 2-(2-Aminopropan-2-yl)-*N*-(4-fluorobenzyl)-5-hydroxy-1-methyl-6-oxo-1,6-dihydropyrimidine-4-carboxamide.
[b] This is a process impurity controlled in the drug substance and not included in total impurities.
[c] (*E*)-2-(2-{[(Dimethylamino)methylidene]amino}propan-2-yl)-*N*-(4-fluorobenzyl)-5-hydroxy-1-methyl-6-oxo-1,6-dihydropyrimidine-4-carboxamide.
[d] 2-[(2-{4-[(4-Fluorobenzyl)carbamoyl]-5-hydroxy-1-methyl-6-oxo-1,6-dihydropyrimidin-2-yl}propan-2-yl)amino]-2-oxoacetic acid.
[e] 2-{2-[2-(2-Acetylhydrazinyl)-2-oxoacetamido]propan-2-yl}-*N*-(4-fluorobenzyl)-5-hydroxy-1-methyl-6-oxo-1,6-dihydropyrimidine-4-carboxamide.

ADDITIONAL REQUIREMENTS
• **PACKAGING AND STORAGE:** Preserve in tight containers. Store at controlled room temperature.
• **USP REFERENCE STANDARDS ⟨11⟩**
USP Raltegravir Potassium RS
USP Raltegravir Related Compound E RS
N-{2-[4-(Benzylcarbamoyl)-5-hydroxy-1-methyl-6-oxo-1,6-dihydropyrimidin-2-yl]propan-2-yl}-5-methyl-1,3,4-oxadiazole-2-carboxamide.
$C_{20}H_{22}N_6O_5$ 426.43

■1S (*USP41*)

Rizatriptan Benzoate Orally Disintegrating Tablets

DEFINITION
Rizatriptan Benzoate Orally Disintegrating Tablets contain an amount of rizatriptan benzoate ($C_{15}H_{19}N_5 \cdot C_7H_6O_2$) equivalent to NLT 90.0% and NMT 110.0% of the labeled amount of rizatriptan ($C_{15}H_{19}N_5$).

IDENTIFICATION
- **A.** The retention times of the major peaks of the *Sample solution* correspond to those of the *Standard solution*, as obtained in the *Assay*.

Add the following:

- ■**B.** The UV spectrum of the major peak of the *Sample solution* corresponds to that of the *Standard solution*, as obtained in the *Assay*.■1S (USP41)

ASSAY

Change to read:

- **PROCEDURE**
  Buffer: Transfer 3.4 g of monobasic potassium phosphate and 2.0 g of 1-heptanesulfonic acid, sodium salt to a 1-L volumetric flask. Add 900 mL of water. Adjust with 50% (w/w) sodium hydroxide to a pH of 7.5, and dilute with water to volume.
  Mobile phase: Acetonitrile and *Buffer* (16:84)
  Diluent: Acetonitrile and 0.025 M monobasic potassium phosphate (10:90)
  Standard solution: 0.07 mg/mL of USP Rizatriptan Benzoate RS in *Diluent*
  Sample stock solution: Nominally 0.5 mg/mL of rizatriptan in *Diluent* prepared as follows. Transfer NLT 10 Tablets to a suitable volumetric flask. Add 25%–50% of the flask volume of *Diluent*, and swirl until the Tablets have disintegrated completely. Dilute with *Diluent* to volume.
  Sample solution: Nominally 0.05 mg/mL of rizatriptan free base from the *Sample stock solution* in *Diluent*
  Chromatographic system
  (See *Chromatography* ⟨621⟩, *System Suitability*.)
  Mode: LC
  Detector: UV 226 nm. ■For *Identification B*, use a diode array detector in the range of 210–400 nm.■1S (USP41)
  Column: 4.6-mm × 25-cm; 5-µm packing L7
  Column temperature: 30°
  Flow rate: 1 mL/min
  Injection volume: 20 µL
  ■**Run time:** NLT 1.5 times the retention time of rizatriptan■1S (USP41)
  System suitability
  Sample: *Standard solution*
  [NOTE—See *Table 1* for relative retention times.]
  Suitability requirements
  Tailing factor: NMT 3.5
  Relative standard deviation: NMT 2.0% for the rizatriptan peak
  Analysis
  Samples: *Standard solution* and *Sample solution*
  Calculate the percentage of the labeled amount of rizatriptan ($C_{15}H_{19}N_5$) in the portion of Tablets taken:

  $$Result = (r_U/r_S) \times (C_S/C_U) \times (M_{r1}/M_{r2}) \times 100$$

  r_U = peak response from the *Sample solution*

r_S = peak response from the *Standard solution*
C_S = concentration of USP Rizatriptan Benzoate RS in the *Standard solution* (mg/mL)
C_U = nominal concentration of rizatriptan in the *Sample solution* (mg/mL)
M_{r1} = molecular weight of rizatriptan free base, 269.35
M_{r2} = molecular weight of rizatriptan benzoate, 391.47
Acceptance criteria: 90.0%–110.0%

PERFORMANCE TESTS

Change to read:

- **DISSOLUTION** ⟨711⟩
  Test 1
  Medium: Water; 900 mL
  Apparatus 2: 50 rpm
  Time: 5 min
  Standard solution: ($L/625$) mg/mL of USP Rizatriptan Benzoate RS in *Medium*, where L is the label claim of rizatriptan in mg/Tablet
  Sample solution: Pass a portion of the solution under test through a suitable membrane filter of 10-µm pore size.
  Instrumental conditions
  Mode: UV
  Analytical wavelengths: 278 and 320 nm
  Analysis
  Samples: *Standard solution* and *Sample solution*
  Calculate the percentage of the labeled amount of rizatriptan ($C_{15}H_{19}N_5$) dissolved:

  $$Result = (A_U/A_S) \times C_S \times V \times (M_{r1}/M_{r2}) \times (1/L) \times 100$$

  A_U = absorbance of rizatriptan from the *Sample solution*, corrected for the absorbance at 320 nm
  A_S = absorbance of rizatriptan from the *Standard solution*, corrected for the absorbance at 320 nm
  C_S = concentration of USP Rizatriptan Benzoate RS in the *Standard solution* (mg/mL)
  V = volume of *Medium*, 900 mL
  M_{r1} = molecular weight of rizatriptan free base, 269.35
  M_{r2} = molecular weight of rizatriptan benzoate, 391.47
  L = label claim of rizatriptan (mg/Tablet)
  Tolerances: NLT 80% (Q) of the labeled amount of rizatriptan ($C_{15}H_{19}N_5$) is dissolved.
  Test 2: If the product complies with this procedure, the labeling indicates that it meets USP *Dissolution Test 2*.
  Medium: Water, deaerated; 900 mL
  Apparatus 2: 50 rpm
  Time: 10 min
  Buffer: Dissolve 2.7 g of monobasic potassium phosphate in 1 L of water. Add 2 mL of triethylamine and adjust with diluted phosphoric acid (1 in 10) to a pH of 5.0.
  Mobile phase: Methanol and *Buffer* (10:90)
  Standard solution: ($L/625$) mg/mL of USP Rizatriptan Benzoate RS in *Medium*, where L is the label claim in mg/Tablet
  Sample solution: Pass a portion of the solution under test through a suitable membrane filter of 0.45-µm pore size.
  Chromatographic system
  (See *Chromatography* ⟨621⟩, *System Suitability*.)

Mode: LC
Detector: UV 225 nm
Column: 4.6-mm × 15-cm; 5-µm packing L7
Column temperature: 40°
Flow rate: 1.5 mL/min
Injection volume: 20 µL
Run time: ■NLT■1S (USP41) 2 times the retention time of rizatriptan
System suitability
Sample: *Standard solution*
Suitability requirements
Tailing factor: NMT 2.0
Relative standard deviation: NMT 2.0%
Analysis
Samples: *Standard solution* and *Sample solution*
Calculate the percentage of the labeled amount of rizatriptan ($C_{15}H_{19}N_5$) dissolved:

$$Result = (r_U/r_S) \times C_S \times (M_{r1}/M_{r2}) \times V \times (1/L) \times 100$$

r_U = peak response from the *Sample solution*
r_S = peak response from the *Standard solution*
C_S = concentration of USP Rizatriptan Benzoate RS in the *Standard solution* (mg/mL)
M_{r1} = molecular weight of rizatriptan, 269.35
M_{r2} = molecular weight of rizatriptan benzoate, 391.47
V = volume of *Medium* (900 mL)
L = label claim (mg/Tablet)
Tolerances: NLT 80% (*Q*) of the labeled amount of rizatriptan ($C_{15}H_{19}N_5$) is dissolved.
- **UNIFORMITY OF DOSAGE UNITS ⟨905⟩:** Meet the requirements

IMPURITIES

Change to read:

- **ORGANIC IMPURITIES**
Mobile phase, Diluent, Standard solution, Sample solution, and **Chromatographic system:** Proceed as directed in the *Assay.*
System suitability stock solution A: Solution containing rizatriptan *N*-oxide prepared as follows. Rinse a suitable flask with hydrogen peroxide. Heat the flask in an oven for about 10 min. Allow the flask to cool and rinse with water. Transfer 5 mL of *Standard solution* to the flask, add 0.2 mL of hydrogen peroxide, and tightly stopper. Mix well and heat in an oven at 60° for about 30 min. Allow to stand for 24 h. [NOTE—This solution is stable for at least 7 days at room temperature.]
System suitability stock solution B: Solution containing an *N*-methyl adduct of rizatriptan prepared as follows. Dissolve 10 mg of USP Rizatriptan Benzoate RS in 1 mL of methanol in a suitable round-bottom flask. Add 1 mL of dimethylcarbonate and mix by swirling. Reflux the resulting solution over a heating mantle at 125° for NLT 2 h. Allow the solution to cool, and dilute 1 mL of the resulting solution with *Diluent* to 100 mL. [NOTE—This solution is stable for 3 months under refrigerated conditions.] Transfer 10 mL of the resulting solution to a suitable container with a stopper. Add 0.2 mL of 6 M sodium hydroxide solution, and allow the solution to remain at room temperature for NLT 2 h. Neutralize the solution with 0.3 mL of 6 M hydrochloric acid.
System suitability solution: *System suitability stock solution A, System suitability stock solution B,* and *Standard solution* (4:4:2)
Sensitivity solution: 0.07 µg/mL of USP Rizatriptan Benzoate RS from the *Standard solution* in *Diluent*

System suitability
Samples: *Standard solution, System suitability solution,* and *Sensitivity solution*
Suitability requirements
Resolution: NLT 2 between *N*-methyl adduct and rizatriptan, *System suitability solution*
Tailing factor: NMT 3.5, *Standard solution*
Signal-to-noise ratio: NLT 10, *Sensitivity solution*
Analysis
Sample: *Sample solution*
Calculate the percentage of each degradation product in the portion of Tablets taken:

$$Result = (r_U/r_T) \times 100$$

r_U = response of each individual degradation product from the *Sample solution*
r_T = sum of all the areas of rizatriptan and all the degradation products excluding the benzoic acid peak and process impurities from the *Sample solution*
Acceptance criteria: See *Table 1.* ■Reporting threshold for the impurities is 0.1%.■1S (USP41)

Table 1

Name	Relative Retention Time	Acceptance Criteria, NMT (%)
Benzoic acid[a]	0.2	—
Rizatriptan *N*-oxide[b]	0.3	0.5
Aspartame[c]	0.4	—
Rizatriptan desmethyl[d]	0.8	0.4
Rizatriptan *N*-methyl adduct[e]	0.9	1.5
Rizatriptan	1.0	—
Any individual unspecified degradation product	—	0.2
Total degradation products[f]	—	2.0

[a] ■This is the counterion. It is not to be reported or included in the total degradation products for the drug product.■1S (USP41)
[b] 2-{5-[(1*H*-1,2,4-Triazol-1-yl)methyl]-1*H*-indol-3-yl}-*N,N*-dimethylethanamine oxide.
[c] Excipient; may not be present in all sample formulations.
[d] 2-{5-[(1*H*-1,2,4-Triazol-1-yl)methyl]-1*H*-indol-3-yl}-*N*-methylethanamine. [NOTE—May not be present in all formulations.]
[e] 2-{5-[(1*H*-1,2,4-Triazol-1-yl)methyl]-1*H*-indol-3-yl}-*N,N,N*-trimethylethan-1-aminium.
[f] ■Process impurities are controlled in the drug substance and are not to be reported or included in the total degradation products for the drug product.■1S (USP41)

ADDITIONAL REQUIREMENTS
- **PACKAGING AND STORAGE:** Preserve in well-closed, light-resistant containers. Store at controlled room temperature.
- **LABELING:** When more than one *Dissolution* test is given, the labeling states the *Dissolution* test used only if *Test 1* is not used.
- **USP REFERENCE STANDARDS ⟨11⟩**
USP Rizatriptan Benzoate RS

Add the following:

▪Rosuvastatin Calcium

Ca(C$_{22}$H$_{27}$FN$_3$O$_6$S)$_2$ 1001.14
6-Heptenoic acid, 7-[4-(4-fluorophenyl)-6-(1-methylethyl)-2-
   [methyl(methylsulfonyl)amino]-5-pyrimidinyl]-3,5-
   dihydroxy-, calcium salt (2:1), (3*R*,5*S*,6*E*);
[*S*-[*R**,*S**-(*E*)]]-7-[4-(4-Fluorophenyl)-6-(1-methylethyl)-2-
   [methyl(methylsulfonyl)amino]-5-pyrimidinyl]-3,5-
   dihydroxy-6-heptenoic acid, calcium salt (2:1);
Calcium (3*R*,5*S*,*E*)-7-(4-(4-fluorophenyl)-6-isopropyl-2-(*N*-
   methylmethylsulfonamido)pyrimidin-5-yl)-3,5-dihydrox-
   yhept-6-enoate salt (1:2) [147098-20-2].

DEFINITION
Rosuvastatin Calcium contains NLT 97.0% and NMT
   103.0% of rosuvastatin calcium [Ca(C$_{22}$H$_{27}$FN$_3$O$_6$S)$_2$], calculated on the anhydrous and solvent-free basis.

IDENTIFICATION
- **A. Infrared Absorption ⟨197K⟩** or ⟨197A⟩
- **B.** The retention time of the major peak of the *Sample
   solution* corresponds to that of the *Standard solution*, as
   obtained in the test for *Enantiomeric Purity*.
- **C. Identification Tests—General ⟨191⟩,** *Chemical Identifi-
   cation Tests, Calcium*
   Sample solution: 8 mg/mL of Rosuvastatin Calcium in a
      mixture of methanol and water (1:1)
   Acceptance criteria: Meets the requirements

ASSAY
- **Procedure**
   Protect all solutions containing rosuvastatin calcium and
      its related compounds from light.
   Solution A: Acetonitrile, 1% (v/v) aqueous trifluoroace-
      tic acid, and water (290:10:700)
   Solution B: Acetonitrile, 1% (v/v) aqueous trifluoroace-
      tic acid, and water (750:10:240)
   Mobile phase: See *Table 1*.

Table 1

Time (min)	Solution A (%)	Solution B (%)
0	100	0
30	100	0
50	60	40
60	0	100
70	0	100
71	100	0
80	100	0

   Diluent: Acetonitrile and water (25:75)
   System suitability solution A: Dissolve 10 mg of
      Rosuvastatin Calcium in 10 mL of 1% trifluoroacetic
      acid in ethyl acetate. Heat at 40° for 1 h. Cool, and
      transfer to a separatory funnel. Add 2 mL of 1 M so-
      dium hydroxide, and shake for 30 s. Allow the layers to
      separate, and discard the lower aqueous layer. Add
      2 mL of water, and shake for 10 s. Allow the layers to
      separate, and discard the aqueous layer. Transfer 2 mL
      of the retained organic layer to a 50-mL standard flask,
      add 12 mL of acetonitrile, and dilute with water to vol-
      ume. This solution contains predominantly rosuvastatin
      lactone.
   System suitability solution B: Dissolve 10 mg of
      Rosuvastatin Calcium in a 50-mL volumetric flask in
      10 mL of 1% trifluoroacetic acid in acetonitrile. Stopper,
      and heat at 40° for 1 h. Cool, add 20 mL of water, and
      neutralize with 1 M sodium hydroxide to a pH of 6–8.
      Dilute with water to volume. This solution contains
      predominantly rosuvastatin diastereomers.
   System suitability solution C: 0.25 mg/mL each of USP
      Rosuvastatin Related Compound A RS and USP Rosuvas-
      tatin Related Compound B RS in a mixture of acetoni-
      trile and water (1:1)
   System suitability solution D: 0.04 mg/mL of USP
      Rosuvastatin Related Compound C RS in a mixture of
      acetonitrile and water (1:1)
   System suitability solution E: Heat 250 mg of Rosuvas-
      tatin Calcium at 50° for 7 days in suitable glassware
      with a porous cover. Dissolve 50 mg of the heated
      rosuvastatin calcium in 11 mL of acetonitrile in a 50-mL
      standard flask. Add 5 mL of *System suitability solution A*,
      3 mL of *System suitability solution B*, 1 mL of *System suit-
      ability solution C*, and 1 mL of *System suitability solution
      D*. Dilute with water to volume.
   Standard solution: 0.7 mg/mL of USP Rosuvastatin Cal-
      cium RS in *Diluent*
   Sample solution: 0.7 mg/mL of Rosuvastatin Calcium in
      Diluent
   Chromatographic system
   (See *Chromatography* ⟨621⟩, *System Suitability*.)
      Mode: LC
      Detector: UV 242 nm
      Column: 3.0-mm × 15-cm; 3-μm packing L1
      Column temperature: 40°
      Flow rate: 0.75 mL/min
      Injection volume: 10 μL
   System suitability
      Samples: *System suitability solution E* and *Standard
         solution*
      [Note—See *Table 2* for relative retention times.]
      Suitability requirements
         Resolution: NLT 2.0 between the rosuvastatin and
            rosuvastatin diastereomer peaks, *System suitability so-
            lution E*
         Tailing factor: NMT 1.5 for the rosuvastatin peak,
            Standard solution
   Analysis
      Samples: *Standard solution* and *Sample solution*
      Calculate the percentage of rosuvastatin calcium
         [Ca(C$_{22}$H$_{27}$FN$_3$O$_6$S)$_2$] in the portion of Rosuvastatin Cal-
         cium taken:

$$\text{Result} = (r_U/r_S) \times (C_S/C_U) \times 100$$

   r_U = peak response of rosuvastatin from the *Sample
         solution*
   r_S = peak response of rosuvastatin from the
         Standard solution
   C_S = concentration of USP Rosuvastatin Calcium RS
         in the *Standard solution* (mg/mL)
   C_U = concentration of Rosuvastatin Calcium in the
         Sample solution (mg/mL)
   Acceptance criteria: 97.0%–103.0% on the anhydrous
      and solvent-free basis

IMPURITIES
- **Organic Impurities**
   Protect all solutions containing rosuvastatin calcium and
      its related compounds from light.
   **Mobile phase, Diluent, System suitability solution E,
      Sample solution, Chromatographic system,** and **Sys-
      tem suitability:** Proceed as directed in the *Assay*.
   Standard solution: 0.0014 mg/mL of USP Rosuvastatin
      Calcium RS in *Diluent*

Analysis

Samples: *Sample solution* and *Standard solution*

Calculate the percentage of each impurity in the portion of Rosuvastatin Calcium taken:

$$Result = (r_U/r_S) \times (C_S/C_U) \times (1/F) \times 100$$

r_U = peak response of each impurity from the *Sample solution*

r_S = peak response of rosuvastatin from the *Standard solution*

C_S = concentration of USP Rosuvastatin Calcium RS in the *Standard solution* (mg/mL)

C_U = concentration of Rosuvastatin Calcium in the *Sample solution* (mg/mL)

F = relative response factor (see *Table 2*)

Acceptance criteria: See *Table 2*. Disregard peaks less than 0.05%.

Table 2

Name	Relative Retention Time	Relative Response Factor	Acceptance Criteria, NMT (%)
Rosuvastatin related compound A	0.9	1.00	0.2
Rosuvastatin	1.0	1.00	—
Rosuvastatin diastereomers[a]	1.1	1.00	0.5
Rosuvastatin ketone[b]	1.5	0.71	0.8
Rosuvastatin lactone[c]	1.7	1.00	0.15
Rosuvastatin related compound B[d]	2.2	1.00	—
Rosuvastatin dehydro analog[e]	1.8	1.00	0.15
Rosuvastatin related compound C[d]	2.6	1.00	—
Any unspecified impurity	—	1.00	0.10
Total impurities	—	—	1.5

[a] (3RS,5RS,E)-7-[4-(4-Fluorophenyl)-6-isopropyl-2-(N-methylmethyl-sulfonamido)pyrimidin-5-yl]-3,5-dihydroxyhept-6-enoic acid.

[b] (R,E)-7-[4-(4-Fluorophenyl)-6-isopropyl-2-(N-methylmethyl-sulfonamido)pyrimidin-5-yl]-3-hydroxy-5-oxohept-6-enoic acid.

[c] N-[4-(4-Fluorophenyl)-5-{(E)-2-[(2S,4R)-4-hydroxy-6-oxotetrahydro-2H-py-ran-2-yl]vinyl}-6-isopropylpyrimidin-2-yl]-N-methylmethanesulfonamide.

[d] Classified as any unspecified impurity.

[e] (S,2ZE,6E)-7-[4-(4-Fluorophenyl)-6-isopropyl-2-(N-methylmethyl-sulfonamido)pyrimidin-5-yl]-5-hydroxyhepta-2,6-dienoic acid.

- **ENANTIOMERIC PURITY**

Prepare all solutions containing rosuvastatin calcium and its related compounds in amber glassware.

Mobile phase: Acetonitrile and 0.1% (v/v) trifluoroacetic acid in water (25:75)

Diluent: Prepare as directed in the *Assay.*

System suitability solution: 1 mg/mL of USP Rosuvastatin Calcium RS and 0.004 mg/mL of USP Rosuvastatin Enantiomer RS in *Diluent*

Standard solution: 0.005 mg/mL of USP Rosuvastatin Calcium RS in *Diluent*

Sample solution: 1 mg/mL of Rosuvastatin Calcium in *Diluent*

Chromatographic system

(See *Chromatography* ⟨621⟩, *System Suitability.*)

Mode: LC

Detector: UV 242 nm

Column: 4.6-mm × 15-cm; 5-µm packing L107

Column temperature: 35°

Flow rate: 0.5 mL/min

Injection volume: 10 µL

System suitability

Sample: *System suitability solution*

[NOTE—The relative retention times for rosuvastatin enantiomer and rosuvastatin are about 0.9 and 1.0, respectively.]

Suitability requirements

Resolution: NLT 1.5 between the rosuvastatin enantiomer and rosuvastatin peaks

Tailing factor: NMT 1.8 for the rosuvastatin peak

Analysis

Samples: *Standard solution* and *Sample solution*

Calculate the percentage of rosuvastatin enantiomer in the portion of Rosuvastatin Calcium taken:

$$Result = (r_U/r_S) \times (C_S/C_U) \times 100$$

r_U = peak response of rosuvastatin enantiomer from the *Sample solution*

r_S = peak response of rosuvastatin from the *Standard solution*

C_S = concentration of USP Rosuvastatin Calcium RS in the *Standard solution* (mg/mL)

C_U = concentration of Rosuvastatin Calcium in the *Sample solution* (mg/mL)

Acceptance criteria: NMT 0.15%

- **LIMIT OF CHLORIDE**

Sample: 150 mg of Rosuvastatin Calcium

Titrimetric system

(See *Titrimetry* ⟨541⟩.)

Mode: Direct titration

Titrant: 0.01 M silver nitrate

Endpoint detection: Potentiometric

Blank: 60 mL of water and 5 mL of 10% (v/v) aqueous nitric acid

Analysis: Dissolve the *Sample* in 60 mL of water, and add 5 mL of 10% (v/v) aqueous nitric acid. Titrate with *Titrant.*

Calculate the percentage of chloride in the portion of Rosuvastatin Calcium taken:

$$Result = \{[(V_S - V_B) \times M \times F]/W\} \times 100$$

V_S = *Titrant* volume consumed by the *Sample* (mL)

V_B = *Titrant* volume consumed by the *Blank* (mL)

M = actual molarity of the *Titrant* (mmol/mL)

F = equivalency factor, 35.45 mg/mmol

W = *Sample* weight (mg)

Acceptance criteria: NMT 0.2%

SPECIFIC TESTS

- **WATER DETERMINATION** ⟨921⟩, *Method I, Method Ia* or *Method Ic*: NMT 6%

ADDITIONAL REQUIREMENTS

- **PACKAGING AND STORAGE:** Preserve in well-closed containers, protected from light. Store at controlled room temperature.
- **USP REFERENCE STANDARDS** ⟨11⟩

USP Rosuvastatin Calcium RS

USP Rosuvastatin Enantiomer RS

Calcium (3S,5R,E)-7-[4-(4-fluorophenyl)-6-isopropyl-2-(N-methylmethylsulfonamido)pyrimidin-5-yl]-3,5-dihydroxyhept-6-enoate salt (1:2).

$Ca(C_{22}H_{27}FN_3O_6S)_2$ 1001.14

USP Rosuvastatin Related Compound A RS

Calcium (3R,5S,E)-7-{4-(4-fluorophenyl)-2-[(2-hydroxy-N,2-dimethylpropyl)sulfonamide]-6-isopropylpyrimidin-5-yl}-3,5-dihydroxyhept-6-enoate salt (1:2).

$Ca(C_{25}H_{33}FN_3O_7S)_2$ 1117.30

USP Rosuvastatin Related Compound B RS
Calcium (3R,5S,E)-7-(4-(4-fluorophenyl)-2-{2-[4-(4-fluorophenyl)-6-isopropyl-2-(N-methylmethyl-sulfonamido)pyrimidin-5-yl]-2-hydroxy-N-methylethyl-sulfonamido}-6-isopropylpyrimidin-5-yl)-3,5-dihydrox-yhept-6-enoate salt (1:2).
Ca(C$_{38}$H$_{45}$F$_2$N$_6$O$_9$S$_2$)$_2$ 1703.93
USP Rosuvastatin Related Compound C RS
tert-Butyl 2-[(4R,6S)-6-{(E)-2-[4-(4-fluorophenyl)-6-iso-propyl-2-(N-methylmethylsulfonamido)pyrimidin-5-yl]vinyl}-2,2-dimethyl-1,3-dioxan-4-yl]acetate.
C$_{29}$H$_{40}$FN$_3$O$_6$S   577.71

■1S (USP41)

Add the following:

▪Rosuvastatin Tablets

DEFINITION
Rosuvastatin Tablets contain NLT 90% and NMT 110% of the labeled amount of rosuvastatin (C$_{22}$H$_{28}$FN$_3$O$_6$S).

IDENTIFICATION
• **A.** The UV absorption spectra of the rosuvastatin peak of the *Sample solution* exhibit maxima and minima at the same wavelengths as those of the corresponding peak of the *Standard solution*, as obtained in the *Assay*.
• **B.** The retention time of the major peak of the *Sample solution* corresponds to that of the *Standard solution*, as obtained in the *Assay*.

ASSAY
• **PROCEDURE**
Protect all solutions containing rosuvastatin from light.
Solution A: 1% trifluoroacetic acid in water
Mobile phase: Acetonitrile, *Solution A*, and water (37:1:62)
Diluent: Acetonitrile and water (25:75)
Standard stock solution: 1 mg/mL of USP Rosuvastatin Calcium RS prepared as follows. To a suitable amount of USP Rosuvastatin Calcium RS in a suitable volumetric flask, add water equal to about 50% of the flask volume. Vigorously mix or sonicate the flask to dissolve the material. Add acetonitrile equal to about 25% of the total volume and then dilute with water to volume.
Standard solution: 25 µg/mL of USP Rosuvastatin Calcium RS in *Diluent* from the *Standard stock solution*
Sample solution: Nominally 25 µg/mL of rosuvastatin prepared as follows. Transfer a suitable number of Tablets, NLT 5 Tablets for 80-mg Tablet strength and NLT 10 Tablets for all other Tablet strengths, into a suitable extraction flask. Add water and vigorously mix to disintegrate the Tablets. Add acetonitrile and mix vigorously. Add more water to obtain a 25:75 composition of acetonitrile and water. Pass the solution through a suitable filter. Dilute the filtrate with *Diluent*, if necessary, to the desired concentration.
Chromatographic system
(See *Chromatography* ⟨621⟩, *System Suitability*.)
Mode: LC
Detector: UV 242 nm. For *Identification A*, use a diode array detector in the range of 200–440 nm.
Column: 3.2-mm × 25-cm; 5-µm packing L1. [NOTE—A suitable guard column may be used.]
Column temperature: 40°
Flow rate: 0.75 mL/min
Injection volume: 10 µL
Run time: NLT 1.3 times the retention time of rosuvastatin

System suitability
Sample: *Standard solution*
Suitability requirements
Tailing factor: NMT 1.8
Relative standard deviation: NMT 2.0%
Analysis
Samples: *Standard solution* and *Sample solution*
Calculate the percentage of the labeled amount of rosuvastatin (C$_{22}$H$_{28}$FN$_3$O$_6$S) in the portion of Tablets taken:

$$\text{Result} = (r_U/r_S) \times (C_S/C_U) \times [M \times (M_{r1}/M_{r2})] \times 100$$

r_U = peak response of rosuvastatin from the *Sample solution*
r_S = peak response of rosuvastatin from the *Standard solution*
C_S = concentration of USP Rosuvastatin Calcium RS in the *Standard solution* (µg/mL)
C_U = nominal concentration of rosuvastatin in the *Sample solution* (µg/mL)
M = number of moles of rosuvastatin per mole of rosuvastatin calcium, 2
M_{r1} = molecular weight of rosuvastatin, 481.54
M_{r2} = molecular weight of rosuvastatin calcium, 1001.14
Acceptance criteria: 90%–110%

PERFORMANCE TESTS
• **DISSOLUTION ⟨711⟩**
Protect all solutions containing rosuvastatin from light.
Test 1
Medium: Citrate buffer, pH 6.6 (prepare a solution of 14.7 g/L of sodium citrate dihydrate and 0.33 g/L of anhydrous citric acid; adjust if necessary with sodium citrate or citric acid to a pH of 6.6); 900 mL
Apparatus 2: 50 rpm
Time: 30 min
Diluent: Acetonitrile and water (25:75)
Mobile phase: Acetonitrile, water, and phosphoric acid (400:600:1)
Standard stock solution: 1 mg/mL of USP Rosuvastatin Calcium RS in *Diluent*
Standard solution: A solution of concentration similar to the *Sample solution* in *Medium* from the *Standard stock solution*
Sample solution: Pass a portion of the solution under test through a suitable filter.
Chromatographic system
(See *Chromatography* ⟨621⟩, *System Suitability*.)
Mode: LC
Detector: UV 242 nm
Column: 4.6-mm × 5-cm; 5-µm packing L1
Flow rate: 1 mL/min
Injection volume: 20 µL
Run time: NLT 2.5 times the retention time of rosuvastatin
System suitability
Sample: *Standard solution*
Suitability requirements
Tailing factor: NMT 1.5
Analysis
Samples: *Standard solution* and *Sample solution*
Calculate the percentage of the labeled amount of rosuvastatin (C$_{22}$H$_{28}$FN$_3$O$_6$S) dissolved:

$$\text{Result} = (r_U/r_S) \times C_S \times V \times (1/L) \times [M \times (M_{r1}/M_{r2})] \times 100$$

r_U = peak response of rosuvastatin from the *Sample solution*
r_S = peak response of rosuvastatin from the *Standard solution*
C_S = concentration of USP Rosuvastatin Calcium RS in the *Standard solution* (mg/mL)
V = volume of *Medium*, 900 mL

L = label claim (mg/Tablet)
M = number of moles of rosuvastatin per mole of rosuvastatin calcium, 2
M_{r1} = molecular weight of rosuvastatin, 481.54
M_{r2} = molecular weight of rosuvastatin calcium, 1001.14

Tolerances: NLT 75% (Q) of the labeled amount of rosuvastatin ($C_{22}H_{28}FN_3O_6S$) is dissolved.

Test 2: If the product complies with this test, the labeling indicates that it meets *Dissolution Test 2*.

Medium: 0.05 M citrate buffer pH 6.6 (to a solution of 10.5 g/L of citric acid monohydrate, add 5.9 g/L of sodium hydroxide and mix; adjust with 0.2 M sodium hydroxide or 0.2 M hydrochloric acid to a pH of 6.6); 900 mL

Apparatus 2: 50 rpm

Time: 30 min

Buffer: Dissolve 2.72 g of potassium dihydrogen phosphate in 1 L of water and add 2 mL of triethylamine. Adjust with phosphoric acid to a pH of 2.5.

Mobile phase: Acetonitrile and *Buffer* (30:70)

Standard stock solution: 0.5 mg/mL of USP Rosuvastatin Calcium RS in *Medium*. Sonication may be necessary for complete dissolution.

Standard solution: (L/900) mg/mL of USP Rosuvastatin Calcium RS in *Medium* from the *Standard stock solution*

Sample solution: Pass a portion of the solution under test through a suitable filter of 0.45-µm pore size.

Chromatographic system
(See *Chromatography* ⟨621⟩, *System Suitability*.)
Mode: LC
Detector: UV 240 nm
Column: 4.6-mm × 10-cm; 5-µm packing L1
Flow rate: 2 mL/min
Injection volume: 20 µL
Run time: NLT 1.5 times the retention time of rosuvastatin

System suitability
Sample: *Standard solution*
Suitability requirements
Tailing factor: NMT 2.0
Relative standard deviation: NMT 2.0%

Analysis
Samples: *Standard solution* and *Sample solution*
Calculate the percentage of the labeled amount of rosuvastatin ($C_{22}H_{28}FN_3O_6S$) dissolved:

$$Result = (r_U/r_S) \times C_S \times V \times (1/L) \times [M \times (M_{r1}/M_{r2})] \times 100$$

r_U = peak response of rosuvastatin from the *Sample solution*
r_S = peak response of rosuvastatin from the *Standard solution*
C_S = concentration of USP Rosuvastatin Calcium RS in the *Standard solution* (mg/mL)
V = volume of *Medium*, 900 mL
L = label claim (mg/Tablet)
M = number of moles of rosuvastatin per mole of rosuvastatin calcium, 2
M_{r1} = molecular weight of rosuvastatin, 481.54
M_{r2} = molecular weight of rosuvastatin calcium, 1001.14

Tolerances: NLT 80% (Q) of the labeled amount of rosuvastatin ($C_{22}H_{28}FN_3O_6S$) is dissolved.

- **UNIFORMITY OF DOSAGE UNITS** ⟨905⟩: Meet the requirements

IMPURITIES
- **ORGANIC IMPURITIES**
  Protect all solutions containing rosuvastatin calcium from light.
  Mobile phase and **Diluent:** Prepare as directed in the *Assay*.

System suitability stock solution: 50 µg/mL each of USP Rosuvastatin Calcium RS and rosuvastatin diastereomers in acidic water prepared as follows. To a suitable amount of USP Rosuvastatin Calcium RS in a suitable volumetric flask, add water equal to about 50% of the flask volume. Add 1 M hydrochloric acid equal to about 10% of the total volume. Heat in a water bath at 60° for 2 h and neutralize by adding 1 M sodium hydroxide. Cool to room temperature and add acetonitrile equal to about 25% of the total volume. Dilute with water to volume.

System suitability solution: 25 µg/mL each of USP Rosuvastatin Calcium RS and rosuvastatin diastereomers prepared by mixing *System suitability stock solution* and *Diluent* (1:1)

Standard solution: 10 µg/mL of USP Rosuvastatin Calcium RS in *Diluent*

Sample solution: Nominally 1 mg/mL of rosuvastatin prepared as follows. Transfer a number of Tablets per *Table 1* into a suitable extraction flask. Add water, and mix vigorously to disintegrate the Tablets. Add acetonitrile and mix vigorously followed by an additional amount of water to obtain a final composition of acetonitrile and water (1:3). Pass the solution through a suitable filter.

Table 1

Tablet Strength (mg)	Number of Tablets	Volumetric Flask Size (mL)	Water (mL)	Acetonitrile (mL)
2.5	40	100	50	25
5	20	100	50	25
10	10	100	50	25
20	10	200	100	50
40	12	500	250	125
80	6	500	250	125

Chromatographic system: Proceed as directed in the *Assay*, except for *Run time*.
Run time: NLT 2.5 times the retention time of rosuvastatin

System suitability
Samples: *System suitability solution* and *Standard solution*
Suitability requirements
Resolution: NLT 1.5 between rosuvastatin and rosuvastatin diastereomers, *System suitability solution*
Tailing factor: NMT 1.8, *Standard solution*
Relative standard deviation: NMT 2.0%, *Standard solution*

Analysis
Samples: *Standard solution* and *Sample solution*
Calculate the percentage of each impurity in the portion of Tablets taken:

$$Result = (r_U/r_S) \times (C_S/C_U) \times [M \times (M_{r1}/M_{r2})] \times (1/F) \times 100$$

r_U = peak response of each impurity from the *Sample solution*
r_S = peak response of rosuvastatin from the *Standard solution*
C_S = concentration of USP Rosuvastatin Calcium RS in the *Standard solution* (mg/mL)
C_U = nominal concentration of rosuvastatin in the *Sample solution* (mg/mL)
M = number of moles of rosuvastatin per mole of rosuvastatin calcium, 2
M_{r1} = molecular weight of rosuvastatin, 481.54
M_{r2} = molecular weight of rosuvastatin calcium, 1001.14
F = relative response factor (see *Table 2*)

Acceptance criteria: See *Table 2*.

Table 2

Name	Relative Retention Time	Relative Response Factor	Acceptance Criteria, NMT (%)
Rosuvastatin related compound A	0.9	—	—
Rosuvastatin	1.0	—	—
Rosuvastatin diastereomers[a,b]	1.1	—	—
Rosuvastatin ketone[c]	1.6	0.71	2.1
Rosuvastatin lactone[d]	2.3	1.0	1.5
Rosuvastatin ethyl ester (if present)[e]	3.8	1.0	0.5
Any unspecified degradation product	—	1.0	0.2
Total degradation products	—	—	3.6

[a] (3RS,5RS,E)-7-[4-(4-Fluorophenyl)-6-isopropyl-2-(N-methylmethyl-sulfonamido)pyrimidin-5-yl]-3,5-dihydroxyhept-6-enoic acid.

[b] Process impurity controlled in the drug substance monograph. Provided for information only; the content is not calculated, not reported, and not included in the total impurities.

[c] (R,E)-7-[4-(4-Fluorophenyl)-6-isopropyl-2-(N-methylmethyl-sulfonamido)pyrimidin-5-yl]-3-hydroxy-5-oxohept-6-enoic acid.

[d] N-[4-(4-Fluorophenyl)-5-{(E)-2-[(2S,4R)-4-hydroxy-6-oxotetrahydro-2H-pyran-2-yl]vinyl}-6-isopropylpyrimidin-2-yl]-N-methylmethanesulfonamide.

[e] Ethyl (3R,5S,E)-7-[4-(4-fluorophenyl)-6-isopropyl-2-(N-methylmethyl-sulfonamido)pyrimidin-5-yl]-3,5-dihydroxyhept-6-enoate.

ADDITIONAL REQUIREMENTS

- **PACKAGING AND STORAGE:** Preserve in well-closed containers. Store at controlled room temperature.
- **LABELING:** When more than one *Dissolution* test is given, the labeling states the *Dissolution* test used only if *Test 1* is not used.
- **USP REFERENCE STANDARDS ⟨11⟩**
  USP Rosuvastatin Calcium RS

■1S *(USP41)*

Salmeterol Xinafoate

C₂₅H₃₇NO₄ · C₁₁H₈O₃   603.75

$C_{25}H_{37}NO_4 \cdot C_{11}H_8O_3$ 603.75

1,3-Benzenedimethanol, 4-hydroxy-α¹-[[[6-(4-phenylbutoxy)hexyl]amino]methyl]-, (±)-, 1-hydroxy-2-naphthalenecarboxylate (salt);
(±)-4-Hydroxy-α¹-[[[6-(4-phenylbutoxy)hexyl]amino]methyl]-m-xylene-α,α'-diol 1-hydroxy-2-naphthoate (salt) [94749-08-3].

DEFINITION

Salmeterol Xinafoate contains NLT 98.0% and NMT 102.0% of salmeterol xinafoate ($C_{25}H_{37}NO_4 \cdot C_{11}H_8O_3$), calculated on the water- and solvent-free basis.

IDENTIFICATION

- **A. INFRARED ABSORPTION ⟨197⟩:** [NOTE—⟨197A⟩, ⟨197K⟩, or ⟨197M⟩ may be used.]
- **B.** The retention time of the major peak of the *Sample solution* corresponds to that of the *Standard solution*, as obtained in the *Assay*.

ASSAY

Change to read:

- **PROCEDURE**
  [NOTE—It is recommended that solutions containing salmeterol be protected from light.]
  Buffer A: 0.1 M sodium dodecyl sulfate
  Buffer B: 0.1 M ammonium acetate
  Mobile phase: Acetonitrile, *Buffer A*, and *Buffer B* (52:24:24). Adjust with glacial acetic acid to a pH of 3.8. [NOTE—This may need as much as 75 mL of glacial acetic acid for each liter.]
  System suitability solution: 0.25 mg/mL of USP Salmeterol Xinafoate RS and 0.02 mg/mL of USP Salmeterol Related Compound B RS in *Mobile phase*
  Standard solution: 0.25 mg/mL of USP Salmeterol Xinafoate RS in *Mobile phase*
  Sample solution: 0.25 mg/mL of Salmeterol Xinafoate in *Mobile phase*
  Chromatographic system
  (See *Chromatography ⟨621⟩, System Suitability*.)
  Mode: LC
  Detector: UV 278 nm
  Column: 4.6-mm × 15-cm; 5-μm packing L1
  Flow rate: 2 mL/min
  Injection volume: 20 μL
  System suitability
  Sample: *System suitability solution*
  [NOTE—The relative retention times for salmeterol related compound B and salmeterol are about 0.9 and 1.0, respectively.]
  Suitability requirements
  Resolution: NLT ●1.0● (RB 1-Aug-2017) between salmeterol and salmeterol related compound B
  Relative standard deviation: NMT 1.0% for salmeterol
  Analysis
  Samples: *Standard solution* and *Sample solution*
  Calculate the percentage of salmeterol xinafoate ($C_{25}H_{37}NO_4 \cdot C_{11}H_8O_3$) in the portion of Salmeterol Xinafoate taken:

$$Result = (r_U/r_S) \times (C_S/C_U) \times 100$$

r_U = peak response from the *Sample solution*
r_S = peak response from the *Standard solution*
C_S = concentration of USP Salmeterol Xinafoate RS in the *Standard solution* (mg/mL)
C_U = concentration of Salmeterol Xinafoate in the *Sample solution* (mg/mL)

Acceptance criteria: 98.0%–102.0% on the water- and solvent-free basis

IMPURITIES

- **RESIDUE ON IGNITION ⟨281⟩:** NMT 0.1%

Change to read:

- **ORGANIC IMPURITIES**
  [NOTE—It is recommended that solutions containing salmeterol be protected from light.]
  Buffer A, Buffer B, and Chromatographic system: Proceed as directed in the *Assay*.
  Diluent: Acetonitrile and water (50:50)
  Solution A: Acetonitrile, *Buffer A*, and *Buffer B* (52:24:24). Adjust with glacial acetic acid to a pH of 3.8.
  Solution B: Acetonitrile
  Mobile phase: See *Table 1*.

Table 1

Time (min)	Solution A (%)	Solution B (%)
0	100	0
16.0	100	0
36.0	30	70
45.0	30	70
45.1	100	0
50[a]	100[a]	0[a]

[a] The required equilibration time may be modified to achieve a stable baseline.

System suitability solution: 5.0 mg/mL of USP Salmeterol Xinafoate RS and 0.3 mg/mL each of USP Salmeterol Related Compound A RS and USP Salmeterol Related Compound B RS in *Diluent*

Sample solution: 5.0 mg/mL of Salmeterol Xinafoate in *Diluent*

System suitability
Sample: *System suitability solution*
[NOTE—See *Table 2* for relative retention times.]
Suitability requirements
Resolution: NLT •1.0• (RB 1-Aug-2017) between salmeterol and salmeterol related compound B
Tailing factor: NMT 2.5 for salmeterol
Analysis
[NOTE—Disregard the peak due to hydroxynaphthoic acid and any peaks from blank injections.]
Sample: *Sample solution*
Calculate the percentage of any individual impurity in the portion of Salmeterol Xinafoate taken:

$$\text{Result} = (r_U/r_T) \times 100$$

r_U = peak response of each impurity from the *Sample solution*
r_T = sum of all the peak responses from the *Sample solution*

Acceptance criteria: See *Table 2*. [NOTE—Calculate the total impurities from the sum of all impurity peaks greater than or equal to 0.05%.]

Table 2

Name	Relative Retention Time	Acceptance Criteria, NMT (%)
Hydroxynaphthoic acid[a]	0.2	—
Salmeterol related compound A	0.3	0.2
Salmeterol-phenylethoxy[b]	0.5	0.1
Salmeterol-phenylpropoxy[c]	0.7	0.1
Salmeterol-O-alkyl[d]	0.8	0.3
Salmeterol related compound B	0.9	0.1
Salmeterol	1.0	—
Salmeterol-deoxy[e]	1.6	0.2
Salmeterol-N-alkyl[f]	2.7	0.2

[a] 1-Hydroxy-naphthalene-2-carboxylic acid. This is the counter ion of salmeterol and is included for identification only.
[b] 4-[1-Hydroxy-2-(6-phenethoxyhexylamino)ethyl]-2-(hydroxymethyl)phenol.
[c] 4-{1-Hydroxy-2-[6-(3-phenylpropoxy)hexylamino]ethyl}-2-(hydroxymethyl)phenol.
[d] 4-{1-Hydroxy-2-[4-{1-hydroxy-2-[6-(4-phenylbutoxy)hexylamino]ethyl}-2-(hydroxymethyl)phenoxy]ethyl}-2-(hydroxymethyl)phenol.
[e] 4-{1-Hydroxy-2-[6-(4-phenylbutoxy)hexylamino]ethyl}-2-methylphenol.
[f] 4-{1-Hydroxy-2-[(2-hydroxy-5-{1-hydroxy-2-[6-(4-phenylbutoxy)hexylamino]ethyl}benzyl)[6-(4-phenylbutoxy)hexyl]amino]ethyl}-2-(hydroxymethyl)phenol.

Table 2 (Continued)

Name	Relative Retention Time	Acceptance Criteria, NMT (%)
Any unspecified impurity	—	0.10
Total impurities	—	0.9

[a] 1-Hydroxy-naphthalene-2-carboxylic acid. This is the counter ion of salmeterol and is included for identification only.
[b] 4-[1-Hydroxy-2-(6-phenethoxyhexylamino)ethyl]-2-(hydroxymethyl)phenol.
[c] 4-{1-Hydroxy-2-[6-(3-phenylpropoxy)hexylamino]ethyl}-2-(hydroxymethyl)phenol.
[d] 4-{1-Hydroxy-2-[4-{1-hydroxy-2-[6-(4-phenylbutoxy)hexylamino]ethyl}-2-(hydroxymethyl)phenoxy]ethyl}-2-(hydroxymethyl)phenol.
[e] 4-{1-Hydroxy-2-[6-(4-phenylbutoxy)hexylamino]ethyl}-2-methylphenol.
[f] 4-{1-Hydroxy-2-[(2-hydroxy-5-{1-hydroxy-2-[6-(4-phenylbutoxy)hexylamino]ethyl}benzyl)[6-(4-phenylbutoxy)hexyl]amino]ethyl}-2-(hydroxymethyl)phenol.

SPECIFIC TESTS
• **WATER DETERMINATION** ⟨921⟩, *Method I*
Sample: 0.5 g
Acceptance criteria: NMT 0.25%

ADDITIONAL REQUIREMENTS
• **PACKAGING AND STORAGE:** Preserve in tight containers. Store at a temperature not exceeding 30°.

Change to read:

• **USP REFERENCE STANDARDS** ⟨11⟩
USP Salmeterol Xinafoate RS
USP Salmeterol Related Compound A RS
4-[1-Hydroxy-2-(4-phenylbutylamino)ethyl]-2-(hydroxymethyl)phenol.
$C_{19}H_{25}NO_3$ 315.41
USP Salmeterol Related Compound B RS
4-{1-Hydroxy-2-[6-(4-phenylbutan-2-yloxy)hexylamino]ethyl}-2-(hydroxymethyl)phenol.
• (RB 1-Aug-2017)
$C_{25}H_{37}NO_4$ 415.57

Scopolamine Hydrobromide

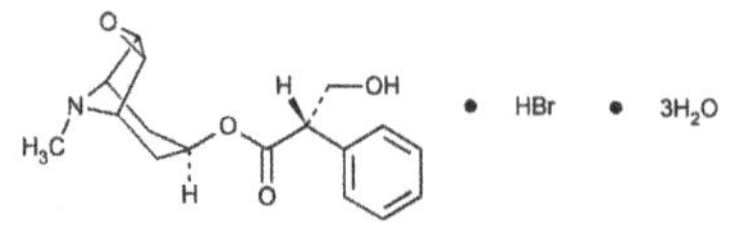

$C_{17}H_{21}NO_4 \cdot HBr \cdot 3H_2O$ 438.31
Benzeneacetic acid, α-(hydroxymethyl)-, 9-methyl-3-oxa-9-azatricyclo[3.3.1.0.^{2,4}]non-7-yl ester, hydrobromide, trihydrate, [7(S)-(1α,2β,4β,5α,7β)]-;
6β,7β-Epoxy-1αH,5αH-tropan-3α-ol (–)-tropate (ester) hydrobromide trihydrate [6533-68-2].
Anhydrous   384.27
[114-49-8].

DEFINITION

Change to read:

Scopolamine Hydrobromide contains NLT ■98.0%■1S (USP41) and NMT 102.0% of scopolamine hydrobromide ($C_{17}H_{21}NO_4 \cdot HBr$), calculated on the anhydrous basis.
[**CAUTION**—Handle scopolamine hydrobromide with exceptional care, because it is highly potent.]

IDENTIFICATION

- **A. INFRARED ABSORPTION ⟨197K⟩**
  Analysis: Dissolve 3 mg in 1 mL of alcohol, and evaporate the solution on a steam bath to dryness. Dissolve the residue in 0.5 mL of chloroform, add 200 mg of potassium bromide, previously dried at 105° for 30 min, and stir frequently for 5 min. Allow the chloroform to evaporate to dryness, and stir frequently to obtain a flowing powder residue. Dry the residue on a steam bath for 5 min, and then immediately compress the residue to a disk.
  Acceptance criteria: Meets the requirements
- **B.**
  Sample solution: 50 mg/mL of alcohol
  Analysis: To 1 mL of *Sample solution* add a few drops of chlorine TS, and shake the mixture with 1 mL of chloroform.
  Acceptance criteria: Brownish color in chloroform layer

Add the following:

■**• C.** The retention time of the scopolamine peak of the *Sample solution* corresponds to that of the *Standard solution*, as obtained in the *Assay*.■1S (USP41)

ASSAY

Change to read:

- **PROCEDURE**
  ■**Buffer solution:** 7.0 g/L of monobasic potassium phosphate in water. Adjust with 0.05 M phosphoric acid to a pH of 3.3.
  Solution A: Dissolve 3.5 g of sodium dodecyl sulfate in 606 mL of *Buffer solution.* Add 320 mL of acetonitrile and mix.
  Solution B: Acetonitrile
  Mobile phase: See *Table 1.*

Table 1

Time (min)	Solution A (%)	Solution B (%)
0	95	5
2.0	95	5
20.0	70	30
20.1	95	5
25.0	95	5

Standard solution: 0.2 mg/mL of USP Scopolamine Hydrobromide RS in *Solution A*
Sample solution: 0.2 mg/mL of Scopolamine Hydrobromide in *Solution A*
Chromatographic system
(See *Chromatography ⟨621⟩, System Suitability.*)
Mode: LC
Detector: UV 210 nm
Column: 4.6-mm × 10-cm; 3-µm packing L1
Flow rate: 1 mL/min
Injection volume: 10 µL
System suitability
Sample: *Standard solution*
Suitability requirements
  Tailing factor: NMT 2.0
  Relative standard deviation: NMT 0.73%
Analysis
Samples: *Standard solution* and *Sample solution*
Calculate the percentage of scopolamine hydrobromide ($C_{17}H_{21}NO_4 \cdot HBr$) in the portion of Scopolamine Hydrobromide taken:

$$Result = (r_U/r_S) \times (C_S/C_U) \times 100$$

r_U = peak response of scopolamine from the *Sample solution*
r_S = peak response of scopolamine from the *Standard solution*
C_S = concentration of USP Scopolamine Hydrobromide RS in the *Standard solution* (mg/mL)
C_U = concentration of Scopolamine Hydrobromide in the *Sample solution* (mg/mL)■1S (USP41)
Acceptance criteria: ■98.0%–■1S (USP41)102.0% on the anhydrous basis

IMPURITIES

Change to read:

- **RESIDUE ON IGNITION ⟨281⟩**
  ■**Sample:** 1 g
  Acceptance criteria: NMT 0.1%■1S (USP41)

Change to read:

- **ORGANIC IMPURITIES**
  ■**Buffer solution, Solution A, Solution B, Mobile phase,** and **Chromatographic system:** Proceed as directed in the *Assay.*
  System suitability solution: 0.2 mg/mL of USP Scopolamine Hydrobromide RS and 0.001 mg/mL of USP Norscopolamine RS in *Solution A*
  Standard solution: 0.002 mg/mL of USP Scopolamine Hydrobromide RS in *Solution A*
  Sample solution: 2.0 mg/mL of Scopolamine Hydrobromide in *Solution A*
  System suitability
  Samples: *System suitability solution* and *Standard solution*
  Suitability requirements
  Resolution: NLT 2.0 between the norscopolamine and scopolamine peaks, *System suitability solution*
  Relative standard deviation: NMT 5.0%, *Standard solution*
  Analysis
  Samples: *Standard solution* and *Sample solution*
  Calculate the percentage of each impurity in the portion of Scopolamine Hydrobromide taken:

$$Result = (r_U/r_S) \times (C_S/C_U) \times 1/F \times 100$$

r_U = peak response of the impurity from the *Sample solution*
r_S = peak response of scopolamine from the *Standard solution*
C_S = concentration of USP Scopolamine Hydrobromide RS in the *Standard solution* (mg/mL)
C_U = concentration of Scopolamine Hydrobromide in the *Sample solution* (mg/mL)
F = relative response factor (see *Table 2*)
Acceptance criteria: See *Table 2.* The reporting threshold is 0.05%. Disregard any peak due to the bromide ion at RRT 0.1 that appears close to the solvent peak.

Table 2

Name	Relative Retention Time	Relative Response Factor	Acceptance Criteria, NMT (%)
Tropic acid[a]	0.19	2.4	0.20
Norscopolamine	0.89	1.4	0.5
Scopolamine	1.0	—	—
Hyoscyamine[b]	1.3	1.3	0.20
Apohyoscine[c]	1.8	2.2	0.20
Apoatropine[d]	2.4	2.3	0.20
Any other individual impurity	—	—	0.10
Total impurities	—	—	0.7

[a] 3-Hydroxy-2-phenylpropanoic acid.

[b] (1R,3r,5S)-8-Methyl-8-azabicyclo[3.2.1]octan-3-yl (S)-3-hydroxy-2-phenyl-propanoate.

[c] (1R,2R,4S,5S,7s)-9-Methyl-3-oxa-9-azatricyclo[3.3.1.0²,⁴]nonan-7-yl 2-phenylacrylate.

[d] (1R,3r,5S)-8-Methyl-8-azabicyclo[3.2.1]octan-3-yl 2-phenylacrylate.

■1S (USP41)

SPECIFIC TESTS

- **OPTICAL ROTATION ⟨781S⟩**, *Procedures, Specific Rotation*
  Sample solution: 50 mg/mL of anhydrous Scopolamine Hydrobromide in water
  Acceptance criteria: −24° to −26°
- **PH ⟨791⟩**
  Sample solution: 50 mg/mL of Scopolamine Hydrobromide in water
  Acceptance criteria: 4.0–5.5
- **WATER DETERMINATION ⟨921⟩**, *Method III*
  Analysis: Dry in two stages (see *Loss on Drying* ⟨731⟩); first at 80° for 2 h, and then at 105° for an additional 3 h.
  Acceptance criteria: NMT 13.0%

ADDITIONAL REQUIREMENTS

- **PACKAGING AND STORAGE:** Preserve in tight, light-resistant containers.

Change to read:

- **USP REFERENCE STANDARDS ⟨11⟩**
  ■USP Norscopolamine RS
  (1R,2R,4S,5S,7s)-3-Oxa-9-azatricyclo[3.3.1.0²,⁴]nonan-7-yl (S)-3-hydroxy-2-phenylpropanoate.
  $C_{16}H_{19}NO_4$ 289.33■1S (USP41)
  USP Scopolamine Hydrobromide RS

Sodium Fluoride Oral Solution

DEFINITION

Sodium Fluoride Oral Solution contains NLT 90.0% and NMT 110.0% of the labeled amount of sodium fluoride (NaF).

IDENTIFICATION

Change to read:

- **A.** ■The retention time of the fluoride peak of the *Sample solution* corresponds to that of the *Standard solution*, as obtained in the *Assay*.■1S (USP41)
- **B. IDENTIFICATION TESTS—GENERAL ⟨191⟩**, *Chemical Identification Tests, Sodium*

Sample solution: 10 mg/mL of sodium in Oral Solution. If necessary, reduce the volume of a portion of Oral Solution by heating on a steam bath.
Acceptance criteria: Meets the requirements

ASSAY

Change to read:

- **PROCEDURE**
  ■[NOTE—Use water with a resistivity of NLT 18 megohm-cm to prepare the solutions.]
  Mobile phase: 150 mg/L of anhydrous sodium carbonate and 1.0 mL/L of 1 N sodium hydroxide in water. Pass through a suitable filter of 0.45-μm pore size.
  System suitability solution: 1.0 μg/mL of USP Sodium Fluoride RS and 0.5 μg/mL of USP Sodium Chloride RS in water
  Standard solution: 1.1 μg/mL of USP Sodium Fluoride RS in water
  Sample solution: Nominally 1.1 μg/mL of sodium fluoride from a portion of Oral Solution in water
  Chromatographic system
  (See *Chromatography* ⟨621⟩, *System Suitability*.)
  Mode: LC
  Detector: Conductivity with suppression
  Columns
  Guard: 4.0-mm × 5-cm; 10-μm packing L46
  Analytical: 4.0-mm × 25-cm; 10-μm packing L46
  Flow rate: 1.0 mL/min
  Injection volume: 20 μL
  [NOTE—It is recommended to use polymethylpentene HPLC vials.]
  Run time: NLT 2 times the retention time of the fluoride peak
  System suitability
  Sample: *System suitability solution*
  [NOTE—The relative retention times for fluoride and chloride ions are 1.0 and 1.2, respectively.]
  Suitability requirements
  Resolution: NLT 1.5 between fluoride and chloride ions
  Tailing factor: NMT 2.0 for fluoride ion
  Relative standard deviation: NMT 2.0% for fluoride ion
  Analysis
  Samples: *Standard solution* and *Sample solution*
  Calculate the percentage of the labeled amount of sodium fluoride (NaF) in the portion of Oral Solution taken:

$$Result = (r_U/r_S) \times (C_S/C_U) \times 100$$

r_U	= peak response of fluoride from the *Sample solution*
r_S	= peak response of fluoride from the *Standard solution*
C_S	= concentration of USP Sodium Fluoride RS in the *Standard solution* (μg/mL)
C_U	= nominal concentration of sodium fluoride in the *Sample solution* (μg/mL)■1S (USP41)

  Acceptance criteria: 90.0%–110.0%

ADDITIONAL REQUIREMENTS

- **PACKAGING AND STORAGE:** Preserve in tight containers; use plastic containers for Oral Solution having a pH below 7.5.
- **LABELING:** Label the Oral Solution in terms of the content of sodium fluoride (NaF) and in terms of the content of fluoride ion.

Change to read:

- **USP Reference Standards ⟨11⟩**
  ■USP Sodium Chloride RS■₁₅ *(USP41)*
  USP Sodium Fluoride RS

Sodium Fluoride and Acidulated Phosphate Topical Solution

DEFINITION
Sodium Fluoride and Acidulated Phosphate Topical Solution contains NLT 90.0% and NMT 110.0% of the labeled amount of fluoride ion.

IDENTIFICATION

Change to read:

- **A.** ■The retention time of the fluoride peak of the *Sample solution* corresponds to that of the *Standard solution*, as obtained in the *Assay*.■₁₅ *(USP41)*

Change to read:

- **B. Identification Tests—General ⟨191⟩,** *Chemical Identification Tests, Phosphate*
  ■**Sample:** A portion of Topical Solution
  [Note—If the *Sample* contains hydrogen peroxide, use of a platinum-coated disc to neutralize hydrogen peroxide is recommended prior to performing the test.]■₁₅ *(USP41)*
  Acceptance criteria: Meets the requirements

ASSAY

Delete the following:

■• **Procedure 1**
  [Note—Store all solutions, except *Buffer*, in plastic containers.]
  Buffer: Dissolve 57 mL of glacial acetic acid, 58 g of sodium chloride, and 4 g of (1,2-cyclohexylenedinitrilo)tetraacetic acid in 500 mL of water. Adjust with 5 N sodium hydroxide to a pH of 5.25 ± 0.25, and dilute with water to 1000 mL.
  Standard solution A: 420 μg/mL of USP Sodium Fluoride RS in water, equivalent to 190 μg/mL of fluoride ion (10^{-2} M)
  Standard solution B: 19 μg/mL of fluoride ion (10^{-3} M) in water, from *Standard solution A*
  Standard solution C: 1.9 μg/mL of fluoride ion (10^{-4} M) in water, from *Standard solution B*
  Sample solution: Nominally 20 μg/mL of fluoride ion from Topical Solution in water
  Analysis
  Samples: *Standard solution A, Standard solution B, Standard solution C,* and *Sample solution*
  Pipet 20 mL of *Standard solution A, Standard solution B, Standard solution C* and *Sample solution* into separate plastic beakers, each containing a plastic-coated stirring bar. Pipet 20 mL of *Buffer* into each beaker. Concomitantly measure the potentials (see *pH ⟨791⟩*), in mV, of each solution with a pH meter capable of a minimum reproducibility of ± 0.2 mV and equipped with a fluoride-specific ion-indicating electrode and a suitable reference electrode.
  [Note—When taking measurements, immerse the electrodes in the solution, stir on a magnetic stirrer having an insulated top until equilibrium is attained (1–2 min), and record the potential. Rinse and dry the electrodes between measurements, taking care to avoid damaging the crystal of the specific-ion electrode.]
  Plot the logarithms of the fluoride-ion concentrations, in μg/mL, of *Standard solution A, Standard solution B,* and *Standard solution C* versus potential, in mV. From the measured potential of the *Sample solution* and the standard response line, determine the concentration, C, in μg/mL, of fluoride ion in the *Sample solution*. Calculate the percentage of the labeled amount of fluoride ion in the Topical Solution taken:

$$\text{Result} = (C/C_U) \times 100$$

C = concentration of fluoride in the *Sample solution* (μg/mL)
C_U = nominal concentration of fluoride ion in the *Sample solution* (μg/mL)
Acceptance criteria: 90.0%–110.0%■₁₅ *(USP41)*

Change to read:

- **Procedure** ■■₁₅ *(USP41)*
  [Note—Use water with a resistivity of NLT 18 megohm-cm to prepare the solutions.]
  Mobile phase: 150 mg/L of anhydrous sodium carbonate and 1.0 mL/L of 1 N sodium hydroxide in water. Pass through a suitable filter of 0.45-μm pore size.
  ■**System suitability solution:** 1.1 μg/mL of USP Sodium Fluoride RS and 0.5 μg/mL of USP Sodium Chloride RS in water■₁₅ *(USP41)*
  Standard solution: ■■₁₅ *(USP41)*1.1 μg/mL of USP Sodium Fluoride RS in water. Pass through a suitable filter of 0.45-μm pore size.
  Sample solution: Nominally 1.1 μg/mL of sodium fluoride from a portion of Topical Solution in water. Pass through a suitable filter of 0.45-μm pore size.
  Chromatographic system
  (See *Chromatography ⟨621⟩, System Suitability*.)
  Mode: LC
  Detector: Conductivity with suppression
  Columns
    Guard: 4.6-mm × 5-cm; ■7-μm packing■₁₅ *(USP41)* L46
    Analytical: 4.6-mm × 25-cm; ■7-μm packing■₁₅ *(USP41)* L46
  Flow rate: 1.0 mL/min
  Injection volume: 20 μL
  [Note—Use of polymethylpentene HPLC vials is recommended.]
  ■**Run time:** NLT 2 times the retention time of the fluoride peak■₁₅ *(USP41)*
  System suitability
    ■**Sample:** *System suitability solution*
    [Note—The relative retention times for fluoride and chloride ions are 1.0 and 1.2, respectively.]■₁₅ *(USP41)*
    Suitability requirements
    Resolution: NLT 1.5 between fluoride and chloride ions
    ■■₁₅ *(USP41)*
    Tailing factor: NMT 2.0 for fluoride ion
    Relative standard deviation: NMT 2.0% for fluoride ion
  Analysis
    Samples: *Standard solution* and *Sample solution*
    Calculate the percentage of the labeled amount of fluoride ion in the portion of Topical Solution taken:

$$\text{Result} = (r_U/r_S) \times (C_S/C_U) \times (A_r/M_r) \times 100$$

r_U = peak response of fluoride from the *Sample solution*
r_S = peak response of fluoride from the *Standard solution*
C_S = concentration of USP Sodium Fluoride RS in the *Standard solution* (μg/mL)

C_U = nominal concentration of sodium fluoride in the *Sample solution* (µg/mL)
A_r = atomic weight of fluoride, 19.00
M_r = molecular weight of sodium fluoride, 41.99
Acceptance criteria: 90.0%–110.0%

SPECIFIC TESTS
- **PH ⟨791⟩**
  Analysis: Place about 40 mL in a plastic beaker, and determine the pH using a suitable electrode system.
  Acceptance criteria: 3.0–4.5

Delete the following:

- ■• **OTHER REQUIREMENTS:** It responds to the *Identification* tests under *Sodium Fluoride and Phosphoric Acid Gel.*
  ■1S (USP41)

ADDITIONAL REQUIREMENTS
- **PACKAGING AND STORAGE:** Preserve in tight, plastic containers.

Change to read:

- **LABELING:** Label the Topical Solution in terms of the content of sodium fluoride (NaF) and in terms of the content of fluoride ion.■■1S (USP41)

Change to read:

- **USP REFERENCE STANDARDS ⟨11⟩**
  ■USP Sodium Chloride RS■1S (USP41)
  USP Sodium Fluoride RS

Somatropin

```
FPTIPLSRLF DNAMLRAHRL HQLAFDTYQE FEEAYIPKEQ KYSFLQNPQT
SLCFSESIPT PSNREETQQK SNLELLRISL LLIQSWLEPV QFLRSVFANS
LVYGASDSNV YDLLKDLEEG IQTLMGRLED GSPRTGQIFK QTYSKFDTNS
HNDDALLKNY GLLYCFRKDM DKVETFLRIV QCRSVEGSCG F
```

$C_{990}H_{1528}N_{262}O_{300}S_7$ 22,124.77
[12629-01-5].

DEFINITION
Somatropin is a protein hormone consisting of 191 amino acid residues, and its structure corresponds to the major component of the growth hormone extracted from human pituitary glands. It is produced as a lyophilized powder or bulk solution by methods based on recombinant DNA technology. The presence of host-cell DNA and host-cell protein impurities in Somatropin is process specific—the limits of these impurities are determined by validated methods. Manufacturers must demonstrate a correlation between the *Assay* and a validated and approved growth-promotion-based bioassay. It may contain excipients.
[NOTE—One mg of anhydrous Somatropin is equivalent to 3.0 USP Somatropin Units.]

IDENTIFICATION
- **A.** The retention time of the somatropin peak of the *Sample solution* corresponds to that of the *Standard solution*, as obtained in the test for *Chromatographic Purity*, except that a *Standard solution* is also chromatographed and prepared by reconstituting a vial of USP Somatropin RS with *Diluent* to obtain a known concentration of about 2 mg/mL.

- **B. PEPTIDE MAPPING**
  Solution A: Trifluoroacetic acid and water (1:999). Filter, and degas.
  Solution B: Water, trifluoroacetic acid, and acetonitrile (100:1:899)
  Solution C: 0.05 M solution of tris(hydroxymethyl)aminomethane (Tris). Adjust with hydrochloric acid to a pH of 7.5.
  Mobile phase: See *Table 1.*

Table 1

Time (min)	Solution A (%)	Solution B (%)
0	100	0
20	80	20
40	75	25
65	50	50
70	20	80
71	100	0
86	100	0

Trypsin solution: 1 mg/mL of trypsin in *Solution C*. Store in a freezer, if necessary.
Standard stock solution: 2.0 mg/mL of USP Somatropin RS in *Solution C*
Standard solution: To 1 mL of the *Standard stock solution* add 30 µL of *Trypsin solution*. Cap the tube, and place it in a water bath at 37° for 4 h. [NOTE—If this solution is not injected immediately, store it in a freezer.]
Sample stock solution: 2.0 mg/mL of Somatropin in *Solution C*
Sample solution: To 1 mL of the *Sample stock solution* add 30 µL of *Trypsin solution*. Cap the tube, and place it in a water bath at 37° for 4 h. [NOTE—If this solution is not injected immediately, store it in a freezer.]
Chromatographic system
(See *Chromatography* ⟨621⟩, *System Suitability*.)
  Mode: LC
  Detector: UV 214 nm
  Column: 4.6-mm × 25-cm; packing L7
  Column temperature: 30°
  Flow rate: 1 mL/min
  Injection volume: 100 µL
Analysis
  Samples: *Standard solution* and *Sample solution*, separately injected
  [NOTE—Condition the chromatographic system by running a blank gradient program before injecting the digests.]
  Acceptance criteria: The chromatographic profile of the *Sample solution* is similar to that of the *Standard solution*.
- **C. SOMATROPIN BIOIDENTITY TESTS ⟨126⟩:** Meets the requirements
  [NOTE—The bioidentity test may be performed either on the Somatropin bulk drug substance or on the finished pharmaceutical product.]

ASSAY
- **SOMATROPIN CONTENT**
  Buffer solution: Dissolve 5.18 g of dibasic sodium phosphate and 3.65 g of monobasic sodium phosphate in 950 mL of water. Adjust with phosphoric acid or sodium hydroxide solution to a pH of 7.0. Dilute with water to 1000 mL.
  Mobile phase: Isopropyl alcohol and *Buffer solution* (3:97). Filter, and degas.
  Diluent: *Buffer solution* and water (1:1.5)
  System suitability solution: Place 1 vial of USP Somatropin RS in an oven at 50° for 12–24 h. Remove from the oven, and dissolve the contents of the vial in *Dilu-*

ent to obtain a solution with a known concentration of about 1 mg/mL and a dimer content of 1%–2%.

Standard solution: Known concentration of about 1 mg/mL of USP Somatropin RS in *Diluent*

Sample solution: About 1 mg/mL of accurately weighed Somatropin in *Diluent*, or by diluting a bulk solution of Somatropin with *Diluent*. [NOTE—If necessary, the amount of protein in the solution can be determined with the test for *Total Protein Content*.]

Chromatographic system
(See *Chromatography* ⟨621⟩, *System Suitability*.)
Mode: LC
Detector: UV 214 nm
Column: 7.8-mm × 30-cm; packing L33
Column temperature: Ambient
Flow rate: 0.6 mL/min
Injection volume: 20 μL
System suitability
Sample: *System suitability solution*
Suitability requirements
Resolution: NMT 0.4 for the ratio of the valley height, between the dimer and the monomer, and the dimer peak height
Tailing factor: NMT 1.7 for the monomer (major) peak

Analysis
Samples: *Standard solution* and *Sample solution*, separately injected
Record the chromatograms for NLT twice the retention time of the somatropin monomer (major) peak, and measure the peak responses for the monomer.
Calculate the concentration, in mg/mL, of somatropin in the *Sample solution* taken:

$$Result = (r_U/r_S) \times C_S$$

r_U = peak response of the monomer from the *Sample solution*
r_S = peak response of the monomer from the *Standard solution*
C_S = concentration of USP Somatropin RS in the *Standard solution* (mg/mL)

Acceptance criteria: NLT 910 μg of somatropin/mg on the anhydrous basis. When prepared as a bulk solution, it contains NLT 910 μg of somatropin/mg of total protein.

IMPURITIES
• **CHROMATOGRAPHIC PURITY**
Diluent: 0.05 M Tris in water. Adjust with hydrochloric acid to a pH of 7.5.
Mobile phase: *n*-Propyl alcohol and degassed *Diluent* (29:71). Filter.
System suitability solution: 2.0 mg/mL of Somatropin in *Diluent*. Pass through a filter to sterilize or add sodium azide to a final concentration of 0.01%, and allow to stand at room temperature for 24 h. [NOTE—Use within 48 h of preparation, or store the solution in a refrigerator until ready to use.]
Sample solution: 2.0 mg/mL of Somatropin in *Diluent*. [NOTE—Maintain the solutions between 2° and 8°, and use within 24 h. If an automatic injector is used, maintain the temperature between 2° and 8°.]
Chromatographic system
(See *Chromatography* ⟨621⟩, *System Suitability*.)

Mode: LC
Detector: UV 220 nm
Column: 4.6-mm × 25-cm; packing L26
Column temperature: 45°
Flow rate: 0.5 mL/min
Injection volume: 20 μL
System suitability
Sample: *System suitability solution*
Suitability requirements
Resolution: NLT 1.0 between somatropin and its adjacent peak
Tailing factor: 0.9–1.8 for the somatropin (major) peak
Analysis
Sample: *Sample solution*
Calculate the percentage of impurities in the portion of Somatropin taken:

$$Result = [A_U/(A_U + A_S)] \times 100$$

A_U = sum of all the peak responses other than the somatropin (major) peak and disregarding any peak due to the solvent from the *Sample solution*
A_S = peak response of somatropin from the *Sample solution*

Acceptance criteria: NMT 6.0% of total impurities

Change to read:

• **LIMIT OF HIGH MOLECULAR WEIGHT PROTEINS**
Buffer solution, Mobile phase, Diluent, System suitability solution, Sample solution, Chromatographic system, and **System suitability:** Proceed as directed in the *Assay*.
Analysis
Sample: ■1S (USP41) *Sample solution*
Measure the areas of the main peak and of the peaks eluting before the main peak, excluding the solvent peaks.
Calculate the percentage of high molecular weight proteins in the portion of Somatropin taken:

$$Result = [A_H/(A_H + A_M)] \times 100$$

A_H = sum of the areas of the high molecular weight peaks
A_M = peak area of the monomer from the *Sample solution*

Acceptance criteria: NMT 4% of high molecular weight proteins

SPECIFIC TESTS

Change to read:

• **TOTAL PROTEIN CONTENT**
(See *Ultraviolet-Visible Spectroscopy* ⟨857⟩.)
■The method is used in the calculation of total protein in the assay of bulk solution.■1S (USP41)
Buffer solution: 0.025 M solution of monobasic potassium phosphate in water. Adjust with sodium hydroxide to a pH of 7.0.
Sample solution: ■Mix a weighed quantity of Somatropin bulk solution with a weighed quantity of■1S (USP41) *Buffer solution* to obtain a solution with an absorbance value between 0.5 and 1.0 at the wavelength of maximum absorbance at 280 nm.
Analysis: Determine the absorbance of the *Sample solution* using a spectrophotometric cell of path length 1 cm, at the wavelength of maximum absorbance around 280 nm and at 320 nm, using *Buffer solution* as the blank.

Calculate the protein content, in mg, in the portion of Somatropin taken:

$$Result = (A_{max} - A_{320}) \times (V/0.82)$$

A_{max} = absorbance value of the *Sample solution* at the wavelength of maximum absorbance
A_{320} = absorbance value of the *Sample solution* at 320 nm
V = volume of the *Sample solution*

- **MICROBIAL ENUMERATION TESTS ⟨61⟩ and TESTS FOR SPECIFIED MICROORGANISMS ⟨62⟩:** The total aerobic microbial count is NMT 3×10^2 cfu/g, the test being performed on 0.2–0.3 g of powder, accurately weighed.
- **WATER DETERMINATION ⟨921⟩,** *Method I, Method Ic*: NMT 10%, when prepared as a lyophilized powder
- **BACTERIAL ENDOTOXINS TEST ⟨85⟩:** NMT 10 USP Endotoxin Units/mg of Somatropin

ADDITIONAL REQUIREMENTS
- **PACKAGING AND STORAGE:** Preserve in tight containers, and store between –10° and –25°.
- **LABELING:** The labeling states that the material is of recombinant DNA origin.

Change to read:

- **USP REFERENCE STANDARDS ⟨11⟩**
    - (CN 1-May-2018)
    USP Somatropin RS

Sumatriptan Nasal Spray

DEFINITION
Sumatriptan Nasal Spray is an aqueous, buffered solution of Sumatriptan. It is supplied in a form suitable for nasal administration. It contains NLT 90.0% and NMT 110.0% of the labeled amount of sumatriptan ($C_{14}H_{21}N_3O_2S$).

IDENTIFICATION
- **A. INFRARED ABSORPTION ⟨197M⟩**
    Sample: To the contents of one vial of Nasal Spray add 1 mL of a saturated sodium chloride solution. Add 1 mL of a saturated solution of sodium carbonate, and shake vigorously for about 30 s. To the solution so obtained add 2 mL of isopropyl alcohol, shake vigorously for about 30 s, and allow to stand until the phases separate. Transfer the organic phase to a suitable glass vial. Repeat the extraction with a second 2-mL portion of isopropyl alcohol, and transfer the organic phase to the same vial. Evaporate the solution under a stream of nitrogen. Dry the residue in an oven at 100° for 30 min, allow to cool to room temperature in a desiccator, and prepare a mull by the addition of 1–2 drops of mineral oil.
    Acceptance criteria: Meets the requirements

Add the following:

- **B.** The retention time of the major peak of the *Sample solution* corresponds to that of the *Standard solution*, as obtained in the *Assay*.■1S (USP41)

ASSAY

Change to read:

- **PROCEDURE**
    Buffer: Dissolve 1.7 mL of dibutylamine, 0.6 mL of phosphoric acid, and 3.9 g of monobasic sodium phos-

phate dihydrate in water. Adjust with a solution of 50% (w/v) sodium hydroxide to a pH of 6.5, and dilute with water to 1 L.
Mobile phase: Acetonitrile and *Buffer* (25:75)
Diluent: Dissolve 3.9 g of monobasic sodium phosphate dihydrate in water. Adjust with a solution of 50% (w/v) sodium hydroxide to a pH of 6.5, and dilute with water to 1 L. Mix 750 mL of the resulting solution with 250 mL of acetonitrile.
System suitability solution: 0.14 mg/mL of USP Sumatriptan Succinate RS and 0.07 mg/mL of USP Sumatriptan Succinate Related Compound C RS in *Diluent*
Standard solution: 0.14 mg/mL of USP Sumatriptan Succinate RS in *Diluent*
Sample solution: Nominally equivalent to 0.1 mg/mL of sumatriptan in *Diluent* from an appropriate volume of Nasal Spray
Chromatographic system
(See *Chromatography* ⟨621⟩, *System Suitability*.)
Mode: LC
Detector: UV 282 nm
Column: 4.6-mm × 20-cm; packing L1
Flow rate: 1.5 mL/min
Injection volume: 10 µL
■Run time: NLT 4 times the retention of sumatriptan■1S (USP41)
System suitability
Samples: *System suitability solution* and *Standard solution*
[NOTE—The relative retention times for sumatriptan succinate related compound C and sumatriptan are 0.9 and 1.0, respectively.]
Suitability requirements
Resolution: NLT 1.5 between sumatriptan succinate related compound C and sumatriptan, *System suitability solution*
Relative standard deviation: NMT 1.5%, *Standard solution*
Analysis
Samples: *Standard solution* and *Sample solution*
Calculate the percentage of the labeled amount of sumatriptan ($C_{14}H_{21}N_3O_2S$) in the portion of Nasal Spray taken:

$$Result = (r_U/r_S) \times (C_S/C_U) \times (M_{r1}/M_{r2}) \times 100$$

r_U = peak response from the *Sample solution*
r_S = peak response from the *Standard solution*
C_S = concentration of USP Sumatriptan Succinate RS in the *Standard solution* (mg/mL)
C_U = nominal concentration of sumatriptan in the *Sample solution* (mg/mL)
M_{r1} = molecular weight of sumatriptan, ■295.40■1S (USP41)
M_{r2} = molecular weight of sumatriptan succinate, ■413.49■1S (USP41)
Acceptance criteria: 90.0%–110.0%

PERFORMANCE TESTS
- **DELIVERABLE VOLUME**
    Analysis: Test 10 vials separately. Weigh each vial before and after actuation, and calculate the individual volume delivered, in µL, then calculate the mean volume delivered:

    $$Result = (W_1 - W_2)/D$$

    W_1 = weight of the individual vial before actuation (mg)
    W_2 = weight of the individual vial after actuation (mg)
    D = density of the nasal solution
    Acceptance criteria: The volume of each spray delivered is between 80 and 120 µL, and the mean volume is between 90 and 110 µL.

IMPURITIES

Change to read:

- **LIMIT OF SUMATRIPTAN RELATED COMPOUND A**
  Buffer: Dissolve 77.1 g of ammonium acetate in 100 mL of water.
  Mobile phase: Methanol and *Buffer* (90:10)
  Diluent: Prepare as directed in the *Assay.*
  Standard solution: ■0.007 mg/mL■1S (USP41) of USP Sumatriptan Succinate Related Compound A RS in *Diluent*
  Sample solution: Nominally equivalent to 1.0 mg/mL of sumatriptan in *Diluent* from an appropriate volume of Nasal Spray
  Chromatographic system
  (See *Chromatography* ⟨621⟩, *System Suitability.*)
  Mode: LC
  Detector: UV 282 nm
  Column: 4.6-mm × 20-cm; packing L3
  Flow rate: 2 mL/min
  Injection volume: 20 µL
  ■**Run time:** NLT 2 times the retention of sumatriptan related compound A■1S (USP41)
  System suitability
  Sample: *Standard solution*
  Suitability requirements
  Relative standard deviation: NMT 5%
  Analysis
  Samples: *Standard solution* and *Sample solution*
  Calculate the percentage of sumatriptan succinate related compound A in the portion of Nasal Spray taken:

$$Result = (r_U/r_S) \times (C_S/C_U) \times (M_{r1}/M_{r2}) \times 100$$

r_U = peak response of sumatriptan related compound A from the *Sample solution*
r_S = peak response of sumatriptan related compound A from the *Standard solution*
C_S = concentration of ■USP Sumatriptan Succinate Related Compound A RS■1S (USP41) in the *Standard solution* (mg/mL)
C_U = nominal concentration of sumatriptan in the *Sample solution* (mg/mL)
M_{r1} = molecular weight of sumatriptan related compound A, ■495.68■1S (USP41)
M_{r2} = molecular weight of sumatriptan succinate related compound A, ■613.77■1S (USP41)
Acceptance criteria: NMT 1.5%

Change to read:

- **ORGANIC IMPURITIES**
  Buffer: Dissolve 1.7 mL of dibutylamine, 0.6 mL of phosphoric acid, and 3.9 g of monobasic sodium phosphate dihydrate in water. Adjust with a solution of 50% (w/v) sodium hydroxide to a pH of 7.5, and dilute with water to 1 L.
  Mobile phase: Acetonitrile and *Buffer* (25:75)
  Diluent: Prepare as directed in the *Assay.*
  System suitability solution: 1.4 mg/mL of USP Sumatriptan Succinate RS and 1 µg/mL of USP Sumatriptan Succinate Related Compound C RS in *Diluent*
  Identification solution: 3 mg/mL of USP Sumatriptan Succinate Related Impurities RS in *Diluent*
  Sample solution: Nominally equivalent to 1 mg/mL of sumatriptan in *Diluent* from an appropriate volume of Nasal Spray
  Chromatographic system: Proceed as directed in the *Assay.* ■1S (USP41)
  System suitability
  Sample: *System suitability solution*
  ■[NOTE—See *Table 1* for the relative retention times.]■1S (USP41)

Suitability requirements
  Resolution: NLT 1.5 between sumatriptan succinate related compound C and sumatriptan
Analysis
  Samples: ■*Identification solution* and■1S (USP41) *Sample solution*
  Calculate the percentage of each ■degradation product■1S (USP41) in the portion of Nasal Spray taken:

$$■Result = (r_U/r_T) \times (1/F) \times 100■1S (USP41)$$

r_U = peak response of each ■degradation product■1S (USP41) from the *Sample solution*
r_T = sum of all the peak responses from the *Sample solution*
F = relative response factor (see *Table 1*)
Acceptance criteria: See *Table 1.*

■**Table 1**

Name	Relative Retention Time	Relative Response Factor	Acceptance Criteria, NMT (%)
Sumatriptan N-oxide[a]	0.3	1.0	1.5
Sumatriptan amino[b]	0.4	1.0	1.5
3-Hydroxy-2-oxo sumatriptan[c]	0.46	0.35	1.5
Sumatriptan monomethyl[d]	0.6	1.0	1.5
Sumatriptan pyrroloindolium analog[e]	0.64	0.22	1.5
Sumatriptan succinate related compound C	0.9	1.0	1.5
Sumatriptan	1.0	1.0	—
Total degradation products[f]	—	—	4.0

[a] N-Methyl-1-{3-[2-(dimethylamino N-oxide)ethyl]-1H-indol-5-yl}methanesulfonamide.
[b] [3-(2-Aminoethyl)-1H-indol-5-yl]-N-methylmethanesulfonamide.
[c] 1-{3-[2-(Dimethylamino)ethyl]-3-hydroxy-2-oxoindolin-5-yl}-N-methylmethanesulfonamide.
[d] N-Methyl-1-{3-[2-(methylamino)ethyl]-1H-indol-5-yl}methanesulfonamide.
[e] 3a-Hydroxy-1,1-dimethyl-5-(N-methylsulfamoylmethyl)-1,2,3,3a,8,8a-hexahydropyrrolo[2,3-b]indol-1-ium sulfate.
[f] Includes the amount of sumatriptan related compound A determined in the test for *Limit of Sumatriptan Related Compound A.*

■1S (USP41)

SPECIFIC TESTS

- **MICROBIAL ENUMERATION TESTS** ⟨61⟩ and **TESTS FOR SPECIFIED MICROORGANISMS** ⟨62⟩: The total aerobic microbial count does not exceed 10^2 cfu/mL, and it meets the requirements of the tests for absence of *Staphylococcus aureus* and *Pseudomonas aeruginosa* in 1 mL.
- **pH** ⟨791⟩: 5.0–6.0

ADDITIONAL REQUIREMENTS

- **PACKAGING AND STORAGE:** Preserve in tight, light-resistant containers, and store between 2° and 30°.

Change to read:

- **USP REFERENCE STANDARDS** ⟨11⟩
  USP Sumatriptan Succinate RS
  USP Sumatriptan Succinate Related Compound A RS
  [3-[2-(Dimethylamino)ethyl]-2-({3-[2-(dimethylamino)ethyl]-1H-indol-5-yl}methyl)-1H-indol-5-yl]-N-methylmethanesulfonamide succinate salt.
  $C_{27}H_{37}N_5O_2S \cdot C_4H_6O_4$ 613.77

USP Sumatriptan Succinate Related Compound C RS
{3-[2-(Dimethylamino)ethyl]-1-(hydroxymethyl)-1H-in-
dol-5-yl}-N-methylmethanesulfonamide succinate salt.
$C_{15}H_{23}N_3O_3S \cdot \frac{1}{2}C_4H_6O_4$ 384.47
USP Sumatriptan Succinate Related Impurities RS
■Mixture of sumatriptan succinate, sumatriptan monomethyl, sumatriptan succinate related compound C,
sumatriptan N-oxide, and sumatriptan amino.
■1S (USP41)

Taurine

Change to read:

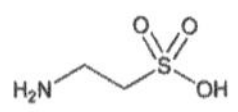

$C_2H_7NO_3S$ 125.15
Taurine
■Ethanesulfonic acid, 2-amino-;
2-Aminoethane-1-sulfonic acid■1S (USP41) [107-35-7].

DEFINITION
Taurine contains NLT 98.0% and NMT 102.0% of taurine
($C_2H_7NO_3S$), calculated on the dried basis.

IDENTIFICATION
• A. INFRARED ABSORPTION ⟨197K⟩

Add the following:

■• B. The retention time of the major peak of the *Sample
solution* corresponds to that of the *Standard solutions*, as
obtained in the *Assay*.■1S (USP41)

ASSAY

Delete the following:

■• NITROGEN DETERMINATION, *Method II* ⟨461⟩
 Analysis: Proceed as directed in the chapter. Each mL
 of 0.01 N sulfuric acid is equivalent to 1.25 mg of
 $C_2H_7NO_3S$.
 Acceptance criteria: 98.5%–101.5% on the dried
 basis■1S (USP41)

Add the following:

■• PROCEDURE
 Solution A: Water adjusted with acetic acid to a pH of
 3.0
 Mobile phase: Acetonitrile and *Solution A* (80:20)
 Standard stock solution: Prepare a solution containing
 1.0 mg/mL of USP Taurine RS in *Mobile phase.*
 Standard solutions: Using the *Standard stock solution*
 prepare three *Standard solutions* with concentrations of
 0.4, 0.5, and 0.6 mg/mL of USP Taurine RS in *Mobile
 phase.*
 Sample solution: 0.5 mg/mL of Taurine in *Mobile phase*
 Chromatographic system
 (See *Chromatography* ⟨621⟩, *System Suitability.*)
 Mode: LC
 Detector: Evaporative light-scattering detector (ELSD)
  Drift tube temperature: 55° or optimize according
   to the manufacturer's recommendations to achieve
   optimal signal-to-noise ratio

 Nebulizer gas: Nitrogen
 Nebulizer gas flow rate: 1.5 L/min or optimize ac-
  cording to the manufacturer's recommendations to
  achieve optimal signal-to-noise ratio
 Column: 3-mm × 10-cm; 2.5-µm packing L104[1]
 Column temperature: 25°
 Flow rate: 0.4 mL/min
 Injection volume: 5 µL
 System suitability
 Sample: *Standard solution* at 0.5 mg/mL
 Suitability requirements
  Column efficiency: NLT 10,000 theoretical plates
  Tailing factor: NMT 1.5
  Relative standard deviation: NMT 2.0%
 Analysis
 Samples: *Standard solutions* and *Sample solution*
 Plot the logarithms of the taurine peak areas against the
  logarithms of taurine concentrations, in mg/mL, in the
  three *Standard solutions* and establish a calibration
  curve by least-squares regression. The correlation coefficient for the regression line is NLT 0.995. Using the
  logarithm of the taurine peak area from the *Sample
  solution*, calculate the logarithm of taurine concentration from the calibration curve and calculate the concentration, C, in mg/mL, of taurine in the *Sample solution* by taking the antilog of the result.
 Calculate the percentage of taurine ($C_2H_7NO_3S$) in the
  portion of Taurine taken:

$$Result = (C/C_U) \times 100$$

C = concentration of Taurine in the *Sample solution*
   (mg/mL), determined from the calibration
   curve
C_U = concentration of Taurine in the *Sample solution*
   (mg/mL)
 Acceptance criteria: 98.0%–102.0% on the dried
 basis■1S (USP41)

IMPURITIES
• RESIDUE ON IGNITION ⟨281⟩: NMT 0.3%
• CHLORIDE AND SULFATE ⟨221⟩, *Chloride*
 Standard: 0.50 mL of 0.020 N hydrochloric acid
 Sample: 0.7 g of Taurine
 Acceptance criteria: NMT 0.05%
• CHLORIDE AND SULFATE ⟨221⟩, *Sulfate*
 Standard: 0.25 mL of 0.020 N sulfuric acid
 Sample: 0.8 g of Taurine
 Acceptance criteria: NMT 0.03%
• IRON ⟨241⟩: NMT 30 ppm

Delete the following:

■• HEAVY METALS, *Method I* ⟨231⟩: NMT 15 ppm• (Official 1-
Jan-2018)
• RELATED COMPOUNDS
 Sample solution: 10 mg/mL of Taurine in water
 Standard solution: 0.05 mg/mL of USP Taurine RS in
  water, an equivalent concentration of about 0.5% of
  the *Sample solution*
 Chromatographic system
 (See *Chromatography* ⟨621⟩, *General Procedures, Thin-
  Layer Chromatography.*)
 Mode: TLC
 Adsorbent: 0.25-mm layer of chromatographic silica
  gel mixture
 Application volume: 5 µL
 Developing solvent system: Butyl alcohol, glacial ace-
  tic acid, and water (3:1:1)
 Spray reagent: 2 mg/mL of ninhydrin in a mixture of
  butyl alcohol and 2 N acetic acid (95:5)

---

[1] COSMOSIL 2.5HILIC (Nacalai). Available from http://www.nacalaiusa.com or
equivalent.

Analysis: Dry the plate at 80° for 30 min. Spray the plate with *Spray reagent,* and heat at 80° for about 10 min. Examine the plate under white light. [NOTE—The R_F value for the taurine spots should be about 0.2.]

Acceptance criteria: No secondary spot of the *Sample solution* is larger or more intense than the principal spot of the *Standard solution.*

Individual impurities: NMT 0.5%

SPECIFIC TESTS
- **LOSS ON DRYING ⟨731⟩**
  Analysis: Dry at 105° for 3 h.
  Acceptance criteria: NMT 0.3%

ADDITIONAL REQUIREMENTS
- **PACKAGING AND STORAGE:** Preserve in well-closed containers.
- **USP REFERENCE STANDARDS ⟨11⟩**
  USP Taurine RS

Delete the following:

▪Terbutaline Sulfate Inhalation Aerosol

» Terbutaline Sulfate Inhalation Aerosol is a suspension of microfine Terbutaline Sulfate in suitable propellants in a pressurized container. It contains not less than 90.0 percent and not more than 110.0 percent of the labeled amount of $(C_{12}H_{19}NO_3)_2 \cdot H_2SO_4$.

Packaging and storage—Preserve in small, nonreactive, light-resistant aerosol containers equipped with metered-dose valves and provided with oral inhalation actuators. Store at controlled room temperature.

USP Reference standards ⟨11⟩—
USP Terbutaline Sulfate RS
USP Terbutaline Related Compound A RS
3,5-Dihydroxy-ω-*t*-butylaminoacetophenone sulfate.

Identification—Chill 10 filled containers to about −75° in a dry ice-acetone mixture for 15 to 20 minutes. Carefully remove the top of each container with a tube cutter, allow to stand for 15 minutes, and pour the contents into a 100-mL beaker. Pour about 5 mL of the combined contents into a 100-mL beaker containing 50 mL of chloroform, shake, and filter through a medium-porosity sintered-glass funnel. Wash the residue with five 10-mL portions of chloroform. Allow the residue to dry by drawing air through the funnel: the IR absorption spectrum of a potassium bromide dispersion of the residue so obtained exhibits maxima only at the same wavelengths as that of a similar preparation of USP Terbutaline Sulfate RS.

Water Determination, *Method I* ⟨921⟩ —Transfer the contents of a weighed container to the titration vessel by attaching the valve stem to an inlet tube. Weigh the empty container, and determine the weight of the specimen taken. The *Water* content, determined by *Method I* ⟨921⟩, is not more than 0.02%.

Delivered dose uniformity over the entire contents: meets the requirements for *Metered-Dose Inhalers* under *Aerosols, Nasal Sprays, Metered-Dose Inhalers, and Dry Powder Inhalers* ⟨601⟩.

PROCEDURE FOR DOSE UNIFORMITY—

4-Aminoantipyrine solution—On the day of use, prepare a solution of 4-aminoantipyrine in water having a concentration of 20 mg per mL.

Potassium ferricyanide solution—On the day of use, prepare a solution of potassium ferricyanide in water having a concentration of 80 mg per mL.

Standard preparation—Dissolve an accurately weighed quantity of USP Terbutaline Sulfate RS in water, and dilute quantitatively and stepwise with water to obtain a solution having a known concentration of about 20 µg of terbutaline sulfate per mL.

Test preparation—Discharge the minimum recommended dose into the sampling apparatus and detach the inhaler as directed. Rinse the apparatus (filter and interior) with four 4.0-mL portions of 0.01 N sulfuric acid, and quantitatively transfer the resulting solutions to a 50-mL centrifuge tube. Wash the apparatus (filter and interior) with 10 mL of chloroform, and add the washing to the solution in the centrifuge tube. Wash the apparatus (filter and interior) with 4.0 mL of 0.01 N sulfuric acid, and quantitatively transfer the resulting liquid to the same centrifuge tube. Shake vigorously for 1 minute, and centrifuge for 10 minutes. Use the clear aqueous phase as the *Test preparation.*

Procedure—Pipet 2 mL of the *Test preparation,* 2 mL of the *Standard preparation,* and 2 mL of water to serve as a reagent blank, into separate 1-cm stoppered cells. To each cell add 0.5 mL of *4-Aminoantipyrine solution,* and mix. Add 0.5 mL of *Potassium ferricyanide solution* to each cell, and mix. Thirty seconds, accurately timed, after the addition of the *Potassium ferricyanide solution,* determine the absorbances of the solutions against the blank, at the wavelength of maximum absorbance at about 550 nm. Calculate the quantity, in µg, of $(C_{12}H_{19}NO_3)_2 \cdot H_2SO_4$ contained in the minimum dose taken by the formula:

$$10CN(A_U / A_S)$$

in which C is the concentration, in µg per mL, of USP Terbutaline Sulfate RS in the *Standard preparation;* N is the number of sprays discharged to obtain the minimum dose; and A_U and A_S are the absorbances of the solutions from the *Test preparation* and the *Standard preparation,* respectively, corrected for the absorbances of the reagent blank solution.

Particle size—Prime the valve of Aerosol container by alternately shaking and firing it several times, and actuate one measured spray onto a clean, dry microscope slide held 5 cm from the end of the oral inhalation actuator, perpendicular to the direction of the spray. Carefully rinse the slide with about 2 mL of carbon tetrachloride, and allow to dry. Prepare four additional slides in the same manner from four additional containers. Examine each slide under a microscope equipped with a calibrated ocular micrometer, using 450× magnification. Focus on the particles of 5 fields of view on each slide, near the center of the test specimen pattern, and note the size of the majority of individual particles. They are less than 5 µm along the longest axis. Record the number and size of all individual crystalline particles (not agglomerates) more than 10 µm in length, measured along the longest axis: not more than 10 such particles are observed.

Assay—

Mobile phase—Prepare a solution containing 750 mL of water, 140 mL of methanol, 110 mL of tetrahydrofuran, and 1.08 g of sodium 1-octanesulfonate. Filter and degas. Make adjustments if necessary (see *System Suitability* under *Chromatography* ⟨621⟩).

Resolution solution—Dissolve suitable quantities of USP Terbutaline Sulfate RS and USP Terbutaline Related Compound A RS in water to obtain a solution containing about 50 µg per mL and 20 µg per mL, respectively.

Standard preparation—Dissolve an accurately weighed quantity of USP Terbutaline Sulfate RS in water to obtain a solution having a known concentration of about 0.3 mg per mL.

Assay preparation—Accurately weigh not fewer than three containers, and separately perform the following procedure for each of the units. Chill in a dry ice–acetone mixture to about −75° for 15 to 20 minutes. Quickly and carefully remove the top of the container with a tube cutter. Allow the propellants to evaporate at room temperature for 10 or 15 minutes. [NOTE—Avoid complete evaporation of the propellants.] Quantitatively transfer the suspension to a 500-mL separatory funnel with the aid of chloroform. Wash all parts of the container alternately with several small portions of chloroform followed by small portions of 0.01 N sulfuric acid. Transfer the washings to the separatory funnel, and adjust the phase volumes to about 100 mL each with chloroform and 0.01 N sulfuric acid, respectively. Dry the container and all of its parts at 105° for 1 hour. Cool to room temperature, and weigh. Shake the separatory funnel for 1 minute, allow the phases to separate, and discard the chloroform layer. Pass the acidic aqueous phase through filter paper into a 250-mL volumetric flask. Wash the separatory funnel with two 10-mL portions of water, and transfer the washings to the volumetric flask. Dilute with water to volume, mix, and filter, discarding the first 2 mL of the filtrate.

Chromatographic system (see *Chromatography* ⟨621⟩)—The liquid chromatograph is equipped with a 280-nm detector, a 0.5-μm precolumn, and a 6.2-mm × 8-cm column that contains 3-μm packing L7. The column temperature is maintained at 40°. The flow rate is about 1.5 mL per minute. Chromatograph the *Resolution solution*, and record the peak responses as directed for *Procedure:* the relative retention times are about 1.0 and 0.83 for terbutaline and terbutaline related compound A, respectively; and the resolution, R, between terbutaline sulfate and terbutaline related compound A is not less than 1.6. Chromatograph the *Standard preparation*, and record the peak responses as directed for *Procedure:* the relative standard deviation for replicate injections is not more than 2.0%.

Procedure—Separately inject equal volumes (about 20 μL) of the *Standard preparation* and the *Assay preparation* into the chromatograph, record the chromatograms, and measure the responses for the major peaks. Calculate the quantity, in mg, of terbutaline sulfate [$(C_{12}H_{19}NO_3)_2 \cdot H_2SO_4$] in each container taken by the formula:

$$250C(r_U / r_S)$$

in which C is the concentration, in mg per mL, of USP Terbutaline Sulfate RS in the *Standard preparation;* and r_U and r_S are the peak responses obtained from the *Assay preparation* and the *Standard preparation*, respectively.

■1 S (USP41)

Tetracycline

$C_{22}H_{24}N_2O_8$　　　444.44
Trihydrate　　　498.49
2-Naphthacenecarboxamide, 4-(dimethylamino)-1,4,4a,5,5a,
　6,11,12a-octahydro-3,6,10,12,12a-pentahydroxy-
　6-methyl-1,11-dioxo-, [4S-(4α,4aα,5aα,6β,12aα)]-;
(4S,4aS,5aS,12aS)-4-(Dimethylamino)-1,4,4a,5,5a,6,11,12a-
　octahydro-3,6,10,12,12a-pentahydroxy-6-methyl-1,11-di-
　oxo-2-naphthacenecarboxamide [60-54-8].
Trihydrate [6416-04-2].

DEFINITION
Tetracycline has a potency equivalent to NLT 975 μg/mg of tetracycline hydrochloride ($C_{22}H_{24}N_2O_8 \cdot HCl$), calculated on the anhydrous basis.

IDENTIFICATION
• **A. ULTRAVIOLET ABSORPTION ⟨197U⟩**
　Sample solution: 20 μg/mL in 0.25 N sodium hydroxide
　Analytical wavelength: 380 nm
　Analysis: Measure the absorptivity 6 min after preparation.
　Acceptance criteria: Absorptivity, calculated on the anhydrous basis and taking into account the potency of the Reference Standard, is between 104.5% and 111.95% of the absorptivity of USP Tetracycline Hydrochloride RS.
• **B.** The retention time of the major peak of the *Sample solution* corresponds to that of the *Standard solution*, as obtained in the *Assay*.

ASSAY
• **PROCEDURE**
　Solution A: Dilute 1 mL of phosphoric acid with water to 1 L.
　Solution B: Acetonitrile
　Mobile phase: See *Table 1*.

Table 1

Time (min)	Solution A (%)	Solution B (%)
0	85	15
7.5	60	40
7.6	85	15
10	85	15

　System suitability solution: 25 μg/mL each of USP Anhydrotetracycline Hydrochloride RS, USP Epitetracycline Hydrochloride RS, and USP 4-Epianhydrotetracycline Hydrochloride RS, and 100 μg/mL of USP Tetracycline Hydrochloride RS in *Solution A*
　Standard solution: 100 μg/mL of USP Tetracycline Hydrochloride RS in *Solution A*
　Sample solution: 90 μg/mL of Tetracycline in *Solution A*
　Chromatographic system
　(See *Chromatography* ⟨621⟩, *System Suitability*.)
　Mode: LC
　Detector: UV 280 nm
　Column: 4.6-mm × 15-cm; 3-μm packing L60.
　　[NOTE—L1 column is also suitable.]
　Temperatures
　　Autosampler: 10°
　　Column: 50°
　Flow rate: 1.0 mL/min
　Injection volume: 10 μL
　System suitability
　　Samples: *System suitability solution* and *Standard solution*
　　Suitability requirements
　　　Resolution: NLT 2.5 between epitetracycline and tetracycline; NLT 2.5 between anhydrotetracycline and 4-epianhydrotetracycline, *System suitability solution*
　　　Tailing factor: NMT 1.5, *Standard solution*
　　　Relative standard deviation: NMT 0.73%, *Standard solution*
　Analysis
　　Samples: *Standard solution* and *Sample solution*
　　Calculate the potency equivalent, in μg/mg, of tetracycline hydrochloride ($C_{22}H_{24}N_2O_8 \cdot HCl$) in the portion of Tetracycline taken:

$$Result = (r_U/r_S) \times (C_S/C_U) \times P$$

r_U = peak response of tetracycline from the *Sample solution*

r_S = peak response of tetracycline from the *Standard solution*

C_S = concentration of USP Tetracycline Hydrochloride RS in the *Standard solution* (µg/mL)

C_U = concentration of Tetracycline in the *Sample solution* (µg/mL)

P = potency of USP Tetracycline Hydrochloride RS (µg/mg)

Acceptance criteria: NLT 975 µg/mg on the anhydrous basis

IMPURITIES

Delete the following:

● **HEAVY METALS,** *Method II* ⟨231⟩: NMT 50 ppm ● (Official 1-Jan-2018)

Change to read:

- **ORGANIC IMPURITIES**
  Solution A, Solution B, Mobile phase, Sample solution, and **Chromatographic system:** Proceed as directed in the *Assay*.
  System suitability solution: 25 µg/mL each of USP Anhydrotetracycline Hydrochloride RS, USP Epitetracycline Hydrochloride RS, USP 4-Epianhydrotetracycline Hydrochloride RS, and USP Tetracycline Hydrochloride RS in *Solution A*
  Standard solution: 0.5 µg/mL of USP Anhydrotetracycline Hydrochloride RS, 3 µg/mL of USP Epitetracycline Hydrochloride RS, 2 µg/mL of USP 4-Epianhydrotetracycline Hydrochloride RS, and 0.1 µg/mL of USP Tetracycline Hydrochloride RS in *Solution A*
  System suitability
  Samples: *System suitability solution* and *Standard solution*
  Suitability requirements
  Resolution: NLT 2.5 between epitetracycline and tetracycline; NLT 2.5 between anhydrotetracycline and 4-epianhydrotetracycline, *System suitability solution*
  Relative standard deviation: NMT 2.8%, *Standard solution*
  Analysis
  Samples: *Standard solution* and *Sample solution*
  Calculate the percentage of ■anhydrotetracycline, epitetracycline, and 4-epianhydrotetracycline■1S (USP41) in the portion of Tetracycline taken:

  $$\text{Result} = (r_U/r_S) \times (C_S/C_U) \times 100$$

  r_U = peak response of ■anhydrotetracycline, epitetracycline, or 4-epianhydrotetracycline■1S (USP41) from the *Sample solution*

  r_S = peak response of the corresponding USP Reference Standard from the *Standard solution*

  C_S = concentration of the corresponding USP Reference Standard in the *Standard solution* (µg/mL)

  C_U = concentration of Tetracycline in the *Sample solution* (µg/mL)

  Calculate the percentage of ■2-acetyl analog or■1S (USP41) any unspecified impurity in the portion of Tetracycline taken:

  $$\text{Result} = (r_U/r_S) \times (C_S/C_U) \times (M_{r1}/M_{r2}) \times 100$$

  r_U = peak response of ■2-acetyl analog or■1S (USP41) any unspecified impurity from the *Sample solution*

r_S = peak response of tetracycline from the *Standard solution*

C_S = concentration of USP Tetracycline Hydrochloride RS in the *Standard solution* (µg/mL)

C_U = concentration of Tetracycline in the *Sample solution* (µg/mL)

M_{r1} = molecular weight of tetracycline, ■444.44■1S (USP41)

M_{r2} = molecular weight of tetracycline hydrochloride, 480.90

Acceptance criteria: See *Table 2*. Disregard any impurity peaks less than 0.05%.

Table 2

Name	Relative Retention Time	Acceptance Criteria, NMT (%)
■4-■1S (USP41)Epitetracycline[a]	0.9	3.0
Tetracycline	1.0	—
■2-Acetyl analog[b]	1.3	2.0■1S (USP41)
4-Epianhydrotetracycline[c]	1.7	2.0
Anhydrotetracycline[d]	1.9	0.5
■Any individual unspecified impurity		0.10■1S (USP41)

[a] (4R,4aS,5aS,6S,12aS)-4-(Dimethylamino)-3,6,10,12,12a-pentahydroxy-6-methyl-1,11-dioxo-1,4,4a,5,5a,6,11,12a-octahydrotetracene-2-carboxamide.

■[b] 2-Acetyl-2-decarbamoyltetracycline; (4S,4aS,5aS,6S,12aS)-2-Acetyl-4-(dimethylamino)-3,6,10,12,12a-pentahydroxy-6-methyl-4a,5a,6,12a-tetrahydrotetracene-1,11(4H,5H)-dione.■1S (USP41)

[c] (4R,4aS,12aS)-4-(Dimethylamino)-3,10,11,12a-tetrahydroxy-6-methyl-1,12-dioxo-1,4,4a,5,12,12a-hexahydrotetracene-2-carboxamide.

[d] (4S,4aS,12aS)-4-(Dimethylamino)-3,10,11,12a-tetrahydroxy-6-methyl-1,12-dioxo-1,4,4a,5,12,12a-hexahydrotetracene-2-carboxamide.

SPECIFIC TESTS

- **OPTICAL ROTATION** ⟨781S⟩, *Procedures, Specific Rotation*
  Sample solution: 5 mg/mL in 0.1 N hydrochloric acid
  Acceptance criteria: −260° to −280° on the anhydrous basis
- **CRYSTALLINITY** ⟨695⟩: Meets the requirements
- **PH** ⟨791⟩
  Sample solution: In an aqueous suspension (1 in 100)
  Acceptance criteria: 3.0–7.0
- **WATER DETERMINATION** ⟨921⟩, *Method I*: NMT 13.0%

ADDITIONAL REQUIREMENTS

- **PACKAGING AND STORAGE:** Preserve in tight, light-resistant containers.
- **LABELING:** Label it to indicate that it is to be used in the manufacture of nonparenteral drugs only.
- **USP REFERENCE STANDARDS** ⟨11⟩
  USP Anhydrotetracycline Hydrochloride RS
  USP 4-Epianhydrotetracycline Hydrochloride RS
  USP Epitetracycline Hydrochloride RS
  USP Tetracycline Hydrochloride RS

Tetrahydrozoline Hydrochloride Ophthalmic Solution

DEFINITION

Tetrahydrozoline Hydrochloride Ophthalmic Solution is a sterile, isotonic solution of Tetrahydrozoline Hydrochloride in water. It contains NLT 90.0% and NMT 110.0% of the labeled amount of tetrahydrozoline hydrochloride ($C_{13}H_{16}N_2 \cdot HCl$).

IDENTIFICATION

Change to read:

- ■A. ULTRAVIOLET ABSORPTION ⟨197U⟩■1S (USP41)
  Diluent: Dilute hydrochloric acid (1 in 100).
  Sample solution: Dilute with *Diluent* (1 in 4000).
  Acceptance criteria: The UV absorption spectrum of
  the *Sample solution* exhibits maxima and minima at the
  same wavelengths as those of a similar solution of USP
  Tetrahydrozoline Hydrochloride RS.

Add the following:

- ■• **B.** The retention time of the major peak of the *Sample
  solution* corresponds to that of the *Standard solution*, as
  obtained in the *Assay*.■1S (USP41)

ASSAY

Change to read:

- PROCEDURE
  ■**Solution A:** 20 mM dibasic ammonium phosphate in
  water. Adjust with ammonium hydroxide to a pH of
  9.0.
  Mobile phase: Acetonitrile and *Solution A* (15:85)
  Standard solution: 0.025 mg/mL of USP Tetrahydrozo-
  line Hydrochloride RS in water
  Sample solution: Nominally 0.025 mg/mL of tetrahy-
  drozoline hydrochloride prepared as follows. Transfer a
  suitable volume of Ophthalmic Solution to a suitable
  volumetric flask. Dilute with water to volume.
  Chromatographic system
  (See *Chromatography* ⟨621⟩, *System Suitability*.)
  Mode: LC
  Detector: UV 210 nm
  Column: 4.6-mm × 15-cm; 3.5-μm packing L1
  Column temperature: 37°
  Flow rate: 1.2 mL/min
  Injection volume: 25 μL
  Run time: NLT 2 times the retention time of
  tetrahydrozoline
  System suitability
  Sample: *Standard solution*
  Suitability requirements
  Tailing factor: 0.8–2.5
  Relative standard deviation: NMT 2.0%
  Analysis
  Samples: *Standard solution* and *Sample solution*
  Calculate the percentage of the labeled amount of tet-
  rahydrozoline hydrochloride ($C_{13}H_{16}N_2 \cdot$ HCl) in the
  portion of Ophthalmic Solution taken:

$$Result = (r_U/r_S) \times (C_S/C_U) \times 100$$

r_U = peak response of tetrahydrozoline from the
　　Sample solution
r_S = peak response of tetrahydrozoline from the
　　Standard solution
C_S = concentration of USP Tetrahydrozoline
　　Hydrochloride RS in the *Standard solution*
　　(mg/mL)
C_U = nominal concentration of tetrahydrozoline
　　hydrochloride in the *Sample solution*
　　(mg/mL)■1S (USP41)

Acceptance criteria: 90.0%–110.0%

IMPURITIES

Add the following:

- ■• ORGANIC IMPURITIES
  Solution A: 20 mM dibasic ammonium phosphate in
  water. Adjust with ammonium hydroxide to a pH of
  9.0.
  Solution B: Acetonitrile
  Mobile phase: See *Table 1*.

Table 1

Time (min)	Solution A (%)	Solution B (%)
0	85	15
11.0	85	15
12.0	60	40
26.0	60	40
27.0	30	70
41.0	30	70
42.0	85	15
50.0	85	15

Standard stock solution: 0.25 mg/mL of USP Tetrahydrozoline Hydrochloride RS in water
Standard solution: 5 μg/mL of USP Tetrahydrozoline
Hydrochloride RS from the *Standard stock solution* in
water
Sensitivity solution: 0.25 μg/mL of USP Tetrahydrozo-
line Hydrochloride RS from the *Standard solution* in
water
Sample solution: Nominally 250 μg/mL of tetrahydro-
zoline hydrochloride in water prepared as follows.
Transfer a suitable volume of Ophthalmic Solution to a
suitable volumetric flask. Dilute with water to volume
and mix.
Chromatographic system
(See *Chromatography* ⟨621⟩, *System Suitability*.)
Mode: LC
Detector: UV 210 nm
Column: 4.6-mm × 15-cm; 3.5-μm packing L1
Column temperature: 37°
Flow rate: 1.2 mL/min
Injection volume: 50 μL
System suitability
Samples: *Standard solution* and *Sensitivity solution*
[NOTE—See *Table 2* for the relative retention times.]
Suitability requirements
Relative standard deviation: NMT 5.0%, *Standard
solution*
Signal-to-noise ratio: NLT 10, *Sensitivity solution*
Analysis
Samples: *Standard solution* and *Sample solution*
Calculate the percentage of each specified and any un-
specified degradation product in the portion of
Ophthalmic Solution taken:

$$Result = (r_U/r_S) \times (C_S/C_U) \times 100$$

r_U = peak response of each specified and any
　　unspecified degradation product from the
　　Sample solution
r_S = peak response of tetrahydrozoline from the
　　Standard solution
C_S = concentration of USP Tetrahydrozoline
　　Hydrochloride RS in the *Standard solution*
　　(mg/mL)
C_U = nominal concentration of tetrahydrozoline
　　hydrochloride in the *Sample solution*
　　(mg/mL)

Acceptance criteria: See *Table 2.*

Table 2

Name	Relative Retention Time	Acceptance Criteria, NMT (%)
Tetrahydrozoline acid[a]	0.8	2.0
Tetrahydrozoline	1.0	—
Tetrahydrozoline amide[b]	1.8	2.0
Tetrahydrozoline related compound A[c]	4.4	2.0
Tetrahydrozoline methyl ester[d]	5.3	2.0
Any unspecified degradation product	—	1.0
Total degradation products	—	3.0

[a] 1,2,3,4-Tetrahydronaphthalene-1-carboxylic acid.
[b] *N*-(2-Aminoethyl)-1,2,3,4-tetrahydronaphthalene-1-carboxamide.
[c] 1,2,3,4-Tetrahydronaphthalene-1-carbonitrile.
[d] Methyl 1,2,3,4-tetrahydronaphthalene-1-carboxylate.

■1S (USP41)

SPECIFIC TESTS
- **STERILITY TESTS ⟨71⟩:** Meets the requirements
- **PH ⟨791⟩:** 5.8–6.5

ADDITIONAL REQUIREMENTS

Change to read:

- **PACKAGING AND STORAGE:** Preserve in tight containers. ■Store at controlled room temperature.■1S (USP41)
- **USP REFERENCE STANDARDS ⟨11⟩**
  USP Tetrahydrozoline Hydrochloride RS

Tiamulin

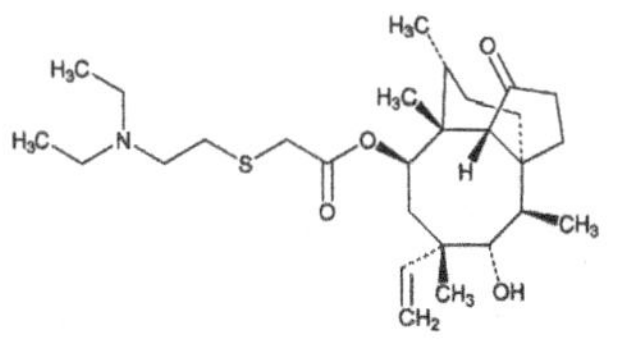

C₂₈H₄₇NO₄S   493.74

$C_{28}H_{47}NO_4S$ 493.74
Acetic acid, [[2-(diethylamino)ethyl]thio]-,
6-ethenyldecahydro-5-hydroxy-4,6,9,10-tetramethyl-
1-oxo-3a,9-propano-3a*H*-cyclopentacycloocten-8-yl ester
[3a*S*-(3aα,4β,5α,6α,8β,9α,9aβ,10*S**)]-;
[[2-(Diethylamino)ethyl]thio]acetic acid 8-ester with (3a*S*,4*R*,
5*S*,6*S*,8*R*,9*R*,9a*R*,10*R*)-octahydro-5,8-dihydroxy-4,6,9,10)-
tetramethyl-6-vinyl-3a,9-propano-3a*H*-cyclopentacyclooc-
ten-1(4*H*)-one [55297-95-5].

DEFINITION
Tiamulin contains NLT 96.5% and NMT 102.0% of tiamulin
($C_{28}H_{47}NO_4S$), calculated on the dried basis.

IDENTIFICATION

Change to read:

- **A. INFRARED ABSORPTION ■⟨197⟩:** [NOTE—Methods described in ⟨197K⟩ or ⟨197A⟩ may be used.]■1S (USP41)
- **B.** The retention time of the major peak of the *Sample solution* corresponds to that of the *Standard solution*, as obtained in the *Assay*.

ASSAY

Change to read:

- **PROCEDURE**
  Buffer: Dissolve 10.0 g of ammonium carbonate in water, add 22 mL of perchloric acid TS, and dilute with water to 1000 mL. Adjust with ammonium hydroxide to a pH of 10.0.
  Mobile phase: Methanol, acetonitrile, and *Buffer* (490:210:300)
  Diluent: Acetonitrile and *Buffer* (1:1)
  Standard solution: 5.0 mg/mL of USP Tiamulin Fumarate RS in *Diluent*
  Sample solution: 4.0 mg/mL of Tiamulin in *Diluent*
  Chromatographic system
  (See *Chromatography* ⟨621⟩, *System Suitability*.)
  Mode: LC
  Detector: UV 212 nm
  Column: 4.6-mm × 15-cm; 5-μm packing L1
  Flow rate: 1 mL/min
  Injection volume: 20 μL
  System suitability
  Sample: *Standard solution*
  Suitability requirements
    Resolution: NLT 2 between tiamulin and its subsequent peak
  Analysis
  Samples: *Standard solution* and *Sample solution*
  Calculate the percentage of tiamulin ($C_{28}H_{47}NO_4S$) in the portion of Tiamulin taken:

$$\blacksquare Result = (r_U/r_S) \times (C_S/C_U) \times (M_{r1}/M_{r2}) \times 100 \blacksquare_{1S \ (USP41)}$$

r_U = peak area from the *Sample solution*
r_S = peak area from the *Standard solution*
C_S = concentration of ■USP Tiamulin Fumarate RS in■1S (USP41) the *Standard solution* (mg/mL)
C_U = concentration Tiamulin in the *Sample solution* (mg/mL)
■M_{r1} = molecular weight of tiamulin, 493.74
M_{r2} = molecular weight of tiamulin fumarate, 609.82■1S (USP41)
Acceptance criteria: 96.5%–102.0% on the dried basis

IMPURITIES

Change to read:

- **LIMIT OF ALCOHOL AND TOLUENE**
  ■Proceed as directed in *Residual Solvents* ⟨467⟩.■1S (USP41)
  Acceptance criteria
    Alcohol: NMT 1.0%
    Toluene: NMT 0.08%
    Sum of alcohol and toluene: NMT 1.0%
- **ORGANIC IMPURITIES**
  Buffer, Mobile phase, Diluent, Standard solution, Sample solution, Chromatographic system, and **System suitability:** Proceed as directed in the *Assay*.
  Toluene solution: Transfer 0.1 mL of toluene to a 100-mL volumetric flask, and dilute with acetonitrile to volume. Transfer 0.1 mL of this solution to another

100-mL volumetric flask, and dilute with *Diluent* to volume.

Diluted sample solution: 0.04 mg/mL of Tiamulin from the *Sample solution* in *Diluent*

Analysis

Samples: *Standard solution*, *Sample solution*, *Toluene solution*, and *Diluted sample solution*

Calculate the area percentage of each impurity, relative to tiamulin, in the portion of Tiamulin taken:

$$Result = (r_U/r_T) \times 100$$

r_U = peak area of each individual impurity from the *Sample solution*

r_T = peak area of tiamulin from the *Diluted sample solution*

Acceptance criteria: See *Table 1*. Disregard the toluene peak and any peak from the *Sample solution* less than 0.1 times the area of the principal peak from the *Diluted sample solution*.

Table 1

Name	Relative Retention Time	Acceptance Criteria, NMT (%)
Mutilin	0.22	1.0
2-(Benzylsulfanyl)-*N,N*-diethylethanamine	0.50	1.0
2,2'-(Disulfane-1,2-diyl)bis(*N,N*-diethylethanamine)	0.66	1.0
Tiamulin	1.0	—
Hydroxy-11-oxo-tiamulin	1.1	1.0
1-Hydroxy-11-oxo-tiamulin	1.6	1.0
11-Oxotiamulin	2.4	1.0
Any individual unspecified impurity	—	0.2
Total impurities	—	3.0

SPECIFIC TESTS
- **BACTERIAL ENDOTOXINS TEST ⟨85⟩:** It contains NMT 0.4 USP Endotoxin Units/mg.
- **LOSS ON DRYING ⟨731⟩**
  Analysis: Dry at 80° to constant weight.
  Acceptance criteria: NMT 1.0%
- **CLARITY AND COLOR OF SOLUTION**
  Sample: 2.5 g
  Instrumental conditions
  (See *Ultraviolet-Visible Spectroscopy ⟨857⟩*.)
  Analytical wavelength: 420 nm
  Analysis: Dissolve the *Sample* in methanol, and dilute with methanol to 50.0 mL.
  Acceptance criteria: The solution is clear, and its absorbance is NMT 0.050.

ADDITIONAL REQUIREMENTS
- **PACKAGING AND STORAGE:** Preserve in well-closed, light-resistant containers, and store at room temperature.
- **LABELING:** Label it to indicate that it is for veterinary use only.

Change to read:

- **USP REFERENCE STANDARDS ⟨11⟩**
  ● (CN 1-May-2018)

USP Tiamulin RS
USP Tiamulin Fumarate RS

Tiamulin Fumarate

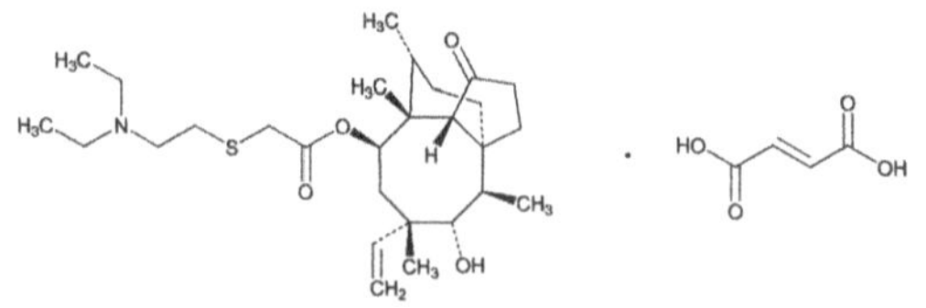

$C_{28}H_{47}NO_4S \cdot C_4H_4O_4$ 609.82

Tiamulin hydrogen fumarate;

Acetic acid, [[2-(diethylamino)ethyl]thio]-, 6-ethenyl-decahydro-5-hydroxy-4,6,9,10-tetramethyl-1-oxo-3a, 9-propano-3a*H*-cyclopentacycloocten-8-yl ester [3a*S*-(3aα, 4β,5α,6α,8β,9α,9aβ,10*S**)]-, (*E*)-2-butenedioate (1:1) (salt);

[[2-(Diethylamino)ethyl]thio]acetic acid 8-ester with (3a*S*, 4*R*,5*S*,6*S*,8*R*,9*R*,9a*R*,10*R*)-octahydro-5,8-dihydroxy-4,6, 9,10-tetramethyl-6-vinyl-3a,9-propano-3a*H*-cyclopentacycloocten-1(4*H*)-one fumarate (1:1) (salt) [55297-96-6].

DEFINITION

Tiamulin Fumarate contains NLT 97.0% and NMT 102.0% of tiamulin fumarate ($C_{28}H_{47}NO_4S \cdot C_4H_4O_4$), calculated on the dried basis.

IDENTIFICATION

Change to read:

- **A. INFRARED ABSORPTION ■⟨197⟩:■**₁S (USP41) [NOTE—■Methods described in ⟨197K⟩ or ⟨197A⟩ may be used. When using ⟨197K⟩,■₁S (USP41) intimately mix Tiamulin Fumarate with potassium bromide, but do not grind.]
- **B.** The retention time of the major peak of the *Sample solution* corresponds to that of the *Standard solution*, as obtained in the *Assay*.

ASSAY

Change to read:

- **PROCEDURE**
  Solution A: 6% perchloric acid
  Buffer: Transfer 10 g of ammonium carbonate to a 1000-mL volumetric flask, and dissolve in 800 mL of water. Add 24 mL of *Solution A*, and dilute with water to volume.
  Mobile phase: Methanol, acetonitrile, and *Buffer* (49:23:28)
  System suitability solution: 0.08 mg/mL of USP Tiamulin Fumarate RS and 0.08 mg/mL of USP Tiamulin Related Compound A RS in *Mobile phase*
  Standard solution: 4 mg/mL of USP Tiamulin Fumarate RS in *Mobile phase*
  Sample solution: 4 mg/mL of Tiamulin Fumarate in *Mobile phase*
  Chromatographic system
  (See *Chromatography ⟨621⟩, System Suitability*.)

Mode: LC
Detector: UV 212 nm
Column: 4.6-mm × 25-cm; 5-µm packing L1
Column temperature: 30 ± 3°
Flow rate: 1.2 mL/min
Injection volume: 20 µL
System suitability
Samples: *System suitability solution* and *Standard solution*
Suitability requirements
[NOTE—The tiamulin related compound A peak elutes before the tiamulin fumarate peak.]
  Resolution: NLT 2.0 between tiamulin related compound A and tiamulin fumarate, *System suitability solution*
  ■1S (USP41)
Tailing factor: NMT 2.0, *Standard solution*
Relative standard deviation: NMT 2.0%, *Standard solution*
Analysis
Samples: *Standard solution* and *Sample solution*
Calculate the percentage of tiamulin fumarate ($C_{28}H_{47}NO_4S \cdot C_4H_4O_4$) in the portion of Tiamulin Fumarate taken:

$$Result = (r_U/r_S) \times (C_S/C_U) \times 100$$

r_U = peak response from the *Sample solution*
r_S = peak response from the *Standard solution*
C_S = concentration of USP Tiamulin Fumarate RS in the *Standard solution* (mg/mL)
C_U = concentration of Tiamulin Fumarate in the *Sample solution* (mg/mL)
Acceptance criteria: 97.0%–102.0% on the dried basis

OTHER COMPONENTS
- **CONTENT OF FUMARATE**
  Sample solution: 450 mg of Tiamulin Fumarate in 60 mL of a mixture of alcohol and water (1:1)
  Analysis: Titrate the *Sample solution* with 0.1 N sodium hydroxide VS, using a glass–calomel electrode (see *Titrimetry* ⟨541⟩). Perform a blank determination, and make any necessary correction. Each milliliter of 0.1 N sodium hydroxide is equivalent to 5.8 mg of fumarate.
  Acceptance criteria: 83.7–87.3 mg

IMPURITIES
- **RESIDUE ON IGNITION** ⟨281⟩: NMT 0.1%

Delete the following:

- **HEAVY METALS**, *Method I* ⟨231⟩: NMT 10 ppm● (Official 1-Jan-2018)

Delete the following:

- **LIMIT OF RESIDUAL SOLVENTS**
  Internal standard solution: Dilute 0.3 mL of *n*-butanol to 1000 mL.
  Standard solution: 0.25 mg/mL each of acetone, ethyl acetate, and isobutyl acetate in *Internal standard solution*
  Sample solution: 50 mg/mL of Tiamulin Fumarate in *Internal standard solution*
  Chromatographic system
  (See *Chromatography* ⟨621⟩, *System Suitability*.)
  Mode: GC
  Detector: Flame ionization
  Column: 0.25-mm × 30-m capillary column; 0.5-µm film of phase G16

Carrier gas: Helium
Flow rate: 1.07 mL/min
Temperature
  Column: 75°
  Injector: 250°
  Detector: 300°
Injection volume: 1.0 µL
Injection type: Split flow ratio, 50:1
System suitability
Samples: *Standard solution*
Suitability requirements
[NOTE—The relative retention times for acetone, ethyl acetate, isobutyl acetate, and *n*-butanol are about 0.34, 0.38, 0.57, and 1.0, respectively.]
  Resolution: NLT 2.0 between acetone and ethyl acetate
Tailing factor: NMT 2 for each of the analyte peaks
Relative standard deviation: NMT 2%
Analysis
Samples: *Standard solution* and *Sample solution*
Calculate the percentages of acetone, ethyl acetate, and isobutyl acetate in the portion of Tiamulin Fumarate taken:

$$Result = (R_U/R_S) \times (W_S/W_U) \times 100$$

R_U = peak response ratio of the solvent of interest to the internal standard of the *Sample solution*
R_S = peak response ratio of the solvent of interest to the internal standard of the *Standard solution*
W_S = weight of the solvent of interest taken to prepare the *Standard solution* (mg)
W_U = weight of Tiamulin Fumarate taken to prepare the *Sample solution* (mg)
Acceptance criteria
Acetone: NMT 0.5%
Ethyl acetate: NMT 0.5%
Isobutyl acetate: NMT 0.5%
Sum of Acetone, Ethyl acetate, and Isobutyl acetate: NMT 0.5%■1S (USP41)

Change to read:

- **ORGANIC IMPURITIES**
  Solution A, Buffer, Mobile phase, System suitability solution, Standard solution, Sample solution, Chromatographic system, and System suitability: Proceed as directed in the *Assay.*
  Analysis
  Sample: *Sample solution*
  Calculate the area percentage of each impurity, relative to tiamulin fumarate, in the portion of Tiamulin Fumarate taken:

$$Result = (r_U/r_T) \times 100$$

r_U = peak response of each impurity from the *Sample solution*
r_T = peak response of tiamulin fumarate from the *Sample solution*
Acceptance criteria: See *Table 1.* ■Disregard the peak due to fumarate at a relative retention time of 0.15.
■1S (USP41)

Table 1

Name	Relative Retention Time	Acceptance Criteria, NMT (%)
Pleuromutilin	0.25	1.0
Mutilin	0.3	1.0

Table 1 (Continued)

Name	Relative Retention Time	Acceptance Criteria, NMT (%)
14-Acetyl mutilin	0.5	1.0
11-Monoacetyl mutilin	0.6	1.0
Tiamulin related compound A	0.8	1.0
Tiamulin	1.0	—
11,14-Diacetyl mutilin	1.1	1.0
8-Dimethylderivative	1.3	1.0
Bisdimethylthioderivative	1.4	1.0
11-Ketoderivative	2.3	1.0
Any individual unspecified impurity	—	0.5
Total impurities	—	3.0

SPECIFIC TESTS

Delete the following:

- **MELTING RANGE OR TEMPERATURE** ⟨741⟩:
  143°–152°■1S (USP41)
- **OPTICAL ROTATION** ⟨781S⟩, *Procedures, Specific Rotation*
  Sample solution: 5.0 mg/mL in dioxane
  Acceptance criteria: +24° to +28°, on the dried basis, measured at 20°
- **PH** ⟨791⟩
  Sample solution: 10 mg/mL
  Acceptance criteria: 3.1–4.1
- **LOSS ON DRYING** ⟨731⟩
  Analysis: Dry under vacuum at 105° for 3 h.
  Acceptance criteria: NMT 0.5%
- **CLARITY AND COLOR OF SOLUTION**
  Sample: 5 g
  Analysis: Transfer the *Sample* to a 100-mL volumetric flask. Dissolve in and dilute with water to volume.
  Acceptance criteria: The solution is clear and colorless, and its absorbances determined in a 1-cm cell at 400 and 650 nm are NMT 0.150 and 0.030 absorbance units, respectively.

ADDITIONAL REQUIREMENTS

- **PACKAGING AND STORAGE:** Preserve in tight, light-resistant containers, and store at room temperature.
- **LABELING:** Label it to indicate that it is for veterinary use only.
- **USP REFERENCE STANDARDS** ⟨11⟩
  USP Tiamulin Fumarate RS
  USP Tiamulin Related Compound A RS
  Tosyl pleuromutilin.

Delete the following:

Tocainide Hydrochloride

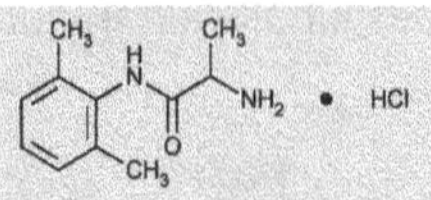

C₁₁H₁₆N₂O · HCl   228.72
Propanamide, 2-amino-N-(2,6-dimethylphenyl)-, hydrochloride, (±)-.
(±)-2-Amino-2′,6′-propionoxylidide hydrochloride.

» Tocainide Hydrochloride contains not less than 98.0 percent and not more than 101.0 percent of C₁₁H₁₆N₂O · HCl, calculated on the dried basis.

Packaging and storage—Preserve in well-closed containers.

USP Reference standards ⟨11⟩—
USP Tocainide Hydrochloride RS

Identification—
  A: *Infrared Absorption* ⟨197K⟩.
  B: It responds to the tests for *Chloride* ⟨191⟩.

Loss on drying ⟨731⟩—Dry it at 105° for 2 hours: it loses not more than 0.5% of its weight.

Residue on ignition ⟨281⟩:   not more than 0.1%.

Delete the following:

•**Heavy metals**, *Method II* ⟨231⟩:   0.002%.● (Official 1-Jan-2018)

Chromatographic purity—
  Adsorbent: 0.25-mm layer of chromatographic silica gel mixture coating on a thin-layer chromatographic plate, previously washed with methanol.
  Test solution: 100 mg per mL, in methanol.
  Standard solutions: 1.0, 0.5, 0.25, and 0.1 mg per mL in methanol to obtain *Standard solutions A, B, C,* and *D,* respectively.
  Application volume: 20 µL.
  Developing solvent system: a freshly prepared mixture of toluene and alcohol (4:1) in a paper-lined equilibrated tank in an atmosphere of ammonia vapors.
  Procedure—Proceed as directed for *Thin-Layer Chromatography* under *Chromatography* ⟨621⟩. Examine the plate under short-wavelength UV light. Expose the plate to iodine vapors, and observe again under white light: the chromatograms show principal spots at about the same R_F value. Estimate the concentration of any spot observed in the chromatogram of the *Test solution*, other than the principal spot and that observed at the origin (which may appear because of the presence of ammonium chloride), by comparison with the principal spots in the chromatograms of *Standard solutions B, C,* and *D:* the intensity of any secondary spot is not greater than that of the principal spot obtained from *Standard solution B* (0.5%), and the sum of all secondary spots is not greater than the intensity of the principal spot obtained from *Standard solution A* (1.0%).

Assay—Dissolve about 180 mg of Tocainide Hydrochloride, accurately weighed, in about 40 mL of glacial acetic acid and 15 mL of a 6 in 100 solution of mercuric acetate in glacial acetic acid, and titrate with 0.1 N perchloric acid VS, determining the endpoint potentiometrically, using a platinum ring electrode and a sleeve-type calomel electrode containing 0.1 N lithium perchlorate in acetic anhydride (see *Titrimetry* ⟨541⟩). Perform a blank determination, and make any necessary correction. Each mL of 0.1 N perchloric acid is equivalent to 22.87 mg of C₁₁H₁₆N₂O · HCl.■1S (USP41)

Delete the following:

Tocainide Hydrochloride Tablets

» Tocainide Hydrochloride Tablets contain not less than 95.0 percent and not more than 105.0 percent of the labeled amount of C₁₁H₁₆N₂O · HCl.

Packaging and storage—Preserve in well-closed containers.

USP Reference standards ⟨11⟩—
USP Tocainide Hydrochloride RS

Identification—

A: Transfer a quantity of finely powdered Tablets, equivalent to about 150 mg of tocainide hydrochloride, to a 100-mL volumetric flask, add 75 mL of water, shake for 15 minutes, dilute with water to volume, and mix. Filter a portion of this solution, and dilute 10 mL of the filtrate with water to 50 mL: the UV absorption spectrum of the solution so obtained exhibits a maximum at the same wavelength as that of a similar solution of USP Tocainide Hydrochloride RS, concomitantly measured.

B: Transfer about 100 mg of finely powdered Tablets to a suitable separator, and add 10 mL of water and 2 mL of 2 M sodium carbonate. Extract with 20 mL of methylene chloride. Add 0.3 mL of filtered methylene chloride extract to 300 mg of potassium bromide, and grind in an agate mortar. Evaporate to dryness under a current of air: the IR absorption spectrum of the potassium bromide dispersion so obtained exhibits maxima only at the same wavelengths as that of a similar preparation of USP Tocainide Hydrochloride RS.

Dissolution ⟨711⟩—

Medium: water; 750 mL.

Apparatus 2: 50 rpm.

Time: 30 minutes.

Procedure—Determine the amount of $C_{11}H_{16}N_2O \cdot HCl$ dissolved from UV absorbances at the wavelength of maximum absorbance at about 263 nm of filtered portions of the solution under test, suitably diluted with *Dissolution Medium*, if necessary, in comparison with a Standard solution having a known concentration of USP Tocainide Hydrochloride RS in the same medium.

Tolerances—Not less than 80% *(Q)* of the labeled amount of $C_{11}H_{16}N_2O \cdot HCl$ is dissolved in 30 minutes.

Uniformity of dosage units ⟨905⟩: meet the requirements.

Procedure for content uniformity—Transfer 1 Tablet to a 100-mL volumetric flask, add 50 mL of water, place in an ultrasonic bath for 20 minutes, dilute with water to volume, and mix. Filter, discarding the first few mL of the filtrate. Transfer an accurately measured volume of the filtrate, equivalent to about 30 mg of tocainide hydrochloride, to a 100-mL volumetric flask, dilute with water to volume, and mix. Dissolve an accurately weighed quantity of USP Tocainide Hydrochloride RS in water, and dilute quantitatively and stepwise with water to obtain a Standard solution having a known concentration of about 300 μg per mL. Concomitantly determine the absorbances of both solutions at the wavelength of maximum absorbance at about 263 nm, with a suitable spectrophotometer, using water as the blank. Calculate the quantity, in mg, of $C_{11}H_{16}N_2O \cdot HCl$ in the Tablet taken by the formula:

$$(TC / D)(A_U / A_S)$$

in which *T* is the labeled quantity, in mg, of tocainide hydrochloride in the Tablet, *C* is the concentration, in μg per mL, of USP Tocainide Hydrochloride RS in the Standard solution, *D* is the concentration, in μg per mL, of tocainide hydrochloride in the solution from the Tablet on the basis of the labeled quantity per Tablet and the extent of dilution, and A_U and A_S are the absorbances of the solution from the Tablet and the Standard solution, respectively.

Assay—

Mobile phase—Dissolve 2.16 g of sodium 1-octanesulfonate in 500 mL of 0.67 N acetic acid, add 500 mL of methanol, and mix. Degas, and filter the solution. Make adjustments if necessary (see *System Suitability* under *Chromatography* ⟨621⟩).

Standard preparation—Dissolve an accurately weighed quantity of USP Tocainide Hydrochloride RS quantitatively in water to obtain a solution having a known concentration of about 0.5 mg per mL.

Assay preparation—Weigh and finely powder not less than 20 Tablets. Transfer an accurately weighed portion of the powder, equivalent to about 100 mg of tocainide hydrochloride, to a 200-mL volumetric flask, add 100 mL of water, and place in an ultrasonic bath for 20 minutes. Dilute with water to volume, and mix. Filter the solution through a membrane filter, and use the filtrate as the *Assay preparation*.

Chromatographic system (see Chromatography ⟨621⟩)—The liquid chromatograph is equipped with a 254-nm detector and a 3.9-mm × 30-cm column that contains packing L1. The flow rate is about 2 mL per minute. Chromatograph the *Standard preparation*, and record the peak responses as directed for *Procedure*: the capacity factor, *k'*, is greater than 1.6, the column efficiency determined from the analyte peak is not less than 1500 theoretical plates, the tailing factor for the analyte peak is not more than 2, and the relative standard deviation for replicate injections is not more than 2.0%.

Procedure—Separately inject equal volumes (about 40 μL) of the *Standard preparation* and the *Assay preparation* into the chromatograph, record the chromatograms, and measure the responses for the major peaks. Calculate the quantity, in mg, of $C_{11}H_{16}N_2O \cdot HCl$ in the portion of Tablets taken by the formula:

$$200C(r_U / r_S)$$

in which *C* is the concentration, in mg per mL, of USP Tocainide Hydrochloride RS in the *Standard preparation*, and r_U and r_S are the peak responses obtained from the *Assay preparation* and the *Standard preparation*, respectively.

∎1S (USP41)

Tolterodine Tartrate

$C_{22}H_{31}NO \cdot C_4H_6O_6$ 475.57

(*R*)-2-[3-[Bis(1-methylethyl)amino]-1-phenylpropyl]-4-methylphenol (2*R*,3*R*)-2,3-dihydroxybutanedioate (1:1) (salt);

(+)-(*R*)-2-[α-[2-(Diisopropylamino)ethyl]benzyl]-*p*-cresol L-tartrate (1:1) (salt);

(*R*)-2-[3-(Diisopropylamino)-1-phenylpropyl]-4-methylphenol tartrate [124937-52-6].

DEFINITION
Tolterodine Tartrate contains NLT 97.0% and NMT 103.0% of tolterodine tartrate ($C_{22}H_{31}NO \cdot C_4H_6O_6$), calculated on the as-is basis.

IDENTIFICATION
- **A. INFRARED ABSORPTION ⟨197K⟩**
- **B.** The retention time of the major peak of the *Sample solution* corresponds to that of the *Standard solution*, as obtained in the *Assay*.

ASSAY
- **PROCEDURE**
  Mobile phase: Acetonitrile, water, and phosphoric acid (330:670:1)

Standard solution: 0.35 mg/mL of USP Tolterodine Tartrate RS in *Mobile phase*

Sample solution: 0.35 mg/mL of Tolterodine Tartrate in *Mobile phase*

Chromatographic system
(See *Chromatography* ⟨621⟩, *System Suitability*.)
 Mode: LC
 Detector: UV 285 nm
 Column: 4.6-mm × 25-cm; 5-µm packing L1
 Flow rate: 1.0 mL/min
 Injection volume: 5 µL

System suitability
 Sample: *Standard solution*
 Suitability requirements
  Relative standard deviation: NMT 1.0% from six replicate injections

Analysis
 Samples: *Standard solution* and *Sample solution*
 Calculate the percentage of tolterodine tartrate ($C_{22}H_{31}NO \cdot C_4H_6O_6$) in the portion of Tolterodine Tartrate taken:

$$Result = (r_U/r_S) \times (C_S/C_U) \times 100$$

r_U = peak response from the *Sample solution*
r_S = peak response from the *Standard solution*
C_S = concentration of USP Tolterodine Tartrate RS in the *Standard solution* (mg/mL)
C_U = concentration of Tolterodine Tartrate in the *Sample solution* (mg/mL)

Acceptance criteria: 97.0%–103.0% on the as-is basis

IMPURITIES
- **RESIDUE ON IGNITION ⟨281⟩:** NMT 0.1%

Change to read:

- **ORGANIC IMPURITIES**
 Solution A: Acetonitrile, water, and perchloric acid (100: 900: 1.5)
 Solution B: Acetonitrile, water, and perchloric acid (500: 500: 1.5)
 Solution C: Acetonitrile
 Mobile phase: See *Table 1*. Return to original conditions, and re-equilibrate the system.

Table 1

Time (min)	Solution A (%)	Solution B (%)	Solution C (%)
0	75	25	0
5	75	25	0
22	0	100	0
47	0	0	100
57	0	0	100

Diluent: Acetonitrile and water (50:50)

System suitability solution: 10 mg/mL of USP Tolterodine System Suitability Mixture RS in *Diluent*. See *Table 2* for relative retention times of the main components of the mixture.

Table 2

Component of USP Tolterodine System Suitability Mixture RS	Relative Retention Time
p-Cresol	0.75
trans-Cinnamic acid	0.81
Monoisopropyl tolterodine	0.88
Tolterodine	1.0

[a] Undefined stereochemistry.

Table 2 (Continued)

Component of USP Tolterodine System Suitability Mixture RS	Relative Retention Time
Diol impurity	1.18
Tolterodine dimer[a]	1.44
6-Methyl-4-phenylchroman-2-ol[a]	1.48
Diol acetate impurity	1.54
6-Methyl-4-phenylchroman-2-one	•1.59• (RB 1-Aug-2017)

[a] Undefined stereochemistry.

Standard solution: 0.01 mg/mL of USP Tolterodine Tartrate RS in *Diluent*

Sensitivity solution: 0.005 mg/mL of USP Tolterodine Tartrate RS in *Diluent* from the *Standard solution*

Sample solution: 10 mg/mL of Tolterodine Tartrate in *Diluent*

Chromatographic system
(See *Chromatography* ⟨621⟩, *System Suitability*.)
 Mode: LC
 Detector: UV 220 nm
 Column: 4.6-mm × 25-cm; 5-µm packing L1
 Column temperature: 65°
 Flow rate: 1.0 mL/min
 Injection volume: 10 µL

System suitability
 Samples: *System suitability solution*, *Standard solution*, and *Sensitivity solution*
 Suitability requirements
  Resolution: • (RB 1-Aug-2017) NLT 1.5 between diol acetate impurity and 6-methyl-4-phenylchroman-2-one, *System suitability solution*
  Relative standard deviation: NMT 3.0%, *Standard solution*
  Signal-to-noise ratio: NLT 10, *Sensitivity solution*

Analysis
 Samples: *Standard solution* and *Sample solution*
 Calculate the percentage of each impurity in the portion of Tolterodine Tartrate taken:

$$Result = (r_U/r_S) \times (C_S/C_U) \times (1/F) \times 100$$

r_U = peak response for each impurity from the *Sample solution*
r_S = peak response of tolterodine from the *Standard solution*
C_S = concentration of USP Tolterodine Tartrate RS in the *Standard solution* (mg/mL)
C_U = concentration of Tolterodine Tartrate in the *Sample solution* (mg/mL)
F = relative response factor (see *Table 3*)

Acceptance criteria: See *Table 3*. Disregard any peak below 0.05% and any peak eluting at retention times of less than 4 min.

Table 3

Name	Relative Retention Time	Relative Response Factor	Acceptance Criteria, NMT (%)
Monoisopropyl tolterodine	0.88	1.6	0.25
Tolterodine	1.0	—	—
6-Methyl-4-phenyl-chroman-2-ol	1.48	1.9	0.25
Any other individual impurity	—	1.0	0.1
Total impurities	—	—	0.5

- **ENANTIOMERIC PURITY**
  Buffer: Prepare pH 7.1 buffer as follows. Transfer 21.0 mL of 1 M solution of monobasic sodium phosphate and 53.3 mL of 0.5 M solution of dibasic sodium phosphate dihydrate to a 1000-mL volumetric flask, and dilute with water to volume. Dilute 100.0 mL of this solution with water to 1000.0 mL.
  Mobile phase: Add 0.97 g of tetrabutylammonium bromide to a mixture of 930 mL of *Buffer* and 70 mL of isobutyl alcohol.
  System suitability solution: 0.02 mg/mL each of USP Tolterodine Tartrate RS and USP Tolterodine *S*-Enantiomer RS in *Mobile phase*
  Standard solution: 0.0004 mg/mL of USP Tolterodine *S*-Enantiomer RS in *Mobile phase*
  Sample solution: 0.04 mg/mL of Tolterodine Tartrate in *Mobile phase*
  Chromatographic system
  (See *Chromatography* ⟨621⟩, *System Suitability*.)
  Mode: LC
  Detector: UV 220 nm
  Column: 2-mm × 10-cm; 5-μm packing L41
  Flow rate: 0.2 mL/min
  Injection volume: 20 μL
  System suitability
  Sample: *System suitability solution*
  [NOTE—The relative retention times for tolterodine *S*-enantiomer and tolterodine are 0.9 and 1.0, respectively.]
  Suitability requirements
  Resolution: NLT 1.4 between tolterodine *S*-enantiomer and tolterodine
  Column efficiency: NLT 1500 theoretical plates for tolterodine
  Relative standard deviation: NMT 3% for each of tolterodine *S*-enantiomer and tolterodine
  Analysis
  Samples: *Standard solution* and *Sample solution*
  Calculate the percentage of tolterodine *S*-enantiomer in the portion of Tolterodine Tartrate taken:

$$\text{Result} = (r_U/r_S) \times (C_S/C_U) \times 100$$

r_U = peak response of tolterodine *S*-enantiomer from the *Sample solution*
r_S = peak response of tolterodine *S*-enantiomer from the *Standard solution*
C_S = concentration of USP Tolterodine *S*-Enantiomer RS in the *Standard solution* (mg/mL)
C_U = concentration of Tolterodine Tartrate in the *Sample solution* (mg/mL)

  Acceptance criteria: NMT 1.0%

SPECIFIC TESTS
- **LOSS ON DRYING** ⟨731⟩
  Analysis: Dry under vacuum at 100° for 2 h.
  Acceptance criteria: NMT 0.5%

ADDITIONAL REQUIREMENTS
- **PACKAGING AND STORAGE:** Preserve in well-closed containers. Store at room temperature.
- **USP REFERENCE STANDARDS** ⟨11⟩
  USP Tolterodine *S*-Enantiomer RS
    (*S*)-2-[3-(Diisopropylamino)-1-phenylpropyl]-4-methylphenol tartrate.
    $C_{22}H_{31}NO \cdot C_4H_6O_6$ 475.57
  USP Tolterodine System Suitability Mixture RS
    The mixture contains tolterodine tartrate and the following impurities (other impurities may also be present):
    p-Cresol.
    C_7H_8O 108.14
    trans-Cinnamic acid.

$C_9H_8O_2$ 148.16
Monoisopropyl tolterodine;
  (*R*)-2-[3-(Isopropylamino)-1-phenylpropyl]-4-methylphenol.
$C_{19}H_{25}NO$ 283.41
Diol impurity;
  2-(3-Hydroxy-1-phenylpropyl)-4-methylphenol.
$C_{16}H_{18}O_2$ 242.32
Tolterodine dimer;
  N,N-Bis[3-(2-hydroxy-5-methylphenyl)-3-phenylpropyl]-*N*-isopropylamine.
$C_{35}H_{41}NO_2$ 507.72
6-Methyl-4-phenylchroman-2-ol.
$C_{16}H_{16}O_2$ 240.30
Diol acetate impurity;
  3-(2-Hydroxy-5-methylphenyl)-3-phenylpropyl acetate.
$C_{18}H_{20}O_3$ 284.35
6-Methyl-4-phenylchroman-2-one.
$C_{16}H_{14}O_2$ 238.29
USP Tolterodine Tartrate RS

Add the following:

▪Tranexamic Acid Injection

DEFINITION
Tranexamic Acid Injection is a sterile solution of Tranexamic Acid in Water for Injection. It contains NLT 90.0% and NMT 110.0% of the labeled amount of tranexamic acid ($C_8H_{15}NO_2$).

IDENTIFICATION
- **A. INFRARED ABSORPTION** ⟨197K⟩
  Sample: Transfer the content of Injection into a beaker and heat on a hot plate at 100° for 30 min, until a paste appears. Then heat it in an oven to complete dryness at 110° for about 30 min.
  Acceptance criteria: Meets the requirements
- **B.** The retention time of the major peak of the *Sample solution* corresponds to that of the *Standard solution*, as obtained in the *Assay*.

ASSAY
- **PROCEDURE**
  Buffer: Dissolve 11 g of monobasic sodium phosphate in 500 mL of water, and add 5 mL of triethylamine. Add 1.4 g of sodium lauryl sulfate, adjust with diluted phosphoric acid (10% w/w) to a pH of 2.5, and dilute with water to 600 mL.
  Mobile phase: Methanol and *Buffer* (40:60)
  Standard solution: 1 mg/mL of USP Tranexamic Acid RS in water
  Sample solution: Nominally 1 mg/mL of tranexamic acid prepared as follows. Transfer an accurately measured volume of Injection from a composite of contents from NLT 3 vials to a suitable volumetric flask, and dilute with water to volume.
  Chromatographic system
  (See *Chromatography* ⟨621⟩, *System Suitability*.)
  Mode: LC
  Detector: UV 220 nm
  Column: 4.6-mm × 25-cm; 5-μm packing L1
  Column temperature: 35°
  Flow rate: 1.5 mL/min
  Injection volume: 20 μL
  Run time: 2 times the retention time of tranexamic acid

System suitability
Sample: *Standard solution*
Suitability requirements
Tailing factor: NMT 2.0
Relative standard deviation: NMT 2.0%
Analysis
Samples: *Standard solution* and *Sample solution*
Calculate the percentage of the labeled amount of tranexamic acid ($C_8H_{15}NO_2$) in the portion of Injection taken:

$$Result = (r_U/r_S) \times (C_S/C_U) \times 100$$

r_U = peak response of tranexamic acid from the *Sample solution*
r_S = peak response of tranexamic acid from the *Standard solution*
C_S = concentration of USP Tranexamic Acid RS in the *Standard solution* (mg/mL)
C_U = nominal concentration of tranexamic acid in the *Sample solution* (mg/mL)
Acceptance criteria: 90.0%–110.0%

IMPURITIES

- **ORGANIC IMPURITIES**
  Buffer and **Mobile phase:** Prepare as directed in the *Assay.*
  System suitability solution: 0.2 mg/mL of USP Tranexamic Acid RS and 2 µg/mL of USP Tranexamic Acid Related Compound C RS in water
  Sensitivity solution: 0.01 mg/mL of USP Tranexamic Acid RS in water
  Standard solution: 0.05 mg/mL of USP Tranexamic Acid RS in water
  Sample solution: Nominally 10 mg/mL of tranexamic acid prepared as follows. Transfer an accurately measured volume of Injection to an appropriate volumetric flask, and dilute with water to volume.
  Chromatographic system
  (See *Chromatography* ⟨621⟩, *System Suitability.*)
  Mode: LC
  Detector: UV 220 nm
  Column: 4.6-mm × 25-cm; 5-µm packing L1
  Flow rate: 1 mL/min
  Injection volume: 20 µL
  Run time: 3.3 times the retention time of tranexamic acid
  System suitability
  Samples: *System suitability solution, Sensitivity solution,* and *Standard solution*
  Suitability requirements
  Resolution: NLT 2.0 between tranexamic acid and tranexamic acid related compound C, *System suitability solution*
  Signal-to-noise ratio: NLT 10, *Sensitivity solution*
  Relative standard deviation: NMT 5.0%, *Standard solution*
  Analysis
  Samples: *Standard solution* and *Sample solution*
  Calculate the percentage of each unspecified impurity in the portion of Injection taken:

  $$Result = (r_U/r_S) \times (C_S/C_U) \times 100$$

  r_U = peak response of each unspecified impurity from the *Sample solution*
  r_S = peak response of tranexamic acid from the *Standard solution*
  C_S = concentration of USP Tranexamic Acid RS in the *Standard solution* (mg/mL)
  C_U = nominal concentration of tranexamic acid in the *Sample solution* (mg/mL)
  Acceptance criteria: See *Table 1.* Disregard any impurity peaks less than 0.03%.

Table 1

Name	Relative Retention Time	Acceptance Criteria, NMT (%)
Tranexamic acid	1.0	—
Tranexamic acid related compound C[a]	1.1	—
Aminomethylbenzoic acid[a,b]	1.3	—
cis-Tranexamic acid[a,c]	1.5	—
Ditranexamic acid amine[a,d]	2.1	—
Any unspecified impurity	—	0.1
Total impurities	—	0.5

[a] For identification only. These are process impurities monitored in the drug substance and are not included in the total impurities.
[b] 4-(Aminomethyl)benzoic acid.
[c] cis-4-(Aminomethyl)cyclohexanecarboxylic acid.
[d] trans,trans-4,4'-[Iminobis(methylene)]dicyclohexanecarboxylic acid.

SPECIFIC TESTS

- **PH ⟨791⟩:** 6.5–8.0
- **PARTICULATE MATTER IN INJECTIONS ⟨788⟩:** It meets the requirements for small-volume injections.
- **STERILITY TESTS ⟨71⟩:** Meets the requirements
- **BACTERIAL ENDOTOXINS TEST ⟨85⟩:** NMT 0.5 USP Endotoxin Units/mg of tranexamic acid
- **OTHER REQUIREMENTS:** It meets the requirements in *Injections and Implanted Drug Products* ⟨1⟩.

ADDITIONAL REQUIREMENTS

- **PACKAGING AND STORAGE:** Preserve in single-dose containers and store at controlled room temperature.
- **USP REFERENCE STANDARDS ⟨11⟩**
  USP Tranexamic Acid RS
  USP Tranexamic Acid Related Compound C RS
  (*RS*)-4-(Aminomethyl) cyclohex-1-enecarboxylic acid.
  $C_8H_{13}NO_2$ 155.19
  ■1S (USP41)

Tranylcypromine Tablets

DEFINITION

Tranylcypromine Tablets contain an amount of tranylcypromine sulfate [($C_9H_{11}N$)$_2 \cdot H_2SO_4$] equivalent to NLT 90.0% and NMT 110.0% of the labeled amount of tranylcypromine ($C_9H_{11}N$).

IDENTIFICATION

Change to read:

- ■**A.**■1S (USP41) The retention time of the major peak of the *Sample solution* corresponds to that of the *Standard solution,* as obtained in the *Assay.*

Add the following:

- ■● **B.** The UV spectrum of the major peak of the *Sample solution* corresponds to that of the *Standard solution,* as obtained in the *Assay.*■1S (USP41)

ASSAY

Change to read:

- **PROCEDURE**
  Buffer: Transfer 3.4 g of monobasic ammonium phosphate into a 1-L volumetric flask containing about 900 mL of water. Adjust the solution with phosphoric acid to a pH of 2.2 ± 0.1. Dilute with water to volume, and mix well.
  Mobile phase: Methanol and *Buffer* (30:70)
  ■1S (USP41)
  Diluent: Methanol, water, and 0.05 N sulfuric acid ■VS■1S (USP41) (20:60:20)
  Standard stock solution: 0.4 mg/mL of USP Tranylcypromine Sulfate RS prepared as follows. Transfer a suitable quantity of USP Tranylcypromine Sulfate RS to a suitable volumetric flask. Add 60% of the flask volume of methanol and 0.05 N sulfuric acid ■VS■1S (USP41) (50:50), sonicate to dissolve, and dilute with *Diluent* to volume.
  Standard solution: 0.04 mg/mL of USP Tranylcypromine Sulfate RS in *Diluent*, from the *Standard stock solution*
  Sample stock solution: Nominally 0.5 mg/mL of tranylcypromine prepared as follows. Transfer a suitable number of Tablets to an appropriate volumetric flask, add 30% of the flask volume of 0.05 N sulfuric acid ■VS,■1S (USP41) and sonicate for 10 min with intermittent shaking. Add 30% of the flask volume of methanol and sonicate for 10 min with intermittent shaking. Shake by mechanical means for 30 min, dilute with *Diluent* to volume, and mix. Centrifuge a portion of the solution and pass the supernatant through a filter of 0.45-μm pore size, discarding the first 2 mL.
  Sample solution: Nominally 0.03 mg/mL of tranylcypromine in *Diluent*, from the *Sample stock solution*
  Chromatographic system
  (See *Chromatography* ⟨621⟩, *System Suitability*.)
  Mode: LC
  Detector: UV 220 nm. ■For *Identification B*, use a diode array detector in the range of 200–400 nm.
  ■1S (USP41)
  Column: 4.6-mm × 25-cm; 4-μm packing L11
  Column temperature: 30°
  Flow rate: 1 mL/min
  Injection volume: 20 μL
  ■**Run time:** NLT 2 times the retention time of tranylcypromine■1S (USP41)
  System suitability
  Sample: *Standard solution*
  Suitability requirements
  Tailing factor: NMT 2.0
  Relative standard deviation: NMT 2.0%
  Analysis
  Samples: *Standard solution* and *Sample solution*
  Calculate the percentage of the labeled amount of tranylcypromine ($C_9H_{11}N$) in the portion of Tablets taken:

$$Result = (r_U/r_S) \times (C_S/C_U) \times [M \times (M_{r1}/M_{r2})] \times 100$$

r_U = peak response from the *Sample solution*
r_S = peak response from the *Standard solution*
C_S = concentration of USP Tranylcypromine Sulfate RS in the *Standard solution* (mg/mL)
C_U = nominal concentration of tranylcypromine in the *Sample solution* (mg/mL)
M = number of moles of tranylcypromine per mole of tranylcypromine sulfate, 2
M_{r1} = molecular weight of tranylcypromine, 133.19
M_{r2} = molecular weight of tranylcypromine sulfate, 364.46

Acceptance criteria: 90.0%–110.0%

PERFORMANCE TESTS

Change to read:

- **DISSOLUTION** ⟨711⟩
  Medium: 0.1 N hydrochloric acid VS; 500 mL, deaerated
  Apparatus 1: 100 rpm
  Time: 45 min
  Buffer: Transfer 6.94 g of sodium perchlorate monohydrate to a 1000-mL volumetric flask containing 900 mL of water and mix until dissolved. Adjust with perchloric acid to a pH of 2.50 and dilute with water to volume.
  Mobile phase: Acetonitrile and *Buffer* (15:85)
  Standard stock solution: 0.54 mg/mL of USP Tranylcypromine Sulfate RS in water. [NOTE—Sonicate as needed.]
  Standard solution: 0.027 mg/mL of USP Tranylcypromine Sulfate RS in *Medium*, from the *Standard stock solution*
  Sample solution: Pass a portion of the solution under test through a suitable filter of 0.45-μm pore size.
  Chromatographic system
  (See *Chromatography* ⟨621⟩, *System Suitability*.)
  Mode: LC
  Detector: UV 220 nm
  Column: 3.9-mm × 15-cm; 5-μm packing L1
  Column temperature: 35°
  Flow rate: 1 mL/min
  Injection volume: 50 μL
  System suitability
  Sample: *Standard solution*
  Suitability requirements
  ■1S (USP41)
  Tailing factor: NMT 2.0
  Relative standard deviation: NMT 2.0%
  Analysis
  Samples: *Standard solution* and *Sample solution*
  Calculate the percentage of the labeled amount of tranylcypromine ($C_9H_{11}N$) dissolved:

$$Result = (r_U/r_S) \times C_S \times V \times [M \times (M_{r1}/M_{r2})] \times (1/L) \times 100$$

r_U = peak response from the *Sample solution*
r_S = peak response from the *Standard solution*
C_S = concentration of USP Tranylcypromine Sulfate RS in the *Standard solution* (mg/mL)
V = volume of *Medium*, 500 mL
M = number of moles of tranylcypromine per mole of tranylcypromine sulfate, 2
M_{r1} = molecular weight of tranylcypromine, 133.19
M_{r2} = molecular weight of tranylcypromine sulfate, 364.46
L = label claim (mg/Tablet)
Tolerances: NLT 75% (Q) of the labeled amount of tranylcypromine ($C_9H_{11}N$) is dissolved.
- **UNIFORMITY OF DOSAGE UNITS** ⟨905⟩: Meet the requirements

IMPURITIES

Change to read:

- **ORGANIC IMPURITIES**
  Buffer ■1S (USP41) and **Diluent:** Prepare as directed in the *Assay*.
  Solution A: Methanol and *Buffer* (15:85)
  Solution B: Methanol and *Buffer* (30:70)
  Mobile phase: See *Table 1*.

Table 1

Time (min)	Solution A (%)	Solution B (%)
0	100	0
20	100	0
25	0	100
37	0	100
39	100	0
45	100	0

Standard stock solution: 70 µg/mL of USP Tranylcypromine Sulfate RS and 280 µg/mL of USP Tranylcypromine Related Compound A RS in *Diluent*. [NOTE—Sonicate as needed.]

Standard solution: 0.7 µg/mL of USP Tranylcypromine Sulfate RS and 2.8 µg/mL of USP Tranylcypromine Related Compound A RS prepared as follows. Transfer a suitable volume of the *Standard stock solution* to a suitable volumetric flask, add 30% each of the flask volume of 0.05 N sulfuric acid ■VS■1S (USP41) and methanol, and dilute with *Diluent* to volume.

Sample solution: Use the *Sample stock solution* prepared as directed in the *Assay*.

Chromatographic system
(See *Chromatography* ⟨621⟩, *System Suitability*.)
Mode: LC
Detector: UV 220 nm
Column: 4.6-mm × 15-cm; 3-µm packing L1
Column temperature: 35°
Flow rate: 1.2 mL/min
Injection volume: 25 µL
System suitability
Sample: *Standard solution*
Suitability requirements
Resolution: NLT 2.0 between tranylcypromine and tranylcypromine related compound A
Tailing factor: NMT 2.0
Relative standard deviation: NMT 6.0%
Analysis
Samples: *Standard solution* and *Sample solution*
Calculate the percentage of each ■degradation product■1S (USP41) in the portion of Tablets taken:

$$Result = (r_U/r_S) \times (C_S/C_U) \times [M \times (M_{r1}/M_{r2})] \times 100$$

r_U = peak response of the ■degradation product■1S (USP41) from the *Sample solution*
r_S = peak response from the *Standard solution*
C_S = concentration of USP Tranylcypromine Sulfate RS in the *Standard solution* (mg/mL)
C_U = nominal concentration of tranylcypromine in the *Sample solution* (mg/mL)
M = number of moles of tranylcypromine per mole of tranylcypromine sulfate, 2
M_{r1} = molecular weight of tranylcypromine, 133.19
M_{r2} = molecular weight of tranylcypromine sulfate, 364.46

Acceptance criteria
Individual ■degradation product:■1S (USP41) NMT 0.2%
Total ■degradation products:■1S (USP41) NMT 1.2%

ADDITIONAL REQUIREMENTS
• **PACKAGING AND STORAGE:** Preserve in well-closed containers, and store at controlled room temperature.
• **USP REFERENCE STANDARDS** ⟨11⟩
USP Tranylcypromine Sulfate RS
USP Tranylcypromine Related Compound A RS
(±)-*cis*-2-Phenylcyclopropanamine hydrochloride;
cis-Tranylcypromine hydrochloride.
$C_9H_{11}N \cdot HCl$ 169.65

Trazodone Hydrochloride Tablets

DEFINITION
Trazodone Hydrochloride Tablets contain NLT 90.0% and NMT 110.0% of the labeled amount of trazodone hydrochloride ($C_{19}H_{22}ClN_5O \cdot HCl$).

IDENTIFICATION

Delete the following:

■• **A. THIN-LAYER CHROMATOGRAPHIC IDENTIFICATION TEST** ⟨201⟩
Standard solution: 20 mg/mL of USP Trazodone Hydrochloride RS in methanol
Sample solution: Nominally 20 mg/mL of trazodone hydrochloride in methanol from a suitable number of Tablets (equivalent to NLT 150 mg) prepared as follows. Place the Tablets in a tube. Add the required amount of methanol, and sonicate until the Tablets have disintegrated. Shake the tube, by hand, for a few seconds to mix, and then filter.
Application volume: 1 µL
Developing solvent system: Cyclohexane, alcohol, toluene, and diethylamine (80:30:20:20)
Analysis
Samples: *Standard solution* and *Sample solution*
Proceed as directed in the chapter, except locate the spots on the plate by examination under long-wavelength UV light.■1S (USP41)

Add the following:

■• **A.** The UV spectrum of the major peak of the *Sample solution* corresponds to that of the *Standard solution*, as obtained in the *Assay*.■1S (USP41)
• **B.** The retention time of the major peak of the *Sample solution* corresponds to that of the *Standard solution*, as obtained in the *Assay*.

ASSAY

Change to read:

• **PROCEDURE**
Buffer: 1.15 g/L of monobasic ammonium phosphate, adjusted with sodium hydroxide to a pH of 6.0
Mobile phase: Methanol and *Buffer* (75:25)
Standard solution: 0.1 mg/mL of USP Trazodone Hydrochloride RS in 0.01 N hydrochloric acid ■TS■1S (USP41)
Sample solution: Nominally 0.1 mg/mL of trazodone hydrochloride from NLT 20 finely powdered Tablets. Transfer a suitable quantity of the powder to a suitable volumetric flask. Dissolve in 0.01 N hydrochloric acid ■TS,■1S (USP41) and dilute with 0.01 N hydrochloric acid ■TS■1S (USP41) to volume. Sonicate for about 30 min, and pass through a ■suitable■1S (USP41) filter of 0.45-µm pore size.
Chromatographic system
(See *Chromatography* ⟨621⟩, *System Suitability*.)
Mode: LC
Detector: UV 246 nm. ■For *Identification A*, use a diode array detector in the range of 200–400 nm. ■1S (USP41)
Column: 5-mm × 10-cm; 4-µm packing L1
Flow rate: 1.5 mL/min
Injection volume: 20 µL
■**Run time:** NLT 4.5 times the retention time of trazodone■1S (USP41)

System suitability
  Sample: *Standard solution*
  Suitability requirements
    Column efficiency: NLT 900 theoretical plates
    Relative standard deviation: NMT 2.0%
Analysis
  Samples: *Standard solution* and *Sample solution*
  Calculate the percentage of the labeled amount of trazodone hydrochloride ($C_{19}H_{22}ClN_5O \cdot HCl$) in the portion of Tablets taken:

$$\text{Result} = (r_U/r_S) \times (C_S/C_U) \times 100$$

r_U = peak response of trazodone from the *Sample solution*
r_S = peak response of trazodone from the *Standard solution*
C_S = concentration of USP Trazodone Hydrochloride RS in the *Standard solution* (mg/mL)
C_U = nominal concentration of trazodone hydrochloride in the *Sample solution* (mg/mL)

Acceptance criteria: 90.0%–110.0%

PERFORMANCE TESTS

Change to read:

- **DISSOLUTION ⟨711⟩**
  Medium: 0.01 N hydrochloric acid ■TS;■₁ₛ (USP41) 900 mL
  Apparatus 2: 50 rpm
  Time: 60 min
  ■Buffer,■₁ₛ (USP41) Mobile phase, Standard solution, Chromatographic system, and System suitability: Proceed as directed in the *Assay*.
  Sample solution: Pass ■a portion of■₁ₛ (USP41) the solution ■under test■₁ₛ (USP41) through a ■suitable■₁ₛ (USP41) filter of 0.45-µm pore size.
  Analysis
    Samples: *Standard solution* and *Sample solution*
    Calculate the percentage of the labeled amount of trazodone hydrochloride ($C_{19}H_{22}ClN_5O \cdot HCl$) dissolved:

$$\text{Result} = (r_U/r_S) \times C_S \times V \times (1/L) \times 100$$

r_U = peak response of trazodone from the *Sample solution*
r_S = peak response of trazodone from the *Standard solution*
C_S = concentration of USP Trazodone Hydrochloride RS in the *Standard solution* (mg/mL)
V = volume of *Medium*, 900 mL
L = label claim (mg/Tablet)
  Tolerances: NLT 80% (Q) of the labeled amount of trazodone hydrochloride ($C_{19}H_{22}ClN_5O \cdot HCl$) is dissolved.

- **UNIFORMITY OF DOSAGE UNITS ⟨905⟩:** Meet the requirements

IMPURITIES

Change to read:

- **ORGANIC IMPURITIES**
  Solution A: 6.75 g/L of monobasic potassium phosphate. Add 1.0 mL of triethylamine for each liter of the solution, and mix.
  Solution B: Acetonitrile
  Mobile phase: See *Table 1*.

Table 1

Time (min)	Solution A (%)	Solution B (%)
0	90	10
5	90	10
30	60	40
35	60	40
60	42	58
63	30	70
78	30	70
78.1	90	10
90	90	10

Diluent: Methanol, water, and hydrochloric acid (650:350:3)
System suitability solution: 0.7 µg/mL of USP Trazodone Hydrochloride RS and 1.5 µg/mL of USP Trazodone Related Compound C RS in *Diluent*
Standard solution: 0.7 µg/mL of USP Trazodone Hydrochloride RS in *Diluent*
Sample solution: Nominally 500 µg/mL of trazodone from finely powdered Tablets (NLT 20) prepared as follows. Transfer a portion of powdered Tablets (NLT 50 mg) to a suitable volumetric flask. Add about 80% of the flask volume of *Diluent*, and sonicate for 10 min. Dilute with *Diluent* to volume. Pass a portion of the solution through a suitable membrane filter of 0.45-µm pore size.
Chromatographic system
  (See *Chromatography ⟨621⟩, System Suitability*.)
  Mode: LC
  Detector: UV 254 nm
  Column: 4.0-mm × 15-cm; 3-µm packing L1
  Flow rate: 0.7 mL/min
  Injection volume: 10 µL
System suitability
  Samples: *System suitability solution* and *Standard solution*
  [NOTE—See *Table 2* for the relative retention times.]
  Suitability requirements
    Resolution: NLT 2.5 between the trazodone related compound C and trazodone peaks, *System suitability solution*
    Tailing factor: NMT 2.0, *Standard solution*
    Relative standard deviation: NMT 5.0%, ■■₁ₛ (USP41) *Standard solution*
Analysis
  Samples: *Standard solution* and *Sample solution*
  Calculate the percentage of each ■degradation product■₁ₛ (USP41) in the portion of Tablets taken:

$$\text{Result} = (r_U/r_S) \times (C_S/C_U) \times 100$$

r_U = peak response of each ■degradation product■₁ₛ (USP41) from the *Sample solution*
r_S = peak response of trazodone from the *Standard solution*
C_S = concentration of USP Trazodone Hydrochloride RS in the *Standard solution* (µg/mL)
C_U = nominal concentration of trazodone in the *Sample solution* (µg/mL)
Acceptance criteria: See *Table 2*.

Table 2

Name	Relative Retention Time	Acceptance Criteria, NMT (%)
Triazolopyridinone[a,b]	0.1	—
Chlorophenylpiperazine[a,c]	0.6	—
Hydroxypropyl chlorophenyl-piperazine[a,d]	0.7	—
Isotrazodone[a,e]	0.8	—
Trazodone related compound C[a]	0.97	—
Trazodone hydrochloride	1.0	—
Trazodone dimer[a,f]	1.5	—
Trazodone related compound F[a,g]	1.6	—
Bispiperazine analog[a,h]	1.8	—
Bis(3-chlorophenyl)piperazine[a,i]	2.2	—
Any individual unspecified degradation product	—	1.0
Total ■degradation products■₁s (USP41)	—	2.0

[a] Process impurity included for identification only. ■Process impurities are controlled in the drug substance, and are not to be reported or included in the total impurities for the drug product.■₁s (USP41)
[b] [1,2,4]Triazolo[4,3-*a*]pyridin-3(2*H*)-one.
[c] 1-(3-Chlorophenyl)piperazine.
[d] 3-[4-(3-Chlorophenyl)piperazin-1-yl]propan-1-ol.
[e] 1-{3-[4-(3-Chlorophenyl)piperazin-1-yl]propyl}-[1,2,4]triazolo[4,3-*a*]pyridin-1-ium-3-olate.
[f] 1,1-Bis{2-chloro-[4-(3-{1,2,4-triazolo[4,3-*a*]pyridin-3-(2*H*)-on-2-yl}propyl)piperazine-1-yl]phenyl}ethane trihydrochloride.
[g] 1-(3-Chlorophenyl)-4-(3-chloropropyl)piperazine.
[h] 1,3-Bis(4-(3-chlorophenyl)piperazin-1-yl)propane.
[i] 1,4-Bis(3-chlorophenyl)piperazine.

ADDITIONAL REQUIREMENTS
- **PACKAGING AND STORAGE:** Preserve in tight, light-resistant containers. Store at controlled room temperature.
- **USP REFERENCE STANDARDS ⟨11⟩**
  USP Trazodone Hydrochloride RS
  USP Trazodone Related Compound C RS
  2-{3-[4-(4-Chlorophenyl)piperazin-1-yl]propyl}-[1,2,4]triazolo[4,3-*a*]pyridin-3(2*H*)-one hydrochloride.
  $C_{19}H_{22}ClN_5O \cdot HCl$ 408.32

Triamterene

Change to read:

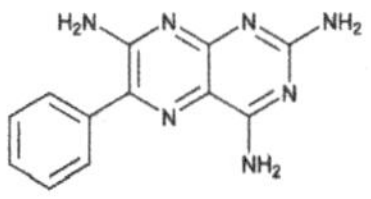

$C_{12}H_{11}N_7$ 253.26
2,4,7-Pteridinetriamine, 6-phenyl-;
2,4,7-Triamino-6-phenylpteridine;
■6-Phenylpteridine-2,4,7-triamine■₁s (USP41) [396-01-0].

DEFINITION
Triamterene contains NLT 98.0% and NMT 102.0% of triamterene ($C_{12}H_{11}N_7$), calculated on the dried basis.

IDENTIFICATION

Change to read:

- **A.** ■**INFRARED ABSORPTION ⟨197⟩:** [NOTE—Procedures described in ⟨197M⟩ or ⟨197A⟩ may be used.]■₁s (USP41)

Change to read:

- **B.** ■The retention time of the major peak of the *Sample solution* corresponds to that of the *Standard solution*, as obtained in the *Assay.*■₁s (USP41)

ASSAY

Change to read:

- **PROCEDURE**
  ■**Mobile phase:** Acetonitrile, methanol, butylamine, and water (140:140:2:720). Sonicate to mix and adjust with acetic acid to a pH of 5.3.
  Standard solution: 0.05 mg/mL of USP Triamterene RS in *Mobile phase*
  Sample solution: 0.05 mg/mL of Triamterene in *Mobile phase*
  Chromatographic system
  (See *Chromatography* ⟨621⟩, *System Suitability*.)
  Mode: LC
  Detector: UV 355 nm
  Column: 4.0-mm × 25-cm; 5-µm packing L7
  Flow rate: 1 mL/min
  Injection volume: 20 µL
  Run time: NLT 3 times the retention time of triamterene
  System suitability
  Sample: *Standard solution*
  Suitability requirements
  Tailing factor: NMT 2.0
  Relative standard deviation: NMT 0.73%
  Analysis
  Samples: *Standard solution* and *Sample solution*
  Calculate the percentage of triamterene ($C_{12}H_{11}N_7$) in the portion of Triamterene taken:

$$Result = (r_U/r_S) \times (C_S/C_U) \times 100$$

r_U	= peak response of triamterene from the *Sample solution*
r_S	= peak response of triamterene from the *Standard solution*
C_S	= concentration of USP Triamterene RS in the *Standard solution* (mg/mL)
C_U	= concentration of Triamterene in the *Sample solution* (mg/mL)■₁s (USP41)

  Acceptance criteria: 98.0%–102.0% on the dried basis

IMPURITIES

Delete the following:

- ■**LIMIT OF 2,4,6-TRIAMINO-5-NITROSOPYRIMIDINE**
  Buffer: 0.01 M monobasic potassium phosphate in water. Adjust to a pH of 3.0.
  Mobile phase: Methanol and *Buffer* (20:80).
  Standard solution: 10 µg/mL of 2,4,6-triamino-5-nitrosopyrimidine in methanol. [NOTE—Heating to 50° and sonication may be used to dissolve the 2,4,6-triamino-5-nitrosopyrimidine.]
  Sample solution: 10,000 µg/mL of Triamterene prepared as follows. Transfer about 1 g of Triamterene into a 250-mL conical flask. Add 100.0 mL of methanol, and stir for 30 min with heating to 50°, cool, and filter.

Chromatographic system
(See *Chromatography* ⟨621⟩, *System Suitability*.)
Mode: LC
Detector: UV 330 nm
Column: 3.9-mm × 30-cm; 10-µm packing L10
Flow rate: 1.5 mL/min
Injection volume: 20 µL
System suitability
Sample: *Standard solution*
[NOTE—The relative retention times for 2,4,6-triamino-5-nitrosopyrimidine and triamterene are about 0.4 and 1.0, respectively.]
Suitability requirements
Tailing factor: NMT 1.5
Relative standard deviation: NMT 2.0%
Analysis
Samples: *Standard solution* and *Sample solution*
Calculate the percentage of 2,4,6-triamino-5-nitrosopyrimidine in the portion of Triamterene taken:

$$Result = (r_U/r_S) \times (C_S/C_U) \times 100$$

r_U = peak response for 2,4,6-triamino-5-nitrosopyrimidine from the *Sample solution*
r_S = peak response for 2,4,6-triamino-5-nitrosopyrimidine from the *Standard solution*
C_S = concentration of 2,4,6-triamino-5-nitrosopyrimidine in the *Standard solution* (µg/mL)
C_U = concentration of Triamterene in the *Sample solution* (µg/mL)
Acceptance criteria: NMT 0.1%■₁ₛ ₍USP41₎

Delete the following:

■● **ORDINARY IMPURITIES** ⟨466⟩
Standard stock solution: 10 mg/mL of USP Triamterene RS in dimethyl sulfoxide
Standard solutions: 0.00025, 0.00125, 0.0025, and 0.005 mg/mL of USP Triamterene RS in methanol from *Standard stock solution*, respectively
Sample stock solution: 10 mg/mL of Triamterene in dimethyl sulfoxide
Sample solution: 0.25 mg/mL of Triamterene in methanol from *Sample stock solution*
Analysis: Separately apply 50 µL of each of the *Standard solutions* and the *Sample solution* to a 0.5-mm thin-layer chromatographic plate that has been preconditioned by heating at 105° for 15 min and allowed to cool at room temperature in a closed chamber.
Eluant: Ethyl acetate, methanol, and 15 M stronger ammonia water (90:10:10)
Visualization: 1■₁ₛ ₍USP41₎

Add the following:

■● **ORGANIC IMPURITIES**
Mobile phase and **Chromatographic system:** Proceed as directed in the *Assay*.
Diluent: To 50 mL of 0.1 N sodium hydroxide in a 500-mL volumetric flask, add 250 mL of acetonitrile and dilute with water to volume.
Standard stock solution 1: 0.25 mg/mL of USP Triamterene RS in *Mobile phase*
Standard stock solution 2: 0.1 mg/mL of USP Triamterene Related Compound A RS in *Diluent*. Sonication may be required for complete dissolution.
Standard stock solution 3: 0.1 mg/mL of USP Triamterene Related Compound B RS in *Diluent*. Sonication may be required for complete dissolution.
Standard stock solution 4: 0.1 mg/mL of USP Triamterene Related Compound C RS in *Diluent*. Sonication may be required for complete dissolution.

System suitability solution: 0.1 mg/mL of USP Triamterene RS from *Standard stock solution 1* and 0.01 mg/mL of USP Triamterene Related Compound B RS from *Standard stock solution 3* in *Mobile phase*
Sensitivity solution: 0.5 µg/mL of USP Triamterene RS in *Mobile phase* from *Standard stock solution 1*
Standard solution: 0.001 mg/mL each of USP Triamterene RS, USP Triamterene Related Compound A RS, USP Triamterene Related Compound B RS, and USP Triamterene Related Compound C RS from the respective *Standard stock solution* in *Mobile phase*
Sample solution: 1 mg/mL of Triamterene in *Mobile phase*. [NOTE—Sonication may be required to aid the dissolution.]
System suitability
Samples: *System suitability solution, Sensitivity solution,* and *Standard solution*
[NOTE—See *Table 1* for the relative retention times for triamterene related compound B and triamterene.]
Suitability requirements
Resolution: NLT 2.0 between triamterene related compound B and triamterene, *System suitability solution*
Relative standard deviation: NMT 5.0%, *Standard solution*
Signal-to-noise ratio: NLT 10, *Sensitivity solution*
Analysis
Samples: *Standard solution* and *Sample solution*
Calculate the percentage of triamterene related compound A, triamterene related compound B, and triamterene related compound C in the portion of Triamterene taken:

$$Result = (r_U/r_S) \times (C_S/C_U) \times 100$$

r_U = peak response of each corresponding specified impurity from the *Sample solution*
r_S = peak response of each corresponding specified impurity from the *Standard solution*
C_S = concentration of each corresponding specified impurity in the *Standard solution* (mg/mL)
C_U = concentration of Triamterene in the *Sample solution* (mg/mL)
Calculate the percentage of any unspecified impurity in the portion of Triamterene taken:

$$Result = (r_U/r_S) \times (C_S/C_U) \times 100$$

r_U = peak response of any unspecified impurity from the *Sample solution*
r_S = peak response of triamterene from the *Standard solution*
C_S = concentration of USP Triamterene RS in the *Standard solution* (mg/mL)
C_U = concentration of Triamterene in the *Sample solution* (mg/mL)
Acceptance criteria: See *Table 1*. Reporting threshold: 0.05%.

Table 1

Name	Relative Retention Time	Acceptance Criteria, NMT (%)
Triamterene related compound A	0.4	0.1
Triamterene related compound B	0.8	0.15
Triamterene	1.0	—
Triamterene related compound C	2.8	0.15
Any unspecified impurity	—	0.10
Total impurities	—	0.5

■1S *(USP41)*

SPECIFIC TESTS
- **LOSS ON DRYING** ⟨731⟩
  Analysis: Dry under vacuum at 105° for 2 h.
  Acceptance criteria: NMT 1.0%

ADDITIONAL REQUIREMENTS
- **PACKAGING AND STORAGE:** Preserve in tight, light-resistant containers.

Change to read:

- **USP REFERENCE STANDARDS** ⟨11⟩
  USP Triamterene RS
  ■USP Triamterene Related Compound A RS
  5-Nitrosopyrimidine-2,4,6-triamine.
  $C_4H_6N_6O$ 154.13
  USP Triamterene Related Compound B RS
  2,7-Diamino-6-phenylpteridin-4-ol.
  $C_{12}H_{10}N_6O$ 254.25
  USP Triamterene Related Compound C RS
  2,4-Diamino-6-phenylpteridin-7-ol.
  $C_{12}H_{10}N_6O$ 254.25■1S *(USP41)*

Verapamil Hydrochloride Extended-Release Tablets

DEFINITION
Verapamil Hydrochloride Extended-Release Tablets contain NLT 90.0% and NMT 110.0% of the labeled amount of verapamil hydrochloride ($C_{27}H_{38}N_2O_4 \cdot HCl$).

IDENTIFICATION

Change to read:

- **A.** ■The retention time of the major peak of the *Sample solution* corresponds to that of the *Standard solution*, as obtained in the *Assay.*■1S *(USP41)*

Add the following:

■• **B.** The UV spectrum of the major peak of the *Diluted sample solution* corresponds to that of the *Diluted standard solution*, as obtained in the *Assay.*■1S *(USP41)*

ASSAY

Change to read:

- **PROCEDURE**
  Buffer: To 0.82 g of sodium acetate, add 33 mL of glacial acetic acid and dilute with water to 1 L.
  Mobile phase: Acetonitrile, 2-aminoheptane, and *Buffer* (60:1:140)
  System suitability solution: 2.5 mg/mL of USP Verapamil Hydrochloride RS and 2.0 mg/mL of USP Verapamil Related Compound B RS in *Mobile phase*
  Standard solution: 1.2 mg/mL of USP Verapamil Hydrochloride RS in *Mobile phase*
  ■**Diluted standard solution:** 0.6 mg/mL of USP Verapamil Hydrochloride RS in *Mobile phase* from the *Standard solution*■1S *(USP41)*
  Sample solution: ■Nominally 1.2 mg/mL of verapamil hydrochloride from Tablets prepared as follows.■1S *(USP41)* Transfer an amount equivalent to 240 mg of verapamil hydrochloride, from NLT 20 powdered Tablets, to a

200-mL volumetric flask, and add about 160 mL of *Mobile phase*. Sonicate for 15 min, stir for 15 min, dilute with *Mobile phase* to volume, and mix. Centrifuge a portion for 20 min, and use the supernatant.
  ■**Diluted sample solution:** Nominally 0.6 mg/mL of verapamil hydrochloride in *Mobile phase* from the *Sample solution*■1S *(USP41)*
  Chromatographic system
  (See *Chromatography* ⟨621⟩, *System Suitability*.)
  Mode: LC
  Detector: UV 278 nm. ■For *Identification B*, use a diode array detector in the range of 200–400 nm.
  ■1S *(USP41)*
  Column: 4.6-mm × 15-cm; ■5-μm■1S *(USP41)* packing L1
  Flow rate: 1 mL/min
  Injection volume: 10 μL
  ■**Run time:** NLT 3 times the retention time of verapamil■1S *(USP41)*
  System suitability
  Samples: *System suitability solution* and *Standard solution*
  ■[NOTE—The relative retention times for verapamil related compound B and verapamil are 0.85 and 1.0, respectively.]■1S *(USP41)*
  Suitability requirements
  Resolution: NLT 1.5 between verapamil and verapamil related compound B, *System suitability solution*
  Relative standard deviation: NMT 2.0%, *Standard solution*
  Analysis
  Samples: *Standard solution*, ■*Diluted standard solution*, ■1S *(USP41)* *Sample solution*, and ■*Diluted sample solution* [NOTE—The *Diluted standard solution* and *Diluted sample solution* are used for *Identification B*.]■1S *(USP41)*
  Calculate the percentage of the labeled amount of verapamil hydrochloride ($C_{27}H_{38}N_2O_4 \cdot HCl$) in the portion of Tablets taken:

$$Result = (r_U/r_S) \times (C_S/C_U) \times 100$$

r_U = peak response of verapamil from the *Sample solution*
r_S = peak response of verapamil from the *Standard solution*
C_S = concentration of USP Verapamil Hydrochloride RS in the *Standard solution* (mg/mL)
C_U = nominal concentration of verapamil hydrochloride in the *Sample solution* (mg/mL)

Acceptance criteria: 90.0%–110.0%

PERFORMANCE TESTS

Change to read:

- **DISSOLUTION** ⟨711⟩
  Test 1: If the product complies with this test, the labeling indicates that it meets USP *Dissolution Test 1*. Proceed as directed in *Dissolution* ⟨711⟩, *Procedure, Apparatus 1 and Apparatus 2, Delayed-Release Dosage Forms, Method B Procedure*.
  Acid stage ■**medium:**■1S *(USP41)* Using 900 mL of simulated gastric fluid TS (without enzyme), conduct this stage of the test for 1 h.
  Buffer stage ■**medium:**■1S *(USP41)* Using 900 mL of simulated intestinal fluid TS (without enzyme), conduct this stage of the test for 7 h.
  Apparatus 2: 50 rpm
  Times
  Acid stage: 1 h
  Buffer stage: 2, 3.5, 5, and 8 h
  Standard solution: USP Verapamil Hydrochloride RS in 0.01 N hydrochloric acid

Sample solution: Pass portions of the solution under test through a suitable filter. Dilute with medium as necessary.

Blank solution: 0.01 N hydrochloric acid

Analysis: Wrap each Tablet in a wire helix to prevent the Tablets from floating. After 1 h in the *Acid stage* ■*medium,*■1 S (USP41) withdraw a specimen for analysis, and carefully transfer the dosage form, including the wire helix, to a vessel containing the *Buffer stage medium,* which has been previously warmed to $37 \pm 0.5°$. At each time interval, pass a portion of the solution under test through a suitable glass microfiber filter paper. Dilute, if necessary, the filtered portions of the solutions under test with water at the 1-h interval and with 0.1 N hydrochloric acid at the 2-, 3.5-, 5-, and 8-h intervals. Determine the percentage of the labeled amount of verapamil hydrochloride ($C_{27}H_{38}N_2O_4 \cdot HCl$) dissolved.

[NOTE—Use only filters that have been shown not to absorb verapamil.]

Detector: UV 278 nm

Tolerances: See *Table 1* and *Table 2*.

Table 1. For Products Labeled to Contain 180 or 240 mg

Time (h)	Amount Dissolved (%)
1	7–15
2	16–30
3.5	31–50
5	51–75
8	NLT 85

Table 2. For Products Labeled to Contain 120 mg

Time (h)	Amount Dissolved (%)
1	10–21
2	18–33
3.5	35–60
5	50–82
8	NLT 85

The percentages of the labeled amount of verapamil hydrochloride ($C_{27}H_{38}N_2O_4 \cdot HCl$) dissolved at the times specified conform to *Dissolution ⟨711⟩, Acceptance Table 2.*

Test 2: If the product complies with this test, the labeling indicates that it meets USP *Dissolution Test 2.* Proceed as directed for *Test 1*, except that in the *Analysis,* the Tablet is not required to be wrapped in a wire helix.

Tolerances: See *Table 3, Table 4,* and *Table 5*.

Table 3. For Products Labeled to Contain 240 mg

Time (h)	Amount Dissolved (%)
1	8–20
2	15–35
3.5	35–65
5	55–85
8	NLT 80

Table 4. For Products Labeled to Contain 180 mg

Time (h)	Amount Dissolved (%)
1	10–25
2	20–40
3.5	40–75
8	NLT 80

Table 5. For Products Labeled to Contain 120 mg

Time (h)	Amount Dissolved (%)
1	10–25
2	20–40
3.5	35–70
5	55–85
8	NLT 80

The percentages of the labeled amount of verapamil hydrochloride ($C_{27}H_{38}N_2O_4 \cdot HCl$) dissolved at the times specified conform to *Dissolution ⟨711⟩, Acceptance Table 2.*

Test 3: If the product complies with this test, the labeling indicates that it meets USP *Dissolution Test 3.* Proceed as directed for *Test 1*.

Tolerances: See *Table 6*.

Table 6

Time (h)	Amount Dissolved (%)
1	8–20
2	15–35
3.5	27–57
5	45–75
8	NLT 80

The percentages of the labeled amount of verapamil hydrochloride ($C_{27}H_{38}N_2O_4 \cdot HCl$) dissolved at the times specified conform to *Dissolution ⟨711⟩, Acceptance Table 2.*

Test 4: If the product complies with this test, the labeling indicates that it meets USP *Dissolution Test 4.*

Medium: Simulated intestinal fluid TS (without enzyme); 50 mL

Apparatus 7: 20 cycles/min (see *Drug Release ⟨724⟩*)

Detector: UV 278 nm

Standard solution: USP Verapamil Hydrochloride RS in *Medium*

Analysis: Scrape about 2 mm × 2 mm of the coating from the side edge of the Tablet under test. Glue the system to a plastic rod sample holder at the area where the color has been removed. Attach each plastic sample holder to an arm of the apparatus, which reciprocates at an amplitude of about 2 cm and 15–30 cycles/min. The Tablet is continuously immersed in tubes containing 50 mL of *Medium* at 37°. At the end of each specified test interval, the systems are transferred to the next row of new test tubes containing 50 mL of fresh *Medium*. Remove the tubes after the last test interval, and allow them to cool to room temperature. Add 2.0 mL of 1.0 M phosphoric acid to each tube, and dilute with water to 50 mL. Stir and mix each tube thoroughly. Determine the percentages of the labeled amount of verapamil hydrochloride ($C_{27}H_{38}N_2O_4 \cdot HCl$) for the filtered portions of the solution under test, suitably diluted with *Medium*.

Tolerances: See *Table 7*.

Table 7

Time (h)	Amount Dissolved (%)
3	NMT 10
6	20–50
9	52.5–82.5
14	NLT 85

The percentages of the labeled amount of verapamil hydrochloride ($C_{27}H_{38}N_2O_4 \cdot HCl$) dissolved at the times specified conform to *Dissolution* ⟨711⟩, *Acceptance Table 2*.

Test 5: If the product complies with this test, the labeling indicates that it meets USP *Dissolution Test 5*.

Phosphate buffer: Dissolve 6.8 g of monobasic potassium phosphate in 250 mL of water. Add 190 mL of 0.2 N sodium hydroxide in 400 mL of water, adjust with 0.2 N sodium hydroxide to a pH of 7.5 ± 0.1, and dilute with water to 1000 mL.

Medium: *Phosphate buffer*; 900 mL

Apparatus 2: 50 rpm

Detector: UV 278 nm

Standard solution: USP Verapamil Hydrochloride RS in *Medium*

Sample solution: Pass portions of the solution under test through a suitable filter. Dilute with *Medium* as necessary.

Analysis: Determine the percentage of the labeled amount of verapamil hydrochloride ($C_{27}H_{38}N_2O_4 \cdot HCl$) dissolved.

Tolerances: See *Table 8*.

Table 8

Time (h)	Amount Dissolved (%)
1	2–12
2	10–25
4	25–50
8	NLT 80

The percentages of the labeled amount of verapamil hydrochloride ($C_{27}H_{38}N_2O_4 \cdot HCl$) dissolved at the times specified conform to *Dissolution* ⟨711⟩, *Acceptance Table 2*.

Test 6: If the product complies with this test, the labeling indicates that it meets USP *Dissolution Test 6*.

Acid stage ■medium,■1S (USP41) **Buffer stage ■medium, ■**1S (USP41) **Apparatus ■2,■**1S (USP41) **Times,** and **Detector:** Proceed as directed for *Test 1*.

Standard solution: 0.04 mg/mL of USP Verapamil Hydrochloride RS in 0.01 N hydrochloric acid

Sample solution: Pass portions of the solution under test through a suitable filter. Dilute with 0.1 N hydrochloric acid to prepare a sample of concentration similar to that of the *Standard solution*.

Analysis

Samples: *Standard solution* and *Sample solution*

Proceed as directed for *Test 1*.

Calculate the concentration (C_i) of verapamil hydrochloride ($C_{27}H_{38}N_2O_4 \cdot HCl$) dissolved in medium (mg/mL) at each time point (i):

$$C_i = (A_U/A_S) \times C_S \times D$$

A_U = absorbance of verapamil from the *Sample solution*

A_S = absorbance of verapamil from the *Standard solution*

C_S = concentration of USP Verapamil Hydrochloride RS in the *Standard solution* (mg/mL)

D = dilution factor

Calculate the percentage of the labeled amount of verapamil hydrochloride ($C_{27}H_{38}N_2O_4 \cdot HCl$) dissolved ($Q_i$), at each time point ($i$):

$$Result_1 = (C_1 \times V) \times (1/L) \times 100$$

$$Result_2 = \{[C_2 \times (V - V_S)] + (C_1 \times V_S)\} \times (1/L) \times 100$$

$$Result_3 = (\{C_3 \times [V - (2 \times V_S)]\} + [(C_2 + C_1) \times V_S]) \times (1/L) \times 100$$

$$Result_4 = (\{C_4 \times [V - (3 \times V_S)]\} + [(C_3 + C_2 + C_1) \times V_S]) \times (1/L) \times 100$$

$$Result_5 = (\{C_5 \times [V - (4 \times V_S)]\} + [(C_4 + C_3 + C_2 + C_1) \times V_S]) \times (1/L) \times 100$$

C_i = concentration of verapamil hydrochloride in the portion of the sample withdrawn at time point i (mg/mL)

V = volume of *Medium*, 900 mL

L = label claim (mg/Tablet)

V_S = volume of the *Sample solution* withdrawn at each time point from the medium in the *Buffer stage* (mL)

Tolerances: See *Table 9*.

Table 9

Time Point (i)	Time (h)	Amount Dissolved (%) Tablet Strength— 240 mg	Tablet Strength— 180 mg	Tablet Strength— 120 mg
1	1	10–25	10–25	15–30
2	2	25–45	27–47	35–55
3	3.5	50–75	55–80	60–85
4	4	70–90	NLT 75	NLT 80
5	8	NLT 85	NLT 85	NLT 85

The percentages of the labeled amount of verapamil hydrochloride ($C_{27}H_{38}N_2O_4 \cdot HCl$) dissolved at the times specified conform to *Dissolution* ⟨711⟩, *Acceptance Table 2*.

Test 7: If the product complies with this test, the labeling indicates that it meets USP *Dissolution Test 7*.

Acid stage medium: Simulated gastric fluid TS (without enzyme); 900 mL

Buffer stage medium: Simulated intestinal fluid TS (without enzyme); 900 mL

Apparatus 2: 50 rpm, with a sinker (see *Dissolution* ⟨711⟩, *Figure 2a*)

Times

Acid stage ■1S (USP41)**:** 1 h

Buffer stage ■1S (USP41)**:** 2, 3.5, 5, and 8 h

Diluent: 0.01 N hydrochloric acid

Dilute phosphoric acid: Dilute 5.0 mL of phosphoric acid with water to 50 mL.

Buffer: 1.74 g/L of dibasic potassium phosphate in water. Adjust to a pH of 7.5 using *Dilute phosphoric acid*.

Mobile phase: Acetonitrile and *Buffer* (650:350)

Standard solution: Prepare the corresponding USP Verapamil Hydrochloride RS solutions in *Diluent* as directed in *Table 10*. Pass through a suitable membrane filter of 0.45-μm pore size.

Table 10

Tablet Strength (mg)	Concentration of USP Verapamil Hydrochloride RS (µg/mL)
240	270
120	135
180	203

Sample solutions: Pass a portion of the solution under test at each time point through a suitable filter of 1-µm pore size, and use the filtrate.

Chromatographic system
(See *Chromatography* ⟨621⟩, *System Suitability*.)
Mode: LC
Detector: UV 278 nm
Column: 4.6-mm × 25-cm; 5-µm packing L7
Column temperature: 30°
Flow rate: 1.5 mL/min
Injection volume: 10 µL
Run time: NLT 1.4 times the retention time of verapamil
System suitability
Sample: *Standard solution*
Suitability requirements
Tailing factor: NMT 2.0
Relative standard deviation: NMT 2.0%
Analysis
Samples: *Standard solution* and *Sample solutions*
After 1 h in the *Acid stage medium*, withdraw 10 mL of the solution under test. Carefully transfer the dosage form including the sinker to a vessel containing the *Buffer stage medium*, previously warmed to $37 \pm 0.5°$.
Calculate the percentage of the labeled amount of verapamil hydrochloride ($C_{27}H_{38}N_2O_4 \cdot HCl$) dissolved in the *Acid stage medium*:

$$\text{Result} = (r_U/r_S) \times C_S \times V \times (1/L) \times 100$$

r_U = peak response of verapamil from the *Sample solutions*
r_S = peak response of verapamil from the *Standard solution*
C_S = concentration of USP Verapamil Hydrochloride RS in the *Standard solution* ■(mg/mL)■1S (USP41)
V = volume of *Acid stage medium*, 900 mL
L = label claim (mg/Tablet)

Calculate the concentration (C_i) of verapamil hydrochloride ($C_{27}H_{38}N_2O_4 \cdot HCl$) in the sample withdrawn from the vessel at each *Buffer stage* time point (*i*):

$$\text{Result}_i = (r_U/r_S) \times C_S$$

r_U = peak response of verapamil from the *Sample solution* at each time point (*i*)
r_S = peak response of verapamil from the *Standard solution*
C_S = concentration of USP Verapamil Hydrochloride RS in the *Standard solution* (mg/mL)

Calculate the percentage of the labeled amount of verapamil hydrochloride ($C_{27}H_{38}N_2O_4 \cdot HCl$) dissolved at each time point (*i*):

$$\text{Result}_1 = C_1 \times V \times (1/L) \times 100$$

$$\text{Result}_2 = \{[C_2 \times (V - V_S)] + (C_1 \times V_S)\} \times (1/L) \times 100$$

$$\text{Result}_3 = (\{C_3 \times [V - (2 \times V_S)]\} + [(C_2 + C_1) \times V_S]) \times (1/L) \times 100$$

$$\text{Result}_4 = (\{C_4 \times [V - (3 \times V_S)]\} + [(C_3 + C_2 + C_1) \times V_S]) \times (1/L) \times 100$$

C_i = concentration of verapamil hydrochloride in the *Sample solution* at the specified time point *i* (mg/mL)
V = volume of *Buffer stage medium*, 900 mL
L = label claim (mg/Tablet)
V_S = volume of the *Sample solution* withdrawn at each time point (mL)
Tolerances: See *Table 11*.

Table 11

Time Point (*i*)	Time (h)	Amount Dissolved (%) Tablet Strength— 240 mg	Amount Dissolved (%) Tablet Strength— 180 mg	Amount Dissolved (%) Tablet Strength— 120 mg
1	1	7–20	7–20	10–21
2	2	15–30	15–30	18–33
3	3.5	31–60	31–60	30–55
4	5	55–85	55–85	50–82
5	8	NLT 85	NLT 85	NLT 85

The percentages of the labeled amount of verapamil hydrochloride ($C_{27}H_{38}N_2O_4 \cdot HCl$) dissolved at the times specified conform to *Dissolution* ⟨711⟩, *Acceptance Table 2*.

• **UNIFORMITY OF DOSAGE UNITS** ⟨905⟩: Meet the requirements

IMPURITIES

Change to read:

• **ORGANIC IMPURITIES**
Buffer, Mobile phase, System suitability solution, Standard solution, Sample solution, Chromatographic system, and **System suitability:** Proceed as directed in the *Assay*.
Analysis
Sample: *Sample solution*
Calculate the percentage of each ■unspecified degradation product■1S (USP41) in the portion of Tablets taken:

$$\text{Result} = (r_U/r_T) \times 100$$

r_U = peak response for each ■unspecified degradation product■1S (USP41) from the *Sample solution*
r_T = sum of all peak responses from the *Sample solution*
Acceptance criteria: ■See *Table 12*.

Table 12

Name	Relative Retention Time	Acceptance Criteria, NMT (%)
Verapamil related compound B[a]	0.85	—
Verapamil	1.0	—
Any unspecified degradation product	—	0.5
Total degradation products	—	1.0

[a] For resolution measurement only. Do not include it in the total.

■1S (USP41)

ADDITIONAL REQUIREMENTS

Change to read:

- **PACKAGING AND STORAGE:** Preserve in tight, light-resistant containers. ■Store at controlled room temperature.■1S (USP41)
- **LABELING:** The labeling indicates the *Dissolution* test with which the product complies.

Change to read:

- **USP REFERENCE STANDARDS ⟨11⟩**
  USP Verapamil Hydrochloride RS
  USP Verapamil Related Compound B RS
    Benzeneacetonitrile, ■4-[(3,4-Dimethox-yphenethyl)(methyl)amino]-2-(3,4-dimethoxyphenyl)-2-isopropylbutanenitrile hydrochloride.■1S (USP41)
    $C_{26}H_{36}N_2O_4 \cdot HCl$ ■477.04■1S (USP41)

Xylazine

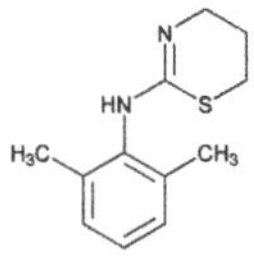

$C_{12}H_{16}N_2S$ 220.33
4*H*-1,3-Thiazin-2-amine, *N*-(2,6-dimethylphenyl)-5,6-dihydro-;
5,6-Dihydro-2-(2,6-xylidino)-4*H*-1,3-thiazine [7361-61-7].

DEFINITION
Xylazine contains NLT 98.0% and NMT 102.0% of xylazine ($C_{12}H_{16}N_2S$).

IDENTIFICATION

Change to read:

- **A. ■INFRARED ABSORPTION ⟨197⟩:** [NOTE—Methods described in ⟨197K⟩ or ⟨197A⟩ may be used.]■1S (USP41)
- **B. ULTRAVIOLET ABSORPTION ⟨197U⟩**
  Sample solution: 5 µg/mL in 0.1 N hydrochloric acid
  Acceptance criteria: Meets the requirements

Delete the following:

- ■• **C. THIN-LAYER CHROMATOGRAPHIC IDENTIFICATION TEST ⟨201⟩**
  Sample solution: 2 mg/mL in chloroform
  Developing solvent system: Acetone, chloroform, and methanol (2:1:1)
  Analysis: Prior to the applications of the *Sample solution* and the *Standard solution*, dry the plate at 105° for NLT 30 min, and allow it to cool in a desiccator. Allow the applications to dry with the aid of a current of warm air, and develop. Examine under short-wavelength UV light.
  Acceptance criteria: Size, intensity, and R_F value of the principal spot from the *Sample solution* correspond to those of the principal spot from the *Standard solution*.■1S (USP41)

ASSAY
- **PROCEDURE**
  Solution A: Dissolve 3.03 g of sodium 1-heptanesulfonate in 800 mL of water, adjust with 2 N sulfuric acid to a pH of 3.0, and dilute with water to 1000 mL. Pass through a filter of 0.5-µm or finer pore size.
  Solution B: Acetonitrile
  Diluent: *Solution A* and *Solution B* (50:50)
  Mobile phase: See *Table 1*. Return to original conditions, and equilibrate the system.

Table 1

Time (min)	Solution A (%)	Solution B (%)
0	70	30
5	70	30
10	60	40
15	60	40

Standard solution: 0.4 mg/mL of USP Xylazine RS in *Diluent*
Sample solution: 0.4 mg/mL of Xylazine in *Diluent*
Chromatographic system
(See *Chromatography ⟨621⟩, System Suitability*.)
  Mode: LC
  Detector: UV 226 nm
  Column: 3.9-mm × 30-cm; packing L1
  Flow rate: 1 mL/min
  Injection volume: 10 µL
System suitability
  Sample: *Standard solution*
  Suitability requirements
    Tailing factor: NMT 2.0
    Relative standard deviation: NMT 2.0%
Analysis
  Samples: *Standard solution* and *Sample solution*
  Calculate the percentage of xylazine ($C_{12}H_{16}N_2S$) in the portion of Xylazine taken:

$$Result = (r_U/r_S) \times (C_S/C_U) \times 100$$

r_U = peak response from the *Sample solution*
r_S = peak response from the *Standard solution*
C_S = concentration of USP Xylazine RS in the *Standard solution* (mg/mL)
C_U = concentration of Xylazine in the *Sample solution* (mg/mL)
Acceptance criteria: 98.0%–102.0%

IMPURITIES
- **RESIDUE ON IGNITION ⟨281⟩:** NMT 0.1%

Delete the following:

- ■• **HEAVY METALS,** *Method II* ⟨231⟩: NMT 20 ppm• (Official 1-Jan-2018)
- **LIMIT OF 3-AMINO-1-PROPANOL**
  Standard solution: 0.5 mg/mL of 3-amino-1-propanol in methanol
  Sample solution: 100 mg/mL of Xylazine in methanol. Sonicate to dissolve.
  Chromatographic system
  (See *Chromatography ⟨621⟩, General Procedures, Thin-Layer Chromatography*.)
    Mode: TLC
    Adsorbent: 0.25-mm layer of chromatographic silica gel
    Application volume: 5 µL
    Developing solvent system: Alcohol and ammonium hydroxide (80:20)

Spray reagent: 2 mg/mL of ninhydrin in alcohol
Analysis
  Samples: *Standard solution* and *Sample solution*
Develop the chromatogram in a saturated chromatographic chamber containing the *Developing solvent system* until the solvent front has moved three-fourths of the length of the plate. Remove the plate from the chromatographic chamber, mark the solvent front, and air-dry the plate. Spray the plate with the *Spray reagent*, and immediately heat the plate in an oven at 105°. When the spots are visible, remove the plate from the oven, and allow to cool.
  Acceptance criteria: The intensity of the spot for 3-amino-1-propanol from the *Sample solution* is not greater than that of the spot for 3-amino-1-propanol from the *Standard solution* (0.5%).

Change to read:

- **LIMIT OF ACETONE AND ISOPROPYL ALCOHOL**
  ■Proceed as directed in *Residual Solvents* ⟨467⟩.■1S (USP41)
  Acceptance criteria
    Acetone: NMT 0.02%
    Isopropyl alcohol: NMT 0.2%

Change to read:

- **ORGANIC IMPURITIES**
  Solution A, Solution B, and **Diluent:** Prepare as directed in the *Assay*.
  Mobile phase: See *Table 2*. Return to original conditions, and equilibrate the system.

Table 2

Time (min)	Solution A (%)	Solution B (%)
0	75	25
8	75	25
35	30	70
40	30	70

  Standard solution: 0.008 mg/mL of USP Xylazine RS in *Diluent*, prepared by diluting the *Standard solution* from the *Assay*
  Sample solution: Transfer 100 mg of Xylazine into a 10-mL volumetric flask, add 5.0 mL of *Solution B*, and swirl to dissolve. Add 4 mL of *Solution A*, and swirl. Dilute with *Solution A* to volume, and mix.
  Chromatographic system
  (See *Chromatography* ⟨621⟩, *System Suitability*.)
  Mode: LC
  Detector: UV 205 nm
  Column: 4.6-mm × 25-cm; packing L7 (use a guard column)
  Flow rate: 1 mL/min
  Injection volume: 10 µL
  System suitability
  Sample: *Standard solution*
  Suitability requirements
    Tailing factor: NMT 1.5
    Relative standard deviation: NMT 5.0%
  Analysis
  Samples: *Standard solution* and *Sample solution*
Calculate the percentage of each impurity in the portion of Xylazine taken:

$$■Result = (r_U/r_S) \times (C_S/C_U) \times (1/F) \times 100■1S (USP41)$$

r_U = peak area of any individual impurity from the *Sample solution* that is not present in the chromatogram of the *Diluent*
r_S = peak area of xylazine from the *Standard solution*
C_S = concentration of USP Xylazine RS in the *Standard solution* (mg/mL)
C_U = concentration of Xylazine in the *Sample solution* (mg/mL)
F = relative response factor (see *Table 3*)
Acceptance criteria: See *Table 3*.

■Table 3

Name	Relative Retention Time	Relative Response Factor	Acceptance Criteria, NMT (%)
2,6-Dimethylaniline	0.8	1.4	0.5
Xylazine	1.0	—	—
Specified unknown	1.3	2.8	0.5
2,6-Dimethylphenyl isothiocyanate	2.0	2.7	0.5
Any individual unspecified impurity	—	1.0	0.5
Total impurities	—	—	1.0

■1S (USP41)

SPECIFIC TESTS

Delete the following:

- ■• **MELTING RANGE OR TEMPERATURE** ⟨741⟩: 136°–142°■1S (USP41)
- **LOSS ON DRYING** ⟨731⟩
  Analysis: Dry under vacuum at 60° for 4 h.
  Acceptance criteria: NMT 0.5%

ADDITIONAL REQUIREMENTS
- **PACKAGING AND STORAGE:** Preserve in tight containers. Store at 25°, excursions permitted between 15° and 30°.
- **LABELING:** Where it is intended for veterinary use only, the label so states.
- **USP REFERENCE STANDARDS** ⟨11⟩
  USP Xylazine RS

Dietary Supplements

Official Monographs

Add the following:

▪Ascorbic Acid Chewable Gels

DEFINITION

Ascorbic Acid Chewable Gels contain ascorbic acid in the form of ascorbic acid ($C_6H_8O_6$), sodium ascorbate ($C_6H_7NaO_6$), calcium ascorbate dihydrate ($C_{12}H_{14}CaO_{12} \cdot 2H_2O$), or their mixture in an amount equivalent to NLT 90.0% and NMT 150.0% of the labeled amount of ascorbic acid ($C_6H_8O_6$).

IDENTIFICATION

- **A.** The retention time of the major peak of the *Sample solution* corresponds to that of the *Standard solution*, as obtained in *Strength*.

STRENGTH

- **PROCEDURE**

  [NOTE—Use amber, low-actinic glassware. Use cryogenic gloves when handling liquid nitrogen.]

  Extracting solution: Dissolve 73 g of metaphosphoric acid in 800 mL of water, add 84 mL of glacial acetic acid, and dilute with water to 1000 mL.

  Mobile phase: 7.8 g/L of monobasic sodium phosphate dihydrate in water. Adjust with phosphoric acid to a pH of 2.5.

  [NOTE—Wash the column periodically with methanol and water using appropriate gradients to eliminate retained substances and avoid carryover interferences.]

  Standard stock solution: 1 mg/mL of USP Ascorbic Acid RS in *Extracting solution*. [NOTE—Sonicate with intermittent shaking to help dissolve, if necessary. Prepare fresh every time.]

  Standard solution: Dilute *Standard stock solution* with *Extracting solution* to obtain a solution containing 0.05 mg/mL of USP Ascorbic Acid RS.

  Sample solution: Immerse 25–30 Chewable Gels in liquid nitrogen in a cryogenic vessel for 10 min. Cool a blender jar by swirling liquid nitrogen for about 1 min and discard the contents. Add frozen Chewable Gels to the cooled blender jar and grind to a fine powder. Transfer a portion of the powder, nominally equivalent to 25 mg of ascorbic acid, into a 25-mL volumetric flask. [NOTE—Proceed to this step immediately or keep the powdered Chewable Gels frozen until use.] Add 15 mL of *Extracting solution*, mix on a vortex mixer until well mixed, and sonicate for 10 min or until the sample has completely dissolved. Cool the solution to room temperature, dilute with *Extracting solution* to volume, and mix well. Quantitatively dilute a portion of the solution with *Extracting solution* to obtain a solution containing 0.05 mg/mL of ascorbic acid. Mix and pass through a 0.45-µm glass microfiber filter, discarding the first few milliliters of the filtrate.

  Chromatographic system

  (See *Chromatography* ⟨621⟩, *System Suitability*.)

  Mode: LC

  Detector: UV 245 nm

  Column: 4.6-mm × 15-cm; 3.5-µm packing L7

  Flow rate: 0.8 mL/min

  Injection volume: 10 µL

  System suitability

  Sample: *Standard solution*

  Suitability requirements

  Relative standard deviation: NMT 2.0%

  Analysis

  Samples: *Standard solution* and *Sample solution*

  Calculate the percentage of vitamin C, as ascorbic acid ($C_6H_8O_6$), in the portion of sample taken:

$$Result = (r_U/r_S) \times (C_S/C_U) \times 100$$

  r_U = peak area of ascorbic acid from the *Sample solution*

  r_S = peak area of ascorbic acid from the *Standard solution*

  C_S = concentration of USP Ascorbic Acid RS in the *Standard solution* (mg/mL)

  C_U = nominal concentration of ascorbic acid in the *Sample solution* (mg/mL)

  Acceptance criteria: 90.0%–150.0%

PERFORMANCE TESTS

- **DISINTEGRATION AND DISSOLUTION** ⟨2040⟩, *Dissolution*

  Medium: 0.1 N hydrochloric acid; 900 mL

  Apparatus 2: 75 rpm

  Time: 15 min

  Sample solution: Withdraw a portion of the solution under test, pass through a 0.45-µm glass microfiber filter, and use the pooled sample as the test specimen.

  Analysis: Proceed as directed in *Strength*, making any necessary modifications.

  Samples: *Standard solution* and *Sample solution*

  Calculate the percentage of the labeled amount of ascorbic acid ($C_6H_8O_6$) dissolved:

$$Result = (r_U/r_S) \times (C_S \times V/L) \times 100$$

  r_U = peak area of ascorbic acid from the *Sample solution*

  r_S = peak area of ascorbic acid from the *Standard solution*

  C_S = concentration of USP Ascorbic Acid RS in the *Standard solution* (mg/mL)

  V = volume of *Medium*, 900 mL

  L = label claim of ascorbic acid (mg/Chewable Gel)

  Tolerances: NLT 75% of the labeled amount of ascorbic acid is dissolved.

- **WEIGHT VARIATION** ⟨2091⟩, *Tablets, Uncoated Tablets and Film-Coated Tablets*: Meet the requirements

SPECIFIC TESTS

- **PH ⟨791⟩**
  Sample solution: Cut the Chewable Gels into small pieces. Transfer about 15 g of the cut Chewable Gels into a 50-mL centrifuge tube, add 15 g of hot (80°–90°) water, close the cap, put the centrifuge tube into a shaker water bath at 55°, and shake for 50–60 min or until all of the Chewable Gels are dissolved. Cool down to 30° and measure the pH.
  Acceptance criteria: NMT 4.5
- **WATER ACTIVITY**
  Procedure: Measure the water activity using the AOAC's *Official Methods of Analysis*, Official Method No. 978.18. [NOTE—Make sure that the sample being measured is homogeneous. If you crush, grind, or slice the sample, be consistent in the procedure used in order to obtain reproducible results. Prepare fresh every time.]
  Acceptance criteria: NMT 0.75

CONTAMINANTS

- **MICROBIAL ENUMERATION TESTS ⟨2021⟩:** The total aerobic microbial count is NMT 10^3 cfu/g, and the total combined yeasts and molds count is NMT 10^2 cfu/g.
- **ABSENCE OF SPECIFIED MICROORGANISMS ⟨2022⟩,** *Test Procedures, Test for Absence of Salmonella Species* and *Test for Absence of Escherichia coli*: Meet the requirements

ADDITIONAL REQUIREMENTS

- **PACKAGING AND STORAGE:** Preserve in tight containers; protect from heat.
- **LABELING:** The label states the quantity of ascorbic acid in mg/Chewable Gel, and the chemical form of ascorbic acid present in the Chewable Gels.
- **USP REFERENCE STANDARDS ⟨11⟩**
  USP Ascorbic Acid RS
  ∎1S *(USP41)*

Add the following:

∎Cholecalciferol Chewable Gels

DEFINITION

Cholecalciferol Chewable Gels contain NLT 90.0% and NMT 140.0% of the labeled amount of cholecalciferol ($C_{27}H_{44}O$).

IDENTIFICATION

- **A.** The retention time of the major peak of the *Sample solution* corresponds to that of the *Standard solution*, as obtained in *Strength*.

STRENGTH

- **PROCEDURE**
  [NOTE—Use amber, low-actinic glassware. Use cryogenic gloves when handling liquid nitrogen.]
  Mobile phase: 1.2% isopropyl alcohol in hexane
  [NOTE—Wash the column periodically with 5% isopropyl alcohol in hexane to eliminate retained substances and avoid carryover interferences.]
  Standard stock solution: 0.3 mg/mL of USP Cholecalciferol RS in 2,2,4-trimethylpentane. Shake on a mechanical shaker for 15 min.
  Standard solution: 1 µg/mL of USP Cholecalciferol RS in 2,2,4-trimethylpentane from the *Standard stock solution*, prepared accurately

Sample solution: Immerse 25–30 Chewable Gels in liquid nitrogen in a cryogenic vessel for 10 min. Cool a blender jar by swirling liquid nitrogen for about 1 min and discard the contents. Add frozen Chewable Gels to the cooled blender jar and grind to a fine powder. Transfer a portion of the powder, nominally equivalent to 10 µg of cholecalciferol, into a 50-mL centrifuge tube. [NOTE—Proceed to this step immediately or keep the powdered Chewable Gels frozen until use.] Add 300 mg of pancreatin and 5 mL of water and shake on a water bath shaker at 55° until complete dissolution (about 20 min). Mix the solution on a vortex mixer to suspend any undissolved solid, add 20 mL of dimethyl sulfoxide, and mix again on a vortex mixer until well mixed. Pipet 10 mL of 2,2,4-trimethylpentane, mix on a vortex mixer until the phases are well mixed, then shake the tube on a horizontal shaker for 20 min, and centrifuge the sample at 2500 rpm for 10 min. Pass a portion of the 2,2,4-trimethylpentane layer through a 0.45-µm glass microfiber filter, discarding the first 2 mL of the filtrate.
Chromatographic system
(See *Chromatography ⟨621⟩, System Suitability.*)
Mode: LC
Detector: UV 265 nm
Column: 4.6-mm × 25-cm; 5-µm packing L3
Flow rate: 1.3 mL/min
Injection volume: 80 µL
System suitability
Sample: *Standard solution*
Suitability requirements
  Relative standard deviation: NMT 3.0%
Analysis
Samples: *Standard solution* and *Sample solution*
Calculate the percentage of the labeled amount of cholecalciferol ($C_{27}H_{44}O$) in the portion of Chewable Gels taken:

$$Result = (r_U/r_S) \times (C_S/C_U) \times 100$$

r_U = peak area of cholecalciferol from the *Sample solution*

r_S = peak area of cholecalciferol from the *Standard solution*

C_S = concentration of cholecalciferol in the *Standard solution* (µg/mL)

C_U = nominal concentration of cholecalciferol in the *Sample solution* (µg/mL)

Acceptance criteria: 90.0%–140.0%

PERFORMANCE TESTS

- **DISINTEGRATION AND DISSOLUTION ⟨2040⟩,** *Dissolution*
  [NOTE—Perform this test under light conditions that minimize photodegradation.]
  Medium: 0.1% (w/v) octoxynol-9 in 0.05 M phosphate buffer pH 6.8; 500 mL
  Apparatus 2: 75 rpm
  Time: 30 min
  Mobile phase: Acetonitrile and water (70:30)
  Standard stock solution: 0.5 mg/mL of USP Cholecalciferol RS in isopropyl alcohol
  Standard solution: Dilute the *Standard stock solution* with *Medium* to obtain the concentration equivalent to that expected in the *Sample solution*.
  Sample solution: Withdraw a portion of the solution under test, pass through a 0.45-µm PVDF filter, and use the pooled sample as the test specimen.
  Chromatographic system
  (See *Chromatography ⟨621⟩, System Suitability.*)

Mode: LC
Detector: UV 265 nm
Column: 4.6-mm × 15-cm; 2.7-µm packing L96
Column temperature: 40°
Flow rate: 1 mL/min
Injection volume: 100 µL
System suitability
Sample: *Standard solution*
Suitability requirements
 Relative standard deviation: NMT 2.0%
Analysis
Samples: *Standard solution* and *Sample solution*
Calculate the percentage of the labeled amount of cholecalciferol dissolved:

$$Result = (r_U/r_S) \times (C_S \times V/L) \times 100$$

r_U = peak area of cholecalciferol from the *Sample solution*
r_S = peak area of cholecalciferol from the *Standard solution*
C_S = concentration of cholecalciferol in the *Standard solution* (µg/mL)
V = volume of *Medium*, 500 mL
L = label claim of cholecalciferol (µg/Chewable Gel)

Tolerances: NLT 75% of the labeled amount of cholecalciferol is dissolved.
• **WEIGHT VARIATION** ⟨2091⟩, *Tablets, Uncoated Tablets and Film-Coated Tablets:* Meet the requirements

SPECIFIC TESTS
• **PH** ⟨791⟩
 Sample solution: Cut the Chewable Gels into small pieces. Transfer about 15 g of the cut Chewable Gels into a 50-mL centrifuge tube, add 15 g of hot water (80°–90°), close the cap, place the centrifuge tube into a shaker water bath at 55°, and shake for 50–60 min or until all of the Chewable Gels are dissolved. Cool down to 30° and measure the pH.
 Acceptance criteria: NMT 4.5
• **WATER ACTIVITY**
 Procedure: Measure the water activity using the AOAC's *Official Methods of Analysis*, Official Method No. 978.18. [NOTE—Make sure that the sample being measured is homogeneous. If you crush, grind, or slice the sample, be consistent in the procedure used in order to obtain reproducible results. Prepare fresh every time.]
 Acceptance criteria: NMT 0.75

CONTAMINANTS
• **MICROBIAL ENUMERATION TESTS** ⟨2021⟩: The total aerobic microbial count is NMT 10^3 cfu/g, and the total combined yeasts and molds count is NMT 10^2 cfu/g.
• **ABSENCE OF SPECIFIED MICROORGANISMS** ⟨2022⟩, *Test Procedures, Test for Absence of Salmonella Species* and *Test for Absence of Escherichia coli:* Meet the requirements

ADDITIONAL REQUIREMENTS
• **PACKAGING AND STORAGE:** Preserve in well-closed containers; protect from heat.
• **LABELING:** Label the Chewable Gels to indicate the content of cholecalciferol, in µg.
• **USP REFERENCE STANDARDS** ⟨11⟩
 USP Cholecalciferol RS
■1S (USP41)

Add the following:

▪Coffee Fruit Dry Extract

DEFINITION
Coffee Fruit Dry Extract is prepared from the dried semi-ripened light red entire fruit of *Coffea arabica* L. (Fam. Rubiaceae) by extraction with hydroalcoholic mixtures. It contains NLT 40% of caffeoylquinic acids, calculated as the sum of neochlorogenic acid, chlorogenic acid, cryptochlorogenic acid, isochlorogenic acid B, isochlorogenic acid A, and isochlorogenic acid C on the dried basis; and NLT 15% of chlorogenic acid on the dried basis.

IDENTIFICATION
• **A. HPTLC FOR ARTICLES OF BOTANICAL ORIGIN** ⟨203⟩
 Standard solution A: 0.2 mg/mL of USP Chlorogenic Acid RS in methanol
 Standard solution B: 4 mg/mL of USP Coffee Fruit Dry Extract RS in methanol. Sonicate for 10 min, centrifuge or filter, and use the supernatant or filtrate.
 Sample solution: 4 mg/mL of Coffee Fruit Dry Extract in methanol. Sonicate for 10 min, centrifuge or filter, and use the supernatant or filtrate.
 Chromatographic system
 Adsorbent: Chromatographic silica gel mixture with an average particle size of 5 µm
 Application volume: 5 µL, as 8-mm bands
 Relative humidity: Condition the plate to a relative humidity of about 33% using a suitable device.
 Temperature: About 25°
 Developing solvent system: The upper layer solution of a mixture of *n*-butyl acetate, formic acid, and water (7:5:5)
 Developing distance: 6 cm
 Derivatization reagent A: 10 mg/mL of 2-aminoethyl diphenylborinate in methanol
 Derivatization reagent B: 50 mg/mL of polyethylene glycol 4000 in alcohol
 Analysis
 Samples: *Standard solution A, Standard solution B*, and *Sample solution*
 Apply the *Samples* as bands and dry in air. Develop in a saturated chamber, remove the plate from the chamber, and dry in air. Treat the plate with *Derivatization reagent A*, and dry in air. Immediately treat the plate with *Derivatization reagent B*, dry in air, and examine under UV light at 366 nm.
 Suitability requirements: Under UV light at 366 nm, *Standard solution A* exhibits a blue fluorescent band due to chlorogenic acid in the lower-third section of the chromatogram. *Standard solution B* exhibits an intense blue fluorescent band corresponding in R_F to chlorogenic acid in *Standard solution A*; a band above chlorogenic acid in deeper blue color; and a blue fluorescent band below chlorogenic acid. In the middle-third section, *Standard solution B* exhibits at least three blue fluorescent bands.
 Acceptance criteria: Under UV light at 366 nm, the *Sample solution* exhibits an intense band corresponding in R_F and color to chlorogenic acid in *Standard solution A*. The *Sample solution* exhibits additional bands corresponding to similar bands in *Standard solution B*, including a band above chlorogenic acid in deeper blue color; a blue fluorescent band below chlorogenic acid; three blue fluorescent bands in the middle-third section with the top one due to isochlorogenic acid A, and below that, a pair of bands corresponding to other isochlorogenic acids; and several faint blue fluorescent bands above isochlorogenic acid A.

- **B. HPLC**
  Analysis: Proceed as directed in the test for *Content of Caffeoylquinic Acids*.
  Acceptance criteria: The chromatogram of the *Sample solution* exhibits the most intense peak corresponding to chlorogenic acid in *Standard solution A*, and peaks corresponding to neochlorogenic acid; cryptochlorogenic acid; 5-*O*-feruloylquinic acid, which typically coelutes with another constituent and sometimes can be resolved into two peaks; isochlorogenic acid B; isochlorogenic acid A; and isochlorogenic acid C in the chromatogram of *Standard solution B*. The peaks of neochlorogenic acid and cryptochlorogenic acid are of comparable medium intensity. The peaks of 5-*O*-feruloylquinic acid, isochlorogenic acid B, isochlorogenic acid A, and isochlorogenic acid C are of lower intensity.

COMPOSITION

- **CONTENT OF CAFFEOYLQUINIC ACIDS**
  Solution A: 2% acetic acid in water
  Solution B: Acetonitrile
  Mobile phase: See *Table 1*.

Table 1

Time (min)	Solution A (%)	Solution B (%)
0	95	5
9	95	5
11.5	91	9
21.5	91	9
60	75	25
75	75	25
75.1	95	5
80	95	5

[NOTE—Protect from light and proceed under low-actinic light. Each *Standard solution* and the *Sample solution* are stable for 24 h at room temperature.]
Solvent: Methanol and water (1:1)
Standard solution A: 0.2 mg/mL of USP Chlorogenic Acid RS in *Solvent*
Standard solution B: 1.0 mg/mL of USP Coffee Fruit Dry Extract RS in *Solvent*. Sonicate for 10 min, and pass through a hydrophilic polypropylene (GHP) membrane filter of 0.45-μm or finer pore size.
Sample solution: Accurately transfer a quantity of Coffee Fruit Dry Extract, equivalent to about 10 mg of total caffeoylquinic acids calculated based on the labeled content, into a 25-mL volumetric flask, and add 15 mL of *Solvent*. Sonicate the sample for 10 min, cool to room temperature, dilute with *Solvent* to volume, and mix. Before injection, pass through a GHP membrane filter of 0.45-μm or finer pore size and discard the first portion of the filtrate.
Chromatographic system
(See *Chromatography* ⟨621⟩, *System Suitability*.)
  Mode: LC
  Detector: UV 325 nm
  Column: 4.6-mm × 15-cm; 5-μm packing L1
  Temperatures
    Autosampler: 4°
    Column: 25°
  Flow rate: 1.0 mL/min
  Injection volume: 20 μL
System suitability
  Samples: *Standard solution A* and *Standard solution B*
  Suitability requirements
    Resolution: NLT 1.5 between the peaks of chlorogenic acid and cryptochlorogenic acid; and peaks of isochlorogenic acid B and isochlorogenic acid A, *Standard solution B*
    Tailing factor: NMT 2.0 for the chlorogenic acid peak, *Standard solution A*

Relative standard deviation: NMT 2.0% for the chlorogenic acid peak in repeated injections, *Standard solution A*
Chromatographic similarity: The chromatogram of *Standard solution B* is similar to the reference chromatogram provided with the lot of USP Coffee Fruit Dry Extract RS being used.
Analysis
  Samples: *Standard solution A*, *Standard solution B*, and *Sample solution*
  Using the chromatograms of *Standard solution A*, *Standard solution B*, and the reference chromatogram provided with the lot of USP Coffee Fruit Dry Extract RS being used, identify the peaks for neochlorogenic acid, chlorogenic acid, cryptochlorogenic acid, 5-*O*-feruloylquinic acid, isochlorogenic acid B, isochlorogenic acid A, and isochlorogenic acid C in the *Sample solution*. [NOTE—See *Table 2* for relative retention times. These values may vary due to differences in the chromatographic conditions allowed by the *Suitability requirements*.]

Table 2

Analyte	Approximate Relative Retention Time	Conversion Factor
Neochlorogenic acid[a]	0.57	1.00
Chlorogenic acid[b]	1.00	1.00
Cryptochlorogenic acid[c]	1.06	1.00
5-*O*-Feruloylquinic acid[d]	1.84	—
Isochlorogenic acid B[e]	2.90	0.84
Isochlorogenic acid A[f]	2.94	0.80
Isochlorogenic acid C[g]	3.20	0.80

[a] (1*R*,3*R*,4*S*,5*R*)-3-{[(*E*)-3-(3,4-Dihydroxyphenyl)acryloyl]oxy}-1,4,5-trihydroxycyclohexane-1-carboxylic acid.
[b] (1*S*,3*R*,4*R*,5*R*)-3-{[(*E*)-3-(3,4-Dihydroxyphenyl)acryloyl]oxy}-1,4,5-trihydroxycyclohexane-1-carboxylic acid.
[c] (1*S*,3*R*,4*S*,5*R*)-4-{[(*E*)-3-(3,4-Dihydroxyphenyl)acryloyl]oxy}-1,3,5-trihydroxycyclohexane-1-carboxylic acid.
[d] (1*S*,3*R*,4*R*,5*R*)-1,3,4-Trihydroxy-5-{[(*E*)-3-(4-hydroxy-3-methoxyphenyl)acryloyl]oxy}cyclohexane-1-carboxylic acid.
[e] (1*S*,3*R*,4*R*,5*R*)-3,4-Bis{[(*E*)-3-(3,4-dihydroxyphenyl)acryloyl]oxy}-1,5-dihydroxycyclohexane-1-carboxylic acid.
[f] (1*S*,3*R*,4*S*,5*R*)-3,5-Bis{[(*E*)-3-(3,4-dihydroxyphenyl)acryloyl]oxy}-1,4-dihydroxycyclohexane-1-carboxylic acid.
[g] (1*R*,3*R*,4*S*,5*R*)-3,4-Bis{[(*E*)-3-(3,4-dihydroxyphenyl)acryloyl]oxy}-1,5-dihydroxycyclohexane-1-carboxylic acid.

[NOTE—These compounds are often referred in the literature as 3-/4-/5-/mono-/di-substituted quinic acids. Due to the confusion in historic and evolving IUPAC ring numbering, that nomenclature is not used in this Pharmacopeia. Instead, the compounds are described by their conformational structures in the *Table 3*.]

Table 3. Graphic Conformational Structures of Caffeoylquinic Acids

Caffeoylquinic Acids	R1	R2	R3
Neochlorogenic acid	Caffeoyl	H	H
Chlorogenic acid	H	H	Caffeoyl
Cryptochlorogenic acid	H	Caffeoyl	H

Table 3. Graphic Conformational Structures of Caffeoylquinic Acids *(Continued)*

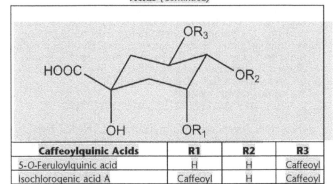

Caffeoylquinic Acids	R1	R2	R3
5-O-Feruloylquinic acid	H	H	Caffeoyl
Isochlorogenic acid A	Caffeoyl	H	Caffeoyl
Isochlorogenic acid B	H	Caffeoyl	Caffeoyl
Isochlorogenic acid C	Caffeoyl	Caffeoyl	H

Separately calculate the percentages of neochlorogenic acid, chlorogenic acid, cryptochlorogenic acid, isochlorogenic acid B, isochlorogenic acid A, and isochlorogenic acid C in the portion of Coffee Fruit Dry Extract taken:

$$Result = (r_U/r_S) \times C_S \times (V/W) \times F \times 100$$

r_U = peak area of the relevant analyte from the *Sample solution*
r_S = peak area of chlorogenic acid from *Standard solution A*
C_S = concentration of USP Chlorogenic Acid RS in *Standard solution A* (mg/mL)
V = volume of the *Sample solution* (mL)
W = weight of Coffee Fruit Dry Extract taken to prepare the *Sample solution* (mg)
F = conversion factor for the analyte (see *Table 2*)

Calculate the content of caffeoylquinic acids as the sum of the percentages of neochlorogenic acid, chlorogenic acid, cryptochlorogenic acid, isochlorogenic acid B, isochlorogenic acid A, and isochlorogenic acid C.
Acceptance criteria: NLT 40% of total caffeoylquinic acids on the dried basis; NLT 15% of chlorogenic acid on the dried basis

CONTAMINANTS
- **ELEMENTAL IMPURITIES—PROCEDURES ⟨233⟩**
  Acceptance criteria
  Arsenic: NMT 2.0 µg/g
  Cadmium: NMT 0.5 µg/g
  Lead: NMT 5.0 µg/g
  Mercury: NMT 0.2 µg/g
- **ARTICLES OF BOTANICAL ORIGIN ⟨561⟩**, *Pesticide Residue Analysis*: Meets the requirements
- **MICROBIAL ENUMERATION TESTS ⟨2021⟩**: The total aerobic bacterial count does not exceed 10^4 cfu/g, and the total combined molds and yeasts count does not exceed 10^3 cfu/g.
- **ABSENCE OF SPECIFIED MICROORGANISMS ⟨2022⟩**, *Test Procedures, Test for Absence of Salmonella Species* and *Test for Absence of Escherichia coli*: Meets the requirements

SPECIFIC TESTS
- **LIMIT OF CAFFEINE**
  Mobile phase: 0.1% perchloric acid in a mixture of water and acetonitrile (9:1)
  Standard solution: 0.05 mg/mL of USP Caffeine RS in *Mobile phase*
  Sample solution: Accurately transfer a quantity of Coffee Fruit Dry Extract, equivalent to 1.0–2.0 mg of caffeine calculated based on the labeled amount, into a 25-mL volumetric flask, and add 15 mL of *Mobile phase*. Sonicate for 10 min, cool to room temperature, dilute with *Mobile phase* to volume, and mix. Transfer 5.0 mL

of the solution into a 15-mL centrifuge tube containing 1 g of PSA (primary and secondary amine) bonded silica. Mix on a vortex mixer for 3 min and allow to sit at room temperature for 10 min. Before injection, pass through a GHP membrane filter of 0.45-µm or finer pore size, and discard the first portion of the filtrate.
  Chromatographic system
  (See *Chromatography* ⟨621⟩, *System Suitability*.)
  Mode: LC
  Detector: UV 275 nm
  Column: 3.0-mm × 15-cm; 2.7-µm packing L11
  Temperatures
  Autosampler: 4°
  Column: 30°
  Flow rate: 0.6 mL/min
  Injection volume: 10 µL
  Run time: 15 min
  System suitability
  Sample: *Standard solution*
  Suitability requirements
  Relative standard deviation: NMT 2.0% for the caffeine peak in repeated injections
  Analysis
  Samples: *Standard solution* and *Sample solution*
  Using the chromatogram of the *Standard solution*, identify the peak corresponding to caffeine in the *Sample solution*.
  Calculate the percentage of caffeine in the portion of Coffee Fruit Dry Extract taken:

$$Result = (r_U/r_S) \times C_S \times (V/W) \times 100$$

r_U = peak area of caffeine from the *Sample solution*
r_S = peak area of caffeine from the *Standard solution*
C_S = concentration of USP Caffeine RS in the *Standard solution* (mg/mL)
V = volume of the *Sample solution* (mL)
W = weight of Coffee Fruit Dry Extract taken to prepare the *Sample solution* (mg)

  Acceptance criteria: NMT 2.0% on the dried basis
- **LOSS ON DRYING ⟨731⟩**
  Sample: 1.0 g of Coffee Fruit Dry Extract
  Analysis: Dry the *Sample* at 105° for 2 h.
  Acceptance criteria: NMT 5.0%

ADDITIONAL REQUIREMENTS
- **PACKAGING AND STORAGE:** Preserve in well-closed containers, protected from light and moisture, and store in a cool place.
- **LABELING:** The label states the Latin binomial of the plant from which the article was prepared following the official name. It meets other labeling requirements in *Botanical Extracts* ⟨565⟩.
- **USP REFERENCE STANDARDS ⟨11⟩**
  USP Caffeine RS
  USP Chlorogenic Acid RS
  USP Coffee Fruit Dry Extract RS
  ■1S *(USP41)*

Add the following:

■Coix Seed

DEFINITION
Coix Seed, also known as Job's tears, consists of the dried ripe caryopsis, freed from the shell, of *Coix lacryma-jobi* var. *ma-yuen* (Rom.Caill.) Stapf (Fam. Poaceae, alt. Gramineae) collected in the fall. It contains NLT 3.5% of triglycerides calculated as the sum of trilinolein ($C_{57}H_{98}O_6$),

1,2-dilinoleoyl-3-palmitin ($C_{55}H_{98}O_6$), 1,2-dilinoleoyl-3-olein ($C_{57}H_{100}O_6$), 1-palmitoyl-2-oleoyl-3-linolein ($C_{55}H_{100}O_6$), 1,2-dioleoyl-3-linolein ($C_{57}H_{102}O_6$), 1,2-dioleoyl-3-palmitin ($C_{55}H_{102}O_6$), and triolein ($C_{57}H_{104}O_6$) on the dried basis.

IDENTIFICATION

• A. HPTLC FOR ARTICLES OF BOTANICAL ORIGIN ⟨203⟩

Standard solution A: 2 mg/mL of USP Oleic Acid RS in methanol

Standard solution B: 40 mg/mL (about 50 µL/mL) of USP Coix Seed Oil Extract RS in methylene chloride

Sample solution: Sonicate 0.5 g of finely powdered Coix Seed in 5 mL of methylene chloride for 10 min. Centrifuge at 5000 rpm for 5 min and use the supernatant.

Chromatographic system and **System suitability**
Use *Identification of Fixed Oils by Thin-Layer Chromatography* ⟨202⟩, *Identification, Method II.*

Derivatization reagent: 25 mg/mL of phosphomolybdic acid in 96% alcohol

Analysis

Samples: *Standard solution A, Standard solution B*, and *Sample solution*

Apply the *Samples* as bands and dry in air. Develop in a saturated chamber up to 7 cm, remove the plate from the chamber, and dry in air. Treat the plate with *Derivatization reagent*, heat at 120° for 3 min, and examine in white light.

Acceptance criteria: The *Sample solution* exhibits, in the upper half, a band corresponding in R_F and color to the oleic acid band in *Standard solution A*. The *Sample solution* exhibits additional bands that correspond to similar bands in *Standard solution B*, including one band right above oleic acid with the same color, a cluster of four blue bands in the lower half, and some faint bands in the middle third.

• B. HPLC

Analysis: Proceed as directed in the test for *Content of Triglycerides*.

Acceptance criteria: The *Sample solution* exhibits a peak with a retention time corresponding to triolein in *Standard stock solution* and peaks due to trilinolein, 1,2-dilinoleoyl-3-palmitin,1,2-dilinoleoyl-3-olein, 1-palmitoyl-2-oleoyl-3-linolein, 1,2-dioleoyl-3-linolein, and 1,2-dioleoyl-3-palmitin at retention times corresponding to the same triglycerides in *Standard solution 6*. The 1,2-dilinoleoyl-3-olein and 1,2-dioleoyl-3-linolein are the most intense peaks; 1-palmitoyl-2-oleoyl-3-linolein and triolein are medium-intensity peaks; trilinolein, 1,2-dilinoleoyl-3-palmitin, and 1,2-dioleoyl-3-palmitin are low-intensity peaks (distinction from *Sorghum bicolor* (L.) Moench, which has similar triglyceride peaks, all of low intensity, and *Hordeum vulgare* L., which has four triglyceride peaks, all of low intensity).

COMPOSITION

• CONTENT OF TRIGLYCERIDES

Mobile phase: Methanol

Standard stock solution: 0.20 mg/mL of USP Triolein RS in methanol. Sonicate to dissolve.

Standard solutions 1–5: Dilute the *Standard stock solution* with methanol to obtain solutions of 0.0125, 0.025, 0.05, 0.10, and 0.20 mg/mL of USP Triolein RS. Pass each through a suitable membrane filter of 0.45-µm or finer pore size.

Standard solution 6: 0.5 mg/mL of USP Coix Seed Oil Extract RS in methanol

Sample solution: Accurately transfer about 500 mg of finely powdered Coix Seed into a suitable flask and add 35 mL of methanol. Sonicate for 30 min and filter under vacuum. Rinse the original flask and the residue left in the flask with 5 mL of methanol, and wash the residue and paper on the filter with the rinsing. Repeat the rinse and wash procedures one more time, and transfer the filtrate from the vacuum flask to a 50-mL volumetric flask. Wash the vacuum flask twice with about 2.5 mL of methanol each time, transfer the washings into the volumetric flask, dilute with methanol to volume, and mix. Before injection, pass through a suitable membrane filter of 0.45-µm or finer pore size, and discard the first portion of the filtrate. [NOTE—Dried filter and vacuum flask should be used.]

Chromatographic system
(See *Chromatography* ⟨621⟩, *System Suitability*.)

Mode: LC

Detector: Evaporative light-scattering. [NOTE—The parameters should be adjusted to achieve the best signal-to-noise ratio, according to the manufacturer's recommendations.]

Column: 3.0-mm × 10-cm; 2.7-µm packing L7

Column temperature: 20°

Flow rate: 0.3 mL/min

Injection volume: 5 µL

System suitability

Samples: *Standard stock solution* and *Standard solutions 1–6*

Suitability requirements

Resolution: NLT 1.5 between the peak of 1,2-dilinoleoyl-3-olein and the small peak following it, *Standard solution 6*

Tailing factor: NMT 1.5 for the triolein peak, *Standard stock solution*

Relative standard deviation: NMT 5.0% for the triolein peak in repeated injections, *Standard stock solution*

Correlation coefficient: NLT 0.995 for the regression line as determined in *Analysis, Standard solutions 1–5*

Signal-to-noise ratio: NLT 15 for the triolein peak, *Standard solution 1* (0.0125 mg/mL)

Chromatogram similarity: The chromatogram of *Standard solution 6* is similar to the reference chromatogram provided with the lot of USP Coix Seed Oil Extract RS being used.

Analysis

Samples: *Standard solutions 1–6* and *Sample solution*

Using the chromatograms of *Standard solutions 5–6* and the reference chromatogram provided with the lot of USP Coix Seed Oil Extract RS being used, identify the retention times of the peaks of the relevant analytes in the *Sample solution*. [NOTE—See *Table 1* for the approximate relative retention times.]

Table 1

Analyte	Approximate Relative Retention Time
Trilinolein	0.61
1,2-Dilinoleoyl-3-palmitin	0.67
1,2-Dilinoleoyl-3-olein	0.71
1-Palmitoyl-2-oleoyl-3-linolein	0.79
1,2-Dioleoyl-3-linolein	0.84
1,2-Dioleoyl-3-palmitin	0.94
Triolein	1.00

Plot the logarithms of peak responses versus the logarithms of concentrations, in mg/mL, of triolein from *Standard solutions 1–5*. Using a least-squares analysis, establish the regression line or determine a linear regression equation.

Determine the concentration (*C*), in mg/mL, of the relevant analytes in the *Sample solution* by using the regression line or linear regression equation.

Separately calculate the percentages of trilinolein, 1,2-dilinoleoyl-3-palmitin, 1,2-dilinoleoyl-3-olein, 1-palmitoyl-2-oleoyl-3-linolein, 1,2-dioleoyl-3-linolein, 1,2-dioleoyl-3-palmitin, and triolein in the portion of Coix Seed taken:

$$Result = C \times (V/W) \times 100$$

C = concentration of the relevant analyte in the *Sample solution* as determined above (mg/mL)

V = volume of the *Sample solution* (mL)

W = weight of Coix Seed taken to prepare the *Sample solution* (mg)

Calculate the content of triglycerides as the sum of the percentages of trilinolein, 1,2-dilinoleoyl-3-palmitin, 1,2-dilinoleoyl-3-olein, 1-palmitoyl-2-oleoyl-3-linolein, 1,2-dioleoyl-3-linolein, 1,2-dioleoyl-3-palmitin, and triolein.

Acceptance criteria: NLT 3.5% on the dried basis

CONTAMINANTS

- **LIMIT OF ZEARALENONE**

  Mobile phase: Acetonitrile and water (1:1)

  Standard stock solution: 250 ng/mL of zearalenone in methanol

  Standard solution: Accurately transfer 1 mL of *Standard stock solution* to a 10-mL volumetric flask and add methanol to volume.

  Sample solution: Accurately transfer about 20 g of finely powdered Coix Seed to a suitable centrifuge tube. Add 4.0 g of sodium chloride, and accurately add 100 mL of 90% acetonitrile. Mix for 2 min with a high speed disperser (NLT 11,000 rpm), and centrifuge for 5 min (4000 rpm). Immediately pipet 10.0 mL of the supernatant into a 50-mL volumetric flask, add water to volume, mix, and centrifuge. Pipet 10.0 mL of the supernatant onto an immunoaffinity column[1] capable of binding zearalenone, and elute at a flow rate of approximately 3 mL/min (60 drops/min). Wash the column with 10 mL of water at a flow rate of approximately 6 mL/min (120 drops/min), let the column run dry, and discard the water eluate. Wash the column with 1.5 mL of methanol at a flow rate of approximately 1 mL/min (20 drops/min), collect the methanol eluate into a 2-mL volumetric flask, and let the column run dry. Add methanol to volume, and mix.

  Chromatographic system

  (See *Chromatography ⟨621⟩, System Suitability.*)

  Mode: LC

  Detector: Fluorometric

   Excitation wavelength: 232 nm

   Emission wavelength: 460 nm

  Column: 4.6-mm × 15-cm; 5-μm packing L1

  Column temperature: 30°

  Flow rate: 1.0 mL/min

  Injection volume: 20 μL of *Sample solution*

  System suitability

  Sample: *Standard solution*

  Suitability requirements

   Column efficiency: NLT 10,000 theoretical plates

   Relative standard deviation: NMT 10.0% for the zearalenone peak

   Correlation coefficient: NLT 0.999 for the regression line as determined in *Analysis*

  Analysis

  Samples: *Standard solution* and *Sample solution*

  Inject the *Standard solution* in volumes of 5, 10, 15, 20, and 25 μL, and measure zearalenone peak areas for each injection. Plot the peak areas versus the amounts, in ng, of zearalenone in the injections, and establish the regression line using a least-squares analysis.

Using the chromatogram of the *Standard solution*, identify the retention time of the peak corresponding to zearalenone in the *Sample solution*.

From the graph, determine the content (C), in ng, of zearalenone in the *Sample solution*.

Calculate content, in ng/g, of zearalenone in the portion of Coix Seed taken:

$$Result = 5000 \times (C/W)$$

C = content of zearalenone as determined above (ng)

W = weight of Coix Seed taken to prepare the *Sample solution* (g)

Acceptance criteria: NMT 60 ng/g on the dried basis

- **ARTICLES OF BOTANICAL ORIGIN ⟨561⟩,** *Limits of Elemental Impurities:* Meets the requirements

- **ARTICLES OF BOTANICAL ORIGIN ⟨561⟩,** *Pesticide Residue Analysis:* Meets the requirements

- **MICROBIAL ENUMERATION TESTS ⟨2021⟩:** The total aerobic bacterial count does not exceed 10^5 cfu/g, the total combined molds and yeasts count does not exceed 10^3 cfu/g, and the bile-tolerant Gram-negative bacteria count does not exceed 10^3 cfu/g.

- **ABSENCE OF SPECIFIED MICROORGANISMS ⟨2022⟩,** *Test Procedures, Test for Absence of Salmonella Species* and *Test for Absence of Escherichia coli:* Meets the requirements

- **ARTICLES OF BOTANICAL ORIGIN ⟨561⟩,** *Test for Aflatoxins:* Meets the requirements

SPECIFIC TESTS

- **BOTANICAL CHARACTERISTICS**

  Macroscopic: Broad ovoid or elongated-elliptical, 4–8 mm long, 3–6 mm wide. Externally milky white, smooth, with yellowish-brown testa occasionally. One end obtusely rounded, the other end relatively broad and slightly dented with one pale, brown dotted hilum. Dorsal surface rounded and protruding; ventral surface with one relatively broad and deep longitudinal furrow. Texture hard, fracture white and starchy.

  Microscopic: The powder contains numerous starch granules usually in clumps, simple granule spherical or polyhedral, 2–20 μm in diameter with a stellate, y-shaped hilum; compound granules rare, usually consisting of two to three simple granules.

- **LOSS ON DRYING ⟨731⟩**

  Analysis: Finely powder and dry at 105° for 2 h.

  Acceptance criteria: NMT 12.0%

- **ARTICLES OF BOTANICAL ORIGIN ⟨561⟩,** *Methods of Analysis, Foreign Organic Matter:* NMT 2.0%

- **ARTICLES OF BOTANICAL ORIGIN ⟨561⟩,** *Methods of Analysis, Alcohol-Soluble Extractives, Method 1:* NLT 5.5%

- **ARTICLES OF BOTANICAL ORIGIN ⟨561⟩,** *Methods of Analysis, Total Ash:* NMT 3.0%

ADDITIONAL REQUIREMENTS

- **PACKAGING AND STORAGE:** Preserve in well-closed containers, protected from light and moisture, and store at 4°–10°.

- **LABELING:** The label states the Latin binomial following the official name of the plant contained in the article.

- **USP REFERENCE STANDARDS ⟨11⟩**

  USP Coix Seed Oil Extract RS

  USP Oleic Acid RS

  USP Triolein RS

  ■1S *(USP41)*

---

[1] Suitable grade of ZearalaTest™. Available from Vicam, Cat. No. G1012 (ZearalaTest) or Cat. No. G1026 (ZearalaTest WB).

Add the following:

▪Coix Seed Powder

DEFINITION
Coix Seed Powder, also known as Job's tears powder, consists of the dried ripe caryopsis, freed from the shell, of *Coix lacryma-jobi* var. *ma-yuen* (Rom.Caill.) Stapf (Fam. Poaceae, alt. Gramineae) collected in the fall and reduced to a fine or very fine powder. It contains NLT 3.5% of triglycerides calculated as the sum of trilinolein ($C_{57}H_{98}O_6$), 1,2-dilinoleoyl-3-palmitin ($C_{55}H_{98}O_6$), 1,2-dilinoleoyl-3-olein ($C_{57}H_{100}O_6$), 1-palmitoyl-2-oleoyl-3-linolein ($C_{55}H_{100}O_6$), 1,2-dioleoyl-3-linolein ($C_{57}H_{102}O_6$), 1,2-dioleoyl-3-palmitin ($C_{55}H_{102}O_6$), and triolein ($C_{57}H_{104}O_6$) on the dried basis.

IDENTIFICATION
- **A. HPTLC FOR ARTICLES OF BOTANICAL ORIGIN ⟨203⟩**
  Standard solution A: 2 mg/mL of USP Oleic Acid RS in methanol
  Standard solution B: 40 mg/mL (about 50 μL/mL) of USP Coix Seed Oil Extract RS in methylene chloride
  Sample solution: Sonicate 0.5 g of Coix Seed Powder in 5 mL of methylene chloride for 10 min. Centrifuge at 5000 rpm for 5 min and use the supernatant.
  Chromatographic system and **System suitability**
  Use *Identification of Fixed Oils by Thin-Layer Chromatography ⟨202⟩, Identification, Method II.*
  Derivatization reagent: 25 mg/mL of phosphomolybdic acid in 96% alcohol
  Analysis
  Samples: *Standard solution A, Standard solution B,* and *Sample solution*
  Apply the *Samples* as bands and dry in air. Develop in a saturated chamber up to 7 cm, remove the plate from the chamber, and dry in air. Treat the plate with *Derivatization reagent,* heat at 120° for 3 min, and examine in white light.
  Acceptance criteria: The *Sample solution* exhibits, in the upper half, a band corresponding in R_F and color to the oleic acid band in *Standard solution A.* The *Sample solution* exhibits additional bands that correspond to similar bands in *Standard solution B,* including one band right above oleic acid with the same color, a cluster of four blue bands in the lower half, and some faint bands in the middle third.
- **B. HPLC**
  Analysis: Proceed as directed in the test for *Content of Triglycerides.*
  Acceptance criteria: The *Sample solution* exhibits a peak with a retention time corresponding to triolein in *Standard stock solution* and peaks due to trilinolein, 1,2-dilinoleoyl-3-palmitin, 1,2-dilinoleoyl-3-olein, 1-palmitoyl-2-oleoyl-3-linolein, 1,2-dioleoyl-3-linolein, and 1,2-dioleoyl-3-palmitin at retention times corresponding to the same triglycerides in *Standard solution 6.* The 1,2-dilinoleoyl-3-olein and 1,2-dioleoyl-3-linolein are the most intense peaks; 1-palmitoyl-2-oleoyl-3-linolein and triolein are medium-intensity peaks; trilinolein, 1,2-dilinoleoyl-3-palmitin, and 1,2-dioleoyl-3-palmitin are low-intensity peaks (distinction from *Sorghum bicolor* (L.) Moench, which has similar triglyceride peaks, all of low intensity, and *Hordeum vulgare* L., which has four triglyceride peaks, all of low intensity).

COMPOSITION
- **CONTENT OF TRIGLYCERIDES**
  Mobile phase: Methanol
  Standard stock solution: 0.20 mg/mL of USP Triolein RS in methanol. Sonicate to dissolve.
  Standard solutions 1–5: Dilute the *Standard stock solution* with methanol to obtain solutions of 0.0125,

0.025, 0.05, 0.10, and 0.20 mg/mL of USP Triolein RS. Pass each through a suitable membrane filter of 0.45-μm or finer pore size.
Standard solution 6: 0.5 mg/mL of USP Coix Seed Oil Extract RS in methanol
Sample solution: Accurately transfer about 500 mg of Coix Seed Powder into a suitable flask and add 35 mL of methanol. Sonicate for 30 min and filter under vacuum. Rinse the original flask and the residue left in the flask with 5 mL of methanol, and wash the residue and paper on the filter with the rinsing. Repeat the rinse and wash procedures one more time, and transfer the filtrate from the vacuum flask to a 50-mL volumetric flask. Wash the vacuum flask twice with about 2.5 mL of methanol each time, transfer the washings into the volumetric flask, dilute with methanol to volume, and mix. Before injection, pass through a suitable membrane filter of 0.45-μm or finer pore size, and discard the first portion of the filtrate. [NOTE—Dried filter and vacuum flask should be used.]
Chromatographic system
(See *Chromatography ⟨621⟩, System Suitability.*)
Mode: LC
Detector: Evaporative light-scattering. [NOTE—The parameters should be adjusted to achieve the best signal-to-noise ratio, according to manufacturer's recommendations.]
Column: 3.0-mm × 10-cm; 2.7-μm packing L7
Column temperature: 20°
Flow rate: 0.3 mL/min
Injection volume: 5 μL
System suitability
Samples: *Standard stock solution* and *Standard solutions 1–6.*
Resolution: NLT 1.5 between the peak of 1,2-dilinoleoyl-3-olein and the small peak following it, *Standard solution 6*
Tailing factor: NMT 1.5 for the triolein peak, *Standard stock solution*
Relative standard deviation: NMT 5.0% for the triolein peak in repeated injections, *Standard stock solution*
Correlation coefficient: NLT 0.995 for the regression line as determined in *Analysis, Standard solutions 1–5*
Signal-to-noise ratio: NLT 15 for the triolein peak, *Standard solution 1* (0.0125 mg/mL)
Chromatogram similarity: The chromatogram of *Standard solution 6* is similar to the reference chromatogram provided with the lot of USP Coix Seed Oil Extract RS being used.
Analysis
Samples: *Standard solutions 1–6* and *Sample solution*
Using the chromatograms of *Standard solutions 5–6* and the reference chromatogram provided with the lot of USP Coix Seed Oil Extract RS being used, identify the retention times of the peaks of the relevant analytes in the *Sample solution.* [NOTE—See *Table 1* for the approximate relative retention times.]

Table 1

Analyte	Approximate Relative Retention Time
Trilinolein	0.61
1,2-Dilinoleoyl-3-palmitin	0.67
1,2-Dilinoleoyl-3-olein	0.71
1-Palmitoyl-2-oleoyl-3-linolein	0.79
1,2-Dioleoyl-3-linolein	0.84
1,2-Dioleoyl-3-palmitin	0.94
Triolein	1.00

Plot the logarithms of peak responses versus the logarithms of concentrations, in mg/mL, of triolein from *Standard solutions 1–5.* Using a least-squares analysis, establish a regression line or determine a linear regression equation.

Determine the concentration (C), in mg/mL, of the relevant analytes in the *Sample solution* by using the regression line or linear regression equation.

Separately calculate the percentages of trilinolein, 1,2-dilinoleoyl-3-palmitin, 1,2-dilinoleoyl-3-olein, 1-palmitoyl-2-oleoyl-3-linolein, 1,2-dioleoyl-3-linolein, 1,2-dioleoyl-3-palmitin, and triolein in the portion of Coix Seed Powder taken:

$$Result = C \times (V/W) \times 100$$

C = concentration of relevant analyte in the *Sample solution* as determined above (mg/mL)
V = volume of the *Sample solution* (mL)
W = weight of Coix Seed Powder taken to prepare the *Sample solution* (mg)

Calculate the content of triglycerides as the sum of the percentages of trilinolein, 1,2-dilinoleoyl-3-palmitin, 1,2-dilinoleoyl-3-olein, 1-palmitoyl-2-oleoyl-3-linolein, 1,2-dioleoyl-3-linolein, 1,2-dioleoyl-3-palmitin, and triolein.

Acceptance criteria: NLT 3.5% on the dried basis

CONTAMINANTS
- **LIMIT OF ZEARALENONE**
  Mobile phase: Acetonitrile and water (1:1)
  Standard stock solution: 250 ng/mL of zearalenone in methanol
  Standard solution: Accurately transfer 1 mL of *Standard stock solution* to a 10-mL volumetric flask and add methanol to volume.
  Sample solution: Accurately transfer about 20 g of Coix Seed Powder to a suitable centrifuge tube. Add 4.0 g of sodium chloride, and accurately add 100 mL of 90% acetonitrile. Mix for 2 min with a high-speed disperser (NLT 11,000 rpm), and centrifuge for 5 min (4000 rpm). Immediately pipet 10.0 mL of the supernatant into a 50-mL volumetric flask, add water to volume, mix, and centrifuge. Pipet 10.0 mL of the supernatant onto an immunoaffinity column[1] capable of binding zearalenone, and elute at a flow rate of approximately 3 mL/min (60 drops/min). Wash the column with 10 mL of water at a flow rate of approximately 6 mL/min (120 drops/min), let the column run dry, and discard the water eluate. Wash the column with 1.5 mL of methanol at a flow rate of approximately 1 mL/min (20 drops/min), collect the methanol eluate into a 2-mL volumetric flask, and let the column run dry. Add methanol to volume, and mix.
  Chromatographic system
  (See *Chromatography* ⟨621⟩, *System Suitability*.)
  Mode: LC
  Detector: Fluorometric
  Excitation wavelength: 232 nm
  Emission wavelength: 460 nm
  Column: 4.6-mm × 15-cm; 5-μm packing L1
  Column temperature: 30°
  Flow rate: 1.0 mL/min
  Injection volume: 20 μL of *Sample solution*
  System suitability
  Sample: *Standard solution*
  Suitability requirements
  Column efficiency: NLT 10,000 theoretical plates
  Relative standard deviation: NMT 10.0% for the zearalenone peak

Correlation coefficient: NLT 0.999 for the regression line as determined in *Analysis*

Analysis
Samples: *Standard solution* and *Sample solution*
Inject the *Standard solution* with volumes of 5, 10, 15, 20, and 25 μL, and measure zearalenone peak areas for each injection. Plot the peak areas versus the amounts, in ng, of zearalenone in the injections, and establish the regression line using a least-squares analysis.
Using the chromatogram of the *Standard solution*, identify the retention time of the peak corresponding to zearalenone in the *Sample solution*.
From the graph, determine the content (C), in ng, of zearalenone in the *Sample solution*.
Calculate content, in ng/g, of zearalenone in the portion of Coix Seed Powder taken:

$$Result = 5000 \times (C/W)$$

C = content of zearalenone as determined above (ng)
W = weight of Coix Seed Powder taken to prepare the *Sample solution* (g)

Acceptance criteria: NMT 60 ng/g on the dried basis
- **ARTICLES OF BOTANICAL ORIGIN** ⟨561⟩, *Limits of Elemental Impurities*: Meets the requirements
- **ARTICLES OF BOTANICAL ORIGIN** ⟨561⟩, *Pesticide Residue Analysis*: Meets the requirements
- **MICROBIAL ENUMERATION TESTS** ⟨2021⟩: The total aerobic bacterial count does not exceed 10^5 cfu/g, the total combined molds and yeasts count does not exceed 10^3 cfu/g, and the bile-tolerant Gram-negative bacteria count does not exceed 10^3 cfu/g.
- **ABSENCE OF SPECIFIED MICROORGANISMS** ⟨2022⟩, *Test Procedures, Test for Absence of Salmonella Species* and *Test for Absence of Escherichia coli*: Meets the requirements
- **ARTICLES OF BOTANICAL ORIGIN** ⟨561⟩, *Test for Aflatoxins*: Meets the requirements

SPECIFIC TESTS
- **BOTANICAL CHARACTERISTICS**
  Macroscopic: Pale, whitish powder
  Microscopic: Starch granules numerous, usually in clumps, simple granules spherical or polyhedral, 2–20 μm in diameter with a stellate, y-shaped hilum; compound granules rare, usually consisting of two to three simple granules.
- **LOSS ON DRYING** ⟨731⟩
  Analysis: Dry at 105° for 2 h.
  Acceptance criteria: NMT 12.0%
- **ARTICLES OF BOTANICAL ORIGIN** ⟨561⟩, *Methods of Analysis, Alcohol-Soluble Extractives, Method 1*: NLT 5.5%
- **ARTICLES OF BOTANICAL ORIGIN** ⟨561⟩, *Methods of Analysis, Total Ash*: NMT 3.0%

ADDITIONAL REQUIREMENTS
- **PACKAGING AND STORAGE:** Preserve in well-closed containers, protected from light and moisture, and store at 4°–10°.
- **LABELING:** The label states the Latin binomial following the official name of the plant contained in the article.
- **USP REFERENCE STANDARDS** ⟨11⟩
  USP Coix Seed Oil Extract RS
  USP Oleic Acid RS
  USP Triolein RS

  ■1S *(USP41)*

---

[1] Suitable grade of ZearalaTest™. Available from Vicam, Cat. No. G1012 (ZearalaTest) or Cat. No. G1026 (ZearalaTest WB).

Flax Seed Oil

[8001-26-1].

DEFINITION

Change to read:

Flax Seed Oil is derived from flaxseed or linseed (*Linum usitatissimum* L.). The oil is extracted from the ■₁ₛ (USP41) seeds by cold pressing. ■₁ₛ (USP41) No solvents or external heat are employed in the extraction process. It contains no added substances.

IDENTIFICATION
- **A.** It meets the requirements in *Specific Tests* for *Fats and Fixed Oils* ⟨401⟩, *Procedures, Fatty Acid Composition*.
- **B. IDENTIFICATION OF FIXED OILS BY THIN-LAYER CHROMATOGRAPHY** ⟨202⟩: The *R_F* values of the principal spots of the *Sample solution* correspond to those of the *Standard solution*.

SPECIFIC TESTS
- **FATS AND FIXED OILS** ⟨401⟩, *Procedures, Acid Value*: NMT 2.0

Change to read:

- **FATS AND FIXED OILS** ⟨401⟩, *Procedures, Peroxide Value*: NMT ■10.0■₁ₛ (USP41)

Change to read:

- **FATS AND FIXED OILS** ⟨401⟩, *Procedures, Iodine Value*: ■160–200■₁ₛ (USP41)

Change to read:

- **FATS AND FIXED OILS** ⟨401⟩, *Procedures, Saponification Value*: 180–■195■₁ₛ (USP41)

Change to read:

- **FATS AND FIXED OILS** ⟨401⟩, *Procedures, Unsaponifiable Matter*: NMT ■1.5■₁ₛ (USP41)
- **FATS AND FIXED OILS** ⟨401⟩, *Procedures, Fatty Acid Composition*: Flax Seed Oil exhibits the composition profile of fatty acids in *Table 1*.

Table 1

Fatty Acid	Shorthand Notation	Percentage (%)
Palmitic acid	16:0	2.0–7.5
Stearic acid	18:0	1.0–6.0
Oleic acid	18:1	12.0–24.0
Linoleic acid	18:2	11.0–23.0
Alpha-linolenic acid	18:3	50.0–65.0

- **REFRACTIVE INDEX** ⟨831⟩: 1.460–1.490 at 20°

ADDITIONAL REQUIREMENTS
- **PACKAGING AND STORAGE:** Preserve in well-closed, tight, light-resistant containers.
- **LABELING:** Where Flax Seed Oil is intended for use in the manufacture of dosage forms, it is so labeled.

Delete the following:

- **USP REFERENCE STANDARDS** ⟨11⟩
  USP Flax Seed Oil RS
  - ● (CN 1-May-2018)

Add the following:

■Menaquinone-4

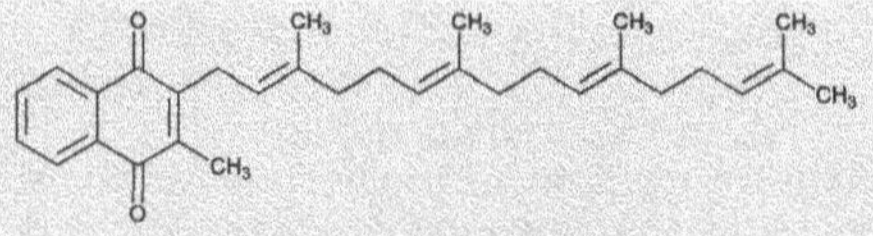

$C_{31}H_{40}O_2$ 444.65
2-Methyl-3-[(2E,6E,10E)-3,7,11,15-tetramethylhexadeca-2,6,10,14-tetraen-1-yl]naphthalene-1,4-dione;
Menatetrenone [863-61-6].

DEFINITION
Menaquinone-4 contains NLT 98.0% and NMT 102.0% of menaquinone-4 ($C_{31}H_{40}O_2$), calculated on the anhydrous basis.

IDENTIFICATION
- **A. INFRARED ABSORPTION** ⟨197A⟩
- **B.** The retention time of the major peak of the *Sample solution* corresponds to that of the *Standard solution*, as obtained in the *Assay*.

ASSAY
- **PROCEDURE**
  Mobile phase: Methanol
  [NOTE—Protect the *Standard solution* and *Sample solution* from light and inject immediately after preparation.]
  Standard solution: 0.05 mg/mL of USP Menaquinone-4 RS in isopropyl alcohol
  System suitability solution: 0.05 mg/mL of USP Phytonadione RS in *Standard solution*
  Sample stock solution: Transfer 50 mg of Menaquinone-4 to a 50-mL volumetric flask. Dissolve in isopropyl alcohol and dilute with the same solvent to volume.
  Sample solution: 0.05 mg/mL of Menaquinone-4 in isopropyl alcohol prepared from the *Sample stock solution*
  Chromatographic system
  (See *Chromatography* ⟨621⟩, *System Suitability*.)
  Mode: LC
  Detector: UV 270 nm
  Column: 4.6-mm × 15-cm; 5-µm packing L1
  Column temperature: 40°
  Flow rate: 1.0 mL/min
  Injection volume: 20 µL
  Run time: NLT 3 times the retention time of menaquinone-4
  System suitability
  Sample: *System suitability solution*
  [NOTE—The relative retention times for menaquinone-4 and phytonadione are 1.0 and 1.7, respectively.]
  Suitability requirements
  Resolution: NLT 4 between menaquinone-4 and phytonadione
  Relative standard deviation: NMT 2.0% for menaquinone-4

Analysis
Samples: *Standard solution* and *Sample solution*
Calculate the percentage of menaquinone-4 ($C_{31}H_{40}O_2$) in the portion of Menaquinone-4 taken:

$$Result = (r_U/r_S) \times (C_S/C_U) \times 100$$

r_U = peak response of menaquinone-4 from the *Sample solution*
r_S = peak response of menaquinone-4 from the *Standard solution*
C_S = concentration of USP Menaquinone-4 RS in the *Standard solution* (mg/mL)
C_U = concentration of Menaquinone-4 in the *Sample solution* (mg/mL)
Acceptance criteria: 98.0%–102.0% on the anhydrous basis

IMPURITIES
- **RESIDUE ON IGNITION ⟨281⟩:** NMT 0.1%
- **ISOMERIC PURITY**
Standard solution: 0.2 mg/mL of USP Menaquinone-4 RS in hexane
Sample solution: 10 mg/mL of Menaquinone-4 in hexane
Chromatographic system
(See *Chromatography ⟨621⟩, General Procedures, Thin-Layer Chromatography*.)
Mode: TLC
Adsorbent: 0.2- to 0.3-mm layer of chromatographic silica gel mixture
Application volume: 10 µL
Developing solvent system: Hexane and butyl ether (17:3)
Analysis
Samples: *Standard solution* and *Sample solution*
[NOTE—The relative R_F values of *cis*-menaquinone-4 and *trans*-menaquinone-4 are about 1.1 and 1.0, respectively.]
Proceed as directed in the chapter and develop the chromatogram until the solvent front has moved about 75% of the length of the plate. Dry the plate in air and examine under short-wavelength UV light.
Acceptance criteria: NMT 2.0%. Any spot corresponding to the relative R_F value of 1.1 in the *Sample solution* is neither larger nor more intense than the principal spot from the *Standard solution*.
- **ORGANIC IMPURITIES**
Mobile phase, System suitability solution, Sample stock solution, Chromatographic system, and **System suitability:** Proceed as directed in the *Assay*.
Standard solution: 1 µg/mL of USP Menaquinone-4 RS in isopropyl alcohol
Sample solution: Use the *Sample stock solution* from the *Assay*.
Analysis
Samples: *Standard solution* and *Sample solution*
Calculate the percentage of each impurity in the portion of Menaquinone-4 taken:

$$Result = (r_U/r_S) \times (C_S/C_U) \times 100$$

r_U = peak response of any impurity from the *Sample solution*
r_S = peak response of menaquinone-4 from the *Standard solution*
C_S = concentration of USP Menaquinone-4 RS in the *Standard solution* (mg/mL)
C_U = concentration of Menaquinone-4 in the *Sample solution* (mg/mL)

Acceptance criteria
Any individual impurity: NMT 0.1%
Total impurities: NMT 1.0%

SPECIFIC TESTS
- **WATER DETERMINATION ⟨921⟩,** *Method I, Method Ia:* NMT 0.5%

ADDITIONAL REQUIREMENTS
- **PACKAGING AND STORAGE:** Store in a tight container in a cool place. Protect from light.
- **USP REFERENCE STANDARDS ⟨11⟩**
USP Menaquinone-4 RS
USP Phytonadione RS

■1S *(USP41)*

Methylcobalamin

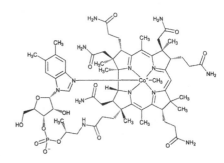

$C_{63}H_{91}CoN_{13}O_{14}P$ 1344.40
Coα-[α-5,6-dimethyl-1*H*-benzoimidazol-1-yl]-Coβ-methylcobamide [13422-55-4].

DEFINITION
Methylcobalamin contains NLT 98.0% and NMT 102.0% of methylcobalamin ($C_{63}H_{91}CoN_{13}O_{14}P$), calculated on the anhydrous basis.

IDENTIFICATION
- **A. ULTRAVIOLET ABSORPTION ⟨197U⟩**
Sample solution: 50 µg/mL in phosphate buffer, pH 7.0
[NOTE—Use low-actinic glassware, and keep the solutions from exposure to light.]
Wavelength range: 200–700 nm
Acceptance criteria: The absorption spectrum exhibits maxima at 267 ± 2 nm, 342 ± 2 nm, and 522 ± 2 nm.
- **B. COBALT**
Sample: 1 mg of Methylcobalamin
Analysis: Fuse the *Sample* with 50 mg of potassium pyrosulfate in a porcelain or silica crucible. Cool, break up the mass with a glass rod, add 3 mL of water, and boil until dissolved. Add 1 drop of phenolphthalein TS, and add 2.5 N sodium hydroxide dropwise until a pink color appears. Add 0.5 g of sodium acetate, 0.5 mL of 1 N acetic acid, and 0.5 mL of a 2-mg/mL solution of nitroso R salt. Add 0.5 mL of hydrochloric acid, and boil for 1 min.
Acceptance criteria: A red or orange-red color appears immediately after the addition of nitroso R salt. The red or orange-red color persists after boiling with the addition of hydrochloric acid.
- **C.** The retention time of the major peak of the *Sample solution* corresponds to that of the *Standard solution*, as obtained in the *Assay*.

ASSAY

Change to read:

- **PROCEDURE**
  Buffer solution: 3.1 g/L of sodium dihydrogen phosphate dihydrate in water. Adjust with phosphoric acid (1 in 100) to a pH of 3.5.
  Mobile phase: To 200 mL of acetonitrile add 800 mL of *Buffer solution*, then add 3.76 g of sodium 1-hexane sulfonate, and mix to dissolve.
  [NOTE—Use low-actinic glassware, and keep the following solutions from exposure to light.]
  System suitability solution: 0.05 mg/mL each of cyanocobalamin and hydroxocobalamin acetate from USP Cyanocobalamin RS and USP Hydroxocobalamin Acetate RS in *Mobile phase* ▪▪1S (USP41)
  Standard solution: 1 mg/mL of USP Methylcobalamin RS in *Mobile phase*
  Sample solution: 1 mg/mL of Methylcobalamin in *Mobile phase*
  Chromatographic system
  (See *Chromatography ⟨621⟩, System Suitability.*)
  Mode: LC
  Detector: UV 266 nm
  Column: 4.6-mm × 25-cm; 5-µm packing L1
  Column temperature: 40°
  Flow rate: 0.6 mL/min, or adjust to have methylcobalamin elute at about 12 min.
  Injection volume: 10 µL
  System suitability
  Samples: *System suitability solution* and *Standard solution*
  [NOTE—The relative retention times for cyanocobalamin and hydroxocobalamin are 0.8 and 1.0, respectively.]
  Suitability requirements
  Resolution: NLT 3 between the cyanocobalamin and hydroxocobalamin peaks, *System suitability solution*
  Column efficiency: NLT 6000 theoretical plates, *Standard solution*
  Relative standard deviation: NMT 2.0%, *Standard solution*
  Analysis
  Samples: *Standard solution* and *Sample solution*
  Calculate the percentage of methylcobalamin ($C_{63}H_{91}CoN_{13}O_{14}P$) in the portion of sample taken:

$$Result = (r_U/r_S) \times (C_S/C_U) \times 100$$

  r_U = peak response from the *Sample solution*
  r_S = peak response from the *Standard solution*
  C_S = concentration of USP Methylcobalamin RS in the *Standard solution* (mg/mL)
  C_U = concentration of Methylcobalamin in the *Sample solution* (mg/mL)
  Acceptance criteria: 98.0%–102.0% on the anhydrous basis

IMPURITIES

Change to read:

- **RELATED COMPOUNDS**
  Buffer solution, Mobile phase, System suitability solution, and Chromatographic system: Proceed as directed in the *Assay* ▪except for the *Run time.*▪1S (USP41)
  [NOTE—Use low-actinic glassware, and keep the following solutions from exposure to light.]
  Sample solution: 1 mg/mL of Methylcobalamin in *Mobile phase*
  Quantitative limit solution: 1 µg/mL of Methylcobalamin in *Mobile phase*, diluted from the *Sample solution*

  ▪**Run time:** NLT 2.5 times the retention time of methylcobalamin▪1S (USP41)
  System suitability
  Samples: *System suitability solution* and *Quantitative limit solution*
  Suitability requirements
  Resolution: NLT 3 between the cyanocobalamin and hydroxocobalamin peaks, *System suitability solution*
  Signal-to-noise ratio: NLT 5.0 for the major peak, *Quantitative limit solution*
  Analysis
  Sample: *Sample solution*
  ▪▪1S (USP41)
  Calculate the percentage of individual impurities in the portion of Methylcobalamin taken:

$$Result = (r_U/r_T) \times 100$$

  r_U = peak response of each impurity from the *Sample solution*
  r_T = sum of all the peak responses from the *Sample solution*
  Acceptance criteria
  Individual impurities: NMT 0.5%
  Total impurities: NMT 2.0%

SPECIFIC TESTS

- **WATER DETERMINATION ⟨921⟩,** *Method I, Method Ia:* NMT 12.0%

ADDITIONAL REQUIREMENTS

- **PACKAGING AND STORAGE:** Preserve in tight, light-resistant containers, and store at controlled room temperature.
- **USP REFERENCE STANDARDS ⟨11⟩**
  USP Cyanocobalamin RS
  USP Hydroxocobalamin Acetate RS
  USP Methylcobalamin RS

Methylcobalamin Tablets

DEFINITION
Methylcobalamin Tablets contain NLT 90.0% and NMT 125.0% of the labeled amount of methylcobalamin ($C_{63}H_{91}CoN_{13}O_{14}P$).

IDENTIFICATION
- **A.** The retention time of the major peak of the *Sample solution* corresponds to that of the *Standard solution*, as obtained in *Strength*.

STRENGTH

Change to read:

- **PROCEDURE**
  Buffer solution: 3.1 g/L of sodium dihydrogen phosphate dihydrate in water. Adjust with phosphoric acid (1 in 100) to a pH of 3.5.
  Mobile phase: Transfer 200 mL of acetonitrile to a 1-L volumetric flask and dilute with *Buffer solution* to volume. Then add 3.76 g of sodium 1-hexane sulfonate, and mix to dissolve.
  [NOTE—Use low-actinic glassware, and keep the following solutions from exposure to light.]
  System suitability solution: 0.05 mg/mL of cyanocobalamin from USP Cyanocobalamin RS and 0.05 mg/mL of USP Hydroxocobalamin Acetate RS in *Mobile phase* ▪▪1S (USP41)
  Standard solution: 100 µg/mL of USP Methylcobalamin RS in *Mobile phase*
  Sample solution: Finely powder NLT 30 Tablets. Transfer a portion of the powder, nominally equivalent to

5 mg of methylcobalamin, to a 50-mL volumetric flask, add a suitable amount of *Mobile phase*, swirl gently, and dilute with *Mobile phase* to volume. Shake vigorously for 10 min and immediately pass through a nylon membrane filter of 0.2-µm pore size.

Chromatographic system
(See *Chromatography* ⟨621⟩, *System Suitability*.)
Mode: LC
Detector: UV 266 nm
Column: 4.6-mm × 25-cm; 5-µm packing L1
Column temperature: 40°
Flow rate: 0.6 mL/min
Injection volume: 50 µL
System suitability
Samples: *System suitability solution* and *Standard solution*
[NOTE—The relative retention times for cyanocobalamin and hydroxocobalamin are 0.8 and 1.0, respectively.]
Suitability requirements
Resolution: NLT 3 between the cyanocobalamin and hydroxocobalamin peaks, *System suitability solution*
Column efficiency: NLT 6000 theoretical plates, *Standard solution*
Relative standard deviation: NMT 2.0%, *Standard solution*
Analysis
Samples: *Standard solution* and *Sample solution*
Calculate the percentage of the labeled amount of methylcobalamin ($C_{63}H_{91}CoN_{13}O_{14}P$) in the portion of Tablets taken:

$$Result = (r_U/r_S) \times (C_S/C_U) \times 100$$

r_U = peak response from the *Sample solution*
r_S = peak response from the *Standard solution*
C_S = concentration of USP Methylcobalamin RS in the *Standard solution* (µg/mL)
C_U = nominal concentration of methylcobalamin in the *Sample solution* (µg/mL)
Acceptance criteria: 90.0%–125.0%

PERFORMANCE TESTS
- **DISINTEGRATION AND DISSOLUTION ⟨2040⟩,** *Disintegration*: Meet the requirements
- **WEIGHT VARIATION ⟨2091⟩:** Meet the requirements

CONTAMINANTS
- **MICROBIAL ENUMERATION TESTS ⟨2021⟩:** The total aerobic microbial count does not exceed 3×10^3 cfu/g, and the total combined molds and yeasts count does not exceed 3×10^2 cfu/g.
- **ABSENCE OF SPECIFIED MICROORGANISMS ⟨2022⟩,** *Test Procedures, Test for Absence of Escherichia coli*: Meet the requirements

ADDITIONAL REQUIREMENTS
- **PACKAGING AND STORAGE:** Preserve in tight, light-resistant containers.
- **USP REFERENCE STANDARDS ⟨11⟩**
  USP Cyanocobalamin RS
  USP Hydroxocobalamin Acetate RS
  USP Methylcobalamin RS

Change to read:

Salix Species Bark
●**(This monograph is postponed indefinitely.)**● (RB 1-Dec-2017)

DEFINITION
Salix Species Bark is prepared from the whole or fragmented dried bark of the young branches, or whole dried pieces of the current-year twigs, obtained from *Salix* species (Fam. Salicaceae). Common in pharmacopeial use are *S. alba* L., *S. babylonica* L., *S. daphnoides* Vill., *S. fragilis* L., *S. chilensis* Molina, *S. pentandra* L., *S. purpurea* L., and a number of other complying willow species and their hybrids. It contains NLT 1.50% of total salicylate derivatives, calculated as salicin ($C_{13}H_{18}O_7$) on the dried basis.

IDENTIFICATION
- **A. HPTLC FOR ARTICLES OF BOTANICAL ORIGIN ⟨203⟩**
  Standard solution A: 1.50 mg/mL of USP Salicin RS in methanol
  Standard solution B: 30 mg/mL of USP *Salix* Species Bark Dry Extract RS in methanol. Sonicate for 10 min, centrifuge, and use the supernatant.
  Sample solution A: Suspend 1000 mg of *Salix* Species Bark, finely powdered, in 10.0 mL of methanol. Sonicate for 10 min, centrifuge, and use the supernatant.
  Sample solution B: Combine 5.0 mL of *Sample solution A* with 1.0 mL of 50-mg/mL anhydrous sodium carbonate. Cap tightly and incubate at 60° for 10 min. Centrifuge and use the supernatant.
  Chromatographic system
  Adsorbent: Chromatographic silica gel with an average particle size of 5 µm (HPTLC plate)[1]
  Application volume: 5.0 µL each of *Standard solution A*, *Standard solution B*, and *Sample solution A* and 6.0 µL of *Sample solution B* as 8-mm bands
  Relative humidity: Condition the plate to a relative humidity of 33%.
  Temperature: Ambient, not to exceed 30°
  Developing solvent system: Ethyl acetate, methanol, and water (77:13:10)
  Developing distance: 6 cm
  Derivatization reagent: Sulfuric acid and methanol (1:9). Slowly add sulfuric acid to ice-cold methanol.
  Analysis
  Samples: *Standard solution A, Standard solution B, Sample solution A,* and *Sample solution B*
  Apply the *Samples* as bands and dry in air. Develop in a saturated chamber, and dry in a current of air for 5 min. Treat with *Derivatization reagent*, heat at 100° for 5 min, and examine under white light.
  System suitability: Under white light, the derivatized chromatogram of *Standard solution B* displays, in the middle third of the plate, three brown bands: the lower corresponds to the salicin band in *Standard solution A*; the one above it is due to salicortin; the top band is due to tremulacin. A faint band, which may appear between the salicortin and tremulacin bands, is due to tremuloidin. Two darker brown bands are seen in the lower third of the plate: one proximate to the application line; another, more intense, above it.
  Acceptance criteria: Under white light, the derivatized chromatogram of *Sample solution A* shows one or several dark bands due to different salicin esters, whose position and intensity are contingent on the *Salix* species being used. The salicylate bands of interest are predominantly located in the middle third of the plate, demarcated by the salicin and tremulacin bands of *Standard solution B*. The salicin band in *Sample solution A*, corresponding to that in *Standard solution A*, may be faint or not visible. Additional bands may be seen in *Sample solution A* and *Sample solution B*. In *Sample solution B*, the bands due to salicin esters are not present, while the salicin band corresponding to that in *Standard solution A* is the principal band observed. The salicin band in *Sample solution A* is of lower intensity than the corresponding band in *Standard solution A*. The salicin band in *Sample solution B* is of comparable or higher intensity than the corresponding band in *Standard solution A*.

---

[1] A suitable commercially available plate is HPTLC Silica Gel 60 F_{254} from EMD Millipore (e.g., Part No. 1.05642.0001).

- **B. HPLC**
  Analysis: Proceed as directed in the test for *Salicylates Profile*.
  Acceptance criteria: The *Sample solution* exhibits peaks at retention times corresponding to those of salicin and salicin derivatives in the *Standard solution*.

COMPOSITION
- **CONTENT OF SALICIN**
  Diluent: Methanol and water (1:1)
  Solution A: 0.01% trifluoroacetic acid
  Solution B: Acetonitrile
  Mobile phase: See *Table 1*.

Table 1

Time (min)	Solution A (%)	Solution B (%)
0	90	10
10	85	15
30	50	50
32	10	90
35	10	90
37	90	10
45	90	10

Standard solution: 0.50 mg/mL of USP Salicin RS in *Diluent*
Sample solution: Reduce to a fine powder and accurately weigh about 1.3 g of *Salix* Species Bark, transfer to a 200-mL round-bottom flask, and add 40 mL of methanol and 3 mL of 1 N sodium hydroxide. Attach the condenser and heat under reflux for 2 h, with intermittent shaking. Allow to cool, neutralize with 3 mL of 1 N hydrochloric acid, and pass through a paper filter into a 100-mL volumetric flask. Wash the round-bottom flask twice with 5-mL aliquots of methanol and filter into the same 100-mL volumetric flask. Adjust with water to volume, mix well, allow to equilibrate to room temperature, and readjust with water. Pass through a PTFE filter of 0.45-μm pore size, discarding the initial 3 mL of the filtrate.
Chromatographic system
(See *Chromatography* ⟨621⟩, *System Suitability*.)
Mode: LC
Detector: UV 270 nm
Column: 4.6-mm × 25-cm; 5-μm base-deactivated packing L1
Column temperature: 30°
Flow rate: 1.0 mL/min
Injection volume: 10 μL
System suitability
Sample: *Standard solution*
Suitability requirements
Tailing factor: 0.8–2.0 for the salicin peak
Relative standard deviation: NMT 2.0% for the salicin peak in replicate injections
Analysis
Samples: *Standard solution* and *Sample solution*
Using the chromatogram of the *Standard solution*, identify the salicin peak in the *Sample solution* chromatogram.
Calculate the percentage of salicin hydrolytically derived from constituent salicylates in the portion of *Salix* Species Bark taken:

$$Result = (r_U/r_S) \times C_S \times (V/W) \times 100$$

r_U = peak area of salicin from the *Sample solution*
r_S = peak area of salicin from the *Standard solution*
C_S = concentration of USP Salicin RS in the *Standard solution* (mg/mL)
V = volume of the *Sample solution* (mL)
W = weight of *Salix* Species Bark taken to prepare the *Sample solution* (mg)
Acceptance criteria: NLT 1.50% of salicin on the dried basis

CONTAMINANTS
- **ARTICLES OF BOTANICAL ORIGIN** ⟨561⟩, *Limits of Elemental Impurities*: Meets the requirements
- **ARTICLES OF BOTANICAL ORIGIN** ⟨561⟩, *Pesticide Residue Analysis*: Meets the requirements
- **MICROBIAL ENUMERATION TESTS** ⟨2021⟩: The total aerobic bacterial count does not exceed 10^5 cfu/g, the total combined yeasts and molds count does not exceed 10^3 cfu/g, and the bile-tolerant Gram-negative bacteria count does not exceed 10^3 cfu/g.
- **ABSENCE OF SPECIFIED MICROORGANISMS** ⟨2022⟩, *Test Procedures, Test for Absence of Salmonella Species* and *Test for Absence of Escherichia coli*: Meets the requirements

SPECIFIC TESTS
- **SALICYLATES PROFILE**
  Diluent, Mobile phase, and **Chromatographic system:** Proceed as directed in the test for *Content of Salicin*.
  Standard solution: 5 mg/mL of USP *Salix* Species Bark Dry Extract RS in *Diluent*. Sonicate for 5 min, mix well, and pass through a PTFE filter of 0.45-μm pore size, discarding the initial 3 mL of the filtrate.
  Sample solution: Reduce to fine powder and accurately weigh about 650 mg of *Salix* Species Bark, transfer to a 50-mL volumetric flask, add 25 mL of methanol, and sonicate for 30 min. Adjust with water to volume, mix well, allow to equilibrate to room temperature, and readjust with water. Pass through a PTFE filter of 0.45-μm pore size, discarding the initial 3 mL of the filtrate.
  System suitability
  Suitability requirements: The chromatogram of the *Standard solution* is similar to the reference chromatogram provided with the lot of USP *Salix* Species Bark Dry Extract RS being used.
  Analysis
  Samples: *Standard solution* and *Sample solution*
  Using the chromatogram of the *Standard solution* and the reference chromatogram provided with the lot of USP *Salix* Species Bark Dry Extract RS being used, identify salicin esters present in the *Sample solution* chromatogram. The approximate relative retention times, with respect to salicin, are provided in *Table 2*.

Table 2

Analyte	Relative Retention Time
Salicin	1.0
Salicortin	3.0
Tremuloidin	3.6
Tremulacin	4.6

  Acceptance criteria: The peak area of salicin is NMT 50% of the combined peak areas of all identified constituent salicylates.
- **BOTANICAL CHARACTERISTICS**
  Macroscopic: The bark is 1–2 cm wide and 1–2 mm thick, and occurs in flexible, elongated, quilled or curved pieces. The outer surface is glossy, smooth or slightly wrinkled longitudinally; greenish yellow in the younger bark to brownish grey in the older bark. The inner surface is smooth or finely striated longitudinally and white, pale yellow or reddish brown, depending on the species. The fracture is short in the outer part and coarsely fibrous in the inner region, and is easily split longitudinally. The diameter of current year twigs is NMT 10 mm. The xylem of young twigs is white or pale yellow.

Microscopic: Two or three rows of poorly developed cork cells with thickened outer walls; cortex of collenchymatous and parenchymatous cells. The latter contains cluster crystals of calcium oxalate, 20–25 μm in diameter, and occasionally tannin. Phloem is characterized by tangential groups of lignified fibers associated with a crystal sheath containing prismatic crystals of calcium oxalate. Simple, rounded starch granules 6–8 μm in diameter in the parenchymatous cells of the phloem and medullary rays.

- **ARTICLES OF BOTANICAL ORIGIN ⟨561⟩,** *Methods of Analysis, Foreign Organic Matter:* NMT 3.0% of twigs with a diameter greater than 10 mm, and NMT 2.0% of other foreign matter
- **LOSS ON DRYING ⟨731⟩**
  Sample: 1.0 g of *Salix* Species Bark, finely powdered
  Analysis: Dry the *Sample* at 105° for 2 h.
  Acceptance criteria: NMT 10.0%
- **ARTICLES OF BOTANICAL ORIGIN ⟨561⟩,** *Methods of Analysis, Total Ash*
  Sample: 2.0 g of *Salix* Species Bark, finely powdered
  Acceptance criteria: NMT 10.0%
- **ARTICLES OF BOTANICAL ORIGIN ⟨561⟩,** *Methods of Analysis, Acid-Insoluble Ash*
  Sample: 2.0 g of *Salix* Species Bark, finely powdered
  Acceptance criteria: NMT 3.0%
- **ARTICLES OF BOTANICAL ORIGIN ⟨561⟩,** *Methods of Analysis, Water-Soluble Extractives*
  Sample: 2.0 g of *Salix* Species Bark, finely powdered
  Acceptance criteria: NLT 10.0%

ADDITIONAL REQUIREMENTS
- **PACKAGING AND STORAGE:** Preserve in well-closed containers, protected from light and moisture, and store at room temperature.
- **LABELING:** The label states the Latin binomial(s) of one or several *Salix* species included in the article.
- **USP REFERENCE STANDARDS ⟨11⟩**
  USP Salicin RS
  USP *Salix* Species Bark Dry Extract RS
  •(This monograph is postponed indefinitely.)• (RB 1-Dec-2017)

Change to read:

Salix Species Bark Dry Extract
•(This monograph is postponed indefinitely.)• (RB 1-Dec-2017)

DEFINITION
Salix Species Bark Dry Extract is prepared from *Salix* Species Bark by extraction with hydroalcoholic, aqueous, or other suitable solvents. It contains NLT 90.0% and NMT 110.0% of the labeled amount of salicylates, calculated as salicin ($C_{13}H_{18}O_7$) on the anhydrous basis. The ratio of starting plant material to extract is between 5:1 and 20:1. It may contain suitable added substances.

IDENTIFICATION
- **A. HPTLC FOR ARTICLES OF BOTANICAL ORIGIN ⟨203⟩**
  Standard solution A: 1.50 mg/mL of USP Salicin RS in methanol
  Standard solution B: 30 mg/mL of USP *Salix* Species Bark Dry Extract RS in methanol. Sonicate for 10 min, centrifuge, and use the supernatant.
  Sample solution A: Suspend the amount of *Salix* Species Bark Dry Extract calculated to contain 15 mg of salicin (post-hydrolysis) in 10.0 mL of methanol. Sonicate for 10 min, centrifuge, and use the supernatant.
  Sample solution B: Combine 5.0 mL of *Sample solution A* with 1.0 mL of 50-mg/mL anhydrous sodium carbon-

ate. Cap tightly and incubate at 60° for 10 min. Centrifuge and use the supernatant.
  Chromatographic system
  Adsorbent: Chromatographic silica gel with an average particle size of 5 μm (HPTLC plate)[1]
  Application volume: 5.0 μL each of *Standard solution A*, *Standard solution B*, and *Sample solution A* and 6.0 μL of *Sample solution B* as 8-mm bands
  Relative humidity: Condition the plate to a relative humidity of 33%.
  Temperature: Ambient, not to exceed 30°
  Developing solvent system: Ethyl acetate, methanol, and water (77:13:10)
  Developing distance: 6 cm
  Derivatization reagent: Sulfuric acid and methanol (1:9). Slowly add sulfuric acid to ice-cold methanol.
  Analysis
  Samples: *Standard solution A*, *Standard solution B*, *Sample solution A*, and *Sample solution B*
  Apply the *Samples* as bands and dry in air. Develop in a saturated chamber, and dry in a current of air for 5 min. Treat with *Derivatization reagent*, heat at 100° for 5 min, and examine under white light.
  System suitability: Under white light, the derivatized chromatogram of *Standard solution B* displays, in the middle third of the plate, three brown bands: the lower corresponds to the salicin band in *Standard solution A*; the one above it is due to salicortin; the top band is due to tremulacin. A faint band, which may appear between the salicortin and tremulacin bands, is due to tremuloidin. Two darker brown bands are seen in the lower third of the plate: one proximate to the application line; another, more intense, above it.
  Acceptance criteria: Under white light, the derivatized chromatogram of *Sample solution A* shows one or several dark bands due to different salicin esters, whose position and intensity are contingent on the *Salix* species being used. The salicylate bands of interest are predominantly located in the middle third of the plate, demarcated by the salicin and tremulacin bands of *Standard solution B*. The salicin band in *Sample solution A*, corresponding to that in *Standard solution A*, may be faint or not visible. Additional bands may be seen in *Sample solution A* and *Sample solution B*. In *Sample solution B*, the bands due to salicin esters are not present, while the salicin band corresponding to that in *Standard solution A* is the principal band observed. The salicin band in *Sample solution A* is of lower intensity than the corresponding band in *Standard solution A*. The salicin band in *Sample solution B* is of comparable or higher intensity than the corresponding band in *Standard solution A*.
- **B. HPLC**
  Analysis: Proceed as directed in the test for *Salicylates Profile and Limit of Free Salicin.*
  Acceptance criteria: The *Sample solution* exhibits peaks at retention times corresponding to those of salicin and salicin derivatives in the *Standard solution.*

COMPOSITION
- **CONTENT OF SALICIN**
  Diluent: Methanol and water (1:1)
  Solution A: 0.01% trifluoroacetic acid
  Solution B: Acetonitrile
  Mobile phase: See *Table 1.*

Table 1

Time (min)	Solution A (%)	Solution B (%)
0	90	10
10	85	15

[1] A suitable commercially available plate is HPTLC Silica Gel 60 F₂₅₄ from EMD Millipore (e.g., Part No. 1.05642.0001).

Table 1 (Continued)

Time (min)	Solution A (%)	Solution B (%)
30	50	50
32	10	90
35	10	90
37	90	10
45	90	10

Standard solution: 0.50 mg/mL of USP Salicin RS in *Diluent*

Sample solution: Accurately weigh the amount of *Salix* Species Bark Dry Extract calculated to contain about 30 mg of salicin, transfer to a 200-mL round-bottom flask, and add 40 mL of methanol and 3 mL of 1 N sodium hydroxide. Attach the condenser and heat under reflux for 2 h, with intermittent shaking. Allow to cool, neutralize with 3 mL of 1 N hydrochloric acid, and pass through a paper filter into a 100-mL volumetric flask. Wash the round-bottom flask twice with 5-mL aliquots of methanol and filter into the same 100-mL volumetric flask. Adjust with water to volume, mix well, allow to equilibrate to room temperature, and readjust with water. Pass through a PTFE filter of 0.45-µm pore size, discarding the initial 3 mL of the filtrate.

Chromatographic system
(See *Chromatography* ⟨621⟩, *System Suitability*.)
Mode: LC
Detector: UV 270 nm
Column: 4.6-mm × 25-cm; 5-µm base-deactivated packing L1
Column temperature: 30°
Flow rate: 1.0 mL/min
Injection volume: 10 µL
System suitability
Sample: *Standard solution*
Suitability requirements
Tailing factor: 0.8–2.0 for the salicin peak
Relative standard deviation: NMT 2.0% for the salicin peak in replicate injections
Analysis
Samples: *Standard solution* and *Sample solution*
Using the chromatogram of the *Standard solution*, identify the salicin peak in the *Sample solution* chromatogram.
Calculate the percentage of salicin hydrolytically derived from constituent salicylates in the portion of *Salix* Species Bark Dry Extract taken:

$$Result = (r_U/r_S) \times C_S \times (V/W) \times 100$$

r_U = peak area of salicin from the *Sample solution*
r_S = peak area of salicin from the *Standard solution*
C_S = concentration of USP Salicin RS in the *Standard solution* (mg/mL)
V = volume of the *Sample solution* (mL)
W = weight of *Salix* Species Bark Dry Extract taken to prepare the *Sample solution* (mg)

Calculate the percentage of the labeled content of salicin in the portion of *Salix* Species Bark Dry Extract taken:

$$Result = (P/L) \times 100$$

P = percentage of salicylates as determined above
L = labeled content of salicin

Acceptance criteria: 90.0%–110.0% of the labeled amount of salicylates calculated as salicin on the anhydrous basis

CONTAMINANTS
• **ARTICLES OF BOTANICAL ORIGIN** ⟨561⟩, *Pesticide Residue Analysis*: Meets the requirements

• **BOTANICAL EXTRACTS** ⟨565⟩, *Preparations*, *General Pharmacopeial Requirements*, *Residual Solvents*: Meets the requirements
• **MICROBIAL ENUMERATION TESTS** ⟨2021⟩: The total aerobic bacterial count does not exceed 10^4 cfu/g, and total combined yeasts and molds count does not exceed 10^3 cfu/g.
• **ABSENCE OF SPECIFIED MICROORGANISMS** ⟨2022⟩, *Test Procedures*, *Test for Absence of Salmonella Species* and *Test for Absence of Escherichia coli*: Meets the requirements

SPECIFIC TESTS
• **SALICYLATES PROFILE AND LIMIT OF FREE SALICIN**[2]
Diluent, Mobile phase, and **Chromatographic system:** Proceed as directed in the test for *Content of Salicin*.
Standard solution: 5 mg/mL of USP *Salix* Species Bark Dry Extract RS in *Diluent*. Sonicate for 5 min, mix well, and pass through a PTFE filter of 0.45-µm pore size, discarding the initial 3 mL of the filtrate.
Sample solution: Weigh the amount of *Salix* Species Bark Dry Extract calculated to contain about 15 mg of salicin, transfer to a 50-mL volumetric flask, add 25 mL of methanol, and sonicate for 5 min. Adjust with water to volume, mix well, allow to equilibrate to room temperature, and readjust with water. Pass through a PTFE filter of 0.45-µm pore size, discarding the initial 3 mL of the filtrate.
System suitability
Suitability requirements: The chromatogram of the *Standard solution* is similar to the reference chromatogram provided with the lot of USP *Salix* Species Bark Dry Extract RS being used.
Analysis
Samples: *Standard solution* and *Sample solution*
Using the chromatogram of the *Standard solution* and the reference chromatogram provided with the lot of USP *Salix* Species Bark Dry Extract RS being used, identify salicin esters present in the *Sample solution* chromatogram. The approximate relative retention times, with respect to salicin, are provided in *Table 2*.

Table 2

Analyte	Relative Retention Time
Salicin	1.0
Salicortin	3.0
Tremuloidin	3.6
Tremulacin	4.6

Acceptance criteria: The peak area of salicin is NMT 50% of the combined peak areas of all identified constituent salicylates.
• **WATER DETERMINATION** ⟨921⟩, *Method I, Method Ia*: NMT 5.0%
• **ARTICLES OF BOTANICAL ORIGIN** ⟨561⟩, *Methods of Analysis, Total Ash*
Sample: 2.0 g of *Salix* Species Bark Dry Extract
Acceptance criteria: NMT 5.0%

ADDITIONAL REQUIREMENTS
• **PACKAGING AND STORAGE:** Preserve in well-closed containers, protected from light and moisture, and store at room temperature.
• **LABELING:** The label states the Latin binomial(s) of one or several *Salix* species from which the article was prepared. The label also indicates the content of salicin, the solvent used in extract preparation, and the ratio of the starting crude plant material to dry extract. It meets the labeling requirements of *Botanical Extracts* ⟨565⟩.

---

[2] Elevated free salicin content may indicate prehydrolysis or fortification with extraneous salicin.

- **USP REFERENCE STANDARDS ⟨11⟩**
  USP Salicin RS
  USP *Salix* Species Bark Dry Extract RS
  •(This monograph is postponed indefinitely.)• (RB 1-Dec-2017)

Change to read:

Salix Species Bark Powder
•(This monograph is postponed indefinitely.)• (RB 1-Dec-2017)

DEFINITION
Salix Species Bark Powder consists of *Salix* Species Bark reduced to fine or very fine powder. It contains NLT 1.50% of total salicylate derivatives, calculated as salicin ($C_{13}H_{18}O_7$) on the dried basis. *Salix* Species Bark Powder contains NMT 1.50% of free salicin, calculated on the dried basis.

IDENTIFICATION
- **A. HPTLC FOR ARTICLES OF BOTANICAL ORIGIN ⟨203⟩**
  Standard solution A: 1.50 mg/mL of USP Salicin RS in methanol
  Standard solution B: 30 mg/mL of USP *Salix* Species Bark Dry Extract RS in methanol. Sonicate for 10 min, centrifuge, and use the supernatant.
  Sample solution A: Suspend 1000 mg of *Salix* Species Bark Powder in 10.0 mL of methanol. Sonicate for 10 min, centrifuge, and use the supernatant.
  Sample solution B: Combine 5.0 mL of *Sample solution A* with 1.0 mL of 50-mg/mL anhydrous sodium carbonate. Cap tightly and incubate at 60° for 10 min. Centrifuge and use the supernatant.
  Chromatographic system
  Adsorbent: Chromatographic silica gel with an average particle size of 5 μm (HPTLC plate)[1]
  Application volume: 5.0 μL each of *Standard solution A*, *Standard solution B*, and *Sample solution A* and 6.0 μL of *Sample solution B* as 8-mm bands
  Relative humidity: Condition the plate to a relative humidity of 33%.
  Temperature: Ambient, not to exceed 30°
  Developing solvent system: Ethyl acetate, methanol, and water (77:13:10)
  Developing distance: 6 cm
  Derivatization reagent: Sulfuric acid and methanol (1:9). Slowly add sulfuric acid to ice-cold methanol.
  Analysis
  Samples: *Standard solution A*, *Standard solution B*, *Sample solution A*, and *Sample solution B*
  Apply the *Samples* as bands and dry in air. Develop in a saturated chamber, and dry in a current of air for 5 min. Treat with *Derivatization reagent*, heat at 100° for 5 min, and examine under white light.
  System suitability: Under white light, the derivatized chromatogram of *Standard solution B* displays, in the middle third of the plate, three brown bands: the lower corresponds to the salicin band in *Standard solution A*; the one above it is due to salicortin; the top band is due to tremulacin. A faint band, which may appear between the salicortin and tremulacin bands, is due to tremuloidin. Two darker brown bands are seen in the lower third of the plate: one proximate to the application line; another, more intense, above it.
  Acceptance criteria: Under white light, the derivatized chromatogram of *Sample solution A* shows one or several dark bands due to different salicin esters, whose position and intensity are contingent on the *Salix* species being used. The salicylate bands of interest are predominantly located in the middle third of the plate, demarcated by the salicin and tremulacin bands of *Standard solution B*. The salicin band in *Sample solution A*, corresponding to that in *Standard solution A*, may be faint or not visible. Additional bands may be seen in *Sample solution A* and *Sample solution B*. In *Sample solution B*, the bands due to salicin esters are not present, while the salicin band corresponding to that in *Standard solution A* is the principal band observed. The salicin band in *Sample solution A* is of lower intensity than the corresponding band in *Standard solution A*. The salicin band in *Sample solution B* is of comparable or higher intensity than the corresponding band in *Standard solution A*.

- **B. HPLC**
  Analysis: Proceed as directed in the test for *Salicylates Profile and Limit of Free Salicin*.
  Acceptance criteria: The *Sample solution* exhibits peaks at retention times corresponding to those of salicin and salicin derivatives in the Standard solutions.

COMPOSITION
- **CONTENT OF SALICIN**
  Diluent: Methanol and water (1:1)
  Solution A: 0.01% trifluoroacetic acid
  Solution B: Acetonitrile
  Mobile phase: See *Table 1*.

Table 1

Time (min)	Solution A (%)	Solution B (%)
0	90	10
10	85	15
30	50	50
32	10	90
35	10	90
37	90	10
45	90	10

  Standard solution A: 0.50 mg/mL of USP Salicin RS in *Diluent*
  Sample solution: Accurately weigh about 1.3 g of *Salix* Species Bark Powder, transfer to a 200-mL round-bottom flask, and add 40 mL of methanol and 3 mL of 1 N sodium hydroxide. Attach the condenser and heat under reflux for 2 h, with intermittent shaking. Allow to cool, neutralize with 3 mL of 1 N hydrochloric acid, and pass through a paper filter into a 100-mL volumetric flask. Wash the round-bottom flask twice with 5-mL aliquots of methanol and filter into the same 100-mL volumetric flask. Adjust with water to volume, mix well, allow to equilibrate to room temperature, and readjust with water. Pass through a PTFE filter of 0.45-μm pore size, discarding the initial 3 mL of the filtrate.
  Chromatographic system
  (See *Chromatography ⟨621⟩, System Suitability*.)
  Mode: LC
  Detector: UV 270 nm
  Column: 4.6-mm × 25-cm; 5-μm base-deactivated packing L1
  Column temperature: 30°
  Flow rate: 1.0 mL/min
  Injection volume: 10 μL
  System suitability
  Sample: *Standard solution A*
  Suitability requirements
  Tailing factor: 0.8–2.0 for the salicin peak
  Relative standard deviation: NMT 2.0% for the salicin peak in replicate injections

[1] A suitable commercially available plate is HPTLC Silica Gel 60 F$_{254}$ from EMD Millipore (e.g., Part No. 1.05642.0001).

Analysis
  Samples: *Standard solution A* and *Sample solution*
  Using the chromatogram of the *Standard solution* A, identify the salicin peak in the *Sample solution* chromatogram.
  Calculate the percentage of salicin hydrolytically derived from constituent salicylates in the portion of *Salix* Species Bark Powder taken:

$$Result = (r_U/r_S) \times C_S \times (V/W) \times 100$$

r_U = peak area of salicin from the *Sample solution*
r_S = peak area of salicin from the *Standard solution* A
C_S = concentration of USP Salicin RS in the *Standard solution A* (mg/mL)
V = volume of the *Sample solution* (mL)
W = weight of *Salix* Species Bark Powder taken to prepare the *Sample solution* (mg)
  Acceptance criteria: NLT 1.50% of salicin on the dried basis

CONTAMINANTS

- **ARTICLES OF BOTANICAL ORIGIN ⟨561⟩**, *Limits of Elemental Impurities*: Meets the requirements
- **ARTICLES OF BOTANICAL ORIGIN ⟨561⟩**, *Pesticide Residue Analysis*: Meets the requirements
- **MICROBIAL ENUMERATION TESTS ⟨2021⟩**: The total aerobic bacterial count does not exceed 10^5 cfu/g, the total combined yeasts and molds count does not exceed 10^3 cfu/g, and the bile-tolerant Gram-negative bacteria count does not exceed 10^3 cfu/g.
- **ABSENCE OF SPECIFIED MICROORGANISMS ⟨2022⟩**, *Test Procedures, Test for Absence of Salmonella Species* and *Test for Absence of Escherichia coli*: Meets the requirements

SPECIFIC TESTS

- **SALICYLATES PROFILE AND LIMIT OF FREE SALICIN[2]**
  Diluent, Mobile phase, Standard solution A, and **Chromatographic system:** Proceed as directed in the test for *Content of Salicin*.
  Standard solution B: 5 mg/mL of USP *Salix* Species Bark Dry Extract RS in *Diluent*. Sonicate for 5 min, mix well, and pass through a PTFE filter of 0.45-μm pore size, discarding the initial 3 mL of the filtrate.
  Sample solution: Accurately weigh about 650 mg of *Salix* Species Bark Powder, transfer to a 50-mL volumetric flask, add 25 mL of methanol, and sonicate for 30 min. Adjust with water to volume, mix well, allow to equilibrate to room temperature, and readjust with water. Pass through a PTFE filter of 0.45-μm pore size, discarding the initial 3 mL of the filtrate.
  System suitability
  Samples: *Standard solution A* and *Standard solution B*
  Suitability requirements
    Tailing factor: 0.8–2.0 for the salicin peak, *Standard solution A*
    Relative standard deviation: NMT 2.0% determined for the salicin peak in replicate injections, *Standard solution A*
    Chromatographic similarity: The chromatogram is similar to the reference chromatogram provided with the lot of USP *Salix* Species Bark Dry Extract RS being used, *Standard solution B*.
  Analysis
  Samples: *Standard solution A, Standard solution B,* and *Sample solution*
  Using the chromatograms of *Standard solution A, Standard solution B,* and the reference chromatogram provided with the lot of USP *Salix* Species Bark Dry Extract RS being used, identify salicin esters present in the *Sample solution* chromatogram. The approximate relative retention times, with respect to salicin, are provided in *Table 2*.

Table 2

Analyte	Relative Retention Time
Salicin	1.0
Salicortin	3.0
Tremuloidin	3.6
Tremulacin	4.6

Calculate the percentage of salicin in the portion of *Salix* Species Bark Powder taken:

$$Result = (r_U/r_S) \times C_S \times (V/W) \times 100$$

r_U = peak area of salicin from the *Sample solution*
r_S = peak area of salicin from *Standard solution A*
C_S = concentration of USP Salicin RS in *Standard solution A* (mg/mL)
V = volume of the *Sample solution* (mL)
W = weight of *Salix* Species Bark Powder taken to prepare the *Sample solution* (mg)
  Acceptance criteria: NMT 1.50% of salicin on the dried basis. The peak area of salicin is NMT 50% of the combined peak areas of all identified constituent salicylates.

- **BOTANICAL CHARACTERISTICS**
  Macroscopic: Pale yellow, greenish-yellow, or light brown powder
  Microscopic: Bundles of narrow fibers, up to about 600 μm long, with very thick walls, lignified, and surrounded by a crystal sheath containing prism crystals of calcium oxalate; parenchyma of the cortex with thick, pitted and deeply beaded walls, and containing large cluster crystals of calcium oxalate; uniseriate medullary rays; thickened and suberized cork cells. Groups of brownish collenchyma from the bud may be present. Twigs show fragments of lignified fibers and vessels from the xylem.

- **LOSS ON DRYING ⟨731⟩**
  Sample: 1.0 g of *Salix* Species Bark Powder
  Analysis: Dry the *Sample* at 105° for 2 h.
  Acceptance criteria: NMT 10.0%

- **ARTICLES OF BOTANICAL ORIGIN ⟨561⟩**, *Methods of Analysis, Total Ash*
  Sample: 2.0 g of *Salix* Species Bark Powder
  Acceptance criteria: NMT 10.0%

- **ARTICLES OF BOTANICAL ORIGIN ⟨561⟩**, *Methods of Analysis, Acid-Insoluble Ash*
  Sample: 2.0 g of *Salix* Species Bark Powder
  Acceptance criteria: NMT 3.0%

- **ARTICLES OF BOTANICAL ORIGIN ⟨561⟩**, *Methods of Analysis, Water-Soluble Extractives*
  Sample: 2.0 g of *Salix* Species Bark Powder
  Acceptance criteria: NLT 10.0%

ADDITIONAL REQUIREMENTS

- **PACKAGING AND STORAGE:** Preserve in well-closed containers, protected from light and moisture, and store at room temperature.
- **LABELING:** The label states the Latin binomial(s) of one or several *Salix* species included in the article.
- **USP REFERENCE STANDARDS ⟨11⟩**
  USP Salicin RS
  USP *Salix* Species Bark Dry Extract RS
  ●(This monograph is postponed indefinitely.)● (RB 1-Dec-2017)

---

[2] Elevated free salicin content may indicate prehydrolysis or fortification with extraneous salicin.

Add the following:

▪Valerian Root Dry Extract Capsules

DEFINITION

Valerian Root Dry Extract Capsules contain dry extract derived from the subterranean parts of *Valeriana officinalis* L. (Fam. Caprifoliaceae, formerly Valerianaceae) including rhizome, root, and stolon. They contain NLT 90% and NMT 120% of the labeled amount of valerenic acids calculated as the sum of hydroxyvalerenic acid ($C_{15}H_{22}O_3$), acetoxyvalerenic acid ($C_{17}H_{24}O_4$), and valerenic acid ($C_{15}H_{22}O_2$).

IDENTIFICATION

- **A. HPTLC FOR ARTICLES OF BOTANICAL ORIGIN ⟨203⟩**
  Standard solution A: 0.25 mg/mL of USP Valerenic Acid RS in methanol
  Standard solution B: 40 mg/mL of USP Powdered Valerian Extract RS in methanol. Sonicate for 10 min, centrifuge, and use the supernatant.
  Sample solution: Transfer a portion of the Capsule contents, equivalent to 400 mg of valerian root dry extract, to a conical flask, add 10 mL of methanol, mix and sonicate for 20 min, centrifuge, and use the supernatant.
  Chromatographic system
  Adsorbent: Chromatographic silica gel mixture with an average particle size of 5 µm (HPTLC plates)
  Application volume: 5 µL, as 8-mm bands
  Relative humidity: Condition the plate to a relative humidity of 33%.
  Temperature: Ambient, not to exceed 30°
  Developing solvent system: Cyclohexane, ethyl acetate, and glacial acetic acid (60:38:2)
  Developing distance: 6 cm
  Derivatization reagent A: Glacial acetic acid and hydrochloric acid (1:4)
  Derivatization reagent B: 0.5 mL of *p*-anisaldehyde, 10 mL of glacial acetic acid, and 5 mL of sulfuric acid. Add to 85 mL of ice-cold methanol, and mix.
  Analysis
  Samples: *Standard solution A, Standard solution B,* and *Sample solution*
  Apply the *Samples* as bands, and dry in air. Develop in a saturated chamber, remove the plate from the chamber, and dry in air. Treat the plate with *Derivatization reagent A,* heat at 120° for 5 min, and examine under white light. Then treat with *Derivatization reagent B,* heat at 100° for 3 min, and examine under white light.
  System suitability: After treatment with *Derivatization reagent A* and heating, *Standard solution A* and *Standard solution B* do not exhibit an intense blue band at about the middle of the chromatogram nor any other significant bands. After treatment with *Derivatization reagent B* and heating, *Standard solution A* exhibits a violet band due to valerenic acid, while *Standard solution B* exhibits a band corresponding in R_F and color to that of valerenic acid in *Standard solution A* as well as a violet band below valerenic acid at about middle of the chromatogram due to acetoxyvalerenic acid and a minor violet band in the lower third of the chromatogram due to hydroxyvalerenic acid.
  Acceptance criteria: After treatment with *Derivatization reagent A* and heating, the *Sample solution* does not exhibit an intense blue band at about the middle of the chromatogram nor any other significant bands [distinction from Mexican valerian (*Valeriana edulis*)], though minor bands may be observed. After treatment with *Derivatization reagent B* and heating, the *Sample solution* exhibits three violet bands in positions and colors similar to those in *Standard solution B*. These bands include a band corresponding in R_F to valerenic acid in *Standard solution A* and *Standard solution B*, a band below valerenic acid at about the middle of the chromatogram due to acetoxyvalerenic acid [distinction from Scouler's valerian (*Valeriana wallichii*)], and a minor violet band in the lower third of the chromatogram due to hydroxyvalerenic acid. Other faint bands may be observed.
- **B. HPLC**
  Analysis: Proceed as directed in the test for *Content of Valerenic Acids.*
  Acceptance criteria: The *Sample solution* exhibits a peak at a retention time corresponding to valerenic acid in *Standard solution A.* The *Sample solution* shows additional peaks corresponding to hydroxyvalerenic acid and acetoxyvalerenic acid.

STRENGTH

- **CONTENT OF VALERENIC ACIDS**
  Extraction solvent: Methanol and a solution of 0.1% phosphoric acid in water (3:1)
  Solution A: Mix 6 mL of 85% phosphoric acid with 900 mL of water, dilute with water to 1000 mL, mix, filter, and degas.
  Solution B: Mix 6 mL of 85% phosphoric acid with 900 mL of methanol, dilute with methanol to 1000 mL, mix, filter, and degas.
  Mobile phase: See *Table 1.*

Table 1

Time (min)	Solution A (%)	Solution B (%)
0	40	60
15	5	95
25	5	95
30	40	60

  Standard solution A: 0.05 mg/mL of USP Valerenic Acid RS in methanol. Sonicate if necessary.
  Standard solution B: Sonicate a portion of USP Powdered Valerian Extract RS in *Extraction solvent* to obtain a solution with a concentration of about 20 mg/mL. Before injection, pass through a membrane filter of 0.45-µm or finer pore size.
  Sample solution: Determine the total weight of 20 Capsules. Empty the Capsules and combine their contents in an appropriate container. Weigh the empty Capsule shells and calculate the average fill weight per Capsule. Transfer a portion of the Capsule contents, equivalent to about 3.0 mg of valerenic acids, to a 25-mL volumetric flask. Add 20 mL of *Extraction solvent* and sonicate for 30 min with occasional shaking. Cool to room temperature, dilute with *Extraction solvent* to volume, mix well, and centrifuge. Pass through a membrane filter of 0.45-µm or finer pore size, discarding the first few milliliters of the filtrate.
  Chromatographic system
  (See *Chromatography* ⟨621⟩, *System Suitability.*)
  Mode: LC
  Detector: UV 225 nm
  Column: 4.6-mm × 25-cm; end-capped, 5-µm, 100-Å packing L1
  Column temperature: 40°
  Flow rate: 1.0 mL/min
  Injection volume: 25 µL
  System suitability
  Samples: *Standard solution A* and *Standard solution B*
  Suitability requirements
  Chromatogram similarity: The chromatogram of *Standard solution B* is similar to the reference chromatogram provided with the lot of USP Powdered Valerian Extract RS being used.
  Tailing factor: NMT 2.0 for the valerenic acid peak, *Standard solution A*
  Relative standard deviation: NMT 2.0%, *Standard solution A*

Analysis

Samples: *Standard solution A, Standard solution B,* and *Sample solution*

Using the chromatograms of *Standard solution B* and the reference chromatogram provided with the lot of USP Powdered Valerian Extract RS being used, identify and measure the areas of the peaks corresponding to hydroxyvalerenic acid, acetoxyvalerenic acid, and valerenic acid in the *Sample solution.*

Calculate the quantity, in mg, of hydroxyvalerenic acid, acetoxyvalerenic acid, and valerenic acid in each Capsule:

$$Result = (r_U/r_S) \times C_S \times (V \times W_{AV}/W) \times F$$

r_U = peak area of the relevant analyte from the *Sample solution*

r_S = peak area of valerenic acid from *Standard solution A*

C_S = concentration of USP Valerenic Acid RS in *Standard solution A* (mg/mL)

V = volume of the solvent taken to prepare the *Sample solution* (mL)

W_{AV} = average Capsule fill weight (mg)

W = weight of the sample taken to prepare the *Sample solution* (mg)

F = conversion factor for analytes (1.10 for hydroxyvalerenic acid, 1.25 for acetoxyvalerenic acid, and 1.00 for valerenic acid)

Calculate the percentage of the labeled amount of valerenic acids, as the sum of hydroxyvalerenic acid, acetoxyvalerenic acid, and valerenic acid in each Capsule:

$$Result = (\Sigma Q_i/L) \times 100$$

Q_i = sum of the quantities of valerenic acids previously determined (mg)

L = labeled amount of valerenic acids (mg)

Acceptance criteria: 90.0%–120.0%

PERFORMANCE TESTS

• **DISINTEGRATION AND DISSOLUTION ⟨2040⟩,** *Disintegration:* Meet the requirements
• **WEIGHT VARIATION ⟨2091⟩:** Meet the requirements

CONTAMINANTS

• **MICROBIAL ENUMERATION TESTS ⟨2021⟩:** The total aerobic bacterial count does not exceed 10^4 cfu/g, and the total combined molds and yeasts count does not exceed 10^3 cfu/g.
• **ABSENCE OF SPECIFIED MICROORGANISMS ⟨2022⟩,** *Test Procedures, Test for Absence of Salmonella Species* and *Test for Absence of Escherichia coli:* Meet the requirements

ADDITIONAL REQUIREMENTS

• **PACKAGING AND STORAGE:** Preserve in well-closed containers, protected from light and moisture, and store at room temperature.
• **LABELING:** The label states the Latin binomial, the official name, and the article from which the Capsules were prepared. The label states the amount of valerenic acids (as the sum of hydroxyvalerenic acid, acetoxyvalerenic acid, and valerenic acid) in mg/Capsule.
• **USP REFERENCE STANDARDS ⟨11⟩**
  USP Valerenic Acid RS
  USP Powdered Valerian Extract RS
  ■1S *(USP41)*

Add the following:

■Valerian Root Powder Capsules

DEFINITION

Valerian Root Powder Capsules contain finely powdered dried subterranean parts of *Valeriana officinalis* L. (Fam. Caprifoliaceae, formerly Valerianaceae) including rhizome, root, and stolon. They contain NLT 0.04% of valerenic acid ($C_{15}H_{22}O_2$) and NLT 0.1% of total valerenic acids, calculated as the sum of hydroxyvalerenic acid ($C_{15}H_{22}O_3$), acetoxyvalerenic acid ($C_{17}H_{24}O_4$) and valerenic acid ($C_{15}H_{22}O_2$), from the labeled amount of valerian root powder.

IDENTIFICATION

• **A. HPTLC FOR ARTICLES OF BOTANICAL ORIGIN ⟨203⟩**
  Standard solution A: 0.25 mg/mL of USP Valerenic Acid RS in methanol
  Standard solution B: 40 mg/mL of USP Powdered Valerian Extract RS in methanol. Sonicate for 10 min, centrifuge, and use the supernatant.
  Sample solution: Transfer a portion of the Capsule contents, equivalent to 0.5 g of valerian root powder, to a centrifuge tube, and add 5 mL of methanol. Sonicate for 10 min, centrifuge, and use the supernatant.
  Chromatographic system
  Adsorbent: Chromatographic silica gel mixture with an average particle size of 5 μm (HPTLC plates)
  Application volume: 5 μL, as 8-mm bands
  Relative humidity: Condition the plate to a relative humidity of about 33% using a suitable device.
  Temperature: Ambient, not to exceed 30°
  Developing solvent system: Cyclohexane, ethyl acetate, and glacial acetic acid (60:38:2)
  Developing distance: 6 cm
  Derivatization reagent A: Glacial acetic acid and hydrochloric acid (1:4)
  Derivatization reagent B: 0.5 mL of *p*-anisaldehyde, 10 mL of glacial acetic acid, and 5 mL of sulfuric acid. Add to 85 mL of ice-cold methanol, and mix.
  Analysis
  Samples: *Standard solution A, Standard solution B,* and *Sample solution*
  Apply the *Samples* as bands and dry in air. Develop in a saturated chamber, remove the plate from the chamber, and dry in air. Treat the plate with *Derivatization reagent A,* heat at 120° for 5 min, and examine under white light. Then treat the plate with *Derivatization reagent B,* heat at 100° for 3 min, and examine under white light.
  System suitability: After treatment with *Derivatization reagent A* and heating, *Standard solution A* and *Standard solution B* do not exhibit an intense blue band at about the middle of the chromatogram nor any other significant bands. After treatment with *Derivatization reagent B* and heating, *Standard solution A* exhibits a violet band due to valerenic acid, while *Standard solution B* exhibits a band corresponding in R_F and color to that of valerenic acid in *Standard solution A* as well as a violet band below valerenic acid at about the middle of the chromatogram due to acetoxyvalerenic acid and a minor violet band in the lower third of the chromatogram due to hydroxyvalerenic acid.
  Acceptance criteria: After treatment with *Derivatization reagent A* and heating, the *Sample solution* does not exhibit an intense blue band at about the middle of the chromatogram nor any other significant bands [distinction from Mexican valerian (*Valeriana edulis*)], though minor bands may be observed. After treatment with *Derivatization reagent B* and heating, the *Sample solution* exhibits three violet bands in positions and colors similar to the bands in *Standard solution B.* These bands

include a band corresponding in R_F to valerenic acid in *Standard solution A* and *Standard solution B*, a band below valerenic acid at about middle of the chromatogram due to acetoxyvalerenic acid [distinction from Scouler's valerian (*Valeriana wallichii*)], and a minor violet band in the lower third of the chromatogram due to hydroxyvalerenic acid. Other minor bands may be observed.

- **B. HPLC**
  Analysis: Proceed as directed in the test for *Content of Valerenic Acids*.
  Acceptance criteria: The chromatogram of the *Sample solution* exhibits peaks at the retention times of those due to valerenic acid, hydroxyvalerenic acid, and acetoxyvalerenic acid in the chromatograms of *Standard solution A* and *Standard solution B*.

STRENGTH

- **CONTENT OF VALERENIC ACIDS**
  Solvent: Methanol and a solution of 0.1% phosphoric acid in water (3:1)
  Solution A: Mix 6 mL of 85% phosphoric acid with 900 mL of water, dilute with water to 1000 mL, mix, filter, and degas.
  Solution B: Mix 6 mL of 85% phosphoric acid with 900 mL of methanol, dilute with methanol to 1000 mL, mix, filter, and degas.
  Mobile phase: See *Table 1*.

Table 1

Time (min)	Solution A (%)	Solution B (%)
0	40	60
15	5	95
25	5	95
30	40	60

Standard solution A: 0.02 mg/mL of USP Valerenic Acid RS in methanol. Sonicate if necessary.
Standard solution B: Sonicate a portion of USP Powdered Valerian Extract RS in *Solvent* to obtain a solution with a concentration of about 20 mg/mL. Before injection, pass through a membrane filter of 0.45-μm or finer pore size.
Sample solution: Determine the total weight of 20 Capsules. Empty the Capsules, combine and mix their contents to obtain a homogenous composite. Weigh the empty Capsule shells and calculate the average fill weight per Capsule. Transfer a portion of the Capsule contents, equivalent to 1.0 g of valerian root powder, to a 50-mL volumetric flask. Add 10.0 mL of water and shake for 2 min while heating in a water bath maintained at about 50°. Sonicate for 15 min, add 35 mL of methanol, and sonicate for 15 min. Cool, dilute with methanol to volume, and mix. Before injection, pass through a membrane filter of 0.45-μm or finer pore size, discarding the first few milliliters of the filtrate.
Chromatographic system
(See *Chromatography* ⟨621⟩, *System Suitability*.)
  Mode: LC
  Detector: UV 225 nm
  Column: 4.6-mm × 25-cm; end-capped, 5-μm, 100-Å packing L1
  Column temperature: 40°
  Flow rate: 1.0 mL/min
  Injection volume: 25 μL
System suitability
  Samples: *Standard solution A* and *Standard solution B*
  Suitability requirements
    Chromatogram similarity: The chromatogram of *Standard solution B* is similar to the reference chromatogram provided with the lot of USP Powdered Valerian Extract RS being used.

Tailing factor: NMT 2.0 for the valerenic acid peak, *Standard solution A*
Relative standard deviation: NMT 2.0%, *Standard solution A*
Analysis
  Samples: *Standard solution A, Standard solution B,* and *Sample solution*
Using the chromatograms of *Standard solution B* and the reference chromatogram provided with the lot of USP Powdered Valerian Extract RS being used, identify and measure the areas of the peaks corresponding to hydroxyvalerenic acid, acetoxyvalerenic acid, and valerenic acid in the *Sample solution*.
Calculate the quantity, in mg, of hydroxyvalerenic acid, acetoxyvalerenic acid, and valerenic acid in each Capsule:

$$\text{Result} = (r_U/r_S) \times C_S \times (V \times W_{AV}/W) \times F$$

r_U = peak area of the relevant analyte from the *Sample solution*
r_S = peak area of valerenic acid from *Standard solution A*
C_S = concentration of USP Valerenic Acid RS in *Standard solution A* (mg/mL)
V = volume of the solvent taken to prepare the *Sample solution* (mL)
W_{AV} = average Capsule fill weight (mg)
W = weight of the sample taken to prepare the *Sample solution* (mg)
F = conversion factor for analytes (1.10 for hydroxyvalerenic acid, 1.25 for acetoxyvalerenic acid, and 1.00 for valerenic acid)

Calculate the percentage of valerenic acid within the labeled amount of valerian rhizome, root, and stolon powder in each Capsule:

$$\text{Result} = (Q/L) \times 100$$

Q = amount of valerenic acid previously determined (mg)
L = labeled amount of valerian rhizome, root, and stolon powder (mg)

Calculate the percentage of valerenic acids, calculated as the sum of hydroxyvalerenic acid, acetoxyvalerenic acid and valerenic acid, within the labeled amount of valerian rhizome, root, and stolon powder in each Capsule:

$$\text{Result} = (\Sigma Q_i/L) \times 100$$

Q_i = sum of the quantities of hydroxyvalerenic acid, acetoxyvalerenic acid, and valerenic acid previously determined (mg)
L = labeled amount of valerian rhizome, root, and stolon powder (mg)

Acceptance criteria: NLT 0.04% of valerenic acid and NLT 0.1% of total valerenic acids

PERFORMANCE TESTS

- **DISINTEGRATION AND DISSOLUTION** ⟨2040⟩, *Disintegration*: Meet the requirements
- **WEIGHT VARIATION** ⟨2091⟩: Meet the requirements

CONTAMINANTS

- **MICROBIAL ENUMERATION TESTS** ⟨2021⟩: The total aerobic bacterial count does not exceed 10^4 cfu/g, and the total combined molds and yeasts count does not exceed 10^3 cfu/g.
- **ABSENCE OF SPECIFIED MICROORGANISMS** ⟨2022⟩, *Test Procedures, Test for Absence of Salmonella Species* and *Test for Absence of Escherichia coli*: Meet the requirements

ADDITIONAL REQUIREMENTS

- **PACKAGING AND STORAGE:** Preserve in well-closed containers, protected from light and moisture, and store at room temperature.
- **LABELING:** The label states the Latin binomial and the official name, and the article from which the Capsules were prepared. The label states the amount of valerian root powder in mg/Capsule.

- **USP REFERENCE STANDARDS ⟨11⟩**
  USP Valerenic Acid RS
  USP Powdered Valerian Extract RS
  ■1S *(USP41)*

Excipients

USP and NF Excipients, Listed by Functional Category

In the following reference table, the grouping of excipients by functional category is intended to summarize commonly identified purposes that these excipients serve in drug product formulations. The association of a functional category with a particular dosage form in this table is not absolute and does not limit the use of an excipient to a single type of dosage form or delivery system.

Adhesive

Dosage Form: Transdermals and "Patches"
Dimethicone
Polyisobutylene

Air Displacement
Carbon Dioxide
Nitrogen

Alcohol Denaturant
Denatonium Benzoate
Methyl Isobutyl Ketone
Sucrose Octaacetate

Antifoaming Agent
Dimethicone
Lauric Acid
Myristic Acid
Palmitic Acid
Simethicone

Antimicrobial Preservative

Dosage Form: Oral Liquids
Alcohol
Benzalkonium Chloride
Benzalkonium Chloride Solution
Benzethonium Chloride
Benzoic Acid
Benzyl Alcohol
Boric Acid
Butylparaben
Calcium Acetate
Calcium Chloride
Calcium Lactate
Calcium Propionate
Cetrimonium Bromide
Cetylpyridinium Chloride
Chlorobutanol
Chlorocresol
Chloroxylenol
Cresol
Dehydroacetic Acid
Erythorbic Acid
Ethylparaben
Ethylparaben Sodium
Glycerin
Imidurea
Mandelic Acid
Methylparaben
Methylparaben Sodium
Monothioglycerol

Pentetic Acid
Phenol
Phenoxyethanol
Phenylethyl Alcohol
Phenylmercuric Acetate
Phenylmercuric Nitrate
Potassium Benzoate
Potassium Metabisulfite
Potassium Sorbate
Propionic Acid
Propylene Glycol
Propylparaben
Propylparaben Sodium
Sodium Acetate
Sodium Benzoate
Sodium Borate
Sodium Dehydroacetate
Sodium Lactate Solution
Sodium Metabisulfite
Sodium Propionate
Sodium Sulfite
Sorbic Acid
Sulfur Dioxide
Thimerosal
Thymol
Zinc Oxide

Dosage Form: Ophthalmic Preparations
Benzalkonium Chloride
Benzyl Alcohol
Chlorobutanol
Propylparaben
Sorbic Acid

Antioxidant

Dosage Form: Oral Liquids
Ascorbic Acid
Ascorbyl Palmitate
Butylated Hydroxyanisole
Butylated Hydroxytoluene
Citric Acid Monohydrate
Erythorbic Acid
Fumaric Acid
Hypophosphorous Acid
Lactobionic Acid
Malic Acid
Methionine
Monothioglycerol
Potassium Metabisulfite
Propionic Acid
Propyl Gallate
Racemethionine
Sodium Ascorbate
Sodium Bisulfite
Sodium Formaldehyde Sulfoxylate
Sodium Metabisulfite

Sodium Sulfite
Sodium Thiosulfate
Stannous Chloride
Sulfur Dioxide
Thymol
Tocopherol
Tocopherols Excipient
Vitamin E
Vitamin E Polyethylene Glycol Succinate

Bulking Agent
Alpha-Lactalbumin
Polydextrose
Polydextrose, Hydrogenated
Pullulan

Dosage Form: Parenterals
Creatinine
Glycine
Mannitol
Trehalose

Capsule Shell

Dosage Form: Tablets and Capsules
Gelatin
Hypromellose
Pullulan

Dosage Form: Dry Powder Inhalers
Gelatin
Hypromellose

Carrier

Dosage Form: Dry Powder Inhalers
Lactose, Anhydrous
Lactose, Monohydrate

Chelating and/or Complexing Agent

Dosage Form: Oral Liquids
Alfadex
Betadex
Betadex Sulfobutyl Ether Sodium
Citric Acid Monohydrate
Edetate Calcium Disodium
Edetate Disodium
Edetic Acid
Galactose
Gamma Cyclodextrin
Hydroxypropyl Betadex
Alpha-Lactalbumin
Malic Acid
Oxyquinoline Sulfate
Pentetic Acid
Potassium Citrate
Sodium Phosphate, Dibasic
Sodium Phosphate, Monobasic

Coating Agent

Dosage Form: Tablets and Capsules
Amino Methacrylate Copolymer
Ammonio Methacrylate Copolymer
Ammonio Methacrylate Copolymer Dispersion
Calcium Carbonate
Carboxymethylcellulose Calcium
Carboxymethylcellulose Sodium
Carboxymethylcellulose Sodium, Enzymatically-Hydrolyzed
Cellaburate
Cellacefate
Cellulose Acetate
Cetyl Alcohol
Chitosan
Coconut Oil
Coconut Oil, Hydrogenated
Copovidone
Corn Syrup Solids
Ethyl Acrylate and Methyl Methacrylate Copolymer Dispersion
Ethylcellulose

Ethylcellulose Aqueous Dispersion
Ethylcellulose Dispersion Type B
Ethylene Glycol and Vinyl Alcohol Graft Copolymer
Gelatin
Glaze, Pharmaceutical
Glucose, Liquid
Glyceryl Behenate
[(Title for this monograph—not to change until December 1, 2019.) (Prior to December 1, 2019, the current practice of labeling the article of commerce with the name Glyceryl Behenate may be continued. Use of the name Glyceryl Dibehenate will be permitted as of December 1, 2014; however, the use of this name will not be mandatory until December 1, 2019. The 60-month extension will provide the time needed by manufacturers and users to make necessary changes.)]
Glyceryl Dibehenate
Hydroxyethyl Cellulose
Hydroxypropyl Cellulose
Hypromellose
Hypromellose Acetate Succinate
Hypromellose Phthalate
Isomalt
Alpha-Lactalbumin
Maltitol
Maltodextrin
Methacrylic Acid and Ethyl Acrylate Copolymer
Methacrylic Acid and Ethyl Acrylate Copolymer Dispersion
Methacrylic Acid and Ethyl Acrylate Copolymer, Partially-Neutralized
Methacrylic Acid and Methyl Methacrylate Copolymer
Methylcellulose
Palm Kernel Oil
Palm Oil
Palm Oil, Hydrogenated
Polydextrose
Polydextrose, Hydrogenated
Polyethylene Glycol
Polyethylene Glycol 3350
Polyethylene Oxide
Polyvinyl Acetate
Polyvinyl Acetate Dispersion
Polyvinyl Acetate Phthalate
Polyvinyl Alcohol
Pullulan
Rapeseed Oil, Fully Hydrogenated
Rapeseed Oil, Superglycerinated Fully Hydrogenated
Shellac
Starch, Pregelatinized Modified
Sucrose
Sugar, Confectioner's
Sunflower Oil
Titanium Dioxide
Wax, Carnauba
Wax, Microcrystalline
Xylitol
Zein
Zinc Oxide

Colloid Stabilizing Agent

Dosage Form: Radiopharmaceuticals
Gelatin

Coloring Agent
Caramel
Ferric Oxide
Ferrosoferric Oxide

Dosage Form: Tablets and Capsules
Aluminum Oxide

Desiccant
Calcium Chloride
Calcium Sulfate
Polyvinyl Acetate
Silicon Dioxide

Diluent
Dosage Form: Tablets and Capsules
  Amino Methacrylate Copolymer
  Ammonio Methacrylate Copolymer
  Ammonio Methacrylate Copolymer Dispersion
  Calcium Carbonate
  Calcium Phosphate, Dibasic, Anhydrous
  Calcium Phosphate, Dibasic, Dihydrate
  Calcium Phosphate, Tribasic
  Calcium Sulfate
  Cellaburate
  Cellulose, Microcrystalline
  Cellulose, Silicified Microcrystalline
  Cellulose, Powdered
  Cellulose Acetate
  Corn Syrup
  Corn Syrup Solids
  Dextrates
  Dextrin
  Dextrose
  Dextrose Excipient
  Erythritol
  Ethyl Acrylate and Methyl Methacrylate Copolymer
    Dispersion
  Fructose
  Invert Sugar
  Isomalt
  Kaolin
  Alpha-Lactalbumin
  Lactitol
  Lactose, Anhydrous
  Lactose, Monohydrate
  Magnesium Carbonate
  Magnesium Oxide
  Maltitol
  Maltodextrin
  Maltose
  Mannitol
  Methacrylic Acid and Ethyl Acrylate Copolymer
  Methacrylic Acid and Ethyl Acrylate Copolymer
    Dispersion
  Methacrylic Acid and Methyl Methacrylate Copolymer
  Polydextrose
  Polyethylene Glycol
  Polyethylene Glycol 3350
  Propylene Glycol Monocaprylate
  Pullulan
  Simethicone
  Sodium Chloride
  Sorbitol
  Starch, Pregelatinized
  Starch, Pregelatinized Modified
  Starch, Corn
  Starch, Hydroxypropyl Corn
  Starch, Pregelatinized Hydroxypropyl Corn
  Starch, Pea
  Starch, Hydroxypropyl Pea
  Starch, Pregelatinized Hydroxypropyl Pea
  Starch, Potato
  Starch, Hydroxypropyl Potato
  Starch, Pregelatinized Hydroxypropyl Potato
  Starch, Tapioca
  Starch, Wheat
  Starch Hydrolysate, Hydrogenated
  Sucrose
  Sugar, Compressible
  Sugar, Confectioner's
  Sugar Spheres
  Sunflower Oil
  Talc
  Trehalose
  Xylitol

Disintegrant
Dosage Form: Tablets and Capsules
  Alginic Acid
  Carboxymethylcellulose Calcium
  Carboxymethylcellulose Sodium
  Cellulose, Microcrystalline
  Cellulose, Silicified Microcrystalline
  Cellulose, Powdered
  Croscarmellose Sodium
  Crospovidone
  Glycine
  Guar Gum
  Hydroxypropyl Cellulose, Low-Substituted
  Magnesium Aluminum Silicate
  Maltose
  Methylcellulose
  Polacrilin Potassium
  Pullulan
  Silicon Dioxide, Colloidal
  Sodium Alginate
  Sodium Starch Glycolate
  Starch, Pregelatinized Modified
  Starch, Corn
  Starch, Hydroxypropyl Corn
  Starch, Pregelatinized Hydroxypropyl Corn
  Starch, Pea
  Starch, Hydroxypropyl Pea
  Starch, Pregelatinized Hydroxypropyl Pea
  Starch, Potato
  Starch, Hydroxypropyl Potato
  Starch, Pregelatinized Hydroxypropyl Potato
  Starch, Tapioca
  Starch, Wheat
  Trehalose

Change to read:

Emollient
Dosage Form: Semisolids, Topicals, and Suppositories
  Alkyl (C12-15) Benzoate
  Almond Oil
  Aluminum Monostearate
  Canola Oil
  Castor Oil
  Cetostearyl Alcohol
  Cholesterol
  Coconut Oil
  Cyclomethicone
  Dimethicone
  Ethylene Glycol Stearates
  Glycerin
  Glyceryl Monooleate
  Glyceryl Monostearate
  ■Isopropyl Isostearate■1S (NF36)
  Isopropyl Myristate
  Isopropyl Palmitate
  ■Isostearyl Isostearate■1S (NF36)
  Hydrogenated Lanolin
  Lecithin
  Mineral Oil
  Mineral Oil, Light
  Myristyl Alcohol
  Octyldodecanol
  Oleyl Alcohol
  Oleyl Oleate
  Petrolatum
  Polydecene, Hydrogenated
  Propylene Glycol Dilaurate
  Propylene Glycol Monolaurate
  Safflower Oil
  Soybean Oil, Hydrogenated
  Sunflower Oil
  Wax, Cetyl Esters

Xylitol
Zinc Acetate

Change to read:

Emulsifying Agent
Dosage Form: Oral Liquids
  Acacia
  Agar
  Behenoyl Polyoxylglycerides
  Benzalkonium Chloride
  Benzyl Benzoate
  Caprylic Acid
  Caprylocaproyl Polyoxylglycerides
  Carbomer Copolymer
  Carbomer Homopolymer
  Carbomer Interpolymer
  Carboxymethylcellulose Calcium
  Cetostearyl Alcohol
  Cetyl Alcohol
  Cetylpyridinium Chloride
  Cholesterol
  Coconut Oil
  Desoxycholic Acid
    [(Title for this monograph—not to change until December 1, 2021.) (Prior to December 1, 2021, the current practice of labeling the article of commerce with the name Desoxycholic Acid may be continued. Use of the name Deoxycholic Acid will be permitted as of December 1, 2016; however, the use of this name will not be mandatory until December 1, 2021. The 60-month extension will provide the time needed by manufacturers and users to make necessary changes.)]
  Deoxycholic Acid
  Diethanolamine (Adjunct)
  Diethylene Glycol Monoethyl Ether
  Diethylene Glycol Stearates
  Egg Phospholipids
  Ethylene Glycol Stearates
  Glyceryl Distearate
  Glyceryl Monocaprylate
  Glyceryl Monocaprylocaprate
  Glyceryl Monolinoleate
  Glyceryl Monooleate
  Glyceryl Monostearate
  ■Glyceryl Tricaprylate■1S (NF36)
  Glyceryl Tristearate
  Hydroxypropyl Cellulose
  Hypromellose
  ■Isopropyl Isostearate■1S (NF36)
  ■Isostearyl Isostearate■1S (NF36)
  Alpha-Lactalbumin
  Lanolin
  Hydrogenated Lanolin
  Lanolin Alcohols
  Lauric Acid
  Lauroyl Polyoxylglycerides
  Lecithin
  Linoleoyl Polyoxylglycerides
  Magnesium Oxide
  Medium-chain Triglycerides
  Methylcellulose
  Mono- and Di-glycerides
  Monoethanolamine (Adjunct)
  Myristic Acid
  Octyldodecanol
  Oleic Acid (Adjunct)
  Oleoyl Polyoxylglycerides
  Oleyl Alcohol (Stabilizer)
  Oleyl Oleate
  Palm Kernel Oil
  Palm Oil
  Palmitic Acid

  Pectin
  Poloxamer
  Polycarbophil
  Polyglyceryl 3 Diisostearate
  Polyglyceryl Dioleate
  Polyoxyl 10 Oleyl Ether
  Polyoxyl 15 Hydroxystearate
  Polyoxyl 20 Cetostearyl Ether
  Polyoxyl 35 Castor Oil
  Polyoxyl 40 Castor Oil, Hydrogenated
  Polyoxyl 40 Stearate
  Polyoxyl Lauryl Ether
  Polyoxyl Stearate
  Polyoxyl Stearyl Ether
  Polysorbate 20
  Polysorbate 40
  Polysorbate 60
  Polysorbate 80
  Potassium Alginate
  Propylene Glycol Alginate
  Propylene Glycol Dicaprylate/Dicaprate
  Propylene Glycol Dilaurate
  Propylene Glycol Monocaprylate
  Propylene Glycol Monolaurate
  Propylene Glycol Monostearate
  Rapeseed Oil, Superglycerinated Fully Hydrogenated
  Sodium Borate
  Sodium Cetostearyl Sulfate
  Sodium Lauryl Sulfate
  Sodium Stearate
  Sorbitan Monolaurate
  Sorbitan Monooleate
  Sorbitan Monopalmitate
  Sorbitan Monostearate
  Sorbitan Sesquioleate
  Sorbitan Trioleate
  Stannous Chloride
  Starch, Hydroxypropyl Corn
  Starch, Hydroxypropyl Pea
  Starch, Hydroxypropyl Potato
  Stearic Acid
  Stearoyl Polyoxylglycerides
  Sucrose Palmitate
  Sucrose Stearate
  Sunflower Oil
  Trolamine
  Vitamin E Polyethylene Glycol Succinate
  Wax, Emulsifying

Film-Forming Agent
Dosage Form: Tablets and Capsules
  Alginic Acid
  Amino Methacrylate Copolymer
  Ammonio Methacrylate Copolymer
  Ammonio Methacrylate Copolymer Dispersion
  Carboxymethylcellulose Calcium
  Carboxymethylcellulose Sodium
  Carboxymethylcellulose Sodium, Enzymatically-Hydrolyzed
  Cellaburate
  Cellacefate
  Cellulose Acetate
  Chitosan
  Copovidone
  Dibutyl Phthalate
  Diethyl Phthalate
  Ethyl Acrylate and Methyl Methacrylate Copolymer Dispersion
  Ethylcellulose
  Ethylcellulose Aqueous Dispersion
  Ethylcellulose Dispersion Type B
  Ethylene Glycol and Vinyl Alcohol Grafted Copolymer
  Gelatin
  Glaze, Pharmaceutical
  Hydroxyethyl Cellulose

Hydroxypropyl Cellulose
Hypromellose
Hypromellose Acetate Succinate
Hypromellose Phthalate
Methacrylic Acid and Ethyl Acrylate Copolymer
Methacrylic Acid and Ethyl Acrylate Copolymer Dispersion
Methacrylic Acid and Ethyl Acrylate Copolymer, Partially-Neutralized
Methacrylic Acid and Methyl Methacrylate Copolymer
Methylcellulose
Polyethylene Glycol 3350
Polyvinyl Acetate
Polyvinyl Acetate Dispersion
Polyvinyl Acetate Phthalate
Polyvinyl Alcohol
Pullulan
Pyroxylin
Shellac
Sodium Alginate

Dosage Form: Transdermals and "Patches"
Chitosan
Dextrin
Gelatin
Hydroxyethyl Cellulose
Hypromellose
Pectin
Polyethylene Glycol
Polyvinyl Alcohol
Pullulan
Sodium Alginate
Xanthan Gum

Filtering Aid
Cellulose, Powdered
Siliceous Earth, Purified

Flavors and Fragrance
Eucalyptus Oil
Isobutyl Alcohol
Sodium Succinate

Dosage Form: Tablets and Capsules
Adipic Acid
Almond Oil
Anethole
Benzaldehyde
Denatonium Benzoate
Ethyl Acetate
Ethyl Maltol
Ethyl Vanillin
Ethylcellulose
Fructose
Fumaric Acid
L-Glutamic Acid, Hydrochloride
Lactitol
Leucine
Malic Acid
Maltol
Menthol
Methionine
Methyl Salicylate
Monosodium Glutamate
Peppermint
Peppermint Oil
Peppermint Spirit
Racemethionine
Rose Oil
Rose Water, Stronger
Sodium Acetate
Sodium Lactate Solution
Tartaric Acid
Thymol
Vanillin

Free Radical Scavenger
Dosage Form: Radiopharmaceuticals
Aminobenzoic Acid
Methylene Blue

Glidant and/or Anticaking Agent
Dosage Form: Tablets and Capsules
Calcium Phosphate, Tribasic
Calcium Silicate
Cellulose, Powdered
Magnesium Oxide
Magnesium Silicate
Magnesium Trisilicate
Silica, Dental-Type
Silica, Hydrophobic Colloidal
Silicon Dioxide, Colloidal
Sodium Stearate
Talc

Humectant
Corn Syrup Solids
Cyclomethicone
Erythritol
Glycerin
Hexylene Glycol
Inositol
Hydrogenated Lanolin
Maltitol
Polydextrose
Polydextrose, Hydrogenated
Propylene Glycol
Sodium Lactate Solution
Sorbitol
Sorbitol Sorbitan Solution
Starch Hydrolysate, Hydrogenated
Tagatose
Triacetin
Xylitol

Change to read:

Lubricant
Dosage Form: Tablets and Capsules
Behenoyl Polyoxylglycerides
Calcium Stearate
Castor Oil, Hydrogenated
Coconut Oil, Hydrogenated
Glyceryl Behenate
[(Title for this monograph—not to change until December 1, 2019.) (Prior to December 1, 2019, the current practice of labeling the article of commerce with the name Glyceryl Behenate may be continued. Use of the name Glyceryl Dibehenate will be permitted as of December 1, 2014; however, the use of this name will not be mandatory until December 1, 2019. The 60-month extension will provide the time needed by manufacturers and users to make necessary changes.)]
Glyceryl Dibehenate
Glyceryl Monocaprylate
Glyceryl Monocaprylocaprate
Glyceryl Monostearate
■Glyceryl Tricaprylate■1S (NF36)
Glyceryl Tristearate
Lauric Acid
Magnesium Stearate
Mineral Oil, Light
Myristic Acid
Palm Oil, Hydrogenated
Palmitic Acid
Poloxamer
Polyethylene Glycol
Polyethylene Glycol 3350
Polyoxyl 10 Oleyl Ether
Polyoxyl 15 Hydroxystearate

Polyoxyl 20 Cetostearyl Ether
Polyoxyl 35 Castor Oil
Polyoxyl 40 Castor Oil, Hydrogenated
Polyoxyl 40 Stearate
Polysorbate 20
Polysorbate 40
Polysorbate 60
Polysorbate 80
Potassium Benzoate
Sodium Benzoate
Sodium Lauryl Sulfate
Sodium Stearate
Sodium Stearyl Fumarate
Sorbitan Monolaurate
Sorbitan Monooleate
Sorbitan Monopalmitate
Sorbitan Monostearate
Sorbitan Sesquioleate
Sorbitan Trioleate
Stearic Acid
Stearic Acid, Purified
Sucrose Stearate
Talc
Vegetable Oil, Hydrogenated, Type I
Zinc Stearate

Ointment Base

Dosage Form: Semisolids, Topicals, and Suppositories
Caprylocaproyl Polyoxylglycerides
Coconut Oil
Diethylene Glycol Monoethyl Ether
Lanolin
Hydrogenated Lanolin
Lanolin Alcohols
Lauroyl Polyoxylglycerides
Linoleoyl Polyoxylglycerides
Ointment, Hydrophilic
Ointment, White
Ointment, Yellow
Oleoyl Polyoxylglycerides
Paraffin
Petrolatum
Petrolatum, Hydrophilic
Petrolatum, White
Polydecene, Hydrogenated
Polyethylene Glycol
Polyethylene Glycol 3350
Polyethylene Glycol Monomethyl Ether
Polyglyceryl 3 Diisostearate
Rose Water Ointment
Squalane
Stearoyl Polyoxylglycerides
Vegetable Oil, Hydrogenated, Type II
Vitamin E Polyethylene Glycol Succinate

Pharmaceutical Water

Dosage Form: Parenterals
Water for Injection
Water for Injection, Bacteriostatic
Water for Injection, Sterile
Water for Irrigation, Sterile
Water Purified
Water Purified, Sterile

pH Modifier (Acidifying Agent/Alkalizing Agent/ Buffering Agent)
Sodium Succinate

Dosage Form: Oral Liquids
Acetic Acid
Acetic Acid, Glacial
Adipic Acid
Ammonia Solution, Strong
Ammonium Carbonate
Ammonium Chloride
Ammonium Phosphate
Boric Acid

Calcium Carbonate
Calcium Hydroxide
Calcium Lactate
Calcium Phosphate, Tribasic
Citric Acid Monohydrate
Citric Acid, Anhydrous
Diethanolamine
Fumaric Acid
Glycine
Hydrochloric Acid
Hydrochloric Acid, Diluted
Alpha-Lactalbumin
Lactic Acid
Lysine Hydrochloride
Maleic Acid
Malic Acid
Methionine
Monoethanolamine
Monosodium Glutamate
Nitric Acid
Phosphoric Acid
Phosphoric Acid, Diluted
Potassium Bicarbonate
Potassium Citrate
Potassium Hydroxide
Potassium Metaphosphate
Potassium Phosphate, Dibasic
Potassium Phosphate, Monobasic
Propionic Acid
Racemethionine
Sodium Acetate
Sodium Bicarbonate
Sodium Borate
Sodium Carbonate
Sodium Citrate
Sodium Hydroxide
Sodium Lactate Solution
Sodium Phosphate, Dibasic
Sodium Phosphate, Monobasic
Succinic Acid
Sulfuric Acid
Tartaric Acid
Trolamine

Plasticizer

Dosage Form: Tablets and Capsules
Acetyltributyl Citrate
Acetyltriethyl Citrate
Benzyl Benzoate
Castor Oil
Chlorobutanol
Diacetylated Monoglycerides
Dibutyl Sebacate
Diethyl Phthalate
Glycerin
Mannitol
Polyethylene Glycol
Polyethylene Glycol 3350
Polyethylene Glycol Monomethyl Ether
Propylene Glycol
Pullulan
Sorbitol
Sorbitol Sorbitan Solution
Triacetin
Tributyl Citrate
Triethyl Citrate
Vitamin E

Polymer Membrane

Dosage Form: Tablets and Capsules
Amino Methacrylate Copolymer
Ammonio Methacrylate Copolymer
Ammonio Methacrylate Copolymer Dispersion
Cellaburate
Cellulose Acetate

Ethyl Acrylate and Methyl Methacrylate Copolymer Dispersion
Ethylcellulose
Ethylcellulose Aqueous Dispersion
Ethylcellulose Dispersion Type B
Pullulan

Polymers for Ophthalmic Use

Dosage Form: Ophthalmic Preparations
Carbomer Copolymer
Carbomer Homopolymer
Carbomer Interpolymer
Carmellose
Guar Gum
Hydroxyethyl Cellulose
Hypromellose
Polyvinyl Alcohol
Povidone
Xanthan Gum

Propellant

Dosage Form: Aerosols
Butane
Carbon Dioxide
Dichlorodifluoromethane
Dichlorotetrafluoroethane
Isobutane
Nitrogen
Nitrous Oxide
Propane
Trichloromonofluoromethane

Reducing Agent

Dosage Form: Radiopharmaceuticals
Stannous Chloride
Stannous Fluoride

Release-Modifying Agent

Dosage Form: Tablets and Capsules
Alginic Acid
Carbomer Copolymer
Carbomer Homopolymer
Carbomer Interpolymer
Carboxymethylcellulose Sodium
Carrageenan
Cellaburate
Ethylcellulose
Ethylcellulose Aqueous Dispersion
Ethylcellulose Dispersion Type B
Glyceryl Monooleate
Glyceryl Monostearate
Guar Gum
Hydroxypropyl Betadex
Hydroxypropyl Cellulose
Hypromellose
Polyethylene Oxide
Polyvinyl Acetate Dispersion
Shellac
Sodium Alginate
Starch, Pregelatinized
Starch, Pregelatinized Modified
Xanthan Gum

Sequestering Agent

Dosage Form: Oral Liquids
Betadex
Betadex Sulfobutyl Ether Sodium
Calcium Acetate
Cyclodextrin, Gamma
Hydroxypropyl Betadex
Pentetic Acid
Pullulan
Sodium Citrate
Sodium Tartrate
Tartaric Acid

Solvent

Acetone
Alcohol
Alcohol, Diluted
Almond Oil
Amylene Hydrate
Benzyl Alcohol
Benzyl Benzoate
Butyl Alcohol
Butylene Glycol
Canola Oil
Caprylocaproyl Polyoxylglycerides
Castor Oil
Corn Oil
Cottonseed Oil
Dibutyl Phthalate
Diethyl Phthalate
Diethylene Glycol Monoethyl Ether
Dimethyl Sulfoxide
Ethyl Acetate
Ethyl Oleate
Glycerin
Hexylene Glycol
Isobutyl Alcohol
Isopropyl Alcohol
Isopropyl Myristate
Isopropyl Palmitate
Lauroyl Polyoxylglycerides
Linoleoyl Polyoxylglycerides
Medium-chain Triglycerides
Methyl Alcohol
Methyl Isobutyl Ketone
Methylene Chloride
Methylpyrrolidone
Mineral Oil
Mineral Oil, Light
Oleoyl Polyoxylglycerides
Peanut Oil
Polydecene, Hydrogenated
Polyethylene Glycol
Polyethylene Glycol 3350
Polyethylene Glycol Monomethyl Ether
Propylene Carbonate
Propylene Glycol
Safflower Oil
Sesame Oil
Soybean Oil
Stearoyl Polyoxylglycerides
Sunflower Oil
Triacetin
Triethyl Citrate
Water for Injection
Water for Injection, Sterile
Water for Irrigation, Sterile
Water, Purified

Sorbent

Cellulose, Powdered
Charcoal, Activated
Siliceous Earth, Purified

Sorbent, Carbon Dioxide

Barium Hydroxide Lime
Soda Lime

Stiffening Agent

Dosage Form: Semisolids, Topicals, and Suppositories
Castor Oil, Hydrogenated
Cetostearyl Alcohol
Cetyl Alcohol
Cetyl Palmitate
Dextrin
Hard Fat
Alpha-Lactalbumin
Paraffin
Paraffin, Synthetic
Rapeseed Oil, Fully Hydrogenated
Rapeseed Oil, Superglycerinated Fully Hydrogenated
Sodium Stearate

Stearyl Alcohol
Wax, Cetyl Esters
Wax, Emulsifying
Wax, Microcrystalline
Wax, White
Wax, Yellow

Suppository Base

Dosage Form: Semisolids, Topicals, and Suppositories
Agar
Cocoa Butter
Hard Fat
Palm Kernel Oil
Polyethylene Glycol
Polyethylene Glycol 3350

Suspending and/or Viscosity-Increasing Agent

Dosage Form: Semisolids, Topicals, and Suppositories
Acacia
Agar
Alamic Acid
Alginic Acid
Aluminum Monostearate
Attapulgite, Activated
Attapulgite, Colloidal Activated
Bentonite
Bentonite, Purified
Bentonite Magma
Carbomer 910
Carbomer 934
Carbomer 934P
Carbomer 940
Carbomer 941
Carbomer 1342
Carbomer Copolymer
Carbomer Homopolymer
Carbomer Interpolymer
Carboxymethylcellulose Calcium
Carboxymethylcellulose Sodium
Carboxymethylcellulose Sodium 12
Carboxymethylcellulose Sodium, Enzymatically-
Hydrolyzed
Carmellose
Carrageenan
Cellulose, Microcrystalline
Cellulose, Microcrystalline, and Carboxymethylcellulose
Sodium
Cellulose, Powdered
Cetostearyl Alcohol
Chitosan
Corn Syrup
Corn Syrup Solids
Cyclomethicone
Dextrin
Egg Phospholipids
Ethylcellulose
Gelatin
Gellan Gum
Glyceryl Behenate
  [(Title for this monograph—not to change until De-
  cember 1, 2019.) (Prior to December 1, 2019, the
  current practice of labeling the article of commerce
  with the name Glyceryl Behenate may be continued.
  Use of the name Glyceryl Dibehenate will be permit-
  ted as of December 1, 2014; however, the use of this
  name will not be mandatory until December 1, 2019.
  The 60-month extension will provide the time needed
  by manufacturers and users to make necessary
  changes.)]
Glyceryl Dibehenate
Guar Gum
Hydroxyethyl Cellulose
Hydroxypropyl Cellulose
Hypromellose
Isomalt
Alpha-Lactalbumin

Kaolin
Magnesium Aluminum Silicate
Maltitol Solution
Maltodextrin
Medium-chain Triglycerides
Methylcellulose
Pectin
Polycarbophil
Polydextrose
Polydextrose, Hydrogenated
Polyethylene Oxide
Polysorbate 20
Polysorbate 40
Polysorbate 60
Polysorbate 80
Polyvinyl Alcohol
Potassium Alginate
Povidone
Propylene Glycol Alginate
Pullulan
Silica, Dental-Type
Silica, Hydrophobic Colloidal
Silicon Dioxide
Silicon Dioxide, Colloidal
Sodium Alginate
Sorbitan Monolaurate
Sorbitan Monooleate
Sorbitan Monopalmitate
Sorbitan Monostearate
Sorbitan Sesquioleate
Sorbitan Trioleate
Starch, Corn
Starch, Hydroxypropyl Corn
Starch, Pregelatinized Hydroxypropyl Corn
Starch, Pea
Starch, Hydroxypropyl Pea
Starch, Pregelatinized Hydroxypropyl Pea
Starch, Potato
Starch, Hydroxypropyl Potato
Starch, Pregelatinized Hydroxypropyl Potato
Starch, Tapioca
Starch, Wheat
Sucrose
Sucrose Palmitate
Tragacanth
Vitamin E Polyethylene Glycol Succinate
Xanthan Gum

Sweetening Agent

Dosage Form: Oral Liquids
Acesulfame Potassium
Aspartame
Aspartame Acesulfame
Corn Syrup
Corn Syrup, High Fructose
Corn Syrup Solids
Dextrates
Dextrose
Dextrose Excipient
Erythritol
Fructose
Galactose
Glucose, Liquid
Glycerin
Inulin
Invert Sugar
Isomalt
Lactitol
Maltitol
Maltitol Solution
Maltose
Mannitol
Neotame
Saccharin
Saccharin Calcium

Saccharin Sodium
Sorbitol
Sorbitol Solution
Starch Hydrolysate, Hydrogenated
Sucralose
Sucrose
Sugar, Compressible
Sugar, Confectioner's
Syrup
Tagatose
Trehalose
Xylitol

Tonicity Agent

Dosage Form: Parenterals
Corn Syrup
Corn Syrup Solids
Dextrose
Glycerin
Mannitol
Potassium Chloride
Sodium Chloride

Transfer Ligand

Dosage Form: Radiopharmaceuticals
Edetate Disodium
Sodium Acetate
Sodium Citrate
Sodium Gluconate
Sodium Tartrate

Change to read:

Vehicle

Dosage Form: Oral Liquids
FLAVORED AND/OR SWEETENED
Aromatic Elixir
Benzaldehyde Elixir, Compound
Corn Syrup Solids
Dextrose
Ethyl Maltol
Peppermint Water
Sorbitol Solution
Syrup
Trehalose
OLEAGINOUS
Alkyl (C12–15) Benzoate
Almond Oil
Canola Oil
Castor Oil
Corn Oil
Cottonseed Oil
Ethyl Oleate
Isopropyl Myristate
Isopropyl Palmitate
Mineral Oil
Mineral Oil, Light
Myristyl Alcohol
Octyldodecanol
Olive Oil
Peanut Oil
Polydecene, Hydrogenated
Polyoxyl 15 Hydroxystearate
Safflower Oil
Sesame Oil
Soybean Oil
Squalane
Sunflower Oil
SOLID CARRIER
Chitosan
Corn Syrup Solids
Alpha-Lactalbumin
■Glyceryl Tricaprylate■1S (NF36)
Propylene Glycol Dicaprylate/Dicaprate

Propylene Glycol Monocaprylate
Sugar Spheres
STERILE
rAlbumin Human
Sodium Chloride Injection, Bacteriostatic
Water for Injection, Bacteriostatic

Water-Repelling Agent
Cyclomethicone
Dimethicone
Simethicone

Wet Binder

Dosage Form: Tablets and Capsules
Acacia
Agar
Alginic Acid
Amino Methacrylate Copolymer
Ammonio Methacrylate Copolymer
Ammonio Methacrylate Copolymer Dispersion
Calcium Carbonate
Calcium Lactate
Carbomer Copolymer
Carbomer Homopolymer
Carbomer Interpolymer
Carboxymethylcellulose Sodium
Cellulose, Microcrystalline
Cellulose, Silicified Microcrystalline
Coconut Oil, Hydrogenated
Copovidone
Corn Syrup
Corn Syrup Solids
Dextrates
Dextrin
Ethyl Acrylate and Methyl Methacrylate Copolymer Dispersion
Ethylcellulose
Ethylene Glycol and Vinyl Alcohol Graft Copolymer
Gelatin
Glucose, Liquid
Glyceryl Behenate
[(Title for this monograph—not to change until December 1, 2019.) (Prior to December 1, 2019, the current practice of labeling the article of commerce with the name Glyceryl Behenate may be continued. Use of the name Glyceryl Dibehenate will be permitted as of December 1, 2014; however, the use of this name will not be mandatory until December 1, 2019. The 60-month extension will provide the time needed by manufacturers and users to make necessary changes.)]
Glyceryl Dibehenate
Guar Gum
Hydroxyethyl Cellulose
Hydroxypropyl Cellulose
Hydroxypropyl Cellulose, Low-Substituted
Hypromellose
Hypromellose Acetate Succinate
Inulin
Invert Sugar
Alpha-Lactalbumin
Lactose, Monohydrate
Maltodextrin
Maltose
Methacrylic Acid and Ethyl Acrylate Copolymer
Methacrylic Acid and Ethyl Acrylate Copolymer Dispersion
Methacrylic Acid and Methyl Methacrylate Copolymer
Methylcellulose
Palm Oil, Hydrogenated
Polycarbophil
Polydextrose, Hydrogenated
Polyethylene Oxide
Polyvinyl Acetate
Povidone
Pullulan

Sodium Alginate
Starch, Pregelatinized
Starch, Pregelatinized Modified
Starch, Corn
Starch, Hydroxypropyl Corn
Starch, Pregelatinized Hydroxypropyl Corn
Starch, Pea
Starch, Hydroxypropyl Pea
Starch, Pregelatinized Hydroxypropyl Pea
Starch, Potato
Starch, Hydroxypropyl Potato
Starch, Pregelatinized Hydroxypropyl Potato
Starch, Tapioca
Starch, Wheat
Starch Hydrolysate, Hydrogenated
Sucrose
Sunflower Oil
Syrup
Trehalose
Vegetable Oil, Hydrogenated
Vitamin E Polyethylene Glycol Succinate
Zein

Wetting and/or Solubilizing Agent
Betadex Sulfobutyl Ether Sodium

Dosage Form: Oral Liquids
Behenoyl Polyoxylglycerides
Benzalkonium Chloride
Benzethonium Chloride
Butylene Glycol
Caprylocaproyl Polyoxylglycerides
Cetylpyridinium Chloride
Docusate Sodium

Egg Phospholipids
Glycine
Lauroyl Polyoxylglycerides
Linoleoyl Polyoxylglycerides
Nonoxynol 9
Octoxynol 9
Oleoyl Polyoxylglycerides
Poloxamer
Polyoxyl 10 Oleyl Ether
Polyoxyl 15 Hydroxystearate
Polyoxyl 20 Cetostearyl Ether
Polyoxyl 35 Castor Oil
Polyoxyl 40 Castor Oil, Hydrogenated
Polyoxyl 40 Stearate
Polyoxyl Lauryl Ether
Polyoxyl Stearate
Polyoxyl Stearyl Ether
Polysorbate 20
Polysorbate 40
Polysorbate 60
Polysorbate 80
Pullulan
Sodium Lauryl Sulfate
Sorbitan Monolaurate
Sorbitan Monooleate
Sorbitan Monopalmitate
Sorbitan Monostearate
Sorbitan Sesquioleate
Sorbitan Trioleate
Stearoyl Polyoxylglycerides
Tyloxapol
Wax, Emulsifying

Official Monographs for NF 36

Ethylcellulose

Portions of the monograph text that are national *USP* text, and are not part of the harmonized text, are marked with symbols (♦♦) to specify this fact.

Cellulose, ethyl ether;
Cellulose ethyl ether [9004-57-3].

DEFINITION

Change to read:

Ethylcellulose is a partly *O*-ethylated cellulose. It contains NLT 44.0% and NMT 51.0% of ethoxy (–OC_2H_5) groups, calculated on the dried basis. ■It may contain a suitable antioxidant.■1S (NF36)

IDENTIFICATION

Change to read:

- **A. INFRARED ABSORPTION** ■⟨197F⟩
  Sample: Dissolve 40 mg in 1 mL of methylene chloride, spread 2 drops of this solution between two sodium chloride plates, then remove one of the plates to evaporate the solvent.
  Acceptance criteria: Meets the requirements■1S (NF36)

ASSAY

Delete the following:

■♦ **PROCEDURE**
  [NOTE—Hydriodic acid and its reaction byproducts are highly toxic. Perform all steps of the *Sample solution* preparation and the *Standard solution* preparation in a properly functioning hood.]
  Internal standard solution: Dilute 120 µL of toluene with *o*-xylene to 10 mL.
  Standard solution: Transfer 100.0 mg of adipic acid, 4.0 mL of the *Internal standard solution*, and 4.0 mL of hydriodic acid into a suitable 10-mL thick-walled reaction vial with a pressure-tight septum closure. Close the vial tightly, and weigh the vial and contents accurately. Afterwards inject 50 µL of iodoethane through the septum with a syringe, weigh the vial again, and calculate the mass of iodoethane added, by difference. Shake well, and allow the layers to separate. Use the upper layer for analysis.
  Sample solution: Transfer 50.0 mg of Ethylcellulose, 50 mg of adipic acid, and 2.0 mL of the *Internal standard solution* into a suitable 5-mL thick-walled reaction vial with a pressure-tight septum closure. Cautiously add 2.0 mL of hydriodic acid, immediately close the vial tightly, and weigh the contents and the vial accurately. Shake the vial for 30 s, heat to 125° for 10 min, allow to cool for 2 min, shake again for 30 s, and heat to 125° for 10 min. Afterwards allow to cool for 2 min, and repeat shaking and heating for a third time. Allow the vial to cool for 45 min, and reweigh. If the loss is greater than 10 mg, discard the mixture, and prepare another. Use the upper layer for analysis.
  Chromatographic system
  (See *Chromatography* ⟨621⟩, *System Suitability.*)
  Mode: GC
  Detector: Flame ionization
  Column: 2-mm × 5.0-m stainless steel packed with 3% G2 on 150–180-µm mesh support S1A
  Temperatures
    Column: 80°
    Injector: 200°
    Detector: 200°
  Carrier gas: Nitrogen
  Flow rate: 15 mL/min
  Injection volume: 1 µL
  System suitability
  Sample: *Standard solution*
  [NOTE—The relative retention times for iodoethane, toluene, and *o*-xylene are 0.6, 1.0, and 2.3, respectively.]
  Suitability requirements
  Resolution: NLT 2.0 between iodoethane and toluene
  Analysis
  Samples: *Standard solution* and *Sample solution*
  Calculate the percentage of ethoxy content of the Ethylcellulose as declared in the labeling:

$$\text{Result} = (451{,}000/312) \times (R_U \times m_2)/[(R_S \times m_1) \times (100 - d)]$$

  R_U = ratio of the iodoethane peak area to the toluene peak area from the *Sample solution*
  m_2 = mass of iodoethane used in the *Standard solution* (mg)
  R_S = ratio of the iodoethane peak area to the toluene peak area from the *Standard solution*
  m_1 = mass of Ethylcellulose used in the *Sample solution* (mg)
  d = loss on drying as a percentage
  Acceptance criteria: 44.0%–51.0% on the dried basis■1S (NF36)

Add the following:

■♦ **PROCEDURE**
  [CAUTION—Hydriodic acid and its reaction byproducts are highly toxic. Perform all steps of the *Standard solution* and the *Sample solution* in a properly functioning hood. Specific safety practices to be followed are to be identified to the analyst performing this test.]
  [NOTE—Prepare the solutions immediately before use.]
  Internal standard solution: To 10 mL of *o*-xylene add 0.5 mL of *n*-octane and dilute to 100.0 mL with *o*-xylene.
  Sample solution: To 30.0 mg of the substance to be examined, previously dried, add 60 mg of adipic acid in a 5-mL pressure-tight reaction vial equipped with a pressure-tight membrane stopper coated with polytetrafluoroethylene and secured with an aluminum crimped cap or any other sealing system providing a sufficient air-tightness. Add 2.00 mL of *Internal standard solution* and 1.0 mL of hydriodic acid and close immediately.

Accurately weigh the vial (total mass before heating). Do not mix the contents of the vial by hand before heating. Place the vial in an oven or heat in a suitable heater, with continuous mechanical agitation, maintaining the internal temperature of the vial at $115 \pm 2°$ for 70 min. Allow to cool and weigh accurately the vial (total mass after heating). If the difference of the total mass before heating to the total mass after heating is more than 10 mg, prepare a new test solution. After phase separation, pierce through the septum of the vial with a cooled syringe and withdraw a sufficient volume of the upper phase as the test solution.

Standard solution: Place 60 mg of adipic acid and 2.00 mL of *Internal standard solution* in another 5-mL reaction vial, add 1.0 mL of hydriodic acid and close immediately. Accurately weigh the vial, then inject 25 µL of iodoethane through the septum in the vial. Weigh again accurately and mix. After phase separation, pierce through the septum of the vial with a cooled syringe and withdraw a sufficient volume of the upper phase as the *Standard solution.*

Chromatographic system
(See *Chromatography* ⟨621⟩, *System Suitability.*)
Mode: GC
Detector: Flame ionization
Column: 0.53-mm × 30-m fused silica coated with 3-µm layer of phase G1. [NOTE—Use a guard column, if necessary.]
Temperatures
Injection port: 250°
Detector: 280°
Column: See *Table 1*.

Table 1

Initial Temperature (°)	Temperature Ramp (°/min)	Final Temperature (°)	Hold Time at Final Temperature (min)
50	0	50	3
50	10	100	0
100	34.9	250	8

Flow rate: 4.2 mL/min
Carrier gas: Helium
Split ratio: 40:1
Injection volume: 1 µL
System suitability
Sample: *Standard solution*
[NOTE—The relative retention time is about 0.6 for iodoethane with reference to *n*-octane (retention time about 10 min).]
Suitability requirements
Resolution: NLT 5.0 between *n*-octane and iodoethane
Relative standard deviation: NMT 2.0%, using the response factor of the principal peak for six injections of the *Standard solution*
Analysis
Sample: *Sample solution*
[NOTE—Measure all of the peak areas, excluding the solvent peak.]
Calculate the response factor (*F*):

$$\text{Result} = (A_1 \times W_1 \times C)/(A_2 \times 100)$$

A_1 = peak area of the internal standard peak from the *Standard solution*
W_1 = weight of iodoethane in the *Standard solution* (mg)
C = content of iodoethane from the certificate of the manufacturer (%)

A_2 = peak area of the iodoethane peak from the *Standard solution*
Calculate the percentage content (m/m) of the ethoxy group:

$$\text{Result} = (A_4 \times F \times M_1 \times 100)/(A_3 \times W_2 \times M_2)$$

A_4 = peak area of iodoethane from the *Sample solution*
F = response factor calculated from above
M_1 = molar mass of ethoxy group, 45.1
A_3 = peak area of the internal standard from the *Sample solution*
W_2 = weight of the sample (dried substance) in the *Sample solution* (mg)
M_2 = molar mass of iodoethane, 156.0
Acceptance criteria: NLT 44.0% and NMT 51.0% of ethoxy groups on the dried basis■₁₅ (NF36)

IMPURITIES
• **RESIDUE ON IGNITION** ⟨281⟩
Sample: 1.0 g
Acceptance criteria: NMT 0.5%

Delete the following:

•• ◆**HEAVY METALS,** *Method II* ⟨231⟩: NMT 20 ppm◆• (Official 1-Jan-2018)
• **CHLORIDES**
Standard stock solution: 0.824 mg/mL of sodium chloride
Standard solution: 8.24 µg/mL of sodium chloride, prepared from the *Standard stock solution.* [NOTE—Prepare immediately before use.]
Sample solution: Disperse 250 mg in 50 mL of water, heat to boiling, and allow to cool, shaking occasionally. Filter, and discard the first 10 mL of the filtrate.
Analysis
Samples: *Standard solution* and *Sample solution*
Separately dilute 10 mL of the *Sample solution* and *Standard solution* with water to 15 mL, add 1 mL of diluted nitric acid (125 g/L), and pour the mixtures as a single addition into test tubes containing 1 mL of 0.1 N silver nitrate VS. Examine the tubes laterally against a black background.
Acceptance criteria: After standing for 5 min protected from light, any opalescence in the *Sample solution* is not more intense than that in the *Standard solution* (0.1%).
• **ACETALDEHYDE**
Solution A: 0.5 mg/mL of methylbenzothiazolone hydrazone hydrochloride
Solution B: 10 mg/mL of ferric chloride and 16 mg/mL of sulfamic acid
Standard stock solution: 10 mg/mL of acetaldehyde in water. [NOTE—Use immediately. Prepare the *Standard solution* and *Sample solution* at the same time.]
Standard solution: 3 µg/mL of acetaldehyde from the *Standard stock solution* in water. [NOTE—Use immediately.]
Sample solution: Dissolve 3.0 g of Ethylcellulose in 10 mL of water, stir by mechanical means for 1 h, allow to stand for 24 h, filter, and dilute the filtrate with water to 100.0 mL.
Analysis
Samples: *Standard solution* and *Sample solution*
Transfer 5.0 mL of the *Sample solution* and *Standard solution* to separate flasks. To each flask add 5 mL of *Solution A*, and heat in a water bath at 60° for 5 min. Add 2 mL of *Solution B*, and heat again at 60° for 5 min. Cool, and dilute with water to 25.0 mL.
Acceptance criteria: The *Sample solution* is not more intensely colored than the *Standard solution*.

SPECIFIC TESTS

- **VISCOSITY—CAPILLARY METHODS ⟨911⟩**
  Solution A: Alcohol and toluene (1:4 w/w)
  Sample solution: Shake a quantity of Ethylcellulose, equivalent to 5.00 g of the dried substance, with 95 g of *Solution A* until the substance is dissolved.
  Analysis: Determine the viscosity using a capillary viscometer.
  Acceptance criteria: The viscosity (mPa · s) determined at 25° is NLT 80.0% and NMT 120.0% of that stated on the label for a nominal viscosity greater than 6 mPa · s; and NLT 75.0% and NMT 140.0% of that stated on the label for a nominal viscosity of NMT 6 mPa · s.
- **ACIDITY OR ALKALINITY**
  Solution A: Dissolve 100 mg of phenolphthalein in 80 mL of alcohol, and dilute with water to 100 mL.
  Solution B: Dilute 50 mg of methyl red with 1.86 mL of 0.1 N sodium hydroxide and 50 mL of alcohol, and dilute with water to 100 mL.
  Sample solution: To 0.5 g of Ethylcellulose add 25 mL of carbon dioxide-free water, and shake for 15 min. Pass through a sintered-glass filter with a maximum diameter of pores between 16 and 40 µm.
  Analysis: To 10 mL of *Sample solution* add 0.1 mL of *Solution A* and 0.5 mL of 0.01 N sodium hydroxide (*Solution C*). To 10 mL of *Sample solution* add 0.1 mL of *Solution B* and 0.5 mL of 0.01 N hydrochloric acid (*Solution D*).
  Acceptance criteria: *Solution C* is pink; *Solution D* is red.
- **LOSS ON DRYING ⟨731⟩**
  Sample: 1 g
  Analysis: Dry at 105° for 2 h.
  Acceptance criteria: It loses NMT 3.0% of its weight.

ADDITIONAL REQUIREMENTS

- **◆PACKAGING AND STORAGE:** Preserve in well-closed containers.◆

Change to read:

- **LABELING:** Label ■■1S (NF36) to indicate its nominal viscosity in mPa · s for a 5% m/m solution. ■The label states the name and amount of any added antioxidant.■1S (NF36)

Change to read:

- **USP REFERENCE STANDARDS ⟨11⟩**
  ◆USP Ethylcellulose RS◆
  ■■1S (NF36)

Add the following:

■Glyceryl Tricaprylate

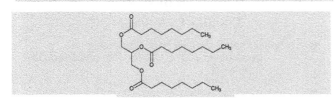

C₂₇H₅₀O₆   470.68
Octanoic acid, 1,1',1''-(1,2,3-propanetriyl) ester;

Octanoic acid, 1,2,3-propanetriyl ester;
1,3-Di(octanoyloxy)propan-2-yl octanoate;
Glyceryl trioctanoate;
Tricapryloylglycerol [538-23-8].

DEFINITION
Glyceryl Tricaprylate contains NLT 90.0% of triglycerides of saturated fatty acids, chiefly glyceryl tricaprylate (C₂₇H₅₀O₆).

IDENTIFICATION
- **A. FATTY ACID COMPOSITION**
  Boron trifluoride methanol solution: 140 mg/mL of boron trifluoride in methanol
  Saturated sodium chloride solution: Mix 1 part of sodium chloride with 2 parts of water, shake intermittently, and allow to stand. Before use, decant the solution from any undissolved substance and filter, if necessary.
  Standard solution 1: 1.0 mg/mL of USP Methyl Caproate RS, 1.0 mg/mL of USP Methyl Caprylate RS, and 2.0 mg/mL of USP Methyl Caprate RS in *n*-heptane
  Standard solution 2: 0.1 mg/mL of USP Methyl Caproate RS, 0.1 mg/mL of USP Methyl Caprylate RS, and 0.2 mg/mL of USP Methyl Caprate RS in *n*-heptane, diluted from *Standard solution 1*
  Standard solution 3: Prepare an ester mixture by mixing a commercially available ester mixture with methyl caprylate and methyl caprate, or prepare an ester mixture by using USP Methyl Caproate RS, USP Methyl Caprylate RS, USP Methyl Caprate RS, and USP Methyl Laurate RS. Dissolve a quantity of the prepared ester mixture containing methyl caproate, methyl caprylate, methyl caprate, and methyl laurate in *n*-heptane to make a solution of about 9.0 mg/mL for methyl caprylate, 0.5 mg/mL for methyl caprate, and 0.1 mg/mL for each of methyl caproate and methyl laurate.
  Sample solution: Transfer 100 mg of Glyceryl Tricaprylate to a 25-mL conical flask fitted with a suitable water-cooled reflux condenser and a magnetic stir bar. Add 2 mL of a 20-mg/mL solution of sodium hydroxide in methanol, mix, and reflux for about 30 min. Add 2 mL of *Boron trifluoride methanol solution* through the condenser and reflux for about 30 min. Add 4 mL of *n*-heptane through the condenser and reflux for 5 min. Cool, remove the condenser, add about 10 mL of *Saturated sodium chloride solution*, shake, add a quantity of *Saturated sodium chloride solution* to bring the upper layer up to the neck of the flask, and allow the layers to separate. Collect 2 mL of the *n*-heptane layer (upper layer); wash with three quantities of water, 2 mL each; and dry the *n*-heptane phase over anhydrous sodium sulfate.
  Chromatographic system
  (See *Chromatography* ⟨621⟩, *System Suitability*.)
  Mode: GC
  Detector: Flame ionization
  Column: 0.53-mm × 30-m capillary bonded with a 1.0-µm layer of phase G16
  Temperatures
  Injection port: 250°
  Detector: 250°
  Column: See *Table 1*.

Table 1

Initial Temperature (°)	Temperature Ramp (°/min)	Final Temperature (°)	Hold Time at Final Temperature (min)
50	20	180	—
180	9	240	12

Carrier gas: Helium
Flow rate: 10 mL/min
Injection volume: 2 μL
Injection type: Split ratio, 4:1
System suitability
Samples: *Standard solution 1* and *Standard solution 2*
[NOTE—The relative retention times for methyl caproate, methyl caprylate, and methyl caprate are about 0.7, 1.0, and 1.4, respectively.]
Suitability requirements
Resolution: NLT 4.0 between the methyl caprylate and methyl caprate peaks, *Standard solution 1*
Signal-to-noise ratio: NLT 10 for the methyl caproate peak, *Standard solution 2*
Analysis
Samples: *Standard solution 3* and *Sample solution*
Measure the peak areas of the methyl esters of the fatty acids. Disregard any peaks with an area less than 0.05% of the total area and any peak due to the solvent. [NOTE—Relative retention times for several methyl esters are summarized in *Table 2.*]

Table 2

Carbon-Chain Length	Number of Double Bonds	Relative Retention Times
6	0	0.7
8	0	1.0
10	0	1.4
12	0	1.7

Take the main component in *Standard solution 3* as a reference component, and calculate the calibration factor (F_{FA}) for each fatty acid methyl ester:

$$F_{FA} = [(F_{MC} \times P_{FA1} \times A_{MC})/(P_{MC} \times A_{FA1})]$$

F_{MC} = factor for the main component, 1
P_{FA1} = percentage by weight of the fatty acid methyl ester in *Standard solution 3*
A_{MC} = peak area for the main component in *Standard solution 3*
P_{MC} = percentage by weight of the main component in *Standard solution 3*
A_{FA1} = peak area for the fatty acid methyl ester in *Standard solution 3*

Calculate the percentage of each fatty acid methyl ester by weight in the portion of Glyceryl Tricaprylate taken:

$$Result = [(A_{FA2} \times F_{FA})/A_T] \times 100$$

A_{FA2} = peak area for the fatty acid methyl ester in the *Sample solution*
F_{FA} = calibration factor, determined previously
A_T = sum of the peak areas for the fatty acid methyl esters in the *Sample solution*
Acceptance criteria: Glyceryl Tricaprylate exhibits the following composition profile of fatty acids shown in *Table 3.*

Table 3

Carbon-Chain Length	Number of Double Bonds	Percentage (w/w)
6	0	≤1.0
8	0	≥90.0
10	0	≤5.0
12	0	≤1.0

• **B. CONTENT OF TRIGLYCERIDES**
Analysis: Proceed as directed in the test for *Content of Triglycerides* in the *Assay*.

Acceptance criteria: NLT 90.0% of triglycerides
• **C. FATS AND FIXED OILS ⟨401⟩,** *Procedures, Saponification Value:* 340–370

ASSAY
• **CONTENT OF TRIGLYCERIDES**
System suitability solution: 20 mg/mL each of 1-monooctanoyl-rac-glycerol and 1-monodecanoyl-rac-glycerol in tetrahydrofuran
Standard solution 1: 50 mg/mL of USP Glyceryl Monocaprylate RS in tetrahydrofuran
Standard solution 2: 50 mg/mL of USP Glyceryl Tricaprylate RS in tetrahydrofuran
Sample solution: 50 mg/mL of Glyceryl Tricaprylate in tetrahydrofuran
Chromatographic system
(See *Chromatography* ⟨621⟩, *System Suitability.*)
Mode: GC
Detector: Flame ionization
Column: 0.32-mm × 10-m bonded with a 0.1-μm layer of phase G27
Temperatures
Injection port: 350°
Detector: 370°
Column: See *Table 4.*

Table 4

Initial Temperature (°)	Temperature Ramp (°/min)	Final Temperature (°)	Hold Time at Final Temperature (min)
60	—	60	3
60	8	340	12

Carrier gas: Helium
Flow rate: 2.3 mL/min
Injection volume: 1 μL
Injection type: Split ratio, 50:1
System suitability
Samples: *System suitability solution, Standard solution 1,* and *Standard solution 2*
[NOTE—The relative retention times for monoglycerides, diglycerides, and triglycerides are 1.0–1.2, 1.5–1.9, and 1.9–2.3, respectively, *Standard solution 1* and *Standard solution 2.*]
Suitability requirements
Resolution: NLT 5.0 between the peaks due to 1-monooctanoyl-rac-glycerol and 1-monodecanoyl-rac-glycerol, *System suitability solution*
Analysis
Samples: *Standard solution 1, Standard solution 2,* and *Sample solution*
Based on the chromatograms from *Standard solution 1* and *Standard solution 2*, identify the peaks due to mono-, di-, and triglycerides in the *Sample solution.* For the calculation of the contents of mono-, di-, and triglycerides, disregard the peaks with a retention time less than that of the monoglycerides, which are due to impurities of the solvent and to the free fatty acids. Calculate the percentage of free fatty acids (C_A) in the portion of Glyceryl Tricaprylate taken:

$$C_A = [(I_A \times F \times M_{r1})/M_{r2}] \times 100$$

I_A = acid value for Glyceryl Tricaprylate, determined in the test for *Fats and Fixed Oils, Acid Value*
F = unit conversion factor, 10^{-3} g/mg
M_{r1} = molecular weight of caprylic acid, 144.21 g/mol
M_{r2} = molecular weight of potassium hydroxide, 56.11 g/mol

Calculate the percentage of triglycerides in the portion of Glyceryl Tricaprylate taken:

$$Result = (r_U/r_T) \times [(100 - C_A - C_W - C_G)/100] \times 100$$

r_U = peak response of the triglycerides from the *Sample solution*

r_T = sum of all the glyceride peak responses from the *Sample solution*

C_A = percentage of free fatty acids, determined previously

C_W = percentage of water, determined in the test for *Water Determination*

C_G = percentage of free glycerin, determined in the test for *Limit of Free Glycerin*

Acceptance criteria: NLT 90.0% of triglycerides

IMPURITIES

- **RESIDUE ON IGNITION ⟨281⟩:** NMT 0.1%
- **ALKALINE IMPURITIES**
  Analysis: Prepare a mixture of 2.0 g of Glyceryl Tricaprylate, 15 mL of alcohol, and 30 mL of ether. Dissolve by gently heating. Add 0.05 mL of bromophenol blue TS, and titrate with 0.01 N hydrochloric acid VS until the mixture turns yellow.
  Acceptance criteria: NMT 0.4 mL of 0.01 N hydrochloric acid is required.
- **LIMIT OF FREE GLYCERIN**
  Sample: 1.2 g
  Periodic acetic acid solution: Dissolve 0.446 g of sodium periodate in 2.5 mL of a 25% (v/v) solution of sulfuric acid, and dilute with glacial acetic acid to 100.0 mL.
  Potassium iodide solution: 75 mg/mL of potassium iodide
  Blank: 25 mL of methylene chloride
  Titrimetric system
  (See *Titrimetry* ⟨541⟩.)
  Mode: Residual titration
  Titrant: 0.1 N sodium thiosulfate VS
  Endpoint detection: Visual
  Analysis: Dissolve the *Sample* in 25 mL of methylene chloride. Heat to about 50°, and allow to cool. Add 100 mL of water. Shake, and add 25 mL of *Periodic acetic acid solution*. Shake again, and allow to stand for 30 min. Add 40 mL of *Potassium iodide solution*, and allow to stand for 1 min. Add 1 mL of starch TS, and titrate the liberated iodine with *Titrant* until the aqueous phase becomes colorless. Perform a blank determination. Calculate the percentage of free glycerol in the portion of Glyceryl Tricaprylate taken:

$$Result = \{[(V_B - V_S) \times N_A \times E \times F]/W\} \times 100$$

V_B = volume of *Titrant* consumed in the blank titration (mL)

V_S = volume of *Titrant* consumed in the *Sample* titration (mL)

N_A = actual normality of the *Titrant* (mEq/mL)

E = equivalent factor for glycerol, 23 mg/mEq

F = conversion factor, 10^{-3} g/mg

W = weight of Glyceryl Triglyceride taken for the titration (g)

Acceptance criteria: NMT 0.5%

SPECIFIC TESTS

- **BACTERIAL ENDOTOXINS TEST ⟨85⟩:** Where the label states that Glyceryl Tricaprylate must be subjected to further processing during the preparation of injectable dosage forms, the level of bacterial endotoxins is such that the requirement in the relevant dosage form monograph(s) in which Glyceryl Tricaprylate is used can be met.
- **FATS AND FIXED OILS ⟨401⟩,** *Procedures, Acid Value*: NMT 0.2
- **FATS AND FIXED OILS ⟨401⟩,** *Procedures, Hydroxyl Value*: NMT 10.0
- **FATS AND FIXED OILS ⟨401⟩,** *Procedures, Peroxide Value*: NMT 1
- **WATER DETERMINATION ⟨921⟩,** *Method I, Method Ia*: NMT 0.2%

ADDITIONAL REQUIREMENTS

- **PACKAGING AND STORAGE:** Preserve in well-closed containers, and store at room temperature. Protect from light and moisture.
- **LABELING:** Where Glyceryl Tricaprylate must be subjected to further processing during the preparation of injectable dosage forms to ensure acceptable levels of bacterial endotoxins, it is so labeled.
- **USP REFERENCE STANDARDS ⟨11⟩**
  USP Glyceryl Monocaprylate RS
  USP Glyceryl Tricaprylate RS
  USP Methyl Caprate RS
  USP Methyl Caproate RS
  USP Methyl Caprylate RS
  USP Methyl Laurate RS
  ■1S *(NF36)*

Add the following:

■Isopropyl Isostearate

Isooctadecanoic acid, 1-methylethyl ester contains mainly isomers of isopropyl branched stearates.

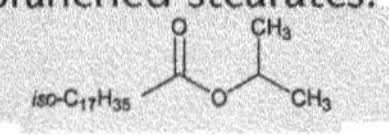

$C_{21}H_{42}O_2$ 326.56
Isooctadecanoic acid, 1-methylethyl ester [68171-33-5].

DEFINITION
Isopropyl Isostearate is obtained by esterification of isostearic acid, which is a mixture mainly of saturated branched 18 carbon-chain (C18) fatty acids and linear hexadecanoic (C16:0) and octadecanoic acids (C18:0), with isopropyl alcohol.

IDENTIFICATION
- **A. INFRARED ABSORPTION ⟨197A⟩ or ⟨197F⟩:** Disregard a weak absorption band at about 1780 cm⁻¹.
- **B.** It meets the requirements of the test for *Content of Isopropyl Fatty Esters*.

ASSAY
- **CONTENT OF ISOPROPYL FATTY ESTERS**
  System suitability solution: 5.0 mg/mL of USP Isopropyl Palmitate RS and 0.5 mg/mL of USP Isopropyl Myristate RS in *n*-hexane
  Reference solution: 2.0 mg/mL of isopropyl stearate in *n*-hexane
  Sample solution: 5.0 mg/mL of Isopropyl Isostearate in *n*-hexane
  Chromatographic system
  (See *Chromatography* ⟨621⟩, *System Suitability*.)
  Mode: GC
  Detector: Flame ionization
  Column: 0.32-mm × 15-m fused silica; coated with a 1.0-µm layer of stationary phase G27
  Temperatures
  Injection port: 240°
  Detector: 280°
  Column: See *Table 1.*

Table 1

Initial Temperature (°)	Temperature Ramp (°/min)	Final Temperature (°)	Hold Time at Final Temperature (min)
150	—	150	1
150	6	230	21

Carrier gas: Helium
Flow rate: 1.5 mL/min
Injection volume: 2.0 µL
Injection type: Split injection, split ratio, 10:1
Run time: About 35 min
System suitability
Samples: *System suitability solution* and *Reference solution*
[NOTE—The relative retention times for isopropyl myristate, isopropyl palmitate, and isopropyl stearate are 0.8, 1.0, and 1.3, respectively.]
Suitability requirements
Resolution: NLT 6.0 between the isopropyl myristate and isopropyl palmitate peaks, *System suitability solution*
Tailing factor: NMT 2 for the isopropyl palmitate peak, *System suitability solution*
Relative standard deviation: NMT 2.0%, *System suitability solution*
Analysis
Samples: *System suitability solution, Reference solution,* and *Sample solution*
Identify the isopropyl fatty ester peaks in the chromatogram of the *Sample solution* by comparing the retention times of these peaks with those obtained in the chromatograms of the *System suitability solution* and *Reference solution,* and measure the peak areas for all of the fatty acid ester peaks in the chromatogram obtained from the *Sample solution.*
Calculate the percentage of each fatty acid ester component in the portion of Isopropyl Isostearate:

$$Result = (r_U/r_T) \times 100$$

r_U = peak area for each individual fatty acid ester component
r_T = sum of the peak areas, excluding the solvent peak, from the *Sample solution*

Acceptance criteria
Sum of the contents of the isopropyl fatty esters eluting between isopropyl palmitate and isopropyl stearate (excluding isopropyl palmitate and isopropyl stearate): NLT 65.0%
Sum of the contents of isopropyl myristate, isopropyl palmitate, and isopropyl stearate: NMT 11.0%

IMPURITIES
- **RESIDUE ON IGNITION ⟨281⟩:** NMT 0.1%

SPECIFIC TESTS
- **FATS AND FIXED OILS ⟨401⟩,** *Procedures, Acid Value:* NMT 1.0, determined on 20.0 g
- **FATS AND FIXED OILS ⟨401⟩,** *Procedures, Hydroxyl Value:* NMT 5.0
- **FATS AND FIXED OILS ⟨401⟩,** *Procedures, Iodine Value:* NMT 3.0, determined on 3.0 g
- **FATS AND FIXED OILS ⟨401⟩,** *Procedures, Peroxide Value:* NMT 5.0
- **FATS AND FIXED OILS ⟨401⟩,** *Procedures, Saponification Value:* 165–180, determined on 2.0 g
- **WATER DETERMINATION ⟨921⟩,** *Method I:* NMT 0.1%, determined on 5.0 g[1]

[1] Hydranal composite 5 is suitable.

ADDITIONAL REQUIREMENTS
- **PACKAGING AND STORAGE:** Preserve in tight containers. Store at room temperature.
- **USP REFERENCE STANDARDS ⟨11⟩**
  USP Isopropyl Isostearate RS
  USP Isopropyl Myristate RS
  USP Isopropyl Palmitate RS
■1S *(NF36)*

Methyl Salicylate

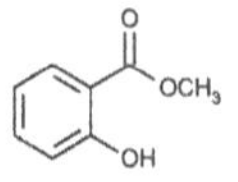

C$_8$H$_8$O$_3$ 152.15
Benzoic acid, 2-hydroxy-, methyl ester;
Methyl salicylate [119-36-8].

DEFINITION

Change to read:

Methyl Salicylate is produced synthetically or is obtained by maceration and subsequent distillation with steam from the leaves of *Gaultheria procumbens* L. (Fam. Ericaceae) or from the bark of *Betula lenta* L. (Fam. Betulaceae). It contains NLT 98.0% and NMT ●102.0%● (RB 1-Aug-2017) of methyl salicylate (C$_8$H$_8$O$_3$).

IDENTIFICATION
- **A. INFRARED ABSORPTION ⟨197F⟩**
- **B. CHROMATOGRAPHIC IDENTITY**
  Analysis: Proceed as directed in the *Assay.*
  Acceptance criteria: The retention time of the major peak of the *Sample solution* corresponds to that of the *Standard solution.*

ASSAY

Change to read:

- **PROCEDURE**
  Mobile phase: Methanol and 0.1% phosphoric acid (55:45)
  Diluent: Methanol
  System suitability solution: 150 µg/mL of USP Methyl Salicylate RS and 3 µg/mL of USP Methyl Salicylate Related Compound A RS in *Diluent*
  Standard solution: 150 µg/mL of USP Methyl Salicylate RS in *Diluent*
  Sample solution: 150 µg/mL of Methyl Salicylate in *Diluent*
  Chromatographic system
  (See *Chromatography* ⟨621⟩, *System Suitability.*)
  Mode: LC
  Detector: UV 237 nm
  Column: 4.6-mm × 7.5-cm; 3.5-µm packing L7
  Column temperature: Ambient
  Flow rate: 1.0 mL/min
  Injection volume: 10 µL
  Run time: 7 min
  System suitability
  Samples: *System suitability solution* and *Standard solution*
  [NOTE—The relative retention times for methyl salicylate and dimethyl 4-hydroxyisophthalate are 1.0 and 1.2, respectively.]

Suitability requirements
 Resolution: NLT 1.5 between methyl salicylate and dimethyl 4-hydroxyisophthalate, *System suitability solution*
 Tailing factor: NMT 1.5 for the methyl salicylate peak, *Standard solution*
 Relative standard deviation: NMT 0.5% for the methyl salicylate peak, *Standard solution*
Analysis
 Samples: *Standard solution* and *Sample solution*
 Calculate the percentage of methyl salicylate in the portion of Methyl Salicylate taken:

$$\text{Result} = (r_U/r_S) \times (C_S/C_U) \times 100$$

r_U = peak response from the *Sample solution*
r_S = peak response from the *Standard solution*
C_S = concentration of USP Methyl Salicylate RS in the *Standard solution* (µg/mL)
C_U = concentration of Methyl Salicylate in the *Sample solution* (µg/mL)
 Acceptance criteria: 98.0%–●102.0%● (RB 1-Aug-2017)

IMPURITIES

Delete the following:

●● **HEAVY METALS,** *Method II* ⟨231⟩: NMT 20 µg/g● (Official 1-Jan-2018)
● **LIMIT OF SALICYLIC ACID AND DIMETHYL 4-HYDROXYISOPHTHALATE**
 Mobile phase, Diluent, Sample solution, and **Chromatographic system:** Proceed as directed in the *Assay*.
 Standard solution: 0.15 µg/mL of USP Salicylic Acid RS, 0.15 µg/mL of USP Methyl Salicylate RS, and 0.75 µg/mL of USP Methyl Salicylate Related Compound A RS in *Diluent*
 System suitability
 Sample: *Standard solution*
 [NOTE—The relative retention times for salicylic acid, methyl salicylate, and dimethyl 4-hydroxyisophthalate are 0.6, 1.0, and 1.2, respectively.]
 Suitability requirements
 Resolution: NLT 4 between salicylic acid and methyl salicylate; NLT 2 between methyl salicylate and dimethyl 4-hydroxyisophthalate
 Relative standard deviation: NMT 3% for all three peaks
 Analysis
 Samples: *Sample solution* and *Standard solution*
 Calculate the percentage of each individual impurity in the portion of Methyl Salicylate taken:

$$\text{Result} = (r_U/r_S) \times (C_S/C_U) \times 100$$

r_U = peak response of salicylic acid or dimethyl 4-hydroxyisophthalate from the *Sample solution*
r_S = peak response of salicylic acid or dimethyl 4-hydroxyisophthalate from the *Standard solution*
C_S = concentration of USP Salicylic Acid RS or USP Methyl Salicylate Related Compound A RS in the *Standard solution* (µg/mL)
C_U = concentration of Methyl Salicylate in the *Sample solution* (µg/mL)
 Acceptance criteria
 Salicylic acid: NMT 0.1%
 Dimethyl 4-hydroxyisophthalate: NMT 0.5%

SPECIFIC TESTS
● **SOLUBILITY IN 70% ALCOHOL:** One volume of synthetic Methyl Salicylate dissolves in seven volumes of 70% alcohol. One volume of natural Methyl Salicylate dissolves in seven volumes of 70% alcohol, the solution shows NMT a slight cloudiness.
● **SPECIFIC GRAVITY** ⟨841⟩: 1.180–1.185 for the synthetic variety; 1.176–1.182 for the natural variety
● **OPTICAL ROTATION** ⟨781A⟩, *Procedures, Angular Rotation*: Synthetic Methyl Salicylate and that from *Betula lenta* are optically inactive. Methyl Salicylate from *Gaultheria procumbens* is slightly levorotatory, the angular rotation not exceeding $-1.5°$ in a 100-mm tube.

ADDITIONAL REQUIREMENTS
● **PACKAGING AND STORAGE:** Preserve in tight containers.
● **LABELING:** Label it to indicate whether it was made synthetically or distilled from either of the plants of *Gaultheria procumbens* or *Betula lenta*.
● **USP REFERENCE STANDARDS** ⟨11⟩
 USP Methyl Salicylate RS
 USP Methyl Salicylate Related Compound A RS
 Dimethyl 4-hydroxyisophthalate.
 $C_{10}H_{10}O_5$ 210.18
 USP Salicylic Acid RS

Polydextrose

[68424-04-4].

DEFINITION
Polydextrose is a randomly branched polymer prepared by melting and subsequent condensation of the ingredients, which consist of approximately 90 parts dextrose, 10 parts sorbitol, and up to 1 part citric acid or 0.1 part phosphoric acid. The 1,6-glycosidic linkage predominates in the polymer but other linkages are present. It contains NLT 90.0% of dextrose polymer units, calculated on the anhydrous and ash-free basis. It contains small quantities of free dextrose, sorbitol, and 1,6-anhydro-D-glucose (levoglucosan), with traces of citric acid or phosphoric acid.

IDENTIFICATION
● **A.** To 1 drop of a solution (1 in 10), add 4 drops of 5% phenol solution, then rapidly add 15 drops of sulfuric acid TS: a deep yellow to orange color is produced.
● **B.** With vigorous swirling, add 1 mL of acetone to 1 mL of a solution (1 in 10): the solution remains clear.
● **C.** With vigorous swirling, add 2 mL of acetone to the solution obtained in *Identification B*: a heavy, milky turbidity develops immediately.
● **D.** To 1 mL of a solution (1 in 50), add 4 mL of alkaline cupric citrate TS. Boil vigorously for 2–4 min. Remove from heat, and allow the precipitate (if any) to settle: the supernatant is blue or blue-green.

Add the following:

■● **E. CHROMATOGRAPHIC IDENTITY**
 Analysis: Proceed as directed in the *Assay*.
 Acceptance criteria: The retention time of the major peak of the *Sample solution* corresponds to that of the *Standard solution*, as obtained in the *Assay*.■1S (NF36)

ASSAY

Change to read:

● **PROCEDURE**
 Mobile phase: 0.001 N sulfuric acid. Pass this solution through a filter of 0.5-µm pore size, and degas.
 Standard solution: 4.0 mg/mL of USP Polydextrose RS ■1S (NF36) in *Mobile phase*

Sample solution: 4.0 mg/mL of Polydextrose, calculated on the anhydrous and ash-free basis, in *Mobile phase*

Chromatographic system

(See *Chromatography* ⟨621⟩, *System Suitability*.)

Mode: LC

Detector: Refractive index

Detector temperature: $35 \pm 0.1°$

Columns

Guard: 4.6-mm × 3.0-cm; packing L17

Analytical: 7.8-mm × 30-cm; packing L17

Flow rate: 0.6 mL/min

Injection volume: 20 µL

System suitability

Sample: *Standard solution*

Suitability requirements

Relative standard deviation: NMT 2.0%

Analysis

Samples: *Standard solution* and *Sample solution*

Calculate the percentage of dextrose polymer units in the portion of Polydextrose taken:

$$\text{Result} = (r_U/r_S) \times (C_S/C_U) \times 100$$

r_U = peak response of dextrose polymer units from the *Sample solution*

r_S = peak response of dextrose polymer units from the *Standard solution*

C_S = concentration of USP Polydextrose RS in the *Standard solution* (mg/mL)

C_U = concentration of Polydextrose in the *Sample solution* (mg/mL)

Acceptance criteria: NLT 90.0%

IMPURITIES

- **RESIDUE ON IGNITION ⟨281⟩:** NMT 0.3%
- **LIMIT OF LEAD**

[NOTE—Use reagent-grade chemicals with as low a lead content as is practicable, as well as high-purity water and gases. Before use in this analysis, rinse all glassware and plasticware twice with 10% nitric acid and twice with 10% hydrochloric acid, and then rinse them thoroughly with Purified Water.]

Matrix modifier solution: Prepare a solution in water containing 100.0 mg of dibasic ammonium phosphate per 10 mL of solution.

Lead nitrate stock solution: Dissolve 159.8 mg of lead nitrate in 100 mL of water to which has been added 1 mL of nitric acid, then dilute with water to 1000 mL. Prepare and store this solution in glass containers free from soluble lead salts.

Standard lead solution: On the day of use, dilute 10.0 mL of *Lead nitrate stock solution* with water to 100.0 mL. Each milliliter of *Standard lead solution* contains the equivalent of 10 µg of lead.

Standard solution A: 0.02 µg/mL of lead, from *Standard lead solution* in water

Standard solution B: 0.05 µg/mL of lead, from *Standard lead solution* in water

Standard solution C: 0.1 µg/mL of lead, from *Standard lead solution* in water

Standard solution D: 0.2 µg/mL of lead, from *Standard lead solution* in water

Standard solution E: 0.5 µg/mL of lead, from *Standard lead solution* in water

Sample solution: Transfer 1.0 g of Polydextrose, weighed and calculated on the anhydrous and ash-free basis, into a 10-mL volumetric flask, and dissolve in and dilute with water to volume.

Spiked sample solution: Transfer 1.0 g of Polydextrose, weighed and calculated on the anhydrous and ash-free basis, into a 10-mL volumetric flask, and dissolve in water. Add 100 µL of the *Standard lead solution*, and dilute with water to volume. This solution contains 0.1 µg/mL of added lead.

Instrumental conditions

(See *Atomic Absorption Spectroscopy* ⟨852⟩.)

Mode: Graphite furnace atomic absorption spectrophotometer, equipped with a pyrolytic tube with a platform

Analytical wavelength: Lead emission line of 283.3 nm

Lamp: A lead hollow-cathode lamp, using a slit width of 0.7 mm (set low) and a deuterium arc lamp for background correction

Autosampler

Sample volume: 10 µL

Alternative volume: 10 µL of *Matrix modifier solution*

Furnace program: For the temperature program, see *Table 1*.

Table 1

Step	Dry	Char	Atomize	Clean	Recharge
Temperature (°)	130	800	2400	2600	20
Ramp time (s)	20	20	0	1	2
Hold time (s)	40	40	6	5	20
Argon flow rate (mL/min)	300	300	50	300	300

Analysis

Samples: 10 µL of the *Matrix modifier solution* was added into each 10-µL aliquot of the five *Standard solutions*, a mixture of 10 µL of the *Matrix modifier solution* and 10 µL of the *Sample solution*, and a mixture of 10 µL of the *Matrix modifier solution* and 10 µL of the *Spiked sample solution*

Concomitantly determine the absorbances of the *Samples* using the *Instrumental conditions* described above. Plot the absorbance of each *Standard solution*, compensated for background correction, versus its content of lead, in µg/mL, and draw the best straight line fitting the five points. From this plot, determine the concentrations, C_T and C_{ST}, in µg/mL, of lead in the *Sample solution* and the *Spiked sample solution*, respectively. Calculate the percentage recovery taken:

$$\text{Result} = [(C_{ST} - C_T)/A] \times 100$$

A = quantity of lead added to the *Spiked sample solution*, 0.1 µg/mL

Calculate the content, in µg/g, of lead in the portion of Polydextrose taken:

$$\text{Result} = (C_T/W) \times V$$

W = weight of Polydextrose taken to prepare the *Sample solution* (g)

V = volume of the *Sample solution*, 10 mL

Acceptance criteria: NMT 0.5 µg/g. The recovery is 80%–120%.

- **ORGANIC IMPURITIES, PROCEDURE 1: LIMIT OF 5-HYDROXYMETHYLFURFURAL AND RELATED COMPOUNDS**

Sample solution: 1.0 g of Polydextrose, weighed and calculated on the anhydrous and ash-free basis, diluted with water to 100 mL

Analysis: Determine the absorbance of the *Sample solution* in a 1-cm quartz cell at 283 nm, with a suitable spectrophotometer, using water as the blank.

Calculate the percentage of 5-hydroxymethylfurfural and related compounds in the Polydextrose taken:

$$\text{Result} = 100 \times (V \times M_r \times A)/(M \times L \times W)$$

V = volume of the *Sample solution*, 0.1 L

M_r = molecular weight of 5-hydroxymethylfurfural, 126 g/mol

A = absorbance of the *Sample solution*

M = molar extinction coefficient of 5-hydroxymethylfurfural at a wavelength of 283 nm, 16,830 L/mol cm

L = path length of the spectrophotometer cell (cm)

W = weight of Polydextrose taken to prepare the *Sample solution* (g)

Acceptance criteria: NMT 0.1%

• **ORGANIC IMPURITIES, PROCEDURE 2: LIMIT OF MONOMERS**

Mobile phase, Sample solution, and **Chromatographic system:** Proceed as directed in the *Assay.*

Standard solution: 0.08 mg/mL each of USP 1,6-Anhydro-D-glucose RS and USP Sorbitol RS, and 0.16 mg/mL of USP Dextrose RS, in *Mobile phase*

System suitability

Sample: *Standard solution*

[NOTE—For relative retention times, see *Table 2.*]

Table 2

Name	Relative Retention Time
Dextrose (glucose)	0.7
Sorbitol	0.8
An isomer of 1,6-anhydro-D-glucose (D-anhydroglucose furanose form)	0.9
1,6-Anhydro-D-glucose (D-anhydroglucose pyranose form)	1.0

Suitability requirements

Resolution: NLT 1.0

Relative standard deviation: NMT 5.0%

Analysis

Samples: *Standard solution* and *Sample solution*

Use peak response of USP 1,6-Anhydro-D-glucose RS in the *Standard solution* for calculation of percentage of the isomer of 1,6-anhydro-D-glucose in the *Sample solution.*

Calculate the percentage of each monomer in the portion of Polydextrose taken:

$$Result = (r_U/r_S) \times (C_S/C_U) \times 100$$

r_U = peak response of the respective monomer from the *Sample solution*

r_S = peak response of the respective monomer from the *Standard solution*

C_S = concentration of the respective standard monomer in the *Standard solution* (mg/mL)

C_U = concentration of Polydextrose in the *Sample solution* (mg/mL)

Acceptance criteria: NMT 4.0% for 1,6-anhydro-D-glucose, NMT 4.0% for dextrose, and NMT 2.0% for sorbitol. [NOTE—In the case of 1,6-anhydro-D-glucose, the peak areas for the pyranose and furanose forms are combined.]

SPECIFIC TESTS

• **MOLECULAR WEIGHT LIMIT**

Mobile phase: Dissolve 35.0 g of sodium nitrate and 1.0 g of sodium azide in 100 mL of water. Dilute with water to 4 L. Pass through a filter of 0.45-μm pore size, and degas by applying an aspirator vacuum for 30 min. The resulting *Mobile phase* is 0.1 N sodium nitrate containing 0.025% sodium azide.

Standard solution: Transfer 20 mg each of USP Dextrose RS, stachyose, and 5800-, 23,700-, and 100,000-molecular weight (MW) pullulan standards into a 10-mL volumetric flask. Dissolve in and dilute with *Mobile phase* to volume. Pass through a syringe filter of 0.45-μm pore size into a suitable autosampler vial, and seal.

Sample solution: Transfer 50 mg of Polydextrose into a 10-mL volumetric flask. Dissolve in and dilute with *Mobile phase* to volume. Pass through a syringe filter of 0.45-μm pore size into a suitable autosampler vial, and seal.

Chromatographic system

(See *Chromatography* ⟨621⟩, *System Suitability.*)

Mode: LC

Detector: Refractive index set at a sensitivity of 4×10^{-6} refractive index units full scale and maintained at a temperature of $35 \pm 0.1°$

Column: 7.8-mm × 30-cm; packing L39

Column temperature: 45°

Flow rate: 0.8 mL/min

[NOTE—After installation of a new column, pump *Mobile phase* through the column overnight at a rate of 0.3 mL/min. Before calibration or analysis, increase the flow slowly over a 1-min period to 0.8 mL/min. Continue to pump *Mobile phase* through the column at this flow rate for at least 1 h before the first injection. Check the flow gravimetrically, and adjust it if necessary. Reduce the flow rate to about 0.1 mL/min when the system is not in use.]

Injection volume: 50 μL

System suitability

Sample: *Standard solution*

[NOTE—The retention times for each component determined on replicate injections agree within ±2 s.]

Chromatograph five replicate injections of the *Standard solution*, allowing 15 min between injections, and record the retention times of the components of the *Standard solution.*

Insert the average retention time along with the molecular weight of each component in the *Standard solution* into the calibration table of the molecular weight distribution software. Check the regression results for a cubic fit of the calibration points, and obtain a *Correlation coefficient R*, for the line.

Suitability requirements

Resolution: Dextrose and stachyose are baseline resolved from one another and from the 5800-MW pullulan standard.

[NOTE—Prominent negative baseline valleys are usually observed between the peaks for the 5800-; 23,700-; and 100,000-MW pullulan standards.]

Correlation coefficient R: NLT 0.9999

Analysis

Samples: *Standard solution* and *Sample solution*

Use the molecular weight distribution software of the data reduction system to generate a molecular weight distribution plot of Polydextrose.

Acceptance criteria: No measurable peak above a molecular weight of 22,000 is found.

• **PH** ⟨791⟩: 2.5–5.0, in a solution (1 in 10)

• **WATER DETERMINATION** ⟨921⟩, *Method I*: NMT 4.0%. Use a mixture of Hydranal solvent and Hydranal formamide dry (2:1) as a solvent. Perform the titration at 50° in a jacketed beaker.

ADDITIONAL REQUIREMENTS

• **PACKAGING AND STORAGE:** Preserve in tight, light-resistant containers. Store in a cool and dry place.

- **USP REFERENCE STANDARDS ⟨11⟩**
  USP 1,6-Anhydro-D-glucose RS
  USP Dextrose RS
  USP Polydextrose RS
  USP Sorbitol RS

Squalane

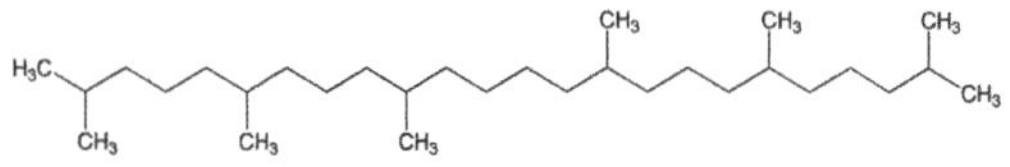

$C_{30}H_{62}$ 422.81
Tetracosane, 2,6,10,15,19,23-hexamethyl-;
2,6,10,15,19,23-Hexamethyltetracosane [111-01-3].

DEFINITION

Change to read:

■Squalane is a saturated hydrocarbon that contains NLT
97.0% and NMT 102.0% of 2,6,10,15,19,23-hex-
amethyltetracosane ($C_{30}H_{62}$). It is obtained either by hydrogenation of squalene, an aliphatic triterpene derived
from certain fish oils, particularly shark liver oil, or from β-
farnesene, a fermentation product of plant sugars.■1S (NF36)

IDENTIFICATION
- **A. INFRARED ABSORPTION ⟨197F⟩**
  Sample: Undried specimen
  Acceptance criteria: Meets the requirements
- **B. CHROMATOGRAPHIC IDENTITY**
  Analysis: Proceed as directed in the *Assay*.
  Acceptance criteria: The retention time of the major
  peak of the *Sample solution*, excluding the solvent peak,
  corresponds to that of the *Standard solution*, as ob-
  tained in the *Assay*.

ASSAY
- **PROCEDURE**
  Diluent: *n*-Heptane
  System suitability solution: 4 mg/mL of USP Squalane
  RS and 4 µL/mL of methyl erucate in *Diluent*
  Standard solution: 4 mg/mL of USP Squalane RS in
  Diluent
  Sample solution: 4 mg/mL of Squalane in *Diluent*
  Chromatographic system
  (See *Chromatography* ⟨621⟩, *System Suitability*.)
  Mode: GC
  Detector: Flame ionization
  Column: 0.32-mm × 30-m fused silica capillary; coated
  with a 1-µm film of phase G2
  Temperatures
  Injection port: 275°
  Detector: 300°
  Column: See *Table 1*.

Table 1

Initial Temperature (°)	Temperature Ramp (°/min)	Final Temperature (°)	Hold Time at Final Temperature (min)
60	5.9	290	11

Carrier gas: Helium
Flow rate: 1.7 mL/min
Injection volume: 1 µL
Injection type: Split; split ratio, 12:1
Liner: General purpose split/splitless liner with deacti-
vated wool
System suitability
Samples: *System suitability solution* and *Standard
solution*
[NOTE—The relative retention times for methyl erucate
and squalane are 0.9 and 1.0, respectively.]
Suitability requirements
Resolution: NLT 5 between the peaks due to methyl
erucate and squalane, *System suitability solution*
Relative standard deviation: NMT 2%, *Standard
solution*
Analysis
Samples: *Standard solution* and *Sample solution*
Calculate the percentage of squalane ($C_{30}H_{62}$) in the
portion of Squalane taken:

$$Result = (r_U/r_S) \times (C_S/C_U) \times 100$$

r_U = peak area from the *Sample solution*
r_S = peak area from the *Standard solution*
C_S = concentration of USP Squalane RS in the
       Standard solution (mg/mL)
C_U = concentration of Squalane in the *Sample
       solution* (mg/mL)
Acceptance criteria: 97.0%–102.0%

IMPURITIES
- **RESIDUE ON IGNITION ⟨281⟩:** NMT 0.5%

SPECIFIC TESTS
- **SPECIFIC GRAVITY ⟨841⟩:** 0.807–0.810 at 20°
- **FATS AND FIXED OILS ⟨401⟩,** *Procedures, Acid Value*: NMT
  0.2
- **FATS AND FIXED OILS ⟨401⟩,** *Procedures, Iodine Value*: NMT
  4
- **FATS AND FIXED OILS ⟨401⟩,** *Procedures, Saponification
  Value*: NMT 2
- **REFRACTIVE INDEX ⟨831⟩:** 1.4510–1.4525 at 20°

ADDITIONAL REQUIREMENTS
- **PACKAGING AND STORAGE:** Preserve in tight containers.

Add the following:

■• **LABELING:** Label to indicate whether it is derived from
animal or plant sources.■1S (NF36)
- **USP REFERENCE STANDARDS ⟨11⟩**
  USP Squalane RS

Reagents, Indicators, And Solutions

1. SCOPE

Reagents required in the tests and assay for *U.S. Pharmacopeia* and *National Formulary* articles and those required only in determining the quality of other reagents are listed in this section, with specifications appropriate to their intended uses.

As stated in *General Notices, 6.70 Reagents*, listing of reagents, indicators, and solutions in the *U.S. Pharmacopeia* in no way implies that they have therapeutic utility; thus, any reference to *USP* or *NF* in their labeling shall include also the term "reagent" or "reagent grade".

Where a particular brand or source of a material, instrument, or piece of equipment, or the name and address of a manufacturer or distributor, is mentioned (ordinarily in a note or footnote), this identification is furnished solely for informational purposes as a matter of convenience, without implication of approval, endorsement, or certification.

1.1 ACS (American Chemical Society) Reagent Grade

Where it is directed to "Use ACS reagent grade", it is intended that a grade meeting the corresponding specifications of the current edition of *Reagent Chemicals*, published by the American Chemical Society (ACS), shall be used.

1.2 Suitable Grade

In the cases where no ACS reagent monograph exists or if the reagent is available in different quality grades, each one specific for a particular application, it is directed to "Use a suitable grade". The intent is that a suitable reagent grade available commercially shall be used.

Occasionally, additional test(s) augment the designation "suitable grade", as indicated in the text. Listed also are some, but not all, reagents that are required only in determining the quality of other reagents. For those reagents that are not listed, satisfactory specifications are available in standard reference publications.

1.3 *USP* or *NF* or *FCC* Grade

In the instances in which a reagent required in a *U.S. Pharmacopeia* or *National Formulary* test or assay meets the requirements in the monograph for that article appearing in this *U.S. Pharmacopeia* or the *National Formulary* or the current edition of the *Food Chemicals Codex* (*FCC*), it suffices to refer to the corresponding monograph in one of the these three compendia. In such cases it is to be understood that the specifications are minimum requirements and that any substance meeting more rigid specifications for chemical purity is suitable.

2. PACKAGING AND STORAGE

Reagents and solutions should be preserved in tight containers made of resistant glass or other suitable material. Directions for storage in light-resistant containers should be carefully observed.

Stoppers and stopcocks brought into contact with substances capable of attacking or penetrating their surfaces may be given a protective coating of a thin film of a suitable lubricant unless specifically interdicted.

3. METAL-ION STANDARD SOLUTIONS

Atomic absorption and flame photometry require the use of a number of metal-ion standard solutions. While the individual monographs usually provide directions for preparation of these solutions, use of commercially prepared standardized solutions of the appropriate ions is permissible, provided that the analyst confirms the suitability of the solutions and has data to support their use.

4. DEFINITIONS

4.1 Reagents: Reagents are substances used either as such or as constituents of solutions.

4.2 Indicators: Indicators are reagents used to determine the specified endpoint in a chemical reaction, to measure hydrogen-ion concentration (pH), or to indicate that a desired change in pH has been effected. They are listed together with indicator test papers.

4.3 Buffer Solutions: Buffer solutions resist changes in the activity of an ion on the addition of substances that are expected to change the activity of that ion.

4.4 Colorimetric Solutions (CS): Colorimetric solutions are solutions used in the preparation of colorimetric standards for comparison purposes.

4.5 Test Solutions (TS): Test solutions are solutions of reagents in such solvents and of such definite concentrations as to be suitable for the specified purposes.

4.6 Volumetric Solutions (VS): Volumetric solutions are solutions of reagents of known concentration intended primarily for use in quantitative determinations.

5. CHROMATOGRAPHIC SOLVENTS AND CARRIER GASES

The chromatographic procedures set forth in the *U.S. Pharmacopeia* may require use of solvents and gases that have been especially purified for such use. The purpose may be (a) to exclude certain impurities that interfere with the proper conduct of the test procedure, or (b) to extend the life of a column by reducing the buildup of impurities on the column. Where solvents and gases are called for in chromatographic procedures, it is the responsibility of the analyst to ensure the suitability of the solvent or gas for the specific use. Solvents and gases suitable for specific high-pressure or other chromatographic uses are available as specialty products from various reagent supply houses, although there is no assurance that similar products from different suppliers are of equivalent suitability in any given procedure.

Reagents

1. DEFINITIONS

1.1 Blank
A blank consists of the same quantities of the same reagents treated in the same manner as the specimen under test.

1.2 Control
A control is a blank to which has been added the limiting quantity of the substance being tested for, or is a specified comparison solution prepared as directed in the particular test.

2. DESCRIPTION OF THE REAGENT ENTRY

See *Figure 1*.

3. VISUAL COMPARISONS

For color and turbidity comparisons, proceed as directed in *Nephelometry, Turbidimetry, and Visual Comparison* ⟨855⟩, *Visual Comparison*. The tubes used in this procedure are frequently called "Nessler tubes".

In making visual comparisons of the densities of turbid fluids, compensate for difference in color, if necessary, by viewing the turbidity through a column of water, the depth of which is determined by the volume specified in the individual reagent specification. Place the water in color-comparison tubes, and hold one of the tubes above the control tube and the other below the specimen tube.

4. RETAIN THE FILTRATE

"Retain the filtrate" is to be understood, unless otherwise indicated, that the washings of the residue are not to be added to the filtrate obtained.

5. EXPRESSION R₂O₃

The expression R_2O_3 is intended to indicate the residue on ignition from compounds precipitated upon the addition of ammonium hydroxide, such as iron oxide (Fe_2O_3) and aluminum oxide (Al_2O_3).

6. GENERAL TESTS FOR REAGENTS

The following general test methods are provided for the examination of reagents to determine their compliance with the specifications of the individual reagents and are to be used unless it is otherwise directed in such specifications.

6.1 Boiling or Distilling Range for Reagents
Use the following procedure for determining the boiling or distilling range of reagents, unless otherwise directed in the individual specifications:

APPARATUS: Use apparatus similar to that specified for *Distilling Range* ⟨721⟩, *Method I*, except that the distilling flask is to be of 250-mL capacity, to have a short neck, and to be connected to the condenser by means of a three-way connecting tube fitted with standard-taper ground joints.

PROCEDURE: Place the distilling flask in an upright position in the perforation in the asbestos board, and connect it to the condenser.

Measure 100 mL of the liquid to be tested in a graduated cylinder, and transfer to the boiling flask together with some device to prevent bumping. Use the cylinder as the receiver for the distillate. Insert the thermometer, and heat so as to distill at the rate of 3–5 mL/min. Make a preliminary trial, if necessary, to determine the adjustment for the proper rate of heating. Read the thermometer when about 20 drops have distilled and thereafter at volumes of distillate of 5, 10, 40, 50, 60, 90, and 95 mL. Continue the distillation until the dry point is reached.

The *Boiling or Distilling Range* is the interval between the temperatures when 1 mL and 95 mL, respectively, have distilled.

6.2 Amino Nitrogen Test in Reagents
Determine the percentage of loss on drying of the sample in appropriate conditions. Transfer about 500 mg of the sample to a 100-mL beaker. Add 20 mL of water. Adjust the pH potentiometrically with 0.1 N hydrochloric acid or 0.2 N sodium hydroxide to 6.0. Add 10 mL of formaldehyde solution. Titrate the solution potentiometrically with 0.2 N sodium hydroxide to a pH of 9.0. Calculate the percentage of amino nitrogen:

$$\% \text{ amino nitrogen} = \frac{V_{NaOH} \times N_{NaOH} \times 14 \times 100 \times f}{\text{mg sample} \times (1.0 - \%LOD/100)}$$

where f is the correction factor obtained in the standardization of 0.2 N sodium hydroxide and %LOD is the percentage of loss on drying.

6.3 Arsenic in Reagents
Select reagents for this test for a low arsenic content, so that a blank test results in either no stain or one that is barely perceptible.

APPARATUS: Prepare a generator by fitting a 1-hole rubber stopper into a wide-mouth bottle of about 60-mL capacity. Through the perforation insert a vertical exit tube about 12 cm in total length and 1 cm in diameter along the entire upper portion (for about 8 cm) and constricted at its lower extremity to a tube about 4 cm in length and about 5 mm in diameter. The smaller portion of the tube should extend to just slightly below the stopper. Place washed sand or a pledget of purified cotton in the upper portion to about 3 cm from the top of the tube. Moisten the sand or cotton uniformly with lead acetate TS, and remove any excess or adhering droplets of the latter from the walls of the tube. Into the upper end of this tube fit a second glass tube 12 cm in length, with an internal diameter of 2.5–3 mm, by means of a rubber stopper. Just before running the test, place a strip of mercuric bromide test paper (see *Indicator and Test Papers*) in this tube, crimping the upper end of the strip so that it will remain in position about 2 cm above the rubber stopper. Clean and dry the tube thoroughly each time it is used.

STANDARD ARSENIC SOLUTION: Use the *Standard Preparation*, prepared as directed in *Arsenic* ⟨211⟩.

TEST PREPARATION: Add 1 mL of sulfuric acid to 5 mL of a solution of the chemical substance (1 in 25), unless another quantity is directed in the individual reagent specification. Omit its addition entirely in the case of inorganic acids. Unless especially directed otherwise, add 10 mL of sulfurous acid. Evaporate the liquid in a small beaker, on a steam bath, until it is free from sulfurous acid and has been reduced to about 2 mL in volume. Dilute with water to 5 mL to obtain the *Test preparation*. Substances subjected to special treatments specified in the individual reagent specification may be used directly as the *Test preparation*. [NOTE—Solutions prepared by the dissolving of the chemical substances in dilute acids are not considered to have undergone special treatment.]

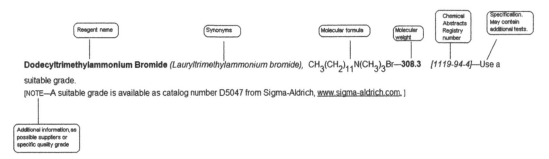

Figure 1. Components of the reagent entry.

STANDARD STAIN: Place in the generator bottle 5 mL of potassium iodide TS, 2.0 mL of *Standard arsenic solution*, 5 mL of acid stannous chloride TS, and 28 mL of water. Add 1.5 g of granulated zinc (in No. 20 powder), and immediately insert the stopper containing the exit tube. Keep the generator bottle immersed in water at 25° during the period of the test to moderate the reaction so that the stain will take the form of a distinctive band to facilitate the comparison of color intensity. When evolution of hydrogen has continued for 1 h, remove the mercuric bromide test paper for comparison. This stain represents 2 µg of arsenic.

PROCEDURE: Pipet into the generator bottle 5 mL of potassium iodide TS and 5 mL of the *Test preparation*, and add 5 mL of acid stannous chloride TS. Set the apparatus aside at room temperature for a period of 10 min, then add 25 mL of water and 1.5 g of granulated zinc (in No. 20 powder), and proceed as directed for the *Standard stain*. Remove the mercuric bromide test paper, and compare the stain upon it with the *Standard stain*: the stain produced by the chemical tested does not exceed the *Standard stain* in length or in intensity of color, indicating NMT 10 parts of arsenic per million parts of the substance being tested. Because light, heat, and moisture cause the stain to fade rapidly, place the papers in clean, dry tubes, and make comparisons promptly.

INTERFERING CHEMICALS: *Antimony*, if present in the substance being tested, produces a gray stain. *Sulfites, sulfides, thiosulfates*, and other compounds that liberate hydrogen sulfide or sulfur dioxide when treated with sulfuric acid must be oxidized by means of nitric acid and then reduced by means of sulfur dioxide as directed for the *Test preparation* before they are placed in the apparatus. Certain *sulfur compounds*, as well as *phosphine*, give a bright yellow band on the test paper. If sulfur compounds are present, the lead acetate-moistened cotton or sand will darken. In that case, repeat the operation as directed for the *Test preparation* upon a fresh portion of the solution being tested, and use greater care in effecting the complete removal of the sulfurous acid. In testing hypophosphites, observe special care to oxidize completely the solution being tested as directed; otherwise the evolution of phosphine may result in a yellow stain that may be confused with the orange-yellow color produced by arsine. The stain produced by phosphine may be differentiated from that given by arsine by means of moistening it with 6 N ammonium hydroxide. A stain caused by arsine becomes dark when so treated, but a stain produced by phosphine does not materially change in color.

6.4 Chloride in Reagents

STANDARD CHLORIDE SOLUTION: Dissolve 165.0 mg of dried sodium chloride in water to make 1000.0 mL. This solution contains the equivalent of 0.10 mg of chlorine (Cl) in each mL.

PROCEDURE: Neutralize, if alkaline, a solution of the quantity of the reagent indicated in the test in 25 mL of water, or a solution prepared as directed in the test, with nitric acid, litmus paper being used as the indicator, and add 3 mL more of nitric acid. Filter the solution, if necessary, through a filter paper previously washed with water until

the paper is free from chloride, and add 1 mL of silver nitrate TS. Mix, and allow to stand for 5 min protected from direct sunlight. Compare the turbidity, if any, with that produced in a control made with the same quantities of the same reagents as in the final test and a volume of *Standard chloride solution* equivalent to the quantity of chloride (Cl) permitted by the test. Adjust the two solutions with water to the same volume before adding the silver nitrate TS, and compare the turbidities.

In *testing barium salts*, neutralize, if alkaline, the solution containing the reagent, with nitric acid, and add only 3 drops more of nitric acid. Conduct the remainder of the test as described previously.

In *testing salts giving colored solutions*, dissolve 2 g of the reagent in 25 mL of water, and add 3 mL of nitric acid. Filter the solution, if necessary, through a filter paper previously washed with water, and divide the filtrate into two equal portions. Treat one portion with 1 mL of silver nitrate TS, allow to stand for 10 min, and, if any turbidity is produced, filter it through a washed filter paper until clear, and use the filtrate as a blank. Treat the other portion with 1 mL of silver nitrate TS, mix, and allow to stand for 5 min protected from direct sunlight. Compare the turbidity with that produced in the blank by the addition of a volume of *Standard chloride solution* equivalent to the quantity of chloride (Cl) permitted in the test, both solutions being adjusted with water to the same volume.

6.5 Flame Photometry for Reagents

The use of flame photometric procedures to determine traces of calcium, potassium, sodium, and strontium is called for in some of the reagent specifications. The suitability of such determinations depends upon the use of adequate apparatus, and several instruments of suitable selectivity are available. The preferred type of flame photometer is one that has a red-sensitive phototube, a multiplier phototube, a monochromator, an adjustable slit-width control, a selector switch, and a sensitivity control. Other types of photometers may be used, provided the operator has proved that the instrument will determine accurately the amount of impurities permitted in the reagent to be tested.

The flame photometric procedures depend upon the use of semi-internal standards, and thus require both a *Sample solution* and a *Control solution*. For the *Sample solution*, a specified weight of specimen is dissolved and diluted to a definite volume. For the *Control solution*, the same amount of specimen is dissolved, the limiting amounts of the suspected impurities are added, and the solution is then diluted to the same definite volume as the *Sample solution*. The flame photometer is set as directed in the general procedures and then adjusted to give an emission reading as near 100% transmittance as is possible with the *Control solution* at the wavelength specified for the particular impurity concerned. With the instrument settings left unchanged, the emission from the *Sample solution* is read at the same wavelength and at a specified background wavelength. The background reading is then used to correct the observed emission of the *Sample solution* for the emission due to the specimen and the solvent. The specimen being tested contains less than the specified limit of impurity if the difference between the observed background and total emissions for the *Sample solution* is less than the difference between the observed emissions for the *Control solution* and the *Sample solution* at the wavelength designated for the particular impurity.

CALCIUM IN REAGENTS

Standard calcium solution: Dissolve 250 mg of calcium carbonate in a mixture of 20 mL of water and 5 mL of diluted hydrochloric acid, and when solution is complete, dilute with water to 1 L. This solution contains 0.10 mg of calcium (Ca) per mL.

Procedure: Use the *Sample solution* and the *Control solution* prepared as directed in the individual test procedure.

Set the slit-width control of a suitable flame photometer at 0.03 mm, and set the selector switch at 0.1. Adjust the instrument to give the maximum emission with the *Control solution* at the 422.7-nm calcium line, and record the transmittance. Without changing any of the instrument settings, record the transmittance for the emission of the *Sample solution* at 422.7 nm. Change the monochromator to the wavelength specified in the individual test procedure, and record the background transmittance for the background emission of the *Sample solution*: the difference between the transmittances for the *Sample solution* at 422.7 nm and at the background wavelength is not greater than the difference between transmittances observed at 422.7 nm for the *Sample solution* and the *Control solution*.

POTASSIUM IN REAGENTS

Standard potassium solution: Dissolve 191 mg of potassium chloride in a few mL of water, and dilute with water to 1 L. Dilute a portion of this solution with water in the ratio of 1:10 to obtain a concentration of 0.01 mg of potassium (K) per mL.

Procedure: Use the *Sample solution* and the *Control solution* prepared as directed in the individual test procedure. [NOTE—In testing calcium salts, use an oxyhydrogen burner.]

Set the slit-width control of a suitable flame photometer equipped with a red-sensitive detector at 0.1 mm, unless otherwise directed, and set the selector switch at 0.1. Adjust the instrument to give the maximum emission with the *Control solution* at the 766.5-nm potassium line, and record the transmittance. Without changing any of the instrument settings, record the transmittance for the emission of the *Sample solution* at 766.5 nm. Change the monochromator to 750 nm, and record the background transmittance for the background emission of the *Sample solution*: the difference between the transmittances for the *Sample solution* at 766.5 and 750 nm is not greater than the difference between transmittances observed at 766.5 nm for the *Sample solution* and the *Control solution*.

SODIUM IN REAGENTS

Standard sodium solution: Dissolve 254 mg of sodium chloride in a few mL of water, and dilute with water to 1 L. Dilute a portion of this solution with water in the ratio of 1:10 to obtain a concentration of 0.01 mg of sodium (Na) per mL.

Procedure: Use the *Sample solution* and the *Control solution* prepared as directed in the individual test procedure.

Set the slit-width control of a suitable flame photometer at 0.01 mm, and set the selector switch at 0.1. Adjust the instrument to give the maximum emission with the *Control solution* at the 589-nm sodium line, and record the transmittance. Without changing any of the instrument settings, record the transmittance for the emission of the *Sample solution* at 589 nm. Change the monochromator to 580 nm, and record the background transmittance for the background emission of the *Sample solution*: the difference between the transmittances for the *Sample solution* at 589 and 580 nm is not greater than the difference between transmittances observed at 589 nm for the *Sample solution* and the *Control solution*.

STRONTIUM IN REAGENTS

Standard strontium solution: Dissolve 242 mg of strontium nitrate in a few mL of water, and dilute with water to 1 L. Dilute a portion of this solution with water in the ratio of 1:10 to obtain a concentration of 0.01 mg of strontium (Sr) per mL.

Procedure: Use the *Sample solution* and the *Control solution* prepared as directed in the individual test procedure.

Set the slit-width control of a suitable flame photometer at 0.03 mm, and set the selector switch at 0.1. Adjust the instrument to give the maximum emission with the *Control solution* at the 460.7-nm strontium line, and record the transmittance. Without changing any of the instrument settings, record the transmittance for the emission of the *Sample solution* at 460.7 nm. Change the monochromator to the wavelength specified in the individual test procedure, and record the background transmittance for the background emission of the *Sample solution*: the difference between the transmittances for the *Sample solution* at 460.7 nm and at the background wavelength is not greater than the difference between transmittances observed at 460.7 nm for the *Sample solution* and the *Control solution*.

6.6 Heavy Metals in Reagents

STANDARD LEAD SOLUTION: Use standard lead solution TS. Each mL of this solution contains the equivalent of 0.01 mg of lead (Pb).

PROCEDURE: Unless otherwise directed, test for heavy metals as follows:

(*a*) If the heavy metals limit is 0.0005% (5 ppm), dissolve 6.0 g of the specimen in water to make 42 mL.

(*b*) If the heavy metals limit is 0.001% (10 ppm) or more, or in the event of limited solubility, use 4 g, and dissolve in water to make 40 mL, warming, if necessary, to aid solution.

For the control, transfer 7 mL of the solution from (*a*) to a color-comparison tube, and add a volume of *Standard lead solution* equivalent to the amount of lead permitted in 4 g of the reagent. Dilute with water to 35 mL, and add diluted acetic acid, or ammonia TS, until the pH is about 3.5, determined potentiometrically, then dilute with water to 40 mL, and mix. Transfer the remaining 35 mL of the solution from (*a*) to a color-comparison tube closely matching that used for the control, and add diluted acetic acid, or ammonia TS, until the pH is about 3.5, determined potentiometrically, then dilute with water to 40 mL, and mix. Then to each tube add 10 mL of hydrogen sulfide TS, mix, and compare the colors by viewing through the color-comparison tube downward against a white surface. The color in the test specimen is not darker than that of the control.

If the solution of the reagent is prepared as in (*b*), use for the control 10 mL of the solution, and add to it a volume of *Standard lead solution* equivalent to the amount of lead permitted in 2 g of the reagent. Dilute the remaining 30 mL of solution (*b*) with water to 35 mL, and proceed as directed in the preceding paragraph, beginning with "add diluted acetic acid, or ammonia TS," in the second sentence.

If the reagent to be tested for heavy metals is a salt of an aliphatic organic acid, substitute 1 N hydrochloric acid for the diluted acetic acid specified in the foregoing method.

6.7 Insoluble Matter in Reagents

Dissolve the quantity of reagent specified in the test in 100 mL of water, heat to boiling unless otherwise directed, in a covered beaker, and warm on a steam bath for 1 h. Filter the hot solution through a tared sintered-glass crucible of fine porosity. Wash the beaker and the filter thoroughly with hot water, dry at 105°, cool in a desiccator, and weigh.

6.8 Loss on Drying for Reagents

Determine as directed in *Loss on Drying* ⟨731⟩.

6.9 Nitrate in Reagents

STANDARD NITRATE SOLUTION: Dissolve 163 mg of potassium nitrate in water, add water to make 100 mL, and dilute 10 mL of this solution with water to 1 L to obtain a solution containing the equivalent of 0.01 mg of nitrate (NO₃) per mL.

BRUCINE SULFATE SOLUTION: Dissolve 600 mg of brucine sulfate in 600 mL of nitrate-free, dilute sulfuric acid (2 in 3) that previously has been cooled to room temperature, and dilute with the acid to 1 L. [NOTE—Prepare the nitrate-free sulfuric acid by adding 4 parts of sulfuric acid to 1 part of water, heating the solution to dense fumes of sulfur trioxide, and cooling. Repeat the dilution and heating three or four times.]

SAMPLE SOLUTION: To the weight of sample specified in the individual reagent specification, dissolved in the designated volume of water, add Brucine sulfate solution to make 50 mL.

CONTROL SOLUTION: To a volume of Standard nitrate solution equivalent to the weight of nitrate (NO₃) specified in the individual reagent specification, add the weight of sample specified in the individual reagent specification, and then add Brucine sulfate solution to make 50 mL.

BLANK SOLUTION: Use 50 mL of Brucine sulfate solution.

PROCEDURE: Heat the Sample solution, Control solution, and Blank solution in a boiling water bath for 10 min, then cool rapidly in an ice bath to room temperature. Adjust a suitable spectrophotometer to zero absorbance at 410 nm with the Blank solution. Determine the absorbance of the Sample solution, note the result, and adjust the instrument to zero absorbance with the Sample solution. Determine the absorbance of the Control solution: the absorbance reading for the Sample solution does not exceed that for the Control solution.

6.10 Nitrogen Compounds in Reagents

PROCEDURE: Unless otherwise directed, test for nitrogen compounds as follows: dissolve the specified quantity of test specimen in 60 mL of ammonia-free water in a Kjeldahl flask connected through a spray trap to a condenser, the end of which dips below the surface of 10 mL of 0.1 N hydrochloric acid. Add 10 mL of freshly boiled sodium hydroxide solution (1 in 10) and 500 mg of aluminum wire, in small pieces, to the Kjeldahl flask, and allow to stand for 1 h, protected from loss of and exposure to ammonia. Distill 35 mL, and dilute the distillate with water to 50 mL. Add 2 mL of freshly boiled sodium hydroxide solution (1 in 10), mix, add 2 mL of alkaline mercuric–potassium iodide TS, and again mix: the color produced is not darker than that of a control containing the amount of added N (as ammonium chloride) specified in the individual test procedure.

6.11 Phosphate in Reagents

STANDARD PHOSPHATE SOLUTION: Dissolve 143.3 mg of dried monobasic potassium phosphate (KH₂PO₄) in water to make 1000.0 mL. This solution contains the equivalent of 0.10 mg of phosphate (PO₄) in each mL.

PHOSPHATE REAGENT A: Dissolve 5 g of ammonium molybdate in 1 N sulfuric acid to make 100 mL.

PHOSPHATE REAGENT B: Dissolve 200 mg of p-methylaminophenol sulfate in 100 mL of water, and add 20 g of sodium bisulfite. Store this reagent in well-filled, tightly stoppered bottles, and use within 1 month.

PROCEDURE: [NOTE—The tests with the specimen and the control are made preferably in matched color-comparison tubes.] Dissolve the quantity of the reagent specified in the test, or the residue obtained after the prescribed treatment, in 20 mL of water, by warming, if necessary, add 2.5 mL of dilute sulfuric acid (1 in 7), and dilute with water to 25 mL. (If preferable, the test specimen or the residue may be dissolved in 25 mL of approximately 0.5 N sulfuric acid.) Then add 1 mL each of Phosphate reagents A and B, mix, and allow to stand at room temperature for 2 h. Compare any blue color produced with that produced in a control made with the same quantities of the same reagents as in the test with the specimen, and a volume of Standard phosphate solution equivalent to the quantity of phosphate (PO₄) designated in the reagent specifications.

6.12 Residue on Ignition in Reagents

PROCEDURE: Unless otherwise directed, determine the residue on ignition as follows: accurately weigh 1–2 g of the substance to be tested in a suitable crucible that previously has been ignited, cooled, and weighed. Ignite the substance, gently and slowly at first and then at a more rapid rate, until it is thoroughly charred, if organic in nature, or until it is completely volatilized, if inorganic in nature. If the use of sulfuric acid is specified, cool the crucible, add the specified amount of acid, and ignite the crucible gently until fumes no longer are evolved. Then ignite the crucible at 800 ± 25°, cool in a suitable desiccator, and weigh. If the use of sulfuric acid is not specified, the crucible need not be cooled but can be ignited directly at 800 ± 25° once the charring or volatilization is complete. Continue the ignition until constant weight is attained, unless otherwise specified.

Conduct the ignition in a well-ventilated hood, but protected from air currents, and at as low a temperature as is possible to effect the complete combustion of the carbon. A muffle furnace may be used, if desired, and its use is recommended for the final ignition at 800 ± 25°.

6.13 Sulfate in Reagents

STANDARD SULFATE SOLUTION: Dissolve 181.4 mg of potassium sulfate (dried at 105° for 2 h) in water to make 1000 mL. This solution contains the equivalent of 0.10 mg of sulfate (SO₄) per mL.

PROCEDURE

Method I: Neutralize, if necessary, a solution of the quantity of the reagent or residue indicated in the test in 25 mL of water, or a solution prepared as directed in the test, with hydrochloric acid or with ammonia TS, litmus paper being used as the indicator, and add 1 mL of 1 N hydrochloric acid. Filter the solution, if necessary, through a filter paper previously washed with water, and add 2 mL of barium chloride TS. Mix, allow to stand for 10 min, and compare the turbidity, if any, with that produced in a control containing the same quantities of the same reagents used in the test and a quantity of Standard sulfate solution equivalent to the quantity of sulfate (SO₄) permitted in the test. Adjust the two solutions with water to the same volume before adding the barium chloride TS.

Method II: Heat the solution to boiling, prepared as directed in the individual test procedure, or the filtrate designated in the procedure, and add 5 mL of barium chloride TS. Then digest the solution on a steam bath for 2 h, and allow to stand overnight. If any precipitate is formed, filter the solution through paper, wash the residue with hot water, and transfer the paper containing the residue to a tared crucible. Char the paper, without burning, and ignite the crucible and its contents to constant weight. Perform a blank determination concurrently with the test specimen determination, and subtract the weight of residue obtained from that obtained in the test specimen determination to obtain the weight of residue attributable to the sulfate content of the specimen.

REAGENT SPECIFICATIONS

Add the following:

■**Ammonium Hydrogen Difluoride,** (NH₄)HF₂—**57.04** [1341-49-7]—Use a suitable grade.■₁S (USP41)

Add the following:

■**Benzil** (Dibenzoyl; Diphenylethanedione), C₁₄H₁₀O₂—**210.23** [134-81-6]—Use a suitable grade with a content of NLT 98%.■₁S (USP41)

Delete the following:

■**Blood Group A₁ Red Blood Cells and Blood Group B Red Blood Cells:** These cells must be obtained from manufacturers or suppliers licensed by the Center for Biologics Evaluation and Research/Food and Drug Administration. The use of reagents from an unlicensed manufacturer or supplier may invalidate the results. Generally, they are available as part of a kit for ABO Blood Group testing. The cells licensed for use in test tubes can also be used in the microtiter plate method described in the monographs of *Red Blood Cells* and *Whole Blood.*

[NOTE—There are many manufacturers and suppliers of these reagents that are licensed by the Center for Biologics Evaluation and Research Food and Drug Administration. Some examples of licensed manufacturers or suppliers are the following: Gamma Biologics, Houston, TX; and Ortho Diagnostics, Raritan, NJ.]■1S (*USP41*)

Change to read:

Cadmium Nitrate, $Cd(NO_3)_2 \cdot 4H_2O$—**308.48** ■[10022-68-1]—Use ACS reagent grade Cadmium Nitrate Tetrahydrate.■1S (*USP41*)

Add the following:

■**2-Chlorobenzophenone,** $C_{13}H_9ClO$—**216.66** [5162-03-8]—Use a suitable grade with a content of NLT 99%.■1S (*USP41*)

Change to read:

2-Chloroethylamine Monohydrochloride ■*(2-Chloroethylamine Hydrochloride; 2-Aminoethyl Chloride Hydrochloride),* ■1S (*USP41*) $C_2H_6ClN \cdot HCl$—**115.99**—Off-white powder.
ASSAY: The area of the 2-chloroethylamine monohydrochloride ($C_2H_6ClN \cdot HCl$) peak is NLT 99% of the total peak area.
Inject an appropriate specimen into a gas chromatograph (see *Chromatography* ⟨621⟩). The following conditions have been found suitable.
Detector: Flame ionization
Column: 0.25-mm × 30-m capillary; ■phase G46■1S (*USP41*)
Temperatures
Injection port: 150°
Column: 50°, programmed to rise 10°/min to 200°
Detector: 300°
Carrier gas: Helium
■■1S (*USP41*)

Delete the following:

■**Cupric Nitrate Hydrate,** $Cu(NO_3)_2 \cdot 2.5H_2O$—**232.59** [19004-19-4]; $Cu(NO_3)_2 \cdot 3H_2O$—**241.60** [10031-43-3]—Use ACS reagent grade.■1S (*USP41*)

Add the following:

■**3-Cyclohexylpropionic Acid** *(3-Cyclohexanepropionic Acid),* $C_9H_{16}O_2$—**156.22** [701-97-3]—Use a suitable grade with a content of NLT 99%.■1S (*USP41*)

Change to read:

L-Cystine, $HOOC(NH_2)CHCH_2S$—$SCH_2CH(NH_2)COOH$—**240.30** ■[56-89-3]■1S (*USP41*)
SPECIFIC ROTATION ⟨781⟩
Sample solution: ■20 mg/mL■1S (*USP41*) of L-cystine, previously dried over silica gel for 4 h ■1S (*USP41*)
Temperature: 20°
Acceptance criteria: −215° to −225°
LOSS ON DRYING ⟨731⟩
Analysis: Dry over silica gel for 4 h.
Acceptance criteria: NMT 0.2%
RESIDUE ON IGNITION (Reagent test): NMT 0.1%

Add the following:

■**Deschloroclotrimazole** *(1-(Triphenylmethyl)imidazole; 1-Tritylimidazole),* $C_{22}H_{18}N_2$—**310.39** [15469-97-3]—Use a suitable grade with a content of NLT 97%. [NOTE—A suitable grade is available as catalog number 524891 from www.sigmaaldrich.com.]■1S (*USP41*)

Add the following:

■**N,N'-Diisopropylethylenediamine,** $C_8H_{20}N_2$—**144.26** [4013-94-9]—Use a suitable grade with a content of NLT 99%.■1S (*USP41*)

Add the following:

■**Dimethylcarbonate** *(Carbonic Acid Dimethyl Ester),* $C_3H_6O_3$—**90.08** [616-38-6]—Use a suitable grade with a content of NLT 99%.■1S (*USP41*)

Add the following:

■**Dimidium Bromide** *(3,8-Diamino-5-methyl-6-phenylphenanthridinium bromide; Trypadine),* $C_{20}H_{18}BrN_3$—**380.28** [518-67-2]—Use a suitable grade with a content of NLT 95%.■1S (*USP41*)

Add the following:

■**2-Ethylhexanoic Acid** *(2-Ethylcaproic Acid),* $C_8H_{16}O_2$—**144.21** [149-57-5]—Use a suitable grade with a content of NLT 99%.■1S (*USP41*)

Add the following:

■**(±)-1-(9-Fluorenyl)ethanol** *(α-Methylfluorene-9-methanol),* $C_{15}H_{14}O$—**210.27** [3023-49-2]—Use a suitable grade with a content of NLT 97.0%.■1S (*USP41*)

Add the following:

■**(+)-1-(9-Fluorenyl)ethyl Chloroformate Solution** *((+)-FLEC),* $C_{16}H_{13}ClO_2$—**272.73** [107474-79-3]—Use a suitable grade with a concentration of NLT 18 mM in acetone.

ENANTIOMERIC PURITY

Mobile phase: Acetonitrile and water (1:1)

Standard solution: 30 µg/mL of (±)-1-(9-fluorenyl)ethanol in alcohol

Sample solution: 18 mM solution of (+)-1-(9-fluorenyl)ethyl chloroformate in acetone

Carbonate buffer solution: Transfer 338 mg of sodium carbonate and 152 mg of sodium bicarbonate to a 100-mL volumetric flask. Dissolve in and dilute with water to volume.

Sodium hydroxide solution: Transfer 30 g of sodium hydroxide to a 100-mL volumetric flask, add 50 mL of water to dissolve, and cool and dilute with water to volume.

Acetate buffer solution: Transfer 0.3 mL of glacial acetic acid to a 100-mL volumetric flask, add 90 mL of water, adjust with *Sodium hydroxide solution* to a pH of 4.2, and dilute with water to volume.

Blank: Water

Procedure: Transfer 20.0 µL each of *Sample solution* and *Blank* to separate 10-mL test tubes. Add 80 µL of *Carbonate buffer solution* to each test tube and cap the tubes tightly. Let each solution react for 24 h at 45° over a water bath. Cool to room temperature, add 5.0 mL of *Acetate buffer solution*, mix by vortex, and transfer to separate vials.

CHROMATOGRAPHIC SYSTEM

(See *Chromatography* ⟨621⟩, *System Suitability*.)

Mode: LC

Detector: Fluorescence

 Excitation wavelength: 260 nm

 Emission wavelength: 315 nm

Column: 4.6-mm × 15-cm; 3.0-µm packing L40

Column temperature: 25°

Flow rate: 0.5 mL/min

Injection volume: 5 µL

Run time: 2 times the retention time of (±)-1-(9-fluorenyl)ethanol

SYSTEM SUITABILITY

Samples: *Standard solution*, hydrolyzed *Sample solution*, and hydrolyzed *Blank*

Suitability requirements

 Relative retention times: About 0.95 for hydrolysate of (–)-1-(9-fluorenyl)ethyl chloroformate and 1.0 for hydrolysate of (+)-1-(9-fluorenyl)ethyl chloroformate

 Resolution: NLT 1.5 between hydrolysate of (–)-1-(9-fluorenyl)ethyl chloroformate and hydrolysate of (+)-1-(9-fluorenyl)ethyl chloroformate. Absence of peaks at the retention times for hydrolysate of (–)-1-(9-fluorenyl)ethyl chloroformate and hydrolysate of (+)-1-(9-fluorenyl)ethyl chloroformate in the hydrolyzed *Blank*.

ANALYSIS

Samples: *Standard solution* and hydrolyzed *Sample solution*

Integrate only peaks at the retention times of (–)-1-(9-fluorenyl)ethanol and (+)-1-(9-fluorenyl)ethanol. Disregard any extraneous peaks in the chromatogram of hydrolyzed *Sample solution*.

Calculate the percentage of (+)-1-(9-fluorenyl)ethyl chloroformate (P_A) in the portion of (+)-1-(9-fluorenyl)ethyl chloroformate taken:

$$Result = r_A/(r_A + r_B) \times 100$$

r_A = peak response of hydrolysate of (+)-1-(9-fluorenyl)ethyl chloroformate from the *Sample solution*

r_B = peak response of hydrolysate of (–)-1-(9-fluorenyl)ethyl chloroformate from the *Sample solution*

Calculate the percentage of (–)-1-(9-fluorenyl)ethyl chloroformate (P_B) in the portion of (+)-1-(9-fluorenyl)ethyl chloroformate taken:

$$Result = 100 - P_A$$

ACCEPTANCE CRITERIA: NLT 99.5% of (+)-1-(9-fluorenyl)ethyl chloroformate and NMT 0.5% of (–)-1-(9-fluorenyl)ethyl chloroformate.∎1S *(USP41)*

Add the following:

■**Fluoroandrostadiene Carboxylic Acid** *(Dexamethasone Acid)*, $C_{21}H_{27}FO_5$—**378.43** [37927-01-8.]—Use a suitable grade.

[NOTE—A suitable grade is available from www.scbt.com or as catalog number D298805 from www.trc-canada.com.]∎1S *(USP41)*

Change to read:

Gadolinium Sulfate, $Gd_2(SO_4)_3 \cdot 8H_2O$—**746.83** ■[13450-87-8]∎1S *(USP41)*—Use a suitable grade with a content of NLT 99.9%. [NOTE—A suitable grade is available as catalog number 41111 from www.gfschemicals.com.]

Add the following:

■**25% Hydrochloric Acid**—Transfer 56.4 mL of hydrochloric acid to a 100-mL volumetric flask containing about 40 mL of water. Cool and dilute with water to volume.∎1S *(USP41)*

Add the following:

■**Isopropyl Stearate** [112-10-7]—A mixture containing isopropyl myristate, isopropyl palmitate, and isopropyl stearate.

[NOTE—A suitable grade is available from www.intlab.org or www.bocsci.com.]∎1S *(USP41)*

Add the following:

■**Isostearic Acid** *(16-Methylheptadecanoic Acid)*, $C_{18}H_{36}O_2$—**284.48** [2724-58-5]—Use a suitable grade with a content of NLT 97%.∎1S *(USP41)*

Change to read:

Lithium Sulfate, $Li_2SO_4 \cdot H_2O$—**127.96** ■[10102-25-7]∎1S *(USP41)*—Use ACS reagent grade.

Add the following:

■**3-Mercaptopropionic Acid**, $C_3H_6O_2S$—**106.14** [107-96-0]—Use a suitable grade with a content of NLT 99%.∎1S *(USP41)*

Add the following:

■**Methyl Isobutyrate**, $C_5H_{10}O_2$—**102.13** [547-63-7]—Use a suitable grade with a content of NLT 99%.∎1S *(USP41)*

Add the following:

■3-Methyl-2-pentanone, $C_6H_{12}O$—**100.16** [565-61-7]—Use a suitable grade with a content of NLT 99%.■1S (*USP41*)

Add the following:

■4-Morpholine Propane Sulfonic Acid (*MOPS; 3-(N-Morpholino) Propanesulfonic Acid; 4-Morpholinepropanesulfonic Acid*), $C_7H_{15}NO_4S$—**209.26** [1132-61-2]—Use a suitable grade with a content of NLT 99%.■1S (*USP41*)

Add the following:

■Nitric Acid, Ultratrace, HNO_3—**63.01** [7697-37-2]—Use ACS reagent grade.■1S (*USP41*)

Add the following:

■Petroleum Ether (*Ligroin; Light Petroleum*), [8032-32-4]—Use ACS reagent grade.■1S (*USP41*)

Add the following:

■Phenylacetic Acid (α-*Toluic Acid;* α-*Tolylic Acid; Benzeneacetic Acid*), $C_8H_8O_2$—**136.15** [103-82-2]—Use a suitable grade with a content of NLT 99%.■1S (*USP41*)

Add the following:

■Sodium Phosphate (*Sodium Orthophosphate; Trisodium Phosphate*), Na_3PO_4—**163.94** [7601-54-9]—Use a suitable grade with a content NLT 95%.■1S (*USP41*)

Add the following:

■Sulfan Blue (*Patent Blue VF; Acid Blue V*), $C_{27}H_{31}N_2NaO_6S_2$—**566.66** [129-17-9]—Use a suitable grade with a dye content of NLT 50%.■1S (*USP41*)

Change to read:

Sulfuric Acid, Diluted■—Transfer 57 mL of sulfuric acid to a 1000-mL volumetric flask containing about 500 mL of water. Cool and dilute with water to volume.■1S (*USP41*)

Add the following:

■1,1,3,3-Tetramethylbutylamine (*tert-Octylamine*), $C_8H_{19}N$—**129.24** [107-45-9]—Use a suitable grade with a content of NLT 95%.■1S (*USP41*)

Add the following:

■Tetramethylethylenediamine (*N,N,N',N'-Tetramethylethylenediamine; 1,2-Bis(dimethylamino)ethane; TEMED; TMEDA*), $C_6H_{16}N_2$—**116.20** [110-18-9]—Use a suitable grade with a content of NLT 99%.■1S (*USP41*)

Delete the following:

■*n*-Tricosane, $C_{23}H_{48}$—**324.63** [638-67-5]—Colorless or white, more or less translucent mass, showing a crystalline structure. Has a slightly greasy feel. Insoluble in water and in alcohol; soluble in chloroform, in ether, in volatile oils, and in most warm fixed oils; slightly soluble in dehydrated alcohol. Boils at about 380°.
MELTING RANGE ⟨741⟩: between 47° and 49°.
SUITABILITY: Determine its suitability for use in the test for *Related Compounds* under *Propoxyphene Hydrochloride* (USP monograph) as follows. Dissolve a suitable quantity in chloroform to yield a solution containing 20 µg per mL. Following the directions given in the test for *Related Compounds* under *Propoxyphene Hydrochloride*, inject a suitable volume of the solution into the chromatograph, and record the chromatogram. Concomitantly record the chromatogram from the *Standard preparation* prepared as directed in the test for *Related compounds:* only one main peak is obtained from the *n*-tricosane solution, and no minor peaks are observed at, or near, the peak positions obtained for propoxyphene, acetoxy, or carbinol in the chromatogram from the *Standard preparation*.■1S (*USP41*)

Change to read:

Water, Ammonia-Free, H_2O—**18.02**—Use ■*Purified Water*.
■1S (*USP41*)

TEST SOLUTIONS (TS)

Add the following:

■4 N Hydrochloric Acid TS—Transfer 331 mL of hydrochloric acid to a 1000-mL volumetric flask containing about 500 mL of water. Cool and dilute with water to volume.
■1S (*USP41*)

Add the following:

■0.1 M Monobasic Sodium Phosphate TS—Transfer 13.8 g of monobasic sodium phosphate to a 1000-mL volumetric flask. Dissolve in and dilute with water to volume.■1S (*USP41*)

Add the following:

■0.05 M Monobasic Sodium Phosphate TS—Transfer 6.9 g of monobasic sodium phosphate to a 1000-mL volumetric flask. Dissolve in and dilute with water to volume.■1S (*USP41*)

Add the following:

■0.1 N Sodium Chloride TS—Transfer 5.84 g of sodium chloride to a 1000-mL volumetric flask. Dissolve in and dilute with water to volume.■1S (*USP41*)

Add the following:

■10 N Sulfuric Acid TS—Transfer 281 mL of sulfuric acid to a 1000-mL volumetric flask containing about 500 mL of water. Cool and dilute with water to volume.■1S (*USP41*)

VOLUMETRIC SOLUTIONS

Change to read:

0.1 N Ceric Sulfate VS Ce(SO$_4$)$_2$, 332.24 ■₁₅ (USP41)
Use commercially available volumetric standard solution.
STANDARDIZATION: Accurately weigh about 0.2 g of sodium oxalate, primary standard, dried according to the label instructions ■or, if this information is not available, dried at 105° for 2 h,■₁₅ (USP41) and dissolve in 75 mL of water. Add, with stirring, 2 mL of sulfuric acid that has previously been mixed with 5 mL of water, mix well, add 10 mL of hydrochloric acid, and heat to between 70° and 75°. Titrate with 0.1 N ceric sulfate to a permanent slight yellow color. Each 6.700 mg of sodium oxalate is equivalent to 1 mL of 0.1 N ceric sulfate.

$$N = \frac{mg\ Na_2C_2O_4}{67.00 \times mL\ Ce(SO_4)_2\ solution}$$

[NOTE—If this volumetric solution is used in a qualitative application such as pH adjustment, dissolution medium, or diluent, its standardization is not required.]

Change to read:

▲**0.01 M Sodium Thiosulfate VS**
Transfer 100 mL of ■0.1 N sodium thiosulfate VS■₁₅ (USP41) to a 1000-mL volumetric flask. Dilute with carbon dioxide-free water to volume.
STANDARDIZATION: Accurately weigh about 21.0 mg of primary standard potassium dichromate, previously pulverized and dried according to the label instructions or, if this information is not available, dried at 120° for 4 h, and dissolve in 100 mL of water in a glass-stoppered, 500-mL flask. Swirl to dissolve the solid, remove the stopper, and quickly add 1 g of potassium iodide, 2 g of sodium bicar-

bonate, and 5 mL of hydrochloric acid. Insert the stopper gently in the flask, swirl to mix, and allow to stand in the dark for exactly 10 min. Rinse the stopper and the inner walls of the flask with water, and titrate the liberated iodine with 0.01 M sodium thiosulfate VS until the solution is yellowish green in color. Add 3 mL of starch TS, and continue the titration until the blue color is discharged. Perform a blank determination. Restandardize the solution as frequently as supported by laboratory stability data. In the absence of such data, restandardize the solution weekly.

$$N = \frac{mg\ K_2Cr_2O_7}{49.04 \times mL\ Na_2S_2O_3}$$

[NOTE—If this volumetric solution is used in a qualitative application such as pH adjustment, dissolution medium, or diluent, its standardization is not required.]▲USP41

Add the following:

■**0.02 N Sulfuric Acid VS** H$_2$SO$_4$, 98.08
Transfer 0.56 mL of sulfuric acid to a 1000-mL volumetric flask containing about 500 mL of water. Cool and dilute with water to volume.
STANDARDIZATION: Accurately weigh about 50 mg of tromethamine, dried according to the label instructions or, if this information is not available, dried at 105° for 3 h. Dissolve in 50 mL of water and add 2 drops of bromocresol green TS. Titrate with the sulfuric acid solution to a pale yellow endpoint. Each 2.423 mg of tromethamine is equivalent to 1 mL of 0.02 N sulfuric acid.

$$N = \frac{mg\ tromethamine}{121.14 \times mL\ H_2SO_4}$$

[NOTE—If this volumetric solution is used in a qualitative application such as pH adjustment, dissolution medium, or diluent, its standardization is not required.]■₁₅ (USP41)

Chromatographic Columns

The following list of packings (L), phases (G), and supports (S) is intended to be a convenient reference for the chromatographer. [NOTE—Particle sizes given in this listing are those generally provided. Where other, usually finer, sizes are required, the individual monograph specifies the desired particle size. Within any category of packings or phases listed below, there may be a wide range of columns available. Where it is necessary to define more specifically the chromatographic conditions, the individual monograph so indicates.]

Change to read:

L52—A strong cation-exchange resin made of porous silica with sulfopropyl ■or sulfoethyl■₁₅ (USP41) groups, ▲1▲USP41–10 µm in diameter. ▲▲USP41

Change to read:

L86—■Fused■₁₅ (USP41) core particles with a highly polar ligand possessing five hydroxyl groups tethered to the silica

gel outer layer, ■1.5–5 µm in diameter.■₁₅ (USP41) [NOTE—A suitable column is Supelco Ascentis Express OH5 from www. sigma-aldrich.com.]

Add the following:

■**L107 (Rosuvastatin Calcium, CHIRALCEL OJ-RH)**—Cellulose tris(4-methylbenzoate)-coated porous spherical particles, 3–5 µm in diameter, for use with reversed-phase mobile phases. [NOTE—A suitable column is Chiralcel OJ-RH from www.chiraltech.com.]■₁₅ (USP41)

Add the following:

■**L110**—A strong anion-exchange resin consisting of highly cross-linked 13-µm (less than 10 Å) particles coated with very low cross-linked latex (0.5%) to provide alkanol quaternary ammonium ion exchange sites.■₁₅ (USP41)

Add the following:

■L112—A hydroxide-selective, strong anion-exchange resin consisting of a highly cross-linked core of 8.5-µm porous particles having a pore size of 2000 Å units and consisting of ethylvinylbenzene cross-linked with 55% divinylbenzene with a latex coating composed of 65-nm diameter microbeads (5% crosslinked) bonded with alkanol quaternary ammonium ions.■1S (USP41)

Reference Tables

CONTAINERS FOR DISPENSING CAPSULES AND TABLETS

The following table is provided as a reminder for the pharmacist engaged in the typical dispensing situation who already is acquainted with the *Packaging and Storage* requirements set forth in the individual monographs. It lists the capsules and tablets that are official in the *United States Pharmacopeia* and indicates the relevant tight (T), well-closed (W), and light-resistant (LR) specifications applicable to containers in which the drug that is repackaged should be dispensed.

This table is not intended to replace, nor should it be interpreted as replacing, the definitive requirements stated in the individual monographs.

Container Specifications for Capsules and Tablets

Monograph Title	Container Specification
Abacavir Tablets	W
Abacavir and Lamivudine Tablets	T, LR
Abiraterone Acetate Tablets	T
Acebutolol Hydrochloride Capsules	T
Acepromazine Maleate Tablets	T, LR
Acetaminophen Capsules	T
Acetaminophen Tablets, Extended-Release	T
Acetaminophen Tablets	T
Acetaminophen and Aspirin Tablets	T
Acetaminophen, Aspirin, and Caffeine Tablets	T
Acetaminophen and Caffeine Tablets	T
Acetaminophen and Salts of Chlorpheniramine, Dextromethorphan, and Pseudoephedrine, Capsules Containing at Least Three of the Following—	T
Acetaminophen and Salts of Chlorpheniramine, Dextromethorphan, and Pseudoephedrine, Tablets Containing at Least Three of the Following—	T
Acetaminophen, Chlorpheniramine Maleate, and Dextromethorphan Hydrobromide Tablets	T
Acetaminophen and Codeine Phosphate Capsules	T, LR
Acetaminophen and Codeine Phosphate Tablets	T, LR
Acetaminophen and Diphenhydramine Citrate Tablets	T
Acetaminophen, Diphenhydramine Hydrochloride, and Pseudoephedrine Hydrochloride Tablets	T
Acetaminophen and Pseudoephedrine Hydrochloride Tablets	T
Acetaminophen and Tramadol Hydrochloride Tablets	T
Acetazolamide Tablets	T
Acetohydroxamic Acid Tablets	T
Acitretin Capsules	W, LR
Acyclovir Capsules	T
Acyclovir Tablets	T
Albendazole Tablets	T
Albuterol Tablets	T, LR
Albuterol Tablets, Extended-Release	T, LR
Alendronate Sodium Tablets	T

Container Specifications for Capsules and Tablets *(Continued)*

Monograph Title	Container Specification
Alfuzosin Hydrochloride Tablets, Extended-Release	LR
Allopurinol Tablets	W
Almotriptan Tablets	T, LR
Alprazolam Tablets	T, LR
Alprazolam Tablets, Extended-Release	T, LR
Alprazolam Tablets, Orally Disintegrating	T
Altretamine Capsules	T, LR
Alumina and Magnesia Tablets	W
Alumina, Magnesia, and Calcium Carbonate Tablets	W
Alumina, Magnesia, Calcium Carbonate, and Simethicone Tablets	W
Alumina, Magnesia, and Simethicone Tablets	W
Alumina and Magnesium Carbonate Tablets	T
Alumina, Magnesium Carbonate, and Magnesium Oxide Tablets	T
Alumina and Magnesium Trisilicate Tablets	W
Aluminum Carbonate Gel, Dried Basic, Capsules	W
Aluminum Carbonate Gel, Dried Basic, Tablets	W
Aluminum Hydroxide Gel, Dried, Capsules	W
Aluminum Hydroxide Gel, Dried, Tablets	W
Amantadine Hydrochloride Capsules	T
Amiloride Hydrochloride Tablets	W
Amiloride Hydrochloride and Hydrochlorothiazide Tablets	W
Aminobenzoate Potassium Capsules	W
Aminobenzoate Potassium Tablets	W
Aminocaproic Acid Tablets	T
Aminoglutethimide Tablets	T, LR
Aminopentamide Sulfate Tablets	W
Aminophylline Tablets	T
Aminophylline Tablets, Delayed-Release	T
Aminosalicylate Sodium Tablets	T, LR
Aminosalicylic Acid Tablets	T, LR
Amitriptyline Hydrochloride Tablets	W
Add the following:	
■Amlodipine and Atorvastatin Tablets	W■1S (USP41)
Amlodipine and Benazepril Hydrochloride Capsules	W
Amlodipine Besylate Tablets	T, LR
Amlodipine and Valsartan Tablets	T
Amlodipine, Valsartan, and Hydrochlorothiazide Tablets	T
Ammonium Chloride Tablets, Delayed-Release	T
Amodiaquine Hydrochloride Tablets	T
Amoxapine Tablets	W
Amoxicillin Capsules	T
Amoxicillin Tablets	T
Amoxicillin and Clavulanate Potassium Tablets	T
Amoxicillin and Clavulanic Acid Tablets, Extended-Release	T
Amphetamine Sulfate Tablets	W
Ampicillin Capsules	T

Container Specifications for Capsules and Tablets (Continued)

Monograph Title	Container Specification
Ampicillin Tablets	T
Anagrelide Capsules	T, LR
Anastrozole Tablets	T
Anileridine Hydrochloride Tablets	T, LR
Apomorphine Hydrochloride Tablets	T, LR
Aprepitant Capsules	T
Arginine Capsules	T, LR
Arginine Tablets	T, LR
Aripiprazole Tablets	T
Aripiprazole Tablets, Orally Disintegrating	T
Ascorbic Acid Tablets	T, LR
Aspirin Capsules	T
Aspirin Capsules, Delayed-Release	T
Aspirin Tablets	T
Aspirin Tablets, Buffered	T
Aspirin Tablets, Delayed-Release	T
Aspirin Tablets, Effervescent for Oral Solution	T
Aspirin Tablets, Extended-Release	T
Aspirin, Alumina, and Magnesia Tablets	T
Aspirin, Alumina, and Magnesium Oxide Tablets	T
Aspirin, Caffeine, and Dihydrocodeine Bitartrate Capsules	T
Aspirin and Codeine Phosphate Tablets	W, LR
Aspirin, Codeine Phosphate, Alumina, and Magnesia Tablets	W, LR
Astemizole Tablets	T
Atenolol Tablets	W
Atenolol and Chlorthalidone Tablets	W
Atomoxetine Capsules	W
Add the following:	
▲Atorvastatin Calcium Tablets	T▲USP41
Atropine Sulfate Tablets	W
Azatadine Maleate Tablets	W
Azathioprine Tablets	LR
Azithromycin Capsules	W
Azithromycin Tablets	T
Bacampicillin Hydrochloride Tablets	T
Baclofen Tablets	W
Balsalazide Disodium Capsules	T
Barium Sulfate Tablets	W
Belladonna Extract Tablets	T, LR
Benazepril Hydrochloride Tablets	W
Bendroflumethiazide Tablets	T
Benzonatate Capsules	T, LR
Benztropine Mesylate Tablets	W
Beta Carotene Capsules	T, LR
Delete the following:	
▲Betamethasone Tablets	T▲USP41
Betaxolol Tablets	T
Bethanechol Chloride Tablets	T
Bicalutamide Tablets	T
Biotin Capsules	T, LR
Biotin Tablets	T, LR
Bisacodyl Tablets	T
Bisacodyl Tablets, Delayed-Release	W
Bismuth Subsalicylate Tablets	T
Bisoprolol Fumarate Tablets	T, LR
Bisoprolol Fumarate and Hydrochlorothiazide Tablets	W

Container Specifications for Capsules and Tablets (Continued)

Monograph Title	Container Specification
Black Cohosh Tablets	T, LR
Borage Seed Oil Capsules	T, LR
Bromocriptine Mesylate Capsules	T, LR
Bromocriptine Mesylate Tablets	T, LR
Brompheniramine Maleate Tablets	T
Bumetanide Tablets	T, LR
Add the following:	
▲Buprenorphine and Naloxone Sublingual Tablets	T▲USP41
Bupropion Hydrochloride Tablets, Extended-Release	W
Buspirone Hydrochloride Tablets	T, LR
Busulfan Tablets	W
Butabarbital Sodium Tablets	T
Butalbital, Acetaminophen, and Caffeine Capsules	T
Butalbital, Acetaminophen, and Caffeine Tablets	T
Butalbital and Aspirin Tablets	T
Butalbital, Aspirin, and Caffeine Capsules	T
Butalbital, Aspirin, and Caffeine Tablets	T
Butalbital, Aspirin, Caffeine, and Codeine Phosphate Capsules	T, LR
Cabergoline Tablets	T, LR
Calcifediol Capsules	T, LR
Calcium with Vitamin D Tablets	T, LR
Calcium Acetate Tablets	W
Calcium Carbonate Tablets	W
Calcium Carbonate and Magnesia Tablets	W
Calcium Carbonate and Magnesia Chewable Tablets	W
Calcium Citrate Tablets	W
Calcium and Magnesium Carbonates Tablets	W
Calcium Gluconate Tablets	W
Calcium L-5-Methyltetrahydrofolate Capsules	T, LR
Calcium L-5-Methyltetrahydrofolate Tablets	T, LR
Calcium Lactate Tablets	T
Calcium Pantothenate Tablets	T
Calcium Phosphate, Dibasic Tablets	W
Candesartan Cilexetil Tablets	T, LR
Candesartan Cilexetil and Hydrochlorothiazide Tablets	T, LR
Capecitabine Tablets	T
Captopril Tablets	T
Captopril and Hydrochlorothiazide Tablets	T
Carbamazepine Tablets	T
Carbamazepine Tablets, Extended-Release	T
Carbenicillin Indanyl Sodium Tablets	T
Change to read:	
Carbidopa and Levodopa Tablets	▲T,▲USP41 LR
Carbidopa and Levodopa Tablets, Extended-Release	W, LR
Carbidopa and Levodopa Tablets, Orally Disintegrating	W, LR
Carbinoxamine Maleate Tablets	T, LR
Urea C14 Capsules	T
Carboxymethylcellulose Sodium Tablets	T
Carisoprodol Tablets	W
Carisoprodol and Aspirin Tablets	W
Carisoprodol, Aspirin, and Codeine Phosphate Tablets	W
Carprofen Tablets	T
Carteolol Hydrochloride Tablets	T

Container Specifications for Capsules and Tablets *(Continued)*

Monograph Title	Container Specification
Carvedilol Tablets	T, LR
Cascara Tablets	T, W
Castor Oil Capsules	T
Cat's Claw Capsules	T, LR
Cat's Claw Tablets	T, LR
Cefaclor Capsules	T
Delete the following:	
▲Cefaclor Tablets, Chewable	T▲*USP41*
Cefaclor Tablets, Extended-Release	T, LR
Cefadroxil Capsules	T
Cefadroxil Tablets	T
Cefdinir Capsules	T, LR
Cefixime Tablets	T
Cefpodoxime Proxetil Tablets	T
Cefprozil Tablets	T
Cefuroxime Axetil Tablets	W
Cephalexin Capsules	T
Cephalexin Tablets	T
Cephradine Capsules	T
Cephradine Tablets	T
Cetirizine Hydrochloride Tablets	W
Cetirizine Hydrochloride Tablets, Orally Disintegrating	T
Cetirizine Hydrochloride and Pseudoephedrine Hydrochloride Tablets, Extended-Release	W
Chloral Hydrate Capsules	T
Chlorambucil Tablets	W, LR
Chloramphenicol Capsules	T
Chloramphenicol Tablets	T
Chlordiazepoxide Tablets	T, LR
Chlordiazepoxide and Amitriptyline Hydrochloride Tablets	T, LR
Chlordiazepoxide Hydrochloride Capsules	T, LR
Chlordiazepoxide Hydrochloride and Clidinium Bromide Capsules	T, LR
Chloroquine Phosphate Tablets	W
Chlorothiazide Tablets	W, LR
Chlorpheniramine Maleate Capsules, Extended-Release	T
Chlorpheniramine Maleate Tablets	T
Chlorpheniramine Maleate and Pseudoephedrine Hydrochloride Capsules, Extended-Release	T, LR
Chlorpromazine Hydrochloride Tablets	W, LR
Chlorpropamide Tablets	W
Chlortetracycline Hydrochloride Tablets	T, LR
Chlorthalidone Tablets	W
Chlorzoxazone Tablets	T
Chlorzoxazone and Acetaminophen Capsules	T
Cholecalciferol Capsules	T, LR
Add the following:	
■Cholecalciferol Tablets	T, LR■*1S (USP41)*
Chondroitin Sulfate Sodium Tablets	T, LR
Chromium Picolinate Tablets	W
Cimetidine Tablets	T, LR
Cilostazol Tablets	T, LR
Ciprofloxacin Tablets	W
Ciprofloxacin Tablets, Extended-Release	T
Citalopram Tablets	W
Clarithromycin Tablets	T

Container Specifications for Capsules and Tablets *(Continued)*

Monograph Title	Container Specification
Clarithromycin Tablets, Extended-Release	W
Clemastine Fumarate Tablets	W
Clindamycin Hydrochloride Capsules	T
Clofazimine Capsules	W
Clofibrate Capsules	W, LR
Clomiphene Citrate Tablets	W
Clomipramine Hydrochloride Capsules	W
Clonazepam Tablets	T, LR
Clonazepam Tablets, Orally Disintegrating	W, LR
Clonidine Hydrochloride Tablets	W
Clonidine Hydrochloride and Chlorthalidone Tablets	W
Clopidogrel Tablets	W
Clorazepate Dipotassium Tablets	T, LR
Clotrimazole Tablets, Vaginal	W
Red Clover Tablets	T, LR
Cloxacillin Sodium Capsules	T
Clozapine Tablets	W
Cyanocobalamin Co 57 Capsules	W, LR
Cyanocobalamin Co 58 Capsules	W, LR
Cocaine Hydrochloride Tablets for Topical Solution	W, LR
Codeine Phosphate Tablets	W, LR
Codeine Sulfate Tablets	W
Colestipol Hydrochloride Tablets	T
Cortisone Acetate Tablets	W
Cromolyn Sodium for Inhalation (in Capsules)	T, LR
Crypthecodinium cohnii Oil Capsules	T, LR
Curcuminoids Capsules	W, LR
Curcuminoids Tablets	W, LR
Cyanocobalamin Tablets	T, LR
Cyclizine Hydrochloride Tablets	T, LR
Cyclobenzaprine Hydrochloride Capsules, Extended-Release	T, LR
Cyclobenzaprine Hydrochloride Tablets	W
Cyclophosphamide Tablets	T
Cycloserine Capsules	T
Cyclosporine Capsules	T
Cyproheptadine Hydrochloride Tablets	W
Danazol Capsules	W
Dantrolene Sodium Capsules	T
Dapsone Tablets	W, LR
Dehydrocholic Acid Tablets	W
Demeclocycline Hydrochloride Capsules	T, LR
Demeclocycline Hydrochloride Tablets	T, LR
Desipramine Hydrochloride Tablets	T
Desloratadine Tablets	T
Desloratadine Tablets, Orally Disintegrating	T
Desogestrel and Ethinyl Estradiol Tablets	W
Dexamethasone Tablets	W
Dexchlorpheniramine Maleate Tablets	T
Dextroamphetamine Sulfate Capsules	T
Dextroamphetamine Sulfate Tablets	W
Diazepam Capsules	T, LR
Diazepam Capsules, Extended-Release	T, LR
Diazepam Tablets	T, LR
Diazoxide Capsules	W
Dichlorphenamide Tablets	W
Diclofenac Potassium Tablets	T, LR
Diclofenac Sodium Tablets, Delayed-Release	T, LR
Diclofenac Sodium Tablets, Extended-Release	W

Container Specifications for Capsules and Tablets (Continued)

Monograph Title	Container Specification
Diclofenac Sodium and Misoprostol Delayed-Release Tablets	T
Dicloxacillin Sodium Capsules	T
Dicyclomine Hydrochloride Capsules	W
Dicyclomine Hydrochloride Tablets	W
Didanosine Capsules, Delayed-Release	W
Didanosine Tablets for Oral Suspension	T
Diethylcarbamazine Citrate Tablets	T
Diethylpropion Hydrochloride Tablets	W
Diethylstilbestrol Tablets	W
Diflunisal Tablets	W
Digitalis Capsules	T
Digitalis Tablets	T
Digitoxin Tablets	W
Digoxin Tablets	T
Dihydrotachysterol Capsules	W, LR
Dihydrotachysterol Tablets	W, LR
Dihydroxyaluminum Sodium Carbonate Tablets	W
Diltiazem Hydrochloride Tablets	T, LR
Diltiazem Hydrochloride Capsules, Extended-Release	T
Dimenhydrinate Tablets	W
Diphenhydramine Citrate and Ibuprofen Tablets	T
Diphenhydramine Hydrochloride Capsules	T
Diphenhydramine Hydrochloride and Ibuprofen Capsules	T
Diphenhydramine and Phenylephrine Hydrochlorides Tablets	T
Diphenhydramine and Pseudoephedrine Capsules	T
Diphenoxylate Hydrochloride and Atropine Sulfate Tablets	W, LR
Dipyridamole Tablets	T, LR
Dirithromycin Tablets, Delayed-Release	T
Disopyramide Phosphate Capsules	W
Disopyramide Phosphate Capsules, Extended-Release	W
Disulfiram Tablets	T, LR
Divalproex Sodium Capsules, Delayed-Release	T, LR
Divalproex Sodium Tablets, Delayed-Release	T, LR
Divalproex Sodium Tablets, Extended-Release	W
Docusate Calcium Capsules	T
Docusate Potassium Capsules	T
Docusate Sodium Capsules	T
Docusate Sodium Tablets	W
Donepezil Hydrochloride Tablets	W
Donepezil Hydrochloride Tablets, Orally Disintegrating	W
Doxazosin Tablets	T
Doxepin Hydrochloride Capsules	W
Doxycycline Capsules	T, LR
Doxycycline Capsules, Extended-Release	T, LR
Doxycycline Hyclate Capsules	T, LR
Doxycycline Hyclate Capsules, Delayed-Release	T, LR
Doxycycline Hyclate Tablets	T, LR
Doxycycline Hyclate Tablets, Delayed-Release	T, LR
Doxycycline Tablets	T, LR
Doxylamine Succinate Tablets	W, LR
Dronabinol Capsules	W, LR
Drospirenone and Ethinyl Estradiol Tablets	W
Duloxetine Capsules, Delayed-Release	T
Dydrogesterone Tablets	W

Container Specifications for Capsules and Tablets (Continued)

Monograph Title	Container Specification
Dyphylline Tablets	T
Dyphylline and Guaifenesin Tablets	T
Echinacea Species Dry Extract Capsules	W
Echinacea Species Dry Extract Tablets	W
Add the following:	
▲*Echinacea* Species Powder Capsules	W▲USP41
Efavirenz Capsules	W
Efavirenz Tablets	W
Eleuthero Root and Rhizome Dry Extract Capsules	W
Eleuthero Root and Rhizome Dry Extract Tablets	W
Eleuthero Root and Rhizome Powder Capsules	W
Enalapril Maleate Tablets	W
Enalapril Maleate and Hydrochlorothiazide Tablets	W
Entacapone Tablets	LR
Entecavir Tablets	T
Ephedrine Sulfate Capsules	T, LR
Ergocalciferol Capsules	T, LR
Ergocalciferol Tablets	T, LR
Ergoloid Mesylates Capsules	T, LR
Ergoloid Mesylates Tablets	T, LR
Ergoloid Mesylates Tablets, Sublingual	T, LR
Ergonovine Maleate Tablets	W
Ergotamine Tartrate Tablets	W, LR
Ergotamine Tartrate Tablets, Sublingual	W, LR
Ergotamine Tartrate and Caffeine Tablets	W, LR
Erythromycin Capsules, Delayed-Release	T
Erythromycin Tablets	T
Erythromycin Tablets, Delayed-Release	T
Erythromycin Estolate Capsules	T
Erythromycin Estolate Tablets	T
Erythromycin Ethylsuccinate Tablets	T
Erythromycin Stearate Tablets	T
Escitalopram Tablets	W
Esomeprazole Magnesium Capsules, Delayed-Release	T
Estazolam Tablets	T, LR
Estradiol Tablets	T, LR
Estradiol and Norethindrone Acetate Tablets	W
Estrogens Tablets, Conjugated	W
Estrogens Tablets, Esterified	W
Estropipate Tablets	W
Eszopiclone Tablets	T
Ethacrynic Acid Tablets	W
Ethambutol Hydrochloride Tablets	W
Ethchlorvynol Capsules	T, LR
Ethinyl Estradiol Tablets	W
Ethionamide Tablets	W
Ethosuximide Capsules	T
Ethotoin Tablets	T
Ethynodiol Diacetate and Ethinyl Estradiol Tablets	W
Ethynodiol Diacetate and Mestranol Tablets	W
Etidronate Disodium Tablets	T
Etodolac Capsules	T
Etodolac Tablets	T
Etodolac Tablets, Extended-Release	W
Evening Primrose Oil Capsules	T, LR
Famotidine Tablets	W, LR

Container Specifications for Capsules and Tablets (Continued)

Monograph Title	Container Specification
Felbamate Tablets	W
Felodipine Tablets, Extended-Release	T
Fenofibrate Capsules	W
Fenofibrate Tablets	W
Fenoprofen Calcium Capsules	W
Fenoprofen Calcium Tablets	W
Ferrous Fumarate Tablets	T
Ferrous Fumarate and Docusate Sodium Tablets, Extended-Release	W
Ferrous Gluconate Capsules	T
Ferrous Gluconate Tablets	T
Ferrous Sulfate Tablets	T
Fexofenadine Hydrochloride Capsules	T, LR
Fexofenadine Hydrochloride Tablets	W
Fexofenadine Hydrochloride and Pseudoephedrine Hydrochloride Tablets, Extended-Release	W
Finasteride Tablets	T, LR
Fish Oil Containing Omega-3 Acids Capsules	T, LR
Fish Oil Containing Omega-3 Acids Capsules, Delayed-Release	T, LR
Flavoxate Hydrochloride Tablets	W, LR
Flax Seed Oil Capsules	T, LR
Flecainide Acetate Tablets	W
Fluconazole Tablets	W
Flucytosine Capsules	T, LR
Fludrocortisone Acetate Tablets	W
Fluoxetine Capsules	T, LR
Fluoxetine Capsules, Delayed-Release	T
Fluoxetine Tablets	T
Fluoxymesterone Tablets	W
Fluphenazine Hydrochloride Tablets	T, LR
Flurazepam Hydrochloride Capsules	T, LR
Flurbiprofen Tablets	W
Flutamide Capsules	W, LR
Fluvastatin Capsules	T, LR
Fluvoxamine Maleate Tablets	T
Folic Acid Tablets	W
Fosinopril Sodium Tablets	T
Fosinopril Sodium and Hydrochlorothiazide Tablets	T
Furazolidone Tablets	T, LR
Furosemide Tablets	W, LR
Gabapentin Capsules	W
Gabapentin Tablets	W
Galantamine Tablets	W
Galantamine Extended-Release Capsules	T, LR
Garlic Tablets, Delayed-Release	T
Gemfibrozil Capsules	T
Gemfibrozil Tablets	T
Ginger Capsules	W
Ginkgo Capsules	T, LR
Ginkgo Tablets	T, LR
American Ginseng Capsules	T, LR
American Ginseng Tablets	T, LR
Asian Ginseng Capsules	T, LR
Asian Ginseng Tablets	T, LR
Glimepiride Tablets	W
Glipizide Tablets	T
Glipizide and Metformin Hydrochloride Tablets	W
Glucosamine Tablets	T, LR
Glucosamine and Chondroitin Sulfate Tablets	T, LR

Container Specifications for Capsules and Tablets (Continued)

Monograph Title	Container Specification
Glucosamine and Methylsulfonylmethane Tablets	T, LR
Glucosamine, Chondroitin Sulfate Sodium, and Methylsulfonylmethane Tablets	T, LR
Glyburide Tablets	W
Glyburide and Metformin Hydrochloride Tablets	T, LR
Glycopyrrolate Tablets	T
Granisetron Hydrochloride Tablets	W, LR
Griseofulvin Capsules	T
Griseofulvin Tablets	T
Griseofulvin Tablets, Ultramicrosize	W
Guaifenesin Capsules	T
Guaifenesin Tablets	T
Guaifenesin and Pseudoephedrine Hydrochloride Capsules	T, LR
Guaifenesin, Pseudoephedrine Hydrochloride, and Dextromethorphan Hydrobromide Capsules	T, LR
Guanabenz Acetate Tablets	T, LR
Guanethidine Monosulfate Tablets	W
Guanfacine Tablets	T, LR
Guggul Tablets	W, LR
Halazone Tablets for Solution	T, LR
Haloperidol Tablets	T, LR
Hexylresorcinol Lozenges	W
Homatropine Methylbromide Tablets	T, LR
Hydralazine Hydrochloride Tablets	T, LR
Hydrochlorothiazide Capsules	W
Hydrochlorothiazide Tablets	W
Hydrocodone Bitartrate Tablets	T, LR
Hydrocodone Bitartrate and Acetaminophen Tablets	T, LR
Hydrocodone Bitartrate and Homatropine Methylbromide Tablets	T, LR
Hydrocortisone Tablets	W
Hydroflumethiazide Tablets	T
Hydromorphone Hydrochloride Tablets	T, LR
Hydroxychloroquine Sulfate Tablets	T, LR
Hydroxyurea Capsules	T
Hydroxyzine Hydrochloride Tablets	T
Hydroxyzine Pamoate Capsules	W
Hyoscyamine Tablets	W, LR
Hyoscyamine Sulfate Tablets	T, LR
Ibuprofen Tablets	W
Ibuprofen and Pseudoephedrine Hydrochloride Tablets	T
Imipramine Hydrochloride Tablets	T
Imipramine Pamoate Capsules	T, LR
Indapamide Tablets	W
Indomethacin Capsules	W
Indomethacin Capsules, Extended-Release	W
Sodium Iodide I 123 Capsules	W
Sodium Iodide I 131 Capsules	W
Iodoquinol Tablets	W
Irbesartan Tablets	W
Irbesartan and Hydrochlorothiazide Tablets	W
Isoniazid Tablets	W, LR
Isopropamide Iodide Tablets	W
Isoproterenol Hydrochloride Tablets	W, LR
Isosorbide Dinitrate Capsules, Extended-Release	W
Isosorbide Dinitrate Tablets	W
Isosorbide Dinitrate Tablets, Chewable	W
Isosorbide Dinitrate Tablets, Extended-Release	W

Container Specifications for Capsules and Tablets (Continued)

Monograph Title	Container Specification
Isosorbide Dinitrate Tablets, Sublingual	W
Isosorbide Mononitrate Tablets	T
Isosorbide Mononitrate Tablets, Extended-Release	T
Isotretinoin Capsules	T
Isoxsuprine Hydrochloride Tablets	T
Isradipine Capsules	T
Ivermectin Tablets	W
Ivermectin and Pyrantel Pamoate Tablets	T, LR
Kanamycin Sulfate Capsules	T
Ketoconazole Tablets	W
Ketoprofen Capsules	T
Ketoprofen Capsules, Extended-Release	T
Ketorolac Tromethamine Tablets	W
Krill Oil Capsules	T
Krill Oil Capsules, Delayed-Release	T
Labetalol Hydrochloride Tablets	T, LR
Lamivudine Tablets	T, LR
Lamivudine and Zidovudine Tablets	W, LR
Lamotrigine Tablets	W
Lamotrigine Tablets, Extended-Release	W
Lamotrigine Tablets for Oral Suspension	T, LR
Lansoprazole Capsules, Delayed-Release	T
Leflunomide Tablets	T, LR
Letrozole Tablets	T
Leucovorin Calcium Tablets	W, LR
Levamisole Hydrochloride Tablets	W
Levetiracetam Tablets	T
Levetiracetam Tablets, Extended-Release	W
Levocarnitine Tablets	T
Levocetirizine Dihydrochloride Tablets	W
Levodopa Capsules	T, LR
Levodopa Tablets	T, LR
Levofloxacin Tablets	T
Levonorgestrel and Ethinyl Estradiol Tablets	W
Levorphanol Tartrate Tablets	W
Levothyroxine Sodium Tablets	T, LR
Lincomycin Hydrochloride Capsules	T
Alpha Lipoic Acid Capsules	W
Alpha Lipoic Acid Tablets	W
Liothyronine Sodium Tablets	T
Liotrix Tablets	T
Lisinopril Tablets	T
Lisinopril and Hydrochlorothiazide Tablets	W
Lithium Carbonate Capsules	W
Lithium Carbonate Tablets	T
Lithium Carbonate Tablets, Extended-Release	W
Lomustine Capsules	W
Loperamide Hydrochloride Capsules	W
Loracarbef Capsules	W
Loratadine Tablets	T
Loratadine Tablets, Chewable	T
Loratadine Tablets, Orally Disintegrating	T
Lorazepam Tablets	T, LR
Losartan Potassium Tablets	T, LR
Losartan Potassium and Hydrochlorothiazide Tablets	T, LR
Lovastatin Tablets	W
Loxapine Capsules	T
Lutein Capsules	T, LR
Lysine Hydrochloride Tablets	W

Container Specifications for Capsules and Tablets (Continued)

Monograph Title	Container Specification
Magaldrate Tablets	W
Magaldrate and Simethicone Tablets	W
Magnesia Tablets	W
Magnesia and Alumina Tablets	W
Magnesium Gluconate Tablets	W
Magnesium Oxide Capsules	W
Magnesium Oxide Tablets	W
Magnesium Salicylate Tablets	T
Magnesium Trisilicate Tablets	W
Maprotiline Hydrochloride Tablets	W
Mazindol Tablets	T
Mebendazole Tablets	W
Mecamylamine Hydrochloride Tablets	W
Meclizine Hydrochloride Tablets	W
Meclofenamate Sodium Capsules	T, LR
Medroxyprogesterone Acetate Tablets	W
Mefenamic Acid Capsules	T
Mefloquine Hydrochloride Tablets	T, LR
Megestrol Acetate Tablets	W
Melatonin Tablets	T, LR
Meloxicam Tablets	W
Melphalan Tablets	W, LR
Memantine Hydrochloride Tablets	T
Menadiol Sodium Diphosphate Tablets	W, LR
Menaquinone-7 Capsules	T, LR
Menaquinone-7 Tablets	T, LR
Meperidine Hydrochloride Tablets	W, LR
Mephenytoin Tablets	W
Mephobarbital Tablets	W
Meprobamate Tablets	W
Mercaptopurine Tablets	W
Mesalamine Capsules, Extended-Release	T, LR
Mesalamine Tablets, Delayed-Release	T
Mesoridazine Besylate Tablets	W, LR
Metaproterenol Sulfate Tablets	W, LR
Metaxalone Tablets	W, LR
Metformin Hydrochloride Tablets	T
Metformin Hydrochloride Tablets, Extended-Release	W, LR
Methacycline Hydrochloride Capsules	T, LR
Methadone Hydrochloride Tablets	W
Methamphetamine Hydrochloride Tablets	T, LR
Methazolamide Tablets	W
Methdilazine Hydrochloride Tablets	T, LR
Methenamine Tablets	W
Methenamine Hippurate Tablets	W
Methenamine Mandelate Tablets	W
Methenamine Mandelate Tablets, Delayed-Release	W
Methimazole Tablets	W, LR
Methocarbamol Tablets	T
Methotrexate Tablets	W
Methoxsalen Capsules	T, LR
Methscopolamine Bromide Tablets	T
Methsuximide Capsules	T
Methyclothiazide Tablets	W
Methylcellulose Tablets	W
Methylcobalamin Tablets	T, LT
Methyldopa Tablets	W
Methyldopa and Chlorothiazide Tablets	W
Methyldopa and Hydrochlorothiazide Tablets	W

Container Specifications for Capsules and Tablets *(Continued)*

Monograph Title	Container Specification
Methylergonovine Maleate Tablets	T, LR
Methylphenidate Hydrochloride Tablets	T
Methylphenidate Hydrochloride Tablets, Extended-Release	T
Methylprednisolone Tablets	T
Methylsulfonylmethane Tablets	T, LR
Methyltestosterone Capsules	W
Methyltestosterone Tablets	W
Methysergide Maleate Tablets	T
Metoclopramide Tablets	T, LR
Metolazone Tablets	T, LR
Metoprolol Succinate Tablets, Extended-Release	T
Metoprolol Tartrate Tablets	T, LR
Metoprolol Tartrate and Hydrochlorothiazide Tablets	T, LR
Metronidazole Capsules	W, LR
Metronidazole Tablets	W, LR
Metronidazole Tablets, Extended-Release	W
Metyrapone Tablets	T, LR
Metyrosine Capsules	W
Mexiletine Hydrochloride Capsules	T
Midodrine Hydrochloride Tablets	W
Minerals Capsules	T, LR
Minerals Tablets	T, LR
Minocycline Hydrochloride Capsules	T, LR
Minocycline Hydrochloride Tablets	T, LR
Minocycline Hydrochloride Tablets, Extended-Release	T
Minoxidil Tablets	T
Mirtazapine Tablets	T, LR
Mirtazapine Tablets, Orally Disintegrating	LR
Mitotane Tablets	T, LR
Modafinil Tablets	T
Moexipril Hydrochloride and Hydrochlorothiazide Tablets	W
Moexipril Hydrochloride Tablets	T, W
Molindone Hydrochloride Tablets	T, LR
Montelukast Sodium Tablets	T
Montelukast Sodium Tablets, Chewable	T
Moricizine Hydrochloride Tablets	T
Morphine Sulfate Capsules, Extended-Release	T, LR
Moxifloxacin Tablets	T
Mycophenolate Mofetil Capsules	W, LR
Mycophenolate Mofetil Tablets	W, LR
Mycophenolic Acid Tablets, Delayed-Release	T
Nabumetone Tablets	W
Nadolol Tablets	T
Nadolol and Bendroflumethiazide Tablets	T
Nafcillin Sodium Capsules	T
Nafcillin Sodium Tablets	T, LR
Nalidixic Acid Tablets	T
Naltrexone Hydrochloride Tablets	T
Naproxen Tablets	W
Naproxen Tablets, Delayed-Release	W
Naproxen Sodium Tablets	W
Naratriptan Tablets	T
Nateglinide Tablets	T
Nefazodone Hydrochloride Tablets	T
Neomycin Sulfate Tablets	T
Neostigmine Bromide Tablets	T
Nevirapine Tablets	W

Container Specifications for Capsules and Tablets *(Continued)*

Monograph Title	Container Specification
Nevirapine Tablets, Extended-Release	W
Niacin Tablets	W
Niacin Tablets, Extended-Release	T
Niacinamide Tablets	T
Nifedipine Capsules	T, LR
Nifedipine Tablets, Extended-Release	T, LR
Nitrofurantoin Capsules	T
Nitrofurantoin Tablets	T, LR
Nitroglycerin Tablets	T
Nitroglycerin Tablets, Sublingual	T
Norethindrone Tablets	W
Norethindrone and Ethinyl Estradiol Tablets	W
Norethindrone and Mestranol Tablets	W
Norethindrone Acetate Tablets	W
Norethindrone Acetate and Ethinyl Estradiol Tablets	W
Norfloxacin Tablets	W
Norgestimate and Ethinyl Estradiol Tablets	W
Norgestrel Tablets	W
Norgestrel and Ethinyl Estradiol Tablets	W
Nortriptyline Hydrochloride Capsules	T
Nystatin Tablets	T, LR
Nystatin Tablets, Vaginal	W, LR
Ofloxacin Tablets	W
Olanzapine Tablets	T, LR
Olanzapine Tablets, Orally Disintegrating	W
Olanzapine and Fluoxetine Capsules	T
Oleovitamin A and D Capsules	T, LR
Olmesartan Medoxomil Tablets	W
Omega-3 Acids Ethyl Esters Capsules	T, LR
Omeprazole Capsules, Delayed-Release	T, LR
Ondansetron Tablets	T, LR
Ondansetron Tablets, Orally Disintegrating	LR
Orbifloxacin Tablets	T
Orlistat Capsules	T
Orphenadrine Citrate, Aspirin, and Caffeine Tablets	T
Orphenadrine Citrate Tablets, Extended-Release	W, LR
Oseltamivir Phosphate Capsules	W
Oxacillin Sodium Capsules	T
Oxandrolone Tablets	T, LR
Oxaprozin Tablets	T, LR
Oxazepam Capsules	W
Oxazepam Tablets	W
Oxcarbazepine Tablets	W
Oxprenolol Hydrochloride Tablets	W, LR
Oxprenolol Hydrochloride Tablets, Extended-Release	W, LR
Oxtriphylline Tablets	T
Oxtriphylline Tablets, Extended-Release	T
Oxybutynin Chloride Tablets	T, LR
Oxybutynin Chloride Tablets, Extended-Release	T
Oxycodone Hydrochloride Tablets	T, LR
Oxycodone Hydrochloride Tablets, Extended-Release	T, LR
Oxycodone and Acetaminophen Capsules	T, LR
Oxycodone and Acetaminophen Tablets	T, LR
Oxycodone and Aspirin Tablets	T, LR
Oxymetholone Tablets	W
Oxymorphone Hydrochloride Tablets	T

Container Specifications for Capsules and Tablets (Continued)

Monograph Title	Container Specification
Oxymorphone Hydrochloride Tablets, Extended-Release	T
Oxytetracycline Tablets	T, LR
Oxytetracycline and Nystatin Capsules	T, LR
Oxytetracycline Hydrochloride Capsules	T, LR
Oxytetracycline Hydrochloride and Polymyxin B Sulfate Tablets, Vaginal	W
Pancreatin Tablets	T
Pancrelipase Capsules	T
Pancrelipase Capsules, Delayed-Release	T
Pancrelipase Tablets	T
Pantoprazole Sodium Tablets, Delayed-Release	W
Papain Tablets for Topical Solution	T, LR
Papaverine Hydrochloride Tablets	T
Paricalcitol Capsules	T
Paromomycin Sulfate Capsules	T
Paroxetine Tablets	T
Paroxetine Tablets, Extended-Release	W
Penbutolol Sulfate Tablets	W, LR
Penicillamine Capsules	T
Penicillamine Tablets	T
Penicillin G Benzathine Tablets	T
Penicillin G Potassium Tablets	T
Penicillin V Tablets	T
Penicillin V Potassium Tablets	T
Pentazocine and Acetaminophen Tablets	T, LR
Pentazocine and Aspirin Tablets	T, LR
Pentazocine and Naloxone Tablets	T, LR
Pentoxifylline Tablets, Extended-Release	W
Perindopril Erbumine Tablets	T
Perphenazine Tablets	T, LR
Perphenazine and Amitriptyline Hydrochloride Tablets	W
Phenazopyridine Hydrochloride Tablets	T
Phendimetrazine Tartrate Capsules	T
Phendimetrazine Tartrate Tablets	W
Phenelzine Sulfate Tablets	T
Phenmetrazine Hydrochloride Tablets	T
Phenobarbital Tablets	W
Phenoxybenzamine Hydrochloride Capsules	W
Phensuximide Capsules	T
Phentermine Hydrochloride Capsules	T
Phentermine Hydrochloride Tablets	T
Phenylbutazone Tablets	T
Phenylephrine Hydrochloride Tablets	T
Phenytoin Chewable Tablets	W
Phenytoin Sodium Capsules, Extended	T
Phenytoin Sodium Capsules, Prompt	T
Phytonadione Tablets	W, LR
Pilocarpine Hydrochloride Tablets	T
Pimozide Tablets	T, LR
Pindolol Tablets	W, LR
Pioglitazone and Glimepiride Tablets	T
Pioglitazone and Metformin Hydrochloride Tablets	T
Pioglitazone Tablets	T
Piperazine Citrate Tablets	T
Piroxicam Capsules	T, LR
Potassium Bicarbonate Effervescent Tablets for Oral Solution	T
Potassium Bicarbonate and Potassium Chloride Effervescent Tablets for Oral Solution	T

Container Specifications for Capsules and Tablets (Continued)

Monograph Title	Container Specification
Potassium and Sodium Bicarbonates and Citric Acid Effervescent Tablets for Oral Solution	T
Potassium Chloride Capsules, Extended-Release	T
Potassium Chloride Tablets, Extended-Release	T
Potassium Chloride, Potassium Bicarbonate, and Potassium Citrate Effervescent Tablets for Oral Solution	T
Potassium Citrate Tablets	W
Potassium Citrate Tablets, Extended-Release	T
Potassium Gluconate Tablets	T
Potassium Iodide Tablets	T
Potassium Iodide Tablets, Delayed-Release	T
Potassium Perchlorate Capsules	T, LR
Pravastatin Sodium Tablets	T
Praziquantel Tablets	T
Prazosin Hydrochloride Capsules	W, LR
Prednisolone Tablets	W
Prednisone Tablets	W
Primaquine Phosphate Tablets	W, LR
Primidone Tablets	W
Probenecid and Colchicine Tablets	W, LR
Probucol Tablets	W, LR
Procainamide Hydrochloride Capsules	T
Procainamide Hydrochloride Tablets	T
Procarbazine Hydrochloride Capsules	T, LR
Prochlorperazine Maleate Tablets	W
Procyclidine Hydrochloride Tablets	T
Promazine Hydrochloride Tablets	T, LR
Promethazine Hydrochloride Tablets	T, LR
Propafenone Hydrochloride Capsules, Extended-Release	T
Propafenone Hydrochloride Tablets	T
Propantheline Bromide Tablets	W
Propranolol Hydrochloride Capsules, Extended-Release	W
Propranolol Hydrochloride Tablets	W, LR
Propranolol Hydrochloride and Hydrochlorothiazide Capsules, Extended-Release	W
Propranolol Hydrochloride and Hydrochlorothiazide Tablets	W
Propylthiouracil Tablets	W
Protriptyline Hydrochloride Tablets	T
Pseudoephedrine Hydrochloride Tablets	T
Pseudoephedrine Hydrochloride Tablets, Extended-Release	T
Pygeum Capsules	T
Pyrazinamide Tablets	W
Pyridostigmine Bromide Tablets	T, LR
Pyridoxine Hydrochloride Tablets	W
Pyrilamine Maleate Tablets	W
Pyrimethamine Tablets	T, LR
Pyrvinium Pamoate Tablets	T, LR
Quazepam Tablets	W
Quetiapine Tablets	W
Quetiapine Tablets, Extended-Release	W
Quinapril Tablets	W
Quinapril and Hydrochlorothiazide Tablets	W, LR
Quinidine Gluconate Tablets, Extended-Release	W, LR
Quinidine Sulfate Capsules	T, LR
Quinidine Sulfate Tablets	W, LR
Quinidine Sulfate Tablets, Extended-Release	W, LR

Container Specifications for Capsules and Tablets (Continued)

Monograph Title	Container Specification
Quinine Sulfate Capsules	T
Quinine Sulfate Tablets	W
Raloxifene Hydrochloride Tablets	T
Add the following:	
▪Raltegravir Tablets	T▪1S (USP41)
Add the following:	
▪Raltegravir Tablets, Chewable	T▪1S (USP41)
Ramipril Capsules	W
Ramipril Tablets	W
Ranitidine Tablets	T, LR
Rauwolfia Serpentina Tablets	T, LR
Reserpine Tablets	T, LR
Reserpine and Chlorothiazide Tablets	T, LR
Reserpine, Hydralazine Hydrochloride, and Hydrochlorothiazide Tablets	T, LR
Rhodiola rosea Capsules	W
Rhodiola rosea Tablets	W
Ribavirin Capsules	W
Ribavirin Tablets	T
Riboflavin Tablets	T, LR
Rifabutin Capsules	W
Rifampin Capsules	T, LR
Rifampin and Isoniazid Capsules	T, LR
Rifampin, Isoniazid, and Pyrazinamide Tablets	T, LR
Rifampin, Isoniazid, Pyrazinamide, and Ethambutol Hydrochloride Tablets	T, LR
Riluzole Tablets	W, LR
Rimantadine Hydrochloride Tablets	T, LR
Risedronate Sodium Tablets	W
Risperidone Tablets, Orally Disintegrating	W, LR
Risperidone Tablets	T, LR
Ritodrine Hydrochloride Tablets	T
Ritonavir Capsules	T, LR
Ritonavir Tablets	T
Rivastigmine Tartrate Capsules	T
Rizatriptan Benzoate Tablets	W, LR
Rizatriptan Benzoate Tablets, Orally Disintegrating	W, LR
Ropinirole Tablets	W
Ropinirole Tablets, Extended-Release	W
Add the following:	
▪Rosuvastatin Tablets	W▪1S (USP41)
Rufinamide Tablets	T
Saccharin Sodium Tablets	W
St. John's Wort Flowering Top Dry Extract Capsules	W
St. John's Wort Flowering Top Dry Extract Tablets	W
Salsalate Capsules	T
Salsalate Tablets	T
Saquinavir Capsules	T
Saw Palmetto Capsules	T, LR
Schizochytrium Oil Capsules	T, LR
Scopolamine Hydrobromide Tablets	T, LR
Secobarbital Sodium Capsules	T
Secobarbital Sodium and Amobarbital Sodium Capsules	W
Selegiline Hydrochloride Capsules	T, LR
Selegiline Hydrochloride Tablets	T, LR

Container Specifications for Capsules and Tablets (Continued)

Monograph Title	Container Specification
Sennosides Tablets	W
Sertraline Tablets	W
Sildenafil Tablets	W
Simethicone Capsules	W
Simethicone Tablets	W
Simvastatin Tablets	T
Sitagliptin Tablets	W
Sodium Bicarbonate Tablets	W
Sodium Chloride Tablets	W
Sodium Chloride Tablets for Solution	W
Sodium Chloride and Dextrose Tablets	W
Sodium Fluoride Tablets	T
Sodium Salicylate Tablets	W
Sotalol Hydrochloride Tablets	W, LR
Soy Isoflavones Capsules	T, LR
Soy Isoflavones Tablets	T, LR
Spironolactone Tablets	T, LR
Spironolactone and Hydrochlorothiazide Tablets	T, LR
Spirulina Tablets	W, LR
Stanozolol Tablets	T, LR
Stavudine Capsules	T
Sulfadiazine Tablets	W, LR
Sulfadimethoxine Tablets	T, LR
Sulfadoxine and Pyrimethamine Tablets	W, LR
Sulfamethizole Tablets	W
Sulfamethoxazole Tablets	W, LR
Sulfamethoxazole and Trimethoprim Tablets	W, LR
Sulfapyridine Tablets	W, LR
Sulfasalazine Tablets	W
Sulfasalazine Tablets, Delayed-Release	W
Sulfinpyrazone Capsules	W
Sulfinpyrazone Tablets	W
Sulfisoxazole Tablets	W, LR
Sulindac Tablets	W
Sumatriptan Tablets	W
Tacrolimus Capsules	T
Tadalafil Tablets	T
Tamoxifen Citrate Tablets	W, LR
Tamsulosin Hydrochloride Capsules	T
Telmisartan Tablets	W
Add the following:	
▲Telmisartan and Amlodipine Tablets	T▲USP41
Telmisartan and Hydrochlorothiazide Tablets	W
Temazepam Capsules	W, LR
Add the following:	
▲Temozolomide Capsules	T▲USP41
Terazosin Capsules	W, LR
Terazosin Tablets	W, LR
Terbinafine Tablets	W, LR
Terbutaline Sulfate Tablets	T
Testolactone Tablets	T
Tetracycline Hydrochloride Capsules	T, LR
Tetracycline Hydrochloride Tablets	T, LR
Tetracycline Hydrochloride and Novobiocin Sodium Tablets	T
Tetracycline Hydrochloride, Novobiocin Sodium, and Prednisolone Tablets	T
Tetracycline Hydrochloride and Nystatin Capsules	T, LR
Thalidomide Capsules	W

Container Specifications for Capsules and Tablets *(Continued)*

Monograph Title	Container Specification
Theophylline Capsules	W
Theophylline Capsules, Extended-Release	W
Theophylline Tablets	W
Theophylline, Ephedrine Hydrochloride, and Phenobarbital Tablets	T
Theophylline and Guaifenesin Capsules	T
Theophylline Sodium Glycinate Tablets	W
Thiabendazole Tablets	T
Thiamine Hydrochloride Tablets	T, LR
Thiethylperazine Maleate Tablets	T, LR
Thioguanine Tablets	T
Thioridazine Hydrochloride Tablets	T, LR
Thiothixene Capsules	W, LR
Thyroid Tablets	T
Ticlopidine Hydrochloride Tablets	W
Tienchi Ginseng Root and Rhizome Dry Extract Capsules	W
Tienchi Ginseng Root and Rhizome Dry Extract Tablets	W
Tienchi Ginseng Root and Rhizome Powder Capsules	W
Tienchi Ginseng Root and Rhizome Powder Tablets	W
Timolol Maleate Tablets	W
Timolol Maleate and Hydrochlorothiazide Tablets	W, LR
Tizanidine Tablets	T
Delete the following:	
■Tocainide Hydrochloride Tablets	W■1S *(USP41)*
Tolazamide Tablets	T
Tolazoline Hydrochloride Tablets	W
Tolbutamide Tablets	W
Tolcapone Tablets	T
Tolmetin Sodium Capsules	T
Tolmetin Sodium Tablets	W
Topiramate Capsules	T
Topiramate Tablets	T
Torsemide Tablets	T
Tramadol Hydrochloride Tablets	T
Tramadol Hydrochloride Tablets, Extended-Release	T
Trandolapril Tablets	T
Add the following:	
▲Trandolapril and Verapamil Hydrochloride Tablets, Extended-Release	W▲USP41
Tranylcypromine Tablets	W
Trazodone Hydrochloride Tablets	T, LR
Triamcinolone Tablets	W
Triamterene Capsules	T, LR
Triamterene and Hydrochlorothiazide Capsules	T, LR
Triamterene and Hydrochlorothiazide Tablets	T, LR
Triazolam Tablets	T, LR
Trichlormethiazide Tablets	T
Trientine Hydrochloride Capsules	T
Trifluoperazine Hydrochloride Tablets	W, LR
Triflupromazine Hydrochloride Tablets	W, LR
Trihexyphenidyl Hydrochloride Capsules, Extended-Release	T
Trihexyphenidyl Hydrochloride Tablets	T
Trimeprazine Tartrate Tablets	W, LR
Trimethobenzamide Hydrochloride Capsules	W

Container Specifications for Capsules and Tablets *(Continued)*

Monograph Title	Container Specification
Trimethoprim Tablets	T, LR
Trioxsalen Tablets	W, LR
Tripelennamine Hydrochloride Tablets	W
Triple Sulfa Tablets, Vaginal	W, LR
Triprolidine Hydrochloride Tablets	T, LR
Triprolidine and Pseudoephedrine Hydrochlorides Tablets	T, LR
Trisulfapyrimidines Tablets	W
Troleandomycin Capsules	T
Trospium Chloride Tablets	T, LR
Ubidecarenone Capsules	T, LR
Ubidecarenone Tablets	T, LR
Ubiquinol Capsules	T, LR
Ursodiol Capsules	W
Ursodiol Tablets	W
Valacyclovir Tablets	T
Valerian Tablets	T, LR
Add the following:	
■Valerian Root Dry Extract Capsules	W■1S *(USP41)*
Add the following:	
■Valerian Root Powder Capsules	W■1S *(USP41)*
Valganciclovir Tablets	T
Valproic Acid Capsules	T
Valsartan Tablets	T
Valsartan and Hydrochlorothiazide Tablets	T
Vancomycin Hydrochloride Capsules	T
Venlafaxine Tablets	W
Verapamil Hydrochloride Capsules, Extended-Release	T, LR
Verapamil Hydrochloride Tablets	T, LR
Verapamil Hydrochloride Tablets, Extended-Release	T, LR
Vigabatrin Tablets	T
Vinpocetine Capsules	T, LR
Vinpocetine Tablets	T, LR
Vitamin A Capsules	T, LR
Vitamin A Tablets	T, LR
Vitamin E Capsules	T
Oil-Soluble Vitamins Capsules	T, LR
Oil-Soluble Vitamins Tablets	T, LR
Oil-Soluble Vitamins with Minerals Capsules	T, LR
Oil-Soluble Vitamins with Minerals Tablets	T, LR
Oil- and Water-Soluble Vitamins Capsules	T, LR
Oil- and Water-Soluble Vitamins Tablets	T, LR
Oil- and Water-Soluble Vitamins with Minerals Capsules	T, LR
Oil- and Water-Soluble Vitamins with Minerals Tablets	T, LR
Water-Soluble Vitamins Capsules	T, LR
Water-Soluble Vitamins Tablets	T, LR
Water-Soluble Vitamins with Minerals Capsules	T, LR
Water-Soluble Vitamins with Minerals Tablets	T, LR
Warfarin Sodium Tablets	T, LR
Zalcitabine Tablets	T, LR
Zaleplon Capsules	LR
Zidovudine Capsules	T, LR
Zidovudine Tablets	T, LR
Zinc Citrate Tablets	W
Zinc Gluconate Tablets	T, LR
Zinc Sulfate Tablets	W

Container Specifications for Capsules and Tablets (Continued)

Monograph Title	Container Specification
Ziprasidone Capsules	W
Zolmitriptan Tablets	W, LR
Zolmitriptan Tablets, Orally Disintegrating	W, LR
Zolpidem Tartrate Tablets	W

Container Specifications for Capsules and Tablets (Continued)

Monograph Title	Container Specification
Zolpidem Tartrate Tablets, Extended-Release	W
Zonisamide Capsules	T, LR

DESCRIPTION AND RELATIVE SOLUBILITY

Description and Relative Solubility of USP and NF Articles

The "description" and "solubility" statements pertaining to an article (formerly included in the individual monograph) are general in nature. The information is provided for those who use, prepare, and dispense drugs, solely to indicate descriptive and solubility properties of an article complying with monograph standards. The properties are not in themselves standards or tests for purity even though they may indirectly assist in the preliminary evaluation of the integrity of an article.

Taste and Odor

Organoleptic characteristics are indicated in many instances because they may be useful and descriptive properties of substances. However, they are not meant to be applied as tests for identifying materials.

The inclusion of odor or taste among other descriptive properties may aid in identifying the causative agent following accidental exposure to or contact with a substance. This information is provided as a warning or to make an individual aware of sensations that may be encountered. The use of odor or taste as a test for identification or content is strongly discouraged.

The characteristic odor of a volatile substance becomes apparent immediately on opening a container of it. The odor may be agreeable (e.g., Peppermint Oil), unpleasant (e.g., Sulfur Dioxide), or potentially hazardous on prolonged exposure (e.g., Coal Tar). Moreover, an unexpected odor may be encountered if the characteristics of a substance are not known or if a container is incorrectly labeled. Consequently, containers of such substances should be opened cautiously, preferably in a well-ventilated fume hood. A characteristic taste or sensation produced in the oral cavity likewise is apparent if traces of residue materials on fingers are inadvertently brought into contact with the tongue or adjacent mucosal tissues.

Solubility

Only where a special, quantitative solubility test is given in the individual monograph, and is designated by a test heading, is it a test for purity.

The approximate solubilities of Pharmacopeial and National Formulary substances are indicated by the descriptive terms in the accompanying table. The term "miscible" as used in this Pharmacopeia pertains to a substance that yields a homogeneous mixture when mixed in any proportion with the designated solvent.

Descriptive Term	Parts of Solvent Required for 1 Part of Solute
Very soluble	Less than 1
Freely soluble	From 1 to 10
Soluble	From 10 to 30
Sparingly soluble	From 30 to 100
Slightly soluble	From 100 to 1000
Very slightly soluble	From 1000 to 10,000
Practically insoluble, or Insoluble	10,000 and over

Soluble Pharmacopeial and National Formulary articles, when brought into solution, may show traces of physical impurities, such as minute fragments of filter paper, fibers, and other particulate matter, unless limited or excluded by definite tests or other specifications in the individual monographs.

Abacavir Sulfate: White to off-white powder. Soluble in water, in ethyl acetate, in absolute alcohol, and in methanol.

Abiraterone Acetate: White to off-white powder. Freely soluble in methylene chloride, in tetrahydrofuran, and in toluene; soluble in methanol, in ethanol, in ethyl acetate, in isobutyl methyl ketone, in *N,N*-dimethylformamide, and in acetone; sparingly soluble in acetonitrile and in dimethyl sulfoxide; slightly soluble in hexane; very slightly soluble in 0.1 N hydrochloric acid; practically insoluble in aqueous media over a wide range of pH values.

Acacia: Is practically odorless and produces a mucilaginous sensation on the tongue. Insoluble in alcohol. Optical rotation varies depending on the source of Acacia. For example, specific rotation values, calculated on the anhydrous basis and determined on a 1.0% (w/v) solution, usually are between −25° and −35° for *Acacia senegal* and between +35° and +60° for *Acacia seyal*. *NF category:* Emulsifying agent; suspending and/or viscosity-increasing agent; wet binder.

Add the following:

▪Acamprosate Calcium: A white or almost-white powder. Freely soluble in water; practically insoluble in alcohol and in methylene chloride.▪1S (USP41)

Acebutolol Hydrochloride: White or almost white, crystalline powder. Soluble in alcohol and in water; very slightly soluble in acetone and in methylene chloride; practically insoluble in ether. Melts at about 141° to 144°.

Acesulfame Potassium: A white, crystalline powder or colorless crystals. Soluble in water; very slightly soluble in acetone and in alcohol. *NF category:* Sweetening agent.

Acetaminophen: White, odorless, crystalline powder, having a slightly bitter taste. Freely soluble in alcohol; soluble in boiling water and in 1 N sodium hydroxide.

Acetazolamide: White to faintly yellowish-white, crystalline, odorless powder. Sparingly soluble in practically boiling water; slightly soluble in alcohol; very slightly soluble in water.

Acetic Acid: Clear, colorless liquid, having a strong, characteristic odor, and a sharply acid taste. Specific gravity is about 1.045. Miscible with water, with alcohol, and with glycerin. *NF category:* pH modifier (acidifying agent/alkalizing agent/buffering agent).

Glacial Acetic Acid: Clear, colorless liquid, having a pungent, characteristic odor and, when well diluted with water, an acid taste. Boils at about 118°. Specific gravity is about 1.05. Miscible with water, with alcohol, and with glycerin. *NF category:* pH modifier (acidifying agent/alkalizing agent/buffering agent).

Acetohydroxamic Acid: White, slightly hygroscopic, crystalline powder. Melts, after drying at about 80° for 2 to 4 hours, at about 88°. Freely soluble in water and in alcohol; very slightly soluble in chloroform.

Acetone: Transparent, colorless, mobile, volatile liquid, having a characteristic odor. A solution (1 in 2) is neutral to litmus. Miscible with water, with alcohol, with ether, with chloroform, and with most volatile oils. *NF category:* Solvent.

Acetylcholine Chloride: White or off-white crystals or crystalline powder. Very soluble in water; freely soluble in alcohol; insoluble in ether. Is decomposed by hot water and by alkalies.

Acetylcysteine: White, crystalline powder, having a slight acetic odor. Freely soluble in water and in alcohol; practically insoluble in chloroform and in ether.

Acetyltributyl Citrate: Clear, practically colorless, oily liquid. Freely soluble in alcohol, in isopropyl alcohol, in acetone, and in toluene; insoluble in water. *NF category:* Plasticizer.

Acetyltriethyl Citrate: Clear, practically colorless, oily liquid. Freely soluble in alcohol, in isopropyl alcohol, in acetone, and in toluene; insoluble in water. *NF category:* Plasticizer.

Acitretin: Yellow or greenish, crystalline powder. Sparingly soluble in tetrahydrofuran; slightly soluble in acetone and in alcohol; very slightly soluble in cyclohexane; practically insoluble in water.

Acyclovir: White to off-white, crystalline powder. Melts at temperatures higher than 250°, with decomposition. Soluble in diluted hydrochloric acid; slightly soluble in water; insoluble in alcohol.

Adapalene: White or almost white powder. Soluble in tetrahydrofuran; sparingly soluble in ethanol; practically insoluble in water.

Ademetionine Disulfate Tosylate: White powder. Freely soluble in water.

Adenine: White crystals or crystalline powder. Is odorless and tasteless. Sparingly soluble in boiling water; slightly soluble in alcohol; very slightly soluble in water; practically insoluble in ether and in chloroform.

Adenosine: White, odorless, crystalline powder. Slightly soluble in water; practically insoluble in alcohol. Melts at about 235°.

Adipic Acid: A white, crystalline powder. Freely soluble in alcohol and in methanol; soluble in boiling water and in acetone; slightly soluble in water. *NF category:* pH modifier (acidifying agent/alkalizing agent/buffering agent); flavors and fragrance.

Agar: Odorless or has a slight odor, and produces a mucilaginous sensation on the tongue. Soluble in boiling water; insoluble in cold water. *NF category:* Suspending and/or viscosity-increasing agent; emulsifying agent; suppository base; wet binder.

Alamic Acid: *NF category:* Suspending and/or viscosity-increasing agent.

Alanine: White, odorless crystals or crystalline powder, having a slightly sweet taste. Freely soluble in water; slightly soluble in 80% alcohol; insoluble in ether.

Albendazole: White to faintly yellowish powder. Freely soluble in anhydrous formic acid; very slightly soluble in ether and in methylene chloride; practically insoluble in alcohol and in water.

Albumin Human: Practically odorless, moderately viscous, clear, brownish fluid.

rAlbumin Human: Clear, slightly viscous, and colorless to yellow amber in color. *NF category:* Vehicle (sterile).

Albuterol: White, crystalline powder. Soluble in alcohol; sparingly soluble in water. Melts at about 156°.

Albuterol Sulfate: White or practically white powder. Freely soluble in water; slightly soluble in alcohol, in chloroform, and in ether.

Alcohol: Clear, colorless, mobile, volatile liquid. Has a characteristic odor and produces a burning sensation on the tongue. Is readily volatilized even at low temperatures, and boils at about 78°. Is flammable. Miscible with water and with practically all organic solvents. *NF category:* Solvent; antimicrobial preservative.

Dehydrated Alcohol: Clear, colorless, mobile, volatile liquid. Has a characteristic odor and produces a burning sensation on the tongue. Is readily volatilized even at low temperatures, and boils at about 78°. Is flammable. Miscible with water and with practically all organic solvents.

Diluted Alcohol: Clear, colorless, mobile liquid, having a characteristic odor and producing a burning sensation on the tongue. *NF category:* Solvent.

Rubbing Alcohol: Transparent, colorless, or colored as desired, mobile, volatile liquid. Has an extremely bitter taste and, in the absence of added odorous constituents, a characteristic odor. Is flammable.

Alendronate Sodium: White, free-flowing powder. Soluble in water; very slightly soluble in dimethyl sulfoxide, in methyl alcohol, and in propylene glycol; practically insoluble in acetone, in acetonitrile, in alcohol, in chloroform, and in isopropyl alcohol.

Alfadex: White or almost white, amorphous or crystalline powder. Freely soluble in water and in propylene glycol; practically insoluble in ethanol and in methylene chloride. *NF category:* Chelating and/or complexing agent.

Alfentanil Hydrochloride: White to almost white powder. Freely soluble in methanol, in alcohol, and in chloroform; soluble in water; sparingly soluble in acetone. Melting point range, crystals from acetone: 136°–143° (anhydrous) and reported as crystals from aqueous hydrochloric acid: 116°–126° (monohydrate).

Alfentanil Injection: Clear, colorless solution.

Alfuzosin Hydrochloride: White to almost white powder, slightly hygroscopic. Freely soluble in water; sparingly soluble in alcohol; practically insoluble in methylene chloride.

Alginic Acid: White to yellowish white, fibrous powder. Is odorless, or practically odorless, and is tasteless. Soluble in alkaline solutions; insoluble in water and in organic solvents. *NF category:* Suspending and/or viscosity-increasing agent; wet binder; disintegrant; film-forming agent; release-modifying agent.

Alkyl (C12-15) Benzoate: Clear, practically colorless, oily liquid. Soluble in acetone, in alcohol, in isopropyl alcohol, in ethyl acetate, in isopropyl myristate, in isopropyl palmitate, in lanolin, in mineral oil, in vegetable oils, and in volatile silicones; insoluble in water, in glycerin, and in propylene glycol. *NF category:* Vehicle (oleaginous); emollient.

Allantoin: White, crystalline powder. Slightly soluble in water; very slightly soluble in alcohol. Melts at about 225°, with decomposition.

Allopurinol: Fluffy white to off-white powder, having only a slight odor. Soluble in solutions of potassium and sodium hydroxides; very slightly soluble in water and in alcohol; practically insoluble in chloroform and in ether.

Allyl Isothiocyanate: Colorless to pale yellow, very refractive, liquid. Pungent irritating odor, acrid taste. [**CAUTION:** *Lachrymator.*] Miscible with alcohol, with carbon disulfide, and with ether. Slightly soluble in water.

Almond Oil: Clear, pale straw-colored or colorless, oily liquid, having a bland taste. Remains clear at −10°, and does not congeal until cooled to almost −20°. Slightly soluble in alcohol. Miscible with ether, with chloroform, with benzene, and with solvent hexane. *NF category:* Flavors and fragrance; vehicle (oleaginous); emollient; solvent.

Almotriptan Malate: White to slightly yellow, crystalline powder. Soluble in water; slightly soluble in methanol and in *N,N*-dimethylformamide; very slightly soluble in acetone, in acetonitrile, in ethanol, in ethyl acetate, in propanol, in tetrahydrofuran, and in toluene; practically insoluble in chloroform and in methylene chloride.

Aloe: Has a characteristic, somewhat sour and disagreeable, odor.

Alprazolam: A white to off-white, crystalline powder. Melts at about 225°. Freely soluble in chloroform; soluble in alcohol; sparingly soluble in acetone; slightly soluble in ethyl acetate; insoluble in water.

Alprostadil: A white to off-white, crystalline powder. Melts at about 110°. Freely soluble in alcohol; soluble in water and in acetone; slightly soluble in ethyl acetate; very slightly soluble in chloroform and in ether.

Altretamine: White, crystalline powder. Soluble in chloroform; insoluble in water.

Ammonium Alum: Large, colorless crystals, crystalline fragments, or white powder. Is odorless, and has a sweetish, strongly astringent taste. Its solutions are acid to litmus. Very soluble in boiling water; freely soluble in water and in glycerin; insoluble in alcohol.

Potassium Alum: Large, colorless crystals, crystalline fragments, or white powder. Is odorless, and has a sweetish, strongly astringent taste. Its solutions are acid to litmus. Very soluble in boiling water; freely soluble in water and in glycerin; insoluble in alcohol.

Aluminum Acetate Topical Solution: Clear, colorless liquid having a faint odor of acetic acid, and a sweetish, astringent taste. Specific gravity is about 1.02.

Aluminum Chloride: White, or yellowish-white, deliquescent, crystalline powder. Is practically odorless, and has a sweet, very astringent taste. Its solutions are acid to litmus. Very soluble in water; freely soluble in alcohol; soluble in glycerin.

Aluminum Hydroxide Gel: White, viscous suspension, from which small amounts of clear liquid may separate on standing.

Dried Aluminum Hydroxide Gel: White, odorless, tasteless, amorphous powder. Soluble in dilute mineral acids and in solutions of fixed alkali hydroxides; insoluble in water and in alcohol.

Aluminum Monostearate: Fine, white to yellowish-white, bulky powder, having a faint, characteristic odor. Insoluble in water, in alcohol, and in ether. *NF category:* Suspending and/or viscosity-increasing agent; emollient.

Aluminum Oxide: Occurs as a white or almost white, amorphous powder. It is very slightly soluble in dilute mineral acids and in solutions of alkali hydroxides. It is practically insoluble in water. *NF category:* Coloring agent.

Aluminum Phosphate Gel: White, viscous suspension from which small amounts of water separate on standing.

Aluminum Subacetate Topical Solution: Clear, colorless or faintly yellow liquid, having an odor of acetic acid and an acid reaction to litmus. Gradually becomes turbid on standing, through separation of a more basic salt.

Aluminum Sulfate: White, crystalline powder, shining plates, or crystalline fragments. Is stable in air. Is odorless, and has a sweet taste, becoming mildly astringent. Freely soluble in water; insoluble in alcohol.

Amantadine Hydrochloride: White or practically white, crystalline powder, having a bitter taste. Freely soluble in water; soluble in alcohol and in chloroform.

Amifostine: White, crystalline powder. Freely soluble in water.

Amikacin: White, crystalline powder. Sparingly soluble in water.

Amikacin Sulfate: White, crystalline powder. Freely soluble in water.

Amiloride Hydrochloride: Yellow to greenish-yellow, odorless or practically odorless powder. Freely soluble in dimethyl sulfoxide; sparingly soluble in methanol; slightly soluble in water; insoluble in ether, in ethyl acetate, in acetone, and in chloroform.

Amino Methacrylate Copolymer: Colorless to yellowish granules. Soluble in acetone, in isopropyl alcohol, and in diluted acids; practically insoluble in water. The solutions are clear to slightly cloudy. *NF category:* Coating agent; polymer membrane; wet binder; diluent; film-forming agent.

Aminobenzoate Potassium: White, crystalline powder. The pH of a 1 in 100 solution in water is about 7. Very soluble in water; soluble in alcohol; practically insoluble in ether.

Aminobenzoic Acid: White or slightly yellow, odorless crystals or crystalline powder. Discolors on exposure to air or light. Freely soluble in alcohol and in solutions of alkali hydroxides and carbonates; sparingly soluble in ether; slightly soluble in water and in chloroform. *NF category:* Free radical scavenger.

Aminobenzoic Acid Topical Solution: Straw-colored solution having the odor of alcohol.

Aminocaproic Acid: Fine, white, crystalline powder. Is odorless, or practically odorless. Its solutions are neutral to litmus. Melts at about 205°. Freely soluble in water, in acids, and in alkalies; slightly soluble in methanol and in alcohol; practically insoluble in chloroform and in ether.

Aminoglutethimide: Fine, white, or creamy white, crystalline powder. Soluble in most organic solvents; very slightly soluble in water. Forms water-soluble salts with strong acids.

Aminohippuric Acid: White, crystalline powder. Discolors on exposure to light. Melts at about 195°, with decomposition. Freely soluble in alkaline solutions, with some decomposition, and in diluted hydrochloric acid; sparingly soluble in water and in alcohol; very slightly soluble in benzene, in carbon tetrachloride, in chloroform, and in ether.

Aminolevulinic Acid Hydrochloride: White to off-white, odorless, crystalline solid. Very soluble in water; slightly soluble in methanol and in ethanol; practically insoluble in chloroform, in hexane, and in mineral oil.

Aminopentamide Sulfate: White, crystalline powder. Freely soluble in water and in alcohol; very slightly soluble in chloroform; practically insoluble in ether.

Aminophylline: White or slightly yellowish granules or powder, having a slight ammoniacal odor and a bitter taste. Upon exposure to air, it gradually loses ethylenediamine and absorbs carbon dioxide with the liberation of free theophylline. Its solutions are alkaline to litmus. One g dissolves in 25 mL of water to give a clear solution; 1 g dissolved in 5 mL of water crystallizes upon standing, but redissolves when a small amount of ethylenediamine is added. Insoluble in alcohol and in ether.

Aminophylline Tablets: May have a faint ammoniacal odor.

Aminosalicylate Sodium: White to cream-colored, crystalline powder. Is practically odorless, and has a sweet, saline taste. Its solutions decompose slowly and darken in color. Freely soluble in water; sparingly soluble in alcohol; very slightly soluble in ether and in chloroform.

Aminosalicylic Acid: White or practically white, bulky powder, that darkens on exposure to light and air. Is odorless, or has a slight acetous odor. Soluble in alcohol; slightly soluble in water and in ether; practically insoluble in benzene.

Amiodarone Hydrochloride: White or almost white, fine, crystalline powder. Freely soluble in methylene chloride; soluble in methanol; sparingly soluble in alcohol; very slightly soluble in water.

Amitriptyline Hydrochloride: White or practically white, odorless or practically odorless, crystalline powder or small crystals. Freely soluble in water, in alcohol, in chloroform, and in methanol; insoluble in ether.

Amlodipine Besylate: A white or almost white powder. Freely soluble in methanol; sparingly soluble in alcohol; slightly soluble in 2-propanol and in water.

Strong Ammonia Solution: Clear, colorless liquid, having an exceedingly pungent, characteristic odor. Specific gravity is about 0.90. *NF category:* pH modifier (acidifying agent/alkalizing agent/buffering agent).

Aromatic Ammonia Spirit: Practically colorless liquid when recently prepared, but gradually acquiring a yellow color on standing. Has the taste of ammonia, has an aromatic and pungent odor, and is affected by light. Specific gravity is about 0.90.

Ammonio Methacrylate Copolymer: Colorless, clear to white-opaque granules or a white powder, both with a faint amine-like odor. Soluble to freely soluble in methanol, in alcohol, and in isopropyl alcohol, each of which contains small amounts of water; soluble to freely soluble in acetone, in ethyl acetate, and in methylene chloride. The solutions are clear to slightly cloudy. Insoluble in petroleum ether and in water. *NF category:* Coating agent; wet binder; polymer membrane; diluent; film-forming agent.

Ammonio Methacrylate Copolymer Dispersion: Milky-white liquids of low viscosity with a faint characteristic odor. Miscible with water in any proportion, the milky-white appearance being retained. A clear or slightly cloudy solution is obtained on mixing one part with five parts of acetone, alcohol, or isopropyl alcohol. When mixed with methanol in a ratio of 1:5, Ammonio Methacrylate Copolymer Dispersion Type A dissolves completely, and Ammonio Methacrylate Copolymer Dispersion Type B dissolves only partially. *NF category:* Coating agent; polymer membrane; wet binder; diluent; film-forming agent.

Ammonium Carbonate: White powder, or hard, white or translucent masses, having a strong odor of ammonia, without empyreuma, and a sharp, ammoniacal taste. Its solutions are alkaline to litmus. On exposure to air, it loses ammonia and carbon dioxide, becoming opaque, and is finally converted into friable lumps or a white powder of ammonium bicarbonate. Freely soluble in water, but is decomposed by hot water. *NF category:* pH modifier (acidifying agent/alkalizing agent/buffering agent).

Ammonium Chloride: Colorless crystals or white, fine or coarse, crystalline powder. Has a cool, saline taste, and is somewhat hygroscopic. Freely soluble in water and in glycerin, and even more so in boiling water; sparingly soluble in alcohol. *NF category:* pH modifier (acidifying agent/alkalizing agent/buffering agent).

Ammonium Glycyrrhizate: White or yellowish-white, hygroscopic powder. It is slightly soluble in water; very slightly soluble in anhydrous ethanol; practically insoluble in acetone. It dissolves in dilute solutions of acids and of alkali hydroxides. *NF category:* Flavors and fragrance; wetting and/or solubilizing agent.

Ammonium Molybdate: Colorless or slightly greenish or yellowish crystals. Soluble in water; practically insoluble in alcohol.

Ammonium Phosphate: Colorless or white granules or powder, having a saline taste. Freely soluble in water; practically insoluble in acetone and in alcohol. *NF category:* pH modifier (acidifying agent/alkalizing agent/buffering agent).

Ammonium Sulfate: Colorless or white crystals or granules that decompose at temperatures above 280°. One g is soluble in about 1.5 mL of water. It is insoluble in alcohol. The pH of a 0.1 M solution is between 4.5 and 6.0.

Amobarbital Sodium: White, friable, granular powder. Is odorless, has a bitter taste, and is hygroscopic. Its solutions decompose on standing, heat accelerating the decomposition. Very soluble in water; soluble in alcohol; practically insoluble in ether and in chloroform.

Amodiaquine: Very pale yellow to light tan-yellow, odorless powder. Sparingly soluble in 1.0 N hydrochloric acid; slightly soluble in alcohol; practically insoluble in water.

Amodiaquine Hydrochloride: Yellow, crystalline powder. Is odorless and has a bitter taste. Soluble in water; sparingly soluble in alcohol; very slightly soluble in benzene, in chloroform, and in ether.

Amoxapine: White to yellowish crystalline powder. Freely soluble in chloroform; soluble in tetrahydrofuran; sparingly soluble in methanol and in toluene; slightly soluble in acetone; practically insoluble in water.

Amoxicillin: White, practically odorless, crystalline powder. Slightly soluble in water and in methanol; insoluble in benzene, in carbon tetrachloride, and in chloroform.

Amphetamine Sulfate: White, odorless, crystalline powder, having a slightly bitter taste. Its solutions are acid to litmus, having a pH of 5 to 6. Freely soluble in water; slightly soluble in alcohol; practically insoluble in ether.

Amphotericin B: Yellow to orange powder; odorless or practically so. Soluble in dimethylformamide, in dimethyl sulfoxide, and in propylene glycol; slightly soluble in methanol; insoluble in water, in anhydrous alcohol, in ether, in benzene, and in toluene.

Amphotericin B for Injection: It yields a colloidal dispersion in water.

Ampicillin: White, practically odorless, crystalline powder. Slightly soluble in water and in methanol; insoluble in benzene, in carbon tetrachloride, and in chloroform.

Ampicillin Sodium: White to off-white, odorless or practically odorless, crystalline powder. Is hygroscopic. Very soluble in water and in isotonic sodium chloride and dextrose solutions.

Amprolium ($C_{14}H_{19}ClN_4 \cdot HCl$): White to light yellow powder. Freely soluble in water, in methanol, in alcohol, and in dimethylformamide; sparingly soluble in dehydrated alcohol; practically insoluble in isopropyl alcohol, in butyl alcohol, and in acetone.

Amyl Nitrite: Clear, yellowish liquid, having a peculiar, ethereal, fruity odor. Is volatile even at low temperatures, and is flammable. Boils at about 96°. Practically insoluble in water. Miscible with alcohol and with ether.

Amylene Hydrate: Clear, colorless liquid, having a camphoraceous odor. Its solutions are neutral to litmus. Freely soluble in water. Miscible with alcohol, with chloroform, with ether, and with glycerin. *NF category:* Solvent.

Anagrelide Hydrochloride: Off-white to pale pinkish powder. Sparingly soluble in dimethylsulfoxide and in dimethylformamide; very slightly soluble in water.

Anastrozole: White to off-white crystalline powder. Very soluble in acetonitrile; freely soluble in methanol, in acetone, in alcohol, and in tetrahydrofuran.

Anethole: Colorless or faintly yellow liquid at or above 23°. Has a sweet taste and the aromatic odor of anise. Is affected by light. Freely soluble in alcohol; very slightly soluble in water. Readily miscible with ether and with chloroform. *NF category:* Flavors and fragrance.

Anileridine: White to yellowish-white, odorless to practically odorless, crystalline powder. Is oxidized on exposure to air and light, becoming darker in color. It exhibits polymorphism, and of two crystalline forms observed, one melts at about 80° and the other at about 89°. Freely soluble in alcohol and in chloroform; soluble in ether, although it may show turbidity; very slightly soluble in water.

Anileridine Hydrochloride: White or nearly white, odorless, crystalline powder. Is stable in air. Melts at about 270°, with decomposition. Freely soluble in water; sparingly soluble in alcohol; practically insoluble in ether, and in chloroform.

Antazoline Phosphate: White to off-white, crystalline powder, having a bitter taste. Soluble in water; sparingly soluble in methanol; practically insoluble in benzene and in ether.

Anthralin: Yellowish-brown, crystalline powder. Is odorless and tasteless. Soluble in chloroform, in acetone, in benzene, and in solutions of alkali hydroxides; slightly soluble in alcohol, in ether, and in glacial acetic acid; insoluble in water.

Anticoagulant Citrate Dextrose Solution: Clear, colorless, odorless liquid. Is dextrorotatory.

Anticoagulant Citrate Phosphate Dextrose Solution: Clear, colorless to slightly yellow, odorless liquid. Is dextrorotatory.

Anticoagulant Sodium Citrate Solution: Clear and colorless liquid.

Antihemophilic Factor: White or yellowish powder. On constitution is opalescent with a slight blue tinge or is a yellowish liquid.

Cryoprecipitated Antihemophilic Factor: Yellowish, frozen solid. On thawing becomes a very viscous, yellow, gummy liquid.

Antimony Potassium Tartrate: Colorless, odorless, transparent crystals, or white powder. The crystals effloresce upon exposure to air and do not readily rehydrate even on exposure to high humidity. Its solutions are acid to litmus. Freely soluble in boiling water; soluble in water and in glycerin; insoluble in alcohol.

Antimony Sodium Tartrate: Colorless, odorless, transparent crystals, or white powder. The crystals effloresce upon exposure to air. Freely soluble in water; insoluble in alcohol.

Antipyrine: Colorless crystals, or white, crystalline powder. Is odorless and has a slightly bitter taste. Its solutions are neutral to litmus. Very soluble in water; freely soluble in alcohol and in chloroform; sparingly soluble in ether.

Antivenin (Crotalidae) Polyvalent: Solid exhibiting the characteristic structure of a freeze-dried solid; light cream in color.

Antivenin (Micrurus Fulvius): Solid exhibiting the characteristic structure of a freeze-dried solid; light cream in color.

Apomorphine Hydrochloride: Minute, white or grayish-white, glistening crystals or white powder. Is odorless. It gradually acquires a green color on exposure to light and air. Its solutions are neutral to litmus. Soluble in water at 80°; sparingly soluble in water and in alcohol; very slightly soluble in chloroform and in ether.

Apraclonidine Hydrochloride: White to off-white, odorless to practically odorless powder. Soluble in methanol; sparingly soluble in water and in alcohol; insoluble in chloroform, in ethyl acetate, and in hexanes.

Aprepitant: White to off-white powder. Sparingly soluble in alcohol; slightly soluble in acetonitrile; practically insoluble in water.

Arginine: White, practically odorless crystals. Freely soluble in water; sparingly soluble in alcohol; insoluble in ether.

Arginine Hydrochloride: White crystals or crystalline powder, practically odorless. Freely soluble in water.

Aripiprazole: A white to off-white, crystalline powder. Freely soluble in dichloromethane; sparingly soluble in toluene; insoluble in methanol and in water.

Aromatic Elixir: *NF category:* Vehicle (flavored and/or sweetened).

Arsanilic Acid: White to off-white, crystalline powder. Melts at about 232°. Soluble in hot water, in amyl alcohol, and in solutions of alkali carbonates; sparingly soluble in concentrated mineral acids; slightly soluble in cold water, in alcohol, and in acetic acid; insoluble in acetone, in benzene, in chloroform, in ether, and in dilute mineral acids.

Articaine Hydrochloride: White or almost white, crystalline powder. Freely soluble in water and in alcohol.

Ascorbic Acid: White or slightly yellow crystals or powder. On exposure to light it gradually darkens. In the dry state, is reasonably stable in air, but in solution rapidly oxidizes. Melts at about 190°. Freely soluble in water; sparingly soluble in alcohol; insoluble in chloroform, in ether, and in benzene. *NF category:* Antioxidant.

Ascorbyl Palmitate: White to yellowish white powder, having a characteristic odor. Soluble in alcohol; very slightly soluble in water and in vegetable oils. *NF category:* Antioxidant.

Asparagine: White crystals or a crystalline powder. Soluble in water; practically insoluble in alcohol and in ether. Its solutions are acid to litmus. It melts at about 234°.

Aspartame: White, odorless, crystalline powder, having a sweet taste. Sparingly soluble in water; slightly soluble in alcohol. Melts at about 246°. The pH of an 8 in 1000 solution is about 5. *NF category:* Sweetening agent.

Aspartame Acesulfame: White, odorless, crystalline powder. Slightly soluble in water and in ethanol. *NF category:* Sweetening agent.

Aspartic Acid: White or almost white, crystalline powder, or colorless crystals. Soluble in dilute solutions of alkali hydroxides and in dilute mineral acids; slightly soluble in water; practically insoluble in alcohol and in ether.

Aspirin: White crystals, commonly tabular or needle-like, or white, crystalline powder. Is odorless or has a faint odor. Is stable in dry air; in moist air it gradually hydrolyzes to salicylic and acetic acids. Freely soluble in alcohol; soluble in chloroform and in ether; sparingly soluble in absolute ether; slightly soluble in water.

Atenolol: White or practically white, odorless powder. Melting point 146°–148° (crystals from ethyl acetate). Freely soluble in methanol; sparingly soluble in alcohol; slightly soluble in water and in isopropanol.

Atomoxetine Hydrochloride: White to practically white solid. Sparingly soluble in water.

Atorvastatin Calcium: White to off-white powder. Soluble to freely soluble in methanol; slightly soluble in alcohol; insoluble to very slightly soluble in distilled water, in pH 7.4 phosphate buffer, and in acetonitrile; insoluble in aqueous solutions of pH 4 and below.

Atovaquone: Yellow powder. Freely soluble in N-methyl-2-pyrrolidone and in tetrahydrofuran; soluble in chloroform; sparingly soluble in acetone, in di-n-butyl adipate, in dimethyl sulfoxide, and in polyethylene glycol 400; slightly soluble in alcohol, in 1,3-butanediol, in ethyl acetate, in glycerin, in octanol, and in polyethylene glycol 200; very slightly soluble in 0.1 N sodium hydroxide; insoluble in water.

Atracurium Besylate: White to yellowish white powder, slightly hygroscopic. Very soluble in acetonitrile, in alcohol, and in methylene chloride; soluble in water.

Atropine: White crystals, usually needle-like, or white, crystalline powder. Its saturated solution is alkaline to phenolphthalein TS. Is optically inactive, but usually contains some levorotatory hyoscyamine. Freely soluble in alcohol and in chloroform; soluble in glycerin and in ether; slightly soluble in water; sparingly soluble in water at 80°.

Atropine Sulfate: Colorless crystals, or white, crystalline powder. Odorless; effloresces in dry air; is slowly affected by light. Very soluble in water; freely soluble in alcohol and even more so in boiling alcohol; freely soluble in glycerin.

Activated Attapulgite: Cream-colored, micronized, nonswelling powder, free from gritty particles. The high heat treatment used in its preparation causes it to yield only moderately viscous aqueous suspensions, its dispersion consisting mainly of particle groups. Insoluble in water. *NF category:* Suspending and/or viscosity-increasing agent.

Colloidal Activated Attapulgite: Cream-colored, micronized, nonswelling powder, free from gritty particles. Yields viscous aqueous suspensions, as a result of dispersion into its constituent ultimate particles. Insoluble in water. *NF category:* Suspending and/or viscosity-increasing agent.

Aurothioglucose: Yellow, odorless or practically odorless powder. Is stable in air. An aqueous solution is unstable on long standing. The pH of its 1 in 100 solution is about 6.3. Freely soluble in water; practically insoluble in acetone, in alcohol, in chloroform, and in ether.

Azatadine Maleate: White to light cream-colored, odorless powder. Melts at about 153°. Freely soluble in water, in alcohol, in chloroform, and in methanol; practically insoluble in benzene and in ether.

Azathioprine: Pale yellow, odorless powder. Soluble in dilute solutions of alkali hydroxides; sparingly soluble in dilute mineral acids; very slightly soluble in alcohol and in chloroform; insoluble in water.

Azathioprine Sodium for Injection: Bright yellow, hygroscopic, amorphous mass or cake.

Azelastine Hydrochloride: White or almost white, crystalline powder. Soluble in ethanol and in methylene chloride; sparingly soluble in water.

Azithromycin: White or almost white powder. Freely soluble in anhydrous ethanol and in methylene chloride; practically insoluble in water.

Aztreonam: White, odorless, crystalline powder. Soluble in dimethylformamide and in dimethyl sulfoxide; slightly soluble in methanol; very slightly soluble in dehydrated alcohol; practically insoluble in ethyl acetate, in chloroform, and in toluene.

Bacampicillin Hydrochloride: White or practically white powder. Is hygroscopic. Freely soluble in alcohol and in chloroform; soluble in methylene chloride and in water; very slightly soluble in ether.

Bacitracin: White to pale buff powder, odorless or having a slight odor. Is hygroscopic. Its solutions deteriorate rapidly at room temperature. Is precipitated from its solutions and is inactivated by salts of many of the heavy metals. Freely soluble in water; soluble in alcohol, in methanol, and in glacial acetic acid, the solution in the organic solvents usually showing some insoluble residue; insoluble in acetone, in chloroform, and in ether.

Bacitracin Zinc: White to pale tan powder, odorless or having a slight odor. Is hygroscopic. Sparingly soluble in water.

Baclofen: White to off-white, crystalline powder. Is odorless or practically so. Slightly soluble in water; very slightly soluble in methanol; insoluble in chloroform.

Balsalazide Disodium: Orange to yellow powder. Freely soluble in water and in isotonic saline; sparingly soluble in methanol and in alcohol; practically insoluble in all other organic solvents.

Adhesive Bandage: The compress of Adhesive Bandage is substantially free from loose threads or ravelings. The adhesive strip may be perforated, and the back may be coated with a water-repellent film.

Gauze Bandage: One continuous piece, tightly rolled, in various widths and lengths and substantially free from loose threads and ravelings.

Barium Hydroxide Lime: White or grayish-white granules. May have a color if an indicator has been added. *NF category:* Sorbent, carbon dioxide.

Barium Sulfate: Fine, white, odorless, tasteless, bulky powder, free from grittiness. Practically insoluble in water, in organic solvents, and in solutions of acids and of alkalies.

Barium Sulfate for Suspension: White or colored, bulky or granular powder.

BCG Vaccine: White to creamy white, dried mass, having the characteristic texture of material dried in the frozen state.

Beclomethasone Dipropionate: White to cream white, odorless powder. Very soluble in chloroform; freely soluble in acetone and in alcohol; very slightly soluble in water.

Behenoyl Polyoxylglycerides: Waxy solid or fine powder. Soluble in methylene chloride; insoluble in alcohol; dispersible in water. *NF category:* Lubricant; emulsifying agent; wetting and/or solubilizing agent.

Belladonna Leaf: When moistened, its odor is slight, somewhat tobacco-like. Its taste is somewhat bitter and acrid.

Benazepril Hydrochloride: White to off-white, crystalline powder. Soluble in water, in methanol, and in alcohol.

Bendroflumethiazide: White to cream-colored, finely divided, crystalline powder. Is odorless, or has a slight odor. Melts at about 220°. Freely soluble in alcohol and in acetone; practically insoluble in water.

Benoxinate Hydrochloride: White, or slightly off-white, crystals or crystalline powder. Is odorless, or has a slight characteristic odor, has a salty taste, and exhibits local anesthetic properties when placed upon the tongue. Its solutions are neutral to litmus, and it melts at about 158°. Very soluble in water; freely soluble in chloroform and in alcohol; insoluble in ether.

Bentonite: Very fine, odorless, pale buff or cream-colored to grayish powder, free from grit. Has a slightly earthy taste. Is hygroscopic. Insoluble in water, but swells to approximately twelve times its volume when added to water; insoluble in, and does not swell in, organic solvents. *NF category:* Suspending and/or viscosity-increasing agent.

Purified Bentonite: Odorless, tasteless, fine (micronized) powder or small flakes that are creamy when viewed on their flat surfaces and tan to brown when viewed on their edges. Insoluble in water and in alcohol. Swells when added to water or glycerin. *NF category:* Suspending and/or viscosity-increasing agent.

Bentonite Magma: *NF category:* Suspending and/or viscosity-increasing agent.

Benzaldehyde: Colorless, strongly refractive liquid. Is affected by light. Slightly soluble in water. Miscible with alcohol, with ether, and with fixed and volatile oils. The specific gravity is 1.041–1.046 at 25° (see *Specific Gravity* ⟨841⟩), and the refractive index is 1.544–1.546 at 20° (see *Refractive Index* ⟨831⟩). *NF category:* Flavors and fragrance.

Benzaldehyde Elixir, Compound: *NF category:* Flavored and/or sweetened vehicle.

Benzalkonium Chloride: White or yellowish-white, thick gel or gelatinous pieces. Usually has a mild, aromatic odor. Its aqueous solution has a bitter taste, foams strongly when shaken, and usually is slightly alkaline. Very soluble in water and in alcohol. Anhydrous form freely soluble in benzene, and slightly soluble in ether. *NF category:* Antimicrobial preservative; wetting and/or solubilizing agent; emulsifying agent.

Benzalkonium Chloride Solution: Clear liquid; colorless or slightly yellow unless a color has been added. Has an aromatic odor and a bitter taste. *NF category:* Antimicrobial preservative.

Benzethonium Chloride: White crystals, having a mild odor. Its solution (1 in 100) is slightly alkaline to litmus. Soluble in water, in alcohol, and in chloroform; slightly soluble in ether. *NF category:* Antimicrobial preservative; wetting and/or solubilizing agent.

Benzethonium Chloride Solution: Odorless, clear liquid, slightly alkaline to litmus.

Benzethonium Chloride Tincture: Clear liquid, having the characteristic odor of acetone and of alcohol.

Benzocaine: Small, white crystals or white, crystalline powder. Is odorless, is stable in air, and exhibits local anesthetic properties when placed upon the tongue. Freely soluble in alcohol, in chloroform, and in ether; sparingly soluble in almond oil and in olive oil; very slightly soluble in water. Dissolves in dilute acids.

Benzoic Acid: White crystals, scales, or needles. Has a slight odor, usually suggesting benzaldehyde or benzoin. Somewhat volatile at moderately warm temperatures. Freely volatile in steam. Freely soluble in alcohol, in chloroform, and in ether; slightly soluble in water. *NF category:* Antimicrobial preservative.

Benzoin: Sumatra Benzoin has an aromatic and balsamic odor. When heated it does not emit a pinaceous odor. When Sumatra Benzoin is digested with boiling water, the odor suggests cinnamates or storax. Its taste is aromatic and slightly acrid. Siam Benzoin has an agreeable, balsamic, vanilla-like odor. Its taste is aromatic and slightly acrid.

Benzonatate: Clear, pale yellow, viscous liquid, having a faint, characteristic odor. Has a bitter taste, and exhibits local anesthetic properties when placed upon the tongue. Miscible with water in all proportions. Freely soluble in chloroform, in alcohol, and in benzene.

Hydrous Benzoyl Peroxide: White, granular powder, having a characteristic odor. Soluble in acetone, in chloroform, and in ether; sparingly soluble in water and in alcohol.

Benzoyl Peroxide Gel: A soft, white gel, having a characteristic odor.

Benzoyl Peroxide Lotion: White, viscous, creamy lotion, having a characteristic odor.

Benztropine Mesylate: White, slightly hygroscopic, crystalline powder. Very soluble in water; freely soluble in alcohol; very slightly soluble in ether.

Benzyl Alcohol: Clear, colorless, oily liquid. Boils at about 206°, without decomposition. Is neutral to litmus. Freely soluble in 50% alcohol; sparingly soluble in water. Miscible with alcohol, with ether, and with chloroform. The specific gravity is between 1.042 and 1.047. *NF category:* Antimicrobial preservative; solvent.

Benzyl Benzoate: Clear, colorless, oily liquid having a slight aromatic odor and producing a sharp, burning sensation on the tongue. Practically insoluble in water and in glycerin. Miscible with alcohol, with ether, and with chloroform. *NF category:* Solvent; emulsifying agent; plasticizer.

Beta Carotene: Red or reddish-brown to violet-brown crystals or crystalline powder. Soluble in carbon disulfide, in benzene, and in chloroform; sparingly soluble in ether, in solvent hexane, and in vegetable oils; practically insoluble in methanol and in alcohol; insoluble in water, in acids, and in alkalies.

Betadex: White, practically odorless, fine crystalline powder having a slightly sweet taste. Sparingly soluble in water. *NF category:* Sequestering agent; chelating and/or complexing agent.

Betadex Sulfobutyl Ether Sodium: White to off-white, amorphous powder. Freely soluble in water; sparingly soluble in methanol; practically insoluble in ethanol, in *n*-hexane, in 1-butanol, in acetonitrile, in 2-propanol, and in ethyl acetate. *NF category:* Chelating and/or complexing agent; sequestering agent; wetting and/or solubilizing agent.

Betahistine Hydrochloride: White to almost yellow, crystalline powder. Very hygroscopic. Melts between 151° and 154°. Very soluble in water; freely soluble in alcohol; practically insoluble in isopropyl alcohol.

Betaine Hydrochloride: White, crystalline powder. Soluble in water and in alcohol; practically insoluble in chloroform and in ether.

Betamethasone: White to practically white, odorless, crystalline powder. Melts at about 240°, with some decomposition. Sparingly soluble in acetone, in alcohol, in dioxane, and in methanol; very slightly soluble in chloroform and in ether; insoluble in water.

Betamethasone Acetate: White to creamy white, odorless powder. Sinters and resolidifies at about 165°, and remelts at about 200° or 220°, with decomposition (see *Melting Range or Temperature* ⟨741⟩). Freely soluble in acetone; soluble in alcohol and in chloroform; practically insoluble in water.

Betamethasone Benzoate: White to practically white, practically odorless powder. Melts at about 220°, with decomposition. Soluble in alcohol, in methanol, and in chloroform; insoluble in water.

Betamethasone Dipropionate: White to cream-white, odorless powder. Freely soluble in acetone and in chloroform; sparingly soluble in alcohol; insoluble in water.

Betamethasone Sodium Phosphate: White to practically white, odorless powder. Is hygroscopic. Freely soluble in water and in methanol; practically insoluble in acetone and in chloroform.

Betamethasone Valerate: White to practically white, odorless powder. Melts at about 190°, with decomposition. Freely soluble in acetone and in chloroform; soluble in alcohol; slightly soluble in benzene and in ether; practically insoluble in water.

Betaxolol Hydrochloride: White, crystalline powder. Freely soluble in water, in alcohol, in chloroform, and in methanol.

Bethanechol Chloride: Colorless or white crystals or white, crystalline powder, usually having a slight, amine-like odor. Is hygroscopic. Exhibits polymorphism, and of two crystalline forms observed, one melts at about 211° and the other melts at about 219°. Freely soluble in water and in alcohol; insoluble in chloroform and in ether.

Bicalutamide: Fine, white to off-white powder. Freely soluble in tetrahydrofuran and in acetone; soluble in acetonitrile; sparingly soluble in methanol; slightly soluble in alcohol.

Biotin: Practically white, crystalline powder. Very slightly soluble in water and in alcohol; insoluble in other common organic solvents.

Biperiden: White, practically odorless, crystalline powder. Freely soluble in chloroform; sparingly soluble in alcohol; practically insoluble in water.

Biperiden Hydrochloride: White, practically odorless, crystalline powder. Melts at about 275°, with decomposition. Is optically inactive. Sparingly soluble in methanol; slightly soluble in water, in ether, in alcohol, and in chloroform.

Bisacodyl: White to off-white, crystalline powder, in which the number of particles having a longest diameter smaller than 50 μm predominate. Soluble in chloroform and in benzene; sparingly soluble in alcohol and in methanol; slightly soluble in ether; practically insoluble in water.

Milk of Bismuth: Thick, white, opaque suspension that separates on standing. Is odorless and practically tasteless. Miscible with water and with alcohol.

Bismuth Citrate: White, amorphous or crystalline powder. Stable in air. Melts at about 300°, with decomposition. Soluble in ammonia TS and in solutions of alkali citrates; insoluble in water and in alcohol.

Bismuth Subcarbonate: White or almost white powder. Practically insoluble in water, in alcohol, and in ether. Dissolves in dilute acids with effervescence.

Bismuth Subgallate: Amorphous, bright yellow powder. Is odorless and tasteless. Is stable in air, but is affected by light. Dissolves readily with decomposition in warm, moderately dilute hydrochloric, nitric, or sulfuric acid; readily dissolved by solutions of alkali hydroxides, forming a clear, yellow liquid that rapidly assumes a deep red color. Practically insoluble in water, in alcohol, in chloroform, and in ether; insoluble in very dilute mineral acids.

Bismuth Subnitrate: White, slightly hygroscopic powder. Practically insoluble in water and in alcohol; readily dissolved by hydrochloric acid or by nitric acid.

Bismuth Subsalicylate: Fine to off-white, microcrystalline, odorless, tasteless powder. Practically insoluble in water, in alcohol, and in ether. Reacts with alkalies and mineral acids.

Bisoprolol Fumarate: White, crystalline powder. Very soluble in water and in methanol; freely soluble in chloroform, in glacial acetic acid, and in alcohol; slightly soluble in acetone and in ethyl acetate.

Bleomycin Sulfate: Cream-colored, amorphous powder. Very soluble in water.

Anti-A Blood Grouping Serum: Liquid Serum is a clear or slightly opalescent fluid unless artificially colored blue.

Dried Serum is light yellow to deep cream color, unless artificially colored as indicated for liquid Serum. The liquid Serum may develop slight turbidity upon storage. The dried Serum may show slight turbidity upon reconstitution for use.

Anti-B Blood Grouping Serum: Liquid Serum is a clear or slightly opalescent fluid unless artificially colored yellow. Dried Serum is light yellow to deep cream color, unless artificially colored as indicated for liquid Serum. The liquid Serum may develop a slight turbidity on storage. The dried Serum may show slight turbidity upon reconstitution for use.

Blood Grouping Serums Anti-D, Anti-C, Anti-E, Anti-c, Anti-e: The liquid Serums are clear, slightly yellowish fluids, that may develop slight turbidity on storage. The dried Serums are light yellow to deep cream color.

Blood Group Specific Substances A, B, and AB: Clear solution that may have a slight odor because of the preservative.

Red Blood Cells: Dark red in color when packed. May show a slight creamy layer on the surface and a small supernatant layer of yellow or opalescent plasma. Also supplied in deep-frozen form with added cryophylactic substance to extend storage time.

Whole Blood: Deep red, opaque liquid from which the corpuscles readily settle upon standing for 24 to 48 hours, leaving a clear, yellowish or pinkish supernatant layer of plasma.

Boric Acid: Colorless, odorless scales of a somewhat pearly luster, or crystals, or white powder that is slightly unctuous to the touch. Is stable in air. Freely soluble in glycerin, in boiling water, and in boiling alcohol; soluble in water and in alcohol. *NF category:* pH modifier (acidifying agent/alkalizing agent/buffering agent); antimicrobial preservative.

Botulism Antitoxin: Transparent or slightly opalescent liquid, practically colorless, and practically odorless or having an odor because of the antimicrobial agent.

Bretylium Tosylate: White, crystalline powder. Is hygroscopic. Freely soluble in water, in methanol, and in alcohol; practically insoluble in ether, in ethyl acetate, and in hexane.

Add the following:

■**Brimonidine Tartrate:** White, or slightly yellowish, or slightly brownish powder. Soluble in water; practically insoluble in anhydrous ethanol and in toluene.■1S (USP41)

Brinzolamide: White or almost white powder. Slightly soluble in alcohol and in methanol; insoluble in water.

Bromocriptine Mesylate: White or slightly colored, fine crystalline powder, odorless or having a weak, characteristic odor.

Bromodiphenhydramine Hydrochloride: White to pale buff, crystalline powder, having no more than a faint odor. Freely soluble in water and in alcohol; soluble in isopropyl alcohol; insoluble in ether and in solvent hexane.

Brompheniramine Maleate: White, odorless, crystalline powder. Freely soluble in water; soluble in alcohol and in chloroform; slightly soluble in ether and in benzene.

Budesonide: White to off-white, odorless, crystalline powder. Freely soluble in chloroform; sparingly soluble in alcohol; practically insoluble in water and in heptane.

Bumetanide: Practically white powder. Soluble in alkaline solutions; slightly soluble in water.

Bupivacaine Hydrochloride: White, odorless, crystalline powder. Melts at about 248°, with decomposition. Freely soluble in water and in alcohol; slightly soluble in chloroform and in acetone.

Bupivacaine Hydrochloride Injection: Clear, colorless solution.

Bupivacaine Hydrochloride and Epinephrine Injection: Clear, colorless solution.

Bupropion Hydrochloride: White powder. Soluble in water, in 0.1 N hydrochloric acid, and in alcohol.

Buspirone Hydrochloride: White crystalline powder. Very soluble in water; freely soluble in methanol and in methylene chloride; sparingly soluble in ethanol and in acetonitrile; very slightly soluble in ethyl acetate; practically insoluble in hexanes.

Busulfan: White, crystalline powder. Sparingly soluble in acetone; slightly soluble in alcohol; very slightly soluble in water.

Butabarbital: White, odorless, crystalline powder. Soluble in alcohol, in chloroform, in ether, and in solutions of alkali hydroxides and carbonates; very slightly soluble in water.

Butabarbital Sodium: White powder, having a bitter taste. Freely soluble in water and in alcohol; practically insoluble in absolute ether.

Butalbital: White, crystalline, odorless powder, having a slightly bitter taste. Is stable in air. Its saturated solution is acid to litmus. Freely soluble in alcohol, in ether, and in chloroform; soluble in boiling water, and in solutions of fixed alkalies and alkali carbonates; slightly soluble in cold water.

Butamben: White, crystalline powder. Is odorless and tasteless. Soluble in dilute acids, in alcohol, in chloroform, in ether, and in fixed oils; very slightly soluble in water. Is slowly hydrolyzed when boiled with water.

Butane: Colorless, flammable gas (boiling temperature is about −0.5°). One volume of water dissolves 0.15 volume, and 1 volume of alcohol dissolves 18 volumes at 17° and 770 mm; 1 volume of ether or chloroform at 17° dissolves 25 or 30 volumes, respectively. Vapor pressure at 21° is about 1620 mm of mercury (17 psig). *NF category:* Propellant.

Butoconazole Nitrate: White to off-white, crystalline powder. Melts at about 160°. Sparingly soluble in methanol; slightly soluble in acetonitrile, in acetone, in dichloromethane, and in tetrahydrofuran; very slightly soluble in ethyl acetate; practically insoluble in water.

Butorphanol Tartrate: White powder. Its solutions are slightly acidic. Melts between 217° and 219°, with decomposition. Soluble in dilute acids; sparingly soluble in water; slightly soluble in methanol; insoluble in alcohol, in chloroform, in ethyl acetate, in ethyl ether, and in hexane.

Butyl Alcohol: Clear, colorless, mobile liquid, having a characteristic, penetrating vinous odor. Soluble in water. Miscible with alcohol, with ether, and with many other organic solvents. *NF category:* Solvent.

Butylene Glycol: Clear, colorless, hygroscopic, viscous liquid. It is miscible with water, with acetone, and with ether in all proportions; immiscible with fixed oils. It dissolves most essential oils and synthetic flavoring substances. *NF category:* Solvent; wetting and/or solubilizing agent.

Butyl Palmitostearate: Colorless or pale yellowish waxy solid at temperatures below 17°–24° or colorless or pale yellowish liquid at temperatures of 17°–24° or above. Soluble in acetone, in alcohol, in ether, in mineral oils, and in vegetable oils; practically insoluble in water and in propylene glycol. *NF category:* Emulsifying and/or solubilizing agent; flavors and fragrance; plasticizer.

Butyl Stearate: Colorless or pale yellowish waxy solid at temperatures below 19°–24° or colorless or pale yellowish liquid at temperatures of 19°–24° or above. Soluble in acetone, in alcohol, in ether, in mineral oils, and in vegetable oils; practically insoluble in water and in propylene glycol. *NF category:* Emulsifying and/or solubilizing agent; flavors and fragrance; plasticizer.

Butylated Hydroxyanisole: White or slightly yellow, waxy solid, having a faint, characteristic odor. Freely soluble in alcohol, in propylene glycol, in chloroform, and in ether; insoluble in water. *NF category:* Antioxidant.

Butylated Hydroxytoluene: White, crystalline solid, having a faint, characteristic odor. Freely soluble in alcohol, in chloroform, and in ether; insoluble in water and in propylene glycol. *NF category:* Antioxidant.

Butylparaben: Small, colorless crystals or white powder. Freely soluble in acetone, in alcohol, in ether, and in propylene glycol; very slightly soluble in water and in glycerin. *NF category:* Antimicrobial preservative.

Cabergoline: White or almost white, crystalline or amorphous powder. Freely soluble in alcohol (96%); slightly soluble in 0.1 M hydrochloric acid; very slightly soluble in hexane; practically insoluble in water.

Caffeine: White powder or white, glistening needles, usually matted together. Is odorless and has a bitter taste. Its solutions are neutral to litmus. The hydrate is efflorescent in air. Freely soluble in chloroform; sparingly soluble in water and in alcohol; slightly soluble in ether.

Calamine: Pink, odorless, practically tasteless, fine powder. Soluble in mineral acids; insoluble in water.

Calcipotriene: White or almost white crystalline powder. Freely soluble in alcohol; slightly soluble in methylene chloride; practically insoluble in water.

Calcitriol: White or almost white crystals. Freely soluble in alcohol; soluble in ether and in fatty oils; practically insoluble in water. It is sensitive to air, heat, and light.

Calcium Acetate: White, odorless or almost odorless, hygroscopic, crystalline powder. When heated to above 160°, it decomposes to calcium carbonate and acetone. Freely soluble in water; slightly soluble in methanol; practically insoluble in acetone, in dehydrated alcohol, and in benzene. *NF category:* Antimicrobial preservative; sequestering agent.

Calcium Ascorbate: White to slightly yellow, practically odorless powder. Freely soluble in water (approximately 50 g per 100 mL); slightly soluble in alcohol; insoluble in ether.

Calcium Carbonate: Fine, white, odorless, tasteless, microcrystalline powder. Is stable in air. Practically insoluble in water. Its solubility in water is increased by the presence of any ammonium salt or of carbon dioxide. The presence of any alkali hydroxide reduces its solubility. Insoluble in alcohol. Dissolves with effervescence in 1 N acetic acid, in 3 N hydrochloric acid, and in 2 N nitric acid. *NF category:* Diluent; pH modifier (acidifying agent/alkalizing agent/buffering agent); coating agent; wet binder.

Calcium Chloride: White, hard, odorless fragments or granules. Is deliquescent. Very soluble in boiling water; freely soluble in water, in alcohol, and in boiling alcohol. *NF category:* Desiccant; antimicrobial preservative.

Calcium Citrate: White, odorless, crystalline powder. Freely soluble in diluted 3 N hydrochloric acid and in diluted 2 N nitric acid; slightly soluble in water; insoluble in alcohol.

Calcium Gluceptate: White to faintly yellow, amorphous powder. Is stable in air, but the hydrous forms may lose part of their water of hydration on standing. Freely soluble in water; insoluble in alcohol and in many other organic solvents.

Calcium Gluconate: White, crystalline, odorless, tasteless granules or powder. Is stable in air. Its solutions are neutral to litmus. Freely soluble in boiling water; sparingly (and slowly) soluble in water; insoluble in alcohol.

Calcium Hydroxide: White powder. Has an alkaline, slightly bitter taste. Soluble in glycerin and in syrup; slightly soluble in water; very slightly soluble in boiling water; insoluble in alcohol. *NF category:* pH modifier (acidifying agent/alkalizing agent/buffering agent).

Calcium Hydroxide Solution: Clear, colorless liquid having an alkaline taste. Is alkaline to litmus.

Calcium Lactate: White, practically odorless granules or powder. The pentahydrate is somewhat efflorescent and at 120° becomes anhydrous. The pentahydrate is soluble in water; it is practically insoluble in alcohol. *NF category:* pH modifier (acidifying agent/alkalizing agent/buffering agent); antimicrobial preservative; wet binder.

Calcium Levulinate: White, crystalline or amorphous, powder, having a faint odor suggestive of burnt sugar. Has a bitter, salty taste. Freely soluble in water; slightly soluble in alcohol; insoluble in ether and in chloroform.

Calcium Pantothenate: Slightly hygroscopic, white powder. Is odorless and has a bitter taste. Freely soluble in water; soluble in glycerin; practically insoluble in alcohol, in chloroform, and in ether.

Racemic Calcium Pantothenate: White, slightly hygroscopic powder, having a faint, characteristic odor, and a bitter taste. Is stable in air. Its solutions are neutral or alkaline to litmus. Is optically inactive. Freely soluble in water; soluble in glycerin; practically insoluble in alcohol, in chloroform, and in ether.

Dibasic Calcium Phosphate: White, odorless, tasteless powder. Is stable in air. Soluble in 3 N hydrochloric acid and in 2 N nitric acid; practically insoluble in water; insoluble in alcohol. *NF category:* Diluent.

Tribasic Calcium Phosphate: White, odorless, tasteless powder. Is stable in air. Freely soluble in 3 N hydrochloric acid and in 2 N nitric acid; practically insoluble in water; insoluble in alcohol. *NF category:* Diluent; pH modifier (acidifying agent/alkalizing agent/buffering solution); glidant and/or anticaking agent.

Calcium Polycarbophil: White to creamy white powder. Insoluble in water, in dilute acids, in dilute alkalies, and in common organic solvents.

Calcium Propionate: Occurs as a white crystalline solid. One g dissolves in about 3 mL of water. *NF category:* Antimicrobial preservative.

Calcium Saccharate: White, odorless, tasteless, crystalline powder. Soluble in dilute mineral acids and in solutions of calcium gluconate; slightly soluble in boiling water; very slightly soluble in alcohol, and in cold water; practically insoluble in ether and in chloroform.

Calcium Silicate: White to off-white, free-flowing powder that remains so after absorbing relatively large amounts of water or other liquids. Insoluble in water. Forms a gel with mineral acids. *NF category:* Glidant and/or anticaking agent.

Calcium Stearate: Fine, white to yellowish-white, bulky powder having a slight, characteristic odor. Is unctuous, and is free from grittiness. Insoluble in water, in alcohol, and in ether. *NF category:* Lubricant.

Calcium Sulfate: Fine, white to slightly yellow-white, odorless powder. Soluble in 3 N hydrochloric acid; slightly soluble in water. *NF category:* Desiccant; diluent.

Calcium Undecylenate: Fine, white powder, having a characteristic odor and no grit. Slightly soluble in hot alcohol; practically insoluble in water, in ether, in chloroform, in acetone, and in cold alcohol.

Camphor: Colorless or white crystals, granules, or crystalline masses; or colorless to white, translucent, tough masses. Has a penetrating, characteristic odor and a pungent, aromatic taste. Specific gravity is about 0.99. Slowly volatilizes at ordinary temperatures. Slightly soluble in water; very soluble in alcohol, in chloroform, and in ether; freely soluble in carbon disulfide, in solvent hexane, and in fixed and volatile oils.

Candelilla Wax: A hard, yellowish-brown-opaque to translucent wax. Its specific gravity is about 0.983. Soluble in chloroform and in toluene; insoluble in water.

Candesartan Cilexetil: White to off-white powder. Sparingly soluble in methanol; practically insoluble in water.

Canola Oil: Clear, pale yellow, slightly viscous liquid. Practically insoluble in water and in alcohol. Miscible with light petroleum (bp: 40° to 60°). *NF category:* Solvent; emollient; vehicle (oleaginous).

Capecitabine: White to off-white crystalline powder. Freely soluble in methanol; soluble in acetonitrile and in alcohol; sparingly soluble in water.

Capreomycin Sulfate: White to practically white, amorphous powder. Freely soluble in water; practically insoluble in most organic solvents.

Caprylic Acid: Clear, colorless or slightly yellowish, oily liquid. Very soluble in acetone and in alcohol; very slightly soluble in water. It dissolves in dilute solutions of alkali hydroxides. *NF category:* Emulsifying agent.

Caprylocaproyl Polyoxylglycerides: Pale yellow, oily liquids. Dispersible in hot water; freely soluble in methylene chloride. *NF category:* Ointment base; solvent; wetting and/or solubilizing agent; emulsifying agent.

Capsaicin: Off-white powder. Melts at about 65°. Soluble in alcohol, in benzene, in chloroform; slightly soluble in carbon disulfide; practically insoluble in cold water.

Capsicum Oleoresin: Dark red, oily liquid. Soluble in alcohol, in acetone, in ether, in chloroform, and in volatile oils; soluble with opalescence in fixed oils.

Captopril: White to off-white, crystalline powder, which may have a characteristic, sulfide-like odor. Melts in the range of 104° to 110°. Freely soluble in water, in methanol, in alcohol, and in chloroform.

Caramel: Thick, dark brown liquid having the characteristic odor of burnt sugar, and a pleasant, bitter taste. One part dissolved in 1000 parts of water yields a clear solution having a distinct yellowish-orange color. The color of this solution is not changed and no precipitate is formed after exposure to sunlight for 6 hours. When spread in a thin layer on a glass plate, it appears homogeneous, reddish-brown, and transparent. Miscible with water. Soluble in dilute alcohol up to 55% (v/v). Immiscible with ether, with chloroform, with acetone, with benzene, and with solvent hexane. *NF category:* Coloring agent.

Carbachol: White powder. Freely soluble in water; sparingly soluble in alcohol; practically insoluble in chloroform and in ether.

Carbamazepine: White to off-white powder. Soluble in alcohol and in acetone; practically insoluble in water.

Carbamide Peroxide Topical Solution: Clear, colorless, viscous liquid, having a characteristic odor and taste.

Carbenicillin Disodium: White to off-white, crystalline powder. Freely soluble in water; soluble in alcohol; practically insoluble in chloroform and in ether.

Carbenicillin Indanyl Sodium: White to off-white powder. Soluble in water and in alcohol.

Carbidopa: White to creamy white, odorless or practically odorless, powder. Freely soluble in 3 N hydrochloric acid; slightly soluble in water, and in methanol; practically insoluble in alcohol, in acetone, in chloroform, and in ether.

Carbinoxamine Maleate: White, odorless, crystalline powder. Very soluble in water; freely soluble in alcohol and in chloroform; very slightly soluble in ether.

Carbol-Fuchsin Topical Solution: Dark purple liquid, which appears purplish red when spread in a thin film.

Carbomer 910:   White, fluffy powder, having a slight, characteristic odor. Is hygroscopic. The pH of a 1 in 100 dispersion is about 3. When neutralized with alkali hydroxides or with amines, it dissolves in water, in alcohol, and in glycerin. *NF category:* Suspending and/or viscosity-increasing agent.

Carbomer 934:   See *Carbomer 910.*

Carbomer 934P: See *Carbomer 910.*

Carbomer 940:   See *Carbomer 910.*

Carbomer 941:   See *Carbomer 910.*

Carbomer 1342:   See *Carbomer 910.*

Carbomer Copolymer: White, hygroscopic powder. It swells in water when a dispersion of it is neutralized with sodium hydroxide to a pH within the range of 7.3 to 7.8. *NF category:* Emulsifying agent; suspending and/or viscosity-increasing agent; wet binder; polymers for ophthalmic use; release-modifying agent.

Carbomer Homopolymer: White, fluffy hygroscopic powder, having a slight, characteristic odor. The pH of a 1 in 100 dispersion in water is about 3. When neutralized with alkali hydroxides or with amines, it swells giving the appearance of dissolving in water; when neutralized with lower amines and alkanolamines, it swells giving the appearance of dissolving in methanol or glycerin; when neutralized with ethoxylated long-chain (C_{14}–C_{18}) amines, it swells giving the appearance of dissolving in ethanol. *NF category:* Wet binder; suspending and/or viscosity-increasing agent; emulsifying agent; polymers for ophthalmic use; release-modifying agent.

Carbomer Interpolymer: White, hygroscopic powder. It swells in water when a dispersion of it is neutralized with sodium hydroxide to a pH within the range of 5.5 to 9. *NF category:* Emulsifying agent; suspending and/or viscosity increasing agent; wet binder; polymers for ophthalmic use; release-modifying agent.

Carbon Dioxide: Odorless, colorless gas. Its solutions are acid to litmus. One L at 0° and at a pressure of 760 mm of mercury weighs 1.977 g. One volume dissolves in about 1 volume of water. *NF category:* Air displacement; propellant.

Carboprost Tromethamine: White to off-white powder. Soluble in water.

Carboxymethylcellulose Calcium: White to yellowish-white powder. Is hygroscopic. Practically insoluble in alcohol, in acetone, in ether, in chloroform, and in benzene. It swells with water to form a suspension; the pH of the suspension, obtained by shaking 1 g with 100 mL of water, is between 4.5 and 6.0. *NF category:* Suspending and/or viscosity-increasing agent; coating agent; emulsifying agent; film-forming agent; disintegrant.

Carboxymethylcellulose Sodium: White to cream-colored powder or granules. The powder is hygroscopic. Is easily dispersed in water to form colloidal solutions. Insoluble in alcohol, in ether, and in most other organic solvents. *NF category:* Coating agent; suspending and/or viscosity-increasing agent; wet binder; film-forming agent; release-modifying agent; disintegrant.

Carboxymethylcellulose Sodium 12:   Colorless or white to off-white powder or granules. Is odorless. Water solubility depends on degree of substitution (easily dispersed in water at all temperatures, forming a clear, colloidal solution). Insoluble in acetone, in alcohol, in ether, and in toluene. *NF category:* Suspending and/or viscosity-increasing agent.

Enzymatically-Hydrolyzed Carboxymethylcellulose Sodium: White or slightly yellowish or grayish, odorless, slightly hygroscopic granular or fibrous powder. Soluble in water; insoluble in alcohol. *NF category:* Coating agent; suspending and/or viscosity-increasing agent; film-forming agent.

Low-Substituted Carboxymethylcellulose Sodium: A white or almost white powder or short fibers. Practically insoluble in acetone, in alcohol, and in toluene. It swells in water to form a gel.

Carisoprodol: White, crystalline powder, having a mild, characteristic odor and a bitter taste. Freely soluble in alcohol, in chloroform, and in acetone; very slightly soluble in water.

Carmellose: White powder. Practically insoluble in ethanol (99.5%). Swells with water to form a suspension. Becomes viscous in sodium hydroxide TS. Is hygroscopic. *NF category:* Suspending and/or viscosity-increasing agent; polymers for ophthalmic use.

Carmustine: Light yellow powder. Freely soluble in ether.

Carprofen: White crystalline powder. Freely soluble in ether, in acetone, in ethyl acetate, and in sodium hydroxide TS or sodium carbonate TS; practically insoluble in water.

Carrageenan: Yellowish or tan to white, coarse to fine powder. Is practically odorless and has a mucilaginous taste. Soluble in water at a temperature of about 80°, forming a viscous, clear or slightly opalescent solution that flows readily. Disperses in water more readily if first moistened with alcohol, with glycerin, or with a saturated solution of sucrose in water. *NF category:* Suspending and/or viscosity-increasing agent; release-modifying agent.

Carvedilol: White or nearly white, crystalline powder. Slightly soluble in alcohol; practically insoluble in water and in dilute acids.

Casanthranol: Light tan to brown, amorphous, hygroscopic powder. Freely soluble in water, with some residue; partially soluble in methanol and in hot isopropyl alcohol; practically insoluble in acetone.

Cascara Sagrada: Has a distinct odor and a bitter and slightly acrid taste.

Castor Oil: Pale yellowish or almost colorless, transparent, viscid liquid. Has a faint, mild odor; is free from foreign and rancid odor; and has a bland, characteristic taste. Soluble in alcohol. Miscible with dehydrated alcohol, with glacial acetic acid, with chloroform, and with ether. *NF category:* Plasticizer; emollient; solvent; vehicle.

Hydrogenated Castor Oil: White, crystalline wax. Insoluble in water and in most common organic solvents. *NF category:* Stiffening agent; lubricant.

Cefaclor: White to off-white, crystalline powder. Slightly soluble in water; practically insoluble in methanol, in chloroform, and in benzene.

Cefadroxil: White to off-white, crystalline powder. Slightly soluble in water; practically insoluble in alcohol, in chloroform, and in ether.

Cefamandole Nafate: White, odorless, crystalline solid. Soluble in water and in methanol; practically insoluble in ether, in chloroform, in benzene, and in cyclohexane.

Cefazolin: White to slightly off-white, odorless, crystalline powder. Melts at about 198° to 200°, with decomposition. Soluble in dimethylformamide and in pyridine; sparingly soluble in acetone; slightly soluble in alcohol, in methanol, and in water; very slightly soluble in ethyl acetate, in isopropyl alcohol, and in methyl isobutyl ketone; practically insoluble in benzene, in chloroform, in ether, and in methylene chloride.

Cefazolin Sodium: White to off-white, practically odorless, crystalline powder, or white to off-white solid. Freely soluble in water, in saline TS, and in dextrose solutions; very slightly soluble in alcohol; practically insoluble in chloroform and in ether.

Cefdinir: White to light-yellow crystalline powder. Sparingly soluble in 0.1 M phosphate buffer (pH 7) solution; practically insoluble in water, in alcohol, and in diethyl ether.

Cefepime Hydrochloride: White to off-white, crystalline, nonhygroscopic solid. Freely soluble in water.

Cefepime for Injection: White to pale yellow powder. Freely soluble in water.

Cefixime: White to light yellow, crystalline powder. Soluble in methanol and in propylene glycol; slightly soluble in alcohol, in acetone, and in glycerin; very slightly soluble in 70% sorbitol and in octanol; practically insoluble in ether, in ethyl acetate, in hexane, and in water.

Cefmenoxime Hydrochloride: White to light orange-yellow crystals or crystalline powder. Freely soluble in formamide; slightly soluble in methanol; very slightly soluble in water; practically insoluble in dehydrated alcohol and in ether.

Cefmetazole Sodium: White solid. Very soluble in water and in methanol; soluble in acetone; practically insoluble in chloroform.

Cefonicid Sodium: White to off-white solid. Freely soluble in water, in 0.9% sodium chloride solution, and in 5% dextrose solution; soluble in methanol; very slightly soluble in dehydrated alcohol.

Cefoperazone Sodium: White to pale buff crystalline powder. Freely soluble in water; soluble in methanol; slightly soluble in dehydrated alcohol; insoluble in acetone, in ethyl acetate, and in ether.

Ceforanide: White to off-white powder. Very soluble in 1 N sodium hydroxide; practically insoluble in water, in methanol, in chloroform, and in ether.

Cefotaxime Sodium: Off-white to pale yellow crystalline powder. Freely soluble in water; practically insoluble in organic solvents.

Cefoxitin Sodium: White to off-white, granules or powder, having a slight characteristic odor. Is somewhat hygroscopic. Very soluble in water; soluble in methanol; sparingly soluble in dimethylformamide; slightly soluble in acetone; insoluble in ether and in chloroform.

Cefpodoxime Proxetil: White to light brownish-white powder. Odorless or having a faint odor, and has a bitter taste. Freely soluble in dehydrated alcohol; soluble in acetonitrile and in methanol; slightly soluble in ether; very slightly soluble in water.

Ceftazidime: White to cream-colored, crystalline powder. Soluble in alkali and in dimethyl sulfoxide; slightly soluble in dimethylformamide, in methanol, and in water; insoluble in acetone, in alcohol, in chloroform, in dioxane, in ether, in ethyl acetate, and in toluene.

Ceftiofur Hydrochloride: White to beige powder. Sparingly soluble in dimethylformamide and in ethanol; slightly soluble in 0.1 N hydrochloric acid; very slightly soluble in tetrahydrofuran; practically insoluble in ethyl acetate.

Ceftiofur Sodium: White to beige powder. Freely soluble in propylene glycol; soluble in water; slightly soluble in tetrahydrofuran, in dehydrated alcohol, and in acetone; insoluble in methylene chloride.

Ceftizoxime Sodium: White to pale yellow crystalline powder. Freely soluble in water.

Ceftriaxone Sodium: White to yellowish-orange crystalline powder. Freely soluble in water; sparingly soluble in methanol; very slightly soluble in alcohol.

Cefuroxime Axetil: White to almost white powder. The amorphous form is freely soluble in acetone; soluble in chloroform, in ethyl acetate, and in methanol; slightly soluble in dehydrated alcohol; insoluble in ether and in water. The crystalline form is freely soluble in acetone; sparingly soluble in chloroform, in ethyl acetate, and in methanol; slightly soluble in dehydrated alcohol; insoluble in ether and in water.

Cefuroxime Sodium: White or faintly yellow powder. Freely soluble in water; soluble in methanol; very slightly soluble in alcohol, in ether, in ethyl acetate, and in chloroform.

Celecoxib: White or almost white, crystalline or amorphous powder. Soluble to freely soluble in ethanol; soluble in methylene chloride; practically insoluble in water.

Cellaburate: Fine white or almost white powder or granules. Available in a range of viscosities, acetyl and butyl contents. Slightly hygroscopic; soluble in acetone, in methylene chloride, in pyridine, and in dimethyl sulfoxide; practically insoluble in water and in alcohol. *NF category:* Coating agent; polymer membrane; film-forming agent; release-modifying agent; diluent.

Cellacefate: Free-flowing, white powder. May have a slight odor of acetic acid. Soluble in acetone and in dioxane; insoluble in water and in alcohol. *NF category:* Coating agent; film-forming agent.

Cellulose Acetate: Fine, white powder or free-flowing pellets. Available in a range of viscosities and acetyl contents. High viscosity, which reflects high molecular weight, decreases solubility slightly. High acetyl content cellulose acetates generally have more limited solubility in commonly used organic solvents than low acetyl content cellulose acetates, but are more soluble in methylene chloride. All acetyl content cellulose acetates are soluble in dioxane and in dimethylformamide; insoluble in alcohol and in water. *NF category:* Coating agent; polymer membrane; film-forming agent; diluent.

Microcrystalline Cellulose: Fine, white or almost white powder. It consists of free-flowing, nonfibrous particles. Practically insoluble in sodium hydroxide solution (1 in 20); insoluble in water, in dilute acids, and in most organic solvents. *NF category:* Diluent; disintegrant; wet binder; suspending and/or viscosity-increasing agent.

Silicified Microcrystalline Cellulose: White or almost white, very fine to moderately fine powder. It is a free-flowing material that may be compacted into self-binding tablets that disintegrate rapidly in water. Slightly soluble in sodium hydroxide solution (1 in 20); practically insoluble in water, in acetone, in ethanol, in toluene, and in diluted acid. *NF category:* Diluent; disintegrant; wet binder.

Microcrystalline Cellulose and Carboxymethylcellulose Sodium: Tasteless, odorless, white to off-white, coarse to fine powder. Swells in water, producing, when dispersed, a white, opaque dispersion or gel. Insoluble in organic solvents and in dilute acids. *NF category:* Suspending and/or viscosity-increasing agent.

Oxidized Cellulose: In the form of gauze or lint. Is slightly off-white in color, is acidic to the taste, and has a slight, charred odor. Soluble in dilute alkalies; insoluble in water and in acids.

Oxidized Regenerated Cellulose: A knit fabric, usually in the form of sterile strips. Slightly off-white, having a slight odor. Soluble in dilute alkalies; insoluble in water and in dilute acids.

Powdered Cellulose: White or almost white powder. Exhibits degrees of fineness ranging from a free-flowing dense powder to a coarse, fluffy, nonflowing material. Slightly soluble in sodium hydroxide solution (1 in 20); insoluble in water, in dilute acids, and in nearly all organic solvents. *NF category:* Filtering aid; sorbent; diluent; disintegrant; glidant and/or anticaking agent; suspending and/or viscosity-increasing agent.

Cellulose Sodium Phosphate: Free-flowing cream-colored, odorless, tasteless powder. Insoluble in water, in dilute acids, and in most organic solvents.

Cephalexin: White to off-white, crystalline powder. Slightly soluble in water; practically insoluble in alcohol, in chloroform, and in ether.

Cephalexin Hydrochloride: White to off-white, crystalline powder. Soluble to the extent of 10 mg per mL in water, in acetone, in acetonitrile, in alcohol, in dimethylformamide, and in methanol; practically insoluble in chloroform, in ether, in ethyl acetate, and in isopropyl alcohol.

Cephalothin Sodium: White to off-white, practically odorless, crystalline powder. Freely soluble in water, in saline TS, and in dextrose solutions; insoluble in most organic solvents.

Cephapirin Benzathine: White, crystalline powder. Soluble in 0.1 N hydrochloric acid; practically insoluble in water, in ether, and in toluene; insoluble in alcohol.

Cephapirin Sodium: White to off-white, crystalline powder, odorless or having a slight odor. Very soluble in water; insoluble in most organic solvents.

Cephradine: White to off-white, crystalline powder. Sparingly soluble in water; very slightly soluble in alcohol and in chloroform; practically insoluble in ether.

Cetirizine Hydrochloride: White to almost white powder. Freely soluble in water; practically insoluble in acetone and in methylene chloride.

Cetostearyl Alcohol: Unctuous, white flakes or granules, having a faint, characteristic odor, and a bland, mild taste. Soluble in alcohol and in ether; insoluble in water. *NF category:* Stiffening agent; emollient; emulsifying agent; suspending and/or viscosity-increasing agent.

Cetrimonium Bromide: A white to creamy white, voluminous, free-flowing powder, with a characteristic faint odor and bitter, soapy taste. Freely soluble in water and in alcohol; practically insoluble in ether. *NF category:* Antimicrobial preservative.

Cetyl Alcohol: Unctuous, white flakes, granules, cubes, or castings. Has a faint characteristic odor and a bland, mild taste. Usually melts in the range between 45° and 50°. Soluble in alcohol and in ether, the solubility increasing with an increase in temperature; insoluble in water. *NF category:* Stiffening agent; coating agent; emulsifying agent.

Cetyl Esters Wax: White to off-white, somewhat translucent flakes, having a crystalline structure and a pearly luster when caked. Has a faint odor and a bland, mild taste, free from rancidity, and has a specific gravity of about 0.83 at 50°. Soluble in boiling alcohol, in ether, in chloroform, and in fixed and volatile oils; slightly soluble in cold solvent hexane; practically insoluble in cold alcohol; insoluble in water. *NF category:* Stiffening agent; emollient.

Cetyl Palmitate: White crystals or flakes. Freely soluble in alcohol and in ether; practically insoluble in water. *NF category:* Stiffening agent.

Cetylpyridinium Chloride: White to almost-white powder, having a slight, characteristic odor. Very soluble in water, in alcohol, and in chloroform; slightly soluble in benzene and in ether. *NF category:* Antimicrobial preservative; wetting and/or solubilizing agent; emulsifying agent.

Cetylpyridinium Chloride Topical Solution: Clear liquid. Is colorless unless a color has been added; has an aromatic odor and a bitter taste.

Activated Charcoal: Fine, black, odorless, tasteless powder, free from gritty matter. *NF category:* Sorbent.

Chitosan: White or almost white powder or granules. Soluble in aqueous solutions of glycolic acid, of formic acid, of acetic acid, of hydrochloric acid, and of lactic acid; practically insoluble in organic solvents and in water. *NF category:* Coating agent; film-forming agent; suspending and/or viscosity-increasing agent; vehicle (solid carrier).

Chloral Hydrate: Colorless, transparent, or white crystals having an aromatic, penetrating, and slightly acrid odor, and a slightly bitter, caustic taste. Melts at about 55°, and slowly volatilizes when exposed to air. Very soluble in water and in olive oil; freely soluble in alcohol, in chloroform, and in ether.

Chlorambucil: Off-white, slightly granular powder. Freely soluble in acetone; soluble in dilute alkali; very slightly soluble in water.

Chloramphenicol: Fine, white to grayish-white or yellowish-white, needle-like crystals or elongated plates. Its solutions are practically neutral to litmus. Is reasonably stable in neutral or moderately acid solutions. Its alcohol solution is dextrorotatory and its ethyl acetate solution is levorotatory. Freely soluble in alcohol, in propylene glycol, in acetone, and in ethyl acetate; slightly soluble in water.

Chloramphenicol Palmitate: Fine, white, unctuous, crystalline powder, having a faint odor and a bland, mild taste. Freely soluble in acetone and in chloroform; soluble in ether; sparingly soluble in alcohol; very slightly soluble in solvent hexane; insoluble in water.

Chloramphenicol Sodium Succinate: Light yellow powder. Freely soluble in water and in alcohol.

Chlordiazepoxide: Yellow, practically odorless, crystalline powder. Is sensitive to sunlight. Melts at about 240°. Sparingly soluble in chloroform and in alcohol; insoluble in water.

Chlordiazepoxide Hydrochloride: White or practically white, odorless, crystalline powder. Is affected by sunlight. Soluble in water; sparingly soluble in alcohol; insoluble in solvent hexane.

Chlorhexidine Acetate: A white or almost white, microcrystalline powder. Soluble in alcohol; sparingly soluble in water; slightly soluble in glycerol and in propylene glycol.

Chlorhexidine Gluconate Solution: Almost colorless or pale yellow, clear liquid. Miscible with glacial acetic acid and with water; miscible with three times its volume of acetone and with five times its volume of dehydrated alcohol; further addition of acetone or dehydrated alcohol yields a white turbidity.

Chlorhexidine Hydrochloride: White or almost white, crystalline powder. Sparingly soluble in propylene glycol and in water; very slightly soluble in alcohol.

Chlorobutanol: Colorless to white crystals, having a characteristic, somewhat camphoraceous, odor and taste. Anhydrous form melts at about 95°, and hydrous form melts at about 76°. Freely soluble in alcohol, in ether, in chloroform, and in volatile oils; soluble in glycerin; slightly soluble in water. *NF category:* Antimicrobial preservative; plasticizer.

Chlorocresol: Colorless or practically colorless crystals or crystalline powder, having a characteristic, nontarry odor. Is volatile in steam. Very soluble in alcohol; soluble in ether, in terpenes, in fixed oils, and in solutions of alkali hydroxides; slightly soluble in water and more soluble in hot water. *NF category:* Antimicrobial preservative.

Chloroprocaine Hydrochloride: White, crystalline powder. Is odorless, and is stable in air. Its solutions are acid to litmus. Exhibits local anesthetic properties when placed upon the tongue. Soluble in water; slightly soluble in alcohol; very slightly soluble in chloroform; practically insoluble in ether.

Chloroquine: White or slightly yellow, crystalline powder. Is odorless, and has a bitter taste. Soluble in dilute acids, in chloroform, and in ether; very slightly soluble in water.

Chloroquine Hydrochloride Injection: Colorless liquid.

Chloroquine Phosphate: White, crystalline powder. Is odorless, has a bitter taste, and is discolored slowly on exposure to light. Its solutions have a pH of about 4.5. Exists in two polymorphic forms, one melting between 193° and 195° and the other between 210° and 215° (see *Melting Range or Temperature ⟨741⟩*); mixture of the forms melts between 193° and 215°. Freely soluble in water; practically insoluble in alcohol, in chloroform, and in ether.

Chlorothiazide: White or practically white, crystalline, odorless powder. Melts at about 340°, with decomposition. Freely soluble in dimethylformamide and in dimethyl sulfoxide; slightly soluble in methanol and in pyridine; practically insoluble in ether, in benzene, and in chloroform; very slightly soluble in water.

Chloroxylenol: White crystals or crystalline powder, having a characteristic odor. Is volatile in steam. Freely soluble in alcohol, in ether, in terpenes, in fixed oils, and in solutions of alkali hydroxides; very slightly soluble in water. *NF category:* Antimicrobial preservative.

Chlorpheniramine Maleate: White, odorless, crystalline powder. Its solutions have a pH between 4 and 5. Freely soluble in water; soluble in alcohol and in chloroform; slightly soluble in ether and in benzene.

Chlorpromazine: White, crystalline solid, having an amine-like odor. Darkens on prolonged exposure to light. Melts at about 60°. Freely soluble in alcohol, in benzene, in chloroform, in ether, and in dilute mineral acids; practically insoluble in water and in dilute alkali hydroxides.

Chlorpromazine Hydrochloride: White or slightly creamy white, odorless, crystalline powder. Darkens on prolonged exposure to light. Very soluble in water; freely soluble in alcohol and in chloroform; insoluble in ether and in benzene.

Chlorpropamide: White, crystalline powder, having a slight odor. Soluble in alcohol; sparingly soluble in chloroform; practically insoluble in water.

Chlortetracycline Hydrochloride: Yellow, crystalline powder. Is odorless, and has a bitter taste. Is stable in air, but is slowly affected by light. Soluble in solutions of alkali hydroxides and carbonates; sparingly soluble in water; slightly soluble in alcohol; practically insoluble in acetone, in chloroform, in dioxane, and in ether.

Chlorthalidone: White to yellowish-white, crystalline powder. Melts at a temperature above 215°, with decomposition. Soluble in methanol; slightly soluble in alcohol; practically insoluble in water, in ether, and in chloroform.

Chlorzoxazone: White or practically white, practically odorless, crystalline powder. Soluble in solutions of alkali hydroxides and ammonia; sparingly soluble in alcohol, in isopropyl alcohol, and in methanol; slightly soluble in water.

Cholecalciferol: White, odorless crystals. Is affected by air and by light. Melts at about 85°. Soluble in alcohol, in chloroform, and in fatty oils; insoluble in water.

Cholesterol: White or faintly yellow, practically odorless, pearly leaflets, needles, powder, or granules. Acquires a yellow to pale tan color on prolonged exposure to light. Soluble in acetone, in chloroform, in dioxane, in ether, in ethyl acetate, in solvent hexane, and in vegetable oils; sparingly soluble in dehydrated alcohol; slightly (and slowly) soluble in alcohol; insoluble in water. *NF category:* Emulsifying agent; emollient.

Cholestyramine Resin: White to buff-colored, hygroscopic, fine powder. Is odorless or has not more than a slight amine-like odor. Insoluble in water, in alcohol, in chloroform, and in ether.

Choline Bitartrate: White, hygroscopic, crystalline powder. Clear, colorless liquid in solution. Melts between 148° and 153°. Is odorless, or may have a faint trimethylamine odor. Freely soluble in water; slightly soluble in alcohol; insoluble in ether and in chloroform.

Choline Chloride: Colorless or white crystals or crystalline powder, usually having a slight odor of trimethylamine. Clear and colorless in solution. Hygroscopic. Soluble in alcohol and in water.

Sodium Chromate Cr 51 Injection: Clear, slightly yellow solution.

Chromic Chloride: Dark green, odorless, slightly deliquescent crystals. Soluble in water and in alcohol; slightly soluble in acetone; practically insoluble in ether.

Chymotrypsin: White to yellowish-white, crystalline or amorphous, odorless, powder. An amount equivalent to 100,000 USP Units is soluble in 10 mL of water and in 10 mL of saline TS.

Ciclopirox: White to slightly yellowish-white, crystalline powder. Freely soluble in ethanol and in methylene chloride; soluble in ether; slightly soluble in water.

Ciclopirox Olamine: White to slightly yellowish-white, crystalline powder. Very soluble in alcohol and in methylene chloride; slightly soluble in water; practically insoluble in cyclohexane.

Cidofovir: White to off-white, crystalline powder. Soluble in 0.1 M sodium hydroxide; sparingly soluble in water; practically insoluble in methanol and in ethanol.

Cilastatin Sodium: White to tan-colored powder. Soluble in water and in methanol.

Cilostazol: White to off-white crystals. Freely soluble in chloroform; slightly soluble in methanol and in alcohol; practically insoluble in water.

Cimetidine: White to off-white, crystalline powder; odorless, or having a slight mercaptan odor. Freely soluble in methanol; soluble in alcohol and in polyethylene glycol 400; sparingly soluble in isopropyl alcohol; slightly soluble in water and in chloroform; practically insoluble in ether.

Cinoxacin: White to yellowish-white, crystalline solid. Is odorless, and has a bitter taste and a lingering aftertaste. Soluble in alkaline solution; insoluble in water and in most common organic solvents.

Ciprofloxacin Hydrochloride: Faintly yellowish to light yellow crystals. Sparingly soluble in water; slightly soluble in acetic acid and in methanol; very slightly soluble in dehydrated alcohol; practically insoluble in acetone, in acetonitrile, in ethyl acetate, in hexane, and in methylene chloride.

Cisapride: White or almost white powder. Freely soluble in dimethylformamide; soluble in methylene chloride; sparingly soluble in methanol; practically insoluble in water.

Cisatracurium Besylate: White to pale yellow powder. Soluble in water; slightly soluble in acetonitrile, in chloroform, in methanol, and in methylene chloride.

Citalopram Hydrobromide: White to almost white, crystalline powder. Soluble in alcohol; sparingly soluble in water and in dehydrated alcohol.

Anhydrous Citric Acid: Colorless, translucent crystals, or white, granular to fine, crystalline powder. Melts at about 153°, with decomposition. Very soluble in water; freely soluble in alcohol; very slightly soluble in ether. *NF category:* pH modifier (acidifying agent/alkalizing agent/buffering agent).

Citric Acid Monohydrate: Colorless, translucent crystals, or white, granular to fine, crystalline powder. Efflorescent in dry air. Very soluble in water; freely soluble in alcohol; very slightly soluble in ether. *NF category:* pH modifier (acidifying agent/alkalizing agent/buffering agent); antioxidant; chelating and/or complexing agent.

Clarithromycin: White to off-white, crystalline powder. Soluble in acetone; slightly soluble in dehydrated alcohol, in methanol, and in acetonitrile, and in phosphate buffer at pH values of 2 to 5; practically insoluble in water.

Clavulanate Potassium: White to off-white powder. Is moisture-sensitive. Freely soluble in water, but stability in aqueous solution is not good, optimum stability at a pH of 6.0 to 6.3; soluble in methanol, with decomposition.

Clemastine Fumarate: White to off-white, odorless powder. Its solutions are acid to litmus. Slightly soluble in methanol; very slightly soluble in water, and in chloroform.

Clenbuterol Hydrochloride: White or almost white, crystalline powder. Soluble in water and in alcohol; slightly soluble in acetone. It melts with decomposition at 173°.

Clidinium Bromide: White to nearly white, practically odorless, crystalline powder. Is optically inactive. Melts at about 242°. Soluble in water and in alcohol; slightly soluble in benzene and in ether.

Clindamycin Hydrochloride: White or practically white, crystalline powder. Is odorless or has a faint mercaptan-like odor. Is stable in the presence of air and light. Its solutions are acidic and are dextrorotatory. Freely soluble in water, in dimethylformamide, and in methanol; soluble in alcohol; practically insoluble in acetone.

Clindamycin Palmitate Hydrochloride: White to off-white amorphous powder, having a characteristic odor. Very soluble in ethyl acetate and in dimethylformamide; freely soluble in water, in benzene, in ether, in chloroform, and in alcohol.

Clindamycin Phosphate: White to off-white, hygroscopic, crystalline powder. Is odorless or practically odorless, and has a bitter taste. Freely soluble in water; slightly solu-

ble in dehydrated alcohol; very slightly soluble in acetone; practically insoluble in chloroform, in benzene, and in ether.

Clioquinol: Voluminous, spongy, yellowish-white to brownish-yellow powder, having a slight, characteristic odor. Darkens on exposure to light. Melts at about 180°, with decomposition. Soluble in hot ethyl acetate and in hot glacial acetic acid; practically insoluble in water and in alcohol.

Clobetasol Propionate: White to cream, crystalline powder. Soluble in acetone, in dimethyl sulfoxide, in chloroform, in methanol, and in dioxane; sparingly soluble in ethanol; slightly soluble in benzene and in diethyl ether; practically insoluble in water.

Clocortolone Pivalate: White to yellowish-white, odorless powder. Melts at about 230°, with decomposition. Freely soluble in chloroform and in dioxane; soluble in acetone; sparingly soluble in alcohol; slightly soluble in benzene and in ether.

Clofazimine: Dark red crystals. Melts at about 217°, with decomposition. Soluble in chloroform and in benzene; sparingly soluble in alcohol, in acetone, and in ethyl acetate; practically insoluble in water.

Clofibrate: Colorless to pale yellow liquid having a characteristic odor. Soluble in acetone, in alcohol, in benzene, and in chloroform; insoluble in water.

Clomiphene Citrate: White to pale yellow, essentially odorless powder. Freely soluble in methanol; sparingly soluble in alcohol; slightly soluble in water and in chloroform; insoluble in ether.

Change to read:

Clomipramine Hydrochloride: White to faintly yellow, crystalline powder. ■Freely■1S (USP41) soluble in water ■and in methylene chloride; soluble in alcohol; practically insoluble in ethyl ether and in hexane.■1S (USP41)

Clonazepam: Light yellow powder, having a faint odor. Sparingly soluble in acetone and in chloroform; slightly soluble in alcohol and in ether; insoluble in water.

Clonidine: White to almost white, crystalline powder. Melting point is about 130°. Freely soluble in methanol and in alcohol.

Clopidogrel Bisulfate: White to off-white powder. Freely soluble at pH 1; practically insoluble at neutral pH.

Cloprostenol Sodium: White or almost white, amorphous powder. Is hygroscopic. Freely soluble in water, in alcohol, and in methanol; practically insoluble in acetone.

Clorazepate Dipotassium: Light yellow, crystalline powder. Darkens on exposure to light. Soluble in water but, upon standing, may precipitate from the solution; slightly soluble in alcohol and in isopropyl alcohol; practically insoluble in acetone, in benzene, in chloroform, in ether, and in methylene chloride.

Clorsulon: White to off-white powder. Freely soluble in acetonitrile and in methanol; slightly soluble in water; very slightly soluble in methylene chloride.

Clotrimazole: White to pale yellow, crystalline powder. Melts at about 142°, with decomposition. Freely soluble in methanol, in acetone, in chloroform, and in alcohol; practically insoluble in water.

Cloxacillin Benzathine: White or almost white, almost odorless, crystals or crystalline powder. Soluble in chloroform and in methanol; sparingly soluble in acetone; slightly soluble in water, in alcohol, and in isopropyl alcohol.

Cloxacillin Sodium: White, odorless, crystalline powder. Freely soluble in water; soluble in alcohol; slightly soluble in chloroform.

Clozapine: Yellow, crystalline powder. Soluble in chloroform, in acetone, and in alcohol; sparingly soluble in acetonitrile; insoluble in water.

Coal Tar: Nearly black, viscous liquid, heavier than water, having a characteristic, naphthalene-like odor, and producing a sharp, burning sensation on the tongue. Slightly soluble in water, to which it imparts its characteristic odor and taste and a faintly alkaline reaction; partially soluble in acetone, in alcohol, in carbon disulfide, in chloroform, in ether, in methanol, and in solvent hexane; soluble in benzene and nitrobenzene.

Cyanocobalamin Co 57 Capsules: May contain a small amount of solid or solids, or may appear empty.

Cyanocobalamin Co 57 Oral Solution: Clear, colorless to pink solution.

Cocaine: Colorless to white crystals or white, crystalline powder. Is levorotatory in 3 N hydrochloric acid solution. Its saturated solution is alkaline to litmus. Very soluble in warm alcohol; freely soluble in alcohol, in chloroform, and in ether; soluble in olive oil; sparingly soluble in mineral oil; slightly soluble in water.

Cocaine Hydrochloride: Colorless crystals or white, crystalline powder. Very soluble in water; freely soluble in alcohol; soluble in chloroform and in glycerin; insoluble in ether.

Coccidioidin: Clear, practically colorless or amber-colored liquid.

Cocoa Butter: Yellowish-white solid, having a faint, agreeable odor, and a bland, chocolate-like taste if the cocoa butter is obtained by pressing. If obtained by extraction, the taste is bland. Is usually brittle at temperatures below 25°. Freely soluble in ether and in chloroform; soluble in boiling dehydrated alcohol; slightly soluble in alcohol. *NF category:* Suppository base.

Coconut Oil: Clear, white to light yellow-tan, viscous liquid. Freely soluble in methylene chloride and in light petroleum (bp: 65° to 70°); very slightly soluble in alcohol; practically insoluble in water. *NF category:* Coating agent; emulsifying agent; emollient; ointment base.

Hydrogenated Coconut Oil: White to yellowish, fatty solid to semi-solid. Freely soluble in ether; very slightly soluble in alcohol; practically insoluble in water. *NF category:* Coating agent; lubricant; wet binder.

Cod Liver Oil: Thin, oily liquid, having a characteristic, slightly fishy but not rancid odor, and a fishy taste. Freely soluble in ether, in chloroform, in carbon disulfide, and in ethyl acetate; slightly soluble in alcohol.

Codeine: Colorless or white crystals or white, crystalline powder. It effloresces slowly in dry air, and is affected by light. In acid or alcohol solutions it is levorotatory. Its saturated solution is alkaline to litmus. Very soluble in chloroform; freely soluble in alcohol; sparingly soluble in ether; slightly soluble in water. When heated in an amount of water insufficient for complete solution, it melts to oily drops that crystallize on cooling.

Codeine Phosphate: Fine, white, needle-shaped crystals, or white, crystalline powder. Is odorless. Is affected by light. Its solutions are acid to litmus. Very soluble in hot water; freely soluble in water; slightly soluble in alcohol but more so in boiling alcohol.

Codeine Sulfate: White crystals, usually needle-like, or white, crystalline powder. Is affected by light. Freely soluble in water at 80°; soluble in water; very slightly soluble in alcohol; insoluble in chloroform and in ether.

Colchicine: Pale yellow to pale greenish-yellow, amorphous scales, or powder or crystalline powder. Is odorless or nearly so, and darkens on exposure to light. Freely soluble in alcohol and in chloroform; soluble in water; slightly soluble in ether.

Colestipol Hydrochloride: Yellow to orange beads. Swells but does not dissolve in water or dilute aqueous solutions of acid or alkali. Insoluble in the common organic solvents.

Colistimethate Sodium: White to slightly yellow, odorless, fine powder. Freely soluble in water; soluble in methanol; insoluble in acetone and in ether.

Colistin Sulfate: White to slightly yellow, odorless, fine powder. Freely soluble in water; slightly soluble in methanol; insoluble in acetone and in ether.

Collodion: Clear, or slightly opalescent, viscous liquid. Is colorless, or slightly yellowish, and has the odor of ether.

Flexible Collodion: Clear, or slightly opalescent, viscous liquid. Is colorless or slightly yellow, and has the odor of ether. The strong odor of camphor becomes noticeable as the ether evaporates.

Copovidone: White to yellowish-white powder or flakes. Is hygroscopic. Freely soluble in water, in alcohol, and in methylene chloride; practically insoluble in ether. *NF category:* Wet binder; coating agent; film-forming agent.

Corn Oil: Clear, light yellow, oily liquid, having a faint, characteristic odor and taste. Slightly soluble in alcohol. Miscible with ether, with chloroform, with benzene, and with solvent hexane. *Specific Gravity* ⟨841⟩: Between 0.914 and 0.921. *NF category:* Solvent; vehicle (oleaginous).

Corn Syrup: Clear, white to light yellow, viscous liquid. Is miscible in all proportions with water. *NF category:* Suspending and/or viscosity-increasing agent; sweetening agent; diluent; wet binder; tonicity agent.

Corn Syrup Solids: Sweet, white to light yellow powder or granules. Soluble in water. *NF category:* Coating agent; vehicle (flavored and/or sweetened and solid carrier); humectant; suspending and/or viscosity-increasing agent; sweetening agent; diluent; wet binder; tonicity agent.

Corticotropin Injection: Colorless or light straw-colored liquid.

Corticotropin for Injection: White or practically white, soluble, amorphous solid having the characteristic appearance of substances prepared by freeze-drying.

Repository Corticotropin Injection: Colorless or light straw-colored liquid, which may be quite viscid at room temperature. Is odorless or has an odor of an antimicrobial agent.

Corticotropin Zinc Hydroxide Injectable Suspension: Flocculent, white, aqueous suspension, free from large particles following moderate shaking.

Cortisone Acetate: White or practically white, odorless, crystalline powder. Is stable in air. Melts at about 240°, with some decomposition (see *Melting Range or Temperature* ⟨741⟩). Freely soluble in chloroform; soluble in dioxane; sparingly soluble in acetone; slightly soluble in alcohol; insoluble in water.

Purified Cotton: White, soft, fine filament-like hairs appearing under the microscope as hollow, flattened, and twisted bands, striate and slightly thickened at the edges. Is practically odorless and practically tasteless. Soluble in ammoniated cupric oxide TS; insoluble in ordinary solvents.

Cottonseed Oil: Pale yellow, oily liquid. Is odorless or nearly so, and has a bland taste. At temperatures below 10° particles of solid fat may separate from the Oil, and at about 0° to −5° the Oil becomes a solid or nearly so. *Specific Gravity* ⟨841⟩: Between 0.915 and 0.921. Slightly soluble in alcohol. Miscible with ether, with chloroform, with solvent hexane, and with carbon disulfide. *NF category:* Solvent; vehicle (oleaginous).

Hydrogenated Cottonseed Oil: A white mass or powder that melts to a clear, pale yellow liquid when heated. Freely soluble in methylene chloride and in toluene; very slightly soluble in alcohol; practically insoluble in water.

Creatinine: White crystals or crystalline powder; odorless. Soluble in water; slightly soluble in alcohol; practically insoluble in acetone, in ether, and in chloroform. *NF category:* Bulking agent.

Cresol: Colorless, or yellowish to brownish-yellow, or pinkish, highly refractive liquid, becoming darker with age and on exposure to light. Has a phenol-like, sometimes empyreumatic odor. A saturated solution of it is neutral or only slightly acid to litmus. Sparingly soluble in water, usually forming a cloudy solution; dissolves in solutions of fixed alkali hydroxides. Miscible with alcohol, with ether, and with glycerin. *NF category:* Antimicrobial preservative.

Cromolyn Sodium: White, odorless, crystalline powder. Is tasteless at first, with a slightly bitter aftertaste. Is hygroscopic. Soluble in water; insoluble in alcohol and in chloroform.

Cromolyn Sodium for Inhalation: White to creamy white, odorless, hygroscopic, and very finely divided powder.

Croscarmellose Sodium: White, free-flowing powder. Partially soluble in water; insoluble in alcohol, in ether, and in other organic solvents. *NF category:* Disintegrant.

Crospovidone: White to creamy-white, hygroscopic powder, having a faint odor. Insoluble in water and in ordinary organic solvents. *NF category:* Disintegrant.

Crotamiton: Colorless to slightly yellowish oil, having a faint amine-like odor. Soluble in alcohol and in methanol.

Cupric Chloride: Bluish green, deliquescent crystals. Freely soluble in water; soluble in alcohol; slightly soluble in ether.

Cupric Sulfate (CuSO$_4$ · 5H$_2$O): Deep blue, triclinic crystals or blue, crystalline granules or powder. It effloresces slowly in dry air. Its solutions are acid to litmus. Very soluble in boiling water; freely soluble in water and in glycerin; slightly soluble in alcohol.

Cupric Sulfate (anhydrous): A white or grayish-white powder. Soluble in water; insoluble in alcohol.

Cyanocobalamin: Dark red crystals or amorphous or crystalline red powder. In the anhydrous form, it is very hygroscopic and when exposed to air it may absorb about 12% of water. Soluble in alcohol; sparingly soluble in water; insoluble in acetone, in chloroform, and in ether.

Cyclandelate: White, crystalline powder. Very soluble in acetonitrile, in alcohol, and in ether; practically insoluble in water. Melts at about 58°.

Cyclizine Hydrochloride: White, crystalline powder or small, colorless crystals. Is odorless or nearly so, and has a bitter taste. Melts indistinctly at about 285°, with decomposition. Sparingly soluble in chloroform; slightly soluble in water and in alcohol; insoluble in ether.

Cyclobenzaprine Hydrochloride: White to off-white, odorless, crystalline powder. Freely soluble in water, in alcohol, and in methanol; sparingly soluble in isopropanol; slightly soluble in chloroform and in methylene chloride; insoluble in hydrocarbons.

Cyclopentolate Hydrochloride: White, crystalline powder, which upon standing develops a characteristic odor. Its solutions are acid to litmus. Melts at about 138°, the melt appearing opaque. Very soluble in water; freely soluble in alcohol; insoluble in ether.

Cyclophosphamide: White, crystalline powder. Liquefies upon loss of its water of crystallization. Soluble in water and in alcohol.

Cyclopropane: Colorless gas having a characteristic odor. Has a pungent taste. One L at a pressure of 760 mm and a temperature of 0° weighs about 1.88 g. One volume dissolves in about 2.7 volumes of water at 15°. Freely soluble in alcohol; soluble in fixed oils.

Cycloserine: White to pale yellow, crystalline powder. Is odorless or has a faint odor. Is hygroscopic and deteriorates upon absorbing water. Its solutions are dextrorotatory. Freely soluble in water.

Cyclosporine: White to almost white powder. Soluble in acetone, in alcohol, in methanol, in ether, in chloroform, and in methylene chloride; slightly soluble in saturated hydrocarbons; practically insoluble in water.

Cyproheptadine Hydrochloride: White to slightly yellow, odorless or practically odorless, crystalline powder. Freely soluble in methanol; soluble in chloroform; sparingly soluble in alcohol; slightly soluble in water; practically insoluble in ether.

Cyromazine: White or off-white, odorless, crystalline powder. Slightly soluble in methanol and in water.

Cysteine Hydrochloride: White crystals or crystalline powder. Soluble in water, in alcohol, and in acetone.

Cytarabine: Odorless, white to off-white, crystalline powder. Freely soluble in water; slightly soluble in alcohol and in chloroform.

Dactinomycin: Bright red, crystalline powder. Is somewhat hygroscopic and is affected by light and by heat. Freely soluble in alcohol; soluble in water at 10° and slightly soluble in water at 37°; very slightly soluble in ether.

Dalfampridine: White powder. Soluble in water, in methanol, in acetone, in tetrahydrofuran, in isopropanol, in acetonitrile, in *N*,*N*-dimethylformamide, in dimethylsulfoxide, and in alcohol.

Danazol: White to pale yellow, crystalline powder. Melts at about 225°, with some decomposition. Freely soluble in chloroform; soluble in acetone; sparingly soluble in alcohol and in benzene; slightly soluble in ether; practically insoluble or insoluble in water and in hexane.

Dantrolene Sodium: Fine orange to orange-brown powder. Sparingly soluble in dimethylformamide and in glycerine; sparingly soluble to practically insoluble in acetone.

Dapsone: White or creamy white, crystalline powder. Is odorless and has a slightly bitter taste. Soluble in acetone and in dilute mineral acids; sparingly soluble in alcohol; very slightly soluble in water.

Daunorubicin Hydrochloride: Orange-red, crystalline, hygroscopic powder. Freely soluble in water and in methanol; slightly soluble in alcohol; very slightly soluble in chloroform; practically insoluble in acetone.

Deferoxamine Mesylate: White to off-white powder. Freely soluble in water; slightly soluble in methanol.

Dehydroacetic Acid: White or nearly white, crystalline powder. Soluble in aqueous solutions of alkalies; very slightly soluble in water. One g of sample dissolves in about 35 mL of alcohol and in 5 mL of acetone. *NF category:* Antimicrobial preservative.

Dehydrocholic Acid: White, fluffy, odorless powder, having a bitter taste. Soluble in glacial acetic acid and in solutions of alkali hydroxides and carbonates; sparingly soluble in chloroform (the solutions in alcohol and in chloroform usually are slightly turbid); slightly soluble in alcohol and in ether; practically insoluble in water.

Demecarium Bromide: White or slightly yellow, slightly hygroscopic, crystalline powder. Freely soluble in water and in alcohol; soluble in ether; sparingly soluble in acetone.

Demeclocycline: Yellow, crystalline, odorless powder, having a bitter taste. Soluble in alcohol; sparingly soluble in water. Dissolves readily in 3 N hydrochloric acid and in alkaline solutions.

Demeclocycline Hydrochloride: Yellow, crystalline, odorless powder, having a bitter taste. Sparingly soluble in water and in solutions of alkali hydroxides and carbonates; slightly soluble in alcohol; practically insoluble in acetone and in chloroform.

Denatonium Benzoate: Very soluble in chloroform and in methanol; freely soluble in water and in alcohol; very slightly soluble in ether. *NF category:* Alcohol denaturant; flavors and fragrance.

Desipramine Hydrochloride: White to off-white, crystalline powder. Melts at about 213°. Freely soluble in methanol and in chloroform; soluble in water and in alcohol; insoluble in ether.

Desloratadine: White to light pink-colored powder. Very soluble in ethanol and in propylene glycol; soluble in dichloromethane; slightly soluble in water.

Desmopressin Acetate: White, fluffy powder. Soluble in water, in alcohol, and in acetic acid.

Desogestrel: White or almost-white, crystalline powder. Very soluble in methanol; freely soluble in anhydrous ethanol and in methylene chloride; practically insoluble in water.

Desonide: White powder or crystal. Soluble in chloroform; sparingly soluble in ethanol and in acetone; practically insoluble in water.

Desoximetasone: White to practically white, odorless, crystalline powder. Freely soluble in alcohol, in acetone, and in chloroform; insoluble in water.

Desoxycholic Acid: [(Title for this monograph is not to change until December 1, 2021.)
   (Prior to December 1, 2021, the current practice of labeling the article of commerce with the name Desoxycholic Acid may be continued. Use of the name Deoxycholic Acid will be permitted as of December 1, 2016; however, the use of this name will not be mandatory until December 1, 2021. The 60-month extension will provide the time needed by manufacturers and users to make necessary changes.)]

Deoxycholic Acid: Occurs as a white, crystalline powder. Freely soluble in alcohol; soluble in acetone and in solutions of alkali hydroxides and carbonates; slightly soluble in chloroform and in ether; practically insoluble in water. *NF category:* Emulsifying agent.

Desoxycorticosterone Acetate: White or creamy white, crystalline powder. Is odorless, and is stable in air. Sparingly soluble in alcohol, in acetone, and in dioxane; slightly soluble in vegetable oils; practically insoluble in water.

Dexamethasone: White to practically white, odorless, crystalline powder. Is stable in air. Melts at about 250°, with some decomposition. Sparingly soluble in acetone, in alcohol, in dioxane, and in methanol; slightly soluble in chloroform; very slightly soluble in ether; practically insoluble in water.

Dexamethasone Acetate: Clear, white to off-white, odorless powder. Freely soluble in methanol, in acetone, and in dioxane; practically insoluble in water.

Dexamethasone Sodium Phosphate: White or slightly yellow, crystalline powder. Is odorless or has a slight odor of alcohol, and is exceedingly hygroscopic. Freely soluble in water; slightly soluble in alcohol; very slightly soluble in dioxane; insoluble in chloroform and in ether.

Dexbrompheniramine Maleate: White, odorless, crystalline powder. Exists in two polymorphic forms, one melting between 106° and 107° and the other between 112° and 113°. Mixtures of the forms may melt between 105° and 113°. The pH of a solution (1 in 100) is about 5. Freely soluble in water; soluble in alcohol and in chloroform.

Dexchlorpheniramine Maleate: White, odorless, crystalline powder. Freely soluble in water; soluble in alcohol and in chloroform; slightly soluble in benzene and in ether.

Dexmedetomidine Hydrochloride: White or almost white powder. Freely soluble in water, and has a pKa of 7.1.

Dexpanthenol: Clear, viscous, somewhat hygroscopic liquid, having a slight, characteristic odor. Some crystallization may occur on standing. Freely soluble in water, in alcohol, in methanol, and in propylene glycol; soluble in chloroform and in ether; slightly soluble in glycerin.

Dextran 1:   A white to off-white powder. Is hygroscopic. Very soluble in water; sparingly soluble in alcohol.

Dextrates: Free-flowing, porous, white, odorless, spherical granules consisting of aggregates of microcrystals, having a sweet taste and producing a cooling sensation in the mouth. May be compressed directly into self-binding tablets. Freely soluble in water (heating increases its solubility in water); soluble in dilute acids and alkalies and in basic organic solvents such as pyridine; insoluble in the common organic solvents. *NF category:* Sweetening agent; diluent; wet binder.

Dextrin: Free-flowing, white, yellow, or brown powder. Its solubility in water varies; it is usually very soluble, but often contains an insoluble portion. *NF category:* Suspending and/or viscosity-increasing agent; diluent; wet binder; film-forming agent; stiffening agent.

Dextroamphetamine Sulfate: White, odorless, crystalline powder. Soluble in water; slightly soluble in alcohol; insoluble in ether.

Dextromethorphan: Practically white to slightly yellow, odorless, crystalline powder. Eleven mg of Dextromethorphan is equivalent to 15 mg of dextromethorphan hydrobromide monohydrate. Freely soluble in chloroform; practically insoluble in water.

Dextromethorphan Hydrobromide: Practically white crystals or crystalline powder, having a faint odor. Melts at about 126°, with decomposition. Freely soluble in alcohol and in chloroform; sparingly soluble in water; insoluble in ether.

Dextrose: Colorless crystals or white, crystalline or granular powder. Is odorless, and has a sweet taste. Very soluble in boiling water; freely soluble in water; soluble in boiling alcohol; slightly soluble in alcohol. *NF category:* Sweetening agent; tonicity agent; vehicle (flavored and/or sweetened); diluent.

Dextrose Excipient: Colorless crystals or white, crystalline or granular powder. Is odorless and sweet-tasting. Very soluble in boiling water; freely soluble in water; sparingly soluble in boiling alcohol; slightly soluble in alcohol. *NF category:* Sweetening agent; diluent.

Diacetylated Monoglycerides: Clear liquid. Very soluble in 80% (w/w) aqueous alcohol, in vegetable oils, and in mineral oils; sparingly soluble in 70% alcohol. *NF category:* Plasticizer.

Diatrizoate Meglumine: White, odorless powder. Freely soluble in water.

Diatrizoate Meglumine Injection: Clear, colorless to pale yellow, slightly viscous liquid.

Diatrizoate Meglumine and Diatrizoate Sodium Injection: Clear, colorless to pale yellow, slightly viscous liquid. May crystallize at room temperature or below.

Diatrizoate Sodium: White, odorless powder. Soluble in water; slightly soluble in alcohol; practically insoluble in acetone and in ether.

Diatrizoate Sodium Injection: Clear, colorless to pale yellow, slightly viscous liquid.

Diatrizoate Sodium Solution: Clear, pale yellow to light brown liquid.

Diatrizoic Acid: White, odorless powder. Soluble in dimethylformamide and in alkali hydroxide solutions; very slightly soluble in water and in alcohol.

Diazepam: Off-white to yellow, practically odorless, crystalline powder. Freely soluble in chloroform; soluble in alcohol; practically insoluble in water.

Diazoxide: White or cream-white crystals or crystalline powder. Very soluble in strong alkaline solutions; freely soluble in dimethylformamide; sparingly soluble to practically insoluble in water and in most organic solvents.

Dibucaine: White to off-white powder, having a slight, characteristic odor. Darkens on exposure to light. Soluble in 1 N hydrochloric acid and in ether; slightly soluble in water.

Dibucaine Hydrochloride: Colorless or white to off-white crystals or white to off-white, crystalline powder. Is odorless, is somewhat hygroscopic, and darkens on exposure to light. Its solutions have a pH of about 5.5. Freely soluble in water, in alcohol, in acetone, and in chloroform.

Dibutyl Phthalate: A clear, oily liquid, colorless or very slightly yellow. Practically insoluble in water. Miscible with alcohol and with ether. *NF category:* Film-forming agent; solvent.

Dibutyl Sebacate: Colorless, oily liquid of very mild odor. Soluble in alcohol, in isopropyl alcohol, and in mineral oil; very slightly soluble in propylene glycol; practically insoluble in water and in glycerin. *NF category:* Plasticizer.

Dichloralphenazone: White, microcrystalline powder. Has a slight odor characteristic of chloral hydrate. Decomposed by dilute alkali, liberating chloroform. Freely soluble in water, in alcohol, and in chloroform; soluble in dilute acids.

Dichlorodifluoromethane: Clear, colorless gas, having a faint, ethereal odor. Its vapor pressure at 25° is about 4880 mm of mercury (80 psig). *NF category:* Propellant.

Dichlorotetrafluoroethane: Clear, colorless gas, having a faint, ethereal odor. Its vapor pressure at 25° is about 1620 mm of mercury (17 psig). Usually contains between 6% and 10% of its isomer, CCl_2F-CF_3. *NF category:* Propellant.

Diclazuril: White to yellow powder. Sparingly soluble in dimethylformamide; practically insoluble in water, in alcohol, and in methylene chloride.

Diclofenac Potassium: White to off-white or slightly yellowish crystalline powder, slightly hygroscopic. Freely soluble in methanol; soluble in alcohol; sparingly soluble in water; slightly soluble in acetone.

Diclofenac Sodium: White to off-white, hygroscopic, crystalline powder. Melts at about 284°. Freely soluble in methanol; soluble in ethanol; sparingly soluble in water; practically insoluble in chloroform and in ether.

Dicloxacillin Sodium: White to off-white, crystalline powder. Freely soluble in water.

Dicyclomine Hydrochloride: Fine, white, crystalline powder. Is practically odorless and has a very bitter taste. Freely soluble in alcohol and in chloroform; soluble in water; very slightly soluble in ether.

Dicyclomine Hydrochloride Injection: Colorless solution, which may have the odor of a preservative.

Didanosine: White to off-white, crystalline powder. Very soluble in dimethyl sulfoxide; practically insoluble or insoluble in acetone and in methanol.

Dienestrol: Colorless, white or practically white, needle-like crystals, or white or practically white, crystalline powder. Is odorless. Soluble in alcohol, in acetone, in ether, in methanol, in propylene glycol, and in solutions of alkali hydroxides; slightly soluble in chloroform and in fatty oils; practically insoluble in water.

Diethanolamine: White or clear, colorless crystals, deliquescing in moist air; or colorless liquid. Miscible with water, with alcohol, with acetone, with chloroform, and with glycerin. Slightly soluble to insoluble in benzene, in ether, and in petroleum ether. *NF category:* Emulsifying agent; pH modifier (acidifying agent/alkalizing agent/buffering agent).

Diethylcarbamazine Citrate: White, crystalline powder. Melts at about 136°, with decomposition. Is odorless or has a slight odor; is slightly hygroscopic. Very soluble in water; sparingly soluble in alcohol; practically insoluble in acetone, in chloroform, and in ether.

Diethylene Glycol Monoethyl Ether: Clear, colorless liquid. Is hygroscopic. Miscible with water, with acetone, and with alcohol; partially miscible with vegetable oils; immiscible with mineral oils. Specific gravity about 0.991. *NF category:* Ointment base; solvent; emulsifying agent.

Diethylene Glycol Stearates: White or almost white, waxy solid. Soluble in acetone and in hot alcohol; practically insoluble in water. *NF category:* Emulsifying agent.

Diethyl Phthalate: Colorless, practically odorless, oily liquid. Insoluble in water. Miscible with alcohol, with ether, and with other usual organic solvents. *NF category:* Plasticizer; film-forming agent; solvent.

Diethyl Sebacate: A colorless to slightly yellow liquid. Miscible with alcohol, with ether, with other organic solvents, and with most fixed oils; insoluble or practically insoluble in water. *NF category:* Flavors and fragrance.

Diethylpropion Hydrochloride: White to off-white, fine crystalline powder. Is odorless, or has a slight characteristic odor. It melts at about 175°, with decomposition. Freely soluble in water, in chloroform, and in alcohol; practically insoluble in ether.

Diethylstilbestrol: White, odorless, crystalline powder. Soluble in alcohol, in chloroform, in ether, in fatty oils, and in dilute alkali hydroxides; practically insoluble in water.

Diethyltoluamide: Colorless liquid, having a faint, pleasant odor. Boils at about 111° under a pressure of 1 mm of mercury. Practically insoluble in water and in glycerin. Miscible with alcohol, with isopropyl alcohol, with ether, with chloroform, and with carbon disulfide.

Diflorasone Diacetate: White to pale yellow, crystalline powder. Soluble in methanol and in acetone; sparingly soluble in ethyl acetate; slightly soluble in toluene; very slightly soluble in ether; insoluble in water.

Diflunisal: White to off-white, practically odorless powder. Freely soluble in alcohol and in methanol; soluble in acetone and in ethyl acetate; slightly soluble in chloroform, in carbon tetrachloride, and in methylene chloride; insoluble in hexane and in water.

Digitoxin: White or pale buff, odorless, microcrystalline powder. Sparingly soluble in chloroform; slightly soluble in alcohol; very slightly soluble in ether; practically insoluble in water.

Digoxin: Clear to white, odorless crystals or white, odorless crystalline powder. Freely soluble in pyridine; slightly soluble in diluted alcohol and in chloroform; practically insoluble in water and in ether.

Dihydroergotamine Mesylate: White to slightly yellowish powder, or off-white to faintly red powder, having a faint odor. Soluble in alcohol; slightly soluble in water and in chloroform.

Dihydrostreptomycin Sulfate: White or almost white, amorphous or crystalline powder. Amorphous form is hygroscopic. Freely soluble in water; practically insoluble in acetone, in chloroform, and in methanol.

Dihydrotachysterol: Colorless or white, odorless crystals, or white, odorless, crystalline powder. Freely soluble in ether and in chloroform; soluble in alcohol; sparingly soluble in vegetable oils; practically insoluble in water.

Dihydroxyacetone: White to off-white crystalline powder. The monomeric form is freely soluble in water, in alcohol, and in ether. The dimeric form is freely soluble in water; soluble in alcohol; and sparingly soluble in ether.

Dihydroxyaluminum Aminoacetate: White, odorless powder having a faintly sweet taste. Soluble in dilute mineral acids and in solutions of fixed alkalies; insoluble in water and in organic solvents.

Dihydroxyaluminum Aminoacetate Magma: White, viscous suspension, from which small amounts of water may separate on standing.

Dihydroxyaluminum Sodium Carbonate: Fine, white, odorless powder. Soluble in dilute mineral acids with the evolution of carbon dioxide; practically insoluble in water and in organic solvents.

Diloxanide Furoate: White or almost white, crystalline powder. Freely soluble in chloroform; slightly soluble in alcohol and in ether; very slightly soluble in water.

Diltiazem Hydrochloride: White, odorless, crystalline powder or small crystals. Freely soluble in chloroform, in formic acid, in methanol, and in water; sparingly soluble in dehydrated alcohol; insoluble in ether. Melts at about 210°, with decomposition.

Dimenhydrinate: White, crystalline, odorless powder. Freely soluble in alcohol and in chloroform; sparingly soluble in ether; slightly soluble in water.

Dimercaprol: Colorless or practically colorless liquid, having a disagreeable, mercaptan-like odor. Soluble in water, in alcohol, in benzyl benzoate, and in methanol.

Dimercaprol Injection: Yellow, viscous solution having a pungent, disagreeable odor. Specific gravity is about 0.978.

Dimethicone: A clear, colorless, and odorless liquid. Soluble in chlorinated hydrocarbons, in benzene, in toluene, in xylene, in *n*-hexane, in petroleum spirits, in ether, and in amyl acetate; very slightly soluble in isopropyl alcohol; insoluble in water, in methanol, in alcohol, and in acetone. *NF category:* Antifoaming agent; water-repelling agent; adhesive; emollient.

Dimethyl Sulfoxide: Clear, colorless, odorless, hygroscopic liquid. Melts at about 18.4°. Boils at about 189°. Soluble in water; practically insoluble in acetone, in alcohol, in benzene, in chloroform, and in ether. *NF category:* Solvent.

Dinoprostone: White to off-white, crystalline powder. Freely soluble in acetone, in alcohol, in ether, in ethyl acetate, in isopropyl alcohol, in methanol, and in methylene chloride; soluble in toluene and in diisopropyl ether; practically insoluble in hexanes.

Dinoprost Tromethamine: White to off-white, crystalline powder. Very soluble in water; freely soluble in dimethylformamide; soluble in methanol; slightly soluble in chloroform.

Dioxybenzone: Yellow powder. Freely soluble in alcohol and in toluene; practically insoluble in water.

Diphenhydramine Hydrochloride: White, odorless, crystalline powder. Slowly darkens on exposure to light. Its solutions are practically neutral to litmus. Freely soluble in water, in alcohol, and in chloroform; sparingly soluble in acetone; very slightly soluble in benzene and in ether.

Diphenoxylate Hydrochloride: White, odorless, crystalline powder. Its saturated solution has a pH of about 3.3. Freely soluble in chloroform; soluble in methanol; sparingly soluble in alcohol and in acetone; slightly soluble in water and in isopropanol; practically insoluble in ether and in solvent hexane.

Diphtheria and Tetanus Toxoids Adsorbed: Turbid, and white, slightly gray, or slightly pink suspension, free from evident clumps after shaking.

Dipivefrin Hydrochloride: White, crystalline powder or small crystals, having a faint odor. Very soluble in water.

Dipyridamole: Intensely yellow, crystalline powder or needles. Very soluble in methanol, in alcohol, and in chloroform; slightly soluble in water; very slightly soluble in acetone and in ethyl acetate.

Dirithromycin: White or practically white powder. Very soluble in methanol and in methylene chloride; very slightly soluble in water.

Disopyramide Phosphate: White or practically white, odorless powder. Melts at about 205°, with decomposition. Freely soluble in water; slightly soluble in alcohol; practically insoluble in chloroform and in ether.

Disulfiram: White to off-white, odorless, crystalline powder. Soluble in acetone, in alcohol, in carbon disulfide, and in chloroform; very slightly soluble in water.

Divalproex Sodium: White to off-white powder. Very soluble in chloroform; freely soluble in methanol and in ethyl ether; soluble in acetone; practically insoluble in acetonitrile.

Dobutamine Hydrochloride: White to practically white, crystalline powder. Soluble in alcohol and in pyridine; sparingly soluble in water and in methanol.

Docetaxel: White or almost white, crystalline powder. Freely soluble in acetone; soluble in methanol; practically insoluble in water.

Docusate Calcium: White, amorphous solid, having the characteristic odor of octyl alcohol. It is free of the odor of other solvents. Very soluble in alcohol, in polyethylene glycol 400, and in corn oil; very slightly soluble in water.

Docusate Potassium: White, amorphous solid, having a characteristic odor suggestive of octyl alcohol. Very soluble in solvent hexane; soluble in alcohol and in glycerin; sparingly soluble in water.

Docusate Sodium: White, wax-like, plastic solid, having a characteristic odor suggestive of octyl alcohol, but no odor of other solvents. Very soluble in solvent hexane; freely soluble in alcohol and in glycerin; sparingly soluble in water. *NF category:* Wetting and/or solubilizing agent.

Dofetilide: White to off-white powder. Soluble in 0.1 N sodium hydroxide, in acetone, and in 0.1 N hydrochloric acid; very slightly soluble in water and in isopropyl alcohol.

Dolasetron Mesylate: White to off-white powder. Freely soluble in water and in propylene glycol; slightly soluble in alcohol and in saline TS.

Donepezil Hydrochloride: White, crystalline powder. Some polymorphic forms are very hygroscopic. Freely soluble in chloroform; soluble in water and in glacial acetic acid; slightly soluble in alcohol and in acetonitrile; practically insoluble in ethyl acetate and in *n*-hexane.

Dopamine Hydrochloride: White to off-white, crystalline powder. May have a slight odor of hydrochloric acid. Melts at about 240°, with decomposition. Freely soluble in water and in aqueous solutions of alkali hydroxides; soluble in methanol; insoluble in ether and in chloroform.

Dorzolamide Hydrochloride: White to off-white, crystalline powder. Soluble in water.

Doxapram Hydrochloride: White to off-white, odorless, crystalline powder. Melts at about 220°. Soluble in water and in chloroform; sparingly soluble in alcohol; practically insoluble in ether.

Doxazosin Mesylate: White to tan-colored powder. Freely soluble in formic acid; very slightly soluble in methanol and in water.

Doxercalciferol: White to off-white powder or crystalline solid. Soluble in *N,N*-dimethylformamide; sparingly soluble in methanol; slightly soluble in acetonitrile; practically insoluble in water.

Doxorubicin Hydrochloride: Red-orange, hygroscopic, crystalline or amorphous powder. Soluble in water, in isotonic sodium chloride solution, and in methanol; practically insoluble in chloroform, in ether, and in other organic solvents.

Doxycycline: Yellow, crystalline powder. Freely soluble in dilute acid and in alkali hydroxide solutions; very slightly soluble in alcohol and in water; practically insoluble in chloroform and in ether.

Doxycycline Hyclate: Yellow, crystalline powder. Soluble in water and in solutions of alkali hydroxides and carbonates; slightly soluble in alcohol; practically insoluble in chloroform and in ether.

Doxylamine Succinate: White or creamy white powder, having a characteristic odor. Very soluble in water and in alcohol; freely soluble in chloroform; very slightly soluble in ether and in benzene.

Dronabinol: Light yellow resinous oil that is sticky at room temperature and hardens upon refrigeration. Insoluble in water.

Add the following:

▲**Dronedarone Hydrochloride:** A white to off-white, fine powder. Freely soluble in methylene chloride and in methanol; practically insoluble in water.▲*USP41*

Droperidol: White to light tan, amorphous or microcrystalline powder. Freely soluble in chloroform; slightly soluble in alcohol and in ether; practically insoluble in water. Melts at about 145°.

Drospirenone: White to off-white powder. Freely soluble in methylene chloride; soluble in acetone and in methanol; sparingly soluble in ethyl acetate and in alcohol; practically insoluble in hexane and in water.

Change to read:

Duloxetine Hydrochloride: White to brownish-white solid. ▪Freely soluble in methanol; sparingly▪1S (USP41) soluble in water; ▪practically insoluble in hexane.▪1S (USP41)

Absorbable Dusting Powder: White, odorless powder.

Dutasteride: White to pale-yellow powder. Soluble in ethanol and methanol; slightly soluble in polyethylene glycol 400; and insoluble in water.

Dyclonine Hydrochloride: White crystals or white crystalline powder, which may have a slight odor. Exhibits local anesthetic properties when placed upon the tongue. Soluble in water, in acetone, in alcohol, and in chloroform.

Dydrogesterone: White to pale yellow, crystalline powder. Sparingly soluble in alcohol; practically insoluble in water.

Dyphylline: White, odorless, extremely bitter, amorphous or crystalline solid. Freely soluble in water; sparingly soluble in alcohol and in chloroform; practically insoluble in ether.

Ecamsule Solution: Clear yellow liquid.

Echothiophate Iodide: White, crystalline, hygroscopic solid having a slight mercaptan-like odor. Its solutions have a pH of about 4. Freely soluble in water and in methanol; soluble in dehydrated alcohol; practically insoluble in other organic solvents.

Echothiophate Iodide for Ophthalmic Solution: White, amorphous powder.

Econazole Nitrate: White or practically white, crystalline powder, having not more than a slight odor. Soluble in methanol; sparingly soluble in chloroform; slightly soluble in alcohol; very slightly soluble in water and in ether.

Edetate Calcium Disodium: White, crystalline granules or white, crystalline powder. Is odorless, is slightly hygroscopic, and has a faint, saline taste. Is stable in air. Freely soluble in water. *NF category:* Chelating and/or complexing agent.

Edetate Disodium: White, crystalline powder. Soluble in water. *NF category:* Chelating and/or complexing agent; transfer ligand.

Edetic Acid: White, crystalline powder. Melts above 220°, with decomposition. Soluble in solutions of alkali hydroxides; very slightly soluble in water. *NF category:* Chelating and/or complexing agent.

Edrophonium Chloride: White, odorless, crystalline powder. Its solution (1 in 10) is practically colorless. Very soluble in water; freely soluble in alcohol; insoluble in chloroform and in ether.

Efavirenz: White to slightly pink crystalline powder. Soluble in methanol; practically insoluble in water.

Emedastine Fumarate: White to faintly yellow, crystalline powder. Soluble in water.

Emetine Hydrochloride: White or very slightly yellowish, odorless, crystalline powder. Is affected by light. Freely soluble in water and in alcohol.

Enalapril Maleate: Off-white, crystalline powder. Melts at about 144°. Freely soluble in methanol and in dimethylformamide; soluble in alcohol; sparingly soluble in water; slightly soluble in semipolar organic solvents; practically insoluble in nonpolar organic solvents.

Enalaprilat: White to nearly white, hygroscopic, crystalline powder. Sparingly soluble in methanol and in dimethyl-

formamide; slightly soluble in water and in isopropyl alcohol; very slightly soluble in acetone, in alcohol, and in hexane; practically insoluble in acetonitrile and in chloroform.

Enflurane: Clear, colorless, stable, volatile liquid, having a mild, sweet odor. Is nonflammable. Slightly soluble in water. Miscible with organic solvents, with fats, and with oils.

Enrofloxacin: Pale yellow to light yellow crystalline powder. Very slightly soluble in water at pH 7.

Entacapone: Greenish yellow to yellow powder. Sparingly soluble in acetone and in methanol; slightly soluble in ethanol, chloroform, isopropanol, and ether; very slightly soluble in toluene; practically insoluble in water.

Entecavir: White to off-white powder. Practically insoluble to slightly soluble in water; practically insoluble in anhydrous ethanol and in heptane.

Ephedrine: Unctuous, practically colorless solid or white crystals or granules. Gradually decomposes on exposure to light. Melts between 33° and 40°, the variability in the melting point being the result of differences in the moisture content, anhydrous Ephedrine having a lower melting point than the hemihydrate of Ephedrine. Its solutions are alkaline to litmus. Soluble in water, in alcohol, in chloroform, and in ether; sparingly and slowly soluble in mineral oil, the solution becoming turbid if the Ephedrine contains more than about 1% of water.

Ephedrine Hydrochloride: Fine, white, odorless crystals or powder. Is affected by light. Freely soluble in water; soluble in alcohol; insoluble in ether.

Ephedrine Sulfate: Fine, white, odorless crystals or powder. Darkens on exposure to light. Freely soluble in water; sparingly soluble in alcohol.

Ephedrine Sulfate Nasal Solution: Clear, colorless solution. Is neutral or slightly acid to litmus.

Epinephrine: White to practically white, odorless, microcrystalline powder or granules, gradually darkening on exposure to light and air. With acids, it forms salts that are readily soluble in water, and the base may be recovered by the addition of ammonia water or alkali carbonates. Its solutions are alkaline to litmus. Very slightly soluble in water and in alcohol; insoluble in ether, in chloroform, and in fixed and volatile oils.

Epinephrine Injection: Practically colorless, slightly acid liquid. Gradually turns dark on exposure to light and air.

Epinephrine Inhalation Solution: Practically colorless, slightly acid liquid. Gradually turns dark on exposure to light and air.

Epinephrine Nasal Solution: Nearly colorless, slightly acid liquid. Gradually turns dark on exposure to light and air.

Epinephrine Ophthalmic Solution: Colorless to faint yellow solution. Gradually turns dark on exposure to light and air.

Epinephrine Bitartrate: White, or grayish-white or light brownish-gray, odorless, crystalline powder. Slowly darkens on exposure to air and light. Its solutions are acid to litmus, having a pH of about 3.5. Freely soluble in water; slightly soluble in alcohol; practically insoluble in chloroform and in ether.

Epinephrine Bitartrate for Ophthalmic Solution: White to off-white solid.

Epinephryl Borate Ophthalmic Solution: Clear, pale yellow liquid, gradually darkening on exposure to light and air.

Epirubicin Hydrochloride: Orange-red powder. Soluble in water and in methanol; slightly soluble in anhydrous ethanol; practically insoluble in acetone.

Eprinomectin: White to off-white powder. Insoluble in cold water.

Ergocalciferol: White, odorless crystals. Is affected by air and by light. Soluble in alcohol, in chloroform, in ether, and in fatty oils; insoluble in water.

Ergocalciferol Oral Solution: Clear liquid having the characteristics of the solvent used in preparing the Solution.

Ergoloid Mesylates: White to off-white, microcrystalline or amorphous, practically odorless powder. Soluble in methanol and in alcohol; sparingly soluble in acetone; slightly soluble in water.

Ergonovine Maleate: White to grayish-white or faintly yellow, odorless, microcrystalline powder. Darkens with age and on exposure to light. Sparingly soluble in water; slightly soluble in alcohol; insoluble in ether and in chloroform.

Ergotamine Tartrate: Colorless crystals or white to yellowish-white, crystalline powder. Is odorless. Melts at about 180°, with decomposition. One g dissolves in about 3200 mL of water; in the presence of a slight excess of tartaric acid 1 g dissolves in about 500 mL of water. Slightly soluble in alcohol.

Erythorbic Acid: White or slightly yellow crystals or powder. It gradually darkens when exposed to light. In the dry state, it is reasonably stable in air, but in solution, it rapidly deteriorates in the presence of air. It melts between 164° and 171° with decomposition. One g is soluble in about 2.5 mL of water and in about 20 mL of alcohol. Slightly soluble in glycerin. *NF category:* Antimicrobial preservative; antioxidant.

Erythritol: White or almost white, crystalline powder or free-flowing granules. It is stable to heat and is nonhygroscopic. Freely soluble in water; very slightly soluble in alcohol. *NF category:* Humectant; sweetening agent; diluent.

Erythromycin: White or slightly yellow, crystalline powder. Is odorless or practically odorless. Soluble in alcohol, in chloroform, and in ether; slightly soluble in water.

Erythromycin Estolate: White, crystalline powder. Is odorless or practically odorless, and is practically tasteless. Soluble in alcohol, in acetone, and in chloroform; practically insoluble in water.

Erythromycin Ethylsuccinate: White or slightly yellow crystalline powder. Is odorless or practically odorless, and is practically tasteless. Freely soluble in alcohol, in chloroform, and in polyethylene glycol 400; very slightly soluble in water.

Erythromycin Gluceptate: Colorless to white crystals. Slightly hygroscopic. Freely soluble in water, in alcohol, in methanol, in dioxane, and in propylene glycol; slightly soluble in acetone and in chloroform; practically insoluble in ether, in carbon tetrachloride, in benzene, and in toluene.

Erythromycin Lactobionate for Injection: White or slightly yellow crystals or powder, having a faint odor. Its solution (1 in 20) is neutral or slightly alkaline. Freely soluble in water, in alcohol, and in methanol; slightly soluble in acetone and in chloroform; practically insoluble in ether.

Erythromycin Stearate: White or slightly yellow crystals or powder. Is odorless or may have a slight, earthy odor, and has a slightly bitter taste. Soluble in alcohol, in chloroform, in methanol, and in ether; practically insoluble in water.

Esmolol Hydrochloride: White to off-white crystalline powder. Very soluble in water; freely soluble in alcohol.

Escitalopram Oxalate: Fine, white to slightly yellow powder. Freely soluble in methanol and in dimethyl sulfoxide; sparingly soluble in water and in alcohol; very slightly soluble in ethyl acetate and in isopropyl alcohol; insoluble in heptane.

Esomeprazole Magnesium: White to slightly colored powder. Soluble in methanol; slightly soluble in water; practically insoluble in heptane.

Esomeprazole Strontium: White to almost-white, crystalline powder. Soluble in water.

Estazolam: White to pale yellowish-white crystal. Soluble in methanol and in acetic anhydride; sparingly soluble in ethanol; practically insoluble in water and in ether.

Estradiol: White or creamy white, small crystals or crystalline powder. Is odorless, and is stable in air. Is hygroscopic. Soluble in alcohol, in acetone, in dioxane, and in solutions of fixed alkali hydroxides; slightly soluble in chloroform; sparingly soluble in vegetable oils; practically insoluble in water.

Estradiol Benzoate: White to off-white, crystalline powder. Soluble in alcohol and in acetone; slightly soluble in diethyl ether; insoluble in water.

Estradiol Cypionate: White to practically white, crystalline powder. Is odorless or has a slight odor. Soluble in alcohol, in acetone, in chloroform, and in dioxane; sparingly soluble in vegetable oils; insoluble in water.

Estradiol Valerate: White, crystalline powder. Is usually odorless but may have a faint, fatty odor. Soluble in castor oil, in methanol, in benzyl benzoate, and in dioxane; sparingly soluble in sesame oil and in peanut oil; practically insoluble in water.

Estriol: White to practically white, odorless, crystalline powder. Melts at about 280°. Soluble in acetone, in chloroform, in dioxane, in ether, and in vegetable oils; sparingly soluble in alcohol; insoluble in water.

Conjugated Estrogens: Conjugated Estrogens obtained from natural sources is a buff-colored, amorphous powder, odorless or having a slight, characteristic odor. The synthetic form is a white to light buff, crystalline or amorphous powder, odorless or having a slight odor.

Synthetic Conjugated Estrogens: A white to light buff, crystalline or amorphous powder that is odorless or has a slight odor.

Esterified Estrogens: White or buff-colored, amorphous powder, odorless or having a slight, characteristic odor.

Estrone: Small, white crystals or white to creamy white, crystalline powder. Is odorless, and is stable in air. Melts at about 260°. Soluble in alcohol, in acetone, in dioxane, and in vegetable oils; slightly soluble in solutions of fixed alkali hydroxides; practically insoluble in water.

Estropipate: White to yellowish-white, fine, crystalline powder. Is odorless, or may have a slight odor. Melts at about 190° to a light brown, viscous liquid, which solidifies on further heating and finally melts at about 245°, with decomposition. Soluble in warm water; very slightly soluble in water, in alcohol, in chloroform, and in ether.

Eszopiclone: White or light-yellow crystalline solid. Freely soluble in methylene chloride; soluble in pH 3.2 phosphate buffer and in dilute mineral acids; slightly soluble in alcohol; very slightly soluble in water.

Ethacrynic Acid: White or practically white, odorless or practically odorless, crystalline powder. Freely soluble in alcohol, in chloroform, and in ether; very slightly soluble in water.

Ethambutol Hydrochloride: White, crystalline powder. Freely soluble in water; soluble in alcohol and in methanol; slightly soluble in ether and in chloroform.

Ethchlorvynol: Colorless to yellow, slightly viscous liquid, having a characteristic pungent odor. Darkens on exposure to light and air. Immiscible with water; miscible with most organic solvents.

Ether: Colorless, mobile, volatile liquid, having a characteristic sweet, pungent odor. Is slowly oxidized by the action of air and light, with the formation of peroxides. It boils at about 35°. Soluble in water and in hydrochloric acid. Miscible with alcohol, with benzene, with chloroform, with solvent hexane, with methylene chloride, and with fixed and volatile oils.

Ethinyl Estradiol: White to creamy white, odorless, crystalline powder. Soluble in alcohol, in chloroform, in ether, in vegetable oils, and in solutions of fixed alkali hydroxides; insoluble in water.

Ethiodized Oil Injection: Straw-colored to amber-colored, oily liquid. It may possess an alliaceous odor. Soluble in acetone, in chloroform, in ether, and in solvent hexane; insoluble in water.

Ethionamide: Bright yellow powder, having a faint to moderate sulfide-like odor. Soluble in methanol; sparingly soluble in alcohol and in propylene glycol; slightly soluble in water, in chloroform, and in ether.

Ethopabate: White to pinkish-white, odorless or practically odorless powder. Soluble in acetonitrile, in acetone, in dehydrated alcohol, and in methanol; sparingly soluble in isopropyl alcohol, in dioxane, in ethyl acetate, and in methylene chloride; slightly soluble in ether; very slightly soluble in water.

Ethosuximide: White to off-white, crystalline powder or waxy solid, having a characteristic odor. Freely soluble in water and in chloroform; very soluble in alcohol and in ether; very slightly soluble in solvent hexane.

Ethotoin: White, crystalline powder. Freely soluble in dehydrated alcohol and in chloroform; soluble in ether; insoluble in water.

Ethyl Acetate: Transparent, colorless liquid, having a fragrant, refreshing, slightly acetous odor, and a peculiar, acetous, burning taste. Soluble in water. Miscible with alcohol, with ether, with fixed oils, and with volatile oils. *NF category:* Flavors and fragrance; solvent.

Ethyl Acrylate and Methyl Methacrylate Copolymer Dispersion: Milky-white liquid of low viscosity with a faint, characteristic odor. It is miscible with water in any proportion; the milky-white appearance is retained. A clear or slightly opalescent, viscous solution is obtained on mixing one part with five parts of acetone, alcohol, or isopropyl alcohol; the polymer substance first precipitates, but then dissolves in the excess organic solvent. When mixed with 1 N sodium hydroxide in a ratio of 1:2, the dispersion does not dissolve; the milky-white appearance is retained. *NF category:* Coating agent; polymer membrane; wet binder; film-forming agent; diluent.

Ethyl Chloride: Colorless, mobile, very volatile liquid at low temperatures or under pressure, having a characteristic, ethereal odor. It boils between 12° and 13°, and its specific gravity at 0° is about 0.921. When liberated at room temperature from its sealed container, it vaporizes immediately. It burns with a smoky, greenish flame, producing hydrogen chloride. Freely soluble in alcohol and in ether; slightly soluble in water.

Ethyl Maltol: White, crystalline powder having a cotton-candy odor and a sweet, fruit-like flavor in dilute solution. One g dissolves in about 55 mL of water, 10 mL of alcohol, 17 mL of propylene glycol, and 5 mL of chloroform. It melts at about 90°. *NF category:* Vehicle (flavored and/or sweetened); flavors and fragrance.

Ethyl Oleate: Mobile, practically colorless liquid, having an agreeable taste. Insoluble in water. Miscible with vegetable oils, with mineral oil, with alcohol, and with most organic solvents. *NF category:* Vehicle (oleaginous); solvent.

Ethyl Vanillin: Fine, white or slightly yellowish crystals. Its taste and odor are similar to the taste and odor of vanillin. Is affected by light. Its solutions are acid to litmus. Freely soluble in alcohol, in chloroform, in ether, and in solutions of alkali hydroxides; sparingly soluble in water at 50°. *NF category:* Flavors and fragrance.

Ethylcellulose: Free-flowing, white to light tan powder. It forms films that have a refractive index of about 1.47. Its aqueous suspensions are neutral to litmus. Ethylcellulose containing less than 46.5% of ethoxy groups is freely soluble in tetrahydrofuran, in methyl acetate, in chloroform, and in mixtures of aromatic hydrocarbons with alcohol; Ethylcellulose containing not less than 46.5% of ethoxy groups is freely soluble in alcohol, in methanol, in toluene, in chloro-

form, and in ethyl acetate; insoluble in water, in glycerin, and in propylene glycol. *NF category:* Coating agent; wet binder; flavors and fragrance; film-forming agent; polymer membrane; release-modifying agent; suspending and/or viscosity-increasing agent.

Ethylcellulose Dispersion Type B: Off-white and slightly viscous liquid. Soluble in alcohol, in methyl alcohol, in tetrahydrofuran, and in ethyl acetate; insoluble in water and in chloroform. *NF category:* Coating agent; film-forming agent; polymer membrane; release-modifying agent.

Ethylenediamine: Clear, colorless or only slightly yellow liquid, having an ammonia-like odor and a strong alkaline reaction. Miscible with water and with alcohol.

Ethylene Glycol Stearates: White or almost white, waxy solid. Soluble in acetone and in hot alcohol; practically insoluble in water. *NF category:* Emulsifying agent; emollient.

Ethylene Glycol and Vinyl Alcohol Graft Copolymer: White or slightly yellowish powder. Very soluble in water; practically insoluble in anhydrous alcohol, and in acetone. It dissolves in dilute acids and dilute solutions of alkali hydroxides. *NF category:* Coating agent; wet binder; film-forming agent.

Ethylparaben: Small, colorless crystals or white powder. Freely soluble in acetone, in alcohol, in ether, and in propylene glycol; slightly soluble in water and in glycerin. *NF category:* Antimicrobial preservative.

Ethylparaben Sodium: White or almost-white, hygroscopic, crystalline powder. Freely soluble in water; soluble in anhydrous alcohol; practically insoluble in methylene chloride. *NF category:* Antimicrobial preservative.

Ethynodiol Diacetate: White, odorless, crystalline powder. Is stable in air. Very soluble in chloroform; freely soluble in ether; soluble in alcohol; sparingly soluble in fixed oils; insoluble in water.

Etidronate Disodium: White powder, which may contain lumps. Freely soluble in water; practically insoluble in alcohol.

Etomidate: White or almost white powder. Freely soluble in alcohol and in methylene chloride; very slightly soluble in water.

Etoposide: Fine, white to off-white, crystalline powder. Sparingly soluble in methanol; slightly soluble in alcohol, in chloroform, in ethyl acetate, and in methylene chloride; very slightly soluble in water.

Eucalyptus Oil: Colorless or pale yellow liquid. One mL of eucalyptus oil dissolves in 5 mL of 70% alcohol. Insoluble in cold water. *NF category:* Flavors and perfumes.

Eugenol: Colorless or pale yellow liquid, having a strongly aromatic odor of clove and a pungent, spicy taste. Upon exposure to air, it darkens and thickens. Is optically inactive. Slightly soluble in water. Miscible with alcohol, with chloroform, with ether, and with fixed oils.

Exemestane: White to slightly yellow, crystalline powder. Freely soluble in *N,N*-dimethylformamide; soluble in methanol; insoluble in water.

Ezetimibe: White powder. Freely soluble in alcohol; soluble in acetonitrile; insoluble in aqueous solvents and nonpolar solvents like hexane.

Famciclovir: A white to pale yellow solid. Freely soluble in methanol and in acetone; sparingly soluble in ethanol and in isopropyl alcohol.

Famotidine: White to pale yellowish-white, crystalline powder. Is sensitive to light. Freely soluble in dimethylformamide and in glacial acetic acid; slightly soluble in methanol; very slightly soluble in water; practically insoluble in acetone, in alcohol, in chloroform, in ether, and in ethyl acetate.

Hard Fat: White mass; almost odorless and free from rancid odor; greasy to the touch. On warming, melts to give a colorless or slightly yellowish liquid. When the molten material is shaken with an equal quantity of hot water, a white emulsion is formed. Freely soluble in ether; slightly soluble in alcohol; practically insoluble in water. *NF category:* Stiffening agent; suppository base.

Felbamate: White to off-white powder. Freely soluble in dimethyl sulfoxide; sparingly soluble in methanol; slightly soluble in acetonitrile; very slightly soluble in water.

Felodipine: Light yellow to yellow, crystalline powder. Freely soluble in acetone and in methanol; very slightly soluble in heptane; insoluble in water.

Fenbendazole: White to off-white powder. Sparingly soluble in dimethylformamide; very slightly soluble in methanol; practically insoluble in water.

Fenofibrate: White or almost white, crystalline powder. Very soluble in methylene chloride; slightly soluble in alcohol; practically insoluble in water.

Fenoldopam Mesylate: White to off-white powder. Soluble in water.

Fenoprofen Calcium: White, crystalline powder. Slightly soluble in *n*-hexanol, in methanol, and in water; practically insoluble in chloroform.

Fentanyl Citrate: White, crystalline powder or white, glistening crystals. Melts at about 150°, with decomposition. Soluble in methanol; sparingly soluble in water; slightly soluble in chloroform.

Ferric Oxide: Powder exhibiting two basic colors (red and yellow), or other shades produced on blending the basic colors. Insoluble in water and in organic solvents; dissolves in hydrochloric acid upon warming, a small amount of insoluble residue usually remaining. *NF category:* Coloring agent.

Ferric Subsulfate Solution: Reddish-brown liquid, odorless or nearly so. Acid to litmus, and is affected by light. Specific gravity is about 1.548.

Ferric Sulfate: Grayish-white or yellowish powder or fawn-colored pearls. Hygroscopic. Slightly soluble in water and in ethanol (96%); practically insoluble in acetone and in ethyl acetate. Hydrolyzes slowly in aqueous solution.

Ferrosoferric Oxide: Black powder. Dissolves in hydrochloric acid upon warming, a small amount of insoluble residue usually remaining; insoluble in water and in organic solvents. *NF category:* Coloring agent.

Ferrous Fumarate: Reddish-orange to red-brown, odorless powder. May contain soft lumps that produce a yellow streak when crushed. Slightly soluble in water; very slightly soluble in alcohol. Its solubility in dilute hydrochloric acid is limited by the separation of fumaric acid.

Ferrous Gluconate: Yellowish-gray or pale greenish-yellow, fine powder or granules, having a slight odor resembling that of burned sugar. Its solution (1 in 20) is acid to litmus. Soluble in water, with slight heating; practically insoluble in alcohol.

Ferrous Sulfate: Pale, bluish-green crystals or granules. Is odorless and is efflorescent in dry air. Oxidizes readily in moist air to form brownish yellow basic ferric sulfate. Its solution (1 in 10) is acid to litmus, having a pH of about 3.7. Very soluble in boiling water; freely soluble in water; insoluble in alcohol.

Dried Ferrous Sulfate: Grayish-white to buff-colored powder, consisting primarily of $FeSO_4 \cdot H_2O$ with varying amounts of $FeSO_4 \cdot 4H_2O$. Slowly soluble in water; insoluble in alcohol.

Ferumoxides Injection: Black to reddish-brown, aqueous colloid. It is stable for 24 hours after dilution.

Fexofenadine Hydrochloride: White to off-white powder. Freely soluble in methanol; very slightly to slightly soluble in water; very slightly soluble in acetone.

Finasteride: White to off-white, crystalline solid. Melts at about 257°. Freely soluble in chloroform and in alcohol; very slightly soluble in water.

Fingolimod Hydrochloride: White to practically white powder. Freely soluble in water and in alcohol. Soluble in propylene glycol.

Fish Oil Containing Omega-3 Acids: Pale yellow liquid. Very soluble in acetone and in heptane; slightly soluble in anhydrous alcohol; practically insoluble in water.

Flavoxate Hydrochloride: White or almost white, crystalline powder. Slightly soluble in alcohol, in water, and in methylene chloride.

Flecainide Acetate: White to slightly off-white, crystalline powder. Freely soluble in alcohol; soluble in water. pK_a is 9.3.

Fluconazole: White or almost white, crystalline powder. Freely soluble in methanol; soluble in alcohol and in acetone; sparingly soluble in isopropanol and in chloroform; slightly soluble in water; very slightly soluble in toluene.

Flucytosine: White to off-white, crystalline powder. Is odorless or has a slight odor. Sparingly soluble in water; slightly soluble in alcohol; practically insoluble in chloroform and in ether.

Fludarabine Phosphate: White to off-white, crystalline, hygroscopic powder. Freely soluble in dimethylformamide; slightly soluble in water and in 0.1 M hydrochloric acid; practically insoluble in ethanol.

Fludrocortisone Acetate: White to pale yellow crystals or crystalline powder. Is odorless or practically odorless. Is hygroscopic. Sparingly soluble in alcohol and in chloroform; slightly soluble in ether; insoluble in water.

Flumazenil: White to off-white powder. Slightly soluble in acidic aqueous solutions; practically insoluble in water.

Flumethasone Pivalate: White to off-white, crystalline powder. Slightly soluble in methanol; very slightly soluble in chloroform and in methylene chloride; insoluble in water.

Flunisolide: White to creamy-white, crystalline powder. Melts at about 245°, with decomposition. Soluble in acetone; sparingly soluble in chloroform; slightly soluble in methanol; practically insoluble in water.

Flunixin Meglumine: White to off-white crystalline powder. Soluble in water, in alcohol, and in methanol; practically insoluble in ethyl acetate.

Fluocinolone Acetonide: White or practically white, odorless, crystalline powder. Is stable in air. Melts at about 270°, with decomposition. Soluble in methanol; slightly soluble in ether and in chloroform; insoluble in water.

Fluocinonide: White to cream-colored, crystalline powder, having not more than a slight odor. Sparingly soluble in acetone and in chloroform; slightly soluble in alcohol, in methanol, and in dioxane; very slightly soluble in ether; practically insoluble in water.

Fluorescein: Yellowish-red to red, odorless powder. Soluble in dilute alkali hydroxides; insoluble in water.

Fluorescein Sodium: Orange-red, hygroscopic, odorless powder. Freely soluble in water; sparingly soluble in alcohol.

Fluorescein Sodium Ophthalmic Strip: Each Strip is a dry, white piece of paper, one end of which is rounded and is uniformly orange-red in color because of the fluorescein sodium impregnated in the paper.

Fluorometholone: White to yellowish-white, odorless, crystalline powder. Melts at about 280°, with some decomposition. Slightly soluble in alcohol; very slightly soluble in chloroform and in ether; practically insoluble in water.

Fluorouracil: White to practically white, practically odorless, crystalline powder. Decomposes at about 282°. Sparingly soluble in water; slightly soluble in alcohol; practically insoluble in chloroform and in ether.

Fluoxetine Hydrochloride: White to off-white crystalline powder. Freely soluble in alcohol and in methanol; sparingly soluble in water and in dichloromethane; practically insoluble in ether.

Fluoxymesterone: White or practically white, odorless, crystalline powder. Melts at about 240°, with some decomposition. Sparingly soluble in alcohol; slightly soluble in chloroform; practically insoluble in water.

Add the following:

■Fluphenazine Decanoate: Pale yellow to yellow-orange, viscous liquid or yellow solid. Slowly crystallizes at room temperature. Melts at about 30°–32°. Very soluble in chloroform, in ether, in cyclohexane, in dehydrated alcohol, and in methylene chloride; freely soluble in methanol; insoluble in water.■₁S (USP41)

Fluphenazine Enanthate: Pale yellow to yellow-orange, clear to slightly turbid, viscous liquid, having a characteristic odor. Is unstable in strong light, but stable to air at room temperature. Freely soluble in alcohol, in chloroform, and in ether; insoluble in water.

Change to read:

Fluphenazine Hydrochloride: White or nearly white, odorless, crystalline powder. Melts, within a range of 5°, at a temperature above 225°. Freely soluble in water; slightly soluble ■₁S (USP41) in alcohol, ■₁S (USP41) in chloroform, ■and in methylene chloride;■₁S (USP41) practically insoluble in benzene and in ether.

Flurandrenolide: White to off-white, fluffy, crystalline powder. Is odorless. Freely soluble in chloroform; soluble in methanol; sparingly soluble in alcohol; practically insoluble in water and in ether.

Flurazepam Hydrochloride: Off-white to yellow, crystalline powder. Is odorless, or has a slight odor, and its solutions are acid to litmus. Melts at about 212°, with decomposition. Freely soluble in water and in alcohol; slightly soluble in isopropyl alcohol and in chloroform.

Flurbiprofen: White, crystalline powder. Freely soluble in acetone, in dehydrated alcohol, in ether, and in methanol; soluble in acetonitrile; practically insoluble in water. Optically inactive (1 in 50 solution in dehydrated alcohol).

Flutamide: Pale yellow, crystalline powder. Freely soluble in acetone, in ethyl acetate, and in methanol; soluble in chloroform and in ether; practically insoluble in mineral oil, in petroleum ether, and in water.

Fluticasone Propionate (micronized): Fine, white powder.

Fluvastatin Sodium: White to pale yellow, brownish-pale yellow, or reddish-pale yellow, hygroscopic powder. Soluble in alcohol, in methanol, and in water.

Fluvoxamine Maleate: White to off-white, crystalline powder. Freely soluble in alcohol and in chloroform; sparingly soluble in water; and practically insoluble in diethyl ether.

Folic Acid: Yellow, yellow-brownish, or yellowish-orange, odorless, crystalline powder. It readily dissolves in dilute solutions of alkali hydroxides and carbonates. Soluble in hot, 3 N hydrochloric acid, in hot, 2 N sulfuric acid, in hydrochloric acid, and in sulfuric acid, yielding very pale yellow solutions; very slightly soluble in water; insoluble in alcohol, in acetone, in chloroform, and in ether.

Folic Acid Injection: Clear, yellow to orange-yellow, alkaline liquid.

Formaldehyde Solution: Clear, colorless or practically colorless liquid, having a pungent odor. The vapor from it irritates the mucous membrane of the throat and nose. On long standing, especially in the cold, it may become cloudy because of the separation of paraformaldehyde. This cloudiness disappears when the solution is warmed. Miscible with water and with alcohol.

Formoterol Fumarate Dihydrate: White or almost white or slightly yellow powder. Freely soluble in dimethyl sulfoxide and in acetic acid; soluble in methanol; slightly soluble in water and in 2-propanol; practically insoluble in acetonitrile and in diethyl ether.

Foscarnet Sodium: White to almost white, crystalline powder. Soluble in water; practically insoluble in alcohol.

Fosphenytoin Sodium: White to pale yellow solid. Freely soluble in water.

Fructose: Colorless crystals or as a white, crystalline powder. Is odorless, and has a sweet taste. Freely soluble in water; soluble in alcohol and in methanol. *NF category:* Sweetening agent; diluent; flavors and fragrance.

Basic Fuchsin: Dark green powder or greenish glistening crystalline fragments, having a bronze-like luster and not more than a faint odor. Soluble in water, in alcohol, and in amyl alcohol; insoluble in ether.

Fulvestrant: White powder. Freely soluble in alcohol.

Fumaric Acid: White, odorless granules or crystalline powder. Soluble in alcohol; slightly soluble in water and in ether; very slightly soluble in chloroform. *NF category:* pH modifier (acidifying agent/alkalizing agent/buffering agent); flavors and fragrance; antioxidant.

Furazolidone: Yellow, odorless, crystalline powder. Is tasteless at first, then a bitter aftertaste develops. Practically insoluble in water, in alcohol, and in carbon tetrachloride.

Furosemide: White to slightly yellow, odorless, crystalline powder. Freely soluble in acetone, in dimethylformamide, and in solutions of alkali hydroxides; soluble in methanol; sparingly soluble in alcohol; slightly soluble in ether; very slightly soluble in chloroform; practically insoluble in water.

Furosemide Injection: Clear, colorless solution.

Gabapentin: White to off-white, crystalline solid. Freely soluble in water and in alkaline and acidic solutions.

Gadodiamide: White, odorless powder. Freely soluble in water and in methanol; soluble in ethyl alcohol; slightly soluble in acetone and in chloroform.

Gadoteridol: White to off-white, crystalline, odorless powder. Freely soluble in water and in methyl alcohol; soluble in isopropyl alcohol. Melts at about 300°.

Gadoversetamide: White, odorless powder. Freely soluble in water.

Galactose: A white, crystalline or finely granulated powder. Soluble in water; very slightly soluble in alcohol. *NF category:* Sweetening agent; chelating and/or complexing agent.

Galantamine Hydrobromide: White to almost white powder. Soluble in 0.1 N sodium hydroxide; sparingly soluble in water; very slightly soluble in alcohol; insoluble in n-propanol.

Gallamine Triethiodide: White, odorless, amorphous powder. Is hygroscopic. Very soluble in water; sparingly soluble in alcohol; very slightly soluble in chloroform.

Gamma Cyclodextrin: White or almost white, amorphous or crystalline powder. Freely soluble in water and in propylene glycol; very slightly soluble in alcohol. *NF category:* Sequestering agent; chelating and/or complexing agent.

Ganciclovir: White to off-white, crystalline powder.

Ganciclovir for Injection: White to off-white powder. Soluble in water.

Petrolatum Gauze: The petrolatum recovered by draining in the *Assay* is a white or faintly yellowish, unctuous mass, transparent in thin layers even after cooling to 0°.

Gelatin: Sheets, flakes, or shreds, or coarse to fine powder. Is faintly yellow or amber in color, the color varying in depth according to the particle size. Has a slight, characteristic bouillon-like odor in solution. Is stable in air when dry, but is subject to microbic decomposition when moist or in solution. Gelatin has any suitable strength that is designated by Bloom Gelometer number. Type A Gelatin exhibits an isoelectric point between pH 7 and pH 9, and Type B Gelatin exhibits an isoelectric point between pH 4.7 and pH 5.2. Soluble in hot water, in 6 N acetic acid, and in a hot mixture of glycerin and water; insoluble in cold water, but swells and softens when immersed in it, gradually absorbing from 5 to 10 times its own weight of water, in alcohol, in chloroform, in ether, and in fixed and volatile oils. *NF category:* Coating agent; suspending and/or viscosity-increasing agent; wet binder; capsule shell; colloid stabilizing agent; film-forming agent.

Absorbable Gelatin Film: Light amber, transparent, pliable film which becomes rubbery when moistened. Insoluble in water.

Absorbable Gelatin Sponge: Light, nearly white, nonelastic, tough, porous, hydrophilic solid. Insoluble in water.

Gellan Gum: Off-white powder. Soluble in hot or in cold deionized water. *NF category:* Suspending and/or viscosity-increasing agent.

Gemcitabine Hydrochloride: White to off-white solid. Soluble in water; slightly soluble in methanol; practically insoluble in alcohol and in polar organic solvents.

Gemfibrozil: White, waxy, crystalline solid. Soluble in alcohol, in methanol, and in chloroform; practically insoluble in water.

Gentamicin Sulfate: White to buff powder. Freely soluble in water; insoluble in alcohol, in acetone, in chloroform, in ether, and in benzene.

Gentamicin Injection: Clear, slightly yellow solution, having a faint odor.

Gentian Violet: Dark green powder or greenish, glistening pieces having a metallic luster, and having not more than a faint odor. Soluble in alcohol, in glycerin, and in chloroform; sparingly soluble in water; insoluble in ether.

Gentian Violet Cream: Dark purple, water-washable cream.

Gentian Violet Topical Solution: Purple liquid, having a slight odor of alcohol. A dilution (1 in 100), viewed downward through 1 cm of depth, is deep purple in color.

Powdered Asian Ginseng Extract: Pale yellow-brown, hygroscopic, powdery or easily pulverizable mass. Soluble in water, forming a slightly cloudy solution.

Glaze, Pharmaceutical: Denatured alcohol solution. *NF category:* Coating agent; film-forming agent.

Glimepiride: White to almost white powder. Soluble in dimethylformamide; sparingly soluble in methylene chloride; slightly soluble in methanol; practically insoluble in water.

Glipizide: White to off-white powder. Freely soluble in dimethylformamide; soluble in 0.1 N sodium hydroxide; slightly soluble in methylene chloride.

Immune Globulin: Transparent or slightly opalescent liquid, either colorless or of a brownish color due to denatured hemoglobin. Is practically odorless. May develop a slight, granular deposit during storage.

Rh₀(D) Immune Globulin: Transparent or slightly opalescent liquid. Is practically colorless and odorless. May develop a slight, granular deposit during storage.

Glucagon: Fine, white or faintly colored, crystalline powder. Is practically odorless and tasteless. Soluble in dilute alkali and acid solutions; insoluble in most organic solvents.

Glucagon for Injection: White, odorless powder.

Gluconolactone: Fine, white, practically odorless, crystalline powder. Melts at about 153°, with decomposition. Freely soluble in water; sparingly soluble in alcohol; insoluble in ether.

Liquid Glucose: Colorless or yellowish, thick, syrupy liquid. Odorless or nearly odorless, and has a sweet taste.

Sparingly soluble in alcohol. Miscible with water. *NF category:* Wet binder; coating agent; sweetening agent.

ʟ-Glutamic Acid Hydrochloride: A white, crystalline powder. 1 g dissolves in about 3 mL of water. It is almost insoluble in alcohol and in ether. Its solutions are acid to litmus. *NF category:* Flavors and fragrance.

Glutamine: White crystals or crystalline powder. Soluble in water; practically insoluble in alcohol and in ether.

Glutaral Concentrate: Clear, colorless or faintly yellow liquid, having a characteristic, irritating odor.

Glycerin: Clear, colorless, syrupy liquid, having a sweet taste. Has not more than a slight characteristic odor, which is neither harsh nor disagreeable. Is hygroscopic. Its solutions are neutral to litmus. Insoluble in chloroform, in ether, and in fixed and volatile oils. Miscible with water and with alcohol. *NF category:* Humectant; plasticizer; solvent; tonicity agent; antimicrobial preservative; emollient; sweetening agent.

Glyceryl Behenate: [(Title for this monograph—not to change until December 1, 2019.)
(Prior to December 1, 2019, the current practice of labeling the article of commerce with the name Glyceryl Behenate may be continued. Use of the name Glyceryl Dibehenate will be permitted as of December 1, 2014; however, the use of this name will not be mandatory until December 1, 2019. The 60-month extension will provide the time needed by manufacturers and users to make necessary changes.)]

Glyceryl Dibehenate: Fine powder, having a faint odor. Melts at about 70°. Soluble in chloroform; practically insoluble in water and in alcohol. *NF category:* Lubricant; coating agent; suspending and/or viscosity-increasing agent; wet binder.

Glyceryl Distearate: Hard, waxy mass or powder or white or almost white flakes. Soluble in methylene chloride and in tetrahydrofuran; slightly soluble in hot alcohol; insoluble in water. *NF category:* Emulsifying agent.

Glyceryl Monocaprylate: Colorless or slightly yellow, oily liquid or semisolid. Very soluble in alcohol; freely soluble in methylene chloride; practically insoluble in water. *NF category:* Lubricant; emulsifying agent.

Glyceryl Monocaprylocaprate: Colorless or slightly yellow, oily liquid or semisolid. Very soluble in alcohol; freely soluble in methylene chloride; practically insoluble in water. *NF category:* Lubricant; emulsifying agent.

Glyceryl Monolinoleate: Amber, oily liquids that may be partially solidified at room temperature. Freely soluble in methylene chloride; soluble in tetrahydrofuran; practically insoluble in water. *NF category:* Emulsifying agent.

Glyceryl Monooleate: Amber, oily liquids that may be partially solidified at room temperature. Freely soluble in methylene chloride; soluble in tetrahydrofuran; practically insoluble in water. *NF category:* Emulsifying agent; emollient; release-modifying agent.

Glyceryl Monostearate: White to yellowish wax-like solid; or white to yellowish wax-like beads, flakes, or powder. Slight, agreeable, fatty odor and taste. Is affected by light. Dissolves in hot organic solvents such as alcohol, minerals or fixed oils, benzene, ether, and acetone. Insoluble in water, but it may be dispersed in hot water with the aid of a small amount of soap or other suitable surface-active agent. *NF category:* Emulsifying agent; emollient; release-modifying agent; lubricant.

Add the following:

■**Glyceryl Tricaprylate:** Clear, colorless to pale-yellow liquid. Very soluble in alcohol; freely soluble in methylene chloride; practically insoluble in water. *NF category:* Lubricant; emulsifying agent; vehicle (solid carrier).■₁ₛ *(NF36)*

Glyceryl Tristearate: White, solid, microcrystalline powder. Soluble in hot alcohol, in acetone, and in chloroform; very slightly soluble in cold alcohol, in ether, and in petroleum ether; insoluble in water. *NF category:* Lubricant; emulsifying agent.

Glycine: White, odorless, crystalline powder, having a sweetish taste. Its solutions are acid to litmus. Freely soluble in water; very slightly soluble in alcohol and in ether. *NF category:* Bulking agent; disintegrant; wetting and/or solubilizing agent; pH modifier (acidifying agent/alkalizing agent/buffering agent).

Glycopyrrolate: White, odorless, crystalline powder. Soluble in water and in alcohol; practically insoluble in chloroform and in ether.

Gonadorelin Acetate: White to slightly yellowish powder. Soluble in water; sparingly soluble in methanol.

Chorionic Gonadotropin: White or practically white, amorphous powder. Freely soluble in water.

Chorionic Gonadotropin for Injection: White or practically white, amorphous solid having the characteristic appearance of substances prepared by freeze-drying.

Gramicidin: White or practically white, odorless, crystalline powder. Soluble in alcohol; insoluble in water.

Add the following:

▲Granisetron: Off-white to pale-yellow powder. Soluble to freely soluble in methanol and in methylene chloride.
▲*USP41*

Granisetron Hydrochloride: White or almost white powder. Freely soluble in water; sparingly soluble in methylene chloride; slightly soluble in methanol.

Green Soap: Soft, unctuous, yellowish-white to brownish or greenish yellow, transparent to translucent mass. Has a slight, characteristic odor, often suggesting the oil from which it was prepared. Its solution (1 in 20) is alkaline to bromothymol blue TS.

Griseofulvin: White to creamy white, odorless powder, in which particles of the order of 4 μm in diameter predominate. Soluble in acetone, in dimethylformamide, and in chloroform; sparingly soluble in alcohol; very slightly soluble in water.

Guaifenesin: White to slightly gray, crystalline powder. May have a slight characteristic odor. Soluble in water, in alcohol, in chloroform, and in propylene glycol; sparingly soluble in glycerin.

Guanabenz Acetate: White or almost white powder having not more than a slight odor. Soluble in alcohol and in propylene glycol; sparingly soluble in water and in 0.1 N hydrochloric acid.

Guanadrel Sulfate: White to off-white, crystalline powder. Melts at about 235°, with decomposition. Soluble in water; sparingly soluble in methanol; slightly soluble in alcohol and in acetone.

Guanethidine Monosulfate: White to off-white, crystalline powder. Very soluble in water; sparingly soluble in alcohol; practically insoluble in chloroform.

Guar Gum: White to yellowish-white, practically odorless powder. Dispersible in hot or cold water, forming a colloidal solution. *NF category:* Suspending and/or viscosity-increasing agent; wet binder; polymers for ophthalmic use; release-modifying agent; disintegrant.

Gutta Percha: Lumps or blocks of variable size; externally brown or grayish-brown to grayish-white in color; internally reddish yellow or reddish gray and having a laminated or fibrous appearance. Is flexible but only slightly elastic. Has a slight, characteristic odor and a slight taste. Soluble in chloroform; partly soluble in benzene, in carbon disulfide, and in turpentine oil; insoluble in water.

Halazone: White, crystalline powder, having a characteristic chlorine-like odor. Is affected by light. Melts at about 194°, with decomposition. Soluble in glacial acetic acid; very slightly soluble in water and in chloroform. Dissolves in solutions of alkali hydroxides and carbonates with the formation of a salt.

Halazone Tablets for Solution: Soluble in water.

Halcinonide: White to off-white, odorless, crystalline powder. Soluble in acetone and in chloroform; slightly soluble in alcohol and in ethyl ether; insoluble in water and in hexanes.

Halobetasol Propionate: White to off-white powder. Freely soluble in dichloromethane and in acetone; practically insoluble in water.

Haloperidol: White to faintly yellowish, amorphous or microcrystalline powder. Its saturated solution is neutral to litmus. Soluble in chloroform; sparingly soluble in alcohol; slightly soluble in ether; practically insoluble in water.

Haloperidol Decanoate: A white or almost white powder. Very soluble in alcohol, in methanol, and in methylene chloride; practically insoluble in water.

Halothane: Colorless, mobile, nonflammable, heavy liquid, having a characteristic odor resembling that of chloroform. Its taste is sweet and produces a burning sensation. Slightly soluble in water. Miscible with alcohol, with chloroform, with ether, and with fixed oils.

Helium: Colorless, odorless, tasteless gas, which is not combustible and does not support combustion. Very slightly soluble in water. At 0° and at a pressure of 760 mm of mercury, 1000 mL of the gas weighs about 180 mg.

Heparin Sodium: White or pale-colored, amorphous powder. Is odorless or practically so, and is hygroscopic. Soluble in water.

Hexachlorophene: White to light tan, crystalline powder. Is odorless or has only a slight, phenolic odor. Freely soluble in acetone, in alcohol, and in ether; soluble in chloroform and in dilute solutions of fixed alkali hydroxides; insoluble in water.

Hexachlorophene Liquid Soap: Clear, amber-colored liquid, having a slight, characteristic odor. Its solution (1 in 20) is clear and has an alkaline reaction.

Hexylene Glycol: Clear, colorless, viscous liquid. Absorbs moisture when exposed to moist air. Miscible with water and with many organic solvents, including alcohol, ether, chloroform, acetone, and hexanes. *NF category:* Humectant; solvent.

Histamine Phosphate: Colorless, odorless, long prismatic crystals. Is stable in air but is affected by light. Its solutions are acid to litmus. Freely soluble in water.

Histidine: White, odorless crystals, having a slightly bitter taste. Soluble in water; very slightly soluble in alcohol; insoluble in ether.

Histoplasmin: Clear, red liquid. Miscible with water.

Homatropine Hydrobromide: White crystals, or white, crystalline powder. Slowly darkens on exposure to light. Freely soluble in water; sparingly soluble in alcohol; slightly soluble in chloroform; insoluble in ether. Melts between 214° and 217°, with slight decomposition.

Homatropine Methylbromide: White, odorless powder. Slowly darkens on exposure to light. Melts at about 190°. Very soluble in water; freely soluble in alcohol and in acetone containing about 20% of water; practically insoluble in ether and in acetone.

Hydralazine Hydrochloride: White to off-white, odorless, crystalline powder. Melts at about 275°, with decomposition. Soluble in water; slightly soluble in alcohol; very slightly soluble in ether.

Hydrochloric Acid: Colorless, fuming liquid having a pungent odor. It ceases to fume when it is diluted with 2 volumes of water. Specific gravity is about 1.18. *NF cate-*

gory: pH modifier (acidifying agent/alkalizing agent/buffering agent).

Diluted Hydrochloric Acid: Colorless, odorless liquid. Specific gravity is about 1.05. *NF category:* pH modifier (acidifying agent/alkalizing agent/buffering agent).

Hydrochlorothiazide: White, or practically white, practically odorless, crystalline powder. Freely soluble in sodium hydroxide solution, in *n*-butylamine, and in dimethylformamide; very slightly soluble in water; sparingly soluble in methanol; insoluble in ether, in chloroform, and in dilute mineral acids.

Hydrocodone Bitartrate: Fine, white crystals or a crystalline powder. Is affected by light. Soluble in water; slightly soluble in alcohol; insoluble in ether and in chloroform.

Hydrocortisone: White to practically white, odorless, crystalline powder. Melts at about 215°, with decomposition. Sparingly soluble in acetone and in alcohol; slightly soluble in chloroform; very slightly soluble in water and in ether.

Hydrocortisone Acetate: White to practically white, odorless, crystalline powder. Melts at about 220°, with decomposition. Slightly soluble in alcohol and in chloroform; insoluble in water.

Hydrocortisone Butyrate: White to practically white, practically odorless, crystalline powder. Freely soluble in chloroform; soluble in methanol, in alcohol, and in acetone; slightly soluble in ether; practically insoluble in water.

Hydrocortisone Sodium Phosphate: White to light yellow, odorless or practically odorless, powder. Is exceedingly hygroscopic. Freely soluble in water; slightly soluble in alcohol; practically insoluble in chloroform, in dioxane, and in ether.

Hydrocortisone Sodium Succinate: White or nearly white, odorless, hygroscopic, amorphous solid. Very soluble in water and in alcohol; very slightly soluble in acetone; insoluble in chloroform.

Hydroflumethiazide: White to cream-colored, finely divided, odorless, crystalline powder. Freely soluble in acetone; soluble in alcohol; very slightly soluble in water.

Hydrogen Peroxide Concentrate: Clear, colorless liquid. Is acid to litmus. Slowly decomposes, and is affected by light.

Hydrogen Peroxide Solution: Clear, colorless liquid, odorless, or having an odor resembling that of ozone. Is acid to litmus and to the taste and produces a froth in the mouth. Rapidly decomposes when in contact with many oxidizing as well as reducing substances. When rapidly heated, it may decompose suddenly. Is affected by light. Specific gravity is about 1.01.

Hydromorphone Hydrochloride: Fine, white or practically white, odorless, crystalline powder. Is affected by light. Freely soluble in water; sparingly soluble in alcohol; practically insoluble in ether.

Hydroquinone: Fine white needles. Darkens upon exposure to light and air. Freely soluble in water, in alcohol, and in ether.

Hydroxocobalamin: Dark red crystals or red crystalline powder. Is odorless, or has not more than a slight acetone odor. The anhydrous form is very hygroscopic. Sparingly soluble in water, in alcohol, and in methanol; practically insoluble in acetone, in ether, in chloroform, and in benzene.

Hydroxyamphetamine Hydrobromide: White, crystalline powder. Its solutions are slightly acid to litmus, having a pH of about 5. Freely soluble in water and in alcohol; slightly soluble in chloroform; practically insoluble in ether.

Hydroxychloroquine Sulfate: White or practically white, crystalline powder. Is odorless, and has a bitter taste. Its solutions have a pH of about 4.5. Exists in two forms, the usual form melting at about 240° and the other form melting at about 198°. Freely soluble in water; practically insoluble in alcohol, in chloroform, and in ether.

Hydroxyethyl Cellulose: White to light tan, practically odorless and tasteless, hygroscopic powder. Soluble in hot water and in cold water, giving a colloidal solution; practically insoluble in alcohol and in most organic solvents. *NF category:* Suspending and/or viscosity-increasing agent; coating agent; film-forming agent; polymers for ophthalmic use; wet binder.

Hydroxyprogesterone Caproate: White or creamy white, crystalline powder. Is odorless or has a slight odor. Soluble in ether; slightly soluble in benzene; insoluble in water.

Hydroxypropyl Betadex: White or almost white, amorphous or crystalline powder. Freely soluble in water and in propylene glycol. *NF category:* Sequestering agent; chelating and/or complexing agent; release-modifying agent.

Hydroxypropyl Cellulose: White to cream-colored, practically odorless and tasteless, granular solid or powder. Is hygroscopic after drying. Soluble in cold water, in alcohol, in chloroform, and in propylene glycol, giving a colloidal solution; insoluble in hot water. *NF category:* Coating agent; suspending and/or viscosity-increasing agent; emulsifying agent; film-forming agent; release-modifying agent; wet binder.

Low-Substituted Hydroxypropyl Cellulose: White to yellowish-white, practically odorless and tasteless, fibrous or granular powder. Is hygroscopic. Practically insoluble in alcohol and in ether. Dissolves in a solution of sodium hydroxide (1 in 10), and produces a viscous solution. Swells in water, in sodium carbonate TS, and in 2 N hydrochloric acid. The pH of the suspension, obtained by shaking 1.0 g with 100 mL of water, is between 5.0 and 7.5. *NF category:* Disintegrant; wet binder.

Hydroxyurea: White to off-white powder. Is somewhat hygroscopic, decomposing in the presence of moisture. Melts at a temperature exceeding 133°, with decomposition. Freely soluble in water and in hot alcohol.

Hydroxyzine Hydrochloride: White, odorless powder. Melts at about 200°, with decomposition. Very soluble in water; soluble in chloroform; slightly soluble in acetone; practically insoluble in ether.

Hydroxyzine Pamoate: Light yellow, practically odorless powder. Freely soluble in dimethylformamide; practically insoluble in water and in methanol.

Hymetellose: A white, yellowish-white or grayish-white powder or granules. Hygroscopic after drying. Dissolves in cold water, giving a colloidal solution. Insoluble in hot water, in acetone, in alcohol, in ether, and in toluene.

Hyoscyamine: White, crystalline powder. Is affected by light. Its solutions are alkaline to litmus. Freely soluble in alcohol, in chloroform, and in dilute acids; sparingly soluble in ether; slightly soluble in water and in benzene.

Hyoscyamine Hydrobromide: White, odorless crystals or crystalline powder. The pH of a solution (1 in 20) is about 5.4. Is affected by light. Freely soluble in water, in alcohol, and in chloroform; very slightly soluble in ether.

Hyoscyamine Sulfate: White or almost white, crystalline powder or colorless needles. Is deliquescent and is affected by light. The pH of a solution (1 in 100) is about 5.3. Very soluble in water; freely soluble in alcohol; practically insoluble in ether. Melts at a temperature not less than 200°.

Hypophosphorous Acid: Colorless or slightly yellow, odorless liquid. Specific gravity is about 1.13. *NF category:* Antioxidant.

Hypromellose: White to slightly off-white, fibrous or granular powder. Swells in water and produces a clear to opalescent, viscous, colloidal mixture. Insoluble in dehydrated alcohol, in ether, and in chloroform. *NF category:* Coating agent; suspending and/or viscosity-increasing agent; wet binder; polymers for ophthalmic use; capsule shell; emulsifying agent; film-forming agent; release-modifying agent.

Hypromellose 2208: White to slightly off-white, fibrous or granular powder. Swells in water and produces a clear to opalescent, viscous, colloidal mixture. Insoluble in dehydrated alcohol, in ether, and in chloroform. *NF category:* Coating agent; suspending and/or viscosity-increasing agent; tablet binder.

Hypromellose 2906: White to slightly off-white, fibrous or granular powder. Swells in water and produces a clear to opalescent, viscous, colloidal mixture. Insoluble in dehydrated alcohol, in ether, and in chloroform. *NF category:* Coating agent; suspending and/or viscosity-increasing agent; tablet binder.

Hypromellose 2910: White to slightly off-white, fibrous or granular powder. Swells in water and produces a clear to opalescent, viscous, colloidal mixture. Insoluble in dehydrated alcohol, in ether, and in chloroform. *NF category:* Coating agent; suspending and/or viscosity-increasing agent; tablet binder.

Hypromellose Acetate Succinate: White to yellowish-white powder or pills. Odorless, or has a faint, acetic acid-like odor, and tasteless. Practically insoluble in water, in dehydrated alcohol, in xylene, and in hexane. On the addition of a mixture of dehydrated alcohol and dichloromethane (1:1) or acetone, a clear or turbid viscous liquid is produced. Dissolves in 1 N sodium hydroxide. Slightly hygroscopic. *NF category:* Coating agent; wet binder; film-forming agent.

Hypromellose Phthalate: White powder or granules. Is odorless and tasteless. Practically insoluble in water, in dehydrated alcohol, and in hexane. Produces a viscous solution in a mixture of methanol and dichloromethane (1:1), or in a mixture of dehydrated alcohol and acetone (1:1). Dissolves in 1 N sodium hydroxide. *NF category:* Coating agent; film-forming agent.

Ibuprofen: White to off-white, crystalline powder, having a slight, characteristic odor. Very soluble in alcohol, in methanol, in acetone, and in chloroform; slightly soluble in ethyl acetate; practically insoluble in water.

Ibutilide Fumarate: White to off-white powder. Freely soluble in water; sparingly soluble in methanol.

Ichthammol: Reddish-brown to brownish-black, viscous fluid, having a strong, characteristic, empyreumatic odor. Miscible with water, with glycerin, and with fixed oils and fats. Partially soluble in alcohol and in ether.

Idarubicin Hydrochloride: Red-orange to red-brown powder. Soluble in methanol; slightly soluble in water; insoluble in acetone and in ethyl ether.

Idoxuridine: White, crystalline, practically odorless powder. Slightly soluble in water and in alcohol; practically insoluble in chloroform and in ether.

Ifosfamide: White, crystalline powder. Melts at about 40°. Very soluble in alcohol, in ethyl acetate, in isopropyl alcohol, in methanol, and in methylene chloride; freely soluble in water; very slightly soluble in hexanes.

Imidurea: White, odorless, tasteless powder. Soluble in water and in glycerin; sparingly soluble in propylene glycol; insoluble in most organic solvents. *NF category:* Antimicrobial preservative.

Imipenem: White to tan-colored crystalline powder. Slightly soluble in water and in methanol.

Imipramine Hydrochloride: White to off-white, odorless or practically odorless, crystalline powder. Freely soluble in water and in alcohol; soluble in acetone; insoluble in ether and in benzene.

Imipramine Pamoate: Fine, yellow powder. Soluble in acetone, in chloroform, in carbon tetrachloride, in ethanol, and in ether; insoluble in water.

Imiquimod: White or almost white, powder or crystalline powder. Very slightly soluble in methanol; practically insoluble in water and in acetone.

Inamrinone: Pale yellow to tan powder. It is odorless or has a faint odor. Slightly soluble in methanol; practically insoluble or insoluble in chloroform and in water.

Indapamide: White to off-white, crystalline powder. Melts between 167° and 170°. Soluble in methanol, in alcohol, in acetonitrile, in glacial acetic acid, and in ethyl acetate; very slightly soluble in ether and in chloroform; practically insoluble in water.

Indigotindisulfonate Sodium: Dusky, purplish-blue powder, or blue granules having a coppery luster. Is affected by light. Its solutions have a blue or bluish purple color. Slightly soluble in water and in alcohol; practically insoluble in most other organic solvents.

Indinavir Sulfate: White or almost white, hygroscopic powder. Freely soluble in water; soluble in methanol; practically insoluble in heptane.

Indocyanine Green: Olive-brown, dark green, blue-green, dark blue, or black powder. Is odorless or has a slight odor. Its solutions are deep emerald-green in color. The pH of a solution (1 in 200) is about 6. Its aqueous solutions are stable for about 8 hours. Soluble in water and in methanol; practically insoluble in most other organic solvents.

Indomethacin: Pale yellow to yellow-tan, crystalline powder, having not more than a slight odor. Is sensitive to light. Melts at about 162°. Exhibits polymorphism. Sparingly soluble in alcohol, in chloroform, and in ether; practically insoluble in water.

Influenza Virus Vaccine: Slightly turbid liquid or suspension, which may have a slight yellow or reddish tinge and may have an odor because of the preservative.

Inositol: White or almost white, crystalline powder. Very soluble in water; practically insoluble in alcohol absolute and in ether. *NF category:* Humectant.

Insulin: White or practically white crystals. Soluble in solutions of dilute acids and alkalies.

Insulin Injection: The Injection containing, in each mL, not more than 100 USP Units is a clear, colorless or almost colorless liquid; the Injection containing, in each mL, 500 Units may be straw-colored. Contains between 0.1% and 0.25% (w/v) of either phenol or cresol. Contains between 1.4% and 1.8% (w/v) of glycerin.

Insulin Lispro: White or practically white crystals. Soluble in solutions of dilute acids and alkalies.

Isophane Insulin Suspension: White suspension of rod-shaped crystals, free from large aggregates of crystals following moderate agitation. Contains either (1) between 1.4% and 1.8% (w/v) of glycerin, between 0.15% and 0.17% (w/v) of metacresol, and between 0.06% and 0.07% (w/v) of phenol; or (2) between 1.4% and 1.8% (w/v) of glycerin and between 0.20% and 0.25% (w/v) of phenol. Contains between 0.15% and 0.25% (w/v) of dibasic sodium phosphate. When examined microscopically, the insoluble matter in the Suspension is crystalline, and contains not more than traces of amorphous material.

Insulin Zinc Suspension: Practically colorless suspension of a mixture of characteristic crystals predominantly between 10 and 40 μm in maximum dimension and many particles that have no uniform shape and do not exceed 2 μm in maximum dimension. Contains between 0.15% and 0.17% (w/v) of sodium acetate, between 0.65% and 0.75% (w/v) of sodium chloride, and between 0.09% and 0.11% (w/v) of methylparaben.

Extended Insulin Zinc Suspension: Practically colorless suspension of a mixture of characteristic crystals the maximum dimension of which is predominantly between 10 and 40 μm. Contains between 0.15% and 0.17% (w/v) of sodium acetate, between 0.65% and 0.75% (w/v) of sodium chloride, and between 0.09% and 0.11% (w/v) of methylparaben.

Prompt Insulin Zinc Suspension: Practically colorless suspension of particles that have no uniform shape and the maximum dimension of which does not exceed 2 μm. Contains between 0.15% and 0.17% (w/v) of sodium acetate, between 0.65% and 0.75% (w/v) of sodium chloride, and between 0.09% and 0.11% (w/v) of methylparaben.

Inulin: White, friable, chalk-like, amorphous, odorless, tasteless powder. Soluble in hot water; slightly soluble in cold water and in organic solvents. *NF category:* Sweetening agent; wet binder.

Invert Sugar: Colorless to pale yellow liquid. Miscible with water, with glycerin, and with glycols. *NF category:* Sweetening agent; diluent; wet binder.

Iodine: Heavy, grayish-black plates or granules, having a metallic luster and a characteristic odor. Freely soluble in carbon disulfide, in chloroform, in carbon tetrachloride, and in ether; soluble in alcohol and in solutions of iodides; sparingly soluble in glycerin; very slightly soluble in water.

Iodine Topical Solution: Transparent, reddish-brown liquid, having the odor of iodine.

Strong Iodine Solution: Transparent liquid having a deep brown color and having the odor of iodine.

Iodine Tincture: Transparent liquid having a reddish-brown color and the odor of iodine and of alcohol.

Sodium Iodide I 123 Capsules: Capsules may contain a small amount of solid or solids, or may appear empty.

Sodium Iodide I 123 Solution: Clear, colorless solution. Upon standing, both the Solution and the glass container may darken as a result of the effects of the radiation.

Iodinated I 125 Albumin Injection: Clear, colorless to slightly yellow solution. Upon standing, both the Albumin and the glass container may darken as a result of the effects of the radiation.

Iodinated I 131 Albumin Injection: Clear, colorless to slightly yellow solution. Upon standing, both the Albumin and the glass container may darken as a result of the effects of the radiation.

Iodinated I 131 Albumin Aggregated Injection: Dilute suspension of white to faintly yellow particles, which may settle on standing. The glass container may darken on standing, as a result of the effects of the radiation.

Sodium Rose Bengal I 131 Injection: Clear, deep-red solution.

Iodohippurate Sodium I 131 Injection: Clear, colorless solution. Upon standing, both the Injection and the glass container may darken as a result of the effects of the radiation.

Sodium Iodide I 131 Capsules: May contain a small amount of solid or solids, or may appear empty.

Sodium Iodide I 131 Solution: Clear, colorless solution. Upon standing, both the Solution and the glass container may darken as a result of the effects of the radiation.

Iodipamide: White, practically odorless, crystalline powder. Slightly soluble in alcohol; very slightly soluble in water, in chloroform, and in ether.

Iodipamide Meglumine Injection: Clear, colorless to pale yellow, slightly viscous liquid.

Iodixanol: White to off-white, amorphous, odorless, hygroscopic powder. Freely soluble in water.

Iodoform: Lustrous greenish yellow powder, or lustrous crystals. It is slightly volatile even at ordinary temperatures, and distills slowly with steam. Freely soluble in ether and in chloroform; soluble in boiling alcohol; sparingly soluble in alcohol, in glycerin, and in olive oil; practically insoluble in water. Melts to a brown liquid at about 115°, and decomposes at a higher temperature, emitting vapors of iodine.

Iodoquinol: Light yellowish to tan, microcrystalline powder not readily wetted by water. Is odorless or has a faint odor; is stable in air. Melts with decomposition. Sparingly soluble in alcohol and in ether; practically insoluble in water.

Iohexol: White to off-white, hygroscopic, odorless powder. Very soluble in water and in methanol; practically insoluble or insoluble in ether and in chloroform.

Iohexol Injection: Clear, colorless to pale yellow liquid.

Iopamidol: Practically odorless, white to off-white powder. Very soluble in water; sparingly soluble in methanol; practically insoluble in alcohol and in chloroform.

Iopanoic Acid: Cream-colored powder. Is tasteless or practically so, and has a faint, characteristic odor. Is affected by light. Soluble in alcohol, in chloroform, and in ether, and in solutions of alkali hydroxides and carbonates; insoluble in water.

Iophendylate: Colorless to pale yellow, viscous liquid, the color darkening on long exposure to air. Is odorless or has a faintly ethereal odor. Freely soluble in alcohol, in benzene, in chloroform, and in ether; very slightly soluble in water.

Iophendylate Injection: Colorless to pale yellow, viscous liquid, the color darkening on long exposure to air. Is odorless or has a faintly ethereal odor. Freely soluble in alcohol, in benzene, in chloroform, and in ether; very slightly soluble in water.

Iopromide: White to slightly yellow powder. Freely soluble in water and in dimethyl sulfoxide; practically insoluble in alcohol, in acetone, and in ether.

Iothalamate Meglumine Injection: Clear, colorless to pale yellow, slightly viscous liquid.

Iothalamate Meglumine and Iothalamate Sodium Injection: Clear, colorless to pale yellow, slightly viscous liquid.

Iothalamate Sodium Injection: Clear, colorless to pale yellow, slightly viscous liquid.

Iothalamic Acid: White, odorless powder. Soluble in solutions of alkali hydroxides; slightly soluble in water and in alcohol.

Ioxilan: White to off-white, practically odorless powder. Soluble in water and in methanol.

Ioxilan Injection: Clear, colorless to pale yellow liquid.

Powdered Ipecac: Pale brown, weak yellow, or light olive-gray powder.

Ipodate Sodium: White to off-white, odorless, fine, crystalline powder. Freely soluble in water, in alcohol, and in methanol; very slightly soluble in chloroform.

Ipratropium Bromide: White to off-white, crystalline powder. Freely soluble in methanol; soluble in water; slightly soluble in alcohol.

Irbesartan: White to off-white, crystalline powder. Slightly soluble in alcohol and in methylene chloride; practically insoluble in water.

Irinotecan Hydrochloride: Pale yellow to yellow crystalline powder. Slightly soluble in water and in organic solvents.

Iron Dextran Injection: Dark brown, slightly viscous liquid.

Iron Sorbitex Injection: Clear liquid, having a dark brown color.

Isobutane: Colorless, flammable gas (boiling temperature is about −11°). Vapor pressure at 21° is about 2950 mm of mercury (31 psig). *NF category:* Propellant.

Isobutyl Alcohol: Clear, colorless, mobile liquid. Soluble in water. Miscible with alcohol, with ether, and with many other organic solvents. *NF category:* Flavors and fragrance; solvent.

Isoetharine Inhalation Solution: Colorless or slightly yellow, slightly acid liquid, gradually turning dark on exposure to air and light.

Isoetharine Hydrochloride: White to off-white, odorless, crystalline solid. Melts between 196° and 208°, with decomposition. Soluble in water; sparingly soluble in alcohol; practically insoluble in ether.

Isoetharine Mesylate: White or practically white, odorless crystals having a salty, bitter taste. Freely soluble in water; soluble in alcohol; practically insoluble in acetone and in ether.

Isoflurane: Clear, colorless, volatile liquid, having a slight odor. Boils at about 49°. Insoluble in water. Miscible with common organic solvents and with fats and oils.

Isoleucine: White, practically odorless crystals, having a slightly bitter taste. Soluble in water; slightly soluble in hot alcohol; insoluble in ether.

Isometheptene Mucate: White, crystalline powder. Freely soluble in water; soluble in alcohol; practically insoluble in chloroform and in ether.

Isoniazid: Colorless or white crystals or white, crystalline powder. Is odorless and is slowly affected by exposure to air and light. Freely soluble in water; sparingly soluble in alcohol; slightly soluble in chloroform; very slightly soluble in ether.

Isoniazid Injection: Clear, colorless to faintly greenish-yellow liquid. Gradually darkens on exposure to air and light. Tends to crystallize at low temperatures.

Isopropamide Iodide: White to pale yellow, crystalline powder, having a bitter taste. Freely soluble in chloroform and in alcohol; sparingly soluble in water; very slightly soluble in benzene and in ether.

Isopropyl Alcohol: Transparent, colorless, mobile, volatile liquid, having a characteristic odor and a slightly bitter taste. Is flammable. Miscible with water, with alcohol, with ether, and with chloroform. *NF category:* Solvent.

Azeotropic Isopropyl Alcohol: Transparent, colorless, mobile, volatile liquid, having a characteristic odor and a slightly bitter taste. Is flammable. Miscible with water, with alcohol, with ether, and with chloroform.

Add the following:

■**Isopropyl Isostearate:** Clear, colorless to pale-yellow liquid. Miscible with alcohol and with fatty oils. Insoluble in water. *NF category:* Emollient; emulsifying agent.■₁ₛ *(NF36)*

Isopropyl Myristate: Clear, practically colorless, oily liquid. Is practically odorless, and congeals at about 5°. Freely soluble in 90% alcohol; insoluble in water, in glycerin, and in propylene glycol. Miscible with most organic solvents and with fixed oils. *NF category:* Vehicle (oleaginous); emollient; solvent.

Isopropyl Palmitate: Colorless, mobile liquid having a very slight odor. Soluble in acetone, in castor oil, in chloroform, in cottonseed oil, in ethyl acetate, in alcohol, and in mineral oil; insoluble in water, in glycerin, and in propylene glycol. *NF category:* Vehicle (oleaginous); emollient; solvent.

Isoproterenol Inhalation Solution: Colorless or practically colorless, slightly acid liquid, gradually turning dark on exposure to air and light.

Isoproterenol Hydrochloride: White to practically white, odorless, crystalline powder, having a slightly bitter taste. Gradually darkens on exposure to air and light. Its solutions become pink to brownish pink on standing exposed to air, doing so almost immediately when rendered alkaline. Its solution (1 in 100) has a pH of about 5. Freely soluble in water; sparingly soluble in alcohol and less soluble in dehydrated alcohol; insoluble in chloroform and in ether.

Isoproterenol Hydrochloride Injection: Colorless or practically colorless liquid, gradually turning dark on exposure to air and light.

Isoproterenol Sulfate: White to practically white, odorless, crystalline powder. It gradually darkens on exposure to air and light. Its solutions become pink to brownish pink on standing exposed to air, doing so almost immediately when rendered alkaline. A solution (1 in 100) has a pH of about 5. Freely soluble in water; very slightly soluble in alcohol, in benzene, and in ether.

Isosorbide Concentrate: Colorless to slightly yellow liquid. Soluble in water and in alcohol.

Diluted Isosorbide Dinitrate: Ivory-white, odorless powder. [NOTE—Undiluted isosorbide dinitrate occurs as white, crystalline rosettes.] Undiluted isosorbide dinitrate is very soluble in acetone; freely soluble in chloroform; sparingly soluble in alcohol; very slightly soluble in water.

Add the following:

■**Isostearyl Isostearate:** Colorless to slightly yellow, oily liquid. *Specific Gravity* ⟨841⟩: 0.840–0.880 at 20°. Soluble in methylene chloride and in mineral oil; insoluble in water and in alcohol. *NF category:* Emollient; emulsifying agent.
■₁ₛ *(NF36)*

Isotretinoin: Yellow crystals. Soluble in chloroform; sparingly soluble in alcohol, in isopropyl alcohol, and in polyethylene glycol 400; practically insoluble in water.

Isoxsuprine Hydrochloride: White, odorless, crystalline powder, having a bitter taste. Melts at about 200°, with decomposition. Sparingly soluble in alcohol; slightly soluble in water.

Isradipine: Yellow, fine crystalline powder.

Itraconazole: A white or almost white powder. Freely soluble in methylene chloride; sparingly soluble in tetrahydrofuran; very slightly soluble in alcohol; practically insoluble in water.

Ivermectin: White to yellowish-white, crystalline powder. Slightly hygroscopic. Freely soluble in methanol and in methylene chloride; soluble in acetone and in acetonitrile; practically insoluble in hexane and in water.

Ixabepilone: White or almost white powder. Slightly soluble in acetonitrile.

Juniper Tar: Dark brown, clear, thick liquid, having a tarry odor and a faintly aromatic, bitter taste. Sparingly soluble in solvent hexane; very slightly soluble in water. One volume dissolves in 9 volumes of alcohol. Dissolves in 3 volumes of ether, leaving only a slight, flocculent residue. Miscible with amyl alcohol, with chloroform, and with glacial acetic acid.

Kanamycin Sulfate: White, odorless, crystalline powder. Freely soluble in water; insoluble in acetone, in ethyl acetate, and in benzene.

Kaolin: Soft, white or yellowish-white powder or lumps. Has an earthy or clay-like taste and, when moistened with water, assumes a darker color and develops a marked clay-like odor. Insoluble in water, in cold dilute acids, and in solutions of alkali hydroxides. *NF category:* Diluent; suspending and/or viscosity-increasing agent.

Ketamine Hydrochloride: White, crystalline powder, having a slight, characteristic odor. Freely soluble in water and in methanol; soluble in alcohol; sparingly soluble in chloroform.

Ketorolac Tromethamine: White to off-white, crystalline powder. Melts between 165° and 170°, with decomposition. Freely soluble in water and in methanol; slightly soluble in alcohol, in dehydrated alcohol, and in tetrahydrofuran; practically insoluble in acetone, in dichloromethane, in toluene, in ethyl acetate, in dioxane, in hexane, in butyl alcohol, and in acetonitrile.

Labetalol Hydrochloride: White to off-white powder. Melts at about 180°, with decomposition. Soluble in water and in alcohol; insoluble in ether and in chloroform.

Alpha-Lactalbumin: Free-flowing, slightly hygroscopic light cream-colored powder. Freely soluble in water; soluble in wide pH ranges; insoluble in methanol, in alcohol, in ether, and in acetone. *NF category:* Bulking agent; coating agent; emulsifying agent; stiffening agent; suspending and/or viscosity-increasing agent; diluent; wet binder; vehicle (solid carrier); pH modifier (acidifying agent/alkalizing agent/buffering agent); chelating and/or complexing agent.

Lactic Acid: Colorless or yellowish, practically odorless, syrupy liquid. Is hygroscopic. When it is concentrated by boiling, lactic acid lactate is formed. Specific gravity is about 1.20. Insoluble in chloroform. Miscible with water, with alcohol, and with ether. *NF category:* pH modifier (acidifying agent/alkalizing agent/buffering agent).

Lactitol: A white or light brown, odorless crystal. Has a mild, sweet taste, and no aftertaste. *NF category:* Flavors and fragrance; diluent; sweetening agent.

Lactobionic Acid: White or almost white, crystalline powder with a melting point of about 125° with decomposition. Freely soluble in water; slightly soluble in glacial acetic acid, in anhydrous ethanol, and in methanol. *NF category:* Antioxidant.

Anhydrous Lactose: White or almost white powder. Freely soluble in water; practically insoluble in alcohol. *NF category:* Diluent; carrier.

Lactose Monohydrate: White, free-flowing powder. Freely but slowly soluble in water; practically insoluble in alcohol. *NF category:* Diluent; carrier; wet binder.

Lactulose Concentrate: Colorless to amber syrupy liquid, which may exhibit some precipitation and darkening upon standing. Miscible with water.

Lamivudine: White to off-white solid. Soluble in water. Melts at about 176°.

Lamotrigine: A white to pale cream-colored powder. Slightly soluble in 0.1 N hydrochloric acid, in acetone, in methanol, and in water.

Lanolin: Yellow, tenacious, unctuous mass, having a slight, characteristic odor. Freely soluble in ether and in chloroform; soluble in hot alcohol; sparingly soluble in cold alcohol; insoluble in water, but mixes without separation with about twice its weight of water. *NF category:* Emulsifying agent; ointment base.

Hydrogenated Lanolin: White or pale yellow, unctuous substance. Soluble in boiling dehydrated alcohol and in light petroleum; insoluble in water. *NF category:* Emulsifying agent; emollient; humectant; ointment base.

Lanolin Alcohols: Hard, waxy, amber solid, having a characteristic odor. Freely soluble in chloroform, in ether, and in petroleum ether; slightly soluble in alcohol; insoluble in water. *NF category:* Emulsifying agent; ointment base.

Lansoprazole: White to brownish-white powder. Freely soluble in dimethylformamide; practically insoluble in water. Melts at about 166°, with decomposition.

Latanoprost: Colorless to slightly yellow oil. Very soluble in acetonitrile; freely soluble in acetone, in ethanol, in ethyl acetate, in isopropanol, in methanol, and in octanol; practically insoluble in water.

Lauric Acid: White or faintly yellow, somewhat glossy, crystalline solid or powder. Very soluble in alcohol, in ether, and in methanol; soluble in acetone; practically insoluble in water. *NF category:* Antifoaming agent; emulsifying agent; lubricant.

Lauroyl Polyoxylglycerides: Pale yellow semi-solids. Freely soluble in methylene chloride. Dispersible in hot water. *NF category:* Ointment base; solvent; emulsifying agent; wetting and/or solubilizing agent.

Lecithin: The consistency of both natural grades and refined grades of lecithin may vary from plastic to fluid, depending upon free fatty acid and oil content, and upon the presence or absence of other diluents. Its color varies from light yellow to brown, depending on the source, on crop variations, and on whether it is bleached or unbleached. It is odorless or has a characteristic, slight nut-like odor and a bland taste. Practically insoluble in water, but it readily hydrates to form emulsions. The oil-free phosphatides are soluble in fatty acids, but are practically insoluble in fixed oils. When all phosphatide fractions are present, lecithin is sparingly soluble in alcohol and practically insoluble in acetone. *NF category:* Emulsifying agent; emollient.

Leflunomide: White to almost white powder. Freely soluble in methanol, in alcohol, in 2-propanol, in ethyl acetate, in acetone, and in acetonitrile; practically insoluble in water.

Letrozole: White to yellowish, crystalline powder. Freely soluble in dichloromethane; slightly soluble in alcohol; practically insoluble in water.

Leucine: White, practically odorless, tasteless crystals. Sparingly soluble in water; insoluble in ether. *NF category:* Flavors and fragrance.

Leucovorin Calcium: Yellowish-white or yellow powder. Slightly soluble to freely soluble in water; practically insoluble in alcohol.

Leucovorin Calcium Injection: Clear, yellowish solution.

Levamisole Hydrochloride: White or almost white, crystalline powder. Freely soluble in water; soluble in alcohol; slightly soluble in methylene chloride; practically insoluble in ether.

Levetiracetam: White to almost white powder. Very soluble in water; soluble in acetonitrile; practically insoluble in hexane.

Levmetamfetamine: Clear, practically colorless liquid.

Levobunolol Hydrochloride: White crystalline, odorless powder. Soluble in water and in methanol; slightly soluble in alcohol and in chloroform.

Levocarnitine: White crystals or crystalline powder. Hygroscopic. Freely soluble in water, and in hot alcohol; practically insoluble in acetone, in ether, and in benzene.

Levocetirizine Dihydrochloride: White to almost white powder. Freely soluble in water and in methanol.

Levodopa: White to off-white, odorless, crystalline powder. In the presence of moisture, is rapidly oxidized by atmospheric oxygen and darkens. Freely soluble in 3 N hydrochloric acid; slightly soluble in water; insoluble in alcohol.

Levofloxacin: Light yellowish-white to yellow-white crystals or crystalline powder. Soluble in dimethylsulfoxide and in acetic acid; sparingly soluble in water, in acetone, and in methanol; practically insoluble in glycerin and in *n*-octanol.

Levonordefrin: White to buff-colored, odorless, crystalline solid. Melts at about 210°. Freely soluble in aqueous solutions of mineral acids; slightly soluble in acetone, in chloroform, in alcohol, and in ether; practically insoluble in water.

Levonorgestrel: White or practically white, odorless powder. Soluble in chloroform; slightly soluble in alcohol; practically insoluble in water.

Levorphanol Tartrate: Practically white, odorless, crystalline powder. Sparingly soluble in water; slightly soluble in alcohol; insoluble in chloroform and in ether. Melts, in a sealed tube, at about 110°, with decomposition.

Levothyroxine Sodium: Light yellow to buff-colored, odorless, tasteless, hygroscopic powder. Is stable in dry air but may assume a slight pink color upon exposure to light. The pH of a saturated solution is about 8.9. Soluble in solutions of alkali hydroxides and in hot solutions of alkali carbonates; slightly soluble in alcohol; very slightly soluble in water; insoluble in acetone, in chloroform, and in ether.

Lidocaine: White or slightly yellow, crystalline powder. Has a characteristic odor and is stable in air. Very soluble in alcohol and in chloroform; freely soluble in benzene and in ether; practically insoluble in water. Dissolves in oils.

Lidocaine Hydrochloride: White, odorless, crystalline powder, having a slightly bitter taste. Very soluble in water and in alcohol; soluble in chloroform; insoluble in ether.

Lime: Hard, white or grayish-white masses or granules, or white or grayish white powder. Is odorless. Slightly soluble in water; very slightly soluble in boiling water.

Lincomycin Hydrochloride: White or practically white, crystalline powder. Is odorless or has a faint odor. Is stable in the presence of air and light. Its solutions are acid and dextrorotatory. Freely soluble in water; soluble in dimethylformamide; very slightly soluble in acetone.

Lincomycin Hydrochloride Injection: Clear, colorless to slightly yellow solution, having a slight odor.

Lincomycin Hydrochloride Soluble Powder: White to off-white, or light tan free-flowing, fine powder.

Lindane: White, crystalline powder, having a slight, musty odor. Freely soluble in chloroform; soluble in dehydrated alcohol; sparingly soluble in ether; slightly soluble in ethylene glycol; practically insoluble in water.

Linezolid: White to off-white or cream-colored, crystalline powder. Sparingly soluble in acetone, in ethanol, and in methanol; very slightly soluble in water.

Linoleoyl Polyoxylglycerides: Amber, oily liquids. May develop deposit after prolonged storage periods at 20°. Freely soluble in methylene chloride; practically insoluble but dispersible in water. *NF category:* Ointment base; solvent; emulsifying agent; wetting and/or solubilizing agent.

Liothyronine Sodium: Light tan, odorless, crystalline powder. Slightly soluble in alcohol; very slightly soluble in water; practically insoluble in most other organic solvents.

Lisinopril: White, crystalline powder. Melts at about 160°, with decomposition. Soluble in water; sparingly soluble in methanol; practically insoluble in alcohol, in acetone, in acetonitrile, and in chloroform.

Lithium Carbonate: White, granular, odorless powder. Sparingly soluble in water; very slightly soluble in alcohol. Dissolves, with effervescence, in dilute mineral acids.

Lithium Citrate: White, odorless, deliquescent powder or granules, having a cooling, faintly alkaline taste. Freely soluble in water; slightly soluble in alcohol.

Lomustine: Yellow crystalline powder. Freely soluble in acetone, and in methylene chloride; soluble in ethanol; practically insoluble in water.

Loperamide Hydrochloride: White to slightly yellow powder. Melts at about 225°, with some decomposition. Freely soluble in methanol and in chloroform; slightly soluble in water and in dilute acids; very slightly soluble in isopropyl alcohol.

Lopinavir: White powder. Freely soluble in methanol and alcohol; soluble in isopropanol; practically insoluble in water.

Loratadine: White to off-white powder. Freely soluble in acetone, in chloroform, in methanol, and in toluene; insoluble in water.

Lorazepam: White or practically white, practically odorless powder. Sparingly soluble in alcohol; slightly soluble in chloroform; insoluble in water.

Losartan Potassium: White to off-white powder. Freely soluble in water; sparingly soluble in isopropyl alcohol; slightly soluble in acetonitrile.

Lovastatin: White to off-white, crystalline powder. Freely soluble in chloroform; soluble in acetone, in acetonitrile, and in methanol; sparingly soluble in alcohol; practically insoluble in hexane; insoluble in water.

Loxapine Succinate: White to yellowish, crystalline powder. Is odorless.

Lufenuron: White or pale yellow powder. Freely soluble in acetonitrile; soluble in dehydrated alcohol; practically insoluble in water.

Lumefantrine: Yellow crystalline powder. Freely soluble in *N,N*-dimethylformamide, in chloroform, and in ethyl acetate; soluble in dichloromethane; slightly soluble in ethanol and in methanol; practically insoluble in water.

Lutein: Red, crystalline powder. Soluble in ethanol, in ethyl acetate, and in methylene chloride; partially soluble in hexane.

Lysine Acetate: White, odorless crystals or crystalline powder, having an acid taste. Freely soluble in water.

Lysine Hydrochloride: White, odorless powder. Freely soluble in water. *NF category:* pH modifier (acidifying agent/alkalizing agent/buffering agent).

Mafenide Acetate: White to pale yellow, crystalline powder. Freely soluble in water.

Magaldrate: White, odorless, crystalline powder. Soluble in dilute solutions of mineral acids; insoluble in water and in alcohol.

Milk of Magnesia: White, opaque, more or less viscous suspension from which varying proportions of water usually separate on standing. pH is about 10.

Magnesium Aluminometasilicate: White powder or granules with an amorphous structure. Very slightly soluble in acids; practically insoluble or insoluble in water, in alcohol, and in alkalies.

Magnesium Aluminosilicate: White powder or granules with an amorphous structure. Very slightly soluble in acids; practically insoluble or insoluble in water, in alcohol, and in alkalies.

Magnesium Aluminum Silicate: Odorless, tasteless, fine (micronized) powder, small cream to tan granules, or small flakes that are creamy when viewed on their flat surfaces and tan to brown when viewed on their edges. Insoluble in water and in alcohol. Swells when added to water or glycerin. *NF category:* Suspending and/or viscosity-increasing agent; disintegrant.

Magnesium Carbonate: Light, white, friable masses or bulky, white powder. Is odorless, and is stable in air. Practically insoluble in water to which, however, it imparts a slightly alkaline reaction; insoluble in alcohol, but is dissolved by dilute acids with effervescence. *NF category:* Diluent.

Magnesium Chloride: Colorless, odorless, deliquescent flakes or crystals, which lose water when heated to 100° and lose hydrochloric acid when heated to 110°. Very soluble in water; freely soluble in alcohol.

Magnesium Citrate Oral Solution: Colorless to slightly yellow, clear, effervescent liquid, having a sweet, acidulous taste and a lemon flavor.

Magnesium Gluconate: Colorless crystals or white powder or granules. Is odorless and tasteless. Freely soluble in water; very slightly soluble in alcohol; insoluble in ether.

Magnesium Hydroxide: Bulky, white powder. Soluble in dilute acids; practically insoluble in water and in alcohol.

Magnesium Oxide: Very bulky, white powder or relatively dense, white powder or granulated powder. Soluble in dilute acids; practically insoluble in water; insoluble in alcohol. *NF category:* Emulsifying agent; glidant and/or anticaking agent; diluent.

Magnesium Phosphate: White, odorless, tasteless powder. Soluble in diluted mineral acids; practically insoluble in water.

Magnesium Salicylate: White, odorless, efflorescent, crystalline powder. Freely soluble in methanol; soluble in alcohol and in water; slightly soluble in ether.

Magnesium Silicate: Fine, white, odorless, tasteless powder, free from grittiness. Insoluble in water and in alcohol. Is readily decomposed by mineral acids. *NF category:* Glidant and/or anticaking agent.

Magnesium Stearate: Very fine, light, white powder, slippery to touch. Insoluble in water, in alcohol, and in ether. *NF category:* Lubricant.

Magnesium Sulfate: Small, colorless crystals, usually needle-like, with a cooling, saline, bitter taste. It effloresces in warm, dry air. Very soluble in boiling water; freely soluble in water; freely (and slowly) soluble in glycerin; sparingly soluble in alcohol.

Magnesium Trisilicate: Fine, white, odorless, tasteless powder, free from grittiness. Insoluble in water and in alcohol. Is readily decomposed by mineral acids. *NF category:* Glidant and/or anticaking agent.

Malathion: Clear, colorless, or slightly yellowish liquid, having a characteristic odor. Congeals at about 2.9°. Slightly soluble in water. Miscible with alcohols, with esters, with ketones, with ethers, with aromatic and alkylated aromatic hydrocarbons, and with vegetable oils.

Maleic Acid: White, crystalline powder. Freely soluble in water and in alcohol; sparingly soluble in ether. *NF category:* pH modifier (acidifying agent/alkalizing agent/buffering agent).

Malic Acid: White or practically white, crystalline powder or granules, having a strongly acid taste. Melts at about 130°. Very soluble in water; freely soluble in alcohol. *NF category:* pH modifier (acidifying agent/alkalizing agent/buffering agent); flavors and fragrance; antioxidant, chelating and/or complexing agent.

Maltitol: White, crystalline powder. Very soluble in water; practically insoluble in ethanol. *NF category:* Humectant; sweetening agent; diluent; coating agent.

Maltodextrin: White, hygroscopic powder or granules. Freely soluble or readily dispersible in water; slightly soluble to insoluble in anhydrous alcohol. *NF category:* Coating agent; suspending and/or viscosity-increasing agent; diluent; wet binder.

Maltol: A white, crystalline powder having a characteristic caramel-butterscotch odor, suggestive of a fruity-strawberry aroma in dilute solution. One g dissolves in about 82 mL of water, in 21 mL of alcohol, in 80 mL of glycerin, and in 28 mL of propylene glycol. *NF category:* Flavors and fragrance.

Maltose: Maltose occurs in either the anhydrous state or as a monohydrate. It is a white, crystalline powder, odorless, and has a sweet taste. Very slightly soluble in ethanol; freely soluble in water; slightly soluble in methanol; practically insoluble in ether. *NF category:* Sweetening agent; diluent; disintegrant; wet binder.

Mandelic Acid: White to light yellow powder or crystalline solid. Soluble in alcohol, in isopropyl alcohol; sparingly soluble in water. *NF category:* Antimicrobial preservative.

Mangafodipir Trisodium: Pale yellow crystals or crystalline powder. Freely soluble in water; sparingly soluble in methanol; slightly soluble in chloroform; very slightly soluble in alcohol and in acetone.

Manganese Chloride: Large, irregular, pink, odorless, translucent crystals. Soluble in water and in alcohol; insoluble in ether.

Manganese Chloride for Oral Solution: Off-white to tan-colored powder with a strawberry odor. Soluble in water.

Manganese Sulfate: Pale red, slightly efflorescent crystals, or purple, odorless powder. Soluble in water; insoluble in alcohol.

Mannitol: White, crystalline powder or free-flowing granules. Is odorless and has a sweet taste. Freely soluble in water; soluble in alkaline solutions; slightly soluble in pyridine; very slightly soluble in alcohol; practically insoluble in ether. *NF category:* Sweetening agent; tonicity agent; bulking agent; diluent; plasticizer.

Maprotiline Hydrochloride: Fine, white to off-white, crystalline powder. Is practically odorless. Freely soluble in methanol and in chloroform; slightly soluble in water; practically insoluble in isooctane.

Mazindol: White to off-white, crystalline powder, having not more than a faint odor. Slightly soluble in methanol and in chloroform; insoluble in water.

Mebendazole: White to slightly yellow powder. Is almost odorless. Melts at about 290°. Freely soluble in formic acid; practically insoluble in water, in dilute solutions of mineral acids, in alcohol, in ether, and in chloroform.

Mechlorethamine Hydrochloride: White, crystalline powder. Is hygroscopic.

Meclizine Hydrochloride: White or slightly yellowish, crystalline powder. Has a slight odor and is tasteless. Slightly soluble in dilute acids and in alcohol; practically insoluble in water and in ether; freely soluble in chloroform, in pyridine, and in acid-alcohol-water mixtures.

Meclofenamate Sodium: A white to creamy white, odorless to almost odorless, crystalline powder. Freely soluble in water, the solution sometimes being somewhat turbid due to partial hydrolysis and absorption of carbon dioxide; soluble in methanol; slightly soluble in chloroform; practically insoluble in ether. The solution is clear above pH 11.5.

Medroxyprogesterone Acetate: White to off-white, odorless, crystalline powder. Melts at about 205°. Is stable in air. Freely soluble in chloroform; soluble in acetone and in dioxane; sparingly soluble in alcohol and in methanol; slightly soluble in ether; insoluble in water.

Mefenamic Acid: White to off-white, crystalline powder. Melts at about 230°, with decomposition. Soluble in solutions of alkali hydroxides; sparingly soluble in chloroform; slightly soluble in alcohol and in methanol; practically insoluble in water.

Mefloquine Hydrochloride: White or slightly yellow, crystalline powder. It exhibits polymorphism. Freely soluble in methanol; soluble in alcohol; very slightly soluble in water.

Megestrol Acetate: White to creamy white, tasteless and essentially odorless, crystalline powder. Very soluble in chloroform; soluble in acetone; sparingly soluble in alcohol; slightly soluble in ether and in fixed oils; insoluble in water. Is unstable under aqueous conditions at pH 7 or above.

Meglumine: White to faintly yellowish-white, odorless crystals or powder. Freely soluble in water; sparingly soluble in alcohol.

Melengestrol Acetate: White to light yellow, crystalline powder. Freely soluble in chloroform and in ethyl acetate; slightly soluble in alcohol; insoluble in water.

Meloxicam: Pale yellow powder. Soluble in dimethylformamide; slightly soluble in acetone; very slightly soluble in methanol and in alcohol; practically insoluble in water.

Melphalan: Off-white to buff powder, having a faint odor. Melts at about 180°, with decomposition. Soluble in dilute mineral acids; slightly soluble in alcohol and in methanol; practically insoluble in water, in chloroform, and in ether.

Memantine Hydrochloride: White to off-white, colored powder. Slightly soluble in water.

Menadiol Sodium Diphosphate: White to pink powder, having a characteristic odor. Is hygroscopic. Its solutions are neutral or slightly alkaline to litmus, having a pH of about 8. Very soluble in water; insoluble in alcohol.

Menadione: Bright yellow, crystalline, practically odorless powder. Is affected by sunlight. Soluble in vegetable oils; sparingly soluble in chloroform and in alcohol; practically insoluble in water.

Menthol: Colorless, hexagonal crystals, usually needle-like, or in fused masses, or crystalline powder. Has a pleasant, peppermint-like odor. Very soluble in alcohol, in chloroform, in ether, and in solvent hexane; freely soluble in glacial acetic acid, in mineral oil, and in fixed and volatile oils; slightly soluble in water. *NF category:* Flavors and fragrance.

Meperidine Hydrochloride: Fine, white, crystalline, odorless powder. The pH of a solution (1 in 20) is about 5. Very soluble in water; soluble in alcohol; sparingly soluble in ether.

Mephobarbital: White, odorless, crystalline powder, having a bitter taste. Its saturated solution is acid to litmus. Soluble in chloroform and in solutions of fixed alkali hydroxides and carbonates; slightly soluble in water, in alcohol, and in ether.

Mepivacaine Hydrochloride: White, odorless, crystalline solid. The pH of a solution (1 in 50) is about 4.5. Freely soluble in water and in methanol; very slightly soluble in chloroform; practically insoluble in ether.

Meprobamate: White powder, having a characteristic odor and a bitter taste. Freely soluble in acetone and in alcohol; slightly soluble in water; practically insoluble or insoluble in ether.

Mercaptopurine: Yellow, odorless or practically odorless, crystalline powder. Melts at a temperature exceeding 308°, with decomposition. Soluble in hot alcohol and in dilute alkali solutions; slightly soluble in 2 N sulfuric acid; insoluble in water, in acetone, and in ether.

Ammoniated Mercury: White, pulverulent pieces or white, amorphous powder. Is odorless, and is stable in air, but darkens on exposure to light. Readily soluble in warm hydrochloric, nitric, and acetic acids; insoluble in water, and in alcohol.

Meropenem: Colorless to white or light yellow crystals or crystalline powder. Soluble in dimethylformamide and in 5% dibasic potassium phosphate solution; sparingly soluble in water and in 5% monobasic potassium phosphate solution; practically insoluble in alcohol, in acetone, in methylene chloride, and in ether.

Mesalamine: Light tan to pink colored, needle-shaped crystals. Color may darken on exposure to air. Is odorless or may have a slight characteristic odor. Soluble in dilute hydrochloric acid and in dilute alkali hydroxides; slightly soluble in water; very slightly soluble in methanol, in dehydrated alcohol, and in acetone; practically insoluble in n-butyl alcohol, in chloroform, in ether, in ethyl acetate, in n-hexane, in methylene chloride, and in n-propyl alcohol.

Mesna: White or slightly yellow crystalline powder; hygroscopic. Freely soluble in water; slightly soluble in alcohol; practically insoluble in cyclohexane.

Mesoridazine Besylate: White to pale yellowish powder, having not more than a faint odor. Melts at about 178°, with decomposition. Freely soluble in water, in chloroform, and in methanol.

Mestranol: White to creamy white, odorless, crystalline powder. Freely soluble in chloroform; soluble in dioxane; sparingly soluble in dehydrated alcohol; slightly soluble in methanol; insoluble in water.

Metaproterenol Sulfate: White to off-white, crystalline powder. Freely soluble in water.

Metaxalone: White to almost-white, crystalline powder. Freely soluble in chloroform; soluble in methanol and in alcohol; practically insoluble in ether and in water.

Metformin Hydrochloride: White, crystalline powder. Freely soluble in water; slightly soluble in alcohol; practically insoluble in acetone and in methylene chloride.

Methacholine Chloride: Colorless or white crystals, or white, crystalline powder. Is odorless or has a slight odor, and is very hygroscopic. Its solutions are neutral to litmus. Very soluble in water; freely soluble in alcohol and in chloroform.

Methacrylic Acid and Ethyl Acrylate Copolymer Dispersion: Milky-white liquid of low viscosity. It is miscible with water in any proportion; the milky-white appearance is retained. A clear or slightly opalescent, viscous solution is obtained on mixing one part with five parts of acetone, alcohol, or isopropyl alcohol; the polymer substance is first precipitated, but then dissolves in the excess organic solvent. A clear or slightly opalescent, viscous solution is obtained on mixing one part with two parts of 1 N sodium hydroxide. *NF category:* Coating agent; film-forming agent; diluent; wet binder.

Methacrylic Acid and Ethyl Acrylate Copolymer: White powder having a faint, characteristic odor. Soluble to freely soluble in methanol, in alcohol, in isopropyl alcohol, and in acetone, each of which contains not less than 3% of water; soluble in diluted alkali, in simulated intestinal fluid TS, and in buffer solutions of pH 7 and above; insoluble in water, in diluted acids, in simulated gastric fluid TS, and in

buffer solutions of up to pH 5. The solubility between pH 5.5 and pH 7 depends on the content of methacrylic acid units in the copolymer. *NF category:* Coating agent; film-forming agent.

Partially-Neutralized Methacrylic Acid and Ethyl Acrylate Copolymer: White or almost white, free-flowing powder. Freely soluble in alcohol, in methanol, and in a 40 g/L solution of sodium hydroxide; soluble in solutions at pH values above pH 5.5 under salt formation; practically insoluble in ethyl acetate and in acidic aqueous solutions. *NF category:* Coating agent; film-forming agent.

Methacrylic Acid and Methyl Methacrylate Copolymer: White powder having a faint, characteristic odor. Soluble to freely soluble in methanol, in alcohol, in isopropyl alcohol, and in acetone, each of which contains not less than 3% of water; soluble in diluted alkali, in simulated intestinal fluid TS, and in buffer solutions of pH 7 and above; insoluble in water, in diluted acids, in simulated gastric fluid TS, and in buffer solutions of up to pH 5. The solubility between pH 5.5 and pH 7 depends on the content of methacrylic acid units in the copolymer. *NF category:* Coating agent; film-forming agent.

Methacycline Hydrochloride: Yellow to dark yellow, crystalline powder. Soluble in water.

Methadone Hydrochloride: Colorless crystals or white, crystalline, odorless powder. Freely soluble in alcohol and in chloroform; soluble in water; practically insoluble in ether and in glycerin.

Methadone Hydrochloride Oral Concentrate: Clear to slightly hazy, syrupy liquid.

Methamphetamine Hydrochloride: White crystals or white, crystalline powder. Is odorless or practically so. Its solutions have a pH of about 6. Freely soluble in water, in alcohol, and in chloroform; very slightly soluble in absolute ether.

Methazolamide: White or faintly yellow, crystalline powder having a slight odor. Melts at about 213°. Soluble in dimethylformamide; slightly soluble in acetone; very slightly soluble in water and in alcohol.

Methdilazine Hydrochloride: Light tan, crystalline powder, having a slight, characteristic odor. Freely soluble in water, in alcohol, and in chloroform.

Methenamine: Colorless, lustrous crystals or white, crystalline powder. Is practically odorless. When brought into contact with fire, it readily ignites, burning with a smokeless flame. It sublimes at about 260°, without melting. Its solutions are alkaline to litmus. Freely soluble in water; soluble in alcohol and in chloroform.

Methenamine Mandelate: White, crystalline powder. Has a sour taste and is practically odorless. Its solutions have a pH of about 4. Melts at about 127°, with decomposition. Very soluble in water; soluble in alcohol and in chloroform; slightly soluble in ether.

Methimazole: White to pale buff, crystalline powder, having a faint, characteristic odor. Its solutions are practically neutral to litmus. Freely soluble in water, in alcohol, and in chloroform; slightly soluble in ether.

Methionine: White crystals, having a characteristic odor and taste. Soluble in water, in warm dilute alcohol, and in dilute mineral acids; insoluble in ether, in absolute alcohol, in benzene, and in acetone (L-form). *NF category:* Flavors and fragrance; pH modifier (acidifying agent/alkalizing agent/buffering agent); antioxidant.

Methocarbamol: White powder, odorless, or having a slight characteristic odor. Melts at about 94°, or, if previously ground to a fine powder, melts at about 90°. Soluble in alcohol only with heating; sparingly soluble in water and in chloroform; insoluble in benzene and in n-hexane.

Methohexital: White to faintly yellowish-white, crystalline, odorless powder. Slightly soluble in alcohol, in chloroform, and in dilute alkalies; very slightly soluble in water.

Methohexital Sodium for Injection: White to off-white, hygroscopic powder. Is essentially odorless.

Methotrexate: Orange-brown, or yellow, crystalline powder. Freely soluble in dilute solutions of alkali hydroxides and carbonates; slightly soluble in 6 N hydrochloric acid; practically insoluble in water, in alcohol, in chloroform, and in ether.

Methotrimeprazine: Fine, white, practically odorless, crystalline powder. Melts at about 126°. Freely soluble in chloroform, in ether, and in boiling alcohol; sparingly soluble in methanol and in alcohol at 25°; practically insoluble in water.

Methoxsalen: White to cream-colored, fluffy, needle-like crystals. Is odorless. Freely soluble in chloroform; soluble in boiling alcohol, in acetone, in acetic acid, in propylene glycol, and in benzene; sparingly soluble in boiling water and in ether; practically insoluble in water.

Methoxsalen Topical Solution: Clear, colorless liquid.

Methoxyflurane: Clear, practically colorless, mobile liquid, having a characteristic odor. Boils at about 105°. Miscible with alcohol, with acetone, with chloroform, with ether, and with fixed oils.

Methsuximide: White to grayish white, crystalline powder. Is odorless, or has not more than a slight odor. Very soluble in chloroform; freely soluble in alcohol and in ether; slightly soluble in hot water.

Methyclothiazide: White or practically white, crystalline powder. Is odorless, or has a slight odor. Freely soluble in acetone and in pyridine; sparingly soluble in methanol; slightly soluble in alcohol; very slightly soluble in water, in chloroform, and in benzene.

Methyl Alcohol: Clear, colorless liquid, having a characteristic odor. Is flammable. Miscible with water, with alcohol, with ether, with benzene, and with most other organic solvents. *NF category:* Solvent.

Methyl Benzylidene Camphor: A white, fine crystalline powder. Very soluble in chloroform; freely soluble in alcohol; practically insoluble in water.

Methyl Isobutyl Ketone: Transparent, colorless, mobile, volatile liquid, having a faint ketonic and camphoraceous odor. Slightly soluble in water. Miscible with alcohol, with ether, and with benzene. *NF category:* Alcohol denaturant; solvent.

Methyl Salicylate: Colorless, yellowish, or reddish liquid, having the characteristic odor and taste of wintergreen. It boils between 219° and 224°, with some decomposition. Soluble in alcohol and in glacial acetic acid; slightly soluble in water. *NF category:* Flavors and fragrance.

Methylbenzethonium Chloride: White, hygroscopic crystals, having a mild odor. Its solutions are neutral or slightly alkaline to litmus. Very soluble in water, in alcohol, and in ether; practically insoluble in chloroform.

Methylcellulose: White, fibrous powder or granules. Its aqueous suspensions are neutral to litmus. It swells in water and produces a clear to opalescent, viscous, colloidal suspension. Soluble in glacial acetic acid and in a mixture of equal volumes of alcohol and chloroform; insoluble in alcohol, in ether, and in chloroform. *NF category:* Coating agent; suspending and/or viscosity-increasing agent; wet binder; emulsifying agent; film-forming agent; disintegrant.

Methyldopa: White to yellowish-white, odorless, fine powder, which may contain friable lumps. Very soluble in 3 N hydrochloric acid; sparingly soluble in water; slightly soluble in alcohol; practically insoluble in ether.

Methyldopate Hydrochloride: White or practically white, odorless or practically odorless, crystalline powder. Freely soluble in water, in alcohol, and in methanol; slightly soluble in chloroform; practically insoluble in ether.

Methylene Blue: Dark green or blue crystals or crystalline powder having a bronze-like luster. Is odorless or practically so, and is stable in air. Its solutions in water and in alcohol are deep blue in color. Slightly soluble in water and in alcohol. *NF category:* Free radical scavenger.

Methylene Chloride: Clear, colorless, mobile liquid, having an odor resembling that of chloroform. Miscible with alcohol, with ether, and with fixed and volatile oils. *NF category:* Solvent.

Methylergonovine Maleate: White to pinkish-tan, microcrystalline powder. Is odorless. Slightly soluble in water and in alcohol; very slightly soluble in chloroform and in ether.

Add the following:

▲**Methylnaltrexone Bromide:** White to almost-white crystalline powder. Freely soluble in dimethylsulfoxide; soluble in dimethylformamide and in water; slightly soluble in methanol; very slightly soluble in ethanol; practically insoluble in toluene.▲*USP41*

Methylparaben: White, crystalline powder or colorless crystals. Freely soluble in alcohol and in methanol; slightly soluble in water. *NF category:* Antimicrobial preservative.

Methylparaben Sodium: White, hygroscopic powder. Freely soluble in water; sparingly soluble in alcohol; insoluble in fixed oils. *NF category:* Antimicrobial preservative.

Methylphenidate Hydrochloride: White, odorless, fine, crystalline powder. Its solutions are acid to litmus. Freely soluble in water and in methanol; soluble in alcohol; slightly soluble in chloroform and in acetone.

Methylprednisolone: White to practically white, odorless, crystalline powder. Melts at about 240°, with some decomposition (see *Melting Range or Temperature* ⟨741⟩). Sparingly soluble in alcohol, in dioxane, and in methanol; slightly soluble in acetone and in chloroform; very slightly soluble in ether; practically insoluble in water.

Methylprednisolone Acetate: White or practically white, odorless, crystalline powder. Melts at about 225°, with some decomposition (see *Melting Range or Temperature* ⟨741⟩). Soluble in dioxane; sparingly soluble in acetone, in alcohol, in chloroform, and in methanol; slightly soluble in ether; practically insoluble in water.

Methylprednisolone Hemisuccinate: White or nearly white, odorless or nearly odorless, hygroscopic solid. Freely soluble in alcohol; soluble in acetone; very slightly soluble in water.

Methylprednisolone Sodium Succinate: White or nearly white, odorless, hygroscopic, amorphous solid. Very soluble in water and in alcohol; very slightly soluble in acetone; insoluble in chloroform.

Methylpyrrolidone: A clear, colorless to very slightly yellow liquid. Miscible with water and with most organic solvents including alcohol, ketones, and aromatic and chlorinated hydrocarbons. Boiling point: about 202°. Refractive index: about 1.469. *NF category:* Solvent.

Methylsulfonylmethane: White powder or flake crystal. Melts at about 109°. Freely soluble in water, in methanol, in alcohol, and in acetone; sparingly soluble in ether.

Methyltestosterone: White or creamy white crystals or crystalline powder. Is odorless and is stable in air, but is slightly hygroscopic. Is affected by light. Soluble in alcohol, in methanol, in ether, and in other organic solvents; sparingly soluble in vegetable oils; practically insoluble in water.

Methysergide Maleate: White to yellowish-white or reddish-white, crystalline powder. Is odorless or has not more than a slight odor. Slightly soluble in water and in alcohol; very slightly soluble in chloroform; practically insoluble in ether.

Metoclopramide Hydrochloride: White or practically white, crystalline, odorless or practically odorless powder. Very soluble in water; freely soluble in alcohol; sparingly soluble in chloroform; practically insoluble in ether.

Metoprolol Succinate: White to off-white powder. Freely soluble in water; soluble in methanol; sparingly soluble in alcohol; slightly soluble in isopropyl alcohol.

Metoprolol Tartrate: White, crystalline powder. Very soluble in water; freely soluble in methylene chloride, in chloroform, and in alcohol; slightly soluble in acetone; insoluble in ether.

Metronidazole: White to pale yellow, odorless crystals or crystalline powder. Is stable in air, but darkens on exposure to light. Soluble in dilute hydrochloric acid (1 in 2); sparingly soluble in water and in alcohol; slightly soluble in ether and in chloroform.

Metronidazole Benzoate: White to slightly yellow, crystalline powder. Freely soluble in methylene chloride; soluble in acetone; slightly soluble in alcohol; very slightly soluble in ethyl ether; practically insoluble in water.

Metyrapone: White to light amber, fine, crystalline powder, having a characteristic odor. Darkens on exposure to light. Soluble in methanol and in chloroform; sparingly soluble in water. It forms water-soluble salts with acids.

Mexiletine Hydrochloride: White powder. Freely soluble in dehydrated alcohol and in water; slightly soluble in acetonitrile; practically insoluble in ether. Optically inactive (1 in 20 solution in water).

Mezlocillin Sodium: White to pale yellow, crystalline powder. Freely soluble in water.

Mibolerone: White to off-white powder. Slightly soluble in chloroform, in dioxane, and in methylene chloride; practically insoluble in water (0.0454 mg per mL at 37°).

Miconazole: White to pale cream powder. Melts in the range of 78° to 88°. May exhibit polymorphism. Freely soluble in alcohol, in methanol, in isopropyl alcohol, in acetone, in propylene glycol, in chloroform, and in dimethylformamide; soluble in ether; insoluble in water.

Miconazole Nitrate: White or practically white, crystalline powder, having not more than a slight odor. Melts in the range of 178° to 183°, with decomposition. Freely soluble in dimethyl sulfoxide; soluble in dimethylformamide; sparingly soluble in methanol; slightly soluble in alcohol, in chloroform, and in propylene glycol; very slightly soluble in water and in isopropyl alcohol; insoluble in ether.

Midazolam: White or yellowish powder. The hydrochloride salt of midazolam is soluble in aqueous solutions. Insoluble in water.

Midodrine Hydrochloride: White crystalline powder. Soluble in water; sparingly soluble in methanol.

Milrinone: White to tan, crystalline solid. Is hygroscopic. Freely soluble in dimethyl sulfoxide; very slightly soluble in methanol; practically insoluble in water and in chloroform.

Mineral Oil: Colorless, transparent, oily liquid, free or practically free from fluorescence. Is odorless and tasteless when cold, and develops not more than a faint odor of petroleum when heated. Soluble in volatile oils; insoluble in water and in alcohol. Miscible with most fixed oils but not with castor oil. *NF category:* Solvent; vehicle (oleaginous); emollient.

Light Mineral Oil: Colorless, transparent, oily liquid, free, or practically free, from fluorescence. Is odorless and tasteless when cold, and develops not more than a faint odor of petroleum when heated. Soluble in volatile oils; insoluble in water and in alcohol. Miscible with most fixed oils, but not with castor oil. *NF category:* Vehicle (oleaginous); lubricant; emollient; solvent.

Minocycline Hydrochloride: Yellow, crystalline powder. Soluble in solutions of alkali hydroxides and carbonates; sparingly soluble in water; slightly soluble in alcohol; practically insoluble in chloroform and in ether.

Minoxidil: White to off-white, crystalline powder. Melts in the approximate range of between 248° and 268°, with decomposition. Soluble in alcohol and in propylene glycol; sparingly soluble in methanol; slightly soluble in water; practically insoluble in chloroform, in acetone, in ethyl acetate, and in hexane.

Mirtazapine: White to creamy white, crystalline powder. Freely soluble in methanol and in toluene; soluble in ethyl ether; sparingly soluble in *n*-hexane; practically insoluble in water.

Misoprostol: Clear, colorless or light yellow viscous liquid. Very slightly soluble in water.

Mitomycin: Blue-violet, crystalline powder. Soluble in acetone, in methanol, in butyl acetate, and in cyclohexanone; slightly soluble in water.

Mitotane: White, crystalline powder, having a slight, aromatic odor. Soluble in alcohol, in ether, in solvent hexane, and in fixed oils and fats; practically insoluble in water.

Mitoxantrone Hydrochloride: Dark blue powder. Sparingly soluble in water; slightly soluble in methanol; practically insoluble in acetone, in acetonitrile, and in chloroform.

Modafinil: White to off-white, crystalline powder. Sparingly soluble in methanol; slightly soluble in absolute alcohol; very slightly soluble in water.

Moexipril Hydrochloride: White to off-white powder. Soluble in water, in alcohol, and in methanol.

Mometasone Furoate: White to off-white powder. Melts at about 220°, with decomposition. Soluble in acetone and in methylene chloride.

Monensin Sodium: Off-white to tan, crystalline powder. Soluble in chloroform and in methanol; slightly soluble in water; practically insoluble in solvent hexane.

Mono- and Di-glycerides: Vary in consistency from yellow liquids, through ivory-colored plastics, to ivory white-colored solids (bead or flake forms). Soluble in alcohol, in ethyl acetate, in chloroform, and in other chlorinated hydrocarbons; insoluble in water. *NF category:* Emulsifying agent.

Monobenzone Ointment: Dispersible with, but not soluble in, water.

Monoethanolamine: Clear, colorless, moderately viscous liquid, having a distinctly ammoniacal odor. Miscible with water, with acetone, with alcohol, with glycerin, and with chloroform. Immiscible with ether, with solvent hexane, and with fixed oils, although it dissolves many essential oils. *NF category:* Emulsifying agent; pH modifier (acidifying agent/alkalizing agent/buffering agent).

Monoglyceride Citrate: Soft white to ivory-colored, waxy solid with a lard-like consistency and bland odor. Dispersible in most common fat solvents and in alcohol. Insoluble in water.

Monosodium Glutamate: White, practically odorless, free-flowing crystals or crystalline powder. Freely soluble in water; sparingly soluble in alcohol. May have either a slightly sweet or a slightly salty taste. *NF category:* Flavors and fragrance; pH modifier (acidifying agent/alkalizing agent/buffering agent).

Monothioglycerol: Colorless or pale yellow, viscous liquid, having a slight sulfidic odor. Is hygroscopic. Freely soluble in water; insoluble in ether. Miscible with alcohol. *NF category:* Antioxidant; antimicrobial preservative.

Montelukast Sodium: White or almost white, hygroscopic powder. Freely soluble to very soluble in alcohol; freely soluble in water and in methylene chloride.

Morantel Tartrate: A white or pale yellow, crystalline powder. Very soluble in water and in alcohol; practically insoluble in ethyl acetate.

Moricizine Hydrochloride: White to off-white, crystalline powder. Melts at about 189°, with decomposition. Soluble in water and in alcohol.

Morphine Sulfate: White, feathery, silky crystals, cubical masses of crystals, or white, crystalline powder. Is odorless, and when exposed to air it gradually loses water of hydration. Darkens on prolonged exposure to light. Freely soluble in hot water; soluble in water; slightly soluble in alcohol but more so in hot alcohol; insoluble in chloroform and in ether.

Moxidectin: White to pale yellow powder. Very soluble in alcohol; slightly soluble in hexane; practically insoluble in water.

Moxifloxacin Hydrochloride: Slightly yellow to yellow powder or crystals. Soluble in 0.1 N sodium hydroxide; sparingly soluble in water and in methanol; slightly soluble in 0.1 N hydrochloric acid, in dimethylformamide, and in alcohol; practically insoluble in methylene chloride, in acetone, in ethyl acetate, and in toluene; insoluble in *tert*-butyl methyl ether and *n*-heptane.

Mumps Skin Test Antigen: Slightly turbid liquid.

Mumps Virus Vaccine Live: Solid having the characteristic appearance of substances dried from the frozen state. The Vaccine is to be constituted with a suitable diluent just prior to use. Constituted vaccine undergoes loss of potency on exposure to sunlight.

Mupirocin: White to off-white, crystalline solid. Freely soluble in acetone, in chloroform, in dehydrated alcohol, and in methanol; slightly soluble in ether; very slightly soluble in water.

Mycophenolate Mofetil: White or almost white, crystalline powder. Its melting range is between 94° and 98°. Freely soluble in acetone; soluble in methanol; sparingly soluble in dehydrated alcohol; slightly soluble in water.

Mycophenolate Sodium: White to off-white crystalline powder. Slightly soluble in water; practically insoluble in 0.1 N hydrochloric acid.

Myristic Acid: Hard, white or faintly yellow, somewhat glossy, crystalline solid or white or yellow-white powder. Soluble in alcohol, in chloroform, and in ether; practically insoluble in water. *NF category:* Antifoaming agent; emulsifying agent; lubricant.

Nabumetone: A white, or almost white, crystalline powder. Freely soluble in acetone; sparingly soluble in alcohol and in methanol; practically insoluble in water.

Nadolol: White to off-white, practically odorless, crystalline powder. Freely soluble in alcohol and in methanol; soluble in water at pH 2; slightly soluble in chloroform, in methylene chloride, in isopropyl alcohol, and in water (between pH 7 and pH 10); insoluble in acetone, in benzene, in ether, in hexane, and in trichloroethane.

Nafcillin Sodium: White to yellowish-white powder, having not more than a slight characteristic odor. Freely soluble in water and in chloroform; soluble in alcohol.

Nalidixic Acid: White to very pale yellow, odorless, crystalline powder. Soluble in chloroform, in methylene chloride, and in solutions of fixed alkali hydroxides and carbonates; slightly soluble in acetone, in alcohol, in methanol, and in toluene; very slightly soluble in ether and in water.

Naloxone Hydrochloride: White to slightly off-white powder. Its aqueous solution is acidic. Soluble in water, in dilute acids, and in strong alkali; slightly soluble in alcohol; practically insoluble in ether and in chloroform.

Naloxone Hydrochloride Injection: Clear, colorless liquid.

Nandrolone Decanoate: Fine, white to creamy white, crystalline powder. Is odorless, or may have a slight odor. Soluble in chloroform, in alcohol, in acetone, and in vegetable oils; practically insoluble in water.

Naphazoline Hydrochloride: White, crystalline powder. Freely soluble in water; soluble in alcohol.

Naproxen: White to off-white, practically odorless, crystalline powder. Soluble in chloroform, in dehydrated alcohol, and in alcohol; sparingly soluble in ether; practically insoluble in water.

Naproxen Sodium: White to creamy crystalline powder. Soluble in water and in methanol; sparingly soluble in alcohol; very slightly soluble in acetone; and practically in-

soluble in chloroform and in toluene. Melts at about 255°, with decomposition.

Narasin: White to off-white, crystalline powder. Melts at about 217°, with decomposition. Soluble in methanol and in water.

Naratriptan Hydrochloride: White to pale yellow solid. Soluble in water.

Natamycin: Off-white to cream-colored powder, which may contain up to 3 moles of water. Soluble in glacial acetic acid and in dimethylformamide; slightly soluble in methanol; practically insoluble in water.

Nateglinide: White powder. Freely soluble in methanol and in alcohol; soluble in ether; sparingly soluble in acetonitrile and in octanol; practically insoluble in water.

Nefazodone Hydrochloride: Nonhygroscopic, white powder. Freely soluble in chloroform; soluble in propylene glycol; slightly soluble in polyethylene glycol and in water.

Neomycin Sulfate: White to slightly yellow powder, or cryodesiccated solid. Is odorless or practically so and is hygroscopic. Its solutions are dextrorotatory. Freely soluble in water; very slightly soluble in alcohol; insoluble in acetone, in chloroform, and in ether.

Netilmicin Sulfate: White to pale yellowish-white powder. Freely soluble in water; practically insoluble in dehydrated alcohol and in ether.

Nevirapine: White to off-white, odorless to nearly odorless, crystalline powder. Slightly soluble in alcohol and in methanol; practically insoluble in water. Hydrous form also slightly soluble in propylene glycol.

Niacin: White crystals or crystalline powder. Is odorless, or has a slight odor. Melts at about 235°. Freely soluble in boiling water, in boiling alcohol, and in solutions of alkali hydroxides and carbonates; sparingly soluble in water; practically insoluble in ether.

Niacinamide: White, crystalline powder. Is odorless or practically so, and has a bitter taste. Its solutions are neutral to litmus. Freely soluble in water and in alcohol; soluble in glycerin.

Nifedipine: Yellow powder. Is affected by exposure to light. Freely soluble in acetone; practically insoluble in water.

Nilutamide: White or almost-white powder. Freely soluble in acetone and in ethyl acetate; soluble in methanol and in dichloromethane; sparingly soluble in absolute alcohol; very slightly soluble in water.

Nimodipine: Light yellow or yellow, crystalline powder, affected by light. Freely soluble in ethyl acetate; sparingly soluble in alcohol; practically insoluble in water. Exhibits polymorphism.

Nitric Acid: Highly corrosive fuming liquid, having a characteristic, highly irritating odor. Stains animal tissues yellow. Boils at about 120°. Specific gravity is about 1.41. *NF category:* pH modifier (acidifying agent/alkalizing agent/buffering agent).

Nitrofurantoin: Lemon-yellow, odorless crystals or fine powder. Has a bitter aftertaste. Soluble in dimethylformamide; very slightly soluble in water and in alcohol.

Nitrofurazone: Lemon yellow, odorless, crystalline powder. Darkens slowly on exposure to light. Melts at about 236°, with decomposition. Soluble in dimethylformamide; slightly soluble in propylene glycol and in polyethylene glycol mixtures; very slightly soluble in alcohol and in water; practically insoluble in chloroform and in ether.

Nitrofurazone Ointment: Yellow, opaque, and water-miscible, and has ointment-like consistency.

Nitrofurazone Topical Solution: Light yellow, clear, somewhat viscous liquid, having a faint characteristic odor. Miscible with water.

Nitrogen: Colorless, odorless, tasteless gas. Is nonflammable and does not support combustion. One L at 0° and at a pressure of 760 mm of mercury weighs about 1.251 g. One volume dissolves in about 65 volumes of water and in about 9 volumes of alcohol at 20° and at a pressure of 760 mm of mercury. *NF category:* Air displacement; propellant.

Diluted Nitroglycerin: When diluted with lactose, it is a white, odorless powder. When diluted with propylene glycol or alcohol, it is a clear, colorless, or pale yellow liquid. [NOTE—Undiluted nitroglycerin occurs as a white to pale yellow, thick, flammable, explosive liquid.] Undiluted nitroglycerin is soluble in methanol, in alcohol, in carbon disulfide, in acetone, in ethyl ether, in ethyl acetate, in glacial acetic acid, in benzene, in toluene, in nitrobenzene, in phenol, in chloroform, and in methylene chloride; slightly soluble in water.

Nitromersol: Brownish yellow to yellow granules or brownish yellow to yellow powder. Is odorless and tasteless and is affected by light. Soluble in solutions of alkalies and of ammonia by opening of the anhydride ring and the formation of a salt; very slightly soluble in water, in alcohol, in acetone, and in ether.

Nitromersol Topical Solution: Clear, reddish-orange solution. Is affected by light.

Nitrous Oxide: Colorless gas, without appreciable odor or taste. One L at 0° and at a pressure of 760 mm of mercury weighs about 1.97 g. One volume dissolves in about 1.4 volumes of water at 20° and at a pressure of 760 mm of mercury. Freely soluble in alcohol; soluble in ether and in oils. *NF category:* Propellant.

Nizatidine: Off-white to buff crystalline solid. Freely soluble in chloroform; soluble in methanol; sparingly soluble in water.

Nonoxynol 9: Clear, colorless to light yellow, viscous liquid. Soluble in water, in alcohol, and in corn oil. *NF category:* Wetting and/or solubilizing agent.

Norepinephrine Bitartrate: White or faintly gray, odorless, crystalline powder. Slowly darkens on exposure to air and light. Its solutions are acid to litmus, having a pH of about 3.5. Freely soluble in water; slightly soluble in alcohol; practically insoluble in chloroform and in ether. Melts between 98° and 104°, without previous drying of the specimen, the melt being turbid.

Norepinephrine Bitartrate Injection: Colorless or practically colorless liquid, gradually turning dark on exposure to air and light.

Norethindrone: White to creamy white, odorless, crystalline powder. Is stable in air. Soluble in chloroform and in dioxane; sparingly soluble in alcohol; slightly soluble in ether; practically insoluble in water.

Norethindrone Acetate: White to creamy white, odorless, crystalline powder. Very soluble in chloroform; freely soluble in dioxane; soluble in ether and in alcohol; practically insoluble in water.

Norfloxacin: White to pale yellow, crystalline powder. Sensitive to light and moisture. Freely soluble in acetic acid; sparingly soluble in chloroform; slightly soluble in acetone, in water, and in alcohol; very slightly soluble in methanol and in ethyl acetate; insoluble in ether.

Norgestimate: White to pale yellow powder. Very to freely soluble in methylene chloride; sparingly soluble in acetonitrile; insoluble in water.

Norgestrel: White or practically white, practically odorless, crystalline powder. Freely soluble in chloroform; sparingly soluble in alcohol; insoluble in water.

Norelgestromin: White to off-white powder. Freely soluble in acetone, in ethanol, in methanol, and in dimethylformamide; sparingly soluble in methylene chloride and in iso-propanol; slightly soluble in acetonitrile; practically insoluble in water.

Nortriptyline Hydrochloride: White to off-white powder, having a slight, characteristic odor. Its solution (1 in 100) has a pH of about 5. Soluble in water and in chloroform; sparingly soluble in methanol; practically insoluble in ether, in benzene, and in most other organic solvents.

Noscapine: Fine, white or practically white, crystalline powder. Freely soluble in chloroform; soluble in acetone; slightly soluble in alcohol and in ether; practically insoluble in water.

Novobiocin Calcium: White or yellowish-white, odorless, crystalline powder. Freely soluble in alcohol and in methanol; sparingly soluble in acetone and in butyl acetate; slightly soluble in water and in ether; very slightly soluble in chloroform.

Novobiocin Sodium: White or yellowish-white, odorless, hygroscopic, crystalline powder. Freely soluble in water, in alcohol, in methanol, in glycerin, and in propylene glycol; slightly soluble in butyl acetate; practically insoluble in acetone, in chloroform, and in ether.

Nystatin: Yellow to light tan powder. Is hygroscopic, and is affected by long exposure to light, heat, and air. Freely soluble in dimethylformamide and in dimethyl sulfoxide; very slightly soluble in methanol; practically insoluble or insoluble in water, in alcohol, in n-propyl alcohol, in n-butyl alcohol, in chloroform, and in ether.

Octoxynol 9: Clear, pale yellow, viscous liquid, having a faint odor and a bitter taste. Soluble in benzene and in toluene; practically insoluble in solvent hexane. Miscible with water, with alcohol, and with acetone. *NF category:* Wetting and/or solubilizing agent.

Octyldodecanol: Clear water-white, free-flowing liquid. Soluble in alcohol and in ether; insoluble in water. *NF category:* Vehicle (oleaginous); emollient; emulsifying agent.

Octyl Methoxycinnamate: Pale yellow oil. Insoluble in water.

Ofloxacin: Pale yellowish-white to light yellowish-white crystals or crystalline powder. Sparingly soluble in chloroform; slightly soluble in alcohol, in methanol, and in water.

Hydrophilic Ointment: *NF category:* Ointment base.

White Ointment: *NF category:* Ointment base.

Yellow Ointment: *NF category:* Ointment base.

Olanzapine: A yellow crystalline solid. Soluble in n-propanol; sparingly soluble in acetonitrile; slightly soluble in methanol and in dehydrated alcohol; practically insoluble in water.

Oleic Acid: Colorless to pale yellow, oily liquid when freshly prepared, but on exposure to air it gradually absorbs oxygen and darkens. Has a characteristic, lard-like odor and taste. When strongly heated in air, it is decomposed with the production of acrid vapors. Practically insoluble in water. Miscible with alcohol, with chloroform, with ether, with benzene, and with fixed and volatile oils. *NF category:* Emulsifying agent.

Oleovitamin A and D: Yellow to red, oily liquid, practically odorless or having a fish-like odor, and having no rancid odor or taste. Is a clear liquid at temperatures exceeding 65°, and may crystallize on cooling. Is unstable in air and in light. Very soluble in ether and in chloroform; soluble in dehydrated alcohol and in vegetable oils; insoluble in water and in glycerin.

Oleovitamin A and D Capsules: The oil contained in Oleovitamin A and D Capsules is a yellow to red, oily liquid, practically odorless or having a fish-like odor, and having no rancid odor or taste. Is a clear liquid at temperatures exceeding 65°, and may crystallize on cooling. Is unstable in air and in light.

Oleoyl Polyoxylglycerides: Amber, oily liquids. May develop deposit after prolonged storage at 20°. Freely soluble in methylene chloride; practically insoluble but dispersible in water. *NF category:* Ointment base; solvent; emulsifying agent; wetting and/or solubilizing agent.

Oleyl Alcohol: Clear, colorless to light yellow, oily liquid. Has a faint characteristic odor and a bland taste. Soluble in alcohol, in ether, in isopropyl alcohol, and in light mineral oil; insoluble in water. *NF category:* Emollient; emulsifying agent.

Oleyl Oleate: Clear, colorless to light yellow liquid. Has a faint characteristic odor. Slightly soluble in alcohol. Miscible with chloroform and with ether. *NF category:* Emollient; emulsifying agent.

Olive Oil: Pale yellow, or light greenish-yellow, oily liquid, having a slight, characteristic odor and taste, with a faintly acrid aftertaste. Slightly soluble in alcohol. Miscible with ether, with chloroform, and with carbon disulfide. *Specific Gravity* ⟨841⟩: Between 0.910 and 0.915. *NF category:* Vehicle (oleaginous).

Olmesartan Medoxomil: White to off-white crystalline powder. Sparingly soluble in methanol; practically insoluble in water.

Olopatadine Hydrochloride: White crystalline powder. Very soluble in formic acid; sparingly soluble in water; very slightly soluble in dehydrated alcohol.

Omeprazole: White to off-white powder. Soluble in dichloromethane; sparingly soluble in methanol and in alcohol; very slightly soluble in water.

Omeprazole Magnesium: White to off-white powder. Sparingly soluble in methanol; slightly soluble in alcohol; very slightly soluble in water and in dichloromethane.

Ondansetron: White to off-white powder. Very soluble in acid solutions; sparingly soluble in water.

Ondansetron Hydrochloride: White to off-white powder. Soluble in methanol; sparingly soluble in water and in alcohol; slightly soluble in isopropyl alcohol and in dichloromethane; very slightly soluble in acetone, in chloroform, and in ethyl acetate.

Opium: Has a very characteristic odor and a very bitter taste.

Powdered Opium: Light brown or moderately yellowish-brown powder.

Orbifloxacin: White to pale yellow crystals or crystalline powder. Odorless. Soluble in acetic acid; very slightly soluble in methanol, in water, and in chloroform; practically insoluble in ethanol and in diethyl ether.

Orlistat: White to off-white fine powder or fine powder with lumps. Freely soluble in chloroform; very soluble in methanol and in alcohol; practically insoluble in water.

Orphenadrine Citrate: White, practically odorless, crystalline powder, having a bitter taste. Sparingly soluble in water; slightly soluble in alcohol; insoluble in chloroform, in benzene, and in ether.

Oseltamivir Phosphate: White to off-white powder. Freely soluble in water; soluble in methanol, in dimethyl sulfoxide, and in propylene glycol; sparingly soluble in dimethylformamide; slightly soluble in alcohol; very slightly soluble in isopropyl alcohol and in polyethylene glycol 400; practically insoluble in acetonitrile, in acetone, in dichloromethane, and in *n*-hexane.

Oxacillin Sodium: Fine, white, crystalline powder, odorless or having a slight odor. Freely soluble in water, in methanol, and in dimethyl sulfoxide; slightly soluble in absolute alcohol, in chloroform, in pyridine, and in methyl acetate; insoluble in ethyl acetate, in ether, in benzene, and in ethylene chloride.

Oxacillin Sodium for Injection: Fine, white, crystalline powder, odorless or having a slight odor. Freely soluble in water, in methanol, and in dimethyl sulfoxide; slightly soluble in absolute alcohol, in chloroform, in pyridine, and in methyl acetate; insoluble in ethyl acetate, in ether, in benzene, and in ethylene chloride.

Oxaliplatin: White to off-white crystalline powder. Slightly soluble in water; very slightly soluble in methanol; practically insoluble in alcohol.

Oxandrolone: White, odorless, crystalline powder. Is stable in air, but darkens on exposure to light. Melts at

about 225°. Freely soluble in chloroform; sparingly soluble in alcohol and in acetone; practically insoluble in water.

Oxaprozin: White to yellowish-white, crystalline powder.

Oxazepam: Creamy white to pale yellow powder. Is practically odorless. Slightly soluble in alcohol and in chloroform; very slightly soluble in ether; practically insoluble in water.

Oxcarbazepine: Light orange to creamish white or off-white powder. Soluble in acetic acid; sparingly soluble in chloroform; practically insoluble in water.

Oxfendazole: White or almost white powder. Slightly soluble in alcohol and in methylene chloride; practically insoluble in water.

Oxprenolol Hydrochloride: White, crystalline powder. Freely soluble in alcohol, in chloroform, and in ether; sparingly soluble in acetone; practically insoluble in water.

Oxtriphylline: White, crystalline powder, having an amine-like odor. A solution (1 in 100) has a pH of about 10.3. Freely soluble in water and in alcohol; very slightly soluble in chloroform.

Oxybenzone: Pale yellow powder. Freely soluble in alcohol and in toluene; practically insoluble in water.

Oxybutynin Chloride: White, crystalline, practically odorless powder. Very soluble in methanol and in chloroform; freely soluble in water and in alcohol; soluble in acetone; slightly soluble in ether; very slightly soluble in hexane.

Oxycodone Hydrochloride: White to off-white, hygroscopic crystals or powder. Is odorless. Soluble in water; slightly soluble in alcohol.

Oxygen: Colorless, odorless, tasteless gas, which supports combustion more energetically than does air. One L at 0° and at a pressure of 760 mm of mercury weighs about 1.429 g. One volume dissolves in about 32 volumes of water and in about 7 volumes of alcohol at 20° and at a pressure of 760 mm of mercury.

Oxymetazoline Hydrochloride: White to practically white, fine crystalline powder. Is hygroscopic. Melts at about 300°, with decomposition. Soluble in water and in alcohol; practically insoluble in benzene, in chloroform, and in ether.

Oxymetholone: White to creamy white, crystalline powder. Is odorless, and is stable in air. Freely soluble in chloroform; soluble in dioxane; sparingly soluble in alcohol; slightly soluble in ether; practically insoluble in water.

Oxymorphone Hydrochloride: White or slightly off-white, odorless powder. Darkens on exposure to light. Its aqueous solutions are slightly acidic. Freely soluble in water; sparingly soluble in alcohol and in ether.

Oxyquinoline Sulfate: Yellow powder. Melts at about 185°. Very soluble in water; freely soluble in methanol; slightly soluble in alcohol; practically insoluble in acetone and in ether. *NF category:* Chelating and/or complexing agent.

Oxytetracycline: Pale yellow to tan, odorless, crystalline powder. Is stable in air, but exposure to strong sunlight causes it to darken. It loses potency in solutions of pH below 2, and is rapidly destroyed by alkali hydroxide solutions. Freely soluble in 3 N hydrochloric acid and in alkaline solutions; sparingly soluble in alcohol; very slightly soluble in water.

Oxytetracycline Calcium: Yellow to light brown, crystalline powder. Insoluble in water.

Oxytetracycline Hydrochloride: Yellow, odorless, crystalline powder, having a bitter taste. Is hygroscopic. Decomposes at a temperature exceeding 180°, and exposure to strong sunlight or to temperatures exceeding 90° in moist air causes it to darken. Its potency is diminished in solutions having a pH below 2, and is rapidly destroyed by alkali hydroxide solutions. Freely soluble in water, but crystals of oxytetracycline base separate as a result of partial hydrolysis of the hydrochloride; sparingly soluble in alcohol and in methanol, and even less soluble in dehydrated alcohol; insoluble in chloroform and in ether.

Paclitaxel: White to off-white powder. Soluble in alcohol; insoluble in water.

Padimate O: A light yellow, mobile liquid having a faint, aromatic odor. Soluble in alcohol, in isopropyl alcohol, and in mineral oil; practically insoluble in water, in glycerin, and in propylene glycol.

Paliperidone: White to yellow powder. Sparingly soluble in 0.1 N hydrochloric acid and in methylene chloride; slightly soluble in N,N-dimethylformamide and in tetrahydrofuran; practically insoluble in water, in 0.1 N sodium hydroxide, and in hexane.

Palm Oil: White to yellowish, fatty solid to semisolid. Insoluble in water. *NF category:* Coating agent; emulsifying agent.

Hydrogenated Palm Oil: White to yellowish, fatty solid to semi-solid. Freely soluble in ether; very slightly soluble in alcohol; practically insoluble in water. *NF category:* Coating agent; lubricant; wet binder.

Palm Kernel Oil: White to yellowish, fatty solid. Insoluble in water. *NF category:* Coating agent; emulsifying agent; suppository base.

Palmitic Acid: Hard, white or faintly yellow, somewhat glossy crystalline solid, or white or yellowish-white powder. It has a slight characteristic odor and taste. Soluble in alcohol, in ether, and in chloroform; practically insoluble in water. *NF category:* Antifoaming agent; emulsifying agent; lubricant.

Palonosetron Hydrochloride: White to off-white, crystalline powder. Freely soluble in water; soluble in propylene glycol; slightly soluble in ethanol; very slightly soluble to slightly soluble in isopropyl alcohol.

Pamidronate Disodium: White, crystalline powder. Soluble in water and in 2 N sodium hydroxide; sparingly soluble in 0.1 N hydrochloric acid and in 0.1 N acetic acid; practically insoluble in organic solvents.

Pancreatin: Cream-colored, amorphous powder, having a faint, characteristic, but not offensive odor. It hydrolyzes fats to glycerol and fatty acids, changes protein into proteoses and derived substances, and converts starch into dextrins and sugars. Its greatest activities are in neutral or faintly alkaline media; more than traces of mineral acids or large amounts of alkali hydroxides make it inert. An excess of alkali carbonate also inhibits its action.

Pancrelipase: Cream-colored, amorphous powder, having a faint, characteristic, but not offensive odor. Pancrelipase hydrolyzes fats to glycerol and fatty acids, changes protein into proteoses and derived substances, and converts starch into dextrins and sugars. Its greatest activities are in neutral or faintly alkaline media; more than traces of mineral acids or large amounts of alkali hydroxides make it inert. An excess of alkali carbonate also inhibits its action.

Pancrelipase Capsules: The contents of Capsules conform to the *Description* under *Pancrelipase*, except that the odor may vary with the flavoring agent used.

Pancuronium Bromide: White, yellowish-white, or slightly pink, crystalline powder. Is hygroscopic. Freely soluble in water, in methylene chloride, and in alcohol.

Panthenol: White to creamy white, crystalline powder having a slight, characteristic odor. Freely soluble in water, in alcohol, and propylene glycol; soluble in chloroform and in ether; slightly soluble in glycerin.

Pantoprazole Sodium: White to off-white powder. Freely soluble in water, in methanol, and in dehydrated alcohol; practically insoluble in hexane and in dichloromethane.

Papain: White to light tan, amorphous powder. Soluble in water, the solution being colorless to light yellow and more or less opalescent; practically insoluble in alcohol, in chloroform, and in ether.

Papaverine Hydrochloride: White crystals or white, crystalline powder. Is odorless, and has a slightly bitter taste. Is optically inactive. Its solutions are acid to litmus. Melts at about 220°, with decomposition. Soluble in water and in chloroform; slightly soluble in alcohol; practically insoluble in ether.

Parachlorophenol: White or pink crystals having a characteristic phenolic odor. When undiluted, it whitens and cauterizes the skin and mucous membranes. Melts at about 42°. Very soluble in alcohol, in glycerin, in chloroform, in ether, and in fixed and volatile oils; soluble in petrolatum; sparingly soluble in water and in liquid petrolatum.

Paraffin: Colorless or white, more or less translucent mass showing a crystalline structure. Is odorless and tasteless, and is slightly greasy to the touch. Freely soluble in chloroform, in ether, in volatile oils, and in most warm fixed oils; slightly soluble in dehydrated alcohol; insoluble in water and in alcohol. *NF category:* Stiffening agent; ointment base.

Synthetic Paraffin: Very hard, white, practically tasteless and odorless wax. Contains mostly long-chain, unbranched, saturated hydrocarbons, with a small amount of branched hydrocarbons. Is represented by the formula C_nH_{2n2}, in which *n* may range from 20 to about 100. The average molecular weight may range from 400 to 1400. Slightly soluble in aromatic and normal paraffinic solvents; very slightly soluble in aliphatic, oxygenated, and halogenated hydrocarbon solvents; insoluble in water. *NF category:* Stiffening agent.

Paraldehyde: Colorless, transparent liquid. Has a strong, characteristic but not unpleasant or pungent odor, and a disagreeable taste. Specific gravity is about 0.99. Soluble in water, but less soluble in boiling water. Miscible with alcohol, with chloroform, with ether, and with volatile oils.

Paricalcitol: White to almost white powder. Soluble in alcohol; insoluble in water.

Paromomycin Sulfate: Creamy white to light yellow powder. Is odorless or practically odorless, and is very hygroscopic. Very soluble in water; insoluble in alcohol, in chloroform, and in ether.

Paroxetine Hydrochloride: White to off-white solid. Soluble in methanol and in alcohol; slightly soluble in water.

Peanut Oil: Colorless or pale yellow, oily liquid with a bland taste. May have a characteristic, nutty odor. Very slightly soluble in alcohol. Miscible with ether, with chloroform, and with carbon disulfide. *Specific Gravity* ⟨841⟩: Between 0.912 and 0.920. *Refractive Index* ⟨831⟩: Between 1.462 and 1.464 at 40°. *NF category:* Solvent; vehicle (oleaginous).

Pectin: Coarse or fine powder, yellowish-white in color, almost odorless, and having a mucilaginous taste. Soluble in 20 parts of water, forming a viscous, opalescent, colloidal solution that flows readily and is acid to litmus; practically insoluble in alcohol or in diluted alcohol and in other organic solvents. Pectin dissolves in water more readily if first moistened with alcohol, glycerin, or simple syrup, or if first mixed with 3 or more parts of sucrose. *NF category:* Suspending and/or viscosity-increasing agent; emulsifying agent; film-forming agent.

Pemetrexed Disodium: White or almost white powder. Freely soluble in water; very slightly soluble in dehydrated alcohol; practically insoluble in methylene chloride.

Penbutolol Sulfate: White to off-white, crystalline powder. Melts at about 217°, with decomposition. Soluble in water and in methanol.

Penicillamine: White or practically white, crystalline powder, having a slight, characteristic odor. Freely soluble in water; slightly soluble in alcohol; insoluble in chloroform and in ether.

Penicillin G Benzathine: White, odorless, crystalline powder. Sparingly soluble in alcohol; very slightly soluble in water.

Penicillin G Potassium: Colorless or white crystals, or white, crystalline powder. Is odorless or practically so, and is moderately hygroscopic. Its solutions are dextrorotatory. Its solutions retain substantially full potency for several days at temperatures below 15°, but are rapidly inactivated by acids, by alkali hydroxides, by glycerin, and by oxidizing agents. Very soluble in water, in saline TS, and in dextrose solutions; sparingly soluble in alcohol.

Penicillin G Procaine: White crystals or white, very fine, microcrystalline powder. Is odorless or practically odorless, and is relatively stable in air. Its solutions are dextrorotatory. Is rapidly inactivated by acids, by alkali hydroxides, and by oxidizing agents. Soluble in alcohol and in chloroform; slightly soluble in water.

Penicillin G Sodium: Colorless or white crystals or white to slightly yellow, crystalline powder. Is odorless or practically odorless, and is moderately hygroscopic. Its solutions are dextrorotatory. It is relatively stable in air, but is inactivated by prolonged heating at about 100°, especially in the presence of moisture. Its solutions lose potency fairly rapidly at room temperature, but retain substantially full potency for several days at temperatures below 15°. Its solutions are rapidly inactivated by acids, by alkali hydroxides, by oxidizing agents, and by penicillinase.

Penicillin V: White, odorless, crystalline powder. Freely soluble in alcohol and in acetone; very slightly soluble in water; insoluble in fixed oils.

Penicillin V Benzathine: Practically white powder, having a characteristic odor. Sparingly soluble in chloroform; slightly soluble in alcohol and in ether; very slightly soluble in water.

Penicillin V Potassium: White, odorless, crystalline powder. Very soluble in water; slightly soluble in alcohol; insoluble in acetone.

Pentamidine Isethionate: White or almost white powder or colorless crystals, hygroscopic. Freely soluble in water; sparingly soluble in alcohol; practically insoluble in methylene chloride.

Pentazocine: White or very pale, tan-colored powder. Freely soluble in chloroform; soluble in alcohol, in acetone, and in ether; sparingly soluble in benzene and in ethyl acetate; practically insoluble in water.

Pentazocine Hydrochloride: White, crystalline powder. It exhibits polymorphism, one form melting at about 254° and the other at about 218°. Freely soluble in chloroform; soluble in alcohol; sparingly soluble in water; very slightly soluble in acetone and in ether; practically insoluble in benzene.

Pentetic Acid: White, odorless or almost odorless powder. Melts with foaming and degradation at 220°. *NF category:* Chelating and/or complexing agent; antimicrobial preservative; sequestering agent.

Pentobarbital: White to practically white, fine, practically odorless powder. May occur in a polymorphic form that melts at about 116°. This form gradually reverts to the more stable higher-melting form upon being heated at about 110°. Very soluble in alcohol, in methanol, in ether, in chloroform, and in acetone; soluble in benzene; very slightly soluble in water and in carbon tetrachloride.

Pentobarbital Sodium: White, crystalline granules or white powder. Is odorless or has a slight characteristic odor, and has a slightly bitter taste. Its solutions decompose on standing, heat accelerating the decomposition. Very soluble in water; freely soluble in alcohol; practically insoluble in ether.

Pentoxifylline: White to almost white crystalline powder. Freely soluble in chloroform and in methanol; soluble in water; sparingly soluble in alcohol; slightly soluble in ether.

Peppermint: Has an aromatic, characteristic odor and a pungent taste, and produces a cooling sensation in the mouth. *NF category:* Flavors and fragrance.

Peppermint Oil: Colorless or pale yellow liquid, having a strong, penetrating, characteristic odor and a pungent taste, followed by a sensation of cold when air is drawn into the mouth. *NF category:* Flavors and fragrance.

Peppermint Spirit: A clear, colorless liquid with a peppermint fragrance. Freely soluble in methanol and in diethyl ether; soluble in water. *NF category:* Flavors and fragrance.

Peppermint Water: *NF category:* Vehicle (flavored and/or sweetened).

Perflubron: Clear, colorless, practically odorless liquid.

Pergolide Mesylate: White to off-white powder. Sparingly soluble in methanol; slightly soluble in water, in dehydrated alcohol, and in chloroform; very slightly soluble in acetone; practically insoluble in ether.

Perindopril Erbumine: White or off-white, crystalline powder; freely soluble in water and in alcohol; sparingly soluble in methylene chloride.

Perphenazine: White to creamy white, odorless powder. Freely soluble in alcohol and in chloroform; soluble in acetone; practically insoluble in water.

Pertussis Immune Globulin: Transparent or slightly opalescent liquid, practically colorless, free from turbidity or particles, and practically odorless. May develop a slight, granular deposit during storage. Is standardized for agglutinating activity with the U.S. Standard Antipertussis Serum.

Petrolatum: Unctuous yellowish to light amber mass, having not more than a slight fluorescence even after being melted. Is transparent in thin layers. Is free or practically free from odor and taste. Freely soluble in benzene, in carbon disulfide, in chloroform, and in turpentine oil; soluble in ether, in solvent hexane, and in most fixed and volatile oils; practically insoluble in cold and hot alcohol and in cold dehydrated alcohol; insoluble in water. *NF category:* Ointment base; emollient.

Hydrophilic Petrolatum: *NF category:* Ointment base.

White Petrolatum: White or faintly yellowish, unctuous mass, transparent in thin layers even after cooling to 0°. Freely soluble in benzene, in carbon disulfide, and in chloroform; soluble in ether, in solvent hexane, and in most fixed and volatile oils; slightly soluble in cold or hot alcohol, and in cold dehydrated alcohol; insoluble in water. *NF category:* Ointment base.

Phenazopyridine Hydrochloride: Light or dark red to dark violet, crystalline powder. Is odorless, or has a slight odor. Melts at about 235°, with decomposition. Slightly soluble in water, in alcohol, and in chloroform.

Phendimetrazine Tartrate: White, odorless, crystalline powder. Freely soluble in water; sparingly soluble in warm alcohol; insoluble in chloroform, in acetone, in ether, and in benzene. Phendimetrazine base is extracted by organic solvents from alkaline solution.

Phenelzine Sulfate: White to yellowish white powder, having a characteristic odor. Freely soluble in water; practically insoluble in alcohol, in chloroform, and in ether.

Pheniramine Maleate: White, crystalline powder having a faint amine-like odor. Soluble in water and in alcohol.

Phenmetrazine Hydrochloride: White to off-white, crystalline powder. Very soluble in water; freely soluble in alcohol and in chloroform.

Phenobarbital: White, odorless, glistening, small crystals, or white, crystalline powder, which may exhibit polymorphism. Is stable in air. Its saturated solution has a pH of about 5. Soluble in alcohol, in ether, and in solutions of fixed alkali hydroxides and carbonates; sparingly soluble in chloroform; very slightly soluble in water.

Phenobarbital Sodium: Flaky crystals, or white, crystalline granules, or white powder. Is odorless, has a bitter taste, and is hygroscopic. Its solutions are alkaline to phenolphthalein TS, and decompose on standing. Very soluble in water; soluble in alcohol; practically insoluble in ether and in chloroform.

Phenol: Colorless to light pink, interlaced or separate, needle-shaped crystals, or white to light pink, crystalline mass. Has a characteristic odor. Is liquefied by warming and by the addition of 10% of water. Boils at about 182°, and its vapor is flammable. Gradually darkens on exposure to light and air. Very soluble in alcohol, in glycerin, in chloroform, in ether, and in fixed and volatile oils; soluble in water; sparingly soluble in mineral oil. *NF category:* Antimicrobial preservative.

Liquefied Phenol: Colorless to pink liquid, which may develop a red tint upon exposure to air or light. Has a characteristic, somewhat aromatic odor. It whitens and cauterizes the skin and mucous membranes. Specific gravity is about 1.065. Miscible with alcohol, with ether, and with glycerin. A mixture of equal volumes of Liquefied Phenol and glycerin is miscible with water.

Camphorated Phenol Topical Gel: Clear, colorless, oily gel.

Phenolsulfonphthalein: A bright-red to dark-red, crystalline powder. Slightly soluble in alcohol; very slightly soluble in water.

Phenoxyethanol: A colorless, slightly viscous liquid. Slightly soluble in water, in peanut oil, and in olive oil. Miscible with acetone, with alcohol, and with glycerol. *NF category:* Antimicrobial preservative.

Phensuximide: White to off-white, crystalline powder. Is odorless, or has not more than a slight odor. Very soluble in chloroform; soluble in alcohol; slightly soluble in water.

Phentermine Hydrochloride: White, odorless, hygroscopic, crystalline powder. Soluble in water and in the lower alcohols; slightly soluble in chloroform; insoluble in ether.

Phentolamine Mesylate: White or off-white, odorless, crystalline powder. Its solutions are acid to litmus, having a pH of about 5, and slowly deteriorate. Melts at about 178°. Freely soluble in water and in alcohol; slightly soluble in chloroform.

Phenylalanine: White, odorless crystals, having a slightly bitter taste. Sparingly soluble in water; very slightly soluble in methanol, in alcohol, and in dilute mineral acids.

Phenylbenzimidazole Sulfonic Acid: White to ivory-colored, odorless powder. Soluble in alcohol; practically insoluble in oily solvents and in water. Its salts are freely soluble in water.

Phenylbutazone: White to off-white, odorless, crystalline powder. Freely soluble in acetone and in ether; soluble in alcohol; very slightly soluble in water.

Phenylephrine Bitartrate: White or almost white powder or colorless crystals. Freely soluble in water.

Phenylephrine Hydrochloride: White or practically white, odorless crystals, having a bitter taste. Freely soluble in water and in alcohol.

Phenylephrine Hydrochloride Nasal Solution: Clear, colorless or slightly yellow, odorless liquid. Is neutral or acid to litmus.

Phenylephrine Hydrochloride Ophthalmic Solution: Clear, colorless or slightly yellow liquid, depending on the concentration.

Phenylethyl Alcohol: Colorless liquid, having a rose-like odor and a sharp, burning taste. Very soluble in alcohol, in fixed oils, in glycerin, and in propylene glycol; sparingly soluble in water; slightly soluble in mineral oil. *NF category:* Antimicrobial preservative.

Phenylmercuric Acetate: White to creamy white, crystalline powder, or small white prisms or leaflets. Is odorless. Soluble in alcohol and in acetone; slightly soluble in water. *NF category:* Antimicrobial preservative.

Phenylmercuric Nitrate: White, crystalline powder. Is affected by light. Its saturated solution is acid to litmus.

Slightly soluble in alcohol and in glycerin; very slightly soluble in water. It is more soluble in the presence of either nitric acid or alkali hydroxides. *NF category:* Antimicrobial preservative.

Phenylpropanolamine Bitartrate: White, crystalline powder.

Phenylpropanolamine Hydrochloride: White, crystalline powder, having a slight aromatic odor. Is affected by light. Freely soluble in water and in alcohol; insoluble in ether.

Phenyltoloxamine Citrate: White, crystalline powder. Very soluble in boiling water; slightly soluble in cold water and in alcohol; practically insoluble in cold acetone, in ethyl ether, and in toluene.

Phenytoin: White, odorless powder. Melts at about 295°. Soluble in hot alcohol; slightly soluble in cold alcohol, in chloroform, and in ether; practically insoluble in water.

Phenytoin Sodium: White, odorless powder. Is somewhat hygroscopic and on exposure to air gradually absorbs carbon dioxide. Freely soluble in water, the solution usually being somewhat turbid due to partial hydrolysis and absorption of carbon dioxide; soluble in alcohol; practically insoluble in ether and in chloroform.

Sodium Phosphate P 32 Solution: Clear, colorless solution. Upon standing, both the Solution and the glass container may darken as a result of the effects of the radiation.

Phosphoric Acid: Colorless, odorless liquid of syrupy consistency. Specific gravity is about 1.71. Miscible with water and with alcohol. *NF category:* pH modifier (acidifying agent/alkalizing agent/buffering agent).

Diluted Phosphoric Acid: Clear, colorless, odorless liquid. Specific gravity is about 1.057. *NF category:* pH modifier (acidifying agent/alkalizing agent/buffering agent).

Physostigmine: White, odorless, microcrystalline powder. Acquires a red tint when exposed to heat, light, air, or contact with traces of metals. Melts at a temperature not lower than 103°. Very soluble in chloroform and in dichloromethane; freely soluble in alcohol; soluble in benzene and in fixed oils; slightly soluble in water.

Physostigmine Salicylate: White, shining, odorless crystals or white powder. Acquires a red tint when exposed to heat, light, air, or contact with traces of metals for long periods. Melts at about 184°. Freely soluble in chloroform; soluble in alcohol; sparingly soluble in water; slightly soluble in ether.

Physostigmine Sulfate: White, odorless, microcrystalline powder. Is deliquescent in moist air and acquires a red tint when exposed to heat, light, air, or contact with traces of metals for long periods. Melts at about 143°. Freely soluble in water; very soluble in alcohol; very slightly soluble in ether.

Phytonadione: Clear, yellow to amber, very viscous, odorless or practically odorless liquid, having a specific gravity of about 0.967. Is stable in air, but decomposes on exposure to sunlight. Soluble in dehydrated alcohol, in benzene, in chloroform, in ether, and in vegetable oils; slightly soluble in alcohol; insoluble in water.

Pilocarpine: A viscous, oily liquid, or crystals melting at about 34°. Exceedingly hygroscopic. Soluble in water, in alcohol, and in chloroform; sparingly soluble in ether and in benzene; practically insoluble in petroleum ether.

Pilocarpine Hydrochloride: Colorless, translucent, odorless, faintly bitter crystals. Is hygroscopic and is affected by light. Its solutions are acid to litmus. Very soluble in water; freely soluble in alcohol; slightly soluble in chloroform; insoluble in ether.

Pilocarpine Nitrate: Shining, white crystals. Is stable in air but is affected by light. Its solutions are acid to litmus. Freely soluble in water; sparingly soluble in alcohol; insoluble in chloroform and in ether.

Pimozide: White, crystalline powder. Freely soluble in chloroform; slightly soluble in ether and in alcohol; insoluble in water.

Pindolol: White to off-white, crystalline powder, having a faint odor. Slightly soluble in methanol; very slightly soluble in chloroform; practically insoluble in water.

Pioglitazone Hydrochloride: White crystals or crystalline powder. Soluble in dimethylformamide; slightly soluble in dehydrated alcohol; very slightly soluble in acetone and in acetonitrile; practically insoluble in water; insoluble in ether.

Piperacillin: White to off-white, crystalline powder. Very soluble in methanol; slightly soluble in isopropyl alcohol; very slightly soluble in ethyl acetate and practically insoluble to very slightly soluble in water.

Piperacillin Sodium: White to off-white solid. Freely soluble in water and in alcohol.

Piperazine: White to slightly off-white lumps or flakes, having an ammoniacal odor. Soluble in water and in alcohol; insoluble in ether.

Piperazine Adipate: White crystalline powder. Soluble in water; practically insoluble in alcohol.

Piperazine Citrate: White, crystalline powder, having not more than a slight odor. Its solution (1 in 10) has a pH of about 5. Soluble in water; insoluble in alcohol and in ether.

Piperazine Dihydrochloride: White crystalline powder. Soluble in water.

Piperazine Phosphate: White crystalline powder. Sparingly soluble in water; practically insoluble in alcohol.

Piroxicam: Off-white to light tan or light yellow, odorless powder. Forms a monohydrate that is yellow. Slightly soluble in alcohol and in aqueous alkaline solutions; very slightly soluble in water, in dilute acids, and in most organic solvents.

Plantago Seed: All varieties are practically odorless and have a bland, mucilaginous taste.

Plicamycin: Yellow, odorless, hygroscopic, crystalline powder. Freely soluble in ethyl acetate; slightly soluble in water and in methanol; very slightly soluble in alcohol.

Podophyllum: Has a slight odor and a disagreeably bitter and acrid taste.

Podophyllum Resin: Amorphous powder, varying in color from light brown to greenish yellow, turning darker when subjected to a temperature exceeding 25° or when exposed to light. Has a slight, peculiar, faintly bitter taste. Its alcohol solution is acid to moistened litmus paper. Soluble in alcohol with a slight opalescence; partially soluble in ether and in chloroform.

Polacrilin Potassium: White to off-white, free-flowing powder. Has a faint odor or is odorless. Insoluble in water and in most liquids. *NF category:* Disintegrant.

Poliovirus Vaccine Inactivated: Clear, reddish-tinged or yellowish liquid, that may have a slight odor because of the preservative.

Poloxalene: Colorless or pale yellow liquid. Soluble in water, in chloroform, and in ethylene dichloride.

Poloxamer: *NF category:* Wetting and/or solubilizing agent; emulsifying agent; lubricant.

Poloxamer 124: Colorless liquid, having a mild odor. When solidified, it melts at about 16°. Freely soluble in water, in alcohol, in isopropyl alcohol, in propylene glycol, and in xylene.

Poloxamer 188: White, prilled or cast solid. Is odorless, or has a very mild odor. Melts at about 52°. Freely soluble in water and in alcohol.

Poloxamer 237: White, prilled or cast solid. Is odorless, or has a very mild odor. Melts at about 49°. Freely soluble in water and in alcohol; sparingly soluble in isopropyl alcohol and in xylene.

Poloxamer 338: White, prilled or cast solid. Is odorless, or has a very mild odor. Melts at about 57°. Freely soluble in water and in alcohol; sparingly soluble in propylene glycol.

Poloxamer 407: White, prilled or cast solid. Is odorless, or has a very mild odor. Melts at about 56°. Freely soluble in water, in alcohol, and in isopropyl alcohol.

Polycarbophil: White to creamy white granules, having a characteristic, ester-like odor. Swells in water to a range of volumes, depending primarily on the pH. Insoluble in water, in dilute acids, in dilute alkalies, and in common organic solvents. *NF category:* Emulsifying agent; suspending and/or viscosity-increasing agent; wet binder.

Hydrogenated Polydecene: Clear, colorless, odorless, tasteless liquid. Very slightly soluble in water. *NF category:* Emollient; ointment base; solvent; vehicle (oleaginous).

Polydextrose: Off-white to light tan-colored solid. Very soluble in water; soluble in alcohol; slightly soluble in glycerin and in propylene glycol. *NF category:* Bulking agent; humectant; coating agent; suspending and/or viscosity-increasing agent; diluent.

Hydrogenated Polydextrose: Off-white to light tan-colored solid. Very soluble in water; soluble in alcohol; slightly soluble in glycerin and in propylene glycol. *NF category:* Bulking agent; coating agent; humectant; suspending and/or viscosity-increasing agent; wet binder.

Polyethylene Glycol: Polyethylene Glycol is usually designated by a number that corresponds approximately to its average molecular weight. As the average molecular weight increases, the water solubility, vapor pressure, hygroscopicity, and solubility in organic solvents decrease, while congealing temperature, specific gravity, flash point, and viscosity increase. Liquid grades occur as clear to slightly hazy, colorless or practically colorless, slightly hygroscopic, viscous liquids, having a slight, characteristic odor, and a specific gravity at 25° of about 1.12. Solid grades occur as practically odorless and tasteless, white, waxy, plastic material having a consistency similar to beeswax, or as creamy white flakes, beads, or powders. The accompanying table states the approximate congealing temperatures that are characteristic of commonly available grades. Liquid grades are miscible with water; solid grades are freely soluble in water; and all are soluble in acetone, in alcohol, in chloroform, in ethylene glycol monoethyl ether, in ethyl acetate, and in toluene; all are insoluble in ether and in hexane. *NF category:* Coating agent; plasticizer; solvent; suppository base; lubricant; film-forming agent; ointment base; diluent.

Nominal Molecular Weight Polyethylene Glycol	Approximate Congealing Temperature (°)
300	−11
400	6
600	20
900	34
1000	38
1450	44
4500	58
8000	60

Polyethylene Glycol 3350: White granular, powder, or flake. Approximate congealing temperature: 56°. Freely soluble in water; soluble in acetone, in alcohol, in chloroform, in ethylene glycol monoethyl ether, in ethyl acetate, and in toluene; insoluble in ether and in hexane. *NF category:* Coating agent; diluent; film-forming agent; lubricant; ointment base; plasticizer; solvent; suppository base.

Polyethylene Glycol Monomethyl Ether: Polyethylene Glycol Monomethyl Ether is usually designated by a number that corresponds approximately to its average molecular weight. As the average molecular weight increases, the water solubility, vapor pressure, hygroscopicity, and solubility in organic solvents decrease, while congealing temperature, specific gravity, flash point, and viscosity increase. Liquid grades occur as clear to slightly hazy, colorless or practically colorless, slightly hygroscopic, viscous liquids, having a slight, characteristic odor, and a specific gravity at 25° of about 1.09–1.10. Solid grades occur as practically odorless and tasteless, white, waxy, plastic material having a consistency similar to beeswax, or as creamy white flakes, beads, or powders. The accompanying table states the approximate congealing temperatures that are characteristic of commonly available grades. Liquid grades are miscible with water; solid grades are freely soluble in water; and all are soluble in acetone, in alcohol, in chloroform, in ethylene glycol monoethyl ether, in ethyl acetate, and in toluene; all are insoluble in ether and in hexane. *NF category:* Ointment base; solvent; plasticizer.

Nominal Molecular Weight Polyethylene Glycol Monomethyl Ether	Approximate Congealing Temperature (°)
350	−7
550	17
750	28
1000	35
2000	51
5000	59
8000	60
10000	61

Polyethylene Oxide: Polyethylene oxide resins are high molecular weight polymers having the common structure:

$$(-O-CH_2CH_2-)_n$$

in which *n*, the degree of polymerization, varies from about 2000 to over 100,000. Polyethylene oxide, being a polyether, strongly hydrogen, bonds with water. It is nonionic and undergoes salting-out effects associated with neutral molecules in solutions of high dielectric media. Salting-out effects manifest themselves in depressing the upper temperature limit of solubility, and in reducing the viscosity of both dilute and concentrated solutions of the polymers. All molecular weight grades are powdered or granular solids. They are soluble in water but, because of the high solution viscosities obtained (see *table*), solutions over 1% in water may be difficult to prepare. The water solubility, hygroscopicity, solubility in organic solvents, and melting point do not vary in the specified molecular weight range. At room temperature polyethylene oxide is miscible with water in all proportions. At concentrations of about 20% polymer in water, the solutions are nontacky, reversible, elastic gels. At higher concentrations, the solutions are tough, elastic materials with the water acting as a plasticizer. Polyethylene oxide is also freely soluble in acetonitrile, in ethylene dichloride, in trichloroethylene, and in methylene chloride. Heating may be required to obtain solutions in many other organic solvents. It is insoluble in aliphatic hydrocarbons, in ethylene glycol, in diethylene glycol, and in glycerol. *NF category:* Suspending and/or viscosity-increasing agent; wet binder; coating agent; release-modifying agent.

Approximate Molecular Weight	Typical Solution Viscosity (cps), 25°	
	5% Solution	1% Solution
100,000	40	
200,000	100	
300,000	800	
400,000	3000	
600,000	6000	
900,000	15,000	
4,000,000		3500
5,000,000		5500

Polyethylene 50 Stearate: *NF category:* Emulsifying and/or solubilizing agent.

Polyglyceryl 3 Diisostearate: Viscous liquid. Soluble in alcohol, in methylene chloride, in mineral oil, and in vegetable oils; insoluble in water. *NF category:* Emulsifying agent; ointment base.

Polyglyceryl Dioleate: Viscous liquid. Soluble in methylene chloride, in mineral oil, and in vegetable oils; sparingly soluble in alcohol; insoluble in water. *NF category:* Emulsifying agent.

Polyisobutylene: Low molecular-weight grades are soft and gummy; high molecular-weight grades are tough and elastic. All grades are light in color, odorless, and tasteless. Soluble in diisobutylene, in toluene, and in chloroform; insoluble in water. *NF category:* Adhesive.

Polymyxin B Sulfate: White to buff-colored powder. Is odorless or has a faint odor. Freely soluble in water; slightly soluble in alcohol.

Polyoxyl Lauryl Ether: A material with 3–5 oxyethylene units per molecule is a colorless liquid. Soluble or dispersible in alcohol; practically insoluble in water and in hexane. A material with 9–23 oxyethylene units per molecule is a white, waxy mass. Soluble or dispersible in water; soluble in alcohol; practically insoluble in hexane. *NF category:* Emulsifying agent; wetting and/or solubilizing agent.

Polyoxyl Oleate: A slightly yellowish, viscous liquid. Dispersible in water and in oils. Soluble in alcohol and in isopropyl alcohol. Miscible with fatty oils and with waxes. Its refractive index is about 1.466.

Polyoxyl 10 Oleyl Ether: White, soft semisolid, or pale yellow liquid, having a bland odor. Soluble in water and in alcohol. Dispersible in mineral oil and in propylene glycol, with possible separation on standing. *NF category:* Emulsifying agent; lubricant; wetting and/or solubilizing agent.

Polyoxyl 15 Hydroxystearate: Yellowish to white waxy mass. Very soluble in water; soluble in alcohol and in 2-propanol; insoluble in mineral oil. It solidifies at 25°. *NF category:* Wetting and/or solubilizing agent; vehicle (oleaginous); lubricant; emulsifying agent.

Polyoxyl 20 Cetostearyl Ether: Cream-colored, waxy, unctuous mass, melting, when heated, to a clear brownish-yellow liquid. Soluble in water, in alcohol, and in acetone; insoluble in solvent hexane. *NF category:* Wetting and/or solubilizing agent; emulsifying agent; lubricant.

Polyoxyl 35 Castor Oil: Yellow, oily liquid, having a faint, characteristic odor and a somewhat bitter taste. Very soluble in water, producing a practically odorless and colorless solution; soluble in alcohol and in ethyl acetate; insoluble in mineral oils. *NF category:* Wetting and/or solubilizing agent; emulsifying agent; lubricant.

Polyoxyl 40 Hydrogenated Castor Oil: White to yellowish paste or pasty liquid, having a faint odor and a slight taste. Very soluble in water, producing a practically tasteless, odorless, and colorless solution; soluble in alcohol and in ethyl acetate; insoluble in mineral oils. *NF category:* Wetting and/or solubilizing agent; emulsifying agent; lubricant.

Polyoxyl 40 Stearate: Waxy, white to light tan solid. Is odorless or has a faint, fat-like odor. Soluble in water, in alcohol, in ether, and in acetone; insoluble in mineral oil and in vegetable oils. *NF category:* Wetting and/or solubilizing agent; emulsifying agent; lubricant.

Polyoxyl Stearate: White or slightly yellowish waxy mass. Soluble in alcohol and in isopropyl alcohol. Polyoxyl stearate corresponding to a product with 6–8 units of ethylene oxide per molecule is soluble in fatty oils and in waxes; practically insoluble in water. Polyoxyl stearate corresponding to a product with 20–100 units of ethylene oxide per molecule is soluble in water; practically insoluble in fatty oils and in waxes. *NF category:* Emulsifying agent; wetting and/or solubilizing agent.

Polyoxyl Stearyl Ether: A white to yellowish-white, waxy, unctuous mass, pellets, microbeads, or flakes. Polyoxyl Stearyl Ether with 2 oxyethylene units per molecule is soluble in alcohol, with heating, and in methylene chloride; practically insoluble in water. Polyoxyl Stearyl Ether with 10 oxyethylene units per molecule is soluble in water and in alcohol. Polyoxyl Stearyl Ether with 20 oxethylene units per molecule is soluble in water, in alcohol, and in methylene chloride. After melting, it solidifies at about 45°. *NF category:* Emulsifying agent; wetting and/or solubilizing agent.

Polysorbate 20: Lemon to amber liquid having a faint characteristic odor. Soluble in water, in alcohol, in ethyl acetate, in methanol, and in dioxane; insoluble in mineral oil. *NF category:* Wetting and/or solubilizing agent; emulsifying agent; lubricant; suspending and/or viscosity-increasing agent.

Polysorbate 40: Yellow liquid having a faint, characteristic odor. Soluble in water and in alcohol; insoluble in mineral oil and in vegetable oils. *NF category:* Wetting and/or solubilizing agent; emulsifying agent; lubricant; suspending and/or viscosity-increasing agent.

Polysorbate 60: Lemon- to orange-colored, oily liquid or semi-gel having a faint, characteristic odor. Soluble in water, in ethyl acetate, and in toluene; insoluble in mineral oil and in vegetable oils. *NF category:* Emulsifying agent; lubricant; suspending and/or viscosity-increasing agent; wetting and/or solubilizing agent.

Polysorbate 80: Lemon- to amber-colored, oily liquid having a faint, characteristic odor and a warm, somewhat bitter taste. Very soluble in water, producing an odorless and practically colorless solution; soluble in alcohol and in ethyl acetate; insoluble in mineral oil. *NF category:* Wetting and/or solubilizing agent; emulsifying agent; lubricant; suspending and/or viscosity-increasing agent.

Polyvinyl Acetate: White or off-white powder or colorless granules or beads. Freely soluble in ethyl acetate; soluble in alcohol, in acetone, and in chloroform; practically insoluble in water. It is hygroscopic and swells in water. *NF category:* Coating agent; desiccant; wet binder; film-forming agent.

Polyvinyl Acetate Dispersion: Opaque, white or off-white, slightly viscous liquid. Miscible with water and with ethanol. It is sensitive to spoilage by microbial contaminants. *NF category:* Coating agent; film-forming agent; release-modifying agent.

Polyvinyl Acetate Phthalate: Free-flowing white powder. May have a slight odor of acetic acid. Soluble in methanol and in alcohol; insoluble in water, in methylene chloride, and in chloroform. *NF category:* Coating agent; film-forming agent.

Polyvinyl Alcohol: White to cream-colored granules, or white to cream-colored powder. Is odorless. Freely soluble in water at room temperature. Solution may be effected more rapidly at somewhat higher temperatures. *NF category:* Suspending and/or viscosity-increasing agent; coating agent; film-forming agent; polymers for ophthalmic use.

Sulfurated Potash: Irregular, liver-brown pieces when freshly made, changing to a greenish yellow. Has an odor of hydrogen sulfide and a bitter, acrid, and alkaline taste, and decomposes on exposure to air. A solution (1 in 10) is light brown in color and is alkaline to litmus. Freely soluble in water, usually leaving a slight residue. Alcohol dissolves only the sulfides.

Potassium Acetate: Colorless, monoclinic crystals or white, crystalline powder having a saline and slightly alkaline taste. Is odorless, or has a faint acetous odor. Deliquesces on exposure to moist air. Very soluble in water; freely soluble in alcohol.

Potassium Alginate: White to yellow, fibrous or granular powder. Dissolves in water to form a viscous, colloidal solution; insoluble in alcohol and in hydroalcoholic solutions in which the alcohol content is greater than 30% by weight;

insoluble in chloroform, in ether, and in acids having a pH lower than about 3. *NF category:* Emulsifying agent; suspending and/or viscosity-increasing agent.

Potassium Benzoate: White, odorless, or practically odorless, granular or crystalline powder. Is stable in air. Freely soluble in water; soluble in 90% alcohol; sparingly soluble in alcohol. *NF category:* Antimicrobial preservative; lubricant.

Potassium Bicarbonate: Colorless, transparent, monoclinic prisms or as a white, granular powder. Is odorless, and is stable in air. Its solutions are neutral or alkaline to phenolphthalein TS. Freely soluble in water; practically insoluble in alcohol. *NF category:* pH modifier (acidifying agent/alkalizing agent/buffering agent).

Potassium Bitartrate: Colorless or slightly opaque crystals, or white, crystalline powder. A saturated solution is acid to litmus. Soluble in boiling water; slightly soluble in water; very slightly soluble in alcohol.

Potassium Bromide: White, crystalline powder or colorless, cubical crystals. Freely soluble in water and in glycerol; slightly soluble in alcohol.

Potassium Chloride: Colorless, elongated, prismatic, or cubical crystals, or white, granular powder. Is odorless, has a saline taste, and is stable in air. Its solutions are neutral to litmus. Freely soluble in water; insoluble in alcohol. *NF category:* Tonicity agent.

Potassium Citrate: Transparent crystals or white, granular powder. Is odorless, has a cooling, saline taste, and is deliquescent when exposed to moist air. Freely soluble in water; very slightly soluble in alcohol. *NF category:* pH modifier (acidifying agent/alkalizing agent/buffering agent); chelating and/or complexing agent.

Potassium Gluconate: White to yellowish-white, crystalline powder or granules. Is odorless, has a slightly bitter taste, and is stable in air. Its solutions are slightly alkaline to litmus. Freely soluble in water; practically insoluble in dehydrated alcohol, in ether, in benzene, and in chloroform.

Potassium Hydroxide: White or practically white, fused masses, or small pellets, or flakes, or sticks, or other forms. Is hard and brittle and shows a crystalline fracture. Exposed to air, it rapidly absorbs carbon dioxide and moisture, and deliquesces. Very soluble in boiling alcohol; freely soluble in water, in alcohol, and in glycerin. *NF category:* pH modifier (acidifying agent/alkalizing agent/buffering agent).

Potassium Iodide: Hexahedral crystals, either transparent and colorless or somewhat opaque and white, or a white, granular powder. Is slightly hygroscopic. Its solutions are neutral or alkaline to litmus. Very soluble in water and even more soluble in boiling water; freely soluble in glycerin; soluble in alcohol.

Potassium Iodide Oral Solution: Clear, colorless, odorless liquid, having a characteristic, strongly salty taste. Is neutral or alkaline to litmus. Specific gravity is about 1.70.

Potassium Metabisulfite: White or colorless, free-flowing crystals, crystalline powder, or granules, usually having an odor of sulfur dioxide. Gradually oxidizes in air to the sulfate. Its solutions are acid to litmus. Soluble in water; insoluble in alcohol. *NF category:* Antioxidant; antimicrobial preservative.

Potassium Metaphosphate: White, odorless powder. Soluble in dilute solutions of sodium salts; insoluble in water. *NF category:* pH modifier (acidifying agent/alkalizing agent/buffering agent).

Potassium Nitrate: White, crystalline powder or colorless crystals. Very soluble in boiling water; freely soluble in water; soluble in glycerin; practically insoluble in alcohol.

Potassium Permanganate: Dark purple crystals, almost opaque by transmitted light and of a blue metallic luster by reflected light. Its color is sometimes modified by a dark bronze-like appearance. Is stable in air. Freely soluble in boiling water; soluble in water.

Dibasic Potassium Phosphate: Colorless or white, somewhat hygroscopic, granular powder. The pH of a solution (1 in 20) is about 8.5 to 9.6. Freely soluble in water; very slightly soluble in alcohol. *NF category:* pH modifier (acidifying agent/alkalizing agent/buffering agent).

Monobasic Potassium Phosphate: Colorless crystals or white, granular or crystalline powder. Is odorless, and is stable in air. The pH of a solution (1 in 100) is about 4.5. Freely soluble in water; practically insoluble in alcohol. *NF category:* pH modifier (acidifying agent/alkalizing agent/buffering agent).

Potassium Sodium Tartrate: Colorless crystals or white, crystalline powder, having a cooling, saline taste. As it effloresces slightly in warm, dry air, the crystals are often coated with a white powder. Freely soluble in water; practically insoluble in alcohol.

Potassium Sorbate: White crystals or powder, having a characteristic odor. Melts at about 270°, with decomposition. Freely soluble in water; soluble in alcohol. *NF category:* Antimicrobial preservative.

Povidone: White to slightly creamy white powder. Is hygroscopic. Freely soluble in water, in methanol, and in alcohol; slightly soluble in acetone; practically insoluble in ether. *NF category:* Suspending and/or viscosity-increasing agent; wet binder; polymers for ophthalmic use.

Povidone-Iodine: Yellowish-brown to reddish-brown, amorphous powder, having a slight, characteristic odor. Its solution is acid to litmus. Soluble in water and in alcohol; practically insoluble in chloroform, in carbon tetrachloride, in ether, in solvent hexane, and in acetone.

Povidone-Iodine Topical Aerosol Solution: The liquid obtained from Povidone-Iodine Topical Aerosol Solution is transparent, having a reddish brown color.

Pralidoxime Chloride: White to pale-yellow, crystalline powder. Is odorless and is stable in air. Freely soluble in water.

Pramipexole Dihydrochloride: White to almost white crystalline powder. Freely soluble in water; soluble in methanol; slightly soluble in alcohol; practically insoluble in methylene chloride.

Pramoxine Hydrochloride: White to practically white, crystalline powder, having a numbing taste. May have a slight aromatic odor. The pH of a solution (1 in 100) is about 4.5. Freely soluble in water and in alcohol; soluble in chloroform; very slightly soluble in ether.

Add the following:

▲**Prasugrel Hydrochloride:** White to almost-white powder. Soluble in water; slightly soluble in acetonitrile; practically insoluble in ethyl acetate.▲*USP41*

Pravastatin Sodium: White to yellowish white, hygroscopic powder. Freely soluble in water and in methanol; soluble in dehydrated alcohol; practically insoluble in acetonitrile and in chloroform.

Praziquantel: White or practically white, crystalline powder; odorless or having a faint characteristic odor. Freely soluble in alcohol and in chloroform; very slightly soluble in water.

Prazosin Hydrochloride: White to tan powder. Slightly soluble in water, in methanol, in dimethylformamide, and in dimethylacetamide; very slightly soluble in alcohol; practically insoluble in chloroform and in acetone.

Prednicarbate: White to almost white, crystalline powder. Freely soluble in acetone and in alcohol; sparingly soluble in propylene glycol; practically insoluble in water.

Prednisolone: White to practically white, odorless, crystalline powder. Melts at about 235°, with some decomposition (see *Melting Range or Temperature* ⟨741⟩). Soluble in methanol and in dioxane; sparingly soluble in acetone and

in alcohol; slightly soluble in chloroform; very slightly soluble in water.

Prednisolone Acetate: White to practically white, odorless, crystalline powder. Melts at about 235°, with some decomposition (see *Melting Range or Temperature* ⟨741⟩). Slightly soluble in acetone, in alcohol, and in chloroform; practically insoluble in water.

Prednisolone Hemisuccinate: Fine, creamy white powder with friable lumps; practically odorless. Melts at about 205°, with decomposition. Freely soluble in alcohol; soluble in acetone; very slightly soluble in water.

Prednisolone Sodium Phosphate: White or slightly yellow, friable granules or powder. Is odorless or has a slight odor. Is slightly hygroscopic. Freely soluble in water; soluble in methanol; slightly soluble in alcohol and in chloroform; very slightly soluble in acetone and in dioxane.

Prednisolone Sodium Succinate for Injection: Creamy white powder with friable lumps, having a slight odor.

Prednisolone Tebutate: White to slightly yellow, free-flowing powder, which may show some soft lumps. Is odorless or has not more than a moderate, characteristic odor. Is hygroscopic. Freely soluble in chloroform and in dioxane; soluble in acetone; sparingly soluble in alcohol and in methanol; very slightly soluble in water.

Prednisone: White to practically white, odorless, crystalline powder. Melts at about 230°, with some decomposition (see *Melting Range or Temperature* ⟨741⟩). Slightly soluble in alcohol, in chloroform, in dioxane, and in methanol; very slightly soluble in water.

Pregabalin: White to off-white, crystalline solid. Freely soluble in water and in both basic and acidic aqueous solutions.

Prilocaine: White or almost white powder or crystal aggregates. Very soluble in alcohol and in acetone; slightly soluble in water.

Prilocaine Hydrochloride: White, odorless, crystalline powder, having a bitter taste. Freely soluble in water and in alcohol; slightly soluble in chloroform; very slightly soluble in acetone; practically insoluble in ether.

Primaquine Phosphate: Orange-red, crystalline powder. Is odorless and has a bitter taste. Its solutions are acid to litmus. Melts at about 200°. Soluble in water; insoluble in chloroform and in ether.

Primidone: White, crystalline powder. Is odorless and has a slightly bitter taste. Slightly soluble in alcohol; very slightly soluble in water and in most organic solvents.

Probucol: White to off-white, crystalline powder. Freely soluble in chloroform and in *n*-propyl alcohol; soluble in alcohol and in solvent hexane; insoluble in water.

Probenecid: White or practically white, fine, crystalline powder. Is practically odorless. Soluble in dilute alkali, in chloroform, in alcohol, and in acetone; practically insoluble in water and in dilute acids.

Procainamide Hydrochloride: White to tan, crystalline powder. Is odorless. Its solution (1 in 10) has a pH between 5 and 6.5. Very soluble in water; soluble in alcohol; slightly soluble in chloroform; very slightly soluble in benzene and in ether.

Procainamide Hydrochloride Injection: Colorless, or having not more than a slight yellow color.

Procaine Hydrochloride: Small, white crystals or white, crystalline powder. Is odorless. Exhibits local anesthetic properties when placed on the tongue. Freely soluble in water; soluble in alcohol; slightly soluble in chloroform; practically insoluble in ether.

Procaine Hydrochloride Injection: Clear, colorless liquid.

Prochlorperazine: Clear, pale yellow, viscous liquid. Is sensitive to light. Freely soluble in alcohol, in chloroform, and in ether; very slightly soluble in water.

Prochlorperazine Edisylate: White to very light yellow, odorless, crystalline powder. Its solutions are acid to litmus. Freely soluble in water; very slightly soluble in alcohol; insoluble in ether and in chloroform.

Prochlorperazine Maleate: White or pale yellow, practically odorless, crystalline powder. Its saturated solution is acid to litmus. Slightly soluble in warm chloroform; practically insoluble in water and in alcohol.

Procyclidine Hydrochloride: White, crystalline powder, having a moderate, characteristic odor. Melts at about 225°, with decomposition. Soluble in water and in alcohol; insoluble in ether and in acetone.

Progesterone: White or creamy white, odorless, crystalline powder. Is stable in air. Soluble in alcohol, in acetone, and in dioxane; sparingly soluble in vegetable oils; practically insoluble in water.

Proguanil Hydrochloride: White, crystalline powder. Sparingly soluble in alcohol; slightly soluble in water; practically insoluble in methylene chloride.

Proline: White, odorless crystals, having a slightly sweet taste. Freely soluble in water and in absolute alcohol; insoluble in ether, in butanol, and in isopropanol.

Promazine Hydrochloride: White to slightly yellow, practically odorless, crystalline powder. It oxidizes upon prolonged exposure to air and acquires a blue or pink color. Freely soluble in water and in chloroform.

Promethazine Hydrochloride: White to faint yellow, practically odorless, crystalline powder. Slowly oxidizes, and acquires a blue color, on prolonged exposure to air. Freely soluble in water, in hot dehydrated alcohol, and in chloroform; practically insoluble in ether, in acetone, and in ethyl acetate.

Propafenone Hydrochloride: White powder. Soluble in methanol and in hot water; slightly soluble in alcohol and in chloroform; very slightly soluble in acetone; insoluble in diethyl ether and in toluene.

Propane: Colorless, flammable gas (boiling temperature is about −42°). One hundred volumes of water dissolves 6.5 volumes at 17.8° and 753 mm pressure; 100 volumes of anhydrous alcohol dissolves 790 volumes at 16.6° and 754 mm pressure; 100 volumes of ether dissolves 926 volumes at 16.6° and 757 mm pressure; 100 volumes of chloroform dissolves 1299 volumes at 21.6° and 757 mm pressure. Vapor pressure at 21° is about 10290 mm of mercury (108 psig). *NF category:* Propellant.

Propanediol: Clear, colorless, hygroscopic liquid. *Specific Gravity* ⟨841⟩, *Method I*: 1.040–1.065. Soluble in water, in alcohol, in methyl alcohol, in isopropyl alcohol, in butyl alcohol, in acetone, in propylene glycol, and miscible with many polar solvents. *NF category:* Humectant; solvent; wetting and/or solubilizing agent.

Propantheline Bromide: White or practically white crystals. Is odorless and has a bitter taste. Melts at about 160°, with decomposition. Very soluble in water, in alcohol, and in chloroform; practically insoluble in ether and in benzene.

Proparacaine Hydrochloride: White to off-white, or faintly buff-colored, odorless, crystalline powder. Its solutions are neutral to litmus. Soluble in water, in warm alcohol, and in methanol; insoluble in ether and in benzene.

Proparacaine Hydrochloride Ophthalmic Solution: Colorless or faint yellow solution.

Propionic Acid: Oily liquid having a slight pungent, rancid odor. Miscible with water and with alcohol and various other organic solvents. *NF category:* pH modifier (acidifying agent/alkalizing agent/buffering agent); antimicrobial preservative; antioxidant.

Propofol: Clear, colorless to slightly yellowish liquid. Very soluble in methanol and in ethanol; slightly soluble in cyclohexane and in isopropyl alcohol; very slightly soluble in water.

Propoxycaine Hydrochloride: White, odorless, crystalline solid, which discolors on prolonged exposure to light and air. The pH of a solution (1 in 50) is about 5.4. Freely soluble in water; soluble in alcohol; sparingly soluble in ether; practically insoluble in acetone and in chloroform.

Propoxyphene Hydrochloride: White, crystalline powder. Is odorless, and has a bitter taste. Freely soluble in water; soluble in alcohol, in chloroform, and in acetone; practically insoluble in benzene and in ether.

Propoxyphene Napsylate: White powder, having essentially no odor, but having a bitter taste. Soluble in methanol, in alcohol, in chloroform, and in acetone; very slightly soluble in water.

Propranolol Hydrochloride: White to off-white, crystalline powder. Is odorless and has a bitter taste. Melts at about 164°. Soluble in water and in alcohol; slightly soluble in chloroform; practically insoluble in ether.

Propyl Gallate: White, crystalline powder having a very slight, characteristic odor. Freely soluble in alcohol; slightly soluble in water. *NF category:* Antioxidant.

Propylene Glycol: Clear, colorless, viscous liquid having a slight, characteristic taste. Is practically odorless. Absorbs moisture when exposed to moist air. Miscible with water, with acetone, and with chloroform. Soluble in ether and will dissolve many essential oils, but is immiscible with fixed oils. *NF category:* Humectant; plasticizer; solvent; antimicrobial preservative.

Propylene Glycol Alginate: White to yellowish fibrous or granular powder. Practically odorless and tasteless. Soluble in water, in solutions of dilute organic acids, and, depending on the degree of esterification, in hydroalcoholic mixture containing up to 60% by weight of alcohol to form stable, viscous colloidal solutions at a pH of 3. *NF category:* Suspending and/or viscosity-increasing agent; emulsifying agent.

Propylene Glycol Dicaprylate/Dicaprate: Clear, colorless or slightly yellow oily liquid at 20°. Soluble in fatty oils and in light petroleum; slightly soluble in dehydrated alcohol; practically insoluble in water. *NF category:* Emulsifying agent; vehicle.

Propylene Glycol Dilaurate: Clear, oily liquid at 20°. Colorless or slightly yellow. Very soluble in alcohol, in methanol, and in methylene chloride; practically insoluble in water. *NF category:* Emollient; emulsifying agent.

Propylene Glycol Monocaprylate: Clear, colorless, or slightly yellow, oily liquid at 20°. Very soluble in alcohol, in chloroform, and in methylene chloride; practically insoluble in water. *NF category:* Vehicle; emulsifying agent; diluent.

Propylene Glycol Monolaurate: Clear, oily liquid at 20°. Colorless or slightly yellow. Very soluble in alcohol, in methanol, and in methylene chloride; practically insoluble in water. *NF category:* Emollient; emulsifying agent.

Propylene Glycol Monostearate: White, wax-like solid or as white, wax-like beads or flakes. Has a slight, agreeable, fatty odor and taste. Soluble in organic solvents such as alcohol, mineral or fixed oils, benzene, ether, and acetone; insoluble in water, but may be dispersed in hot water with the aid of a small amount of soap or other suitable surface-active agent. *NF category:* Emulsifying agent.

Propylhexedrine: Clear, colorless liquid, having a characteristic, amine-like odor. Volatilizes slowly at room temperature. Absorbs carbon dioxide from the air, and its solutions are alkaline to litmus. Boils at about 205°. Very slightly soluble in water. Miscible with alcohol, with chloroform, and with ether.

Propyliodone: White or almost white, crystalline powder. Is odorless or has a faint odor. Soluble in acetone, in alcohol, and in ether; practically insoluble in water.

Propylparaben: Small, colorless crystals or white powder. Freely soluble in alcohol and in ether; slightly soluble in boiling water; very slightly soluble in water. *NF category:* Antimicrobial preservative.

Propylparaben Sodium: White powder. Is odorless and hygroscopic. Freely soluble in water; sparingly soluble in alcohol; insoluble in fixed oils. *NF category:* Antimicrobial preservative.

Propylthiouracil: White, powdery, crystalline substance. Is starch-like in appearance and to the touch, and has a bitter taste. Soluble in ammonium hydroxide and in alkali hydroxides; sparingly soluble in alcohol; slightly soluble in water, in chloroform, and in ether.

Protamine Sulfate Injection: Colorless solution, which may have the odor of a preservative.

Protamine Sulfate for Injection: White, odorless powder, having the characteristic appearance of solids dried from the frozen state.

Protein Hydrolysate Injection: Yellowish to reddish-amber, transparent liquid.

Protriptyline Hydrochloride: White to yellowish powder. Is odorless, or has not more than a slight odor. Melts at about 168°. Freely soluble in water, in alcohol, and in chloroform; practically insoluble in ether.

Pseudoephedrine Hydrochloride: Fine, white to off-white crystals or powder, having a faint characteristic odor. Very soluble in water; freely soluble in alcohol; slightly soluble in chloroform.

Pseudoephedrine Sulfate: White crystals or crystalline powder. Is odorless. Freely soluble in alcohol.

Pullulan: White powder. Freely soluble in water; practically insoluble in dehydrated alcohol. *NF category:* Coating agent; plasticizer; polymer membrane; sequestering agent; suspending and/or viscosity-increasing agent; wetting and/or solubilizing agent; bulking agent; diluent; disintegrant; wet binder; capsule shell; film-forming agent.

Pumice: Very light, hard, rough, porous, grayish masses or gritty, grayish powder. Is odorless and tasteless, and is stable in air. Practically insoluble in water; is not attacked by acids.

Pyrantel Pamoate: Yellow to tan solid. Soluble in dimethyl sulfoxide; slightly soluble in dimethylformamide; practically insoluble in water and in methanol.

Pyrazinamide: White to practically white, odorless or practically odorless, crystalline powder. Sparingly soluble in water; slightly soluble in alcohol, in ether, and in chloroform.

Pyrethrum Extract: Pale yellow liquid having a bland, flowery odor. Soluble in mineral oil and in most organic solvents; insoluble in water. *Pyrethrins I* denotes the group containing pyrethrin 1, cinerin 1, and jasmolin 1; *Pyrethrins II* denotes the group containing pyrethrin 2, cinerin 2, and jasmolin 2.

Pyridostigmine Bromide: White or practically white, crystalline powder, having an agreeable, characteristic odor. Is hygroscopic. Freely soluble in water, in alcohol, and in chloroform; slightly soluble in solvent hexane; practically insoluble in ether.

Pyridoxine Hydrochloride: White to practically white crystals or crystalline powder. Is stable in air, and is slowly affected by sunlight. Its solutions have a pH of about 3. Freely soluble in water; slightly soluble in alcohol; insoluble in ether.

Pyrilamine Maleate: White, crystalline powder, usually having a faint odor. Its solutions are acid to litmus. Very soluble in water; freely soluble in alcohol and in chloroform; slightly soluble in ether and in benzene.

Pyrimethamine: White, odorless, crystalline powder. Slightly soluble in acetone, in alcohol, and in chloroform; practically insoluble in water.

Pyrvinium Pamoate: Bright orange or orange-red to practically black, crystalline powder. Freely soluble in glacial acetic acid; slightly soluble in chloroform and in methoxyethanol; very slightly soluble in methanol; practically insoluble in water and in ether.

Pyrvinium Pamoate Oral Suspension: Dark red, opaque suspension of essentially very fine, amorphous particles or aggregates, usually less than 10 μm in size. Larger particles, some of which may be crystals, up to 100 μm in size also may be present.

Quazepam: Off-white to yellowish powder.

Quetiapine Fumarate: White to off-white crystalline powder. Soluble in 0.1 N hydrochloric acid; slightly soluble in water, in alcohol, and in methanol.

Quinapril Hydrochloride: White to off-white powder, with a pink cast at times. Freely soluble in aqueous solvents.

Quinidine Gluconate: White powder. Is odorless and has a very bitter taste. Freely soluble in water; slightly soluble in alcohol.

Quinidine Sulfate: Fine, needle-like, white crystals, frequently cohering in masses, or fine, white powder. Is odorless, and darkens on exposure to light. Its solutions are neutral or alkaline to litmus. Soluble in alcohol; sparingly soluble in chloroform; slightly soluble in water; insoluble in ether.

Quinine Sulfate: White, fine, needle-like crystals, usually lusterless, making a light and readily compressible mass. Is odorless. It darkens on exposure to light. Its saturated solution is neutral or alkaline to litmus. Freely soluble in alcohol at 80°, and in a mixture of 2 volumes of chloroform and 1 volume of dehydrated alcohol; sparingly soluble in water at 100°; slightly soluble in water, in alcohol, and in chloroform; very slightly soluble in ether.

Rabies Immune Globulin: Transparent or slightly opalescent liquid, practically colorless and practically odorless. May develop a slight, granular deposit during storage.

Rabies Vaccine: White to straw-colored, amorphous pellet, which may or may not become fragmented when shaken.

Racemethionine: Almost white, crystalline powder or small flakes. Sparingly soluble in water; very slightly soluble in alcohol. It dissolves in dilute acids and in dilute solutions of alkali hydroxides. It melts at about 270°. *NF category:* Antioxidant; pH modifier (acidifying agent/alkalizing agent/buffering agent); flavors and fragrance.

Racepinephrine: White to nearly white, crystalline, odorless powder, gradually darkening on exposure to light and air. With acids, it forms salts that are readily soluble in water, and the base may be recovered by the addition of ammonium hydroxide. Very slightly soluble in water and in alcohol; insoluble in ether, in chloroform, and in fixed and volatile oils.

Racepinephrine Hydrochloride: Fine, white, odorless powder. Darkens on exposure to light and air. Its solutions are acid to litmus. Melts at about 157°. Freely soluble in water; sparingly soluble in alcohol.

Raloxifene Hydrochloride: Almost white to pale yellow powder. Freely soluble in dimethylsulfoxide; slightly soluble to sparingly soluble in methanol; practically insoluble to very slightly soluble in water; practically insoluble in ether and in ethyl acetate.

Add the following:

▲**Raltegravir Potassium:** White to off-white powder. Soluble in water; slightly soluble in methanol; very slightly soluble in acetonitrile and in ethanol; insoluble in isopropyl alcohol.▲USP41

Ramipril: White to almost white crystalline powder. Freely soluble in methanol; sparingly soluble in water.

Ranitidine Hydrochloride: White to pale yellow, crystalline, practically odorless powder. Is sensitive to light and moisture. Melts at about 140°, with decomposition. Very soluble in water; sparingly soluble in alcohol.

Fully Hydrogenated Rapeseed Oil: White, waxy solid. Insoluble in water and in alcohol. *NF category:* Coating agent; stiffening agent.

Superglycerinated Fully Hydrogenated Rapeseed Oil: White solid. Insoluble in water and in alcohol. *NF category:* Coating agent; emulsifying agent; stiffening agent.

Purified Rayon: White, lustrous or dull, fine, soft, filamentous fibers, appearing under the microscope as round, oval, or slightly flattened translucent rods, straight or crimped, striate and with serrate cross-sectional edges. Is practically odorless and practically tasteless. Very soluble in ammoniated cupric oxide TS and in dilute sulfuric acid (3 in 5); insoluble in ordinary solvents.

Repaglinide: White to off-white solid. Melts at about 132° to 136°. Soluble in methanol.

Reserpine: White or pale buff to slightly yellowish, odorless, crystalline powder. Darkens slowly on exposure to light, but more rapidly when in solution. Freely soluble in acetic acid and in chloroform; slightly soluble in benzene; very slightly soluble in alcohol and in ether; insoluble in water.

Resorcinol: White, or practically white, needle-shaped crystals or powder. Has a faint, characteristic odor and a sweetish, followed by a bitter, taste. Acquires a pink tint on exposure to light and air. Its solution (1 in 20) is neutral or acid to litmus. Freely soluble in water, in alcohol, in glycerin, and in ether; slightly soluble in chloroform.

Ribavirin: White, crystalline powder. Freely soluble in water; slightly soluble in dehydrated alcohol.

Riboflavin: Yellow to orange-yellow, crystalline powder having a slight odor. Melts at about 280°. Its saturated solution is neutral to litmus. When dry, it is not appreciably affected by diffused light, but when in solution, light induces quite rapid deterioration, especially in the presence of alkalies. Soluble in dilute solutions of alkalies; very slightly soluble in water, in alcohol, and in isotonic sodium chloride solution; insoluble in ether and in chloroform.

Riboflavin 5′-Phosphate Sodium: Fine, orange-yellow, crystalline powder, having a slight odor. Sparingly soluble in water. When dry, it is not affected by diffused light, but when in solution, light induces deterioration rapidly. Is hygroscopic.

Rifabutin: Amorphous red-violet powder. Soluble in chloroform and in methanol; sparingly soluble in alcohol; very slightly soluble in water.

Rifampin: Red-brown, crystalline powder. Freely soluble in chloroform; soluble in ethyl acetate and in methanol; very slightly soluble in water.

Riluzole: White to slightly yellow powder or crystalline powder. Freely soluble in acetonitrile, in alcohol, and in methylene chloride; slightly soluble in hexane; very slightly soluble in water.

Rimexolone: White to off-white powder. Freely soluble in chloroform; sparingly soluble in methanol.

Risedronate Sodium: White to off-white powder. Soluble in water and in aqueous solutions; insoluble in common organic solvents.

Risperidone: White or almost white powder. Soluble in methylene chloride; sparingly soluble in alcohol; practically insoluble in water.

Ritodrine Hydrochloride: White to nearly white, odorless or practically odorless, crystalline powder. Melts at about 200°. Freely soluble in water and in alcohol; soluble in *n*-propyl alcohol; practically insoluble in ether.

Ritonavir: White to light tan powder. Freely soluble in methanol and in methylene chloride; very slightly soluble in acetonitrile; practically insoluble in water.

Rivastigmine Tartrate: White to off-white powder. Very soluble in water and in methanol; very slightly soluble in ethyl acetate.

Rizatriptan Benzoate: White to almost white crystalline powder. Soluble in water; sparingly soluble in alcohol; slightly soluble in methylene chloride.

Rocuronium Bromide: Almost white or pale yellow. Slightly hygroscopic powder. Freely soluble in water and in dehydrated alcohol.

Ropinirole Hydrochloride: Pale cream to yellow powder. Soluble in water.

Ropivacaine Hydrochloride: White, crystalline powder. Soluble in water.

Rose Oil: Colorless or yellow liquid, having the characteristic odor and taste of rose. At 25° is a viscous liquid. Upon gradual cooling, changes to a translucent, crystalline mass, easily liquefied by warming. *NF category:* Flavors and fragrance.

Rose Water Ointment: *NF category:* Ointment base.

Stronger Rose Water: Practically colorless and clear, having the pleasant odor and taste of fresh rose blossoms. Is free from empyreuma, mustiness, and fungal growths. *NF category:* Flavors and fragrance.

Rosiglitazone Maleate: White to off-white solid. Sparingly soluble in alcohol; slightly soluble in methylene chloride; practically insoluble to very slightly soluble in water.

Roxarsone: Pale yellow, crystalline powder. Freely soluble in acetic acid, in acetone, in alkalies, in methanol, and in dehydrated alcohol; soluble in boiling water; sparingly soluble in dilute mineral acids; slightly soluble in cold water; insoluble in ether and in ethyl acetate. Puffs up and deflagrates on heating.

Rubella Virus Vaccine Live: Solid having the characteristic appearance of substances dried from the frozen state. Undergoes loss of potency on exposure to sunlight. The Vaccine is to be constituted with a suitable diluent just prior to use.

Rufinamide: White, crystalline neutral powder. Slightly soluble in tetrahydrofuran and in methanol; very slightly soluble in alcohol and in acetonitrile; practically insoluble in water.

Saccharin: White crystals or white, crystalline powder. Is odorless or has a faint, aromatic odor. In dilute solution, it is intensely sweet. Its solutions are acid to litmus. Soluble in boiling water; sparingly soluble in alcohol; slightly soluble in water, in chloroform, and in ether. Is readily dissolved by dilute solutions of ammonia, by solutions of alkali hydroxides, and by solutions of alkali carbonates with the evolution of carbon dioxide. *NF category:* Sweetening agent.

Saccharin Calcium: White crystals or white, crystalline powder. Is odorless, or has a faint, aromatic odor, and has an intensely sweet taste even in dilute solutions. Its dilute solution is about 300 times as sweet as sucrose. Freely soluble in water. *NF category:* Sweetening agent.

Saccharin Sodium: White crystals or white, crystalline powder. Is odorless, or has a faint, aromatic odor, and has an intensely sweet taste even in dilute solutions. Its dilute solution is about 300 times as sweet as sucrose. When in powdered form, it usually contains about one-third the theoretical amount of water of hydration as a result of efflorescence. Freely soluble in water; sparingly soluble in alcohol. *NF category:* Sweetening agent.

Saccharin Sodium Oral Solution: Clear, colorless, odorless liquid, having a sweet taste.

Safflower Oil: Light yellow oil. Thickens and becomes rancid on prolonged exposure to air. Insoluble in water. Miscible with ether and with chloroform. *NF category:* Vehicle (oleaginous); emollient; solvent.

Salicylamide: White, practically odorless, crystalline powder. Freely soluble in ether and in solutions of alkalies; soluble in alcohol and in propylene glycol; slightly soluble in water and in chloroform.

Salicylic Acid: White crystals, usually in fine needles, or fluffy, white, crystalline powder. Has a sweetish, followed by an acrid, taste and is stable in air. The synthetic form is white and odorless. When prepared from natural methyl salicylate, it may have a slightly yellow or pink tint, and a faint, mint-like odor. Freely soluble in alcohol and in ether; soluble in boiling water; sparingly soluble in chloroform; slightly soluble in water and in benzene.

Salmeterol Xinafoate: White to off-white powder. Soluble in methanol; slightly soluble in alcohol, in isopropanol, and in chloroform; practically insoluble in water (pH 8), and in saline solution (0.9% w/w).

Scopolamine Hydrobromide: Colorless or white crystals or white, granular powder. Melts at about 197°, with decomposition. Is odorless, and slightly efflorescent in dry air. Freely soluble in water; soluble in alcohol; slightly soluble in chloroform; insoluble in ether.

Secobarbital: White, amorphous or crystalline, odorless powder, having a slightly bitter taste. Its saturated solution has a pH of about 5.6. Freely soluble in alcohol, in ether, and in solutions of fixed alkali hydroxides and carbonates; soluble in chloroform; very slightly soluble in water.

Secobarbital Sodium: White powder. Is odorless, has a bitter taste, and is hygroscopic. Its solutions decompose on standing, heat accelerating the decomposition. Very soluble in water; soluble in alcohol; practically insoluble in ether.

Selegiline Hydrochloride: White, odorless, crystalline powder. Freely soluble in water, in chloroform, and in methanol.

Selenium Sulfide: Reddish-brown to bright orange powder, having not more than a faint odor. Practically insoluble in water and in organic solvents.

Sennosides: Brownish powder.

Serine: White, odorless crystals, having a sweet taste. Soluble in water; practically insoluble in absolute alcohol and in ether.

Sertraline Hydrochloride: White or off-white crystalline powder. Sparingly soluble or slightly soluble in absolute alcohol; slightly soluble in water and in isopropanol; and slightly or very slightly soluble in acetone.

Sesame Oil: Pale yellow, oily liquid. Is practically odorless, and has a bland taste. Slightly soluble in alcohol. Miscible with ether, with chloroform, with solvent hexane, and with carbon disulfide. *NF category:* Solvent, vehicle (oleaginous).

Sevoflurane: Clear, colorless, volatile, nonflammable liquid. Slightly soluble in water. Miscible with alcohol, with chloroform, and with ether.

Shellac: *Orange Shellac*—Thin, hard, brittle, transparent, pale lemon-yellow to brownish orange flakes, having little or no odor; *Bleached Shellac*—Opaque, amorphous cream to yellow granules or coarse powder, having little or no odor. Soluble (very slowly) in alcohol, 85% to 95% (w/w), in ether, 13% to 15%, in benzene, 10% to 20%, in petroleum ether, 2% to 6%; soluble in aqueous solutions of ethanolamines, alkalies, and borax; sparingly soluble in oil of turpentine; insoluble in water. *NF category:* Coating agent; film-forming agent; release-modifying agent.

Sibutramine Hydrochloride Monohydrate: White to cream crystalline powder. Slightly soluble in pH 5.2 water.

Sildenafil Citrate: White or almost white slightly hygroscopic crystalline powder. Slightly soluble in water and in methanol; practically insoluble in hexane.

Dental-Type Silica: Fine, white, hygroscopic, odorless, amorphous powder, in which the diameter of the average particles ranges between 0.5 and 40 μm. Soluble in hot solutions of alkali hydroxides; insoluble in water, in alcohol, and in acid (except hydrofluoric acid). *NF category:* Glidant and/or anticaking agent; suspending and/or viscosity-increasing agent.

Hydrophobic Colloidal Silica: Light, fine, white or almost white, amorphous powder, not wettable by water. Dissolves slowly in hot solutions of alkali hydroxides. Practically insoluble in water and in mineral acids, except hydrofluoric acid. *NF category:* Glidant and/or anticaking agent; suspending and/or viscosity-increasing agent.

Purified Siliceous Earth: Very fine, white, light gray, or pale buff mixture of amorphous powder and lesser amounts of crystalline polymorphs, including quartz and cristobalite. Is gritty, readily absorbs moisture, and retains about four times its weight of water without becoming fluid. Insoluble in water, in acids, and in dilute solutions of the alkali hydroxides. *NF category:* Filtering aid; sorbent.

Silicon Dioxide: Fine, white, hygroscopic, odorless, amorphous powder, in which the diameter of the average particles ranges between 2 and 10 μm. Soluble in hot solutions of alkali hydroxides; insoluble in water, in alcohol, and in other organic solvents. *NF category:* Desiccant; suspending and/or viscosity-increasing agent.

Colloidal Silicon Dioxide: Light, white, nongritty powder of extremely fine particle size (about 15 nm). Soluble in hot solutions of alkali hydroxides; insoluble in water and in acid (except hydrofluoric). *NF category:* Glidant and/or anticaking agent; suspending and/or viscosity-increasing agent; disintegrant.

Silver Nitrate: Colorless or white crystals. The pH of its solutions is about 5.5. On exposure to light in the presence of organic matter, it becomes gray or grayish black. Very soluble in water and even more so in boiling water; freely soluble in boiling alcohol; sparingly soluble in alcohol; slightly soluble in ether.

Toughened Silver Nitrate: White, crystalline masses generally molded as pencils or cones. It breaks with a fibrous fracture. Its solutions are neutral to litmus. It becomes gray or grayish black upon exposure to light. Soluble in water to the extent of its nitrate content (there is always a residue of silver chloride); partially soluble in alcohol; slightly soluble in ether.

Simethicone: Translucent, gray, viscous fluid. The liquid phase is soluble in chloroform, in ether, and in benzene, but silicon dioxide remains as a residue in these solvents. Insoluble in water and in alcohol. *NF category:* Antifoaming agent; water-repelling agent; diluent.

Simvastatin: White to off-white powder. Freely soluble in chloroform, in methanol, and in alcohol; sparingly soluble in propylene glycol; very slightly soluble in hexane; practically insoluble in water.

Sitagliptin Phosphate: White or almost white powder. Soluble in water; very slightly soluble in anhydrous ethanol; practically insoluble in heptane.

Smallpox Vaccine: Liquid Vaccine is a turbid, whitish to greenish suspension, which may have a slight odor due to the antimicrobial agent. Dried Vaccine is a yellow to grayish pellet, which may or may not become fragmented when shaken.

Soda Lime: White or grayish-white granules. May have a color if an indicator has been added. *NF category:* Sorbent, carbon dioxide.

Sodium Acetate: Colorless, transparent crystals, or white, granular crystalline powder, or white flakes. Is odorless or has a faint acetous odor, and has a slightly bitter, saline taste. Is efflorescent in warm, dry air. Very soluble in water; soluble in alcohol. *NF category:* Flavors and fragrance; pH modifier (acidifying agent/alkalizing agent/buffering agent); antimicrobial preservative; transfer ligand.

Sodium Alginate: Practically odorless and tasteless, coarse or fine powder, yellowish white in color. Soluble in water, forming a viscous, colloidal solution; insoluble in alcohol and in hydroalcoholic solutions in which the alcohol content is greater than about 30% by weight, in chloroform, in ether, and in acids when the pH of the resulting solution becomes lower than about 3. *NF category:* Suspending and/or viscosity-increasing agent; film-forming agent; release-modifying agent; disintegrant; wet binder.

Sodium Ascorbate: White or very faintly yellow crystals or crystalline powder. Is odorless or practically odorless. Is relatively stable in air. On exposure to light it gradually darkens. Freely soluble in water; very slightly soluble in alcohol; insoluble in chloroform and in ether. *NF category:* Antioxidant.

Sodium Benzoate: White, odorless or practically odorless, granular or crystalline powder. Is stable in air. Freely soluble in water; soluble in 90% alcohol; sparingly soluble in alcohol. *NF category:* Antimicrobial preservative; lubricant.

Sodium Bicarbonate: White, crystalline powder. Is stable in dry air, but slowly decomposes in moist air. Its solutions, when freshly prepared with cold water, without shaking, are alkaline to litmus. The alkalinity increases as the solutions stand, as they are agitated, or as they are heated. Soluble in water; insoluble in alcohol. *NF category:* pH modifier (acidifying agent/alkalizing agent/buffering agent).

Sodium Bisulfite: White, crystalline powder. Freely soluble in cold water and in hot water; sparingly soluble in alcohol. *NF category:* Antioxidant.

Sodium Borate: Colorless, transparent crystals or white, crystalline powder. Is odorless. Its solutions are alkaline to phenolphthalein TS. As it effloresces in warm, dry air, the crystals are often coated with white powder. Freely soluble in boiling water and in glycerin; soluble in water; insoluble in alcohol. *NF category:* pH modifier (acidifying agent/alkalizing agent/buffering agent); antimicrobial preservative; emulsifying agent.

Sodium Bromide: White, crystalline powder or colorless, cubical crystals. Freely soluble in water; soluble in alcohol.

Sodium Butyrate: Clear, colorless, hygroscopic powder. Soluble in water and in methanol. Melting range is about 250° to 253°.

Sodium Caprylate: A white, crystalline powder. Very soluble or freely soluble in water; freely soluble in acetic acid; sparingly soluble in alcohol; practically insoluble in acetone.

Sodium Carbonate: Colorless crystals, or white, crystalline powder or granules. Is stable in air under ordinary conditions. When exposed to dry air above 50°, the hydrous salt effloresces and, at 100°, becomes anhydrous. Very soluble in boiling water; freely soluble in water. *NF category:* pH modifier (acidifying agent/alkalizing agent/buffering agent).

Sodium Cetostearyl Sulfate: A white or pale yellow, amorphous or crystalline powder. Soluble in hot water giving an opalescent solution; slightly soluble in alcohol; practically insoluble in cold water. *NF category:* Emulsifying agent.

Sodium Chloride: Colorless, cubic crystals or white crystalline powder. Has a saline taste. Freely soluble in water; soluble in glycerin; slightly soluble in alcohol. *NF category:* Tonicity agent; diluent.

Sodium Chloride Inhalation Solution: Clear, colorless solution.

Bacteriostatic Sodium Chloride Injection: Clear, colorless solution, odorless or having the odor of the bacteriostatic substance. *NF category:* Vehicle (sterile).

Sodium Chloride Irrigation: Clear, colorless solution.

Sodium Citrate: Colorless crystals, or white, crystalline powder. Hydrous form very soluble in boiling water; freely soluble in water; insoluble in alcohol. *NF category:* pH modifier (acidifying agent/alkalizing agent/buffering agent); sequestering agent; transfer ligand.

Sodium Citrate and Citric Acid Oral Solution: Clear solution having the color of any added preservative or flavoring agents.

Sodium Dehydroacetate: White or practically white, odorless powder, having a slight characteristic taste. Freely soluble in water, in propylene glycol, and in glycerin. *NF category:* Antimicrobial preservative.

Sodium Fluoride: White, odorless powder. Soluble in water; insoluble in alcohol.

Sodium Formaldehyde Sulfoxylate: White crystals or hard, white masses, having the characteristic odor of garlic. Freely soluble in water; slightly soluble in alcohol, in ether, in chloroform, and in benzene. *NF category:* Antioxidant.

Sodium Hydroxide: White, or practically white, fused masses, in small pellets, in flakes, or sticks, and in other forms. Is hard and brittle and shows a crystalline fracture. Exposed to the air, it rapidly absorbs carbon dioxide and moisture. Freely soluble in water and in alcohol. *NF category:* pH modifier (acidifying agent/alkalizing agent/buffering agent).

Sodium Hypochlorite Solution: Clear, pale greenish-yellow liquid, having the odor of chlorine. Is affected by light.

Sodium Iodide: Colorless, odorless crystals, or white, crystalline powder. Is deliquescent in moist air, and develops a brown tint upon decomposition. Very soluble in water; freely soluble in alcohol and in glycerin.

Sodium Lactate Solution: Clear, colorless or practically colorless, slightly viscous liquid, odorless or having a slight, not unpleasant odor. Miscible with water. *NF category:* pH modifier (acidifying agent/alkalizing agent/buffering agent); antimicrobial preservative; humectant; flavors and fragrance.

Sodium Lauryl Sulfate: Small, white or light yellow crystals having a slight, characteristic odor. Freely soluble in water, forming an opalescent solution. *NF category:* Emulsifying agent; lubricant; wetting and/or solubilizing agent.

Sodium Metabisulfite: White crystals or white to yellowish, crystalline powder, having the odor of sulfur dioxide. Freely soluble in water and in glycerin; slightly soluble in alcohol. *NF category:* Antioxidant; antimicrobial preservative.

Sodium Monofluorophosphate: White to slightly gray, odorless powder. Freely soluble in water.

Sodium Nitrite: White to slightly yellow, granular powder, or white or practically white, opaque, fused masses or sticks. Has a mild, saline taste and is deliquescent in air. Its solutions are alkaline to litmus. Freely soluble in water; sparingly soluble in alcohol.

Sodium Nitrite Injection: Clear, colorless liquid.

Sodium Nitroprusside: Reddish-brown, practically odorless, crystals or powder. Freely soluble in water; slightly soluble in alcohol; very slightly soluble in chloroform; insoluble in benzene.

Dibasic Sodium Phosphate (*dried*): White powder that readily absorbs moisture. Freely soluble in water; insoluble in alcohol. *NF category:* pH modifier (acidifying agent/alkalizing agent/buffering agent); chelating and/or complexing agent.

Dibasic Sodium Phosphate (*heptahydrate*): Colorless or white, granular or caked salt. Effloresces in warm, dry air. Its solutions are alkaline to phenolphthalein TS, a 0.1 M solution having a pH of about 9. Freely soluble in water; very slightly soluble in alcohol. *NF category:* Buffering agent.

Monobasic Sodium Phosphate: Colorless crystals or white, crystalline powder. Is odorless and is slightly deliquescent. Its solutions are acid to litmus and effervesce with sodium carbonate. Freely soluble in water; practically insoluble in alcohol. *NF category:* pH modifier (acidifying agent/alkalizing agent/buffering agent); chelating and/or complexing agent.

Tribasic Sodium Phosphate: The formula for a crystalline material is approximately $4(Na_3PO_4 \cdot 12H_2O)NaOH$. It occurs as white, odorless crystals or granules or as a crystalline powder. Freely soluble in water; insoluble in alcohol. The pH of a 1 in 100 solution is between 11.5 and 12.0.

Sodium Picosulfate: White or almost white crystalline powder. Freely soluble in water; slightly soluble in alcohol.

Sodium Polystyrene Sulfonate: Golden brown, fine powder. Is odorless and has a characteristic taste. Insoluble in water.

Sodium Propionate: Colorless, transparent crystals or granular, crystalline powder. Is odorless, or has a faint acetic-butyric odor and is deliquescent in moist air. Very soluble in water; soluble in alcohol. *NF category:* Antimicrobial preservative.

Sodium Salicylate: Amorphous or microcrystalline powder or scales. Is colorless, or has not more than a faint, pink tinge. Is odorless, or has a faint, characteristic odor, and is affected by light. A freshly made solution (1 in 10) is neutral or acid to litmus. Very soluble in boiling water and in boiling alcohol; freely (and slowly) soluble in water and in glycerin; slowly soluble in alcohol.

Sodium Starch Glycolate: White, tasteless, odorless, relatively free-flowing powder; available in several different viscosity grades. A 2% (w/v) dispersion in cold water settles, on standing, in the form of a highly hydrated layer. *NF category:* Disintegrant.

Sodium Stearate: Fine, white powder, soapy to the touch, usually having a slight, tallow-like odor. Is affected by light. Its solutions are alkaline to phenolphthalein TS. Slowly soluble in cold water and in cold alcohol; readily soluble in hot water and in hot alcohol. *NF category:* Emulsifying agent; glidant and/or anticaking agent; stiffening agent; lubricant.

Sodium Stearyl Fumarate: Fine, white powder. Slightly soluble in methanol; practically insoluble in water. *NF category:* Lubricant.

Sodium Succinate: White crystals or white powder. Freely soluble in water. *NF category:* Flavors and fragrance; pH modifier.

Sodium Sulfate: Large, colorless, odorless, transparent crystals, or a granular powder. Effloresces rapidly in air, liquefies in its water of hydration at about 33°, and loses all of its water of hydration at about 100°. Freely soluble in water; soluble in glycerin; insoluble in alcohol.

Sodium Sulfite: Colorless crystals. Freely soluble in water; very slightly soluble in alcohol. *NF category:* Antioxidant; antimicrobial preservative.

Sodium Tartrate: Transparent, colorless, odorless crystals. Freely soluble in water; insoluble in alcohol. *NF category:* Sequestering agent; transfer ligand.

Sodium Thiosulfate: Large, colorless crystals or coarse, crystalline powder. Is deliquescent in moist air and effloresces in dry air at temperatures exceeding 33°. Its solutions are neutral or faintly alkaline to litmus. Very soluble in water; insoluble in alcohol. *NF category:* Antioxidant.

Add the following:

■**Solifenacin Succinate:** White to pale, yellowish-white crystal or crystalline powder. Freely soluble in water and in methanol.■1S *(USP41)*

Sorbic Acid: Free-flowing, white, crystalline powder, having a characteristic odor. Soluble in alcohol and in ether; slightly soluble in water. *NF category:* Antimicrobial preservative.

Sorbitan Monolaurate: Yellow to amber-colored, oily liquid, having a bland, characteristic odor. Soluble in mineral oil; slightly soluble in cottonseed oil and in ethyl acetate; insoluble in water. *NF category:* Emulsifying agent; lubricant; suspending and/or viscosity-increasing agent; wetting and/or solubilizing agent.

Sorbitan Monooleate: Viscous, yellow to amber-colored, oily liquid, having a bland, characteristic odor. Insoluble in water and in propylene glycol. Miscible with mineral and vegetable oils. *NF category:* Emulsifying agent; lubricant; suspending and/or viscosity-increasing agent; wetting and/or solubilizing agent.

Sorbitan Monopalmitate: Cream-colored, waxy solid having a faint fatty odor. Soluble in warm absolute alcohol; soluble, with haze, in warm peanut oil and in warm mineral oil; insoluble in water. *NF category:* Emulsifying agent; lubricant; suspending and/or viscosity-increasing agent; wetting and/or solubilizing agent.

Sorbitan Monostearate: Cream-colored to tan, hard, waxy solid, having a bland odor and taste. Soluble, with haze, above 50° in mineral oil and in ethyl acetate; insoluble in cold water and in acetone. Dispersible in warm water. *NF category:* Emulsifying agent; lubricant; suspending and/or viscosity-increasing agent; wetting and/or solubilizing agent.

Sorbitan Sesquioleate: Viscous, yellow to amber-colored, oily liquid. Soluble in alcohol, in isopropyl alcohol, in cottonseed oil, and in mineral oil; insoluble in water and in propylene glycol. *NF category:* Emulsifying agent; lubricant; suspending and/or viscosity-increasing agent; wetting and/or solubilizing agent.

Sorbitan Trioleate: Yellow to amber-colored, oily liquid. Soluble in methyl alcohol, in alcohol, in isopropyl alcohol, in corn oil, in cottonseed oil, and in mineral oil; insoluble in water, in ethylene glycol, and in propylene glycol. *NF category:* Emulsifying agent; lubricant; suspending and/or viscosity-increasing agent; wetting and/or solubilizing agent.

Sorbitol: D-Sorbitol occurs as white granules, powder, or crystalline masses. Is odorless, and has a sweet taste with a cold sensation. Very soluble in water; sparingly soluble in alcohol; and practically insoluble in ethyl ether. Is hygroscopic. *NF category:* Humectant; sweetening agent; diluent; plasticizer.

Sorbitol Solution: Clear, colorless, syrupy liquid. Is odorless and has a sweet taste. It sometimes separates into crystalline masses. Miscible with water, with alcohol, with glycerin, and with propylene glycol. Is neutral to litmus. *NF category:* Sweetening agent; vehicle (flavored and/or sweetened).

Sorbitol Sorbitan Solution: A clear, colorless to pale yellow, syrupy liquid. Is odorless and has a sweet taste. Insoluble in mineral oil and in vegetable oil. Miscible with water, with alcohol, with glycerin, and with propylene glycol. *NF category:* Humectant; plasticizer.

Sotalol Hydrochloride: White to off-white powder. Freely soluble in water; soluble in alcohol; very slightly soluble in chloroform.

Soybean Oil: Clear, pale yellow, oily liquid having a characteristic odor and taste. Insoluble in water. Miscible with ether and with chloroform. *Specific Gravity* ⟨841⟩: between 0.916 and 0.922. *Refractive Index* ⟨831⟩: between 1.465 and 1.475. *NF category:* Vehicle (oleaginous); solvent.

Hydrogenated Soybean Oil: A white mass or powder that melts to a clear, pale yellow liquid when heated. Freely soluble in methylene chloride, in hexane after heating, and in toluene; very slightly soluble in alcohol; practically insoluble in water. *NF category:* Emollient.

Spectinomycin Hydrochloride: White to pale-buff crystalline powder. Freely soluble in water; practically insoluble in alcohol, in chloroform, and in ether.

Spironolactone: Light cream-colored to light tan, crystalline powder. Has a faint to mild mercaptan-like odor; is stable in air. Freely soluble in benzene and in chloroform; soluble in ethyl acetate and in alcohol; slightly soluble in methanol and in fixed oils; practically insoluble in water.

Squalane: Colorless, practically odorless transparent oil. Slightly soluble in acetone; very slightly soluble in absolute alcohol; insoluble in water. Miscible with ether and with chloroform. *NF category:* Ointment base; vehicle (oleaginous).

Stannous Chloride: White, crystalline powder or colorless crystals, efflorescent in air. Freely soluble in water (the solution becomes cloudy after standing or on dilution) and in alcohol. Dissolves in dilute hydrochloric acid. *NF category:* Emulsifying agent; antioxidant; reducing agent.

Stannous Fluoride: White, crystalline powder, having a bitter, salty taste. Melts at about 213°. Freely soluble in water; practically insoluble in alcohol, in ether, and in chloroform. *NF category:* Reducing agent.

Stanozolol: Odorless, crystalline powder, occurring in two forms: as needles, melting at about 155°, and as prisms, melting at about 235°. Soluble in dimethylformamide; sparingly soluble in alcohol and in chloroform; slightly soluble in ethyl acetate and in acetone; very slightly soluble in benzene; insoluble in water.

Corn Starch: Irregular, angular, white masses (which may be bleached) or fine powder. Is odorless, and has a slight, characteristic taste. Insoluble in cold water and in alcohol. *NF category:* Diluent; disintegrant; wet binder; suspending and/or viscosity-increasing agent.

Hydroxypropyl Corn Starch: White or slightly yellowish powder. Practically insoluble in cold water and in alcohol. *NF category:* Diluent; disintegrant; wet binder; emulsifying agent; suspending and/or viscosity-increasing agent.

Pregelatinized Hydroxypropyl Corn Starch: White or slightly yellowish powder. It swells in water and produces a clear or translucent, viscous, colloidal mixture. *NF category:* Suspending and/or viscosity-increasing agent; diluent; disintegrant; wet binder; emulsifying agent.

Pea Starch: White or almost white, very fine powder. Practically insoluble in cold water and in alcohol. *NF category:* Suspending and/or viscosity-increasing agent; diluent; disintegrant; wet binder.

Hydroxypropyl Pea Starch: White or slightly yellowish powder. Practically insoluble in cold water and in alcohol. *NF category:* Suspending and/or viscosity-increasing agent; diluent; disintegrant; wet binder; emulsifying agent.

Pregelatinized Hydroxypropyl Pea Starch: White or slightly yellowish powder. It swells in water and produces a clear or translucent, viscous, colloidal mixture. *NF category:* Suspending and/or viscosity-increasing agent; wet binder; diluent; disintegrant.

Potato Starch: Irregular, angular, white masses (which may be bleached) or fine powder. Is odorless, and has a slight, characteristic taste. Insoluble in cold water and in alcohol. *NF category:* Suspending and/or viscosity-increasing agent; diluent; disintegrant; wet binder.

Hydroxypropyl Potato Starch: White or slightly yellowish powder. Practically insoluble in cold water and in alcohol. *NF category:* Suspending and/or viscosity-increasing agent; diluent; disintegrant; wet binder; emulsifying agent.

Pregelatinized Hydroxypropyl Potato Starch: White or slightly yellowish powder. It swells in water and produces a clear or translucent, viscous, colloidal mixture. *NF category:* Suspending and/or viscosity-increasing agent; wet binder; diluent; disintegrant.

Pregelatinized Starch: Moderately coarse to fine, white to off-white powder. Is odorless and has a slight, characteristic taste. Slightly soluble to soluble in cold water; insoluble in alcohol. *NF category:* Wet binder; diluent; disintegrant; release-modifying agent.

Pregelatinized Modified Starch: Moderately coarse to fine, white to off-white powder. Is odorless and has a slight, characteristic taste. Soluble to slightly soluble in cold water; insoluble in alcohol. *NF category:* Coating agent; diluent; disintegrant; wet binder; release-modifying agent.

Tapioca Starch: Irregular, angular, white to pale yellow masses (which may be bleached) or fine powder. Insoluble in cold water and in alcohol. *NF category:* Suspending and/or viscosity-increasing agent; diluent; disintegrant; wet binder.

Wheat Starch: Irregular, angular, white masses (which may be bleached) or fine powder. Is odorless and has a slight, characteristic taste. Insoluble in cold water and in alcohol. *NF category:* Suspending and/or viscosity-increasing agent; diluent; disintegrant; wet binder.

Hydrogenated Starch Hydrolysate: Concentrated, aqueous solution or spray-dried or dried powder. Very soluble in water; insoluble in alcohol. *NF category:* Sweetening agent; humectant; diluent; wet binder.

Stavudine: White to off-white, crystalline powder. Soluble in water, in dimethylacetamide, and in dimethyl sulfoxide; sparingly soluble in methanol, in alcohol, and in acetonitrile; slightly soluble in dichloromethane; insoluble in hexane.

Stearic Acid: Hard, white or faintly yellowish, somewhat glossy and crystalline solid, or white or yellowish-white powder. Its odor and taste are slight, suggesting tallow. Freely soluble in chloroform and in ether; soluble in alcohol; practically insoluble in water. *NF category:* Emulsifying agent; lubricant.

Purified Stearic Acid: Hard, white or faintly yellowish, somewhat glossy and crystalline solid, or white or yellowish-white powder. Its odor and taste are slight, suggesting tallow. Freely soluble in chloroform and in ether; soluble in alcohol; practically insoluble in water. *NF category:* Lubricant.

Stearoyl Polyoxylglycerides: Pale yellow, waxy solids. Dispersible in warm water and in warm paraffin. Freely soluble in methylene chloride; soluble in warm methanol. *NF category:* Ointment base; solvent; emulsifying agent; wetting and/or solubilizing agent.

Stearyl Alcohol: Unctuous, white flakes or granules. Has a faint, characteristic odor and a bland, mild taste. Soluble in alcohol and in ether; insoluble in water. *NF category:* Stiffening agent.

Storax: Semiliquid, grayish to grayish-brown, sticky, opaque mass depositing on standing a heavy dark brown layer (Levant Storax); or semisolid, sometimes a solid mass, softened by gently warming (American Storax). Is transparent in thin layers, has a characteristic odor and taste, and is more dense than water. Soluble, usually incompletely, in an equal weight of warm alcohol, in acetone, in carbon disulfide, and in ether, some insoluble residue usually remaining; insoluble in water.

Streptomycin Sulfate: White or practically white powder. Is odorless or has not more than a faint odor. Is hygroscopic, but is stable in air and on exposure to light. Its solutions are acid to practically neutral to litmus. Freely soluble in water; very slightly soluble in alcohol; practically insoluble in chloroform.

Streptomycin Sulfate Injection: Clear, colorless to yellow, viscous liquid. Is odorless or has a slight odor.

Strontium Chloride: Colorless, odorless crystals or white granules. Effloresces in air; deliquesces in moist air. Very soluble in water; soluble in alcohol.

Succinic Acid: White, odorless crystals. Freely soluble in boiling water; soluble in water, in alcohol, and in glycerin. *NF category:* pH modifier (acidifying agent/alkalizing agent/buffering agent).

Succinylcholine Chloride: White, odorless, crystalline powder. Its solutions have a pH of about 4. The dihydrate form melts at about 160°; the anhydrous form melts at about 190°, and is hygroscopic. Freely soluble in water; slightly soluble in alcohol and in chloroform; practically insoluble in ether.

Sucralose: White to off-white, crystalline powder. Freely soluble in water, in methanol, and in alcohol; slightly soluble in ethyl acetate. *NF category:* Sweetening agent.

Sucrose: White, crystalline powder or lustrous, dry, colorless or white crystals. Very soluble in water; slightly soluble in alcohol; practically insoluble in dehydrated alcohol. *NF category:* Coating agent; sweetening agent; diluent; suspending and/or viscosity-increasing agent; wet binder.

Sucrose Palmitate: White or almost white, unctuous powder. Sparingly soluble in ethanol (96%); very slightly soluble in water. *NF category:* Suspending and/or viscosity-increasing agent; emulsifying agent.

Sucrose Octaacetate: White, practically odorless powder, having an intensely bitter taste. Is hygroscopic. Very soluble in methanol and in chloroform; soluble in alcohol and in ether; very slightly soluble in water. *NF category:* Alcohol denaturant.

Sucrose Stearate: White or almost white, unctuous powder. Sparingly soluble in ethanol (96%); very slightly soluble in water. *NF category:* Emulsifying agent; lubricant.

Sufentanil Citrate: White powder. Freely soluble in methanol; soluble in water; sparingly soluble in acetone, in alcohol, and in chloroform. Melts between 133° and 140°.

Compressible Sugar: Practically white, crystalline, odorless powder, having a sweet taste. Is stable in air. The sucrose portion of Compressible Sugar is very soluble in water. *NF category:* Sweetening agent; diluent.

Confectioner's Sugar: Fine, white, odorless powder, having a sweet taste. Is stable in air. The sucrose portion of Confectioner's Sugar is soluble in cold water. Confectioner's Sugar is freely soluble in boiling water. *NF category:* Sweetening agent; diluent; coating agent.

Sugar Spheres: Hard, brittle, free-flowing, spherical masses ranging generally in size from 10- to 60-mesh. Usually white, but may be colored. Solubility in water varies according to the sugar-to-starch ratio. *NF category:* Vehicle (solid carrier); diluent.

Sulbactam Sodium: White to off-white, crystalline powder. Freely soluble in water and in dilute acid; sparingly soluble in acetone, in ethyl acetate, and in chloroform.

Sulconazole Nitrate: White to off-white, crystalline powder. Melts at about 130°, with decomposition. Freely soluble in pyridine; sparingly soluble in methanol; slightly soluble in alcohol, in chloroform, in acetone, and in methylene chloride; very slightly soluble in water, in toluene, and in dioxane.

Sulfabenzamide: Fine, white, practically odorless powder. Soluble in alcohol, in acetone, and in sodium hydroxide TS; insoluble in water and in ether.

Sulfacetamide: White, crystalline powder, odorless and having a characteristic sour taste. Its aqueous solutions are sensitive to light, and are unstable when acidic or strongly alkaline. Freely soluble in dilute mineral acids and in solutions of potassium and sodium hydroxides; soluble in alcohol; slightly soluble in water and in ether; very slightly soluble in chloroform; practically insoluble in benzene.

Sulfacetamide Sodium: White, crystalline powder. Is odorless and has a bitter taste. Freely soluble in water; sparingly soluble in alcohol; practically insoluble in chloroform and in ether.

Sulfadiazine: White or slightly yellow powder. Is odorless or nearly odorless and is stable in air, but slowly darkens on exposure to light. Freely soluble in dilute mineral acids, in solutions of potassium and sodium hydroxides, and in ammonia TS; sparingly soluble in alcohol and in acetone; slightly soluble in human serum at 37°; practically insoluble in water.

Silver Sulfadiazine: White to creamy-white, crystalline powder, odorless to having a slight odor. Is stable in air, but turns yellow on exposure to light. Freely soluble in 30% ammonium solution; slightly soluble in acetone; practically insoluble in alcohol, in chloroform, and in ether. Decomposes in moderately strong mineral acids.

Sulfadiazine Sodium: White powder. On prolonged exposure to humid air it absorbs carbon dioxide with the liberation of sulfadiazine and becomes incompletely soluble in water. Its solutions are alkaline to phenolphthalein. Is affected by light. Freely soluble in water; slightly soluble in alcohol.

Sulfadimethoxine: Practically white, crystalline powder. Soluble in 2 N sodium hydroxide; sparingly soluble in 2 N hydrochloric acid; slightly soluble in alcohol, in ether, in chloroform, and in hexane; practically insoluble in water.

Sulfamethazine: White to yellowish-white powder, which may darken on exposure to light. Has a slightly bitter taste and is practically odorless. Soluble in acetone; slightly soluble in alcohol; very slightly soluble in water and in ether.

Sulfamethizole: White crystals or powder, having a slightly bitter taste. Is practically odorless, and has no odor of hydrogen sulfide. Freely soluble in solutions of ammonium, potassium, and sodium hydroxides; soluble in dilute mineral acids and in acetone; sparingly soluble in alcohol; very slightly soluble in water, in chloroform, and in ether; practically insoluble in benzene.

Sulfamethoxazole: White to off-white, practically odorless, crystalline powder. Freely soluble in acetone and in dilute solutions of sodium hydroxide; sparingly soluble in alcohol; practically insoluble in water, in ether, and in chloroform.

Sulfapyridine: White or faintly yellowish-white crystals, granules, or powder. Is odorless or practically odorless, and is stable in air, but slowly darkens on exposure to light. Freely soluble in dilute mineral acids and in solutions of potassium and sodium hydroxides; sparingly soluble in acetone; slightly soluble in alcohol; very slightly soluble in water.

Sulfasalazine: Bright yellow or brownish-yellow, odorless, fine powder. Melts at about 255°, with decomposition. Soluble in aqueous solutions of alkali hydroxides; very slightly soluble in alcohol; practically insoluble in water, in ether, in chloroform, and in benzene.

Sulfathiazole: Fine, white or faintly yellowish-white, practically odorless powder. Soluble in acetone, in dilute mineral acids, in solutions of alkali hydroxides, and in 6 N ammonium hydroxide; slightly soluble in alcohol; very slightly soluble in water.

Sulfinpyrazone: White to off-white powder. Soluble in alcohol and in acetone; sparingly soluble in dilute alkali; practically insoluble in water and in solvent hexane.

Sulfisoxazole: White to slightly yellowish, odorless, crystalline powder. Soluble in boiling alcohol and in 3 N hydrochloric acid; very slightly soluble in water.

Sulfisoxazole Acetyl: White or slightly yellow, crystalline powder. Sparingly soluble in chloroform; slightly soluble in alcohol; practically insoluble in water.

Precipitated Sulfur: Very fine, pale yellow, amorphous or microcrystalline powder. Is odorless and tasteless. Very soluble in carbon disulfide; slightly soluble in olive oil; very slightly soluble in alcohol; practically insoluble in water.

Sublimed Sulfur: Fine, yellow, crystalline powder, having a faint odor and taste. Sparingly soluble in olive oil; practically insoluble in water and in alcohol.

Sulfur Dioxide: Colorless, nonflammable gas, possessing a strong, suffocating odor characteristic of burning sulfur. Under pressure, it condenses readily to a colorless liquid that boils at −10° and has a density of approximately 1.5. At 20° and at standard pressure, approximately 36 volumes dissolve in 1 volume of water and approximately 114 volumes dissolve in 1 volume of alcohol. Soluble also in ether and in chloroform. *NF category:* Antioxidant; antimicrobial preservative.

Sulfuric Acid: Clear, colorless, oily liquid. Miscible with water and with alcohol with the generation of much heat. Is very caustic and corrosive. Specific gravity is about 1.84. *NF category:* pH modifier (acidifying agent/alkalizing agent/buffering agent).

Sulindac: Yellow, crystalline powder, which is odorless or practically so. Slightly soluble in methanol, in alcohol, in acetone, and in chloroform; very slightly soluble in isopropanol and in ethyl acetate; practically insoluble in hexane and in water.

Sulisobenzone: Light tan powder, with a melting point of about 145°. Freely soluble in methanol, in alcohol, and in water; sparingly soluble in ethyl acetate.

Sumatriptan: White to pale yellow powder. Very slightly soluble in water.

Sumatriptan Succinate: White or almost white powder. Freely soluble in water; sparingly soluble in methanol; practically insoluble in methylene chloride.

Sunflower Oil: Clear, light yellow liquid. It is miscible with petroleum at a boiling point of 40°–60°. Practically insoluble in water and in alcohol. *Refractive Index* ⟨831⟩: 1.472–1.474 at 25°. *Specific Gravity* ⟨841⟩: 0.914–0.924 at 20°. *NF category*: Coating agent; emollient; solvent; diluent; vehicle (oleaginous).

Suprofen: White to off-white powder, odorless to having a slight odor. Sparingly soluble in water.

Syrup: *NF category*: Sweetening agent; wet binder; vehicle.

Tacrine Hydrochloride: White powder. Freely soluble in water, in 0.1 N hydrochloric acid, in pH 4.0 acetate buffer, in phosphate buffer (pH between 7.0 and 7.4), in methanol, in dimethylsulfoxide, in alcohol, and in propylene glycol; sparingly soluble in linoleic acid and in polyethylene glycol 400.

Tacrolimus: White crystals or white crystalline powder. Very soluble in methanol; freely soluble in N,N-dimethylformamide, and in alcohol; practically insoluble in water.

Tadalafil: White or almost white powder. Freely soluble in dimethyl sulfoxide; slightly soluble in methylene chloride; practically insoluble in water.

Tagatose: White or almost white crystals, having a sweet taste. Very soluble in water; very slightly soluble in alcohol. *NF category*: Sweetening agent; humectant.

Talc: Very fine, white or grayish-white, crystalline powder. Is unctuous, adheres readily to the skin, and is free from grittiness. *NF category*: Glidant and/or anticaking agent; lubricant; diluent.

Tamoxifen Citrate: White, fine, crystalline powder. Soluble in methanol; very slightly soluble in water, in acetone, in chloroform, and in alcohol. Melts at about 142°, with decomposition.

Tamsulosin Hydrochloride: White or almost white crystalline powder. Melts with decomposition at approximately 230°. Freely soluble in formic acid; sparingly soluble in methanol; slightly soluble in water and in dehydrated alcohol; practically insoluble in ether.

Tannic Acid: Amorphous powder, glistening scales, or spongy masses, varying in color from yellowish-white to light brown. Is odorless or has a faint, characteristic odor, and has a strongly astringent taste. Very soluble in water, in acetone, and in alcohol; freely soluble in diluted alcohol; slightly soluble in dehydrated alcohol; practically insoluble in benzene, in chloroform, in ether, and in solvent hexane; 1 g dissolves in about 1 mL of warm glycerin.

Tartaric Acid: Colorless or translucent crystals or white, fine to granular, crystalline powder. Is odorless, has an acid taste, and is stable in air. Very soluble in water; freely soluble in alcohol. *NF category*: pH modifier (acidifying agent/alkalizing agent/buffering agent); flavors and fragrance; sequestering agent.

Taurine: White crystals or crystalline powder. Soluble in water.

Tazobactam: White to pale yellow, nonhygroscopic, crystalline powder. Soluble in dimethylformamide; slightly soluble in water, in methanol, in acetone, and in alcohol; very slightly soluble in ethyl acetate, in ethyl ether, and in chloroform; insoluble in hexane.

Technetium Tc 99m Aggregated Albumin Injection: Milky suspension, from which particles settle upon standing.

Technetium Tc 99m Pentetate Injection: Clear, colorless solution.

Sodium Pertechnetate Tc 99m Injection: Clear, colorless solution.

Technetium Tc 99m (Pyro- and trimeta-) Phosphates Injection: Clear solution.

Technetium Tc 99m Sulfur Colloid Injection: Colloidal dispersion. Slightly opalescent, colorless to light tan liquid.

Telmisartan: White or slightly yellowish, crystalline powder. Sparingly soluble in methylene chloride; slightly soluble in methanol; practically insoluble in water. It dissolves in 1 M sodium hydroxide.

Temazepam: White or nearly white, crystalline powder. Sparingly soluble in alcohol; very slightly soluble in water. Melts between 157° and 163°, within a 3° range.

Temozolomide: White to light pink/light tan powder. Soluble in dimethyl sulfoxide; sparingly soluble in water; practically insoluble in toluene.

Teniposide: White to off-white, crystalline powder. Very soluble in acetone and in dimethylformamide; slightly soluble in methanol; insoluble in water and in ether.

Terazosin Hydrochloride: White to pale yellow, crystalline powder. Freely soluble in isotonic saline solution; soluble in methanol and in water; slightly soluble in alcohol and in 0.1 N hydrochloric acid; very slightly soluble in chloroform; practically insoluble in acetone and in hexanes.

Terbinafine Hydrochloride: White or off-white powder. Freely soluble in dehydrated alcohol and in methanol; slightly soluble in acetone; very slightly or slightly soluble in water.

Terbutaline Sulfate: White to gray-white, crystalline powder. Is odorless or has a faint odor of acetic acid. Soluble in water and in 0.1 N hydrochloric acid; slightly soluble in methanol; insoluble in chloroform.

Terconazole: White to off-white powder. Freely soluble in methylene chloride; soluble in acetone; sparingly soluble in alcohol; practically insoluble in water. It exhibits polymorphism.

Terpin Hydrate: Colorless, lustrous crystals or white powder. Has a slight odor, and effloresces in dry air. A hot solution (1 in 100) is neutral to litmus. When dried in vacuum at 60° for 2 hours, it melts at about 103°. Very soluble in boiling alcohol; soluble in alcohol; sparingly soluble in boiling water; slightly soluble in water, in chloroform, and in ether.

Testolactone: White to off-white, practically odorless, crystalline powder. Melts at about 218°. Soluble in alcohol and in chloroform; slightly soluble in water and in benzyl alcohol; insoluble in ether and in solvent hexane.

Testosterone: White or slightly creamy white crystals or crystalline powder. Is odorless, and is stable in air. Freely soluble in dehydrated alcohol and in chloroform; soluble in dioxane and in vegetable oils; slightly soluble in ether; practically insoluble in water.

Testosterone Cypionate: White or creamy white, crystalline powder. Is odorless or has a slight odor, and is stable in air. Freely soluble in alcohol, in chloroform, in dioxane, and in ether; soluble in vegetable oils; insoluble in water.

Testosterone Enanthate: White or creamy white, crystalline powder. Is odorless or has a faint odor characteristic of heptanoic acid. Very soluble in ether; soluble in vegetable oils; insoluble in water.

Testosterone Propionate: White or creamy white crystals or crystalline powder. Is odorless and is stable in air. Freely soluble in alcohol, in dioxane, in ether, and in other organic solvents; soluble in vegetable oils; insoluble in water.

Tetanus Immune Globulin: Transparent or slightly opalescent liquid, practically colorless and practically odorless. May develop a slight granular deposit during storage.

Tetanus Toxoid: Clear, colorless to brownish-yellow, or slightly turbid liquid, free from evident clumps or particles, having a characteristic odor or an odor of formaldehyde.

Tetanus Toxoid Adsorbed: Turbid, white, slightly gray, or slightly pink suspension, free from evident clumps after shaking.

Tetanus and Diphtheria Toxoids Adsorbed for Adult Use: Turbid, white, slightly gray, or cream-colored suspension, free from evident clumps after shaking.

Tetracaine: White or light yellow, waxy solid. Soluble in alcohol, in ether, in benzene, and in chloroform; very slightly soluble in water.

Tetracaine Hydrochloride: Fine, white, crystalline, odorless powder. Has a slightly bitter taste followed by a sense of numbness. Its solutions are neutral to litmus. Melts at about 148°, or may occur in either of two other polymorphic modifications that melt at about 134° and 139°, respectively. Mixtures of the forms may melt within the range of 134° to 147°. Is hygroscopic. Very soluble in water; soluble in alcohol; insoluble in ether and in benzene.

Tetracycline: Yellow, odorless, crystalline powder. Is stable in air, but exposure to strong sunlight causes it to darken. It loses potency in solutions of pH below 2, and is rapidly destroyed by alkali hydroxide solutions. Freely soluble in dilute acid and in alkali hydroxide solutions; sparingly soluble in alcohol; very slightly soluble in water; practically insoluble in chloroform and in ether.

Tetracycline Hydrochloride: Yellow, odorless, crystalline powder. Is moderately hygroscopic. Is stable in air, but exposure to strong sunlight in moist air causes it to darken. It loses potency in solution at a pH below 2, and is rapidly destroyed by alkali hydroxide solutions. Soluble in water and in solutions of alkali hydroxides and carbonates; slightly soluble in alcohol; practically insoluble in chloroform and in ether.

Tetrahydrozoline Hydrochloride: White, odorless solid. Melts at about 256°, with decomposition. Freely soluble in water and in alcohol; very slightly soluble in chloroform; practically insoluble in ether.

Thalidomide: White to off-white powder. Very soluble in dimethyl sulfoxide; sparingly soluble in ethanol and in water.

Theophylline: White, odorless, crystalline powder, having a bitter taste. Is stable in air. Freely soluble in solutions of alkali hydroxides and in ammonia; sparingly soluble in alcohol, in chloroform, and in ether; slightly soluble in water, but more soluble in hot water.

Theophylline Sodium Glycinate: White, crystalline powder having a slight ammoniacal odor and a bitter taste. Freely soluble in water; very slightly soluble in alcohol; practically insoluble in chloroform.

Thiabendazole: White to practically white, odorless or practically odorless powder. Slightly soluble in acetone and in alcohol; very slightly soluble in chloroform and in ether; practically insoluble in water.

Thiacetarsamide: White to yellowish, crystalline powder. Soluble in warm dehydrated alcohol and in warm methanol; sparingly soluble in cold dehydrated alcohol, in cold methanol, and in cold water; more soluble in water above 90°; insoluble in warm isopropyl alcohol. pK$_a$ is 4.

Thiamine Hydrochloride: White crystals or crystalline powder, usually having a slight, characteristic odor. When exposed to air, the anhydrous product rapidly absorbs about 4% of water. Melts at about 248°, with some decomposition. Freely soluble in water; soluble in glycerin; slightly soluble in alcohol; insoluble in ether and in benzene.

Thiamine Mononitrate: White crystals or crystalline powder, usually having a slight, characteristic odor. Sparingly soluble in water; slightly soluble in alcohol; very slightly soluble in chloroform.

Thiethylperazine Maleate: Yellowish, granular powder. Is odorless or has not more than a slight odor. Melts at about 183°, with decomposition. Slightly soluble in methanol; practically insoluble in water and in chloroform.

Thimerosal: Light cream-colored, crystalline powder, having a slight characteristic odor. Is affected by light. The pH of a solution (1 in 100) is about 6.7. Freely soluble in water; soluble in alcohol; practically insoluble in ether. *NF category:* Antimicrobial preservative.

Thimerosal Topical Solution: Clear liquid, having a slight characteristic odor. Is affected by light.

Thimerosal Tincture: Transparent, mobile liquid, having the characteristic odor of alcohol and acetone. Is affected by light.

Thioguanine: Pale yellow, odorless or practically odorless, crystalline powder. Freely soluble in dilute solutions of alkali hydroxides; insoluble in water, in alcohol, and in chloroform.

Thiopental Sodium: White to off-white, crystalline powder, or yellowish-white to pale greenish-yellow, hygroscopic powder. May have a disagreeable odor. Its solutions are alkaline to litmus. Its solutions decompose on standing, and on boiling precipitation occurs. Soluble in water and in alcohol; insoluble in benzene, in absolute ether, and in solvent hexane.

Thiopental Sodium for Injection: White to off-white, crystalline powder, or yellowish-white to pale greenish-yellow, hygroscopic powder. May have a disagreeable odor. Its solutions are alkaline to litmus. Its solutions decompose on standing, and on boiling precipitation occurs.

Thioridazine: White to slightly yellow, crystalline or micronized powder, odorless or having a faint odor. Very soluble in chloroform; freely soluble in dehydrated alcohol and in ether; practically insoluble in water.

Thioridazine Hydrochloride: White to slightly yellow, granular powder, having a faint odor and a very bitter taste. Freely soluble in water, in methanol, and in chloroform; insoluble in ether.

Thiostrepton: White to off-white, crystalline solid. Soluble in glacial acetic acid, in chloroform, in dimethylformamide, in dimethyl sulfoxide, in dioxane, and in pyridine; practically insoluble in water, in the lower alcohols, in nonpolar organic solvents, and in dilute aqueous acids or alkali.

Thiotepa: Fine, white, crystalline flakes, having a faint odor. Freely soluble in water, in alcohol, in chloroform, and in ether.

Thiotepa for Injection: White powder.

Thiothixene: White to tan, practically odorless crystals. Is affected by light. Very soluble in chloroform; slightly soluble in methanol and in acetone; practically insoluble in water.

Thiothixene Hydrochloride: White, or practically white, crystalline powder, having a slight odor. Is affected by light. Soluble in water; slightly soluble in chloroform; practically insoluble in benzene, in acetone, and in ether.

Threonine: White, odorless crystals, having a slightly sweet taste. Freely soluble in water; insoluble in absolute alcohol, in ether, and in chloroform.

Thrombin: White to grayish, amorphous substance dried from the frozen state.

Thymol: Colorless, often large, crystals, or white, crystalline powder, having an aromatic, thyme-like odor and a pungent taste. Is affected by light. Its alcohol solution is neutral to litmus. Freely soluble in alcohol, in chloroform, in ether, and in olive oil; soluble in glacial acetic acid and in fixed and volatile oils; very slightly soluble in water. *NF category:* Antimicrobial preservative; flavors and fragrance; antioxidant.

Thyroid: Yellowish to buff-colored, amorphous powder, having a slight, characteristic, meat-like odor and a saline taste.

Tiagabine Hydrochloride: White to off-white powder. Freely soluble in methanol and in alcohol; soluble in isopropanol; very slightly soluble in chloroform; sparingly soluble in water; practically insoluble in *n*-heptane.

Tiamulin: A sticky, translucent yellowish mass, slightly hygroscopic. Very soluble in dichloromethane; freely soluble in dehydrated alcohol; practically insoluble in water.

Ticarcillin Disodium: White to pale yellow powder, or white to pale yellow solid. Freely soluble in water.

Ticlopidine: White or almost white crystalline powder. Sparingly soluble in water and in alcohol; very slightly soluble in ethyl acetate.

Tigecycline: Orange powder. Freely soluble in water; soluble in 1-octanol; slightly soluble in methanol, in ethanol, and in isopropyl alcohol.

Tiletamine Hydrochloride: White to off-white, crystalline powder. Freely soluble in water and in 0.1 N hydrochloric acid; soluble in methanol; slightly soluble in chloroform; practically insoluble in ether.

Tilmicosin: White to off-white, amorphous solid. Slightly soluble in water and in *n*-hexane.

Timolol Maleate: White to practically white, odorless or practically odorless powder. Soluble in water, in alcohol, and in methanol; sparingly soluble in chloroform and in propylene glycol; insoluble in ether and in cyclohexane.

Tinidazole: Almost white or pale yellow, crystalline powder. Soluble in acetone and in methylene chloride; sparingly soluble in methanol; practically insoluble in water.

Titanium Dioxide: White, odorless, tasteless powder. Its 1 in 10 suspension in water is neutral to litmus. Insoluble in water, in hydrochloric acid, in nitric acid, and in 2 N sulfuric acid. Dissolves in hydrofluoric acid and in hot sulfuric acid. Is rendered soluble by fusion with potassium bisulfate or with alkali carbonates or hydroxides. *NF category:* Coating agent.

Tizanidine Hydrochloride: Almost white to slightly yellow, crystalline powder. Slightly soluble in water and in methanol.

Tobramycin: White to off-white, hygroscopic powder. Freely soluble in water; very slightly soluble in alcohol; practically insoluble in chloroform and in ether.

Tobramycin Sulfate Injection: Clear, colorless solution.

Tocainide Hydrochloride: Fine, white, odorless powder. Freely soluble in water and in alcohol; practically insoluble in chloroform and in ether.

Tocopherol: Clear, colorless to yellow, yellowish-brown, or greenish-yellow, viscous oil. Is odorless. Soluble in oils, in fats, in acetone, in alcohol, in chloroform, in ether, and in alcohol; insoluble in water. *NF category:* Antioxidant.

Tocopherols Excipient: Brownish-red to red, clear, viscous oil, having a mild, characteristic odor and taste. May show a slight separation of waxlike constituents in microcrystalline form. Oxidizes and darkens slowly in air and on exposure to light, particularly in alkaline media. Soluble in alcohol; insoluble in water. Miscible with acetone, with chloroform, with ether, and with vegetable oils. *NF category:* Antioxidant.

Tolazamide: White to off-white, crystalline powder, odorless or having a slight odor. Melts with decomposition in the approximate range of 161° to 173°. Freely soluble in chloroform; soluble in acetone; slightly soluble in alcohol; very slightly soluble in water.

Tolazoline Hydrochloride: White to off-white, crystalline powder. Its solutions are slightly acid to litmus. Freely soluble in water and in alcohol.

Tolbutamide: White, or practically white, crystalline powder. Is slightly bitter and practically odorless. Soluble in alcohol and in chloroform; practically insoluble in water.

Tolbutamide Sodium: White to off-white, practically odorless, crystalline powder, having a slightly bitter taste. Freely soluble in water; soluble in alcohol and in chloroform; very slightly soluble in ether.

Tolcapone: Yellow, fine powder or fine powder with lumps. Freely soluble in acetone and in tetrahydrofuran; soluble in methanol and ethyl acetate; sparingly soluble in chloroform and in dichloromethane; insoluble in water and in *n*-hexane.

Tolmetin Sodium: Light yellow to light orange, crystalline powder. Freely soluble in water and in methanol; slightly soluble in alcohol; very slightly soluble in chloroform.

Tolnaftate: White to creamy white, fine powder, having a slight odor. Freely soluble in acetone and in chloroform; sparingly soluble in ether; slightly soluble in alcohol; practically insoluble in water.

Tolterodine Tartrate: White or almost white, crystalline powder. Sparingly soluble in water; slightly soluble in anhydrous ethanol; practically insoluble in heptane.

Tolu Balsam: Brown or yellowish-brown, plastic solid, transparent in thin layers and brittle when old, dried, or exposed to cold temperatures. Has a pleasant, aromatic odor resembling that of vanilla, and a mild, aromatic taste. Soluble in alcohol, in chloroform, and in ether, sometimes with slight residue or turbidity; practically insoluble in water and in solvent hexane. *NF category:* Flavors and perfumes.

Topiramate: White to off-white powder. Freely soluble in dichloromethane.

Torsemide: White to off-white, crystalline powder. Slightly soluble in 0.1 N sodium hydroxide, in 0.1 N hydrochloric acid, in alcohol, and in methanol; very slightly soluble in acetone and in chloroform; practically insoluble in water and in ether.

Tragacanth: Is odorless, and has an insipid, mucilaginous taste. *NF category:* Suspending and/or viscosity-increasing agent.

Tramadol Hydrochloride: White, crystalline powder. Freely soluble in water and in methanol; very slightly soluble in acetone.

Trandalopril: White or almost white powder. Freely soluble in methylene chloride; sparingly soluble in absolute alcohol; practically insoluble in water.

Tranexamic Acid: White, crystalline powder. Freely soluble in water and in glacial acetic acid; practically insoluble in acetone and in alcohol.

Tranylcypromine Sulfate: White or almost white crystalline powder. Freely soluble in water; very slightly soluble in alcohol and in ether; practically insoluble in chloroform.

Travoprost: Clear, colorless, viscous oil. Insoluble in water.

Trazodone Hydrochloride: White to off-white, crystalline powder. Sparingly soluble in chloroform and in water. Melts between 231° and 234° when the melting point determination is carried out in an evacuated capillary tube; otherwise melts with decomposition over a broad range below 230°.

Trehalose: White, odorless, nonhygroscopic crystalline powder. Soluble in water, solubility increases with temperature; practically insoluble in dehydrated alcohol. Trehalose is typically used in the dihydrate form. *NF category:* Bulking agent; sweetening agent; diluent; disintegrant; wet binder; vehicle.

Tretinoin: Yellow to light-orange, crystalline powder. Slightly soluble in alcohol, in chloroform, and in methanol; insoluble in water.

Triacetin: Colorless, somewhat oily liquid having a slight, fatty odor and a bitter taste. Soluble in water; slightly soluble in carbon disulfide. Miscible with alcohol, with ether, and with chloroform. *NF category:* Plasticizer; humectant; solvent.

Triamcinolone: White or practically white, odorless, crystalline powder. Slightly soluble in alcohol and in methanol; very slightly soluble in water, in chloroform, and in ether.

Triamcinolone Acetonide: White to cream-colored, crystalline powder, having not more than a slight odor. Sparingly soluble in dehydrated alcohol, in chloroform, and in methanol; practically insoluble in water.

Triamcinolone Diacetate: Fine, white to off-white, crystalline powder, having not more than a slight odor. Soluble in chloroform; sparingly soluble in alcohol and in methanol; slightly soluble in ether; practically insoluble in water.

Triamcinolone Hexacetonide: White to cream-colored powder. Soluble in chloroform; slightly soluble in methanol; practically insoluble in water.

Triamterene: Yellow, odorless, crystalline powder. Soluble in formic acid; sparingly soluble in methoxyethanol; very slightly soluble in acetic acid, in alcohol, and in dilute mineral acids; practically insoluble in water, in benzene, in chloroform, in ether, and in dilute alkali hydroxides.

Triazolam: White to off-white, practically odorless, crystalline powder. Soluble in chloroform; slightly soluble in alcohol; practically insoluble in ether and in water.

Tributyl Citrate: Clear, practically colorless, oily liquid. Freely soluble in alcohol, in isopropyl alcohol, in acetone, and in toluene; insoluble in water. *NF category:* Plasticizer.

Trichlorfon: White crystalline powder. Very soluble in methylene chloride; freely soluble in acetone, in alcohol, in benzene, in chloroform, in ether, and in water; very slightly soluble in hexane and in pentane. Decomposed by alkali. Melts at about 78° with decomposition.

Trichlormethiazide: White or practically white, crystalline powder. Is odorless, or has a slight characteristic odor. Melts at about 274°, with decomposition. Freely soluble in acetone; soluble in methanol; sparingly soluble in alcohol; very slightly soluble in water, in ether, and in chloroform.

Trichloromonofluoromethane: Clear, colorless gas, having a faint, ethereal odor. Its vapor pressure at 25° is about 796 mm of mercury (1 psig). *NF category:* Propellant.

Triclocarban: White powder. Freely soluble in ethanol, in acetone, and in polyethylene glycol; slightly soluble in acetonitrile and in propylene glycol; insoluble in water.

Triclosan: Fine, whitish, crystalline powder. Melts at about 57°. Soluble in methanol, in alcohol, and in acetone; slightly soluble in hexane; practically insoluble in water.

Trientine Hydrochloride: White to pale yellow, crystalline powder. Melts at about 117°. Freely soluble in water; soluble in methanol; slightly soluble in alcohol; insoluble in chloroform and in ether.

Triethyl Citrate: Practically colorless, oily liquid. Soluble in water. Miscible with alcohol and with ether. *NF category:* Plasticizer; solvent.

Trifluoperazine Hydrochloride: White to pale yellow, crystalline powder. Is practically odorless, and has a bitter taste. Melts at about 242°, with decomposition. Freely soluble in water; soluble in alcohol; sparingly soluble in chloroform; insoluble in ether and in benzene.

Triflupromazine: Viscous, light amber-colored, oily liquid, which crystallizes on prolonged standing into large, irregular crystals. Practically insoluble in water.

Triflupromazine Hydrochloride: White to pale tan, crystalline powder, having a slight, characteristic odor. Melts between 170° and 178°. Soluble in water, in alcohol, and in acetone; insoluble in ether.

Trifluridine: Odorless, white powder appearing under the microscope as rodlike crystals; melts at 175°, with sublimation.

Medium-Chain Triglycerides: Colorless or slightly yellowish, oily liquid. Practically insoluble in water. Miscible with alcohol, with methylene chloride, with hexane, and with fatty oils. *NF category:* Emulsifying agent; solvent; suspending and/or viscosity-increasing agent.

Trihexyphenidyl Hydrochloride: White or slightly off-white, crystalline powder, having not more than a very faint odor. Melts at about 250°. Soluble in alcohol and in chloroform; slightly soluble in water.

Trimeprazine Tartrate: White to off-white, odorless, crystalline powder. Freely soluble in water and in chloroform; soluble in alcohol; very slightly soluble in ether and in benzene.

Trimethobenzamide Hydrochloride: White, crystalline powder having a slight phenolic odor. Soluble in water and in warm alcohol; insoluble in ether and in benzene.

Trimethoprim: White to cream-colored, odorless crystals, or crystalline powder. Soluble in benzyl alcohol; sparingly soluble in chloroform and in methanol; slightly soluble in alcohol and in acetone; very slightly soluble in water; practically insoluble in ether and in carbon tetrachloride.

Trimethoprim Sulfate: White to off-white, crystalline powder. Soluble in water, in alcohol, in dilute mineral acids, and in fixed alkalies.

Trimipramine Maleate: White to almost white crystalline powder. Slightly soluble in water and in alcohol.

Trioxsalen: White to off-white or grayish, odorless, crystalline solid. Melts at about 230°. Sparingly soluble in chloroform; slightly soluble in alcohol; practically insoluble in water.

Tripelennamine Hydrochloride: White, crystalline powder. Slowly darkens on exposure to light. Its solutions are practically neutral to litmus. Freely soluble in water, in alcohol, and in chloroform; slightly soluble in acetone; insoluble in benzene, in ether, and in ethyl acetate.

Triprolidine Hydrochloride: White, crystalline powder, having no more than a slight, but unpleasant, odor. Its solutions are alkaline to litmus, and it melts at about 115°. Soluble in water, in alcohol, and in chloroform; insoluble in ether.

Trolamine: Colorless to pale yellow, viscous, hygroscopic liquid having a slight, ammoniacal odor. Soluble in chloroform. Miscible with water and with alcohol. *NF category:* Emulsifying agent; pH modifier (acidifying agent/alkalizing agent/buffering agent).

Troleandomycin: White, odorless, crystalline powder. Freely soluble in alcohol; soluble in chloroform; slightly soluble in ether and in water.

Tromethamine: White, crystalline powder, having a slight, characteristic odor. Freely soluble in water.

Tropicamide: White or practically white, crystalline powder, odorless or having not more than a slight odor. Freely soluble in chloroform and in solutions of strong acids; slightly soluble in water.

Trospium Chloride: Colorless or white to slightly yellow crystalline powder. Very soluble in water; freely soluble in methanol.

Crystallized Trypsin: White to yellowish white, odorless, crystalline or amorphous powder.

Tryptophan: White to slightly yellowish-white crystals or crystalline powder, having a slightly bitter taste. Soluble in hot alcohol and in dilute hydrochloric acid.

Tuberculin: Old Tuberculin is a clear, brownish liquid, which is readily miscible with water and has a characteristic odor. Purified Protein Derivative (PPD) of Tuberculin is a very slightly opalescent, colorless solution. Old Tuberculin and PPD concentrates contain 50% of glycerin for use with various application devices. Old Tuberculin and PPD are also dried on the tines of multiple-puncture devices.

Tubocurarine Chloride: White or yellowish-white to grayish-white, crystalline powder. Melts at about 270°, with decomposition. Soluble in water; sparingly soluble in alcohol.

Tylosin: White to buff-colored powder. Freely soluble in methanol; soluble in alcohol, in amyl acetate, in chloroform, and in dilute mineral acids; slightly soluble in water.

Tylosin Tartrate: Almost white or slightly yellow, hygroscopic powder. Freely soluble in water and in dichloromethane; slightly soluble in alcohol. It dissolves in dilute solutions of mineral acids.

Tyloxapol: Viscous, amber liquid, having a slight, aromatic odor. May exhibit a slight turbidity. Slowly but freely miscible with water. Soluble in glacial acetic acid, in benzene, in toluene, in carbon tetrachloride, in chloroform, and in carbon disulfide. *NF category:* Wetting and/or solubilizing agent.

Tyrosine: White, odorless, tasteless crystals or crystalline powder. Very slightly soluble in water; insoluble in alcohol and in ether.

Ubidecarenone: Yellow to orange, crystalline powder. Melts at about 48°. Soluble in ether; very slightly soluble in dehydrated alcohol; practically insoluble in water.

Undecylenic Acid: Clear, colorless to pale yellow liquid having a characteristic odor. Practically insoluble in water. Miscible with alcohol, with chloroform, with ether, with benzene, and with fixed and volatile oils.

Urea: Colorless to white, prismatic crystals, or white, crystalline powder, or small white pellets. Is practically odorless, but may gradually develop a slight odor of ammonia upon long standing. Its solutions are neutral to litmus. Freely soluble in water and in boiling alcohol; practically insoluble in chloroform and in ether.

Urea C 13: See *Urea.*

Ursodiol: White or almost white, crystalline powder. Freely soluble in alcohol and in glacial acetic acid; sparingly soluble in chloroform; slightly soluble in ether; practically insoluble in water.

Vaccinia Immune Globulin: Transparent or slightly opalescent liquid. Is practically colorless and practically odorless. May develop a slight, granular deposit during storage.

Valacyclovir Hydrochloride: White to off-white powder. Soluble in water; insoluble in dichloromethane.

Powdered Valerian Extract: Brown, hygroscopic, powdery or easily pulverizable mass. Soluble in water to form a slightly cloudy solution; sparingly soluble in 70 percent alcohol; practically insoluble in alcohol.

Valganciclovir Hydrochloride: White to off-white powder. Very slightly soluble in alcohol; practically insoluble in 2-propanol, in hexane, in acetone, and in ethyl acetate.

Valine: White, odorless, tasteless crystals. Soluble in water; practically insoluble in ether, in alcohol, and in acetone.

Valproic Acid: Colorless to pale yellow, slightly viscous, clear liquid, having a characteristic odor. Refractive index: about 1.423 at 20°. Freely soluble in 1 N sodium hydroxide, in methanol, in alcohol, in acetone, in chloroform, in benzene, in ether, and in *n*-heptane; slightly soluble in water and in 0.1 N hydrochloric acid.

Valrubicin: Orange to orange-red, crystalline powder. Soluble in methylene chloride, in dehydrated alcohol, in methanol, and in acetone; very slightly soluble in water, in hexane, and in petroleum ether.

Valsartan: White or almost white, hygroscopic powder. Freely soluble in anhydrous ethanol; sparingly soluble in methylene chloride; practically insoluble in water.

Vancomycin Hydrochloride: White, almost white, or tan to brown, free-flowing powder, odorless, and having a bitter taste. Freely soluble in water; insoluble in ether and in chloroform.

Vanillin: Fine, white to slightly yellow crystals, usually needle-like, having an odor and taste suggestive of vanilla. Is affected by light. Its solutions are acid to litmus. Freely soluble in alcohol, in chloroform, in ether, and in solutions of the fixed alkali hydroxides; soluble in glycerin and in hot water; slightly soluble in water. *NF category:* Flavors and fragrance.

Vardenafil Hydrochloride: White or slightly brown or yellow powder. Freely soluble in anhydrous alcohol; slightly soluble in water; practically insoluble in heptane.

Vasopressin Injection: Clear, colorless or practically colorless liquid, having a faint, characteristic odor.

Vecuronium Bromide: White or creamy white crystals, or a crystalline powder. Sparingly soluble in alcohol; slightly soluble in water and in acetone.

Hydrogenated Vegetable Oil: Type I Hydrogenated Vegetable Oil—Fine, white powder, beads, or small flakes. Type II Hydrogenated Vegetable Oil—Plastic (semi-solid) or flakes having a softer consistency than Type I. Soluble in hot isopropyl alcohol, in hexane, and in chloroform; insoluble in water. *NF category:* Hydrogenated Vegetable Oil—Wet binder; Type I Hydrogenated Vegetable Oil—Lubricant; Type II Hydrogenated Vegetable Oil—Ointment base.

Venlafaxine Hydrochloride: Off-white to white crystalline powder. Soluble in methanol and in water.

Verapamil Hydrochloride: White or practically white, crystalline powder. Is practically odorless and has a bitter taste. Freely soluble in chloroform; soluble in water; sparingly soluble in alcohol; practically insoluble in ether.

Vidarabine: White to off-white powder. Slightly soluble in dimethylformamide; very slightly soluble in water.

Vigabatrin: White or almost white powder. Freely soluble in water; slightly soluble in methanol; very slightly soluble in alcohol and in chloroform; practically insoluble in methylene chloride; insoluble in hexane and in toluene.

Vinblastine Sulfate: White or slightly yellow, odorless, amorphous or crystalline powder. Is hygroscopic. Freely soluble in water.

Vincristine Sulfate: White to slightly yellow, odorless, amorphous or crystalline powder. Is hygroscopic. Freely soluble in water; soluble in methanol; slightly soluble in alcohol.

Vincristine Sulfate for Injection: Yellowish-white solid, having the characteristic appearance of products prepared by freeze-drying.

Vinorelbine Tartrate: White to yellow or light brown, amorphous powder. Freely soluble in water.

Vitamin A: In liquid form, a light-yellow to red oil that may solidify upon refrigeration. In solid form, has the appearance of any diluent that has been added. May be practically odorless or may have a mild fishy odor, but has no rancid odor or taste. Is unstable to air and light. In liquid form, very soluble in chloroform and in ether; soluble in absolute alcohol and in vegetable oils; insoluble in water and in glycerin. In solid form, may be dispersible in water.

Vitamin E: Practically odorless and tasteless. The alpha tocopherols and alpha tocopheryl acetates occur as clear, yellow, or greenish yellow, viscous oils. *d*-Alpha tocopheryl acetate may solidify in the cold. Alpha tocopheryl acid succinate occurs as a white powder; the *d*-isomer melts at about 75°, and the *dl*-form melts at about 70°. The alpha tocopherols are unstable to air and light, particularly when in alkaline media. The esters are stable to air and light, but are unstable to alkali; the acid succinate is also unstable when held molten. Alpha tocopheryl acid succinate is very soluble in chloroform; soluble in alcohol, in ether, in acetone, and in vegetable oils; slightly soluble in alkaline solutions; insoluble in water. The other forms of Vitamin E are insoluble in water; soluble in alcohol; miscible with ether, with acetone, with vegetable oils, and with chloroform. *NF category:* Antioxidant; plasticizer.

Vitamin E Preparation: The liquid forms are clear, yellow to brownish red, viscous oils. The solid forms are white to tan-white granular powders. The liquid forms are soluble in alcohol; insoluble in water. Miscible with ether, with acetone, with vegetable oils, and with chloroform. The solid forms disperse in water to give cloudy suspensions.

Voriconazole: White to almost white powder. Freely soluble in acetone and in methylene chloride; very slightly soluble in water.

Warfarin Sodium: White, odorless, amorphous or crystalline powder, having a slightly bitter taste. Is discolored by light. Very soluble in water; freely soluble in alcohol; very slightly soluble in chloroform and in ether.

Water for Injection: Clear, colorless, odorless liquid. *NF category:* Solvent; pharmaceutical water.

Bacteriostatic Water for Injection: Clear, colorless liquid, odorless or having the odor of the antimicrobial substance. *NF category:* Vehicle (sterile); pharmaceutical water.

Sterile Water for Inhalation: Clear, colorless solution.

Sterile Water for Injection: Clear, colorless, odorless liquid. *NF category:* Solvent; pharmaceutical water.

Sterile Water for Irrigation: Clear, colorless, odorless liquid. *NF category:* Solvent; pharmaceutical water.

Purified Water: Clear, colorless, odorless liquid. *NF category:* Solvent; pharmaceutical water.

Carnauba Wax: Light brown to pale yellow, moderately coarse powder or flakes, possessing a characteristic bland odor, and free from rancidity. Specific gravity is about 0.99. Freely soluble in warm benzene; soluble in warm chloroform and in warm toluene; slightly soluble in boiling alcohol; insoluble in water. *NF category:* Coating agent.

Emulsifying Wax: Creamy white, wax-like solid, having a mild, characteristic odor. Freely soluble in ether, in chloroform, in most hydrocarbon solvents, and in aerosol propellants; soluble in alcohol; insoluble in water. *NF category:* Emulsifying agent; wetting and/or solubilizing agent; stiffening agent.

Microcrystalline Wax: White or cream-colored, odorless, waxy solid. Soluble in chloroform, in ether, in volatile oils, and in most warm fixed oils; sparingly soluble in dehydrated alcohol; insoluble in water. *NF category:* Coating agent; stiffening agent.

White Wax: Yellowish-white solid, somewhat translucent in thin layers. Has a faint, characteristic odor, and is free from rancidity. Specific gravity is about 0.95. Sparingly soluble in cold alcohol; insoluble in water. Boiling alcohol dissolves the cerotic acid and a portion of the myricin, which are constituents of White Wax. Completely soluble in chloroform, in ether, and in fixed and volatile oils. Partly soluble in cold benzene and in cold carbon disulfide; completely soluble in these liquids at about 30°. *NF category:* Stiffening agent.

Yellow Wax: Solid varying in color from yellow to grayish brown. Has an agreeable, honey-like odor. Is somewhat brittle when cold, and presents a dull, granular, noncrystalline fracture when broken. It becomes pliable from the heat of the hand. Specific gravity is about 0.95. Sparingly soluble in cold alcohol; insoluble in water. Boiling alcohol dissolves the cerotic acid and a portion of the myricin, that are constituents of Yellow Wax. Soluble in chloroform, in ether, in fixed oils, and in volatile oils; sparingly soluble in cold benzene and in cold carbon disulfide; soluble in these liquids at about 30°. *NF category:* Stiffening agent.

Wheat Bran: Light tan powder having a characteristic aroma. Practically insoluble in cold water and in alcohol. Available in a variety of particle sizes depending upon the degree of milling to which it is subjected. Color and flavor development variable, depending on the extent to which it is heat-stabilized.

Xanthan Gum: Cream-colored powder. Its solutions in water are neutral to litmus. Soluble in hot or cold water. *NF category:* Suspending and/or viscosity-increasing agent; film-forming agent; polymers for ophthalmic use; release-modifying agent.

Xenon Xe 127: Clear, colorless gas.

Xenon Xe 133 Injection: Clear, colorless solution.

Xylazine: Colorless to white crystals. Sparingly soluble in dilute acid, in acetone, and in chloroform; insoluble in dilute alkali.

Xylazine Hydrochloride: Colorless to white crystals. Sparingly soluble in dilute acid, in acetone, and in methanol; insoluble in dilute alkali.

Xylitol: White crystals or crystalline powder. It has a sweet taste and produces a cooling sensation in the mouth. One g dissolves in about 0.65 mL of water. Sparingly soluble in alcohol. Crystalline xylitol has a melting range between 92° and 96°. *NF category:* Coating agent; emollient; humectant; sweetening agent; diluent.

Xylometazoline Hydrochloride: White to off-white, odorless, crystalline powder. Melts above 300°, with decomposition. Freely soluble in alcohol; soluble in water; sparingly soluble in chloroform; practically insoluble in benzene and in ether.

Xylose: Colorless needles or white, crystalline powder. Is odorless, and has a slightly sweet taste. Very soluble in water; slightly soluble in alcohol.

Yellow Fever Vaccine: Slightly dull, light-orange colored, flaky or crustlike, desiccated mass.

Yohimbine Hydrochloride: White to yellow powder. Melts at about 295°, with decomposition. Soluble in boiling water; slightly soluble in water and in alcohol.

Yttrium Chloride: Colorless, deliquescent crystals. Soluble in water and in alcohol.

Zalcitabine: White to off-white, crystalline powder. Soluble in water and in methanol; sparingly soluble in alcohol, in acetonitrile, in chloroform, and in methylene chloride; slightly soluble in cyclohexane.

Zaleplon: White to off-white powder. Sparingly soluble in alcohol; slightly soluble in propylene glycol; practically insoluble in water.

Zanamivir: White, crystalline powder. Sparingly soluble in water; insoluble in acetone, in acetonitrile, in alcohol, and in isopropyl alcohol.

Zein: White to yellow powder. Soluble in aqueous alcohols, in glycols, in ethylene glycol ethyl ether, in furfuryl alcohol, in tetrahydrofurfuryl alcohol, in aqueous alkaline solutions of pH 11.5 or greater, and in acetone-water mixtures between the limits of 60% and 80% of acetone by volume; insoluble in water, in acetone, and in all anhydrous alcohols except methanol. *NF category:* Coating agent; wet binder.

Zidovudine: White to yellowish powder. Melts at about 124°. Exhibits polymorphism. Soluble in alcohol; sparingly soluble in water.

Zileuton: White to off-white powder.

Zinc Acetate: White crystals or granules, having a slight acetous odor and an astringent taste. Is slightly efflorescent. Freely soluble in water and in boiling alcohol; slightly soluble in alcohol. *NF category:* Emollient.

Zinc Chloride: White or practically white, odorless, crystalline powder, or white or practically white crystalline granules. May also be in porcelain-like masses or molded into cylinders. Is very deliquescent. A solution (1 in 10) is acid to litmus. Very soluble in water; freely soluble in alcohol and in glycerin. Its solution in water or in alcohol is usually slightly turbid, but the turbidity disappears when a small quantity of hydrochloric acid is added.

Zinc Gluconate: White or practically white powder or granules. Soluble in water; very slightly soluble in alcohol.

Zinc Oxide: Very fine, odorless, amorphous, white or yellowish white powder, free from gritty particles. It gradually absorbs carbon dioxide from air. Soluble in dilute acids; insoluble in water and in alcohol. *NF category:* Antimicrobial preservative; coating agent.

Zinc Stearate: Fine, white, bulky powder, free from grittiness. Has a faint, characteristic odor. Is neutral to moistened litmus paper. Insoluble in water, in alcohol, and in ether. *NF category:* Lubricant.

Zinc Sulfate: Colorless, transparent prisms, or small needles. May occur as a white, granular, crystalline powder. Is odorless and is efflorescent in dry air. Its solutions are acid to litmus. Very soluble in water (heptahydrate); freely soluble in water (monohydrate) and in glycerin (heptahydrate); practically insoluble in alcohol (monohydrate); insoluble in alcohol (heptahydrate).

Zinc Undecylenate: Fine, white powder. Practically insoluble in water and in alcohol.

Ziprasidone Hydrochloride (anhydrous): White to slightly pink powder. Soluble in anhydrous formic acid; insoluble in *n*-hexane.

Ziprasidone Hydrochloride (monohydrate): White to slightly pink powder. Slightly soluble in methanol and in methylene chloride; practically insoluble in water.

Zolazepam Hydrochloride: White to off-white, crystalline powder. Freely soluble in water and in 0.1 N hydrochloric acid; soluble in methanol; slightly soluble in chloroform; practically insoluble in ether.

Zolmitriptan: White to off-white, crystalline powder. Freely soluble to soluble in methanol; soluble in water; sparingly soluble in dichloromethane; practically insoluble in toluene.

Zolpidem Tartrate: White to off-white powder, hygroscopic. Sparingly soluble in methanol; slightly soluble in water; practically insoluble in methylene chloride.

Zonisamide: White to off-white powder. Freely soluble in dimethylformamide; soluble in methanol.

Chapter Charts

Chart Guide—USP General Chapters[1]

Official Articles
- • Chemical Medicines Drug Substances—Universal Tests: See *Chart 1a*
- • Chemical Medicines Drug Substances—Specific Tests: See *Chart 1b*
- • Biologics Drug Substances: See *Chart 2*
- • Excipients—Universal Tests: See *Chart 3a*
- • Excipients—Specific Tests: See *Chart 3b*
- • Chemical Medicines Drug Products—Universal Tests: See *Chart 4a*
- • Chemical Medicines Drug Products—Specific Tests: See *Chart 4b*
- • Biologics Drug Products: See *Chart 5*
- • Vaccines: See *Chart 6*
- • Blood and Blood Products: See *Chart 7*
- • Cell, Gene, and Tissue Based Products: See *Chart 8*
- • Dietary Supplement Ingredients: See *Chart 11*
- • Dietary Supplement Products: See *Chart 12*
- • Compounding—Substance/Preparation/Practice: See *Chart 13*
- • Medical Devices
  - • ⟨691⟩ *Cotton*
  - • ⟨861⟩ *Sutures—Diameter*
  - • ⟨871⟩ *Sutures—Needle Attachment*

Generally Applicable
- • Basic Elements
  - • ⟨1010⟩ *Analytical Data—Interpretation and Treatment*
  - • ⟨1029⟩ *Good Documentation Guidelines*
  - • ⟨1039⟩ *Chemometrics*
  - • ⟨1058⟩ *Analytical Instrument Qualification*
  - • ⟨1097⟩ *Bulk Powder Sampling Procedures*
  - • ⟨1151⟩ *Pharmaceutical Dosage Forms*
  - • ⟨1210⟩ *Statistical Tools for Procedure Validation*
  - • ⟨1224⟩ *Transfer of Analytical Procedures*
  - • ⟨1225⟩ *Validation of Compendial Procedures*
  - • ⟨1226⟩ *Verification of Compendial Procedures*
- • Drug Product Distribution: See *Chart 9*
- • Microbiology—Nonsterile Products: See *Chart 10a*
- • Microbiology—Sterile Products: See *Chart 10b*

---

[1] This table and the *Charts 1–13* that follow are intended as a guide to the chapters in this publication. They may not be all-inclusive, and they are not intended to describe expectations for articles or limit the application of tests to any article in the *USP–NF*.

Chart 1a. Chemical Medicines Drug Substances—Universal Tests

Chapter	Description	Identification	Assay	Impurities		
				Organic	**Inorganic**	**Residual Solvents**
⟨7⟩ Labeling	♦					
⟨11⟩ USP Reference Standards			♦			
⟨81⟩ Antibiotics—Microbial Assays			♦			
⟨181⟩ Identification Organic Nitrogenous Bases		♦				
⟨191⟩ Identification Tests—General		♦				
⟨193⟩ Identification Tests—Tetracyclines		♦				
⟨197⟩ Spectrophotometric Identification Test		♦				
⟨201⟩ Thin-Layer Chromatographic Identification Test		♦				
⟨202⟩ Identification of Fixed Oils by Thin-Layer Chromatography		♦				
⟨203⟩ High-Performance Thin-Layer Chromatography Procedure for Identification of Articles of Botanical Origin		♦				
⟨206⟩ Aluminum					♦	
⟨211⟩ Arsenic					♦	
⟨221⟩ Chloride and Sulfate					♦	
⟨223⟩ Dimethylaniline				♦		
⟨231⟩ Heavy Metals					♦	
⟨232⟩ Elemental Impurities—Limits					♦	
⟨233⟩ Elemental Impurities—Procedures					♦	
⟨241⟩ Iron					♦	
⟨251⟩ Lead					♦	
⟨261⟩ Mercury					♦	
⟨281⟩ Residue on Ignition					♦	
⟨291⟩ Selenium					♦	
⟨351⟩ Assay for Steroids			♦			
⟨391⟩ Epinephrine Assay			♦			
⟨401⟩ Fats and Fixed Oils		♦				
⟨425⟩ Iodometric Assay—Antibiotics			♦			
⟨451⟩ Nitrate Titration			♦			
⟨461⟩ Nitrogen Determination				♦		
⟨466⟩ Ordinary Impurities				♦		
⟨467⟩ Residual Solvents						♦
⟨471⟩ Oxygen Flask Combustion					♦	
⟨511⟩ Single-Steroid Assay			♦			
⟨541⟩ Titrimetry		♦	♦			
⟨621⟩ Chromatography		♦	♦	♦		♦
⟨659⟩ Packaging and Storage Requirements	♦					
⟨730⟩ Plasma Spectrochemistry					♦	
⟨731⟩ Loss on Drying		♦				♦
⟨733⟩ Loss on Ignition					♦	
⟨735⟩ X-Ray Fluorescence Spectrometry		♦	♦		♦	
⟨736⟩ Mass Spectrometry		♦	♦			
⟨761⟩ Nuclear Magnetic Resonance Spectroscopy		♦				
⟨781⟩ Optical Rotation		♦		♦		
⟨801⟩ Polarography			♦	♦		
⟨852⟩ Atomic Absorption Spectroscopy		♦	♦	♦		
⟨853⟩ Fluorescence Spectroscopy		♦	♦	♦		

Chart 1a. Chemical Medicines Drug Substances—Universal Tests *(Continued)*

Chapter	Description	Identification	Assay	Impurities Organic	Inorganic	Residual Solvents
⟨854⟩ Mid-Infrared Spectroscopy		♦	♦	♦		
⟨855⟩ Nephelometry, Turbidimetry, and Visual Comparison		♦		♦		
⟨857⟩ Ultraviolet-Visible Spectroscopy		♦	♦	♦		
⟨941⟩ Characterization of Crystalline and Partially Crystalline Solids by X-Ray Powder Diffraction (XRPD)		♦				
⟨1064⟩ Identification of Articles of Botanical Origin by High-Performance Thin-Layer Chromatography Procedure		♦				
⟨1086⟩ Impurities in Drug Substances and Drug Products				♦		
⟨1119⟩ Near-Infrared Spectroscopy		♦				
⟨1120⟩ Raman Spectroscopy		♦	♦			
⟨1223.1⟩ Validation of Alternative Methods to Antibiotic Microbial Assays			♦			
⟨1730⟩ Plasma Spectrochemistry—Theory and Practice		♦	♦			
⟨1735⟩ X-Ray Fluorescence Spectrometry—Theory and Practice		♦	♦			
⟨1736⟩ Applications of Mass Spectrometry		♦	♦			
⟨1761⟩ Applications of Nuclear Magnetic Resonance Spectroscopy		♦				
⟨1852⟩ Atomic Absorption Spectroscopy—Theory and Practice		♦	♦	♦		
⟨1853⟩ Fluorescence Spectroscopy—Theory and Practice		♦	♦	♦		
⟨1854⟩ Mid-Infrared Spectroscopy—Theory and Practice		♦	♦	♦		
⟨1857⟩ Ultraviolet-Visible Spectroscopy—Theory and Practice		♦	♦	♦		

Chart 1b. Chemical Medicines Drug Substances—Specific Tests

Chapter	Physicochemical Characterization	Equipment	Water Content
⟨31⟩ Volumetric Apparatus		♦	
⟨41⟩ Balances		♦	
⟨268⟩ Porosity by Nitrogen Adsorption–Desorption	♦		
⟨301⟩ Acid-Neutralizing Capacity	♦		
⟨429⟩ Light Diffraction Measurement of Particle Size	♦		
⟨541⟩ Titrimetry			♦
⟨616⟩ Bulk Density and Tapped Density	♦		
⟨631⟩ Color and Achromicity	♦		
⟨641⟩ Completeness of Solution	♦		
⟨651⟩ Congealing Temperature	♦		
⟨695⟩ Crystallinity	♦		
⟨699⟩ Density of Solids	♦		
⟨721⟩ Distilling Range	♦		
⟨731⟩ Loss on Drying	♦		♦
⟨735⟩ X-Ray Fluorescence Spectrometry	♦		
⟨741⟩ Melting Range or Temperature	♦		
⟨761⟩ Nuclear Magnetic Resonance Spectroscopy	♦		
⟨776⟩ Optical Microscopy	♦		
⟨781⟩ Optical Rotation	♦		

Chart 1b. Chemical Medicines Drug Substances—Specific Tests (Continued)

Chapter	Physicochemical Characterization	Equipment	Water Content
⟨782⟩ Vibrational Circular Dichroism Spectroscopy	♦		
⟨785⟩ Osmolality and Osmolarity	♦		
⟨786⟩ Particle Size Distribution Estimation by Analytical Sieving	♦		
⟨791⟩ pH	♦		
⟨811⟩ Powder Fineness	♦		
⟨831⟩ Refractive Index	♦		
⟨841⟩ Specific Gravity	♦		
⟨846⟩ Specific Surface Area	♦		
⟨881⟩ Tensile Strength	♦		
⟨891⟩ Thermal Analysis			♦
⟨911⟩ Viscosity—Capillary Methods	♦		
⟨912⟩ Viscosity—Rotational Methods	♦		
⟨913⟩ Viscosity—Rolling Ball Method	♦		
⟨921⟩ Water Determination			♦
⟨941⟩ Characterization of Crystalline and Partially Crystalline Solids by X-Ray Powder Diffraction (XRPD)	♦		
⟨1051⟩ Cleaning Glass Apparatus		♦	
⟨1119⟩ Near-Infrared Spectroscopy	♦		
⟨1120⟩ Raman Spectroscopy	♦		
⟨1251⟩ Weighing on an Analytical Balance		♦	
⟨1730⟩ Plasma Spectrochemistry—Theory and Practice	♦		
⟨1735⟩ X-Ray Fluorescence Spectrometry—Theory and Practice	♦		
⟨1761⟩ Applications of Nuclear Magnetic Resonance Spectroscopy	♦		
⟨1782⟩ Vibrational Circular Dichroism Spectroscopy—Theory and Practice	♦		
⟨1911⟩ Rheometry	♦		

Chart 2. Biologics Drug Substances

Chapter	Description	Identification	Safety	Assay	Physicochemical	Equipment	Impurities Process Related	Impurities Product Related	Characterization
⟨7⟩ Labeling	♦								
⟨11⟩ USP Reference Standards		♦	♦	♦	♦		♦	♦	
⟨31⟩ Volumetric Apparatus						♦			
⟨41⟩ Balances						♦			
⟨61⟩ Microbiological Examination of Nonsterile Products: Microbial Enumeration Tests			♦						
⟨63⟩ Mycoplasma Tests			♦				♦		
⟨71⟩ Sterility Tests			♦						
⟨81⟩ Antibiotics—Microbial Assays							♦		
⟨85⟩ Bacterial Endotoxins Test			♦						
⟨87⟩ Biological Reactivity Tests, In Vitro			♦						
⟨88⟩ Biological Reactivity Tests, In Vivo			♦						
⟨111⟩ Design and Analysis of Biological Assays				♦			♦	♦	♦
⟨121⟩ Insulin Assays		♦		♦					
⟨121.1⟩ Physicochemical Analytical Procedures for Insulins		♦			♦		♦	♦	♦
⟨126⟩ Somatropin Bioidentity Tests		♦							

Chart 2. Biologics Drug Substances *(Continued)*

Chapter	Description	Identification	Safety	Assay	Physico-chemical	Equipment	Impurities Process Related	Impurities Product Related	Characterization
⟨129⟩ Analytical Procedures for Recombinant Therapeutic Monoclonal Antibodies					♦			♦	♦
⟨191⟩ Identification Tests—General		♦							
⟨197⟩ Spectrophotometric Identification Tests		♦							
⟨208⟩ Anti-factor Xa and Anti-factor IIA Assays for Unfractionated and Low Molecular Weight Heparins				♦					
⟨209⟩ Low Molecular Weight Heparin Molecular Weight Determinations		♦							
⟨210⟩ Monosaccharide Analysis					♦			♦	♦
⟨212⟩ Oligosaccharide Analysis					♦			♦	♦
⟨231⟩ Heavy Metals							♦		
⟨232⟩ Elemental Impurities—Limits							♦		
⟨233⟩ Elemental Impurities—Procedures							♦		
⟨467⟩ Residual Solvents							♦		
⟨503⟩ Acetic Acid in Peptides							♦		
⟨503.1⟩ Trifluoroacetic Acid (TFA) in Peptides							♦		
⟨507⟩ Protein Determination Procedures					♦				♦
⟨541⟩ Titrimetry				♦			♦		
⟨621⟩ Chromatography		♦		♦	♦		♦	♦	♦
⟨631⟩ Color and Achromicity	♦								
⟨695⟩ Crystallinity	♦								
⟨730⟩ Plasma Spectrochemistry							♦		
⟨731⟩ Loss on Drying							♦		
⟨736⟩ Mass Spectrometry		♦		♦	♦		♦	♦	♦
⟨761⟩ Nuclear Magnetic Resonance Spectroscopy		♦		♦	♦		♦	♦	♦
⟨781⟩ Optical Rotation				♦					
⟨782⟩ Vibrational Circular Dichroism Spectroscopy				♦					
⟨786⟩ Particle Size Distribution Estimation by Analytical Sieving					♦				
⟨831⟩ Refractive Index					♦				
⟨852⟩ Atomic Absorption Spectroscopy		♦		♦	♦		♦		♦
⟨853⟩ Fluorescence Spectroscopy		♦		♦	♦		♦		♦
⟨854⟩ Mid-Infrared Spectroscopy		♦		♦	♦		♦		♦
⟨855⟩ Nephelometry, Turbidimetry, and Visual Comparison				♦	♦		♦		♦
⟨857⟩ Ultraviolet-Visible Spectroscopy		♦		♦	♦		♦		♦
⟨921⟩ Water Determination							♦		
⟨1025⟩ Pancreatin	♦	♦	♦	♦	♦		♦	♦	♦
⟨1030⟩ Biological Assay Chapters—Overview and Glossary		♦		♦					♦
⟨1032⟩ Design and Development of Biological Assays		♦		♦					♦
⟨1033⟩ Biological Assay Validation		♦		♦					♦
⟨1034⟩ Analysis of Biological Assays		♦		♦					♦
⟨1041⟩ Biologics	♦								

Chart 2. Biologics Drug Substances *(Continued)*

Chapter	Descrip-tion	Identifica-tion	Safety	Assay	Physico-chemical	Equip-ment	Impurities Process Related	Impurities Product Related	Charac-teriza-tion
⟨1044⟩ Cryopreservation of Cells				♦					♦
⟨1048⟩ Quality of Biotechnological Products: Analysis of the Expression Construct in Cells Used for Production of r-DNA Derived Protein Products									♦
⟨1050.1⟩ Design, Evaluation, and Characterization of Viral Clearance Procedures			♦						
⟨1052⟩ Biotechnology-Derived Arti-cles—Amino Acid Analysis		♦		♦	♦		♦		♦
⟨1053⟩ Capillary Electrophoresis		♦		♦	♦		♦		♦
⟨1054⟩ Biotechnology-Derived Arti-cles—Isoelectric Focusing		♦		♦	♦		♦		♦
⟨1055⟩ Biotechnology-Derived Arti-cles—Peptide Mapping		♦		♦	♦		♦		♦
⟨1056⟩ Biotechnology-Derived Arti-cles—Polyacrylamide Gel Electropho-resis		♦		♦	♦		♦		♦
⟨1057⟩ Biotechnology-Derived Arti-cles—Total Protein Assay		♦		♦	♦		♦		♦
⟨1065⟩ Ion Chromatography					♦				
⟨1084⟩ Glycoprotein and Glycan Analy-sis—General Considerations							♦		♦
⟨1102⟩ Immunological Test Methods—General Considerations		♦		♦			♦	♦	♦
⟨1103⟩ Immunological Test Methods—Enzyme-Linked Immunosorbent Assay (ELISA)		♦		♦			♦	♦	♦
⟨1104⟩ Immunological Test Methods—Immunoblot Analysis		♦					♦	♦	♦
⟨1105⟩ Immunological Test Methods—Surface Plasmon Resonance				♦					♦
⟨1113⟩ Microbial Characterization, Identification, and Strain Typing			♦						
⟨1121⟩ Nomenclature	♦								
⟨1125⟩ Nucleic Acid-Based Techni-ques—General		♦							♦
⟨1126⟩ Nucleic Acid-Based Techni-ques—Extraction, Detection, and Se-quencing		♦							♦
⟨1127⟩ Nucleic Acid-Based Techni-ques—Amplification		♦							♦
⟨1128⟩ Nucleic Acid-Based Techni-ques—Microarray									♦
⟨1129⟩ Nucleic Acid-Based Techni-ques—Genotyping									♦
⟨1130⟩ Nucleic Acid-Based Techni-ques—Approaches for Detecting Trace Nucleic Acids (Residual DNA Testing)			♦				♦		♦
⟨1132⟩ Residual Host Cell Protein Measurement in Biopharmaceuticals			♦				♦		
⟨1180⟩ Human Plasma			♦						
⟨1181⟩ Scanning Electron Microscopy									♦
⟨1211⟩ Sterility Assurance			♦						
⟨1228⟩ Depyrogenation			♦						
⟨1228.1⟩ Dry Heat Depyrogenation			♦						
⟨1228.3⟩ Depyrogenation by Filtration			♦						

Chart 2. Biologics Drug Substances *(Continued)*

Chapter	Descrip-tion	Identifica-tion	Safety	Assay	Physico-chemical	Equip-ment	Impurities		Charac-teriza-tion
							Process Related	Product Related	
⟨1228.5⟩ *Endotoxin Indicators for De-pyrogenation*			♦						
⟨1229⟩ *Sterilization of Compendial Arti-cles*			♦						
⟨1229.4⟩ *Sterilizing Filtration of Liquids*			♦						
⟨1229.14⟩ *Sterilization Cycle Develop-ment*			♦						
⟨1229.15⟩ *Sterilizing Filtration of Gases*			♦			♦			
⟨1251⟩ *Weighing on an Analytical Bal-ance*						♦			
⟨1736⟩ *Applications of Mass Spectrom-etry*		♦	♦						
⟨1761⟩ *Applications of Nuclear Mag-netic Resonance Spectroscopy*		♦		♦	♦		♦	♦	♦
⟨1782⟩ *Vibrational Circular Dichroism Spectroscopy—Theory and Practice*					♦				
⟨1852⟩ *Atomic Absorption Spectrosco-py—Theory and Practice*		♦		♦	♦		♦		♦
⟨1853⟩ *Fluorescence Spectroscopy—Theory and Practice*		♦		♦	♦		♦		♦
⟨1854⟩ *Mid-Infrared Spectroscopy—Theory and Practice*		♦		♦	♦		♦		♦
⟨1857⟩ *Ultraviolet-Visible Spectrosco-py—Theory and Practice*		♦		♦	♦		♦		♦

Chart 3a. Excipients—Universal Tests

Chapter	Description	Identification	Assay	Impurities		
				Organic	Inorganic	Residual Solvents
⟨7⟩ *Labeling*	♦					
⟨11⟩ *USP Reference Standards*		♦	♦	♦		
⟨181⟩ *Identification—Organic Nitrogenous Bases*		♦				
⟨191⟩ *Identification Tests—General*		♦				
⟨197⟩ *Spectrophotometric Identification Tests*		♦				
⟨201⟩ *Thin-Layer Chromato-graphic Identification Test*		♦				
⟨202⟩ *Identification of Fixed Oils by Thin-Layer Chroma-tography*		♦				
⟨203⟩ *High-Performance Thin-Layer Chromatography Procedure for Identification of Articles of Botanical Ori-gin*		♦				
⟨206⟩ *Aluminum*					♦	
⟨211⟩ *Arsenic*					♦	
⟨221⟩ *Chloride and Sulfate*					♦	
⟨226⟩ *4-Epianhydrotetracy-cline*				♦		
⟨228⟩ *Ethylene Oxide and Di-oxane*						♦
⟨231⟩ *Heavy Metals*					♦	
⟨232⟩ *Elemental Impurities—Limits*					♦	

Chart 3a. Excipients—Universal Tests *(Continued)*

Chapter	Description	Identification	Assay	Impurities Organic	Impurities Inorganic	Residual Solvents
⟨233⟩ Elemental Impurities—Procedures					♦	
⟨241⟩ Iron					♦	
⟨251⟩ Lead					♦	
⟨261⟩ Mercury					♦	
⟨281⟩ Residue on Ignition					♦	
⟨291⟩ Selenium					♦	
⟨311⟩ Alginates Assay			♦			
⟨345⟩ Assay for Citric Acid/Citrate and Phosphate			♦			
⟨401⟩ Fats and Fixed Oils		♦				
⟨425⟩ Iodometric Assay—Antibiotics			♦			
⟨431⟩ Methoxy Determination			♦			
⟨461⟩ Nitrogen Determination				♦		
⟨466⟩ Ordinary Impurities				♦		
⟨467⟩ Residual Solvents						♦
⟨469⟩ Ethylene Glycol, Diethylene Glycol, and Triethylene Glycol in Ethoxylated Substances				♦		
⟨471⟩ Oxygen Flask Combustion					♦	
⟨541⟩ Titrimetry			♦			
⟨621⟩ Chromatography		♦	♦	♦		♦
⟨730⟩ Plasma Spectrochemistry					♦	
⟨731⟩ Loss on Drying		♦				♦
⟨733⟩ Loss on Ignition					♦	
⟨735⟩ X-Ray Fluorescence Spectrometry		♦			♦	
⟨736⟩ Mass Spectrometry		♦				
⟨781⟩ Optical Rotation		♦		♦		
⟨801⟩ Polarography			♦	♦		
⟨852⟩ Atomic Absorption Spectroscopy		♦	♦	♦		
⟨853⟩ Fluorescence Spectroscopy		♦	♦	♦		
⟨854⟩ Mid-Infrared Spectroscopy		♦	♦	♦		
⟨855⟩ Nephelometry, Turbidimetry, and Visual Comparison			♦	♦		
⟨857⟩ Ultraviolet-Visible Spectroscopy		♦	♦	♦		
⟨941⟩ Characterization of Crystalline and Partially Crystalline Solids by X-Ray Powder Diffraction (XRPD)		♦				
⟨1064⟩ Identification of Articles of Botanical Origin by High-Performance Thin-Layer Chromatography Procedure		♦				

Chart 3a. Excipients—Universal Tests (Continued)

Chapter	Description	Identification	Assay	Impurities		
				Organic	**Inorganic**	**Residual Solvents**
⟨1086⟩ Impurities in Drug Substances and Drug Products				♦		
⟨1091⟩ Labeling of Inactive Ingredients	♦					
⟨1119⟩ Near-Infrared Spectroscopy		♦				
⟨1730⟩ Plasma Spectrochemistry—Theory and Practice		♦	♦			
⟨1735⟩ X-Ray Fluorescence Spectrometry—Theory and Practice		♦	♦			
⟨1736⟩ Applications of Mass Spectrometry		♦				
⟨1852⟩ Atomic Absorption Spectroscopy—Theory and Practice		♦	♦	♦		
⟨1853⟩ Fluorescence Spectroscopy—Theory and Practice		♦	♦	♦		
⟨1854⟩ Mid-Infrared Spectroscopy—Theory and Practice		♦	♦	♦		
⟨1857⟩ Ultraviolet-Visible Spectroscopy—Theory and Practice		♦	♦	♦		

Chart 3b. Excipients—Specific Tests

Chapter	Physicochemical Characterization	Equipment	Pharmaceutical Water	Functionality/Safety/GMPs
⟨31⟩ Volumetric Apparatus		♦		
⟨41⟩ Balances		♦		
⟨61⟩ Microbiological Examination of Nonsterile Products: Microbial Enumeration Tests				♦
⟨62⟩ Microbiological Examination of Nonsterile Products: Tests For Specified Microorganisms				♦
⟨85⟩ Bacterial Endotoxins Test				♦
⟨268⟩ Porosity by Nitrogen Adsorption–Desorption	♦			
⟨301⟩ Acid-Neutralizing Capacity				♦
⟨429⟩ Light Diffraction Measurement of Particle Size	♦			
⟨541⟩ Titrimetry			♦	
⟨616⟩ Bulk Density and Tapped Density	♦			
⟨631⟩ Color and Achromicity	♦			
⟨641⟩ Completeness of Solution	♦			
⟨643⟩ Total Organic Carbon			♦	
⟨645⟩ Water Conductivity			♦	
⟨651⟩ Congealing Temperature	♦			
⟨695⟩ Crystallinity	♦			
⟨699⟩ Density of Solids	♦			

Chart 3b. Excipients—Specific Tests *(Continued)*

Chapter	Physicochemical Characterization	Equipment	Pharmaceutical Water	Functionality/Safety/GMPs
⟨721⟩ Distilling Range	♦			
⟨731⟩ Loss on Drying	♦			
⟨735⟩ X-Ray Fluorescence Spectrometry	♦			
⟨741⟩ Melting Range or Temperature	♦			
⟨761⟩ Nuclear Magnetic Resonance Spectroscopy	♦			
⟨776⟩ Optical Microscopy	♦			
⟨781⟩ Optical Rotation	♦			
⟨782⟩ Vibrational Circular Dichroism Spectroscopy	♦			
⟨785⟩ Osmolality and Osmolarity	♦			
⟨786⟩ Particle Size Distribution Estimation by Analytical Sieving	♦			
⟨791⟩ pH	♦		♦	
⟨811⟩ Powder Fineness	♦			
⟨831⟩ Refractive Index	♦			
⟨841⟩ Specific Gravity	♦			
⟨846⟩ Specific Surface Area	♦			
⟨881⟩ Tensile Strength	♦			
⟨891⟩ Thermal Analysis			♦	
⟨911⟩ Viscosity—Capillary Methods	♦			
⟨912⟩ Viscosity—Rotational Methods	♦			
⟨913⟩ Viscosity—Rolling Ball Method	♦			
⟨914⟩ Viscosity—Pressure Driven Methods	♦			
⟨921⟩ Water Determination			♦	
⟨941⟩ Characterization of Crystalline and Partially Crystalline Solids by X-Ray Powder Diffraction (XRPD)	♦			
⟨1051⟩ Cleaning Glass Apparatus		♦		
⟨1059⟩ Excipient Performance				♦
⟨1063⟩ Shear Cell Methodology for Powder Flow Testing	♦	♦		
⟨1074⟩ Excipient Biological Safety Evaluation Guidelines				♦
⟨1078⟩ Good Manufacturing Practices for Bulk Pharmaceutical Excipients				♦
⟨1080⟩ Bulk Pharmaceutical Excipients—Certificate of Analysis				♦
⟨1097⟩ Bulk Powder Sampling Procedures				♦
⟨1119⟩ Near-Infrared Spectroscopy	♦			
⟨1174⟩ Powder Flow	♦			♦

Chart 3b. Excipients—Specific Tests *(Continued)*

Chapter	Physicochemical Characterization	Equipment	Pharmaceutical Water	Functionality/Safety/ GMPs
⟨1195⟩ Significant Change Guide for Bulk Pharmaceutical Excipients				♦
⟨1197⟩ Good Distribution Practices for Bulk Pharmaceutical Excipients				♦
⟨1230⟩ Water for Hemodialysis Applications			♦	
⟨1231⟩ Water for Pharmaceutical Purposes			♦	
⟨1251⟩ Weighing on an Analytical Balance		♦		
⟨1644⟩ Theory and Practice of Electrical Conductivity Measurements of Solutions			♦	
⟨1730⟩ Plasma Spectrochemistry—Theory and Practice	♦			
⟨1735⟩ X-Ray Fluorescence Spectrometry—Theory and Practice	♦			
⟨1761⟩ Applications of Nuclear Magnetic Resonance Spectroscopy	♦			
⟨1782⟩ Vibrational Circular Dichroism Spectroscopy—Theory and Practice	♦			
⟨1911⟩ Rheometry	♦			

Chart 4a. Chemical Medicines Drug Products—Universal Tests

Chapter	Description	Identification	Assay	Impurities		
				Organic	Inorganic	Residual Solvents
⟨1⟩ Injections and Implanted Drug Products (Parenterals)—Product Quality Tests	♦	♦	♦	♦	♦	♦
⟨2⟩ Oral Drug Products—Product Quality Tests	♦	♦	♦	♦	♦	♦
⟨3⟩ Topical and Transdermal Drug Products—Product Quality Tests	♦	♦	♦	♦	♦	♦
⟨4⟩ Mucosal Drug Products—Product Quality Tests	♦	♦	♦	♦	♦	♦
⟨5⟩ Inhalation and Nasal Drug Products—General Information and Product Quality Checks	♦	♦	♦	♦	♦	♦
⟨7⟩ Labeling	♦					
⟨81⟩ Antibiotics—Microbial Assays			♦			
⟨191⟩ Identification Tests—General		♦				
⟨197⟩ Spectrophotometric Identification Tests		♦				
⟨201⟩ Thin-Layer Chromatographic Identification Test		♦				
⟨202⟩ Identification of Fixed Oils by Thin-Layer Chromatography		♦				
⟨203⟩ High-Performance Thin-Layer Chromatography Procedure for Identification of Articles of Botanical Origin		♦				

Chart 4a. Chemical Medicines Drug Products—Universal Tests (Continued)

Chapter	Description	Identification	Assay	Organic	Inorganic	Residual Solvents
				Impurities		
⟨227⟩ 4-Aminophenol in Acetaminophen-Containing Drug Products				♦		
⟨232⟩ Elemental Impurities—Limits					♦	
⟨233⟩ Elemental Impurities—Procedures					♦	
⟨281⟩ Residue on Ignition					♦	
⟨341⟩ Antimicrobial Agents—Content			♦			
⟨351⟩ Assay for Steroids			♦			
⟨391⟩ Epinephrine Assay			♦			
⟨413⟩ Impurities Testing in Medical Gases				♦		
⟨415⟩ Medical Gases Assay			♦			
⟨451⟩ Nitrate Titration			♦			
⟨461⟩ Nitrogen Determination				♦		
⟨466⟩ Ordinary Impurities				♦		
⟨467⟩ Residual Solvents						♦
⟨501⟩ Salts of Organic Nitrogenous Bases		♦	♦			
⟨541⟩ Titrimetry			♦			
⟨611⟩ Alcohol Determination			♦			
⟨621⟩ Chromatography		♦	♦	♦		♦
⟨730⟩ Plasma Spectrochemistry					♦	
⟨733⟩ Loss on Ignition					♦	
⟨735⟩ X-Ray Fluorescence Spectrometry		♦			♦	
⟨736⟩ Mass Spectrometry		♦				
⟨781⟩ Optical Rotation				♦		
⟨801⟩ Polarography			♦	♦		
⟨821⟩ Radioactivity		♦	♦	♦	♦	♦
⟨823⟩ Positron Emission Tomography Drugs for Compounding, Investigational, and Research Uses		♦	♦	♦	♦	♦
⟨852⟩ Atomic Absorption Spectroscopy		♦	♦	♦		
⟨853⟩ Fluorescence Spectroscopy		♦	♦	♦		
⟨854⟩ Mid-Infrared Spectroscopy		♦	♦	♦		
⟨855⟩ Nephelometry, Turbidimetry, and Visual Comparison			♦	♦		
⟨857⟩ Ultraviolet-Visible Spectroscopy		♦	♦	♦		
⟨1064⟩ Identification of Articles of Botanical Origin by High-Performance Thin-Layer Chromatography Procedure		♦				
⟨1065⟩ Ion Chromatography			♦			
⟨1086⟩ Impurities in Drug Substances and Drug Products				♦		
⟨1121⟩ Nomenclature	♦					
⟨1223.1⟩ Validation of Alternative Methods to Antibiotic Microbial Assays			♦			

Chart 4a. Chemical Medicines Drug Products—Universal Tests *(Continued)*

Chapter	Description	Identification	Assay	Impurities		
				Organic	**Inorganic**	**Residual Solvents**
⟨1730⟩ *Plasma Spectrochemistry—Theory and Practice*		♦	♦			
⟨1735⟩ *X-Ray Fluorescence Spectrometry—Theory and Practice*		♦	♦			
⟨1736⟩ *Applications of Mass Spectrometry*		♦				
⟨1821⟩ *Radioactivity—Theory and Practice*	♦					
⟨1823⟩ *Positron Emission Tomography Drugs—Information*	♦					
⟨1852⟩ *Atomic Absorption Spectroscopy—Theory and Practice*		♦	♦	♦		
⟨1853⟩ *Fluorescence Spectroscopy—Theory and Practice*		♦	♦	♦		
⟨1854⟩ *Mid-Infrared Spectroscopy—Theory and Practice*		♦	♦	♦		
⟨1857⟩ *Ultraviolet-Visible Spectroscopy—Theory and Practice*		♦	♦	♦		

Chart 4b. Chemical Medicines Drug Products—Specific Tests

Chapter	Equipment	Water Content	Performance Tests						Mucosal (7 membrane surfaces)
			Mucosal		Parenteral	Oral	Topical	Inhalational	
			Ophthalmic[1]	Nasal					
⟨31⟩ *Volumetric Apparatus*	♦								
⟨41⟩ *Balances*	♦								
⟨71⟩ *Sterility Tests*					♦				
⟨85⟩ *Bacterial Endotoxins Test*					♦				
⟨87⟩ *Biological Reactivity Tests, In Vitro*					♦				
⟨88⟩ *Biological Reactivity Tests, In Vivo*					♦				
⟨151⟩ *Pyrogen Test*					♦				
⟨301⟩ *Acid-Neutralizing Capacity*						♦			
⟨381⟩ *Elastomeric Closures for Injections*					♦				
⟨541⟩ *Titrimetry*		♦							
⟨601⟩ *Inhalation and Nasal Drug Products: Aerosols, Sprays, and Powders—Performance Quality Tests*				♦				♦	
⟨602⟩ *Propellants*								♦	
⟨603⟩ *Topical Aerosols*							♦		
⟨604⟩ *Leak Rate*				♦			♦	♦	
⟨697⟩ *Container Content for Injections*					♦				
⟨701⟩ *Disintegration*						♦			
⟨705⟩ *Quality Attributes of Tablets Labeled as Having a Functional Score*						♦			
⟨711⟩ *Dissolution*						♦			
⟨724⟩ *Drug Release*						♦	♦		

[1] See *Microbiology (Chart 10)*.

Chart 4b. Chemical Medicines Drug Products—Specific Tests *(Continued)*

Chapter	Equipment	Water Content	Mucosal Ophthalmic[1]	Nasal	Parenteral	Oral	Topical	Inhalational	Mucosal (7 membrane surfaces)
(729) Globule Size Distribution in Lipid Injectable Emulsions					♦				
(731) Loss on Drying		♦							
(771) Ophthalmic Products—Quality Tests			♦						
(785) Osmolality and Osmolarity			♦						
(787) Subvisible Particulate Matter in Therapeutic Protein Injections					♦				
(788) Particulate Matter in Injections					♦				
(789) Particulate Matter in Ophthalmic Solutions			♦						
(790) Visible Particulates in Injections					♦				
(791) pH			♦	♦	♦		♦	♦	
(891) Thermal Analysis		♦							
(905) Uniformity of Dosage Units			♦	♦	♦	♦	♦		♦
(921) Water Determination		♦							
(1004) Mucosal Drug Products—Performance Tests									♦
(1005) Acoustic Emission						♦			
(1051) Cleaning Glass Apparatus	♦								
(1087) Apparent Intrinsic Dissolution—Dissolution Testing Procedures for Rotating Disk and Stationary Disk						♦			
(1088) In Vitro and In Vivo Evaluation of Dosage Forms						♦			
(1090) Assessment of Drug Product Performance—Bioavailability, Bioequivalence, and Dissolution						♦			
(1092) The Dissolution Procedure: Development and Validation						♦			
(1094) Capsules—Dissolution Testing and Related Quality Attributes						♦			
(1113) Microbial Characterization, Identification, and Strain Typing					♦				
(1211) Sterility Assurance					♦				
(1216) Tablet Friability						♦			
(1217) Tablet Breaking Force						♦			
(1228) Depyrogenation					♦				
(1228.1) Dry Heat Depyrogenation					♦				

[1] See *Microbiology (Chart 10)*.

Chart 4b. Chemical Medicines Drug Products—Specific Tests (Continued)

Chapter	Equipment	Water Content	Performance Tests							Mucosal (7 membrane surfaces)
			Mucosal		Parenteral	Oral	Topical	Inhalational		
			Ophthalmic[1]	Nasal						
⟨1228.3⟩ Depyrogenation by Filtration					♦					
⟨1228.5⟩ Endotoxin Indicators for Depyrogenation					♦					
⟨1229⟩ Sterilization of Compendial Articles					♦					
⟨1229.2⟩ Moist Heat Sterilization of Aqueous Liquids					♦					
⟨1229.3⟩ Monitoring of Bioburden					♦					
⟨1229.4⟩ Sterilizing Filtration of Liquids					♦					
⟨1229.13⟩ Sterilization-in-Place	♦									
⟨1229.14⟩ Sterilization Cycle Development					♦					
⟨1229.15⟩ Sterilizing Filtration of Gases	♦				♦					
⟨1251⟩ Weighing on an Analytical Balance	♦									
⟨1601⟩ Products for Nebulization—Characterization Tests								♦		
⟨1602⟩ Spacers and Valved Holding Chambers Used With Inhalation Aerosols—Characterization Tests								♦		
⟨1724⟩ Semisolid Drug Products—Performance Tests							♦			
⟨1771⟩ Ophthalmic Products—Performance Tests			♦							
⟨1788⟩ Methods for the Determination of Particulate Matter in Injections and Ophthalmic Solutions					♦					
⟨1787⟩ Measurement of Subvisible Particulate Matter in Therapeutic Protein Injections					♦					

[1] See *Microbiology* (Chart 10).

Chart 5. Biologics Drug Products

Chapter	Identification	Characterization	Equipment	Misc. Tests	Description	Safety	Assay	Physicochemical	Impurities	
									Process Related	Product Related
⟨1⟩ Injections and Implanted Drug Products (Parenterals)—Product Quality Tests				♦						
⟨7⟩ Labeling				♦						
⟨11⟩ USP Reference Standards	♦					♦	♦	♦	♦	♦
⟨31⟩ Volumetric Apparatus			♦							
⟨41⟩ Balances			♦							

Chart 5. Biologics Drug Products *(Continued)*

Chapter	Identification	Characterization	Equipment	Misc. Tests	Description	Safety	Assay	Physicochemical	Impurities Process Related	Product Related
⟨61⟩ Microbiological Examination of Nonsterile Products: Microbial Enumeration Tests						♦			♦	
⟨62⟩ Microbiological Examination of Nonsterile Products: Tests for Specified Microorganisms						♦			♦	
⟨63⟩ Mycoplasma Tests						♦			♦	
⟨71⟩ Sterility Tests						♦				
⟨85⟩ Bacterial Endotoxins Test						♦				
⟨87⟩ Biological Reactivity Tests, In Vitro						♦				
⟨88⟩ Biological Reactivity Tests, In Vivo						♦				
⟨89⟩ Enzymes Used as Ancillary Materials in Pharmaceutical Manufacturing	♦	♦			♦	♦	♦		♦	
⟨89.1⟩ Collagenase I	♦	♦			♦	♦	♦		♦	
⟨89.2⟩ Collagenase II	♦	♦			♦	♦	♦		♦	
⟨90⟩ Fetal Bovine Serum—Quality Attributes and Functionality Tests									♦	
⟨111⟩ Design and Analysis of Biological Assays		♦					♦		♦	♦
⟨121⟩ Insulin Assays	♦						♦			
⟨121.1⟩ Physicochemical Analytical Procedures for Insulins	♦	♦						♦	♦	♦
⟨123⟩ Glucagon Bioidentity Tests	♦									
⟨124⟩ Erythropoietin Bioassays		♦					♦			
⟨126⟩ Somatropin Bioidentity Tests	♦									
⟨129⟩ Analytical Procedures for Recombinant Therapeutic Monoclonal Antibodies		♦						♦		♦
⟨130⟩ Protein A Quality Attributes									♦	
⟨151⟩ Pyrogen Test						♦				
⟨191⟩ Identification Tests—General	♦									
⟨197⟩ Spectrophotometric Identification Tests	♦									
⟨208⟩ Anti-factor Xa and Anti-factor IIa Assays for Unfractionated and Low Molecular Weight Heparins		♦					♦			
⟨209⟩ Low Molecular Weight Heparin Molecular Weight Determinations		♦								

Chart 5. Biologics Drug Products (Continued)

Chapter	Identification	Characterization	Equipment	Misc. Tests	Description	Safety	Assay	Physicochemical	Impurities Process Related	Impurities Product Related
⟨212⟩ Oligosaccharide Analysis		♦						♦		♦
⟨231⟩ Heavy Metals									♦	
⟨232⟩ Elemental Impurities—Limits									♦	
⟨233⟩ Elemental Impurities—Procedures									♦	
⟨341⟩ Antimicrobial Agents—Content						♦				
⟨467⟩ Residual Solvents									♦	
⟨503⟩ Acetic Acid in Peptides									♦	
⟨507⟩ Protein Determination Procedures		♦						♦		
⟨541⟩ Titrimetry							♦		♦	
⟨621⟩ Chromatography	♦	♦					♦	♦	♦	♦
⟨631⟩ Color and Achromicity					♦					
⟨660⟩ Containers—Glass				♦						
⟨661⟩ Plastic Packaging Systems and Their Materials of Construction				♦						
⟨661.1⟩ Plastic Materials of Construction				♦						
⟨661.2⟩ Plastic Packaging Systems for Pharmaceutical Use				♦						
⟨671⟩ Containers—Performance Testing				♦						
⟨695⟩ Crystallinity					♦					
⟨697⟩ Container Content for Injections				♦						
⟨730⟩ Plasma Spectrochemistry									♦	
⟨731⟩ Loss on Drying									♦	
⟨736⟩ Mass Spectrometry	♦	♦					♦	♦	♦	♦
⟨761⟩ Nuclear Magnetic Resonance Spectroscopy	♦	♦					♦	♦	♦	♦
⟨781⟩ Optical Rotation							♦			
⟨782⟩ Vibrational Circular Dichroism Spectroscopy							♦			
⟨785⟩ Osmolality and Osmolarity								♦		
⟨786⟩ Particle Size Distribution Estimation by Analytical Sieving								♦		
⟨787⟩ Subvisible Particulate Matter in Therapeutic Protein Injections				♦						
⟨788⟩ Particulate Matter in Injections				♦						
⟨791⟩ pH					♦			♦		
⟨821⟩ Radioactivity	♦	♦	♦			♦	♦		♦	♦
⟨831⟩ Refractive Index								♦		

Chart 5. Biologics Drug Products (Continued)

Chapter	Identification	Characterization	Equipment	Misc. Tests	Description	Safety	Assay	Physicochemical	Impurities Process Related	Product Related
⟨852⟩ Atomic Absorption Spectroscopy	◆	◆					◆	◆	◆	
⟨853⟩ Fluorescence Spectroscopy	◆	◆					◆	◆	◆	
⟨854⟩ Mid-Infrared Spectroscopy	◆	◆					◆	◆	◆	
⟨855⟩ Nephelometry, Turbidimetry, and Visual Comparison		◆					◆	◆	◆	
⟨857⟩ Ultraviolet-Visible Spectroscopy	◆	◆					◆	◆	◆	
⟨921⟩ Water Determination									◆	
⟨1024⟩ Bovine Serum									◆	
⟨1025⟩ Pancreatin	◆	◆			◆	◆	◆	◆	◆	◆
⟨1030⟩ Biological Assay Chapters—Overview and Glossary	◆	◆					◆			
⟨1032⟩ Design and Development of Biological Assays	◆	◆					◆			
⟨1033⟩ Biological Assay Validation	◆	◆					◆			
⟨1034⟩ Analysis of Biological Assays	◆	◆					◆			
⟨1041⟩ Biologics					◆					
⟨1044⟩ Cryopreservation of Cells		◆					◆			
⟨1050⟩ Viral Safety Evaluation of Biotechnology Products Derived from Cell Lines of Human or Animal Origin						◆				
⟨1050.1⟩ Design, Evaluation, and Characterization of Viral Clearance Procedures						◆				
⟨1052⟩ Biotechnology Derived Articles—Amino Acid Analysis	◆	◆					◆	◆	◆	
⟨1053⟩ Capillary Electrophoresis	◆	◆					◆	◆	◆	
⟨1054⟩ Biotechnology Derived Articles—Isoelectric Focusing	◆	◆					◆	◆	◆	
⟨1055⟩ Biotechnology Derived Articles—Peptide Mapping	◆	◆					◆	◆	◆	
⟨1056⟩ Biotechnology Derived Articles—Polyacrylamide Gel Electrophoresis	◆	◆					◆	◆	◆	
⟨1057⟩ Biotechnology Derived Articles—Total Protein Assay	◆	◆					◆	◆	◆	
⟨1065⟩ Ion Chromatography										◆

Chart 5. Biologics Drug Products *(Continued)*

Chapter	Identifica-tion	Charac-terization	Equip-ment	Misc. Tests	Descrip-tion	Safety	Assay	Physico-chemical	Impurities	
									Proc-ess Rela-ted	Prod-uct Re-lated
⟨1084⟩ *Glycoprotein and Glycan Analysis—General Considerations*		♦						♦	♦	
⟨1102⟩ *Immunological Test Methods—General Considerations*	♦	♦					♦		♦	♦
⟨1103⟩ *Immunological Test Methods—Enzyme-Linked Immunosorbent Assay (ELISA)*	♦	♦					♦		♦	♦
⟨1104⟩ *Immunological Test Methods—Immuno-blot Analysis*	♦	♦							♦	♦
⟨1105⟩ *Immunological Test Methods—Surface Plasmon Resonance*		♦					♦			
⟨1106⟩ *Immunogenicity Assays—Design and Vali-dation of Immunoassays to Detect Anti-Drug Anti-bodies*						♦				
⟨1106.1⟩ *Immunogenicity Assays—Design and Vali-dation of Assays to De-tect Anti-Drug Neutraliz-ing Antibody*						♦				
⟨1111⟩ *Microbiological Ex-amination of Nonsterile Products: Acceptance Cri-teria for Pharmaceutical Preparations and Sub-stances for Pharmaceuti-cal Use*						♦				
⟨1113⟩ *Microbial Charac-terization, Identification, and Strain Typing*						♦			♦	
⟨1121⟩ *Nomenclature*					♦					
⟨1125⟩ *Nucleic Acid-Based Techniques—General*							♦		♦	
⟨1126⟩ *Nucleic Acid-Based Techniques—Extraction, Detection, and Sequenc-ing*							♦		♦	
⟨1127⟩ *Nucleic Acid-Based Techniques—Amplifica-tion*							♦		♦	
⟨1128⟩ *Nucleic Acid-Based Techniques—Microarray*									♦	
⟨1129⟩ *Nucleic Acid-Based Techniques—Genotyping*							♦		♦	
⟨1130⟩ *Nucleic Acid-Based Techniques—Approaches for Detecting Trace Nu-cleic Acids (Residual DNA Testing)*						♦			♦	
⟨1132⟩ *Residual Host Cell Protein Measurement in Biopharmaceuticals*						♦			♦	

Chart 5. Biologics Drug Products (Continued)

Chapter	Identifica-tion	Charac-terization	Equip-ment	Misc. Tests	Descrip-tion	Safety	Assay	Physico-chemical	Impurities Process Related	Product Related
⟨1181⟩ *Scanning Electron Microscopy*		♦								
⟨1211⟩ *Sterility Assurance*						♦				
⟨1228⟩ *Depyrogenation*						♦				
⟨1228.1⟩ *Dry Heat Depyrogenation*						♦				
⟨1228.3⟩ *Depyrogenation by Filtration*						♦				
⟨1228.5⟩ *Endotoxin Indicators for Depyrogenation*						♦				
⟨1229⟩ *Sterilization of Compendial Articles*						♦				
⟨1229.4⟩ *Sterilizing Filtration of Liquids*						♦				
⟨1229.13⟩ *Sterilization-in-Place*			♦							
⟨1229.14⟩ *Sterilization Cycle Development*						♦				
⟨1229.15⟩ *Sterilizing Filtration of Gases*			♦			♦				
⟨1251⟩ *Weighing on an Analytical Balance*			♦							
⟨1660⟩ *Evaluation of the Inner Surface Durability of Glass Containers*				♦						
⟨1661⟩ *Evaluation of Plastic Packaging Systems and Their Materials of Construction with Respect to Their User Safety Impact*				♦						
⟨1663⟩ *Assessment of Extractables Associated with Pharmaceutical Packaging/Delivery Systems*				♦						
⟨1664⟩ *Assessment of Drug Product Leachables Associated with Pharmaceutical Packaging/Delivery Systems*				♦						
⟨1736⟩ *Applications of Mass Spectrometry*	♦	♦					♦	♦	♦	♦
⟨1761⟩ *Applications of Nuclear Magnetic Resonance Spectroscopy*	♦	♦					♦	♦	♦	♦
⟨1782⟩ *Vibrational Circular Dichroism Spectroscopy—Theory and Practice*								♦		
⟨1787⟩ *Measurement of Subvisible Particulate Matter in Therapeutic Protein Injections*				♦						

Chart 5. Biologics Drug Products (*Continued*)

Chapter	Identification	Characterization	Equipment	Misc. Tests	Description	Safety	Assay	Physicochemical	Impurities Process Related	Product Related
⟨1788⟩ *Methods for the Determination of Particulate Matter in Injections and Ophthalmic Solutions*				♦						
⟨1821⟩ *Radioactivity—Theory and Practice*					♦					
⟨1852⟩ *Atomic Absorption Spectroscopy—Theory and Practice*	♦	♦					♦	♦	♦	
⟨1853⟩ *Fluorescence Spectroscopy—Theory and Practice*	♦	♦					♦	♦	♦	
⟨1854⟩ *Mid-Infrared Spectroscopy—Theory and Practice*	♦	♦					♦	♦	♦	
⟨1857⟩ *Ultraviolet-Visible Spectroscopy—Theory and Practice*	♦	♦					♦	♦	♦	

Chart 6. Vaccines

Chapter	Identification	Characterization	Equipment	Misc. Tests	Description	Safety	Assay	Physicochemical	Impurities Process Related	Product Related
⟨1⟩ *Injections and Implanted Drug Products (Parenterals)—Product Quality Tests*				♦						
⟨11⟩ *USP Reference Standards*						♦				
⟨31⟩ *Volumetric Apparatus*			♦							
⟨41⟩ *Balances*			♦							
⟨63⟩ *Mycoplasma Tests*						♦				
⟨71⟩ *Sterility Tests*						♦				
⟨81⟩ *Antibiotics—Microbial Assays*									♦	
⟨85⟩ *Bacterial Endotoxins Test*						♦				
⟨88⟩ *Biological Reactivity Tests, In Vivo*						♦				
⟨90⟩ *Fetal Bovine Serum—Quality Attributes and Functionality Tests*						♦			♦	
⟨111⟩ *Design and Analysis of Biological Assays*		♦					♦		♦	♦
⟨151⟩ *Pyrogen Test*						♦				
⟨198⟩ *Nuclear Magnetic Resonance Spectroscopy Identity Testing of Bacterial Polysaccharides Used in Vaccine Manufacture*	♦									
⟨341⟩ *Antimicrobial Agents—Content*						♦				
⟨507⟩ *Protein Determination Procedures*		♦						♦		

Chart 6. Vaccines *(Continued)*

Chapter	Identifica-tion	Charac-terization	Equip-ment	Misc. Tests	Descrip-tion	Safety	Assay	Physico-chemical	Impurities Process Related	Impurities Product Related
⟨621⟩ Chromatography	♦	♦					♦	♦	♦	♦
⟨660⟩ Containers—Glass				♦						
⟨661⟩ Plastic Packaging Systems and Their Materials of Construction				♦						
⟨661.1⟩ Plastic Materials of Construction				♦						
⟨661.2⟩ Plastic Packaging Systems for Pharmaceutical Use				♦						
⟨671⟩ Containers—Performance Testing				♦						
⟨695⟩ Crystallinity										
⟨697⟩ Container Content for Injections				♦						
⟨731⟩ Loss on Drying									♦	
⟨736⟩ Mass Spectrometry	♦	♦					♦	♦	♦	♦
⟨761⟩ Nuclear Magnetic Resonance Spectroscopy	♦	♦					♦	♦	♦	♦
⟨786⟩ Particle Size Distribution Estimation by Analytical Sieving								♦		
⟨787⟩ Subvisible Particulate Matter in Therapeutic Protein Injections				♦						
⟨788⟩ Particulate Matter in Injections				♦						
⟨790⟩ Visible Particulates in Injections				♦						
⟨791⟩ pH					♦			♦		
⟨852⟩ Atomic Absorption Spectroscopy							♦	♦		
⟨853⟩ Fluorescence Spectroscopy							♦	♦		
⟨854⟩ Mid-Infrared Spectroscopy							♦	♦		
⟨855⟩ Nephelometry, Turbidimetry, and Visual Comparison							♦	♦		
⟨857⟩ Ultraviolet-Visible Spectroscopy							♦	♦		
⟨921⟩ Water Determination									♦	
⟨1024⟩ Bovine Serum						♦			♦	
⟨1030⟩ Biological Assay Chapters—Overview and Glossary	♦	♦					♦			
⟨1032⟩ Design and Development of Biological Assays	♦	♦					♦			
⟨1033⟩ Biological Assay Validation	♦	♦					♦			
⟨1034⟩ Analysis of Biological Assays	♦	♦					♦			
⟨1041⟩ Biologics					♦					

Chart 6. Vaccines *(Continued)*

Chapter	Identifica-tion	Charac-terization	Equip-ment	Misc. Tests	Descrip-tion	Safety	Assay	Physico-chemical	Impurities	
									Proc-ess Rela-ted	Prod-uct Re-lated
⟨1044⟩ *Cryopreservation of Cells*		♦					♦			
⟨1052⟩ *Biotechnology Derived Articles—Amino Acid Analysis*	♦	♦					♦	♦	♦	
⟨1053⟩ *Capillary Electrophoresis*	♦	♦					♦	♦	♦	
⟨1054⟩ *Biotechnology Derived Articles—Isoelectric Focusing*	♦	♦					♦	♦	♦	
⟨1055⟩ *Biotechnology Derived Articles—Peptide Mapping*	♦	♦					♦	♦	♦	
⟨1056⟩ *Biotechnology Derived Articles—Polyacrylamide Gel Electrophoresis*	♦	♦					♦	♦	♦	
⟨1057⟩ *Biotechnology Derived Articles—Total Protein Assay*	♦	♦					♦	♦	♦	
⟨1065⟩ *Ion Chromatography*								♦		
⟨1084⟩ *Glycoprotein and Glycan Analysis—General Considerations*		♦						♦	♦	
⟨1102⟩ *Immunological Test Methods—General Considerations*	♦	♦							♦	♦
⟨1103⟩ *Immunological Test Methods—Enzyme-Linked Immunosorbent Assay (ELISA)*	♦	♦							♦	♦
⟨1104⟩ *Immunological Test Methods—Immunoblot Analysis*	♦	♦							♦	♦
⟨1105⟩ *Immunological Test Methods—Surface Plasmon Resonance*		♦					♦			
⟨1113⟩ *Microbial Characterization, Identification, and Strain Typing*						♦				
⟨1121⟩ *Nomenclature*						♦				
⟨1126⟩ *Nucleic Acid-Based Techniques—Extraction, Detection, and Sequencing*	♦	♦							♦	
⟨1127⟩ *Nucleic Acid-Based Techniques—Amplification*	♦	♦							♦	
⟨1128⟩ *Nucleic Acid-Based Techniques—Microarray*	♦									
⟨1129⟩ *Nucleic Acid-Based Techniques—Genotyping*	♦									
⟨1130⟩ *Nucleic Acid-Based Techniques—Approaches for Detecting Trace Nucleic Acids (Residual DNA Testing)*									♦	

Chart 6. Vaccines *(Continued)*

Chapter	Identification	Characterization	Equipment	Misc. Tests	Description	Safety	Assay	Physicochemical	Impurities Process Related	Product Related
⟨1211⟩ Sterility Assurance						♦				
⟨1228⟩ Depyrogenation						♦				
⟨1228.1⟩ Dry Heat Depyrogenation						♦				
⟨1228.3⟩ Depyrogenation by Filtration						♦				
⟨1228.5⟩ Endotoxin Indicators for Depyrogenation						♦				
⟨1229⟩ Sterilization of Compendial Articles						♦				
⟨1229.4⟩ Sterilizing Filtration of Liquids						♦				
⟨1229.13⟩ Sterilization-in-Place			♦							
⟨1229.14⟩ Sterilization Cycle Development						♦				
⟨1229.15⟩ Sterilizing Filtration of Gases			♦			♦				
⟨1234⟩ Vaccines for Human Use—Polysaccharide and Glycoconjugate Vaccines	♦	♦				♦	♦	♦	♦	♦
⟨1235⟩ Vaccines for Human Use—General Considerations	♦	♦					♦			♦
⟨1237⟩ Virology Test Methods						♦	♦		♦	♦
⟨1238⟩ Vaccines for Human Use—Bacterial Vaccines	♦	♦					♦	♦	♦	♦
⟨1251⟩ Weighing on an Analytical Balance			♦							
⟨1660⟩ Evaluation of the Inner Surface Durability of Glass Containers				♦						
⟨1661⟩ Evaluation of Plastic Packaging Systems and Their Materials of Construction with Respect to Their User Safety Impact				♦						
⟨1663⟩ Assessment of Extractables Associated with Pharmaceutical Packaging/Delivery Systems				♦						
⟨1664⟩ Assessment of Drug Product Leachables Associated with Pharmaceutical Packaging/Delivery Systems				♦						
⟨1736⟩ Applications of Mass Spectrometry	♦	♦					♦	♦	♦	♦
⟨1761⟩ Applications of Nuclear Magnetic Resonance Spectroscopy	♦	♦					♦		♦	♦

Chart 6. Vaccines *(Continued)*

Chapter	Identification	Characterization	Equipment	Misc. Tests	Description	Safety	Assay	Physicochemical	Impurities Process Related	Product Related
⟨1787⟩ *Measurement of Subvisible Particulate Matter in Therapeutic Protein Injections*				♦						
⟨1788⟩ *Methods for the Determination of Particulate Matter in Injections and Ophthalmic Solutions*				♦						
⟨1852⟩ *Atomic Absorption Spectroscopy—Theory and Practice*							♦	♦		
⟨1853⟩ *Fluorescence Spectroscopy—Theory and Practice*							♦	♦		
⟨1854⟩ *Mid-Infrared Spectroscopy—Theory and Practice*							♦	♦		
⟨1857⟩ *Ultraviolet-Visible Spectroscopy—Theory and Practice*							♦	♦		

Chart 7. Blood and Blood Products

Chapter	Identification	Characterization	Equipment	Misc. Tests	Description	Safety	Assay	Physicochemical	Impurities Process Related	Product Related
⟨1⟩ *Injections and Implanted Drug Products (Parenterals)—Product Quality Tests*				♦						
⟨11⟩ *USP Reference Standards*	♦					♦	♦	♦	♦	♦
⟨31⟩ *Volumetric Apparatus*			♦							
⟨41⟩ *Balances*			♦							
⟨51⟩ *Antimicrobial Effectiveness Testing*						♦				
⟨61⟩ *Microbiological Examination of Nonsterile Products: Microbial Enumeration Tests*						♦				
⟨62⟩ *Microbiological Examination of Nonsterile Products: Tests for Specified Microorganisms*						♦				
⟨71⟩ *Sterility Tests*						♦				
⟨85⟩ *Bacterial Endotoxins Test*						♦				
⟨87⟩ *Biological Reactivity Tests, In Vitro*						♦				
⟨88⟩ *Biological Reactivity Tests, In Vivo*						♦				
⟨111⟩ *Design and Analysis of Biological Assays*		♦					♦		♦	♦
⟨151⟩ *Pyrogen Test*						♦				
⟨191⟩ *Identification Tests—General*	♦									

Chart 7. Blood and Blood Products *(Continued)*

Chapter	Identifica-tion	Charac-terization	Equip-ment	Misc. Tests	Descrip-tion	Safety	Assay	Physico-chemical	Impurities Process Related	Impurities Product Re-lated
⟨197⟩ Spectrophotometric Identification Tests	♦									
⟨208⟩ Anti-factor Xa and Anti-factor IIa Assays for Unfractionated and Low Molecular Weight Heparins							♦			
⟨209⟩ Low Molecular Weight Heparin Molecular Weight Determinations	♦									
⟨341⟩ Antimicrobial Agents—Content						♦				
⟨507⟩ Protein Determination Procedures		♦						♦		
⟨621⟩ Chromatography	♦	♦					♦	♦	♦	♦
⟨631⟩ Color and Achromicity					♦					
⟨660⟩ Containers—Glass				♦						
⟨661⟩ Plastic Packaging Systems and Their Materials of Construction				♦						
⟨661.1⟩ Plastic Materials of Construction				♦						
⟨661.2⟩ Plastic Packaging Systems for Pharmaceutical Use				♦						
⟨671⟩ Containers—Performance Testing				♦						
⟨695⟩ Crystallinity					♦					
⟨697⟩ Container Content for Injections				♦						
⟨731⟩ Loss on Drying									♦	
⟨736⟩ Mass Spectrometry	♦	♦					♦	♦	♦	♦
⟨761⟩ Nuclear Magnetic Resonance Spectroscopy	♦	♦					♦	♦	♦	♦
⟨785⟩ Osmolality and Osmolarity								♦		
⟨787⟩ Subvisible Particulate Matter in Therapeutic Protein Injections				♦						
⟨788⟩ Particulate Matter in Injections				♦						
⟨790⟩ Visible Particulates in Injections				♦						
⟨791⟩ pH					♦			♦		
⟨852⟩ Atomic Absorption Spectroscopy	♦	♦					♦	♦	♦	
⟨853⟩ Fluorescence Spectroscopy	♦	♦					♦	♦	♦	
⟨854⟩ Mid-Infrared Spectroscopy	♦	♦					♦	♦	♦	
⟨855⟩ Nephelometry, Turbidimetry, and Visual Comparison		♦					♦	♦	♦	

Chart 7. Blood and Blood Products (Continued)

Chapter	Identification	Characterization	Equipment	Misc. Tests	Description	Safety	Assay	Physico-chemical	Impurities Process Related	Impurities Product Related
⟨857⟩ Ultraviolet-Visible Spectroscopy	♦	♦					♦	♦	♦	
⟨921⟩ Water Determination									♦	
⟨1030⟩ Biological Assay Chapters—Overview and Glossary	♦	♦					♦			
⟨1032⟩ Design and Development of Biological Assays	♦	♦					♦			
⟨1033⟩ Biological Assay Validation	♦	♦					♦			
⟨1034⟩ Analysis of Biological Assays	♦	♦					♦			
⟨1041⟩ Biologics					♦					
⟨1044⟩ Cryopreservation of Cells		♦								
⟨1052⟩ Biotechnology Derived Articles—Amino Acid Analysis	♦	♦					♦	♦	♦	
⟨1053⟩ Capillary Electrophoresis	♦	♦					♦	♦	♦	
⟨1054⟩ Biotechnology Derived Articles—Isoelectric Focusing	♦	♦					♦	♦	♦	
⟨1055⟩ Biotechnology Derived Articles—Peptide Mapping	♦	♦					♦	♦	♦	
⟨1056⟩ Biotechnology Derived Articles—Polyacrylamide Gel Electrophoresis	♦	♦					♦	♦	♦	
⟨1057⟩ Biotechnology Derived Articles—Total Protein Assay	♦	♦					♦	♦	♦	
⟨1065⟩ Ion Chromatography	♦									
⟨1102⟩ Immunological Test Methods—General Considerations	♦	♦							♦	♦
⟨1103⟩ Immunological Test Methods—Enzyme-Linked Immunosorbent Assay (ELISA)	♦	♦							♦	♦
⟨1104⟩ Immunological Test Methods—Immunoblot Analysis	♦	♦							♦	♦
⟨1105⟩ Immunological Test Methods—Surface Plasmon Resonance		♦					♦			
⟨1106⟩ Immunogenicity Assays—Design and Validation of Immunoassays to Detect Anti-Drug Antibodies						♦				

Chart 7. Blood and Blood Products *(Continued)*

Chapter	Identifica-tion	Charac-terization	Equip-ment	Misc. Tests	Descrip-tion	Safety	Assay	Physico-chemical	Impurities Process Related	Product Related
⟨1106.1⟩ Immunogenicity Assays—Design and Validation of Assays to Detect Anti-Drug Neutralizing Antibody						♦				
⟨1111⟩ Microbiological Examination of Nonsterile Products: Acceptance Criteria for Pharmaceutical Preparations and Substances for Pharmaceutical Use						♦				
⟨1113⟩ Microbial Characterization, Identification, and Strain Typing						♦				
⟨1116⟩ Microbiological Control and Monitoring of Aseptic Processing Environments						♦				
⟨1121⟩ Nomenclature					♦					
⟨1125⟩ Nucleic Acid-Based Techniques—General		♦								
⟨1130⟩ Nucleic Acid-Based Techniques—Approaches for Detecting Trace Nucleic Acids (Residual DNA Testing)		♦								
⟨1180⟩ Human Plasma						♦				
⟨1211⟩ Sterility Assurance						♦				
⟨1228⟩ Depyrogenation						♦				
⟨1228.1⟩ Dry Heat Depyrogenation						♦				
⟨1228.3⟩ Depyrogenation by Filtration						♦				
⟨1228.5⟩ Endotoxin Indicators for Depyrogenation						♦				
⟨1229⟩ Sterilization of Compendial Articles						♦				
⟨1229.4⟩ Sterilizing Filtration of Liquids						♦				
⟨1229.5⟩ Biological Indicators for Sterilization						♦				
⟨1229.13⟩ Sterilization-in-Place			♦							
⟨1229.14⟩ Sterilization Cycle Development						♦				
⟨1229.15⟩ Sterilizing Filtration of Gases			♦			♦				
⟨1237⟩ Virology Test Methods						♦				
⟨1240⟩ Virus Testing of Human Plasma for Further Manufacture						♦				
⟨1251⟩ Weighing on an Analytical Balance			♦							

Chart 7. Blood and Blood Products (Continued)

Chapter	Identifica-tion	Charac-terization	Equip-ment	Misc. Tests	Descrip-tion	Safety	Assay	Physico-chemical	Impurities Process Related	Product Related
⟨1660⟩ Evaluation of the Inner Surface Durability of Glass Containers				♦						
⟨1661⟩ Evaluation of Plastic Packaging Systems and Their Materials of Construction with Respect to Their User Safety Impact				♦						
⟨1663⟩ Assessment of Extractables Associated with Pharmaceutical Packaging/Delivery Systems				♦						
⟨1664⟩ Assessment of Drug Product Leachables Associated with Pharmaceutical Packaging/Delivery Systems				♦						
⟨1736⟩ Applications of Mass Spectrometry	♦	♦					♦	♦	♦	♦
⟨1761⟩ Applications of Nuclear Magnetic Resonance Spectroscopy	♦	♦					♦	♦	♦	♦
⟨1787⟩ Measurement of Subvisible Particulate Matter in Therapeutic Protein Injections				♦						
⟨1788⟩ Methods for the Determination of Particulate Matter in Injections and Ophthalmic Solutions				♦						
⟨1852⟩ Atomic Absorption Spectroscopy—Theory and Practice	♦	♦					♦	♦	♦	
⟨1853⟩ Fluorescence Spectroscopy—Theory and Practice	♦	♦					♦	♦	♦	
⟨1854⟩ Mid-Infrared Spectroscopy—Theory and Practice	♦	♦					♦	♦	♦	
⟨1857⟩ Ultraviolet-Visible Spectroscopy—Theory and Practice	♦	♦					♦	♦	♦	

Chart 8. Cell, Gene, and Tissue Based Products

Chapter	Universal Tests Identifica-tion	Assay	Specific Tests[1,2] Biocompati-bility	Microbial/ Sterility Issues	Produc-tion Issues	Product Issues	Equip-ment	Characteri-zation
⟨1⟩ Injections and Implanted Drug Products (Parenterals)—Product Quality Tests					♦			
⟨11⟩ USP Reference Standards	♦							
⟨31⟩ Volumetric Apparatus							♦	
⟨41⟩ Balances							♦	

[1] For Functionality test, see ⟨881⟩ Tensile Strength.
[2] For Water test, see ⟨1231⟩ Water for Pharmaceutical Purposes.

Chart 8. Cell, Gene, and Tissue Based Products (Continued)

Chapter	Universal Tests		Specific Tests[1,2]					
	Identification	Assay	Biocompatibility	Microbial/ Sterility Issues	Production Issues	Product Issues	Equipment	Characterization
⟨61⟩ Microbiological Examination of Nonsterile Products: Microbial Enumeration Tests				♦				
⟨62⟩ Microbiological Examination of Nonsterile Products: Tests for Specified Microorganisms				♦				
⟨63⟩ Mycoplasma Tests				♦				
⟨71⟩ Sterility Tests				♦				
⟨85⟩ Bacterial Endotoxins Test				♦				
⟨87⟩ Biological Reactivity Tests, In Vitro			♦					
⟨88⟩ Biological Reactivity Tests, In Vivo			♦					
⟨90⟩ Fetal Bovine Serum— Quality Attributes and Functionality Tests					♦			
⟨92⟩ Growth Factors and Cytokines Used in Cell Therapy Manufacturing					♦			
⟨111⟩ Design and Analysis of Biological Assays								♦
⟨151⟩ Pyrogen Test				♦				
⟨161⟩ Medical Devices—Bacterial Endotoxin and Pyrogen Tests				♦				
⟨381⟩ Elastomeric Closures for Injections						♦		
⟨507⟩ Protein Determination Procedures								♦
⟨621⟩ Chromatography		♦						♦
⟨785⟩ Osmolality and Osmolarity								♦
⟨787⟩ Subvisible Particulate Matter in Therapeutic Protein Injections								♦
⟨788⟩ Particulate Matter in Injections								♦
⟨791⟩ pH								♦
⟨797⟩ Pharmaceutical Compounding—Sterile Preparations					♦			
⟨905⟩ Uniformity of Dosage Units								♦
⟨911⟩ Viscosity—Capillary Methods								♦
⟨912⟩ Viscosity—Rotational Methods								♦
⟨913⟩ Viscosity—Rolling Ball Method								♦
⟨1024⟩ Bovine Serum					♦			
⟨1027⟩ Flow Cytometry								♦

[1] For Functionality test, see ⟨881⟩ *Tensile Strength*.
[2] For Water test, see ⟨1231⟩ *Water for Pharmaceutical Purposes*.

Chart 8. Cell, Gene, and Tissue Based Products *(Continued)*

Chapter	Universal Tests		Specific Tests[1,2]					
	Identifica-tion	Assay	Biocompati-bility	Microbial/ Sterility Issues	Produc-tion Issues	Product Issues	Equip-ment	Characteri-zation
⟨1030⟩ *Biological Assay Chapters—Overview and Glossary*	♦	♦						♦
⟨1031⟩ *The Biocompatibility of Materials Used in Drug Containers, Medical Devices, and Implants*			♦					
⟨1032⟩ *Design and Develop-ment of Biological Assays*	♦	♦						♦
⟨1033⟩ *Biological Assay Vali-dation*	♦	♦						♦
⟨1034⟩ *Analysis of Biological Assays*	♦	♦						♦
⟨1041⟩ *Biologics*					♦			
⟨1043⟩ *Ancillary Materials for Cell, Gene, and Tissue-Engi-neered Products*					♦			
⟨1044⟩ *Cryopreservation of Cells*	♦	♦			♦			♦
⟨1046⟩ *Cellular and Tissue-Based Products*					♦	♦		♦
⟨1047⟩ *Gene Therapy Prod-ucts*					♦			
⟨1048⟩ *Quality of Biotechnol-ogy Products: Analysis of the Expression Construct in Cells Used for Production of r-DNA Derived Protein Prod-ucts*								♦
⟨1049⟩ *Quality of Biotechno-logical Products: Stability Testing of Biotechnological/ Biological Products*								♦
⟨1050⟩ *Viral Safety Evalua-tion of Biotechnology Prod-ucts Derived from Cell Lines of Human or Animal Origin*				♦				
⟨1051⟩ *Cleaning Glass Appa-ratus*							♦	
⟨1052⟩ *Biotechnology Derived Articles—Amino Acid Analy-sis*								♦
⟨1053⟩ *Capillary Electropho-resis*								♦
⟨1054⟩ *Biotechnology Derived Articles—Isoelectric Focusing*								♦
⟨1055⟩ *Biotechnology Derived Articles—Peptide Mapping*								♦
⟨1056⟩ *Biotechnology Derived Articles—Polyacrylamide Gel Electrophoresis*								♦
⟨1057⟩ *Biotechnology Derived Articles—Total Protein Assay*								♦
⟨1074⟩ *Excipient Biological Safety Evaluation Guidelines*					♦			

[1] For Functionality test, see ⟨881⟩ *Tensile Strength.*
[2] For Water test, see ⟨1231⟩ *Water for Pharmaceutical Purposes.*

Chart 8. Cell, Gene, and Tissue Based Products *(Continued)*

Chapter	Universal Tests		Specific Tests[1,2]					
	Identification	Assay	Biocompatibility	Microbial/ Sterility Issues	Production Issues	Product Issues	Equipment	Characterization
⟨1084⟩ *Glycoprotein and Glycan Analysis—General Considerations*								♦
⟨1086⟩ *Impurities in Drug Substances and Drug Products*						♦		
⟨1102⟩ *Immunological Test Methods—General Considerations*	♦	♦						♦
⟨1103⟩ *Immunological Test Methods—Enzyme-Linked Immunosorbent Assay (ELISA)*	♦	♦						♦
⟨1104⟩ *Immunological Test Methods—Immunoblot Analysis*	♦							♦
⟨1113⟩ *Microbial Characterization, Identification, and Strain Typing*				♦				
⟨1116⟩ *Microbiological Control and Monitoring of Aseptic Processing Environments*				♦				
⟨1121⟩ *Nomenclature*						♦		
⟨1126⟩ *Nucleic Acid-Based Techniques—Extraction, Detection, and Sequencing*					♦			♦
⟨1127⟩ *Nucleic Acid-Based Techniques—Amplification*					♦			♦
⟨1128⟩ *Nucleic Acid-Based Techniques—Microarray*								♦
⟨1129⟩ *Nucleic Acid-Based Techniques—Genotyping*								♦
⟨1130⟩ *Nucleic Acid-Based Techniques—Approaches for Detecting Trace Nucleic Acids (Residual DNA Testing)*								♦
⟨1151⟩ *Pharmaceutical Dosage Forms*						♦		
⟨1184⟩ *Sensitization Testing*			♦					
⟨1208⟩ *Sterility Testing—Validation of Isolator Systems*				♦				
⟨1211⟩ *Sterility Assurance*				♦				
⟨1227⟩ *Validation of Microbial Recovery from Pharmacopeial Articles*				♦				
⟨1228⟩ *Depyrogenation*				♦				
⟨1228.1⟩ *Dry Heat Depyrogenation*				♦				
⟨1228.3⟩ *Depyrogenation by Filtration*				♦				
⟨1228.5⟩ *Endotoxin Indicators for Depyrogenation*				♦				
⟨1229⟩ *Sterilization of Compendial Articles*				♦				

[1] For Functionality test, see ⟨881⟩ *Tensile Strength*.
[2] For Water test, see ⟨1231⟩ *Water for Pharmaceutical Purposes*.

Chart 8. Cell, Gene, and Tissue Based Products *(Continued)*

Chapter	Universal Tests		Specific Tests[1,2]					
	Identification	Assay	Biocompatibility	Microbial/ Sterility Issues	Production Issues	Product Issues	Equipment	Characterization
⟨1229.3⟩ Monitoring of Bioburden				♦				
⟨1229.4⟩ Sterilizing Filtration of Liquids				♦				
⟨1229.13⟩ Sterilization-in-Place							♦	
⟨1229.14⟩ Sterilization Cycle Development				♦				
⟨1229.15⟩ Sterilizing Filtration of Gases				♦			♦	
⟨1237⟩ Virology Test Methods					♦			♦
⟨1251⟩ Weighing on an Analytical Balance							♦	
⟨1285⟩ Preparation of Biological Specimens for Histologic and Immunohistochemical Analysis	♦				♦			♦
⟨1285.1⟩ Hematoxylin and Eosin Staining of Sectioned Tissue for Microscopic Examination	♦				♦			♦
⟨1787⟩ Measurement of Subvisible Particulate Matter in Therapeutic Protein Injections								♦
⟨1788⟩ Methods for the Determination of Particulate Matter in Injections and Ophthalmic Solutions								♦

[1] For Functionality test, see ⟨881⟩ *Tensile Strength.*
[2] For Water test, see ⟨1231⟩ *Water for Pharmaceutical Purposes.*

Chart 9. Drug Product Distribution

Chapter	Manufacturer	Shipper	Wholesaler	Sample Distribution	Repackager	Pharmacy	Practitioner
⟨7⟩ Labeling	♦						
⟨17⟩ Prescription Container Labeling						♦	
⟨87⟩ Biological Reactivity Tests, In Vitro	♦				♦	♦	
⟨88⟩ Biological Reactivity Tests, In Vivo	♦				♦	♦	
⟨381⟩ Elastomeric Closures for Injections	♦					♦	
⟨659⟩ Packaging and Storage Requirements	♦				♦	♦	
⟨660⟩ Containers—Glass	♦				♦	♦	
⟨661⟩ Plastic Packaging Systems and Their Materials of Construction	♦				♦	♦	
⟨661.1⟩ Plastic Materials of Construction	♦				♦	♦	
⟨661.2⟩ Plastic Packaging Systems for Pharmaceutical Use	♦				♦	♦	
⟨670⟩ Auxiliary Packaging Components	♦						
⟨671⟩ Containers—Performance Testing	♦				♦	♦	

Chart 9. Drug Product Distribution (*Continued*)

Chapter	Manufac- turer	Shipper	Wholesaler	Sample Distribution	Repackager	Phar- macy	Practi- tioner
⟨698⟩ *Deliverable Volume*	♦				♦		
⟨735⟩ *X-Ray Fluorescence Spectrometry*	♦				♦		
⟨755⟩ *Minimum Fill*	♦				♦		
⟨1066⟩ *Physical Environments That Promote Safe Medication Use*					♦	♦	♦
⟨1079⟩ *Good Storage and Distribution Practices for Drug Products*	♦	♦	♦	♦	♦	♦	
⟨1079.1⟩ *Storage and Transportation of Investigational Drug Products*	♦						
⟨1118⟩ *Monitoring Devices— Time, Temperature, and Humidity*	♦	♦	♦	♦	♦	♦	
⟨1136⟩ *Packaging and Repackaging—Single-Unit Containers*	♦				♦	♦	
⟨1151⟩ *Pharmaceutical Dosage Forms*	♦						
⟨1152⟩ *Animal Drugs for Use in Animal Feeds*	♦						♦
⟨1177⟩ *Good Packaging Practices*	♦	♦	♦	♦	♦	♦	
⟨1178⟩ *Good Repackaging Practices*					♦		
⟨1191⟩ *Stability Considerations in Dispensing Practice*	♦					♦	♦
⟨1265⟩ *Written Prescription Drug Information—Guidelines*						♦	
⟨1660⟩ *Evaluation of the Inner Surface Durability of Glass Containers*	♦				♦	♦	
⟨1661⟩ *Evaluation of Plastic Packaging Systems and Their Materials of Construction with Respect to Their User Safety Impact*	♦				♦	♦	
⟨1663⟩ *Assessment of Extractables Associated with Pharmaceutical Packaging/Delivery Systems*	♦						
⟨1664⟩ *Assessment of Drug Product Leachables Associated with Pharmaceutical Packaging/Delivery Systems*	♦						

Chart 10a. Microbiology—Nonsterile Products

Chapter	Microbial Enumeration	Absence of Objectionable Microorganisms
⟨61⟩ *Microbiological Examination of Nonsterile Products: Microbial Enumeration Tests*	♦	
⟨62⟩ *Microbiological Examination of Nonsterile Products: Tests for Specified Microorganisms*		♦
⟨63⟩ *Mycoplasma Tests*		♦
⟨610⟩ *Alternative Microbiological Sampling Methods for Nonsterile Inhaled and Nasal Products*	♦	♦
⟨1111⟩ *Microbiological Examination of Nonsterile Products: Acceptance Criteria for Pharmaceutical Preparations and Substances for Pharmaceutical Use*	♦	♦

Chart 10a. Microbiology—Nonsterile Products *(Continued)*

Chapter	Microbial Enumeration	Absence of Objectionable Microorganisms
⟨1113⟩ *Microbial Characterization, Identification, and Strain Typing*		◆
⟨1115⟩ *Bioburden Control of Nonsterile Drug Substances and Products*		◆
⟨2021⟩ *Microbial Enumeration Tests—Nutritional and Dietary Supplements*	◆	
⟨2022⟩ *Microbiological Procedures for Absence of Specified Microorganisms—Nutritional and Dietary Supplements*		◆
⟨2023⟩ *Microbiological Attributes for Nonsterile Nutritional and Dietary Supplements*	◆	

Chart 10b. Microbiology—Sterile Products[1]

Chapter	Sterility Tests	Mycoplasma	Aseptic Processing	Filtration	Assembly[2] Assembly	Assembly[2] Other	Terminal Sterilization Terminal Sterilization	Terminal Sterilization Moist Heat	Terminal Sterilization Dry Heat	Terminal Sterilization Radiation	Terminal Sterilization EtO	Terminal Sterilization Liquid Phase	Terminal Sterilization Vapor Phase
⟨55⟩ *Biological Indicators—Resistance Performance Tests*								◆	◆	◆	◆		
⟨63⟩ *Mycoplasma Tests*		◆											
⟨71⟩ *Sterility Tests*	◆												
⟨151⟩ *Pyrogen Tests*						◆							
⟨1072⟩ *Disinfectants and Antiseptics*						◆							
⟨1112⟩ *Application of Water Activity Determination to Nonsterile Pharmaceutical Products*						◆							
⟨1113⟩ *Microbial Characterization, Identification, and Strain Typing*	◆	◆	◆										
⟨1116⟩ *Microbiological Control and Monitoring of Aseptic Processing Environments*			◆		◆	◆							
⟨1117⟩ *Microbiological Best Laboratory Practices*						◆							

[1] For endotoxins limits, see ⟨85⟩ *Bacterial Endotoxins Test*.

[2] For BFS, FFS, and SFS, see ⟨1116⟩ *Microbiological Control and Monitoring of Aseptic Processing Environments*.

Chart 10b. Microbiology—Sterile Products[1] *(Continued)*

| Chapter | Sterility Tests | Myco-plasma | Aseptic Pro-cessing | Filtra-tion | Assembly[2] | | Terminal Sterilization | | | | | | |
					As-sem-bly	Other	Termi-nal Steri-liza-tion	Moist Heat	Dry Heat	Radia-tion	EtO	Liquid Phase	Vapor Phase
⟨1207⟩ Pack-age Integrity Evalua-tion—Sterile Products					◆								
⟨1207.1⟩ Package Integrity Test-ing in the Product Life Cycle—Test Method Se-lection and Validation					◆								
⟨1207.2⟩ Package In-tegrity Leak Test Tech-nologies					◆								
⟨1207.3⟩ Package Seal Quality Test Tech-nologies					◆								
⟨1208⟩ Sterili-ty Testing—Validation of Isolator Sys-tems	◆		◆										
⟨1211⟩ Sterili-ty Assurance			◆	◆				◆	◆	◆	◆		
⟨1222⟩ Ter-minally Sterilized Pharma-ceutical Products—Parametric Release							◆						
⟨1223⟩ Vali-dation of Al-ternative Microbiolog-ical Methods						◆							
⟨1228⟩ De-pyrogena-tion			◆	◆	◆		◆	◆	◆	◆	◆		
⟨1228.1⟩ Dry Heat Depyr-ogenation			◆		◆		◆		◆				
⟨1228.3⟩ De-pyrogena-tion by Fil-tration			◆	◆						◆			

[1] For endotoxins limits, see ⟨85⟩ *Bacterial Endotoxins Test*.
[2] For BFS, FFS, and SFS, see ⟨1116⟩ *Microbiological Control and Monitoring of Aseptic Processing Environments*.

Chart 10b. Microbiology—Sterile Products[1] *(Continued)*

| Chapter | Sterility Tests | Myco-plasma | Aseptic Pro-cessing | Filtra-tion | Assembly[2] | | Terminal Sterilization | | | | | | |
					As-sem-bly	Other	Termi-nal Steri-liza-tion	Moist Heat	Dry Heat	Radia-tion	EtO	Liquid Phase	Vapor Phase
⟨1228.5⟩ En-dotoxin Indi-cators for Depyroge-nation			◆	◆	◆		◆		◆				
⟨1229⟩ Sterili-zation of Compendial Articles			◆	◆	◆		◆	◆	◆	◆	◆		
⟨1229.1⟩ Steam Steri-lization by Direct Con-tact								◆					
⟨1229.2⟩ Moist Heat Sterilization of Aqueous Liquids								◆					
⟨1229.3⟩ Monitoring of Bioburden			◆	◆				◆		◆			
⟨1229.4⟩ Sterilizing Filtration of Liquids			◆	◆									
⟨1229.5⟩ Bio-logical Indi-cators for Sterilization								◆	◆	◆	◆		
⟨1229.6⟩ Liq-uid-Phase Sterilization					◆							◆	
⟨1229.7⟩ Gaseous Sterilization											◆		
⟨1229.8⟩ Dry Heat Sterili-zation									◆				
⟨1229.9⟩ Physico-chemical In-tegrators and Indica-tors for Ster-ilization								◆			◆		
⟨1229.10⟩ Radiation Sterilization										◆			
⟨1229.11⟩ Vapor Phase Sterilization					◆								◆
⟨1229.12⟩ New Sterili-zation Methods			◆				◆						

[1] For endotoxins limits, see ⟨85⟩ *Bacterial Endotoxins Test*.
[2] For BFS, FFS, and SFS, see ⟨1116⟩ *Microbiological Control and Monitoring of Aseptic Processing Environments*.

Chart 10b. Microbiology—Sterile Products[1] *(Continued)*

Chapter	Sterility Tests	Myco-plasma	Aseptic Pro-cessing	Filtra-tion	Assembly[2]		Terminal Sterilization						
					As-sem-bly	Other	Terminal Sterili-zation	Moist Heat	Dry Heat	Radia-tion	EtO	Liquid Phase	Vapor Phase
⟨1229.13⟩ Sterilization-in-Place							♦	♦	♦		♦	♦	♦
⟨1229.14⟩ Sterilization Cycle Devel-opment			♦	♦			♦	♦	♦	♦	♦	♦	♦
⟨1229.15⟩ Sterilizing Filtration of Gases					♦								

[1] For endotoxins limits, see ⟨85⟩ *Bacterial Endotoxins Test*.
[2] For BFS, FFS, and SFS, see ⟨1116⟩ *Microbiological Control and Monitoring of Aseptic Processing Environments*.

Chart 11. Dietary Supplement Ingredients

Chapter	Botanicals						Nonbo-tanicals[1,2]
	Description	Identifica-tion	Con-tent	Safety/ Purity	Physicochemical Characterization	Other	Vitamin Assays[3]
⟨7⟩ *Labeling*	♦						
⟨91⟩ *Calcium Pantothenate Assay*							♦
⟨115⟩ *Dexpanthenol Assay*							♦
⟨171⟩ *Vitamin B₁₂ Activity Assay*							♦
⟨197⟩ *Spectrophotometric Identification Tests*		♦					
⟨201⟩ *Thin-Layer Chromatographic Iden-tification Test*		♦					
⟨202⟩ *Identification of Fixed Oils by Thin-Layer Chromatography*		♦					
⟨203⟩ *High-Performance Thin-Layer Chromatography Procedure for Identifi-cation of Articles of Botanical Origin*		♦					
⟨211⟩ *Arsenic*				♦			
⟨231⟩ *Heavy Metals*				♦			
⟨233⟩ *Elemental Impurities—Procedures*				♦			
⟨251⟩ *Lead*				♦			
⟨261⟩ *Mercury*				♦			
⟨281⟩ *Residue on Ignition*				♦			
⟨401⟩ *Fats and Fixed Oils*					♦		
⟨411⟩ *Folic Acid Assay*							♦
⟨441⟩ *Niacin or Niacinamide Assay*							♦
⟨451⟩ *Nitrate Titration*				♦			
⟨461⟩ *Nitrogen Determination*				♦			
⟨467⟩ *Residual Solvents*				♦			
⟨481⟩ *Riboflavin Assay*							♦
⟨531⟩ *Thiamine Assay*							♦
⟨541⟩ *Titrimetry*			♦				
⟨551⟩ *Vitamin E Assay*							♦
⟨561⟩ *Articles of Botanical Origin*	♦	♦	♦	♦	♦		

[1] For complex see *Biologics Drug Substances (Chart 2)*.
[2] For noncomplex Minerals, Amino Acids, and Metabolites, see *Chemical Medicines Drug Substances (Chart 1a and 1b)*.
[3] See also *Chemical Medicines Drug Substances—Universal Tests (Chart 1a)*.

Chart 11. Dietary Supplement Ingredients (Continued)

Chapter	Botanicals						Nonbotanicals[1,2]
	Description	Identification	Content	Safety/Purity	Physicochemical Characterization	Other	Vitamin Assays[3]
⟨563⟩ *Identification of Articles of Botanical Origin*	♦	♦					
⟨565⟩ *Botanical Extracts*	♦			♦			
⟨571⟩ *Vitamin A Assay*							♦
⟨581⟩ *Vitamin D Assay*							♦
⟨591⟩ *Zinc Determination*							♦
⟨611⟩ *Alcohol Determination*				♦			
⟨621⟩ *Chromatography*		♦	♦		♦		
⟨730⟩ *Plasma Spectrochemistry*				♦			
⟨731⟩ *Loss on Drying*				♦			
⟨733⟩ *Loss on Ignition*				♦			
⟨735⟩ *X-Ray Fluorescence Spectrometry*		♦		♦	♦		♦
⟨736⟩ *Mass Spectrometry*					♦		
⟨761⟩ *Nuclear Magnetic Resonance Spectroscopy*					♦		
⟨776⟩ *Optical Microscopy*	♦	♦					
⟨791⟩ *pH*					♦		
⟨852⟩ *Atomic Absorption Spectroscopy*			♦		♦		
⟨853⟩ *Fluorescence Spectroscopy*			♦		♦		
⟨854⟩ *Mid-Infrared Spectroscopy*			♦		♦		
⟨855⟩ *Nephelometry, Turbidimetry, and Visual Comparison*					♦		
⟨857⟩ *Ultraviolet-Visible Spectroscopy*			♦		♦		
⟨1064⟩ *Identification of Articles of Botanical Origin by High-Performance Thin-Layer Chromatography Procedure*		♦					
⟨1065⟩ *Ion Chromatography*					♦		
⟨1113⟩ *Microbial Characterization, Identification, and Strain Typing*				♦			
⟨1181⟩ *Scanning Electron Microscopy*	♦	♦					
⟨1225⟩ *Validation of Compendial Procedures*						♦	
⟨1226⟩ *Verification of Compendial Procedures*						♦	
⟨1736⟩ *Applications of Mass Spectrometry*					♦		
⟨1761⟩ *Applications of Nuclear Magnetic Resonance Spectroscopy*					♦		
⟨1852⟩ *Atomic Absorption Spectroscopy—Theory and Practice*			♦		♦		
⟨1853⟩ *Fluorescence Spectroscopy—Theory and Practice*			♦		♦		
⟨1854⟩ *Mid-Infrared Spectroscopy—Theory and Practice*			♦		♦		
⟨1857⟩ *Ultraviolet-Visible Spectroscopy—Theory and Practice*			♦		♦		
⟨2021⟩ *Microbial Enumeration Tests—Nutritional and Dietary Supplements*				♦			
⟨2022⟩ *Microbiological Procedures for Absence of Specified Microorganisms—Nutritional and Dietary Supplements*				♦			

[1] For complex see *Biologics Drug Substances (Chart 2)*.
[2] For noncomplex Minerals, Amino Acids, and Metabolites, see *Chemical Medicines Drug Substances (Chart 1a and 1b)*.
[3] See also *Chemical Medicines Drug Substances—Universal Tests (Chart 1a)*.

Chart 11. Dietary Supplement Ingredients (Continued)

Chapter	Botanicals						Nonbo-tanicals[1,2]
	Description	Identifica-tion	Con-tent	Safety/ Purity	Physicochemical Characterization	Other	Vitamin Assays[3]
⟨2023⟩ *Microbiological Attributes of Nonsterile Nutritional and Dietary Supplements*				♦			
⟨2030⟩ *Supplemental Information for Articles of Botanical Origin*						♦	
⟨2232⟩ *Elemental Contaminants in Dietary Supplements*				♦			
⟨2250⟩ *Detection of Irradiated Dietary Supplements*				♦			

[1] For complex see *Biologics Drug Substances (Chart 2).*
[2] For noncomplex Minerals, Amino Acids, and Metabolites, see *Chemical Medicines Drug Substances (Chart 1a and 1b).*
[3] See also *Chemical Medicines Drug Substances—Universal Tests (Chart 1a).*

Chart 12. Dietary Supplement Products

Chapter	Universal Tests						Specific Tests		
	De-scrip-tion	Identifica-tion	Assay/ Content	Impurities			Equip-ment	Perform-ance Tests	Safety/ Purity
				Organ-ic	Inorgan-ic	Residual Solvents			
⟨7⟩ *Labeling*	♦								
⟨31⟩ *Volumetric Apparatus*							♦		
⟨41⟩ *Balances*							♦		
⟨91⟩ *Calcium Pantothenate Assay*			♦						
⟨171⟩ *Vitamin B₁₂ Assay*			♦						
⟨191⟩ *Identification Tests— General*		♦							
⟨197⟩ *Spectrophotometric Identification Tests*		♦							
⟨201⟩ *Thin-Layer Chromato-graphic Identification Test*		♦							
⟨202⟩ *Identification of Fixed Oils by Thin-Layer Chroma-tography*		♦							
⟨203⟩ *High-Performance Thin-Layer Chromatography Procedure for Identification of Articles of Botanical Origin*		♦							
⟨211⟩ *Arsenic*									♦
⟨231⟩ *Heavy Metals*									♦
⟨251⟩ *Lead*									♦
⟨261⟩ *Mercury*									♦
⟨281⟩ *Residue on Ignition*				♦					
⟨411⟩ *Folic Acid Assay*			♦						
⟨441⟩ *Niacin or Niacinamide Assay*			♦						
⟨451⟩ *Nitrate Titration*									♦
⟨466⟩ *Ordinary Impurities*				♦					
⟨467⟩ *Residual Solvents*						♦			
⟨531⟩ *Thiamine Assay*			♦						
⟨541⟩ *Titrimetry*			♦						
⟨551⟩ *Vitamin E Assay*			♦						
⟨561⟩ *Articles of Botanical Origin*			♦						♦

Chart 12. Dietary Supplement Products (Continued)

Chapter	Universal Tests						Specific Tests		
	De-scrip-tion	Identifica-tion	Assay/ Content	Organ-ic	Inorgan-ic	Residual Solvents	Equip-ment	Perform-ance Tests	Safety/ Purity
				Impurities					
⟨563⟩ Identification of Articles of Botanical Origin		◆							
⟨565⟩ Botanical Extracts									◆
⟨571⟩ Vitamin A Assay			◆						
⟨581⟩ Vitamin D Assay			◆						
⟨621⟩ Chromatography		◆	◆	◆		◆			
⟨730⟩ Plasma Spectrochemistry			◆		◆				◆
⟨733⟩ Loss on Ignition					◆				
⟨735⟩ X-Ray Fluorescence Spectrometry		◆	◆		◆				◆
⟨736⟩ Mass Spectrometry		◆							
⟨776⟩ Optical Microscopy		◆							
⟨781⟩ Optical Rotation				◆					
⟨782⟩ Vibrational Circular Dichroism Spectroscopy				◆					
⟨801⟩ Polarography				◆					
⟨852⟩ Atomic Absorption Spectroscopy		◆	◆	◆					
⟨853⟩ Fluorescence Spectroscopy		◆	◆	◆					
⟨854⟩ Mid-Infrared Spectroscopy		◆	◆	◆					
⟨855⟩ Nephelometry, Turbidimetry, and Visual Comparison			◆	◆					
⟨857⟩ Ultraviolet-Visible Spectroscopy		◆	◆	◆					
⟨1051⟩ Cleaning Glass Apparatus							◆		
⟨1064⟩ Identification of Articles of Botanical Origin by High-Performance Thin-Layer Chromatography Procedure		◆							
⟨1065⟩ Ion Chromatography		◆							
⟨1086⟩ Impurities in Drug Substances and Drug Products				◆					
⟨1094⟩ Capsules—Dissolution Testing and Related Quality Attributes								◆	
⟨1113⟩ Microbial Characterization, Identification, and Strain Typing									◆
⟨1151⟩ Pharmaceutical Dosage Forms	◆								
⟨1216⟩ Tablet Friability								◆	
⟨1251⟩ Weighing on an Analytical Balance							◆		
⟨1736⟩ Applications of Mass Spectrometry		◆							
⟨1782⟩ Vibrational Circular Dichroism Spectroscopy—Theory and Practice				◆					

Chart 12. Dietary Supplement Products (Continued)

Chapter	Universal Tests						Specific Tests		
	De-scrip-tion	Identifica-tion	Assay/Content	Impurities			Equip-ment	Perform-ance Tests	Safety/Purity
				Organ-ic	Inorgan-ic	Residual Solvents			
⟨1852⟩ *Atomic Absorption Spectroscopy—Theory and Practice*		♦	♦	♦					
⟨1853⟩ *Fluorescence Spectro-scopy—Theory and Practice*		♦	♦	♦					
⟨1854⟩ *Mid-Infrared Spectro-scopy—Theory and Practice*		♦	♦	♦					
⟨1857⟩ *Ultraviolet-Visible Spectroscopy—Theory and Practice*		♦	♦	♦					
⟨2021⟩ *Microbiological Enu-meration Tests—Nutritional and Dietary Supplements*									♦
⟨2022⟩ *Microbiological Proce-dures for Absence of Speci-fied Microorganisms—Nutri-tional and Dietary Supple-ments*									♦
⟨2023⟩ *Microbiological Attrib-utes of Nonsterile Nutrition-al and Dietary Supplements*									♦
⟨2030⟩ *Supplemental Infor-mation for Articles of Botani-cal Origin*									♦
⟨2040⟩ *Disintegration and Dissolution of Dietary Sup-plements*								♦	
⟨2091⟩ *Weight Variation of Dietary Supplements*								♦	
⟨2232⟩ *Elemental Contami-nants in Dietary Supple-ments*					♦				♦
⟨2250⟩ *Detection of Irradi-ated Dietary Supplements*					♦				
⟨2750⟩ *Manufacturing Practi-ces for Dietary Supplements*							♦	♦	♦

Chart 13. Compounding—Substance/Preparation/Practice

Chapter	Global	Descrip-tion	Identifi-cation	Assay	Packag-ing	Physico-chemical Charac-terization	Safety	Equip-ment	Impurities	
									Process Related	Product Related
⟨7⟩ *Labeling*		♦								
⟨11⟩ *USP Ref-erence Standards*			♦	♦		♦	♦		♦	♦
⟨31⟩ *Volumet-ric Appara-tus*								♦		
⟨41⟩ *Balances*								♦		
⟨61⟩ *Micro-biological Examination of Nonsterile Products: Microbial Enumeration Tests*							♦			

Chart 13. Compounding—Substance/Preparation/Practice (Continued)

Chapter	Global	Descrip-tion	Identifi-cation	Assay	Packag-ing	Physico-chemical Charac-terization	Safety	Equip-ment	Impurities Process Related	Impurities Product Related
⟨62⟩ Micro-biological Examination of Nonsterile Products: Tests for Specified Mi-croorgan-isms							♦			
⟨71⟩ Sterility Tests							♦			
⟨81⟩ Antibiot-ics—Micro-bial Assays									♦	
⟨85⟩ Bacterial Endotoxins Test							♦			
⟨87⟩ Biologi-cal Reactivi-ty Tests, In Vitro							♦			
⟨88⟩ Biologi-cal Reactivi-ty Tests, In Vivo							♦			
⟨111⟩ Design and Analysis of Biological Assays									♦	♦
⟨191⟩ Identi-fication Tests—Gen-eral			♦							
⟨197⟩ Spec-trophoto-metric Iden-tification Tests			♦					♦		
⟨201⟩ Thin-Layer Chro-matographic Identifica-tion Test			♦							
⟨202⟩ Identi-fication of Fixed Oils by Thin-Layer Chromatog-raphy			♦							
⟨203⟩ High-Performance Thin-Layer Chromatog-raphy Proce-dure for Identifica-tion of Arti-cles of Bota-nical Origin			♦							
⟨231⟩ Heavy Metals									♦	

Chart 13. Compounding—Substance/Preparation/Practice (Continued)

Chapter	Global	Descrip-tion	Identifi-cation	Assay	Packag-ing	Physico-chemical Charac-terization	Safety	Equip-ment	Impurities Process Related	Impurities Product Related
〈541〉 Titrimetry				◆					◆	
〈621〉 Chromatography			◆	◆		◆		◆	◆	◆
〈659〉 Packaging and Storage Requirements					◆					
〈660〉 Containers—Glass					◆					
〈661〉 Plastic Packaging Systems and Their Materials of Construction					◆					
〈661.1〉 Plastic Materials of Construction					◆					
〈661.2〉 Plastic Packaging Systems for Pharmaceutical Use					◆					
〈671〉 Containers—Performance Testing					◆					
〈730〉 Plasma Spectrochemistry								◆	◆	
〈731〉 Loss on Drying									◆	
〈736〉 Mass Spectrometry			◆	◆		◆		◆	◆	◆
〈761〉 Nuclear Magnetic Resonance Spectroscopy			◆	◆		◆		◆	◆	◆
〈781〉 Optical Rotation				◆						
〈786〉 Particle Size Distribution Estimation by Analytical Sieving						◆				
〈795〉 Pharmaceutical Compounding—Nonsterile Preparations	◆	◆			◆		◆	◆		
〈797〉 Pharmaceutical Compounding—Sterile Preparations	◆	◆			◆		◆	◆		

Chart 13. Compounding—Substance/Preparation/Practice *(Continued)*

Chapter	Global	Descrip-tion	Identifi-cation	Assay	Packag-ing	Physico-chemical Charac-terization	Safety	Equip-ment	Impurities Process Related	Impurities Product Related
⟨800⟩ Hazardous Drugs—Handling in Healthcare Settings	♦				♦		♦	♦		
⟨823⟩ Positron Emission Tomography Drugs for Compounding, Investigational, and Research Uses	♦									
⟨831⟩ Refractive Index						♦				
⟨852⟩ Atomic Absorption Spectroscopy			♦	♦		♦		♦	♦	
⟨853⟩ Fluorescence Spectroscopy			♦	♦		♦		♦	♦	
⟨854⟩ Mid-Infrared Spectroscopy			♦	♦		♦		♦	♦	
⟨855⟩ Nephelometry, Turbidimetry, and Visual Comparison				♦		♦		♦	♦	
⟨857⟩ Ultraviolet-Visible Spectroscopy			♦	♦		♦		♦	♦	
⟨921⟩ Water Determination									♦	
⟨1031⟩ The Biocompatibility of Materials Used in Drug Containers, Medical Devices, and Implants							♦			
⟨1052⟩ Biotechnology-Derived Articles—Amino Acid Analysis								♦	♦	
⟨1053⟩ Capillary Electrophoresis								♦	♦	

Chart 13. Compounding—Substance/Preparation/Practice *(Continued)*

Chapter	Global	Descrip-tion	Identifi-cation	Assay	Packag-ing	Physico-chemical Charac-terization	Safety	Equip-ment	Impurities Process Related	Impurities Product Related
⟨1054⟩ Bio-technology-Derived Arti-cles—Iso-electric Fo-cusing								♦	♦	
⟨1055⟩ Bio-technology-Derived Arti-cles—Pep-tide Map-ping								♦	♦	
⟨1056⟩ Bio-technology-Derived Arti-cles—Polya-crylamide Gel Electro-phoresis								♦	♦	
⟨1057⟩ Bio-technology-Derived Arti-cles—Total Protein As-say								♦	♦	
⟨1064⟩ Iden-tification of Articles of Botanical Origin by High-Per-formance Thin-Layer Chromatog-raphy Proce-dure			♦							
⟨1065⟩ Ion Chromatog-raphy			♦							
⟨1066⟩ Physi-cal Environ-ments That Promote Safe Medi-cation Use							♦			
⟨1113⟩ Mi-crobial Characteri-zation, Iden-tification, and Strain Typing							♦			
⟨1121⟩ No-menclature		♦								
⟨1136⟩ Pack-aging and Repackag-ing—Single-Unit Con-tainers					♦					
⟨1151⟩ Phar-maceutical Dosage Forms	♦									

Chart 13. Compounding—Substance/Preparation/Practice *(Continued)*

Chapter	Global	Descrip-tion	Identifi-cation	Assay	Packag-ing	Physico-chemical Charac-terization	Safety	Equip-ment	Impurities Process Related	Impurities Product Related
⟨1152⟩ Animal Drugs for Use in Animal Feeds	♦									
⟨1160⟩ Pharmaceutical Calculations in Pharmacy Practice	♦						♦			
⟨1163⟩ Quality Assurance in Pharmaceutical Compounding	♦	♦		♦	♦		♦	♦		
⟨1176⟩ Prescription Balances and Volumetric Apparatus Used in Compounding	♦	♦					♦	♦		
⟨1191⟩ Stability Considerations in Dispensing Practice					♦					
⟨1228⟩ Depyrogenation							♦			
⟨1228.1⟩ Dry Heat Depyrogenation							♦			
⟨1228.3⟩ Depyrogenation by Filtration							♦			
⟨1228.5⟩ Endotoxin Indicators for Depyrogenation							♦			
⟨1229⟩ Sterilization of Compendial Articles							♦			
⟨1229.2⟩ Moist Heat Sterilization of Aqueous Liquids							♦			
⟨1229.3⟩ Monitoring of Bioburden							♦			
⟨1229.4⟩ Sterilizing Filtration of Liquids							♦			

Chart 13. Compounding—Substance/Preparation/Practice *(Continued)*

Chapter	Global	Descrip-tion	Identifi-cation	Assay	Packag-ing	Physico-chemical Charac-terization	Safety	Equip-ment	Impurities	
									Process Related	Product Related
⟨1229.6⟩ Liq-uid-Phase Sterilization							♦			
⟨1229.7⟩ Gaseous Sterilization							♦			
⟨1229.8⟩ Dry Heat Sterili-zation							♦			
⟨1229.10⟩ Radiation Sterilization							♦			
⟨1229.11⟩ Vapor Phase Sterilization							♦			
⟨1229.12⟩ New Sterili-zation Methods							♦			
⟨1229.13⟩ Sterilization-in-Place							♦			
⟨1229.14⟩ Sterilization Cycle Devel-opment							♦			
⟨1229.15⟩ Sterilizing Filtration of Gases					♦		♦	♦		
⟨1231⟩ Water for Pharma-ceutical Pur-poses	♦									
⟨1251⟩ Weighing on an Analyti-cal Balance								♦		
⟨1265⟩ Writ-ten Prescrip-tion Drug Informa-tion—Guidelines	♦									
⟨1660⟩ Evalu-ation of the Inner Sur-face Dura-bility of Glass Con-tainers					♦					

Chart 13. Compounding—Substance/Preparation/Practice (Continued)

Chapter	Global	Description	Identification	Assay	Packaging	Physicochemical Characterization	Safety	Equipment	Impurities Process Related	Impurities Product Related
⟨1661⟩ Evaluation of Plastic Packaging Systems and their Materials of Construction with Respect to Their User Safety Impact					♦					
⟨1663⟩ Assessment of Extractables Associated with Pharmaceutical Packaging/Delivery Systems					♦					
⟨1664⟩ Assessment of Drug Product Leachables Associated with Pharmaceutical Packaging/Delivery Systems					♦					
⟨1736⟩ Applications of Mass Spectrometry			♦	♦		♦		♦	♦	♦
⟨1761⟩ Applications of Nuclear Magnetic Resonance Spectroscopy			♦	♦		♦		♦	♦	♦
⟨1852⟩ Atomic Absorption Spectroscopy—Theory and Practice			♦	♦		♦		♦	♦	
⟨1853⟩ Fluorescence Spectroscopy—Theory and Practice			♦	♦		♦		♦	♦	
⟨1854⟩ Mid-Infrared Spectroscopy—Theory and Practice			♦	♦		♦		♦	♦	
⟨1857⟩ Ultraviolet-Visible Spectroscopy—Theory and Practice			♦	♦		♦		♦	♦	

General Chapters

General Tests and Assays

Biological Tests and Assays

⟨123⟩ GLUCAGON BIOIDENTITY TESTS

INTRODUCTION

Change to read:

Glucagon is a ▪peptide▪₁ₛ ₍USP41₎ hormone that increases blood glucose levels via release of liver glycogen stores. ▪A robust and precise physicochemical chromatographic procedure is used in the glucagon assay to assign potency on a mass basis. Bioidentity is still required in *Glucagon for Injection*, and two procedure options are presented here: an in vivo procedure based on release of glucose from freshly prepared rat liver cells (hepatocytes) stimulated with glucagon ex vivo, or production of cyclic adenosine monophosphate (cAMP) in vitro in response to glucagon stimulation of the glucagon receptor cell line. To meet the acceptance criteria of the bioidentity test, only one of these bioidentity tests is required.▪₁ₛ ₍USP41₎

PROCEDURE

Change to read:

- ▪**A.**▪₁ₛ ₍USP41₎ **PRIMARY LIVER CELL** ▪**BIOIDENTITY TEST**▪₁ₛ ₍USP41₎
  [NOTE—All buffers are oxygenated, prepared with either *Sterile Water for Injection* or *Sterile Water for Irrigation*, warmed to 37°, and adjusted to a final pH of 7.4 unless otherwise indicated. At least two independent assays (replicates) must be performed utilizing two rat livers for each lot of glucagon. *Figure 1* demonstrates the process used to generate one replicate value. A minimum of two replicates are combined according to the *Calculations* section. The concentration range of the *Standard preparations* and *Assay preparations* may be modified to fall within the linear range of the *Assay*, and the calculations can be adjusted accordingly. Alternatively, full curve analysis using validated nonlinear statistical methods can be used, provided that similarity is demonstrated when analysts compare the responses of the *Standard preparations* and *Assay preparations*.]

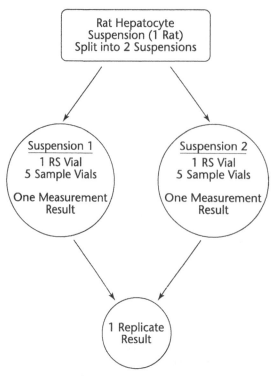

Figure 1. Rat hepatocyte assay method flow diagram (RS = Reference Standard).

Hepatocyte preparation

Calcium-free perfusion buffer with dextrose: Prepare a solution containing 7.92 g/L of sodium chloride, 0.35 g/L of potassium chloride, 1.80 g/L of dextrose, 0.19 g/L of edetic acid (EDTA), and 2.38 g/L of 4-(2-hydroxyethyl)-1-piperazineethanesulfonic acid (HEPES). Oxygenate before use.

Collagenase buffer: Prepare a solution containing 3.62 g/L of sodium chloride, 23.83 g/L of HEPES, 0.35 g/L of potassium chloride, 0.52 g/L of calcium chloride, and 1.8 g/L of dextrose. Adjust to a pH of 7.6. Immediately before perfusion, dissolve a quantity of collagenase in this solution to obtain a concentration of 0.02%–0.05%. The exact concentration of collagenase is determined empirically for each new lot of enzyme and is the amount that can consistently dissociate the tissue within 10 min of buffer entry and produce a viable cell concentration of NLT 3×10^6 cells/mL.

Wash buffer: Prepare a solution containing 7.92 g/L of sodium chloride, 0.35 g/L of potassium chloride, 0.19 g/L of EDTA, 2.38 g/L of HEPES, 0.11 g/L of calcium chloride, and 0.06 g/L of magnesium sulfate.

Incubation buffer: Prepare a solution containing 6.19 g/L of sodium chloride, 0.35 g/L of potassium chloride, 0.22 g/L of calcium chloride, 0.12 g/L of magnesium sulfate, 0.16 g/L of monobasic potassium phosphate, 11.915 g/L of HEPES, and 10 g/L of bovine serum albumin (1% BSA). Adjust to a pH of 7.5.

Test animals: Male Sprague-Dawley rats are maintained on a standard rat chow diet, given water ad libitum, and allowed to adjust to their new housing before testing. On the morning of the test, select a healthy rat weighing approximately 300–400 g, and administer 100 units of *Heparin Sodium* subcutaneously.

Procedure: [NOTE—Conduct this procedure in the morning to ensure that the rat has optimal glycogen in its liver and so that the procedure can be completed in 1 day.] Anesthetize the rat with an appropriate anesthetic. Open the abdominal cavity and isolate the portal vein. Insert an angiocatheter and tie into the portal vein at the general location of the lienal branch and then connect to a perfusion pump. Start the perfusion (25 mL/min) in situ with the previously warmed, oxygenated, *Calcium-free perfusion buffer with dextrose*. As the liver enlarges, cut the inferior vena cava to allow pressure equilibrium. [NOTE—About 300 mL of the perfusate is needed to clear the liver of red blood cells at a flow rate of 25–60 mL/min.] Then circulate *Collagenase buffer* at an appropriate flow rate so that the liver leaks perfusate out of the lobes in approximately 10 min (typically 25–60 mL/min). When the liver significantly increases in size, changes color and consistency, and starts to leak perfusate out of the lobes, change the system to the oxygenated prewarmed *Wash buffer*. About 100 mL of *Wash buffer* is needed to wash the liver of collagenase at a flow rate of 25 mL/min. Surgically remove the liver from the animal, and place in a prewarmed Petri dish containing a small amount of oxygenated *Wash buffer* (37°). Gently comb the liver with a stainless steel, fine-toothed comb to free the hepatocytes. Filter and wash the hepatocytes with *Wash buffer*, through prewetted cheesecloth (three layers thick, or through a 150-µm mesh polyethylene net) into a beaker. Transfer the cells to two centrifuge tubes and spin for about 1 min at 600 rpm. Discard the supernatant fractions and resuspend the two pellets in *Incubation buffer*. Combine the two pellets in a suitable container and add sufficient *Incubation buffer* to make 150 mL.

System suitability of cell preparation: The cell yield may vary because of the collagenase activity and the viability of the hepatocytes. To check cell viability and to determine viable cell concentration, dilute a 100-µL aliquot of the cell suspension with 400 µL of *Wash buffer* and 500 µL of isotonic 0.4% trypan blue solution. Load aliquots of the cell suspension into both chambers of a hemocytometer and count all eight quadrants. To meet system suitability of the cell preparation method, a viable cell concentration of 3×10^6 cells/mL (acceptable range of 2.5×10^6 to 3.4×10^6 cells/mL) must be obtained to proceed with the bioassay. If the viable cell concentration exceeds the upper limit, additional *Incubation buffer* may be added to the cells to adjust the concentration to 3×10^6 cells/mL. In this case, the cells are counted again in a hemocytometer, as described above to verify the concentration. [NOTE—Viable cells are those cells that exclude the trypan blue.]

Glucose determination

Negative control solution: Prepare a solution containing 0.5% BSA using *Sterile Water for Injection* or *Sterile Water for Irrigation*.

Incubation flasks: Use specially prepared 25-mL conical flasks, the bottoms of which have been heated and pushed inward to form a conically raised center, or similar flasks that allow sufficient mixing when swirling. Place the *Incubation flasks* in an orbital shaker water bath at 35°.

Standard preparations: On the day of the assay, dissolve two vials of USP rGlucagon RS■₁S (USP41) in 0.01 N hydrochloric acid or other suitable diluent (volume based on the potency of the Reference Standard lot) to obtain two solutions each containing 1 USP rGlucagon Unit/mL. All dilutions thereafter are made using *Negative control solution*. Accurately dilute measured volumes of each solution with *Negative control solution* to obtain an intermediate concentration of 400 µU/mL, and then dilute the intermediate to produce five concentrations: 200, 100, 50, 25, and 12.5 µU/mL (*Standard preparations*). Pipet 0.1 mL of each *Standard preparation* into separate *Incubation flasks*. Pipet 0.1 mL of *Negative control solution* into each of two flasks (*Negative control solutions 1* and *2*).

Assay preparations: Using accurately weighed quantities of glucagon samples, proceed as directed for *Standard preparations* or, if testing *Glucagon for Injection*, reconstitute 10 vials by slowly adding the contents of the accompanying prefilled syringes containing an appropriate glucagon diluent. Gently mix each vial until the glucagon is dissolved. Using the same syringes, withdraw the contents of five vials and place the solutions in a 25-mL volumetric flask. Repeat for the second five vials, transferring the contents to a second 25-mL volumetric flask. Dilute each flask with 0.01 N hydrochloric acid to volume. Dilute an accurate amount of each solution with 0.5% BSA to yield a concentration of 400 µU/mL, and dilute the intermediate to produce five *Assay preparation* concentrations: 200, 100, 50, 25, and 12.5 µU/mL. Then proceed as directed for the *Standard preparations*.

Reference stock solution: Dry USP Dextrose RS, and then transfer 1.0 g, accurately weighed, to a 100-mL volumetric flask. Dissolve in and dilute with saturated benzoic acid solution to volume.

Reference solutions: Transfer suitable quantities of *Reference stock solution* to four flasks, and dilute with saturated benzoic acid solution to obtain *Reference solutions* having concentrations of 100, 500, 1000, and 1500 mg/L.

Potassium ferrocyanide solution: Dissolve 1.25 g of trihydrate potassium ferrocyanide in 125 mL of *Sterile Water for Injection*, or use an appropriate commercial source.

System suitability: Analyze the *Potassium ferrocyanide solution*, the *Reference solutions*, and an additional 5 replicates of either the 500- or 1000-mg/L *Reference solution* in an appropriate glucose analyzer. [NOTE—*Potassium ferrocyanide solutions* are only appropriate standards for glucose analyzers that measure glucose oxidase activity. The procedure can also be performed using alternative platforms.] Prepare a standard curve using the *Reference solutions* as directed for the *Standard preparations*. The square root of the residual error mean square from the regression divided by the average of the response multiplied by 100% (line %RSD) must be NMT 2.0%. In addition, the response of the *Potassium ferrocyanide solution* must be NMT 30 mg/L, and the relative standard deviation must be NMT 2.0% for the replicate analyses of the middle *Reference solution*.

Procedure: Dispense 5 mL of *Hepatocyte preparation* into the *Incubation flasks* in sequence from high glucagon concentration to low glucagon concentration, alternating the *Standard preparations* with the *Assay preparations*. Swirl the flasks in an orbiting water bath at 125 rpm at 30°–35° for approximately 30 min. Following incubation, remove 1.0-mL aliquots from each *Incubation flask*, transfer to labeled microcentrifuge tubes, and centrifuge at 13,000 rpm for 15 s. Place each supernatant fraction in a labeled sampling tube for a glucose analyzer, and determine the glucose concentration (mg/L) of each *Standard preparation* and *Assay preparation*. Measure the background reading of *Negative control solutions 1* and *2*, and calculate the average of the two responses.

To conform to the linear range of the instrument being used, analysts may find it necessary to adjust by dilution each of the *Standard preparations* and *Assay preparations*. Use a glucose analyzer that has demonstrated appropriate specificity, accuracy, precision, and linear response over the range of concentrations being determined. Determine the increase in glucose concentration for each *Standard preparation* and *Assay preparation* compared to the average value of the *Negative control solution*.

Calculations

Calculate the relative potency of the glucagon samples using statistical methods for parallel-line assays, comparing the Reference Standard curve (from the *Standard preparations*) to the glucagon sample curve (from the *Assay preparations*). No dose–response reversals may occur within a run for the 25, 50, or 100 µU/mL *Standard preparations* and *Assay preparations*. [NOTE—Either the low- or high-dose level, but not both, may be excluded from the calculation in order to meet

8630 ⟨123⟩ / Biological Tests

First Supplement to USP 41–NF 36

linearity requirements.] Because a minimum of two valid assays (rats) are required, the estimated potencies are combined using the procedures in *Design and Analysis of Biological Assays* ⟨111⟩, *Combination of Independent Assays*, and the width, *L*, of a 95% confidence interval for the estimated logarithm of the relative potency is calculated. If *L* is NMT 0.1938, the results are valid. If *L* is >0.1938, additional assays may be performed and combined until a valid *L* term results, and the relative potency is then calculated from all valid independent runs. Calculate the potency of the glucagon samples in USP rGlucagon Units/mg by multiplying the relative potency result by the potency of USP rGlucagon RS.

■**Acceptance criteria:**   NLT 0.80 USP rGlucagon Units/mg■1S (USP41)

Add the following:

- ■**B. IN VITRO CELL-BASED BIOIDENTITY TEST**
   Medium A: Dulbecco's Modified Eagle Medium (DMEM) containing 4.5 mg/mL of D-glucose and sodium pyruvate, 4 mM L-alanine-L-glutamine[1] or L-glutamine, 10% (v/v) fetal bovine serum,[2] and 0.5 mg/mL G418[3]
   Buffer A: Hank's balanced salt solution[4] containing 5.3 mM potassium chloride, 0.4 mM potassium phosphate monobasic, 4.2 mM sodium bicarbonate, 137.9 mM sodium chloride, 0.3 mM sodium phosphate dibasic anhydrous, and 5.6 mM dextrose
   Cell culture preparation: Remove glucagon receptor cell line[5] from cryostorage and immediately thaw at 37° until the cell suspension has just thawed. Aseptically transfer the cell suspension from the cryotube into a sterile test tube containing 10 mL of warmed *Medium A*. Mix and then pellet the cells by centrifugation for 5 min at 125 × g. Remove the supernate and resuspend the cells in fresh, warmed *Medium A*. Measure the quantity of cells contained in an aliquot of the suspension by suitable methods and adjust the cell concentration with *Medium A* such that the cell suspension is $0.5–5 \times 10^3$ cells/cm² of tissue culture flask surface. Inoculate tissue culture flasks[6] and store in a humidified incubator at 37° containing 5% carbon dioxide. Cells should be passaged 2–3 times/week when they are NMT 90% confluent but never trypsinized 2 days in a row. If cells are not ready for passaging after 3 days of culture, the medium should be replaced with fresh *Medium A*. Cells are passaged by first removing the medium from the cell flasks, followed by adding sufficient *Buffer A* prewarmed to room temperature to cover the surface of the flasks. The flasks are gently rocked to wash the cells. This wash fluid is discarded and then sufficient trypsin[7] is added to the cell flasks to cover the surface, followed by gentle rocking and placement back in the incubator. After 3–5 min, the trypsinized cells are aseptically collected from the flasks and transferred to a sterile centrifuge tube, then a volume of *Medium A* is added that is a minimum of 2 times the volume of trypsinized cells, and an aliquot is counted. The cell suspension is further diluted with fresh *Medium A* to a final cell concentration of $0.5–5 \times 10^3$ cells/cm² of tissue culture flask surface. After a minimum of 8 passages post-thaw but NMT 25 passages, the cells can be used in the assay. The day before an assay, follow the cell passaging instructions above but resuspend the cells in fresh, warmed *Medium A* to a final cell concentration of $4–5 \times 10^4$ cells/mL. [NOTE—Three identical, independent 96-well white plates[8] are needed for measurement of two test samples ("A" and "B") analyzed on each. All wells must be loaded with cells within 40 min of resuspension following trypsinization and counting in order to keep a homogeneous cell suspension.] Using constant, gentle mixing without foaming, each well is loaded with 0.1 mL of cell suspension and incubated overnight at 37° and 5% carbon dioxide (approximately 24 h ± 4 h) prior to starting the *Procedure*. [NOTE—All remaining solutions should be prepared on the day of the *Procedure*.]
   Medium B: Kreb's salt solution containing 0.3% (v/v) human serum albumen, 25 mM HEPES, 1.7 mM 3-isobutyl-1-methyl-xanthine, 0.2 mg/mL of glucose, 650 KIU/mL of aprotinin, and 0.0003% (v/v) polysorbate 80, pH 7.4
   Medium C: Kreb's salt solution containing 0.3% (v/v) human serum albumen and 25 mM HEPES, pH 7.4
   Standard stock solution: Reconstitute USP rGlucagon RS in *Water for Injection* or another suitable diluent to a concentration of 4 mg/mL by gently mixing on a rotator for 10 min or until completely clear. Dilute this material 1:1000 with *Medium B* to a concentration of 0.4 µg/mL and then 1:200 with *Medium B* to 20 ng/mL.
   Standard solutions: Within an hour of use, dilute the 20 ng/mL *Standard stock solution* with *Medium B* to make a 1:5 concentration series of 4 ng/mL (R8), 0.8 ng/mL (R7), 160 pg/mL (R6), 32 pg/mL (R5), 6.4 pg/mL (R4), and 1.3 pg/mL (R3). A final dilution is made from R3 in *Medium B* to make 65 fg/mL (R2). [NOTE—Alternative suitable concentrations can be similarly prepared if necessary and validated.] R1 is a blank solution of *Medium B*. [NOTE—For these *Standard solutions*, as well as the *Sample solutions* and *cAMP standard solutions* described below, it may be helpful to prepare these dilutions in a dilution microplate that mimics the assay plate layout to easily and quickly transfer the materials to the wells of the assay plate.]
   Sample solutions: Reconstitute two independent preparations of glucagon from the same lot of material in *Water for Injection* or the same suitable diluent used to prepare the *Standard stock solution* to a concentration of 4 mg/mL. Prepare by

---

[1] Invitrogen catalog #31966-021 or suitable equivalent.
[2] Gibco catalog #10082-147 or suitable equivalent.
[3] Calbiochem catalog #345812 or suitable equivalent.
[4] Invitrogen catalog #14175 or suitable equivalent.
[5] Available from ATCC.
[6] Corning catalog #3151 or suitable equivalent.
[7] Gibco catalog #12563-011 or suitable equivalent.
[8] PerkinElmer catalog #6005680 or suitable equivalent.

diluting this material further with *Medium B* to prepare a concentration series similar to that suggested for the *Standard solutions*. One preparation series is *Sample solution* A8–A2 and the other preparation series is *Sample solution* B8–B2.

cAMP standard solutions: Prepare a 5 mM cAMP[9] solution in water, and then prepare further solutions by dilution with *Medium B* as shown in *Table 1*. [NOTE—To conform to the linear range of the instrument being used, analysts may find it necessary to adjust by dilution each of the *Standard solutions*, *cAMP standard solutions*, and *Assay solutions*. Alternative suitable concentrations can be similarly prepared if necessary and validated.]

Table 1. Preparation of cAMP Standard Solutions

Starting cAMP Solution	Fold Dilution with Medium B	Final cAMP Solution	Final cAMP Standard Solution Name
5 mM	1:10	0.5 mM	—
0.5 mM	1:20	25 µM	C1
25 µM	1:3.3	7.5 µM	C2
25 µM	1:10	2.5 µM	C3
7.5 µM	1:10	0.75 µM	C4
2.5 µM	1:10	250 nM	C5
0.75 µM	1:10	75 nM	C6
250 nM	1:10	25 nM	C7
75 nM	1:10	7.5 nM	C8
Medium B only	—	No cAMP	C9

Donor biotin-cAMP beads: Dissolve 10 nmol biotinylated cAMP in 0.5 mL of phosphate-buffered saline, pH 7.4. Add 80 µL of this biotinylated cAMP solution to 33.8 mL of a 5 mM HEPES lysis buffer containing 0.1% (w/v) BSA and 0.3% (v/v) polysorbate 20, pH 7.4.[9] Add 270 µL of donor beads and 2.4 mL of 120 mM $MgCl_2$ solution.

Procedure: Remove the plates seeded with cells the day before, and discard the *Medium A* in each well. Wash the cells with 350 µL/well of *Medium C*, then discard the wash solution. Rapidly add 20 µL/well of diluted 1× anti-cAMP-acceptor beads. Add 30 µL/well of each *Standard solution*, *Sample solution*, *Medium B*, or *cAMP standard solution* as indicated in the plate layouts shown in *Tables 2* and *3*. [NOTE—The white plate for the *cAMP standard solutions* does not contain cells.] Cover the plate,[10] protecting it from light and evaporation, and incubate for 35–60 min in an incubator at 37° with gentle shaking. Next, dispense 60 µL of *Donor biotin-cAMP beads* per well, mix well, then cover[9] the plate again and wrap it with foil. [NOTE—The beads are light sensitive so plates should be kept dark or under green light conditions.] Gently rotate the plate on a shaker for at least 30 min at room temperature. Keep the plate in the dark, at room temperature, without shaking for 16–30 h before measuring the top luminescence from the plate wells on a suitable plate reader[11] and detection mode (excitation wavelength of about 680 nm; emission of 520–620 nm).

Table 2. Schematic Representation of the Standard and Sample Assay Plate

	1	2	3	4	5	6	7	8	9	10	11	12
A	R1	R2	A2	B2	R3	A3	B3	R4	A4	B4	R8	—
B	R1	R2	A2	B2	R3	A3	B3	R4	A4	B4	R8	—
C	R1	R2	A2	B2	R3	A3	B3	R4	A4	B4	R8	—
D	R1	R2	A2	B2	R3	A3	B3	R4	A4	B4	R8	—
E	R5	A5	B5	R6	A6	B6	R7	A7	B7	A8	B8	C9
F	R5	A5	B5	R6	A6	B6	R7	A7	B7	A8	B8	C6
G	R5	A5	B5	R6	A6	B6	R7	A7	B7	A8	B8	C4
H	R5	A5	B5	R6	A6	B6	R7	A7	B7	A8	B8	C1

LEGEND:

A2–A8 = Dilution series of *Sample solution* A (same solution is used on three plates, with 4 ng/mL as starting concentration).

R1–R8 = Dilution series of *Standard solution* for each test plate, with 4 ng/mL as starting concentration; as a result, each *Sample solution* is only compared to the *Standard solution* on that plate.

B2–B8 = Dilution series of *Sample solution* B (same solution is used on three plates, with 4 ng/mL as starting concentration).

— = No glucagon (contains 30 µL *Medium B* instead), but cells are present.

C = cAMP standard controls, no glucagon. C1 contains 25 µM cAMP, C4 contains 0.75 µM cAMP, C6 contains 75 nM cAMP, and C9 contains no cAMP.

---

[9] PerkinElmer catalog #6760635D or suitable equivalent.
[10] PerkinElmer catalog #6050195 or suitable equivalent.
[11] PerkinElmer catalog #2300-0000 or suitable equivalent.

Table 3. Schematic Representation of the cAMP Standards Assay Plate

	1	2	3	4	5	6	7	8	9	10	11	12
A	—	—	—	—	—	—	—	—	—	—	—	—
B	—	—	—	—	—	—	—	—	—	—	—	—
C	C1	C2	C3	C4	C5	C6	C7	C8	C9	—	—	—
D	C1	C2	C3	C4	C5	C6	C7	C8	C9	—	—	—
E	C1	C2	C3	C4	C5	C6	C7	C8	C9	—	—	—
F	—	—	—	—	—	—	—	—	—	—	—	—
G	—	—	—	—	—	—	—	—	—	—	—	—
H	—	—	—	—	—	—	—	—	—	—	—	—

LEGEND:
C1–C9 = Dilution series of cAMP standard controls starting with C1, which contains 25 µM cAMP, through C9, which does not contain cAMP.

System suitability criteria: The lower asymptote of the 4-parameter logistic curves generated from *Sample solutions* A2–A8 and B2–B8 and *Standard solutions* R1–R8 must be above the lower limit (defined as C3) of the *cAMP standard solutions*. NLT 3-fold difference between the signals obtained in the wells of cells treated without glucagon (R1) versus those with the maximal amount of glucagon (R8). NMT 4 technical outliers may be omitted per standard curve. Any plate that fails one or more of these criteria is rejected and must be repeated. If either *Sample solutions* A or B fail one of these criteria, then only the passing series can be used for the calculations. [NOTE—The upper asymptotes of the 4-parameter logistic standard curves generated from *Sample solutions* A2–A8 and B2–B8 and *Standard solutions* R1–R8 should be approximately equal to or less than the C8 response of the *cAMP standard solutions* and within the linear range of the instrument used.]

Calculations: A series of two independent *Sample solution* preparations must be used for each test sample across three plates (assays). Outliers identified by Grubbs' test (see ⟨111⟩; but NMT 4/curve and NMT 1 data point from a replicate set) are omitted, and then the same number of *Standard solution* and *Sample solution* dose responses, including the 50% response (EC_{50}) of the standard/test sample within this range, are used to calculate the relative potency of the glucagon sample using statistical methods for parallel-curve analysis with a 4-parameter logistic fit using all replicate values. For each individual *Sample solution* compared to the *Standard solution*, the statistical tests for slope and parallelism must pass at the 95% level. Calculate the relative potency of the glucagon samples by comparing the Reference Standard curve (from the *Standard solutions*) to the glucagon sample curve (from the *Sample solutions*). Because a minimum of three valid assays are required, the estimated potencies are combined using the procedures in *Design and Analysis of Biological Assays* ⟨111⟩, *Combination of Independent Assays*, and the confidence interval is calculated using suitable statistical methods. If the confidence limits are between 64% and 156%, the results are valid. If not, up to two more assay plates may be performed and combined until a valid confidence interval results, and the relative potency is then calculated from all valid independent runs. Calculate the potency of the glucagon samples in USP rGlucagon Units/mg by multiplying the relative potency result by the potency of USP rGlucagon RS.

Acceptance criteria: NLT 0.80 USP rGlucagon Units/mg■1S (USP41)

ADDITIONAL REQUIREMENTS
- **USP REFERENCE STANDARDS ⟨11⟩**
  USP Dextrose RS
  USP rGlucagon RS

Chemical Tests and Assays

IDENTIFICATION TESTS

Add the following:

■⟨198⟩ NUCLEAR MAGNETIC RESONANCE SPECTROSCOPY IDENTITY TESTING OF BACTERIAL POLYSACCHARIDES USED IN VACCINE MANUFACTURE

1. INTRODUCTION AND SCOPE

This chapter describes the application of nuclear magnetic resonance (NMR) spectroscopy to the identity testing of bacterial polysaccharides used in vaccine manufacture. The identity of the saccharide component in polysaccharide and glycoconjugate vaccines should be confirmed at various stages of the manufacturing process, including bulk monovalent polysaccharide, blended polysaccharide bulk, activated polysaccharide (if isolated), bulk monovalent conjugate, blended conjugate bulks, and final fills. NMR is an appropriate method to confirm the identity of polysaccharides, although it is most useful for bulk monovalent polysaccharides and activated polysaccharides (if isolated). This chapter describes the use of NMR spectroscopy for this purpose, but alternative validated approaches may also be suitable.

For additional information on NMR, including its general principles and applications, see *Applications of Nuclear Magnetic Resonance Spectroscopy* ⟨1761⟩. More specific information on instrument qualification, procedure validation, and Reference Standards are included in *Nuclear Magnetic Resonance Spectroscopy* ⟨761⟩.

1.1 NMR Spectra

NMR spectra for identity testing are typically collected for samples dissolved in deuterated water (D_2O) or a combination of deuterated water and small amounts of one or more internal standards for chemical shift calibration, quantification, or other purposes. The chemical shift of the resonance from residual water in deuterated solvent (HOD) is more temperature sensitive than other solvent resonances. The spectral separation and resolution of the HOD resonance may be optimized by the choice of temperature at which the spectrum is obtained.

1.2 -Acetylated Polysaccharides

For those polysaccharides that are *O*-acetylated, the consistency of the degree of *O*-acetylation is considered part of the identity test. This could be evaluated through the use of the spectrum of a reference polysaccharide with an acceptable degree of *O*-acetylation, quantification of resonances characteristic of the *O*-acetylation in the spectrum of the intact polysaccharide, or chemical de-*O*-acetylation and relative quantification of the resulting acetate anion compared to the polysaccharide (see *2.4 Experimental Procedures*). The implementation of any given approach is likely to be product specific.

For some polysaccharides, a quantitative specification for the minimum degree of *O*-acetylation may exist; the approaches described in this chapter, appropriately validated, can be used to perform that assay. Requirements for the *O*-acetyl content of polysaccharides are typically quoted as a minimum quantity of "*O*-acetyl residues" (measured by a Hestrin assay) in millimoles per gram of dry weight of polysaccharide. This NMR assay method described in this chapter reports a value based on the average number of *O*-acetyl groups per repeat unit. A method to calibrate between the two approaches should be developed during method validation.

2. PROCEDURE

2.1 Equipment Requirements

A description of a typical NMR spectrometer is given in ⟨1761⟩, and approaches to installation, performance, and operational qualification are given in ⟨761⟩. This section, and the rest of the chapter, refers to specific requirements for the identity testing of bacterial polysaccharides.

NMR SPECTROMETER

An NMR spectrometer with a minimal nominal field strength corresponding to a proton resonance frequency of NLT 400 MHz and with control of the sample temperature should be used. Temperature calibration within ±3° of the desired temperature is sufficient, provided a consistent sample temperature between the test and reference samples is achieved (or demonstrated in method validation), with temperature stability within a run of NMT 0.5°. NMR probes optimized for proton detection and suitable for 5-mm (outside diameter) NMR tubes should be used. Other probe options are possible but should be proven suitable before use.

PROCESSING PARAMETERS

A weighting function may be applied to the free induction decay (FID) before Fourier transform: a suitable line broadening function may be applied, and in some cases 0.3 Hz has been found suitable. After transform of the FID, the phase is adjusted to pure adsorption phase. Baseline correction should be applied consistently.

NMR TUBES

These should be of a quality suitable for use in high-field spectrometers and qualified for use in the assay.

2.2 Reagents for Vaccine Polysaccharide Sample Solutions

SOLVENTS

Deuterated solvents subject to proton exchange with the polysaccharide [e.g., deuterated water (D_2O)] must be selected with the highest deuterium proportion (e.g., >99.9 atom % D).

CHEMICAL SHIFT REFERENCE COMPOUNDS

Sodium 2,2-dimethyl-2-silapentane-5-sulfonate (DSS; preferred), sodium trimethylsilylpropionate (TSP), or a deuterated analogue (TSP–d_4) are classically used and set to 0 ppm for the methyl signals. The reference material is usually added at low amounts [0.1%–0.01% (w/v) has been found to be appropriate] to the deuterated water used to dissolve the final sample. [NOTE—Deuterated water >99.96% ^2H containing 0.01% DSS (w/v) is commercially available.]

SODIUM DEUTEROXIDE

Forty percent w/v (10 M) sodium deuteroxide (NaOD) in deuterated water (>99 atom % D) is commonly used to induce the de-*O*-acetylation of polysaccharides.

2.3 Sample Requirements

An aliquot of bulk purified polysaccharide or appropriate process intermediates in solid or liquid state containing 0.5–20 mg of saccharide content is suitable for preparation of NMR analytical samples. To obtain a solid aliquot, the relevant amount of material in liquid solution is dried under vacuum (using a freeze-drier, lyophilizer, or other solvent evaporator).

REFERENCE SPECTRA FOR ANTICIPATED IMPURITIES

Reference spectra for anticipated process-related impurities (e.g., ethanol, antifoaming agents, phenol, cetyl trimethylammonium bromide) should be obtained under the same experimental conditions as those used to analyze the test sample and at concentrations found similar to those in routine test samples. These spectra provide evidence for those resonances that may be excluded from further consideration when assigning the identity of the samples.

REFERENCE SPECTRA FOR POLYSACCHARIDES

Reference spectra for the polysaccharides samples being tested should be obtained by collecting spectra of authentic samples under identical sample preparation and spectrometer acquisition and data processing conditions to those used for test samples. Comparison of the spectra of test samples with these reference spectra allows the identity of the test samples to be confirmed.

2.4 Experimental Procedures

Two experimental protocols are described below. The first protocol is suitable for samples in which a single one-dimensional ¹H NMR spectrum will produce all of the required information. The second protocol includes in situ base-catalyzed de-*O*-acetylation of the polysaccharide to release *O*-acetyl groups as acetate anions, both simplifying the spectrum of the polysaccharide and allowing quantification of the degree of *O*-acetylation. A second one-dimensional ¹H NMR spectrum is collected after the de-*O*-acetylation step. The choice of which protocol to adopt will depend upon the product being tested and the information required; many stages in these two protocols are similar (e.g., sample preparation).

SAMPLE PREPARATION

NMR analytical samples of polysaccharide and its derivatives can be prepared as either solid- or liquid-state aliquots. NMR analytical samples are usually prepared by dissolving the solid aliquot in about 0.7 mL of deuterated solvent or, more rarely, by adding at least 10% (v/v) of deuterated solvent to the liquid aliquot. The solution is mixed to obtain a uniform concentration and is subsequently transferred to a 5-mm NMR tube. [NOTE—NMR instrument design may allow or require the use of smaller volumes; users should confirm this for their instrument configuration.]

DEUTERIUM EXCHANGE

With suitable method validation, lyophilization from deuterium oxide ("deuterium exchange") may be used to reduce the intensity of the resonance from residual water (H_2O)/HOD.

PH

Under some circumstances, control of the pH of the sample may be appropriate.

2.5 Procedure 1a

This procedure uses visual comparison with a reference spectra and/or comparison of test chemical shifts with reference chemical shift values.

SCOPE

This approach is compatible with polysaccharides that lack *O*-acetylation, such as *Haemophilus influenzae* type b or many pneumococcal polysaccharides, or with *O*-acetylated polysaccharides, such as *Neisseria meningitidis* or many pneumococcal polysaccharides where the product and spectral consistency allow identity to be established through direct comparison of test and reference spectra.

NMR SPECTRUM OF THE TEST SAMPLE

The NMR spectrum of the test sample is acquired under the same instrument operational and data processing parameters to those used to obtain the reference spectrum. Confirmation of identity can be based on visual comparison of the test and product-specific reference spectra, comparing resonance position, line width, relative intensity, and multiplicity. The complete spectrum, distinctive regions of the spectrum, or a series of at least five resonances (or three distinctive resonances in polysaccharides with monosaccharide or disaccharide repeat units) can be used in this comparison (as long as these are shown to be diagnostic).

RESONANCES

In a well-understood assay, resonances assigned as deriving from process-related impurities that are known to be removed at a later stage in the manufacturing process or otherwise proven not to impact product quality can be excluded from determination of identity.

2.6 Procedure 1b

This procedure uses analytical samples in deuterated water (D_2O) and a comparison with a reference spectrum by calculation of a correlation coefficient.

This approach is compatible with *Streptococcus pneumoniae* polysaccharides where the consistency of the product and the spectrum allow identity to be established through direct mathematical comparison of test and reference spectra.

With mathematical comparisons, a distinctive region of each spectrum (e.g., 4.64–5.89 ppm) is compared to spectra generated for designated reference samples for each polysaccharide of interest. The similarity of two spectral profiles for a test and reference sample acquired under identical conditions and in the same matrix is evaluated using a correlation coefficient (ρ). A positive identification of the sample polysaccharide is achieved when ρ is NLT 0.95 (or another validated value) between the sample and reference spectra.

2.7 Procedure 2

The procedure is in-tube base-catalyzed de-*O*-acetylation and quantification of the acetate content.

SCOPE

In some cases, the degree of *O*-acetylation and their position, accompanied by spontaneous *O*-acetyl migration in solution, can complicate the NMR profile. Base-catalyzed de-*O*-acetylation of the polysaccharide in the NMR tube has proven useful for the *Salmonella typhi* Vi and the meningococcal Groups A, C, W135, and Y polysaccharides. Adding a base may also reduce line widths.

SAMPLE HANDLING

The sample is prepared as in *Sample Preparation* in *2.4 Experimental Procedures* and a one-dimensional ¹H NMR spectrum is acquired as in *2.5 Procedure 1a*. This spectrum provides information on the presence/amount of acetate anion in the native sample. Sodium deuteroxide (NaOD) in deuterated water (D_2O) is added to the sample in the NMR tube to a final concentration of approximately 200 mM [equivalent to adding 14 μL of 10 M sodium deuteroxide (NaOD) in deuterated water (D_2O) to a 0.7-mL sample]. De-*O*-acetylation is very rapid for almost all polysaccharides, but appropriate conditions should be evaluated in method development and validation. The NMR spectrum of the sample is reacquired after de-*O*-acetylation using acquisition conditions appropriate for quantitative spectroscopy. The spectrum of the de-*O*-acetylated material is characteristic of the polysaccharide backbone, and the degree of *O*-acetylation in the original sample is calculated from the integrals of the acetate anion and an appropriate resonance arising from the saccharide backbone. If the amount of acetate anion in the native sample is low, for example <5%, correction of the intensity of the acetate anion resonance in the de-*O*-acetylated sample is not necessary.

2.8 Assay Criteria

TEMPERATURE

The temperature of the sample should be the same, within limits established during method validation, as that of the Reference Standard, and the sample temperature can be determined by the chemical shift difference between the HOD resonance and the internal chemical shift Reference Standard. For example, when using TSP-d_4 as the Reference Standard, calculate the actual temperature using the following equation based on the chemical shift of the HOD signal:

$$\delta = 5.051 - 0.0111(T)$$

where δ is the chemical shift of the HOD peak, and T is the temperature in Celsius (°).

Other equations apply when different chemical shift Reference Standards are used. Consistency in the chemical shift difference between the HOD and chemical shift Reference Standard is a surrogate for sample temperature.

CHEMICAL SHIFT REFERENCE STANDARD

The full width half-height (*fwhh*) line width of a defined resonance from a small molecule (e.g., the chemical shift Reference Standard) in the test sample should be within limits set during method validation to indicate both acceptable shimming of the magnet and sample temperature stability during the analysis. The signal-to-noise ratio of a defined signal within the spectrum of the polysaccharide material should exceed the specification established during method validation.

2.9 System Suitability

SYSTEM SUITABILITY SOLUTION

Dissolve 1 vial of USP PS NMR System Suitability RS in deuterated water (>99.9% D, 1 mL) containing 0.01% DSS with brief mixing. [NOTE—For example, for 10 s using a rotary mixer.] Transfer 0.7 mL of this solution into an NMR tube (5-mm outside diameter). [NOTE—NMR instrument design may allow or require the use of smaller volumes; users should confirm this for their instrument configuration.]

SYSTEM SUITABILITY: PROCEDURE

Using an NMR spectrometer operating at NLT 400 MHz nominal frequency for ^{1}H, acquire an FID using NLT 64 scans with a 90° pulse, a spectral width of 12 ppm, a recycle delay of NLT 30 s, a number of data points NLT 64,000, and with the spectral window centered at 4 ppm. Record the ^{1}H NMR spectra of the *System suitability solution* at a stable temperature of 25 ± 3°. Obtain the spectrum using the above parameters. Transform the data after exponential multiplication (0.3 Hz line broadening). The DSS methyl signal should be set to 0.00 ppm.

ACCEPTANCE CRITERIA

- The chemical shifts for the N-acetyl, GlcA H-2, and GlcNAc H-1 anomeric resonances in the *System suitability solution* should be observed at 2.01 ± 0.05, 3.33 ± 0.05, and 5.15 ± 0.05 ppm, respectively.
- The line width (*fwhh*) of the N-acetyl resonance at 2.01 ppm should be NMT 3.5 Hz.

2.10 USP Reference Standards ⟨11⟩

USP PS NMR System Suitability RS
■1S *(USP41)*

Physical Tests and Determinations

⟨724⟩ DRUG RELEASE

SCOPE

This test is provided to determine compliance with drug release or dissolution requirements where stated in the individual monographs for transdermal systems (TDS) and other dosage forms. From the types of apparatus described herein, use the one specified in the individual monograph.

Change to read:

GENERAL DRUG RELEASE STANDARDS

Apparatus 5 (Paddle over Disk)

APPARATUS

Use the paddle and vessel assembly as described in *Dissolution* ⟨711⟩, *Apparatus, Apparatus 2*, with the addition of a disk assembly designed to hold the TDS at the bottom of the vessel. This disk assembly is designed to minimize any "dead" volume between the assembly and the bottom of the vessel. The disk assembly holds the TDS flat and is positioned such that the release surface is parallel with the bottom of the paddle blade (see *Figure 1a, Figure 1b,* and *Figure 1c*). A distance of 25 ± 2 mm between the paddle blade and the surface of the disk assembly is maintained during the test. Other appropriate devices may be used (see *Figure 2*), provided they do not sorb, react with, or interfere with the specimen being tested. ■[NOTE—A suitable device is catalog number TRANDE-SC from www.qla-llc.com.]■1S *(USP41)*

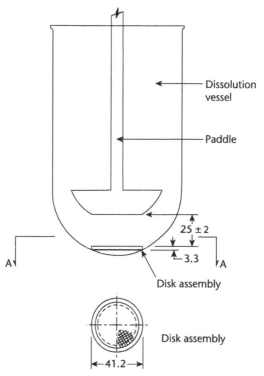

Figure 1a. Paddle over disk. (All measurements are expressed in mm unless noted otherwise.)

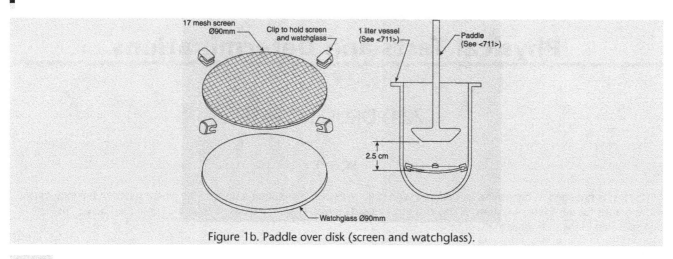

Figure 1b. Paddle over disk (screen and watchglass).

■1S *(USP41)*

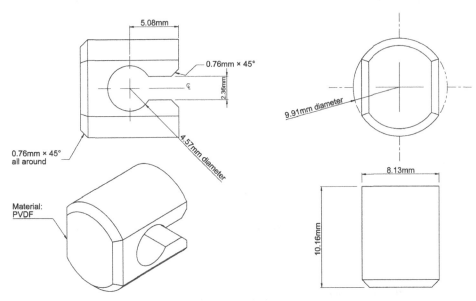

Figure 1c. Clip to hold screen and watchglass.

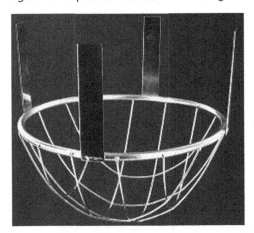

Figure 2. Holding wire screen.

APPARATUS SUITABILITY

Proceed as directed for *Apparatus 2* in *Dissolution ⟨711⟩*, *Apparatus, Apparatus 4, Apparatus Suitability, Performance verification test, Apparatus 1 and Apparatus 2*.

MEDIUM

Proceed as directed for *Dissolution medium* in *Dissolution ⟨711⟩*, *Procedure, Apparatus 1 and Apparatus 2, Immediate-Release Dosage Forms*.

PROCEDURE

Place the stated volume of *Medium* in the vessel, and equilibrate to $32 \pm 0.5°$.

Apply the TDS to the disk assembly, assuring that the release surface is as smooth as possible and the TDS is completely and firmly attached to the disk. The TDS, with release surface side up, may be attached to the disk by an appropriate and validated procedure such as use of an adhesive, double-face adhesive tape, screen, or membrane. Care must be taken to avoid the presence of air bubbles between the membrane, if used, and the TDS, or the presence of wrinkles on the surface of the TDS. Carefully remove the protective liner from the TDS without causing damage to the surface of the TDS.

Place the disk assembly flat at the bottom of the vessel with the release surface facing up and parallel to the edge of the paddle blade and surface of the *Medium*. Ensure that the surface of the TDS is devoid of air bubbles. The bottom edge of the paddle is 25 ± 2 mm from the surface of the disk assembly. The vessel may be covered during the test to minimize evaporation.

Immediately operate the apparatus at the rate specified in the monograph.

At each sampling time interval, withdraw a specimen from a zone midway between the surface of the *Medium* and the top of the blade, not less than 1 cm from the vessel wall.

Perform the analysis on each sample aliquot as directed in the individual monograph, correcting for any volume losses, as necessary. Repeat the test with additional TDS as needed.

TIME

The test time points, at least three, are expressed in hours. Specimens are to be withdrawn within a tolerance of ±15 min or ±2% of the stated time, selecting the tolerance that results in the narrowest time interval.

INTERPRETATION

Unless otherwise specified in the individual monograph, the requirements are met if the quantities of active ingredient released from the system conform to *Acceptance Table 1* below. Continue testing through the three levels unless the results conform at either L_1 or L_2.

Acceptance Table 1

Level	Number Tested	Criteria
L_1	6	No individual value lies outside the stated range.
L_2	6	The average value of the 12 units ($L_1 + L_2$) lies within the stated range. No individual value is outside the stated range by more than 10% of the average of the stated range.
L_3	12	The average value of the 24 units ($L_1 + L_2 + L_3$) lies within the stated range. Not more than 2 of the 24 units are outside the stated range by more than 10% of the average of the stated range; and none of the units is outside the stated range by more than 20% of the average of the stated range.

Apparatus 6 (Cylinder)

APPARATUS

Use the vessel assembly as described in *Dissolution* ⟨711⟩, *Apparatus, Apparatus 1*, except replace the basket and shaft with a stainless steel cylinder stirring element with the specifications shown in *Figure 3*. This cylinder stirring element is composed of two parts, one comprising the shaft and the upper cylinder, and the other being the extension cylinder. Since both parts are serially numbered, it is recommended that they be kept paired because the friction fitting is done individually for each cylinder, allowing a very tight fit. The distance between the inside bottom of the vessel and the cylinder is maintained at 25 ± 2 mm during the test.

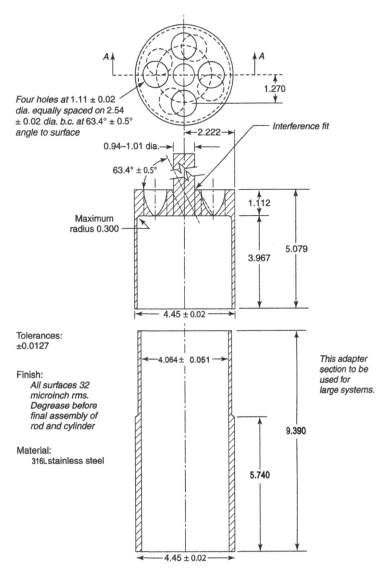

Four holes at 1.11 ± 0.02 dia. equally spaced on 2.54 ± 0.02 dia. b.c. at 63.4° ± 0.5° angle to surface

Interference fit

0.94–1.01 dia.

63.4° ± 0.5°

2.222

1.270

1.112

5.079

3.967

Maximum radius 0.300

4.45 ± 0.02

Tolerances:
±0.0127

4.064 ± 0.051

This adapter section to be used for large systems.

Finish:
All surfaces 32 microinch rms. Degrease before final assembly of rod and cylinder

9.390

Material:
316L stainless steel

5.740

4.45 ± 0.02

Figure 3. Cylinder stirring element.
(All measurements are expressed in cm unless noted otherwise.)

MEDIUM

See *Dissolution medium* in *Dissolution* ⟨711⟩, *Procedure, Apparatus 1 and Apparatus 2, Immediate-Release Dosage Forms.*

PROCEDURE

Place the stated volume of *Medium* in the vessel, and equilibrate to 32 ± 0.5°.

Apply the TDS to the cylinder, assuring that the release surface is as smooth as possible and the TDS is completely and firmly attached to the cylinder. The TDS, with release side facing the *Medium,* may be attached to the cylinder by an appropriate and validated procedure such as use of an adhesive, double-face adhesive tape, membrane, or nylon net. Care must be taken to avoid the presence of air bubbles between the membrane, if used, and the TDS, or the presence of wrinkles on the surface of the TDS. Carefully remove the protective liner from the TDS without causing damage to the surface. If additional reinforcement of the TDS to the cylinder is needed, inert metal wire or a polymer ring may be used.

Place the cylinder in the apparatus, and immediately rotate at the rate specified in the individual monograph. The vessel may be covered during the test to minimize evaporation.

At each sampling time interval, withdraw a specimen from a zone midway between the surface of the *Medium* and the top of the rotating cylinder, not less than 1 cm from the vessel wall.

Perform the analysis on each sample aliquot as directed in the individual monograph, correcting for any volume losses, as necessary. Repeat the test with additional TDS, as needed.

TIME

The test time points, at least three, are expressed in hours. Specimens are to be withdrawn within a tolerance of ±15 min or ±2% of the stated time, selecting the tolerance that results in the narrowest time interval.

INTERPRETATION

Unless otherwise specified in the individual monograph, the requirements are met if the quantities of active ingredient released from the system conform to *Acceptance Table 1* above. Continue testing through the three levels unless the results conform at either L_1 or L_2.

Apparatus 7 (Reciprocating Holder)

APPARATUS

The assembly consists of (1) a set of volumetrically calibrated or tared solution containers made of glass or other suitable inert material that should not sorb, react with, or interfere with the specimen being tested; (2) a motor and drive assembly to reciprocate the system vertically and to index the system horizontally to a different row of vessels, automatically if desired; and (3) a set of suitable sample holders (see *Figure 4*, *Figure 5a*, *Figure 5b*, *Figure 5c*, and *Figure 5d*).

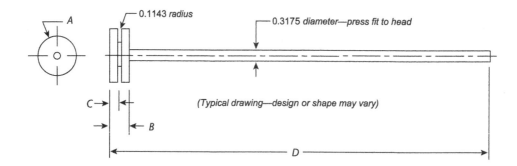

Dimensions are in centimeters.

Systemᵃ	A (Diameter)	B	C	Materialᵇ	D	Materialᶜ	(not shown)
	HEAD				**ROD**		**O-RING**
1.6 cm²	1.428	0.9525	0.4750	SS/VT	30.48	SS/P	Parker 2–113–V884–75
2.5 cm²	1.778	0.9525	0.4750	SS/VT	30.48	SS/P	Parker 2–016–V884–75
5 cm²	2.6924	0.7620	0.3810	SS/VT	8.890	SS/P	Parker 2–022–V884–75
7 cm²	3.1750	0.7620	0.3810	SS/VT	30.48	SS/P	Parker 2–124–V884–75
10 cm²	5.0292	0.6350	0.3505	SS/VT	31.01	SS/P	Parker 2–225–V884–75

ᵃ Typical system sizes.
ᵇ SS/VT=Either stainless steel or virgin Teflon.
ᶜ SS/P=Either stainless steel or Plexiglas.

Figure 4. Reciprocating disk sample holder.

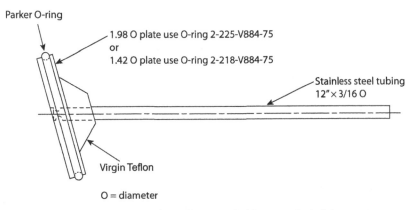

Figure 5a. Transdermal system holder—angled disk.

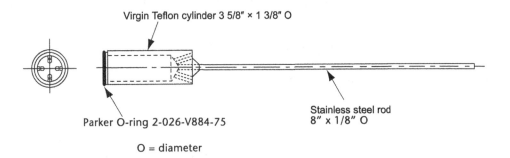

Figure 5b. Transdermal system holder—cylinder.

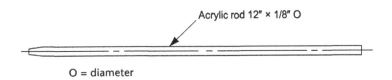

Figure 5c. Oral extended-release tablet holder—rod, pointed for gluing.

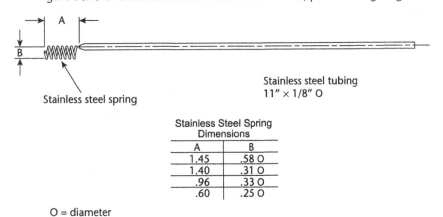

Stainless Steel Spring Dimensions	
A	B
1.45	.58 O
1.40	.31 O
.96	.33 O
.60	.25 O

O = diameter

Figure 5d. Oral extended-release tablet holder—spring holder.

During the test, the solution containers are partially immersed in a suitable water bath of any convenient size that permits maintaining the temperature inside the containers at $32 \pm 0.5°$ for TDS or at $37 \pm 0.5°$ for other dosage forms during the test.

No part of the assembly, including the environment in which the assembly is placed, contributes significant motion, agitation, or vibration beyond that due to the smooth, vertically reciprocating sample holder.

Apparatus that permits observation of the system and holder during the test is preferable.

Use the size container and sample holder as specified in the individual monograph.

MEDIUM

See *Dissolution medium* in *Dissolution* ⟨711⟩, *Procedure, Apparatus 1 and Apparatus 2, Immediate-Release Dosage Forms.*

SAMPLE PREPARATION A (FOR OSMOTIC PUMP TABLETS)

Attach each unit to be tested to a suitable holder by an appropriate and validated procedure such as use of an adhesive to adhere the edge of the tablet to a holder (e.g., *Figure 5c*), the spring holder (*Figure 5d*), a small nylon net bag, or a membrane.

SAMPLE PREPARATION B (FOR TDS)

Apply the TDS to the appropriate holder, assuring that the release surface is as smooth as possible and the TDS is completely and firmly attached to the holder. The TDS, with release side facing the *Medium*, may be attached to the holder by an appropriate and validated procedure such as use of an adhesive, double-face adhesive tape, membrane, or nylon net. Care must be taken to avoid the presence of air bubbles between the membrane, if used, and the TDS, or the presence of wrinkles on the surface of the TDS. Carefully remove the protective liner from the TDS without causing damage to the surface of the TDS. If additional reinforcement of the TDS to the holder is needed, inert metal wire or a polymer ring may be used.

SAMPLE PREPARATION C (FOR OTHER DOSAGE FORMS)

Attach each dosage form to be tested to a suitable holder.

PROCEDURE

Place the stated volume of *Medium* in the solution containers, and equilibrate to the test temperature.
Suspend each prepared sample holder from a vertically reciprocating shaker such that each system is continuously immersed in *Medium* during the entire test.
Reciprocate at a frequency of about 30 cycles/min with an amplitude of about 2 cm, or as specified in the individual monograph, for the specified time.
At each sampling time interval, remove the solution containers from the bath, cool to room temperature, and add sufficient solvent (i.e., water in most cases) to correct for evaporative losses.
Perform the analysis on each sample as directed in the individual monograph. Repeat the test with additional TDS, as needed.

TIME

The test time points, at least three, are expressed in hours. Specimens are to be withdrawn within a tolerance of ±15 min or ±2% of the stated time, selecting the tolerance that results in the narrowest time interval.

INTERPRETATION

Unless otherwise specified in the individual monograph, the requirements are met if the quantities of active ingredient released from the TDS conform to *Acceptance Table 1* above, or the appropriate acceptance table in ⟨711⟩ for other dosage forms. Continue testing through the three levels unless the results conform at either L_1 or L_2.

⟨741⟩ MELTING RANGE OR TEMPERATURE

Change to read:

■The terms melting range, melting point, or melting temperature are all used in pharmacopeial contexts. Most substances exhibit a melting transition, spanning the temperatures at which the first detectable change of phase or liquid phase is detected to the temperature at which no solid phase is apparent. The transition may appear instantaneous for a highly pure material, but usually a range is observed from the beginning to the end of the process. Factors influencing this transition include the sample size, the particle size, the efficiency of heat diffusion within the sample, and the heating rate, among other variables, that are controlled by procedure instructions.

For pharmacopeial purposes, the temperatures of the beginning (onset temperature) and end of transition (clear temperature) represent the melting range, except as defined otherwise for *Procedure for Class II* and *Procedure for Class III* below. The terms melting point and melting temperature are considered to be equivalent.

Substances which melt with no decomposition or chemical change are known to melt congruently. In these cases, the melting point is taken to be the end of the melting range, i.e., the temperature at which no solid phase is apparent. In some articles, the melting process is accompanied by simultaneous decomposition, which is visually evidenced as a side event like darkening of the material, charring, bubbling, or other incident. These transitions are known to be non-congruent. The visual impact of this side reaction frequently obscures the end of the melting process, which may be impossible to accurately determine. In those circumstances, only the beginning of the melting can be accurately established, and it is to be reported as the melting point.

Since there may be a thermal lag between the heating medium and the sample within the capillary tube, in order to achieve consistency and repeatability, it is important to perform the melting determination at a heating rate, also referred to as ramp rate, of 1°/min.■₁s *(USP41)*

The accuracy of the apparatus to be used as described below should be checked at suitable intervals by the use of one or more of the available USP Melting Point Standards, preferably those that melt nearest the melting temperatures of the compounds being tested (see *USP Reference Standards* ⟨11⟩). ■The USP Melting Point Standards are intended to check the accuracy of the device and may be suitable to calibrate.■₁s *(USP41)*

Eight procedures for the determination of melting range or temperature are given herein, varying in accordance with the nature of the substance. When no class is designated in the monograph, use the *Procedure for Class Ia* for crystalline or amorphous substances and the *Procedure for Class II* for waxy substances.

The procedure known as the mixed-melting point determination, whereby the melting range or temperature of a solid under test is compared with that of an intimate mixture of equal parts of the solid and an authentic specimen of it, e.g., the corresponding USP Reference Standard, if available, may be used as a confirmatory identification test. Agreement of the observations on the original and the mixture constitutes reliable evidence of chemical identity.

Change to read:

APPARATUS

Apparatus with cameras or other computerized equipment ■to improve■₁s *(USP41)* accuracy, sensitivity, or precision may be used provided that the apparatus is properly qualified.

Apparatus I

An example of a suitable melting range *Apparatus I* consists of a glass container for a bath of transparent fluid, a suitable stirring device, an accurate thermometer, and a controlled source of heat. The bath fluid is selected with a view to the temperature required, but light paraffin is used generally and certain liquid silicones are well adapted to the higher temperature ranges. The fluid is deep enough to permit immersion of the thermometer to its specified immersion depth so that the bulb is still about 2 cm above the bottom of the bath. The heat may be supplied by an open flame or electrically. The capillary tube is about 10 cm long and 0.8–1.2 mm in internal diameter with walls 0.2–0.3 mm in thickness.

Apparatus II

An instrument may be used in the *Procedure for Class I, Procedure for Class Ia,* and *Procedure for Class Ib*. An example of a suitable melting range *Apparatus II* consists of a block of metal that may be heated at a controlled rate, with its temperature being monitored by a sensor. The block accommodates the capillary tube containing the test substance and permits monitoring of the melting process, typically by means of a beam of light and a detector. The detector signal may be processed by a microcomputer to determine and display the melting point or range, or the detector signal may be plotted to allow visual estimation of the melting point or range. ■Some approaches broadly used by automated systems employ optical methods such as light absorption or bulk reflection.■₁s *(USP41)*

Change to read:

PROCEDURES

Procedure for Class I, Apparatus I

Reduce the substance under test to a very fine powder, and, unless otherwise directed, render it anhydrous when it contains water of hydration by drying it at the temperature specified in the monograph, or, when the substance contains no water of hydration, dry it over a suitable desiccant for NLT 16 h (or at the conditions stated in *Loss on Drying* ⟨731⟩, if appropriate).

Charge a capillary glass tube, one end of which is sealed, with a sufficient amount of the dry powder to form a column in the bottom of the tube ■to a nominal height of■₁ₛ ₍ᵤₛₚ₄₁₎ 3 mm high when packed down as closely as possible by moderate tapping on a solid surface. Due to the instrument design, alternative sample sizes may be ■used as■₁ₛ ₍ᵤₛₚ₄₁₎ instructed by the instrument manufacturer.

Heat the bath until the temperature is about 10° below the expected melting point. Remove the thermometer, and quickly attach the capillary tube to the thermometer by wetting both with a drop of the liquid of the bath or otherwise, and adjust its height so that the material in the capillary is level with the thermometer bulb. Replace the thermometer, and continue the heating, with constant stirring, sufficiently to ■achieve the ramp■₁ₛ ₍ᵤₛₚ₄₁₎ rate of about 3°/min. When the temperature is about 3° below the lower limit of the expected melting range, reduce the heating so that the ■ramp■₁ₛ ₍ᵤₛₚ₄₁₎ rate of about 1°/min ■is achieved.■₁ₛ ₍ᵤₛₚ₄₁₎ Continue heating until melting is complete.

The temperature at which the column of the substance under test is observed to collapse definitely against the side of the tube at any point indicates the beginning of melting, and the temperature at which the test substance becomes liquid throughout corresponds to the end of melting or the melting point. The two temperatures fall within the limits of the melting range. If melting occurs with decomposition, the melting temperature corresponding to the beginning of the melting ■(melting point)■₁ₛ ₍ᵤₛₚ₄₁₎ is within the range specified.

Procedure for Class Ia, Apparatus I

Prepare the test substance and charge the capillary as directed in *Procedure for Class I, Apparatus I*. Heat the bath until the temperature is about 10° below the expected melting point and is rising at a rate of about 1°/min. Insert the capillary as directed in *Procedure for Class I, Apparatus I* when the temperature is about 5° below the lower limit of the expected melting range, and continue heating until melting is complete. Record the melting range as directed in *Procedure for Class I, Apparatus I*.

Procedure for Class Ib, Apparatus I

Place the test substance in a closed container and cool to 10°, or lower, for at least 2 h. Without ■■₁ₛ ₍ᵤₛₚ₄₁₎ powdering, charge the cooled material into the capillary tube as directed in *Procedure for Class I, Apparatus I*, then immediately place the charged tube in a vacuum desiccator and dry at a pressure not exceeding 20 mm of mercury for 3 h. Immediately upon removal from the desiccator, fire-seal the open end of the tube, and as soon as practicable proceed with the determination of the melting range as follows. Heat the bath until the temperature is about 10° below the expected melting range, then introduce the charged tube, and heat at a rate of rise of about 1°/min until melting is complete. Record the melting range as directed in *Procedure for Class I, Apparatus I*.

If the particle size of the material is too large for the capillary, precool the test substance as directed above, then with as little pressure as possible gently crush the particles to fit the capillary, and immediately charge the tube.

Procedure for Class I, Apparatus II

Prepare the substance under test and charge the capillary tube as directed in *Procedure for Class I, Apparatus I*. Operate the apparatus according to the manufacturer's instructions. Heat the block until the temperature is about 10° below the expected melting point. Insert the capillary tube into the heating block, and continue heating at a rate of temperature increase of about 1°/min until melting is complete.

The temperature at which the detector signal first leaves its initial value indicates the beginning of melting, and the temperature at which the detector signal reaches its final value corresponds to the end of melting, or the melting point. The two temperatures fall within the limits of the melting range. If melting occurs with decomposition, the melting temperature corresponding to the beginning of the melting ■(melting point)■₁ₛ ₍ᵤₛₚ₄₁₎ is within the range specified.

Procedure for Class Ia, Apparatus II

Prepare the test substance and charge the capillary as directed in *Procedure for Class I, Apparatus I*. Operate the apparatus according to the manufacturer's instructions. Heat the block until the temperature is about ■5°■₁ₛ ₍ᵤₛₚ₄₁₎ below the expected melting point and is rising at a rate of about 1°/min. Insert the capillary as directed in *Procedure for Class I, Apparatus I*, ■■₁ₛ ₍ᵤₛₚ₄₁₎ and continue heating until melting is complete. Record the melting range as directed in *Procedure for Class I, Apparatus I*. If melting occurs with decomposition, the melting temperature corresponding to the beginning of the melting ■(melting point)■₁ₛ ₍ᵤₛₚ₄₁₎ is within the range specified.

Procedure for Class Ib, Apparatus II

Place the test substance in a closed container and cool to 10°, or lower, for at least 2 h. Without previous powdering, charge the cooled material into the capillary tube as directed in *Procedure for Class I, Apparatus I*, then immediately place the charged tube in a vacuum desiccator, and dry at a pressure not exceeding 20 mm of mercury for 3 h. Immediately upon removal from the desiccator, fire-seal the open end of the tube, and as soon as practicable proceed with the determination of the melting range as follows. Operate the apparatus according to the manufacturer's instructions. Heat the block until the temperature is about 10° below the expected melting range, then introduce the charged tube, and heat at a rate of rise of about 1°/min until melting is complete. Record the melting range as directed in *Procedure for Class I, Apparatus I*.

If the particle size of the material is too large for the capillary, precool the test substance as directed above, then with as little pressure as possible gently crush the particles to fit the capillary, and immediately charge the tube.

Procedure for Class II

Carefully melt the material to be tested at as low a temperature as possible, and draw it into a capillary tube, which is left open at both ends, to a depth of about 10 mm. Cool the charged tube at 10°, or lower, for 24 h, or in contact with ice for at least 2 h. Then attach the tube to the thermometer by suitable means, adjust it in a water bath so that the upper edge of the material is 10 mm below the water level, and heat as directed in *Procedure for Class I, Apparatus I* except, within 5° of the expected melting temperature, to regulate the rate of rise of temperature of about 1.0°/min. The temperature at which the material is observed to rise in the capillary tube is the melting temperature.

Procedure for Class III

■While stirring, melt■₁ₛ (USP41) a quantity of the test substance slowly ■₁ₛ (USP41) until it reaches a temperature of 90°–92°. Remove the source of the heat, and allow the molten substance to cool to a temperature of 8°–10° above the expected melting point. Chill the bulb of a suitable thermometer to 5°, wipe it dry, and while it is still cold dip it into the molten substance so that approximately the lower half of the bulb is submerged. Withdraw it immediately, and hold it vertically away from the heat until the wax surface dulls, then dip it for 5 min into a water bath having a temperature NMT 16°.

Fix the thermometer securely in a test tube so that the lower point is 15 mm above the bottom of the test tube. Suspend the test tube in a water bath adjusted to about 16°, and raise the temperature of the bath at the rate of about 2°/min to 30°, then change to a rate of about 1°/min, and note the temperature at which the first drop of melted substance leaves the thermometer. Repeat the determination twice on a freshly melted portion of the test substance. If the variation of three determinations is less than 1°, take the average of the three as the melting point. If the variation of three determinations is 1° or greater than 1°, make two additional determinations and take the average of the five.

General Chapters

General Information

General Information

The chapters in this section are information, and aside from excerpts given herein from Federal Acts and regulations that may be applicable, they contain no standards, tests, assays, nor other mandatory specifications, with respect to any Pharmacopeial articles. The excerpts from pertinent Federal Acts and regulations included in this section are placed here inasmuch as they are not of Pharmacopeial authorship. Revisions of the federal requirements that affect these excerpts will be included in *USP Supplements* as promptly as practical. The official requirements for Pharmacopeial articles are set forth in the *General Notices,* the individual monographs, and the *General Tests and Assays* chapters of this *Pharmacopeia.*

〈1151〉 PHARMACEUTICAL DOSAGE FORMS

Change to read:

GENERAL CONSIDERATIONS

This chapter provides general descriptions of and definitions for drug products, or dosage forms, commonly used to administer the drug substance (active pharmaceutical ingredient; API). It discusses general principles involved in the manufacture or compounding of these dosage forms. A glossary is provided as a nomenclature resource.

A dosage form is a combination of drug substance(s) and/or excipient(s) to facilitate dosing, administration, and delivery of the medicine to the patient. The design, materials, manufacturing, and testing of all dosage forms target drug product quality.[1] A testing protocol must consider not only the physical, chemical, and biological properties of the dosage form as appropriate, but also the administration route and desired dosing regimen. The interrelationships of dosage forms and routes of administration have been summarized in the compendial taxonomy for pharmaceutical dosage forms (see *Figure 1*).[2] The organization of this general information chapter is mainly focused on the physical attributes of each particular dosage form (*Tier Two*), generally without specific reference to the route of administration. Those dosage form terms with asterisk notation (*) are not preferred and should not be used for new drug product titles. Information specific to the route of administration is given when needed.

---

[1] In the United States, a drug with a name recognized in *USP–NF* must comply with compendial identity standards or be deemed adulterated, misbranded, or both. To avoid being deemed adulterated, such drugs must also comply with compendial standards for strength, quality, and purity, unless labeled to show all respects in which the drug differs. See the Federal Food, Drug, and Cosmetic Act (FDCA), §501(b) and §502(e)(3)(b), and Food and Drug Administration (FDA) regulations at 21 CFR §299.5. In addition, to avoid being deemed misbranded, drugs recognized in *USP–NF* must also comply with compendial standards for packaging and labeling, FDCA Section 502(g). "Quality" is used herein as suitable shorthand for all such compendial requirements. This approach is also consistent with U.S. and FDA participation in the International Conference on Harmonisation (ICH). The ICH guideline on specifications, Q6A, notes that "specifications are chosen to confirm the quality of the drug substance and drug product..." and defines "quality" as "The suitability of either a drug substance or drug product for its intended use. This term includes such attributes as identity, strength, and purity."

[2] Marshall K, Foster TS, Carlin HS, & Williams RL. Development of a compendial taxonomy and glossary for pharmaceutical dosage forms. *Pharm Forum.* 2003;29(5):1742–1752.

TIER **ONE**
ROUTE OF ADMINISTRATION

INJECTION/IMPLANTATION   GASTRO-INTESTINAL   TOPICAL/DERMAL   MUCOSAL   INHALATION

TIER **TWO**
DOSAGE FORM

AEROSOLS   CAPSULES   CREAMS   EMULSIONS   FILMS   FOAMS   GASES   GELS
GRANULES   GUMS   IMPLANTS   INJECTIONS   INSERTS   IRRIGATIONS   LIQUIDS   LOTIONS
LOZENGES   OINTMENTS   PASTES   PELLETS   PILLS   PLASTERS*   POWDERS
SOAPS/SHAMPOOS   SOLUTIONS   SPRAYS   STRIPS   SUPPOSITORIES
SUSPENSIONS   SYSTEMS   TABLETS   TAPES*

TIER **THREE**
RELEASE PATTERN

IMMEDIATE   EXTENDED   DELAYED

Figure 1. Compendial taxonomy for pharmaceutical dosage forms.

Tests to ensure compliance with *USP* standards for dosage form performance fall into one of the following areas.

Dose Uniformity

(See also *Uniformity of Dosage Units* ⟨905⟩.) Consistency in dosing for a patient or consumer requires that the variation in the drug substance content of each dosage unit be accurately controlled throughout the manufactured batch or compounded lot of drug product. Uniformity of dosage units typically is demonstrated by one of two procedures: content uniformity or weight variation. The procedure for content uniformity requires the appropriate assay of the drug substance content of individual units. The procedure for weight variation uses the weight of the individual units to estimate their content. Weight variation may be used where the underlying distribution of the drug substance in the blend is presumed to be uniform and well-controlled, as in solutions. In such cases, the content of the drug substance may be adequately estimated by the net weight. Content uniformity does not rely on the assumption of blend uniformity and can be applied in all cases. Successful development and manufacture of dosage forms requires careful evaluation of the drug substance particle or droplet size, incorporation techniques, and excipient properties.

Stability

Drug product stability involves the evaluation of chemical stability, physical stability, and performance over time. The chemical stability of the drug substance in the dosage form matrix must support the expiration dating for the commercially prepared dosage forms and a beyond-use date for a compounded dosage form. Test procedures for potency must be stability indicating (see *Validation of Compendial Procedures* ⟨1225⟩). Degradation products should be quantified. In the case of dispersed or emulsified systems, consideration must be given to the potential for settling or separation of the formulation components. Any physical changes to the dosage form must be easily reversed (e.g., by shaking) prior to dosing or administration. For tablets, capsules, oral suspensions, and implants, in vitro release test procedures such as dissolution and disintegration provide a measure of continuing consistency in performance over time (see *Dissolution* ⟨711⟩, *Disintegration* ⟨701⟩, and *Drug Release* ⟨724⟩).

Bioavailability

(See also *In Vitro and In Vivo Evaluation of Dosage Forms* ⟨1088⟩ and *Assessment of Drug Product Performance—Bioavailability, Bioequivalence, and Dissolution* ⟨1090⟩.) Bioavailability is influenced by factors such as the method of manufacture or compounding, particle size, crystal form (polymorph) of the drug substance, the properties of the excipients used to formulate the dosage form, and physical changes as the drug product ages. Assurance of consistency in bioavailability over time (bioequivalence) requires close attention to all aspects of the production (or compounding) and testing of the dosage form. With proper justification, in vitro release testing (e.g., disintegration and dissolution) may be used as a surrogate to demonstrate consistent availability of the drug substance from the formulated dosage.

▪Release Profile

Two principal categories of drug release are recognized: immediate-release and modified-release.

"Immediate-release" is observed when no deliberate effort has been made to modify the drug substance release profile. For example, capsules and tablets are considered immediate-release even if a disintegrating agent or a lubricant has been used.

"Modified-release" is a term used when the rate and/or time of release of the drug substance is altered as compared to what would be observed or anticipated for an immediate-release product. Two modified-release profiles are recognized, delayed-release and extended-release. The term "modified-release" is not used for official article titles.

"Delayed-release" is when deliberate formulation achieves a delay in the release of the drug substance for some period of time after initial administration. For oral products, expressions such as "enteric-coated" or "gastro-resistant" have also been used where release of the drug substance is prevented in the gastric environment but promoted in the intestinal environment. However, the term "delayed-release" is used for official article titles.

"Extended-release" is when the deliberate formulation achieves prolongation of drug substance release compared to that observed or anticipated for an immediate-release dosage form. Expressions such as "prolonged-release", "repeat-action", "controlled-release", "long-acting", and "sustained-release" have also been used to describe such dosage forms. However, the term "extended-release" is used for official article titles.

The *Nomenclature Guidelines*[3] should be consulted for naming conventions for products with a single drug substance or for products with a combination of more than one drug substance displaying the combination of release profiles of immediate-release and extended-release, immediate-release and delayed-release, or extended-release and delayed-release.∎1S *(USP41)*

Manufacture

Although detailed instructions about the manufacture of any of these dosage forms are beyond the scope of this general information chapter, general manufacturing principles have been included.[4] Information relative to extemporaneous compounding of dosage forms can be found in *Pharmaceutical Compounding—Nonsterile Preparations* ⟨795⟩ and *Pharmaceutical Compounding—Sterile Preparations* ⟨797⟩.

Route of Administration

The primary routes of administration for pharmaceutical dosage forms can be defined as parenteral (see *Injections and Implanted Drug Products* ⟨1⟩), gastrointestinal (see *Oral Drug Products—Product Quality Tests* ⟨2⟩), topical/dermal (see *Topical and Transdermal Drug Products—Product Quality Tests* ⟨3⟩), mucosal, and inhalation (see *Inhalation and Nasal Drug Products—General Information and Product Quality Tests* ⟨5⟩), and each has subcategories as needed. Many tests used to ensure quality generally are applied across all of the administration routes, but some tests are specific for individual routes. For example, products intended for injection must be evaluated using *Sterility Tests* ⟨71⟩, *Bacterial Endotoxins Test* ⟨85⟩, or *Pyrogen Test* ⟨151⟩, and the manufacturing process (and sterilization technique) employed for parenterals (by injection) should ensure compliance with these tests. Tests for particulate matter may be required for certain dosage forms depending on the route of administration (e.g., by injection—*Particulate Matter in Injections* ⟨788⟩, or mucosal—*Particulate Matter in Ophthalmic Solutions* ⟨789⟩). Additionally, dosage forms intended for the inhalation route of administration must be monitored for particle size and spray pattern (for a metered-dose inhaler or dry powder inhaler) and droplet size (for nasal sprays). Further information regarding administration routes and suggested testing can be found in the *Guide to General Chapters, Chapter Charts, Charts 4–8, 10,* and *13.*

An appropriate manufacturing process and testing regimen help ensure that a dosage form can meet the appropriate quality attributes for the intended route of administration.

Packaging and Storage

Suitable packaging is determined for each product. For additional information about meeting packaging requirements listed in the individual labeling, refer to *Packaging and Storage Requirements* ⟨659⟩, *Containers—Performance Testing* ⟨671⟩, *Good Packaging Practices* ⟨1177⟩, and *Good Repackaging Practices* ⟨1178⟩. Product labeling must specify storage requirements that describe environmental conditions, limitations, and restrictions. For instance, exposure to excessive temperature, humidity, and light can influence the ability of the packaging to protect the product.

Labeling Statements

Some dosage forms or articles have mandatory labeling statements that are given in the *Code of Federal Regulations* (e.g., 21 CFR §201.320 and 21 CFR §369.21). The text of 21 CFR should be consulted to determine the current recommendations.

Change to read:

PRODUCT QUALITY TESTS, GENERAL

ICH Guidance Q6A (available at www.ich.org) recommends specifications (list of tests, references to analytical procedures, and acceptance criteria) to ensure that drug products are safe and effective at the time of release and over their shelf life. Tests that are universally applied to ensure safety, efficacy, strength, quality, and purity include description, identification, assay, and impurities.

Description

The *Definition* section (see ●*General Notices, 4.10 Monographs*)● (CN 1-May-2018) in a *USP* monograph describes the drug product and specifies the range of acceptable assayed content of the drug substance(s) present in the dosage form. For certain prod-

---

[3] *Nomenclature Guidelines*, http://www.usp.org/health-quality-safety/compendial-nomenclature.
[4] The terms "manufacture" and "preparation" are used interchangeably in this general chapter.

ucts, the *Definition* includes any relevant additional information, such as the presence or absence of other components, excipients, or adjuvants, cautionary statements on toxicity and stability, etc. While appearance information to aid in identification is used in a regulatory submission (e.g., a qualitative description of size, shape, color, etc.) it is typically not required as part of a *USP* monograph. This information is drug product specific.

Identification

Identification tests are discussed in the ●*General Notices, 5.40 Identification.*● (CN 1-May-2018) Identification tests should establish the identity of the drug substance(s) present in the drug product and should discriminate between compounds of closely related structure that are likely to be present. Identification tests should be specific for the drug substance(s). For example, the infrared absorption spectrum is often used (see *Mid-Infrared Spectroscopy* ⟨854⟩ and *Spectrophotometric Identification Tests* ⟨197⟩). If no suitable infrared spectrum can be obtained, other analytical methods can be used. Near-infrared (NIR) or Raman spectrophotometric methods could also be acceptable as the sole identification method of the drug product formulation (see *Near-Infrared Spectroscopy* ⟨1119⟩ and *Raman Spectroscopy* ⟨1120⟩). Identification by a chromatographic retention time from a single procedure is not regarded as specific. The use of retention times from two chromatographic procedures for which the separation is based on different principles or a combination of tests in a single procedure can be acceptable (see *Chromatography* ⟨621⟩ and *Thin-Layer Chromatographic Identification Test* ⟨201⟩).

Assay

A specific and stability-indicating test should be used to determine the strength (drug substance content) of the drug product. Some examples of these procedures are *Antibiotics—Microbial Assays* ⟨81⟩, ⟨621⟩, or *Assay for Steroids* ⟨351⟩. In cases when the use of a nonspecific assay is justified (e.g., *Titrimetry* ⟨541⟩), other supporting analytical procedures should be used to achieve specificity. When evidence of excipient interference with a nonspecific assay exists, a procedure with demonstrated specificity should be used.

Impurities

Process impurities, synthetic byproducts, and other inorganic and organic impurities may be present in the drug substance and excipients used in the manufacture of the drug product. These impurities are evaluated by tests in the drug substance and excipients monographs. Impurities arising from degradation of the drug substance or from the drug-product manufacturing process should be monitored. *Residual Solvents* ⟨467⟩ is applied to all products where relevant.

In some cases, testing for heavy metal impurities is appropriate. ●● (Official 1-Jan-2018)

In addition to the universal tests listed, the following tests may be considered on a case-by-case basis.

Physicochemical Properties

Examples include *pH* ⟨791⟩, *Viscosity—Capillary Methods* ⟨911⟩ or *Viscosity—Rotational Methods* ⟨912⟩, and *Specific Gravity* ⟨841⟩.

Particle Size

For some dosage forms, particle size can have a significant effect on dissolution rates, bioavailability, therapeutic outcome, and stability. Procedures such as those found in *Inhalation and Nasal Drug Products: Aerosols, Sprays, and Powders—Performance Quality Tests* ⟨601⟩ and *Particle Size Distribution Estimation by Analytical Sieving* ⟨786⟩ could be used.

Uniformity of Dosage Units

See the discussion of *Dose Uniformity* in the *General Considerations* section.

Water Content

A test for water content is included when appropriate (see *Water Determination* ⟨921⟩).

Microbial Limits

The type of microbial test(s) and acceptance criteria are based on the nature of the nonsterile drug product, method of manufacture, and the route of administration (see *Microbial Enumeration Tests* ⟨61⟩, *Tests for Specified Microorganisms* ⟨62⟩, and *Microbiological Examination of Nonsterile Products: Acceptance Criteria for Pharmaceutical Preparations and Substances for Pharmaceutical Use* ⟨1111⟩).

Antimicrobial Preservative Content

Acceptance criteria for preservative content in multidose products should be established. They are based on the levels of antimicrobial preservative necessary to maintain the product's microbiological quality at all stages throughout its proposed usage and shelf life (see *Antimicrobial Effectiveness Testing* ⟨51⟩).

Antioxidant Content

If antioxidants are present in the drug product, tests of their content should be performed to maintain the product's quality at all stages throughout its proposed usage and shelf life.

Sterility

Depending on the route of administration (e.g., ophthalmic preparations, implants, aqueous-based preparations for oral inhalation, and injections) sterility of the product is demonstrated as appropriate (see ⟨71⟩).

Dissolution

A test to measure the release of the drug substance(s) from the drug product normally is included for dosage forms such as tablets, capsules, suspensions, granules for suspensions, implants, transdermal delivery systems, and medicated chewing gums. Single-point measurements typically are used for immediate-release dosage forms. For modified-release dosage forms, appropriate test conditions and sampling procedures are established as needed (see ⟨711⟩ and ⟨724⟩). In some cases, dissolution testing may be replaced by disintegration testing (see ⟨701⟩).

Breaking Force and Friability

These parameters are evaluated as in-process controls. Acceptance criteria depend on packaging, supply chain, and intended use (see *Tablet Friability* ⟨1216⟩ and *Tablet Breaking Force* ⟨1217⟩).

Leachables

When evidence exists that leachables from the container–closure systems (e.g., rubber stopper, cap liner, or plastic bottle) have an impact on the safety or efficacy of the drug product, a test is included to evaluate the presence of leachables.

Other Tests

Depending on the type and composition of the dosage form, other tests such as alcohol content, redispersibility, particle size distribution, rheological properties, reconstitution time, endotoxins/pyrogens, particulate matter, functionality testing of delivery systems, delivered dose uniformity, viscosity, and osmolarity may be necessary.

Change to read:

DOSAGE FORMS

Aerosols

Aerosols are dosage forms packaged under pressure and contain therapeutic agent(s) and a propellant that are released upon actuation of an appropriate valve system. Upon actuation of the valve system, the drug substance is released as a plume of fine particles or droplets. Only one dose is released from the preparation upon actuation of a metered valve. In the case of topical products and depending on the nature of the drug substance and the conditions being treated, actuation of the valve may result in a metered release of a controlled amount of the formulation or the continuous release of the formulation as long as the valve is depressed.

The aerosol dosage form refers only to those products packaged under pressure that release a fine mist of particles or droplets when actuated (see *Glossary*). Other products that produce dispersions of fine droplets or particles will be covered in subsequent sections (e.g., *Powders* and *Sprays*).

TYPICAL COMPONENTS

Typical components of aerosols are the formulation containing one or more drug substance(s) and propellant, the container, the valve, and the actuator. Each component plays a role in determining various characteristics of the emitted plume, such as droplet or particle size distribution, uniformity of delivery of the therapeutic agent, delivery rate, and plume velocity and geometry. The metering valve and actuator act in tandem to generate the plume of droplets or particles. The metering valve delivers an accurate volume of the pressurized liquid formulation from the container. The actuator directs the metered volume to a small orifice that is open to the atmosphere. Upon actuation, the formulation is forced through the opening, forming the fine mist of particles that are directed to the site of administration.

Aerosol preparations may consist of either a two-phase (gas and liquid) or a three-phase (gas, liquid, and solid or liquid) formulation. The two-phase formulation consists of drug substance(s) dissolved in liquefied propellant. Co-solvents such as alcohol may be added to enhance the solubility of the drug substance(s). Three-phase inhalation and nasal aerosol systems consist of suspended drug substance(s) in propellant(s), co-solvents, and potentially other suitable excipients. The suspension or emulsion of the finely divided drug substance is typically dispersed in the liquid propellant with the aid of suitable biocompatible surfactants or other excipients.

Propellants for aerosol formulations are typically low molecular weight hydrofluorocarbons or hydrocarbons that are liquid when constrained in the container, exhibit a suitable vapor pressure at room temperature, and are biocompatible and nonirritating. Compressed gases do not supply a constant pressure over use and typically are not used as propellants.

Metal containers can withstand the vapor pressure produced by the propellant. Excess formulation may be added to the container to ensure that the full number of labeled doses can be accurately administered. The container and closure must be able to withstand the pressures anticipated under normal use conditions as well as when the system is exposed to elevated temperatures.

TYPES OF AEROSOL DOSAGE FORMS

Aerosol dosage forms can be delivered via various routes. The container, actuator, and metering valve, as well as the formulation, are designed to target the site of administration.

Inhalation aerosols, commonly known as metered-dose inhalers (MDIs), are intended to produce fine particles or droplets for inhalation through the mouth and deposition in the pulmonary tree. The design of the delivery system is intended to release measured mass and appropriate quality of the active substance with each actuation.

Nasal aerosols, commonly known as nasal MDIs, produce fine particles or droplets for delivery through the nasal vestibule and deposition in the nasal cavity. Each actuation of the valve releases a measured mass of the drug substance with appropriate quality characteristics.

Lingual aerosols are intended to produce fine particles or droplets for deposition on the surface of the tongue. The design of the delivery system releases one dose with each actuation.

Topical aerosols produce fine particles or droplets for application to the skin.

LABELING FOR PROPER USE

Refer to 21 CFR §201.320 and 21 CFR §369.21.

Capsules

Capsules are solid dosage forms in which the drug substance and/or excipients are enclosed within a soluble container or shell or coated on the capsule shell. The shells may be composed of two pieces (a body and a cap), or they may be composed of a single piece. Two-piece capsules are commonly referred to as hard-shell capsules, and one-piece capsules are often referred to as soft-shell capsules. This two-piece and one-piece capsule distinction, although imprecise, reflects differing levels of plasticizers in the two compositions and the fact that one-piece capsules typically are more pliable than two-piece capsules.

The shells of capsules are usually made from gelatin. However, they may also be made from cellulose polymers or other suitable material. Most capsules are designed for oral administration. When no deliberate effort has been made to modify the drug substance release rate, capsules are referred to as immediate-release.

TWO-PIECE OR HARD-SHELL CAPSULES

Two-piece capsules consist of two telescoping cap and body pieces in a range of standard sizes.

ONE-PIECE OR SOFT-SHELL CAPSULES

One-piece capsules typically are used to deliver a drug substance as a solution or suspension. Liquid formulations placed into one-piece capsules may offer advantages by comparison with dry-filled capsules and tablets in achieving content uniformity of potent drug substance(s) or acceptable dissolution of drug substance(s) with poor aqueous solubility. Because the contact between the shell wall and its liquid contents is more intimate than in dry-filled capsules, undesired interactions may be more likely to occur (including gelatin crosslinking and pellicle formation).

MODIFIED-RELEASE CAPSULES

The release of drug substance(s) from capsules can be modified in several ways. There are two categories of modified-release capsule formulations recognized by USP.

Delayed-release capsules: Capsules are sometimes formulated to include enteric-coated granules to protect acid-labile drug substances from the gastric environment or to prevent adverse events such as irritation. Enteric-coated multiparticulate capsule dosage forms may reduce variability in bioavailability associated with gastric emptying times for larger particles (i.e., tablets) and to minimize the likelihood of a therapeutic failure when coating defects occur during manufacturing. Alternatively, a coating may be applied to the capsule shell to achieve delayed release of the contents.

Extended-release capsules: Extended-release capsules are formulated in such a manner as to make the contained drug substance available over an extended period of time following ingestion. ■1S *(USP41)* Requirements for dissolution (see ⟨711⟩) are typically specified in the individual monograph.

Methods for modifying drug substance release from capsules include coating the filled capsule shells or the contents, in the case of dry-filled capsules.

PREPARATION

Two-piece capsules: Two-piece gelatin capsules are usually formed from blends of gelatins that have relatively high gel strength in order to optimize shell clarity and toughness or from hypromellose. They may also contain colorants such as D&C and FD&C dyes[5] or various pigments, opaquing agents such as titanium dioxide, dispersing agents, plasticizers, and preservatives. Gelatin capsule shells normally contain between 12% and 16% water.

The shells are manufactured in one set of operations and later filled in a separate manufacturing process. Two-piece shell capsules are made by a process that involves dipping shaped pins into gelatin or hypromellose solutions, followed by drying, cutting, and joining steps.

Powder formulations for two-piece gelatin capsules generally consist of the drug substance and at least one excipient. Both the formulation and the method of filling can affect release of the drug substance. In the filling operation, the body and cap of the shell are separated before filling. Following the filling operation, the machinery rejoins the body and cap and ensures satisfactory closure of the capsule by exerting appropriate force on the two pieces. The joined capsules can be sealed after filling by a band at the joint of the body and cap or by a designed locking joint between the cap and body. In compounding prescription practice, two-piece capsules may be hand-filled. This permits the prescriber the choice of selecting either a single drug substance or a combination of drug substances at the exact dose level considered best for an individual patient.

One-piece capsules: One-piece capsules are formed, filled, and sealed in a single process on the same machine and are available in a wide variety of sizes, shapes, and colors. The most common type of one-piece capsule is that produced by a rotary die process that results in a capsule with a seam. The soft gelatin shell is somewhat thicker than that of two-piece capsules and is plasticized by the addition of polyols such as glycerin, sorbitol, or other suitable materials. The ratio of the plasticizer to the gelatin can be varied to change the flexibility of the shell depending on the nature of the fill material, its intended usage, or environmental conditions.

In most cases, one-piece capsules are filled with liquids. Typically, drug substances are dissolved or suspended in a liquid vehicle. Classically, an oleaginous vehicle such as a vegetable oil was used. However, nonaqueous, water-miscible liquid vehicles such as the lower molecular weight polyethylene glycols are now more common. The physicochemical properties of the vehicle can be chosen to ensure stability of the drug substance as well as to influence the release profile from the capsule shell.

Creams

(See *Emulsions*.)

Emulsions

An emulsion is a dispersed colloidal system consisting of two immiscible liquid phases generally stabilized with one or more suitable agents.

Typical pharmaceutical emulsions are prepared from immiscible aqueous and organic (oil) liquids. Complex multiple-phase systems may exist in an emulsion. Whether the organic or the aqueous phase is the dispersed phase depends on the volumes of the two phases, the emulsifier chosen, and the method of preparation. When an oil phase is dispersed in an aqueous phase, the emulsion is termed an oil-in-water (O/W) emulsion and water is referred to as the continuous phase. When water is dis-

---

[5] In 1960 Congress enacted the Color Additive Amendments, requiring the FDA to regulate dyes, pigments, or other coloring agents in foods, drugs, and cosmetics separately from food additives. Under the law, color additives are deemed unsafe unless they are used in compliance with FDA regulations. The law provides a framework for the listing and certification of color additives. See FDCA §721; see FDA regulations at 21 CFR Part 70. Colors must also be listed in pertinent FDA regulations for specific uses; the list of color additives for drugs that are exempt from certification is published at 21 CFR Part 73, Subpart B. FDA also conducts a certification program for batches of color additives that are required to be certified before sale; see 21 CFR Part 74 (Subpart B re: drugs). Regulations regarding certification procedures, general specifications, and the listing of certified provisionally listed colors are at 21 CFR Part 80. FDA maintains a color additives website with links to various legal and regulatory resources at: http://www.fda.gov; search by document title.

persed in oil, the emulsion is referred to as a water-in-oil (W/O) emulsion. Emulsions have dispersed phases typically ranging from 0.1 to 100 μm. Emulsions are opaque while microemulsions are usually transparent or translucent. Microemulsions have dispersed phases less than 0.1 μm.

Emulsions may exhibit three types of instability: flocculation, creaming, and coalescence. Flocculation describes the process by which the dispersed phase comes out of suspension in the form of flakes. Coalescence is another form of instability—small droplets within the media continuously combine to form progressively larger droplets. Emulsions can also undergo creaming, where one of the phases migrates to the top (or the bottom, depending on the relative densities of the two phases) of the emulsion. To prevent flocculation, creaming, and coalescence of the emulsions, manufacturers commonly add surfactants, pH-modifying agents, or emulsifying agents to increase the stability of emulsions so that the emulsion does not change significantly with time.

Emulsions are widely used as pharmaceutical dosage forms. Oral emulsions have been prepared to improve taste, solubility, stability, or bioavailability. Emulsions for topical administration are referred to as creams, lotions, and sometimes ointments. Parenteral emulsions have been used for anesthetics, parenteral nutrition, and to deliver poorly water-soluble drugs.

CREAMS

Creams are semisolid emulsion dosage forms. They often contain more than 20% water and volatiles, and/or typically contain less than 50% hydrocarbons, waxes, or polyols as the vehicle for the drug substance. Creams are generally intended for external application to the skin or to the mucous membranes. Creams have a relatively soft, spreadable consistency and can be formulated as either a W/O emulsion (e.g., *Cold Cream* or *Fatty Cream* as in the *European Pharmacopoeia*) or as an oil-in-water emulsion (e.g., *Betamethasone Valerate Cream*). Creams are generally described as either nonwashable or washable, reflecting the fact that an emulsion with an aqueous external continuous phase is more easily removed than one with a nonaqueous external phase (W/O emulsion).

LOTIONS

Lotions are an emulsified liquid dosage form intended for external application to the skin. Historically, some topical suspensions such as calamine lotion have been called lotions but that nomenclature is not currently preferred. Lotions share many characteristics with creams. The distinguishing factor is that they are more fluid than semisolid and thus pourable. Due to their fluid character, lotions are more easily applied to large skin surfaces than semisolid preparations. Lotions may contain antimicrobial agents as preservatives.

INJECTABLE EMULSIONS

Injectable emulsions are sterile liquid dosage forms of drug substances dissolved or dispersed in a suitable emulsion medium. Injectable emulsions are for parenteral administration of poorly water-soluble drugs.

OINTMENTS

Ointments are sometimes semisolid emulsion dosage forms (see *Dosage Forms, Ointments*).

PREPARATION

Chapter ⟨795⟩ provides general information regarding the preparation of emulsions.

Creams: Creams may be formulated from a variety of oils, both mineral and vegetable, and from fatty alcohols, fatty acids, and fatty esters. Emulsifying agents include nonionic surfactants, detergents, and soaps. Soaps are usually formed in situ during the preparation of creams from a fatty acid in the oil phase hydrolyzed by a base dissolved in the aqueous phase.

Preparation usually involves separating the formula components into two portions: lipid and aqueous. The lipid portion contains all water-insoluble components and the aqueous portion contains the water-soluble components. Both phases are heated to a temperature above the melting point of the highest melting component. The phases are then mixed and the mixture is stirred until reaching ambient temperature or until the mixture has congealed. Mixing is generally continued during the cooling process to promote uniformity. Traditionally, the aqueous phase is added to the lipid phase, but comparable results have been obtained with the reverse procedure. High-shear homogenization may be employed to reduce particle or droplet size and to improve the physical stability of the resultant dosage form.

The drug substance(s) can be added to the phase in which it is soluble at the beginning of the manufacturing process, or it can be added after the cream is prepared by a suitable dispersion process such as levigation or milling with a roller mill. Creams usually require the addition of a preservative(s) unless they are compounded immediately prior to use and intended to be consumed in a relatively short period of time.

Lotions: Lotions are usually prepared by dissolving or dispersing the drug substance into the more appropriate phase (oil or water), adding the appropriate emulsifying or suspending agents, and mixing the oil and water phases to form a uniform fluid emulsion.

Injectable emulsions: Chapter ⟨1⟩ provides guidance on sterile preparations. Emulsions intended for parenteral administration can be formulated using the same principles as creams and lotions. The formulation should be designed for ease of administration. The particle size of the dispersed phase can vary by route of administration. For example, emulsions intended for intravenous administration should comply with *Globule Size Distribution in Lipid Injectable Emulsions* ⟨729⟩. The procedure to assure sterility should be validated by media fills. Preservatives are generally not used in injectable emulsions.

Ointments: (See *Dosage Forms, Ointments*.)

Films

Films are thin sheets that are placed in the oral cavity. They contain one or more layers. A layer may or may not contain the drug substance. Typically, these thin sheets are formed by casting or extrusion that results in a dispersion of the components through the film. Films are classified by the site of application. "Oral films" can be formulated to deliver medication to the mouth such as oral hygiene products or to deliver medication to the gastrointestinal tract for absorption. "Buccal films" and "sublingual films" are formulated to facilitate absorption through the proximal mucosal membranes avoiding first pass metabolism or degradation in the gastrointestinal tract and providing a quick onset of action.

Films can be formulated with edible polymers such as pullulan or with water-soluble polymers such as modified cellulose, edible gums, and copolymers. The dissolution rate of the film is controlled to facilitate incorporation of the medication into saliva or for absorption by the proximal mucosa. These films must be substantial enough to maintain their integrity during manufacture and packaging, and permit handling by the patient. Because of the rapid dissolution, taste and mouth feel are important considerations.

Foams

Foams are preparations that comprise gas bubbles distributed in a liquid. The liquid contains the drug substance and suitable excipients. Medicated foams may be packaged in pressurized containers or in other special dispensing devices. For medicated foams dispensed from nonpressurized containers, the use of mechanical force is required to generate the foam. Foams are intended for application to the skin or mucous membranes. The medicated foam is formed at the time of application. Surfactants are used to ensure the distribution of the gas in the liquid and to stabilize the foam. Medicated foams have a semisolid consistency and can be formulated to quickly break down into liquid or to remain as foam to ensure prolonged contact.

Medicated foams intended to treat severely injured skin or open wounds must be sterile.

PREPARATION

A foam may contain one or more drug substances, surfactants, and aqueous or nonaqueous liquids, and is produced with or without the aid of propellants. When a propellant is not used, mechanical work is required to generate the foam. If the propellant is in the internal (discontinuous) phase, a stable foam is discharged. If the propellant is in the external (continuous) phase, a quick-breaking foam is discharged. Quick-breaking foams formulated with alcohol create a cooling sensation after application to the skin and may have antimicrobial properties.

Gases

Medical gases are products that are administered directly as a gas. A medical gas has a direct pharmacological action or acts as a diluent for another medical gas. Gases used as excipients for administration of aerosol products, as an adjuvant in packaging, or produced by other dosage forms, are not included in this definition.

COMPONENTS

Medical gases may be single components or defined mixtures of components. Mixtures can also be extemporaneously prepared at the point of use.

ADMINISTRATION

Medical gases may be administered to the patient using several methods: nasal cannulas, face masks, atmospheric tents, and endotracheal tubes for the pulmonary route; hyperbaric chambers for the pulmonary and dermal routes of administration; jetted tubes that are directed at dental tissue to promote drying in preparation for fillings and crowns; tubes for expanding the intestines to facilitate medical imaging during colonoscopy; tubes for expanding the pelvis via transuterine inflation in preparation for fallopian tubal ligation; and tubes for expanding angioplasty devices. The dose of medical gas is typically metered by a volume rate of flow under ambient temperature and pressure conditions. Administration of a highly compressed gas generally requires a regulator to decrease the pressure, a variable-volume flow controller, and suitable tubing to conduct the gas to the patient. For pulmonary administration, the gas flow will be directed to the nose or mouth by a suitable device or into the trachea through a mechanical ventilator. When medical gases are administered chronically, provision for humidification is common. Care should be exercised to avoid microbial contamination.

SPECIAL CONSIDERATIONS

The container and system fittings should be appropriate for the medical gas. Adaptors should not be used to connect containers to patient-use supply system piping or equipment. Large quantities of gases such as oxygen or nitrogen can be stored in the liquid state in a cryogenic container and converted into a gas, as needed, by evaporation. Additional rules concerning the construction and use of cryogenic containers are promulgated by governmental agencies (e.g., U.S. Department of Commerce).

Containers, tubing, and administration masks employed for gases containing oxygen are free of any compound that would be sensitive to oxidation or that would be irritating to the respiratory tract.

A significant fraction of the dose of a medical gas may be released into the general vicinity of the patient due to incomplete absorption. Adequate ventilation may be necessary to protect health care workers and others from exposure to the gas (e.g., nitrous oxide).

Gels

■A gel is solid or semisolid. Gels can be classified in two groups, chemical and physical gels. Chemical gels are usually covalently crosslinked gels, while physical gels consist of small molecules or molecular chains that are physically crosslinked into networks, or solutions, or colloidal dispersions that are stiffened by a gelling agent. Typically, gels hold their form being self-supporting. Some gels may exhibit a range of behavior under mechanical forces. Gels may be thixotropic, forming semisolids on standing and becoming less viscous on agitation. Like emulsions, gels can be characterized as having a continuous phase as well as a dispersed phase. A variety of routes are available for gel administration such as topical, mucosal, or oral. In veterinary medicine, gels can also be administered via mammary infusion.

Gels may consist of a network of small discrete particles (e.g., *Aluminum Hydroxide Gel, Bentonite Magma,* or *Psyllium Hemicellulose*). As these gels may be thixotropic, forming semisolids on standing and becoming less viscous on agitation, they should be shaken before use to ensure homogeneity and should be so labeled.

Gels can consist of organic macromolecules uniformly distributed throughout a liquid in such a manner that no apparent boundaries exist between the dispersed macromolecules and the liquid continuous phase. These gels may be made from natural or synthetic macromolecules (e.g., carbomer, hypromellose, or starch) or natural gums (e.g., tragacanth). Although these gels are commonly aqueous based, alcohols and oils may be used as the continuous phase.

Chewable gels are used to deliver drug substances or dietary supplements via the oral route. Chewable gels can consist of all or some of the following components—gelling agent(s), sugars, water, sweeteners, and flavoring agents. The sweeteners and flavoring are intended to enhance patient acceptance and mask the taste of the delivered labeled drug substance or dietary supplement. Chewable gels maintain their molded shape, are elastic, and yield to mastication. They are intended to be chewed before swallowing. Chewable gels are also known as "gummies" in the confectionary and dietary supplement industries but that term is not used in official article titles.■1S (USP41)

PREPARATION

■Gels may be formed by dispersing the gelling agent in the continuous phase (e.g., by heating starch), by crosslinking the dispersed phase gelling agent, by changing the pH (as for *Carbomer Copolymer*), or by reducing the continuous phase by heat or vacuum (as for gels formed with sucrose).

Care should be taken to ensure uniformity of the drug substances by dispersing them by vigorous mixing or milling, or by shaking if the preparation is less viscous.

Chewable gels are formulated with one or more gelling agents (such as gelatin or starch), sugars (such as sucrose or corn syrup), flavoring agents, sweeteners, colorants, and water. The ingredients are blended and heated to form a viscous solution that is poured into molds (e.g., corn starch molds). After cooling, the individual units are separated from the molds.■1S (USP41)

Granules

Granules are solid dosage forms that are composed of agglomerations of smaller particles. These multicomponent compositions are prepared for oral administration and are used to facilitate flexible dosing regimens as granules or as suspensions, address stability challenges, allow taste masking, or facilitate flexibility in administration (for instance, to pediatric patients, geriatric patients, or animals). Granular dosage forms may be formulated for direct oral administration and may facilitate compounding of multiple drug substances by allowing compounding pharmacists to blend various granular compositions in the retail or hospital pharmacy. More commonly, granules are reconstituted to a suspension by the addition of water or a supplied liquid diluent immediately prior to delivery to the patient. Effervescent granules are formulated to liberate gas (carbon dioxide) upon addition of water. Common examples of effervescent granules include antacid and potassium supplementation preparations. Common therapeutic classes formulated as granule dosage forms include antibiotics, certain laxatives (such as senna extract products), electrolytes, and various cough and cold remedies that contain multiple drug substances.

PREPARATION

Granules are often the precursors used in tablet compression or capsule filling. Although this application represents a pharmaceutical intermediate and not a final dosage form, numerous commercial products are based on granules. In the typical manufacture of granules, the drug substance(s) is blended with excipients (processing aids) and wetted with an appropriate pharmaceutical binding solution, solvent, or blend of solvents to promote agglomeration. This composition is dried and sized to yield the desired material properties.

Frequently, granules are used because the drug substance is unstable in aqueous environments and cannot be exposed to water for periods sufficient to accommodate manufacture, storage, and distribution in a suspension. Preparation of the liquid dosage form from the granules immediately prior to dispensing allows acceptable stability for the duration of use. Granules manufactured for this purpose are packaged in quantities sufficient for a limited time period—usually one course of therapy that typically does not exceed 2 weeks. In addition to the drug substances, other ingredients may be added to ensure acceptable stability (e.g., buffers, antioxidants, or chelating agents) or to provide color, sweetness, and flavor; and for suspensions, to provide acceptable viscosity to ensure adequate suspension of the particulate to enable uniform dosing.

Effervescent granules are typically formulated from sodium or potassium bicarbonate and an acid such as citric or tartaric acid. To prevent untimely generation of carbon dioxide, manufacturers should take special precautions to limit residual water in the product due to manufacture and to select packaging that protects the product from moisture. The manufacture of effervescent granules can require specialized facilities designed to maintain very low humidity (approximately 10% relative humidity). Effervescent powder mixtures are purposely formed into relatively course granules to reduce the rate of dissolution and provide a more controlled effervescence.

Reconstitution of granules must ensure complete wetting of all ingredients and sufficient time and agitation to allow the soluble components to dissolve. Specific instructions for reconstitution provided by the manufacturer should be carefully followed.

Reconstituted suspensions should be thoroughly mixed or shaken before use to resuspend the dispersed particulates. This is especially true of suspension preparations dosed from multiple-dose containers. For particularly viscous suspensions prone to air entrapment, instructions may advise the user how to shake the preparation to resuspend settled particulates while minimizing air entrapment.

For granules reconstituted to form suspensions for oral administration, acceptable suspension of the particulate phase depends on the particle size of the dispersed phase as well as the viscosity of the vehicle. Temperature can influence the viscosity, which influences suspension properties and the ease of removal of the dose from the bottles. In addition, temperature cycling can lead to changes in the particle size of the dispersed phase via Ostwald ripening. Thus, clear instructions should be provided regarding the appropriate storage temperature for the product.

Gums

Medicated gum is a pliable dosage form that is designed to be chewed rather than swallowed. Medicated gums release the drug substance(s) into the saliva. Medicated gums can deliver therapeutic agents for local action in the mouth or for systemic absorption via the buccal or gastrointestinal routes (e.g., nicotine or aspirin). Most gums are manufactured using the conventional melting process derived from the confectionary industry or alternatively may be directly compressed from gum powder. Medicated gums are formulated from insoluble synthetic gum bases such as polyisoprene, polyisobutylene, isobutyleneisoprene copolymer, styrene butadiene rubber, polyvinyl acetate, polyethylene, ester gums, or polyterpenes. Plasticizers and softeners such as propylene glycol, glycerin, oleic acid, or processed vegetable oils are added to keep the gum base pliable and to aid in the incorporation of the drug substance(s), sweeteners, and flavoring agents. Sugars as well as artificial sweeteners and flavorings are incorporated to improve taste, and dyes may be used to enhance appearance. Some medicated gums are coated with magnesium stearate to reduce tackiness and improve handling during packaging. A preservative may be added.

PREPARATION

Melted gum: The gum base is melted at a temperature of about 115° until it has the viscosity of thick syrup and, at that point, is filtered through a fine-mesh screen. This molten gum base is transferred to mixing tanks where the sweeteners, plasticizers, and typically the drug substance are added and mixed. Colorings, flavorings, and preservatives are added and mixed while the melted gum is cooling. The cooled mixture is shaped by extrusion or rolling and cutting. Dosage units of the desired shape and potency are packaged individually. Additional coatings such as powder coatings to reduce tackiness or film or sugar coatings may be added to improve taste or facilitate bulk packaging.

Directly compressed gum: The gum base is supplied in a free-flowing granular powder form. The powder gum base is then dry blended with sweeteners, flavors, the drug substance, and lubricant. The blend is then processed through a conventional tablet press and tableted into desired shapes. The resulting medicated gum tablets can be further coated with sugar or sugar-free excipients. These tablets can be packaged in blisters or bottles as needed.

SPECIAL CONSIDERATIONS

Medicated gums are typically dispensed in unit-dose packaging. The patient instructions also may include a caution to avoid excessive heat.

Implants

Implants are long-acting dosage forms that provide continuous release of the drug substance often for periods of months to years. They are administered by the parenteral route. For systemic delivery they may be placed subcutaneously, or for local delivery they can be placed in a specific region in the body (e.g., in the sinus, in an artery, in the eye, in the brain, etc.).

Several types of implants are available. Pellet implants are small, sterile, solid masses composed of a drug substance with or without excipients. They are usually administered by means of a suitable special injector (e.g., trocar) or by surgical incision. Release of the drug substance from pellets is typically controlled by diffusion and dissolution kinetics. The size of the pellets and rate of erosion will influence the release rate, which typically follows first-order kinetics. Drug substance release from pellets for periods of 6 months or more is possible.

Resorbable microparticles are a type of implant that provides extended release of a drug substance over periods varying from a few weeks to months. They can be administered subcutaneously or intramuscularly for systemic delivery, or they may be deposited in a desired location in the body for site-specific delivery. Injectable resorbable microparticles (or microspheres) generally range from 20 to 100 µm in diameter. They are composed of a drug substance dispersed within a biocompatible, bioresorbable polymeric excipient (matrix). Poly(lactide-co-glycolide) polymers have been used frequently. These excipients typically resorb by hydrolysis of ester linkages. The microparticles are administered by suspension in an aqueous vehicle followed by injection with a conventional syringe and needle. Release of the drug substance from the microparticles begins after physiological fluid enters the polymer matrix, dissolving some of the drug substance that is then released by a diffusion-controlled process. Drug release also can occur as the matrix erodes.

Polymer implants can be formed as a single-shaped mass such as a cylinder. The polymer matrix must be biocompatible (see *The Biocompatibility of Materials Used in Drug Containers, Medical Devices, and Implants* ⟨1031⟩), but it can be either biodegradable or nonbiodegradable. Shaped polymer implants are administered by means of a suitable special injector. Release kinetics are typically not zero-order, but zero-order kinetics are possible. Drug substance release can be controlled by the diffusion of the drug substance from the bulk polymer matrix or by the properties of a rate-limiting polymeric membrane coating. Polymer implants are used to deliver potent small molecules like steroids (e.g., estradiol for cattle) and large molecules like peptides [e.g., luteinizing hormone-releasing hormone (LHRH)]. Example durations of drug substance release are 2 and 3 months for biodegradable implants and up to 3 years for nonbiodegradable implants. An advantage of biodegradable implants is that they do not require removal after the release of all drug substance content. Nonbiodegradable polymer implants can be removed before or after a drug substance release is complete or may be left in situ. An implant can have a tab with a hole in it to facilitate suturing it in place (e.g., for an intravitreal implant for local ocular delivery). Such implants may provide therapeutic release for periods as long as 2.5 years.

Drug substance-eluting stents combine the mechanical effect of the stent to maintain arterial patency with the prolonged pharmacologic effect of the incorporated drug substance (to reduce restenosis, inhibit clot formation, or combat infection). As an example, a metal stent can be coated with a nonbiodegradable or biodegradable polymer-containing drug substance. The resultant coating is a polymeric matrix that controls the extended release of the drug substance.

In veterinary medicine, drug substance(s) in pellets may be implanted subcutaneously in the animal's ear (cattle).

PREPARATION

Pellet implants are made by drug substance compression or molding. Cylindrical polymeric implants are typically made by melt extrusion of a blend of drug substance and polymer, resulting in a rod that is cut into shorter lengths. Polymer implants can also be made by injection molding. Still other implants are assembled from metal tubes and injection-molded plastic components.

Sterility can be achieved by terminal sterilization or by employing aseptic manufacturing procedures.

Injections

(See *Emulsions*, *Powders*, *Solutions*, and *Suspensions*.)

Injections are not treated as a dosage form in this chapter. Chapter ⟨1⟩ provides quality and other information about injectable products. Information on specific dosage form terminology can be found in the *Glossary*. For appropriate injection nomenclature, see *Nomenclature* ⟨1121⟩.

Excess volume in injections: Each container of an injection is filled with a volume in slight excess of the labeled "size" or the volume that is to be withdrawn. The excess volumes recommended in *Table 1* are usually sufficient to permit withdrawal and administration of the labeled volumes.

Table 1

Labeled Size (mL)	Recommended Excess Volume	
	For Mobile Liquids (mL)	For Viscous Liquids (mL)
0.5	0.10	0.12
1.0	0.10	0.15
2.0	0.15	0.25
5.0	0.30	0.50
10.0	0.50	0.70
20.0	0.60	0.90
30.0	0.80	1.20
50.0 or more	2%	3%

Inserts

Inserts are solid dosage forms that are inserted into a naturally occurring (nonsurgical) body cavity other than the mouth or rectum (see *Suppositories*). The drug substance in inserts is delivered for local or systemic action. Vaginal inserts are usually globular or oviform and weigh about 5 g each. Inserts intended to dissolve in vaginal secretions are usually made from water-soluble or water-miscible vehicles such as polyethylene glycol or glycerinated gelatin.

PREPARATION

For general considerations, see ⟨795⟩. Inserts vary considerably in their preparation. Inserts may be molded (using technology similar to that used to prepare lozenges, suppositories, or plastics), compressed from powders (as in tableting), or formulated as special applications of capsules (soft gelatin capsules and hard gelatin capsules have been employed for extemporaneously compounded preparations). Inserts may be formulated to melt at body temperature or disintegrate upon insertion. Design of the dosage form should take into consideration the fluid volume available at the insertion site and minimize the potential to cause local irritation. Most inserts are formulated to ensure retention at the site of administration.

Irrigations

(See *Solutions*.)

Liquids

As a dosage form, a liquid consists of a pure chemical in its liquid state. Examples include mineral oil, isoflurane, and ether. This dosage form term is not applied to solutions.

Lotions

(See *Emulsions*.)

Lozenges

Lozenges are solid oral dosage forms that are designed to dissolve or disintegrate slowly in the mouth. They contain one or more drug substances that are slowly liberated from the, typically, flavored and sweetened base. They are frequently intended to provide local action in the oral cavity or the throat but also include those intended for systemic absorption after dissolution. The typical therapeutic categories of drug substances delivered in lozenges are antiseptics, analgesics, decongestants, antitussives, and antibiotics. Molded lozenges are called cough drops or pastilles but these terms are not used in ▪official article titles.▪1S (USP41) Lozenges prepared by compression or by stamping or cutting from a uniform bed of paste are sometimes known as troches (a term not used in ▪official article titles).▪1S (USP41) Compressed or stamped lozenges are often produced in a circular shape.

Lozenges can be made using sugars such as sucrose and dextrose, or can provide the benefits of a sugar-free formulation that is usually based on sorbitol or mannitol. Polyethylene glycols and hypromellose are sometimes included to slow the rate of dissolution.

PREPARATION

Excipients used in molded lozenge manufacture include gelatin, fused sucrose, sorbitol, or another carbohydrate base.

Molded lozenges using a sucrose or sorbitol base containing drug substances such as phenol, dextromethorphan, fentanyl, dyclonine hydrochloride, and menthol are prepared by cooking the sugar (sucrose, corn syrup, and sorbitol) and water at about 150° to reduce the water content to less than 2%. The molten sugar solution is transferred to a cooling belt or cooling table, and medicaments, flavorings, and colorings are added and thoroughly mixed while cooling. Individual dosage units of the desired shape are formed by filling the molten mass into molds. These lozenges are quickly cooled in the molds to trap the base in the glassy state. Once formed, the lozenges are removed from the molds and packaged. Care is taken to avoid excessive moisture during storage to prevent crystallization of the sugar base.

Compressed lozenges are made using excipients that may include a filler, binder, sweetening agent, flavoring agent, and lubricant. Sugars such as sucrose, sorbitol, and mannitol are often included because they can act as a filler and binder as well as serve as sweetening agents. Approved FD&C and D&C dyes or lakes (dyes adsorbed onto insoluble aluminum hydroxide) may also be present.

The manufacturing of compressed lozenges is essentially the same as that for conventional tableting, with the exception that a tablet press capable of making larger tablets and exerting greater force to produce harder tablets may be required (see *Tablets*).

The paste used to produce lozenges manufactured by stamping or cutting contains a moistening agent, sucrose, and flavoring and sweetening agents. The homogenous paste is spread as a bed of uniform thickness, and the lozenges are cut or stamped from the bed and are allowed to dry. Some lozenges are prepared by forcing dampened powders under low pressure into mold cavities and then ejecting them onto suitable trays for drying at moderate temperatures.

Ointments

Ointments are semisolid preparations generally intended for external application to the skin or mucous membranes. Drug substances delivered in ointments are intended for local action or for systemic absorption. Ointments usually contain less than 20% water and volatiles, and more than 50% hydrocarbons, waxes, or polyols as the vehicle. Ointment bases recognized for use as vehicles fall into four general classes: hydrocarbon bases, absorption bases, water-removable bases, and water-soluble bases.

HYDROCARBON BASES

Also known as oleaginous ointment bases, hydrocarbon bases allow the incorporation of only small amounts of an aqueous component. Ointments prepared from hydrocarbon bases act as occlusive dressings and provide prolonged contact of the drug substance with the skin. They are difficult to remove and do not change physical characteristics upon aging.

ABSORPTION BASES

Allow the incorporation of aqueous solutions. Such bases include only anhydrous components (e.g., *Hydrophilic Petrolatum*) or W/O emulsions (e.g., *Lanolin*). Absorption bases are also useful as emollients.

WATER-REMOVABLE BASES

O/W emulsions (e.g., *Hydrophilic Ointment*) are sometimes referred to as creams (see *Emulsions*). Water-removable bases may be readily washed from the skin or clothing with water, making them acceptable for cosmetic reasons. Other advantages of the water-removable bases are that they can be diluted with water and that they favor the absorption of serous discharges in dermatological conditions.

WATER-SOLUBLE BASES

Also known as greaseless ointment bases, they are formulated entirely from water-soluble constituents. *Polyethylene Glycol Ointment* is the only official preparation in this group. Water-soluble bases offer many of the advantages of the water-removable bases and, in addition, contain no water-insoluble substances such as petrolatum, anhydrous lanolin, or waxes. They are more correctly categorized as gels (see *Gels*).

The choice of an ointment base depends on the action desired, the characteristics of the incorporated drug substance, and the latter's bioavailability if systemic action is desired. The product's stability may require the use of a base that is less than ideal in meeting other quality attributes. Drug substances that hydrolyze rapidly, for example, are more stable in hydrocarbon bases than in bases that contain water.

PREPARATION

Ointments are typically prepared by either direct incorporation into a previously prepared ointment base or by fusion (heating during the preparation of the ointment). A levigating agent is often added to facilitate the incorporation of the medicament into the ointment base by the direct incorporation procedure. In the fusion method, the ingredients are heated. Homogenization is often necessary. The rate of cooling is an important manufacturing detail because rapid cooling can impart increased structure to the product of the fusion method.

Pastes

Pastes are semisolid preparations of stiff consistency and contain a high percentage (20%–50%) of finely dispersed solids. Pastes are intended for application to the skin, oral cavity, or mucous membranes. Pastes ordinarily do not flow at body temperature and thus can serve as occlusive, protective coatings. As a consequence, pastes are more often used for protective action than are ointments.

Fatty pastes that have a high proportion of hydrophilic solids appear less greasy and are more absorptive than ointments. They are used to absorb serous secretions and are often preferred for acute lesions that have a tendency toward crusting, vesiculation, or oozing.

Dental pastes are applied to the teeth. Other orally administered pastes may be indicated for adhesion to the mucous membrane for a local effect.

In veterinary medicine, pastes are typically administered orally and are intended for systemic delivery of drug substances. The paste is squeezed into the mouth of the animal, generally at the back of the tongue, or is spread inside the mouth.

Pellets

Pellets are dosage forms composed of small, solid particles of uniform shape sometimes called beads, although the use of the term "beads" as a dosage form is not preferred. Typically, pellets are nearly spherical but this is not required. Pellets may be administered by the oral (gastrointestinal) or by the injection route (see also *Implants*). Pellet formulations may provide several advantages, including physical separation for chemically or physically incompatible materials, extended release of the drug substance, or delayed release to protect an acid-labile drug substance from degradation in the stomach or to protect stomach tissues from irritation. Extended-release pellet formulations may be designed with the drug substance dispersed in a matrix, or the pellet may be coated with an appropriate polymer coating that modifies the drug-release characteristics. Alternatively, the pellet design may combine these two approaches. In the case of delayed-release formulations, the coating polymer is chosen to resist dissolution at the lower pH of the gastric environment but to dissolve in the higher pH intestinal environment. Injected or surgically administered pellet preparations (see *Implants*) are often used to provide continuous therapy for periods of months or years.

Pellet dosage forms may be designed as single or multiple entities. Often, implanted pellets will contain the desired drug substance content in one or several units. Oral pellets are typically contained within hard gelatin capsules for administration. Although there are no absolute requirements for size, the useful size range of pellets is governed by the practical constraints of the volume of commonly used capsules and the need to include sufficient numbers of pellets in each dose to ensure uniform dosing of the drug substance. As a result, many pellets used for oral administration fall within a size range of 710 μm to 2.5 mm. Pellet formulations are sometimes used to minimize variability associated with gastric retention of larger dosage forms.

Delayed-release pellet formulations and some extended-release formulations are prepared by applying a coating to the formulated particles. The coating must be applied as a continuous film over the entire surface of each particle. Because a small population of imperfectly coated particles may be unavoidable, oral pellets are designed to require the administration of a large number in a single dose to minimize any adverse influence of imperfectly coated pellets on drug delivery.

PREPARATION

The desired performance characteristics determine the manufacturing method chosen. In general, pellet dosage forms are manufactured by wet extrusion processes followed by spheronization, by wet or dry coating processes, or by compression. Manufacture of pellets by wet coating usually involves the application of successive coatings upon nonpareil seeds. This manufacturing process is frequently conducted in fluid-bed processing equipment. Dry powder coating or layering processes are often performed in specialized rotor granulation equipment. The extent of particle growth achievable in wet coating processes is generally more limited than the growth that can be obtained with dry powder layering techniques, but either method allows the formulator to develop and apply multiple layers of coatings to achieve the desired release profile. The manufacture of pellets by compression is largely restricted to the production of material for subcutaneous implantation. This method of manufacture provides the necessary control to ensure dose uniformity and is generally better suited to aseptic processing requirements.

Alternatively, microencapsulation techniques can be used to manufacture pellets. Coacervation coating techniques typically produce coated particles that are much smaller than those made by other techniques.

Pills

Pills are drug substance-containing small, spherical, solid bodies intended for oral administration. The pill dosage form has been largely replaced by compressed tablets and by capsules. Unlike tablets, pills are usually prepared by a wet massing, piping, and molding technique. This term is frequently incorrectly used as a general term to describe solid oral dosage forms, such as tablets and capsules.

PREPARATION

Excipients are selected on the basis of their ability to produce a mass that is firm and plastic. The drug substance is triturated with powdered excipients in serial dilutions to attain a uniform mixture. Liquid excipients that act to bind and provide plasticity to the mass are subsequently added to the dry materials. The mass is formed by kneading. The properties of firmness and plasticity are necessary to permit the mass to be worked and retain the shape produced. Cylindrical pill pipes are produced from portions of the mass. The pill pipe is cut into individual lengths corresponding to the intended pill size, and the pills are rolled to form the final shape. Pill-making machines can automate the preparation of the mass, production of pill piping, and the cutting and rolling of pills.

Plasters

A plaster is a semisolid substance for external application that is supplied on a support material. Plasters are applied for prolonged periods to provide protection, support, or occlusion (maceration). This term is not preferred and should not be used for new drug product titles. Plasters consist of an adhesive layer that may contain active substances. This layer is spread uniformly on an appropriate support that is usually made of a rubber base or synthetic resin. Unmedicated plasters are designed to provide protection or mechanical support to the site of application. Plasters are available in a range of sizes or cut to size to effectively provide prolonged contact to the site of application. They adhere firmly to the skin but can be peeled off the skin without causing injury.

Powders

Powders are defined as a single solid or a mixture of solids in a finely divided state. Powders used as pharmaceutical dosage forms may contain one or more drug substances and can be used as is or can be mixed with a suitable vehicle for administration. ■1S (USP41) Powders can be intended for internal or external use. Powders for external use are typically dusted onto the skin or applied to bandages or clothing. Powders for internal use can be applied to accessible mucous membranes with suitable applicators or are entrained in air streams for application to the nose or lungs.

The performance of powder dosage forms can be affected by the physical characteristics of the powder. ■Selection of relevant and appropriate powder characteristics depends on the dosage form and its route of administration.■1S (USP41) For example, particle size can influence the dissolution rate of the particles and thus the bioavailability and/or effectiveness at the site of action. Externally applied powders should have a particle size of 150 μm or less (typically in the 50- to 100-μm range to prevent a gritty feel on the skin that could further irritate traumatized skin). The particle size of powders delivered to the lung or nose influences where the powder is deposited. Particle size ■may■1S (USP41) influence the mixing, segregation, and aggregation of the particles, which can affect the delivery and uniformity of the dosage form. ■For more information see *Powder Fineness* ⟨811⟩ and ⟨5⟩.■1S (USP41)

In veterinary medicine, a powder that needs to be reconstituted prior to administration has been called a concentrate (e.g., drug products administered via drinking water). Such use of the term "concentrate" is no longer preferred.

INHALATION POWDERS AND NASAL POWDERS

Inhalation powders and nasal powders consist of an appropriately finely divided solid and a suitable container–closure delivery system. For additional information, see ⟨5⟩ and ⟨601⟩.

PREPARATION

Powder dosage forms can be produced by the combination of multiple components into a uniform blend. This preparation can also involve particle size reduction, a process referred to as comminution. Milling, spray drying, supercritical fluid, high-pressure homogenization, precipitation technologies, and porous microparticle fabrication techniques may be used to reduce the particle size of powders. As the particle size is decreased, the number of particles and the surface area increase, which can increase the dissolution rate and bioavailability, and/or the rate and extent of local action, of the drug substance.

Blending of powders may be accomplished by different techniques. Industrial processes may employ sifting or tumbling the powders in a rotating container. One of the most common tumble blenders is a V-blender, which is available in a variety of sizes suitable for small-scale and large-scale compounding and industrial production. Depending on the particle size of the drug substance, a random mixture of powders may be employed. Blending techniques for powders include those used in compounding pharmacy such as spatulation and trituration (see ⟨795⟩).

Powder flow can be influenced by both particle size and shape. Larger particles generally flow more freely than do fine particles. Powder flow is an important attribute that can affect the packaging or dispensing of a powder.

Soaps and Shampoos

Soaps and shampoos are solid or liquid preparations intended for topical application to the skin or scalp followed by subsequent rinsing with water. Soaps and shampoos are emulsions, suspensions, or surface-active compositions that readily form emulsions, micelles, or foams upon the addition of water followed by rubbing. Incorporation of drug substances in soaps and shampoos combines the cleansing/degreasing abilities of the vehicle and facilitates the topical application of the drug substance to affected areas, even large areas, of the body. The surface-active properties of the vehicle facilitate contact of the drug substance with the skin or scalp. Medicated soap and shampoo formulations frequently contain suitable antimicrobial agents to protect against bacteria, yeast, and mold contamination.

PREPARATION

The preparation of medicated soaps and shampoos follows techniques frequently used for the preparation of emulsified systems. To ensure uniformity, the drug substance(s) must be added to the vehicle prior to congealing (in the case of soaps) followed by thorough mixing. If the medication is present as a suspension, the particle size must be controlled to promote uniform distribution of the drug substance and possibly optimize performance. Because soap manufacture frequently involves processing the ingredients at an elevated temperature, care must be exercised to avoid excessive degradation of the drug substance during processing.

Solutions

A solution is a preparation that contains one or more dissolved chemical substances in a suitable solvent or mixture of mutually miscible solvents. Because molecules of a drug substance in solution are uniformly dispersed, the use of solutions as dosage forms generally provides assurance of uniform dosage upon administration and good accuracy when the solution is diluted or otherwise mixed.

Substances in solutions are more susceptible to chemical instability than they are in the solid state and, dose-for-dose, are generally heavier and more bulky than solid dosage forms. These factors increase the cost of packaging and shipping relative to that of solid dosage forms. Solution dosage forms can be administered by injection, inhalation, and the mucosal, topical/dermal, and gastrointestinal routes. A solution administered by injection is officially titled "injection" (see ⟨1⟩).

Some solutions are designed to form a mass in situ. These solutions comprise polymer, drug substance, and solvent for the polymer. The polymer solvent can be water or an organic solvent. After administration of the solution to a patient by subcutaneous or intramuscular administration, it forms a gel or a solid polymeric matrix that traps the drug substance and extends the drug substance release for days or months.

Solutions intended for oral administration usually contain flavorings and colorants to make the medication more attractive and palatable for the patient or consumer. When needed, they also may contain stabilizers to maintain chemical and physical stability and preservatives to prevent microbial growth.

Solutions are sometimes placed on devices such as swabs, cloths, or sponges, that aid application.

In veterinary medicine, a solution that needs to be diluted prior to administration has been called a concentrate (e.g., drug products administered via drinking water). Such use of the term "concentrate" is no longer preferred.

Sprays

Spray preparations may deliver either accurately metered or nonmetered amounts of formulation.

A spray drug product is a dosage form that contains a drug substance in the liquid state as a solution or suspension and is intended for administration as a mist. Sprays are distinguished from aerosols in that spray containers are not pressurized. Most of the sprays are generated by manually squeezing a flexible container or actuation of a pump that generates the mist by discharging the contents through a nozzle.

Depending on the design of the formulation and the valve system, the droplets generated may be intended for immediate inhalation through the mouth and deposition in the pulmonary tree, or for inhalation into the nose and deposition in the nasal cavity.

The mechanism for droplet generation and the intended use of the preparation distinguish various classes of sprays. A spray may be composed of a pump, container, actuator, valve, nozzle, or mouthpiece in addition to the formulation containing the drug(s), solvent(s), and any excipient(s). The design of each component plays a role for the appropriate performance of the drug product and in determining the critical characteristics of the droplet size distribution. Droplet and particle size distributions, delivered dose uniformity, plume geometry, and droplet velocity are critical parameters that influence the efficiency of drug delivery. When the preparation is supplied as a multidose container, the addition of a suitable antimicrobial preservative may be necessary. Spray formulations intended for local or systemic effect typically have an aqueous base and may contain excipients to control pH and viscosity. In addition, depending on the route of administration, the formulation may be isotonic. For additional information, see ⟨5⟩ and ⟨601⟩.

LABELING AND USE

Refer to the Center for Drug Evaluation and Research (CDER) *Guidance for Industry: Nasal Spray and Inhalation Solution, Suspension, and Spray Drug Products—Chemistry, Manufacturing, and Controls Documentation.*

Strips

A strip is a dosage form or device in the shape of a long, narrow, thin, absorbent, solid material such as filter paper. Typically it is sterile and it may be impregnated with a compound or be gauged to allow measurements for diagnostic purposes, such as in measuring tear production. The term "strip" should not be used when another term such as "film" is more appropriate.

Suppositories

Suppositories are dosage forms adapted for application into the rectum. They melt, soften, or dissolve at body temperature. A suppository may have a local protectant or palliative effect, or may deliver a drug substance for systemic or local action.

Suppository bases typically include cocoa butter, glycerinated gelatin, hydrogenated vegetable oils, mixtures of polyethylene glycols of various molecular weights, and fatty acid esters of polyethylene glycol. The suppository base can have a notable influence on the release of the drug substance(s). Although cocoa butter melts quickly at body temperature, it is immiscible with body fluids and this inhibits the diffusion of fat-soluble drug substances to the affected sites. Polyethylene glycol is a suitable base for some antiseptics. In cases when systemic action is desired, incorporating the ionized rather than the nonionized form of the drug substance may help maximize bioavailability. Although nonionized drug substances partition more readily out of water-miscible bases such as glycerinated gelatin and polyethylene glycol, the bases themselves tend to dissolve very slowly, which slows drug substance release. Cocoa butter and its substitutes (e.g., *Hard Fat*) perform better than other bases for allaying irritation in preparations intended for treating internal hemorrhoids. Suppositories for adults are tapered at one or both ends and usually weigh about 2 g each.

PREPARATION

Cocoa butter suppositories have cocoa butter as the base and can be made by incorporating the finely divided drug substance into the solid oil at room temperature and suitably shaping the resulting mass, or by working with the oil in the melted state and allowing the resulting suspension to cool in molds. A suitable quantity of hardening agents may be added to counteract the tendency of some drug substances (such as chloral hydrate and phenol) to soften the base. The finished suppository melts at body temperature.

A variety of vegetable oils, such as coconut or palm kernel, modified by esterification, hydrogenation, or fractionation, are used as cocoa butter substitutes to obtain products that display varying compositions and melting temperatures (e.g., *Hydrogenated Vegetable Oil* and *Hard Fat*). These products can be designed to reduce rancidity while incorporating desired characteristics such as narrow intervals between melting and solidification temperatures, and melting ranges to accommodate formulation and climatic conditions.

Drug substances can be incorporated into glycerinated gelatin bases by addition of the prescribed quantities to a vehicle consisting of about 70 parts of glycerin, 20 parts of gelatin, and 10 parts of water.

Several combinations of polyethylene glycols that have melting temperatures that are above body temperature are used as suppository bases. Because release from these bases depends on dissolution rather than on melting, there are significantly fewer problems in preparation and storage than is the case for melting-type vehicles. However, high concentrations of higher molecular weight polyethylene glycols may lengthen dissolution time, resulting in problems with retention.

Several nonionic surface-active agents closely related chemically to the polyethylene glycols can be used as suppository vehicles. Examples include polyoxyethylene sorbitan fatty acid esters and the polyoxyethylene stearates. These surfactants are used alone or in combination with other suppository vehicles to yield a wide range of melting temperatures and consistencies. A notable advantage of such vehicles is their water dispersibility. However, care must be taken with the use of surfactants because they may either increase the rate of drug substance absorption or interact with the drug substance to reduce therapeutic activity.

Compounding suppositories using a suppository base typically involves melting the suppository base and dissolution or dispersion of the drug substance in the molten base (see ⟨795⟩). When compounding suppositories, the compounding professional prepares an excess amount of total formulation to allow the prescribed quantity to be accurately dispensed. In compounding suppositories, avoid caustic or irritating ingredients, carefully select a base that will allow the drug substance to provide the intended effect, and in order to minimize abrasion of the rectal membranes, reduce solid ingredients to the smallest reasonable particle size.

Suspensions

A suspension is a biphasic preparation consisting of solid particles dispersed throughout a liquid phase. Suspension dosage forms may be formulated for specific routes of administration such as oral, topical, inhalation, ophthalmic, otic, and injection. Some suspensions are prepared and ready for use, and others are prepared as solid mixtures intended for reconstitution with an appropriate vehicle just before use.

Inhalation suspensions (see ⟨5⟩), ophthalmic suspensions, injectable suspensions, and some otic suspensions are prepared in sterile form. Suspensions are generally not injected intravenously, epidurally, or intrathecally unless the product labeling clearly specifies these routes of administration.

Some liposomal drug products are referred to as suspensions because they can settle and require resuspension prior to administration (see ⟨1⟩).

Some suspensions are designed to form a mass in situ. These suspensions comprise polymer, drug substance, and solvent for the polymer. The polymer solvent can be water or an organic solvent. After administration of the suspension to a patient by subcutaneous or intramuscular administration, it forms a gel or a solid polymeric matrix that traps the drug substance and extends the drug substance release for days or months.

Historically, the term "milk" was sometimes used for suspensions in aqueous vehicles intended for oral administration (e.g., *Milk of Magnesia*). The term "magma" is often used to describe suspensions of inorganic solids, such as clays in water, that display a tendency toward strong hydration and aggregation of the solid, giving rise to gel-like consistency and thixotropic rheological behavior (e.g., *Bentonite Magma*). In the past, the term "lotion" referred to both topical suspensions and topical emulsions. Now the term only refers to topical emulsions (see *Emulsions*).

Limited aqueous solubility of the drug substance(s) is the most common rationale for developing a suspension. Other potential advantages of an oral suspension include taste masking and improved patient compliance because of the more convenient dosage form. When compared to solutions, suspensions can have improved chemical stability. Ideally, a suspension should contain small uniform particles that are readily suspended and easily redispersed following settling. Unless the dispersed solid is colloidal, the particulate matter in a suspension will likely settle to the bottom of the container upon standing. Such sedimentation may lead to caking and solidification of the sediment and difficulty in redispersing the suspension upon agitation. To prevent such problems, manufacturers commonly add ingredients to increase viscosity and the gel state of the suspension or flocculation, including clays, surfactants, polyols, polymers, or sugars. Frequently, thixotropic vehicles are used to counter particle-settling tendencies, but these vehicles must not interfere with pouring or redispersal. Additionally, the density of the dispersed phase and continuous phase may be modified to further control settling rate. For topical suspensions, rapid drying upon application is desirable.

Temperature can influence the viscosity (and thus suspension properties and the ease of removing the dose from the bottle), and temperature cycling can lead to changes in the particle size of the dispersed phase via Ostwald ripening. When manufacturers conduct stability studies to establish product shelf life and storage conditions, they should cycle conditions (freeze/thaw) to investigate temperature effects.

Unless studies confirm that the formulation will not support microbial growth, suspension preparations packaged to provide multiple doses should contain suitable antimicrobial agents to protect against bacterial, yeast, and mold contamination (see ⟨51⟩) or other appropriate measures should be taken to avoid microbial contamination.

Suspensions for reconstitution are dry powder or granular mixtures that require the addition of water or a supplied formulated diluent before administration. This formulation approach is frequently used when the chemical or physical stability of the drug substance or suspension does not allow sufficient shelf life for a preformulated suspension. Typically, these suspensions are refrigerated after reconstitution to increase their shelf life. For this type of suspension, the powder blend is uniform and the powder readily disperses when reconstituted.

Injectable suspensions are generally intended for either subcutaneous or intramuscular routes of administration and should have a controlled particle size, typically in the range of 5 μm or smaller. The rationale for the development of injectable suspensions may include poor drug substance solubility, improved chemical stability, prolonged duration of action, and avoidance of first-pass metabolism. Care is needed in selecting the sterilization technique because it may affect product stability or alter the physical properties of the material.

In veterinary medicine, a suspension that needs to be diluted prior to administration has been called a concentrate (e.g., drug products administered via drinking water). Such use of the term "concentrate" is no longer preferred.

PREPARATION

Suspensions are prepared by adding suspending agents or other excipients and purified water or oil to solid drug substances and mixing to achieve uniformity. In the preparation of a suspension, the characteristics of both the dispersed phase and the dispersion medium should be considered. During development, manufacturers should define an appropriate particle size distribution for the suspended material to achieve the desired effectiveness and to minimize the likelihood of particle size changes during storage.

In some instances, the dispersed phase has an affinity for the vehicle and is readily wetted upon its addition. For some materials, the displacement of air from the solid surface is difficult, and the solid particles may clump together or float on top of the vehicle. In the latter case, a wetting agent may be used for certain types of suspensions to facilitate displacement of air from the powder surface. Surfactants, alcohol, glycerin, and other hydrophilic liquids can be used as wetting agents when an aqueous vehicle will be used as the dispersion phase. These agents function by displacing the air in the crevices of the particles and dispersing the particles. In the large-scale preparation of suspensions, wetting of the dispersed phase may be aided by the use of high-energy mixing equipment such as colloid mills or other rotor–stator mixing devices.

After the powder has been wetted, the dispersion medium (containing the soluble formulation components such as colorants, flavorings, and preservatives) is added in portions to the powder, and the mixture is thoroughly blended before subsequent additions of the vehicle. A portion of the vehicle is used to wash the mixing equipment free of suspended material, and this portion is used to bring the suspension to final volume and ensure that the suspension contains the desired concentration of solid matter. The final product may be passed through a colloid mill or other blender or mixing device to ensure uniformity.

Suspensions are resuspended before the dose is dispensed. Because of the viscosity of many suspension vehicles, air entrainment may occur during dosing. The formulation process allows evaluation of this possibility; adjustments in vehicle viscosity or the incorporation of low levels of antifoaming agents are common approaches to minimize air entrainment. Alternatively, specific instructions for resuspending the formulation may be provided to minimize air incorporation and ensure accurate dosing.

Systems

Systems are preparations of drug substance(s) in carrier devices, often containing adhesive backing, that are applied topically or inserted into body cavities. The drug substance is designed to be released in a controlled manner over a specified period of time or the drug substance is released based on its concentration in the formulation. Unless otherwise stated in the labeling, the carrier device is removed after use. The term "system" should not be used when another dosage form term is more appropriate (e.g., inserts and implants).

The notation of strength is either defined in terms of the amount of the drug substance released from the system over a specific period of time or as the drug concentration within the formulation (e.g., the percentage of the drug). Various routes of administration are possible, so the route must always be indicated in the compendial name when a specific location for application is essential for proper use (e.g., "intrauterine", "ocular", or "periodontal" as the route of administration). For example, systems applied to the eye are called ocular systems. The route is named "transdermal" when, for example, systemic absorption of the drug substance may take place through the dermis without specifying the region of the body to which the system is applied.

The term "patch" has sometimes been used but is not preferred for use in drug product monograph nomenclature when referring to a system.

Intrauterine systems are intended for placement in the uterus. Release of the drug substance can be up to 5 years.

Ocular systems are intended for placement in the lower conjunctival fornix from which the drug diffuses through a membrane at a constant rate.

Periodontal systems are intended for placement in the pocket between the tooth and the gum. In some cases, periodontal systems may be formed in situ in the periodontal pocket and release the drug substance(s) for several weeks.

Transdermal systems (TDS) are placed onto intact skin to deliver the drug to the systemic circulation. They are designed for prolonged release (up to 7 days). Specific quality tests for TDSs are found in ⟨3⟩.

Tablets

Tablets are solid dosage forms in which the drug substance is generally blended with excipients and compressed into the final dosage. Tablets are the most widely used dosage form in the United States. Tablet presses use steel punches and dies to prepare compacted tablets by the application of high pressures to powder blends or granulations. Tablets can be produced in a wide variety of sizes, shapes, and surface markings. Capsule-shaped tablets are commonly referred to as caplets, although the term is not ■used in official article titles.■₁₅ (USP41) Specialized tablet presses may be used to produce tablets with multiple layers or with specially formulated core tablets placed in the interior of the final dosage form. These specialized tablet presentations can delay or extend the release of the drug substance(s) or physically separate incompatible drug substances. Tablets may be coated by a variety of techniques to provide taste masking, protection of photo-labile drug substance(s), extended or delayed release, or unique appearance (colors). When no deliberate effort has been made to modify the drug substance release rate, tablets are referred to as immediate-release.

BUCCAL TABLETS

Intended to be inserted in the buccal pouch, where the drug substance is absorbed directly through the oral mucosa. Few drug substances are readily absorbed in this way (examples are nitroglycerin and certain steroid hormones).

CHEWABLE TABLETS

Formulated and manufactured to produce a pleasant-tasting residue in the mouth and to facilitate swallowing. Hard chewable tablets are typically prepared by compaction, usually utilizing mannitol, sorbitol, or sucrose as binders and fillers, and contain colors and flavors to enhance their appearance and taste. Soft chewable tablets are typically made by a molding or extrusion process, frequently with more than 10% water to help maintain a pliable, soft product. Hard chewable tablets in veterinary medicine often have flavor enhancers like brewer's yeast or meat/fish-based flavors.

Tablets for human use that include "chewable" in the title must be chewed or crushed prior to swallowing to ensure reliable release of the drug substance(s) or to facilitate swallowing. If tablets are designed so that they may be chewed (but chewing is not required for drug substance release or ease of swallowing), the title should not include a reference to "chewable". In that case, the product may still be described as "chewable" in the ancillary labeling statement.

Tablets for veterinary use that are intended to be chewed will include "Chewable" in the title. However, it is understood that for veterinary products it is not possible to ensure that tablets are chewed prior to ingestion. Chewable tablets may be broken into pieces and fed to animals that normally swallow treats whole.

EFFERVESCENT TABLETS

Prepared by compaction and contain, in addition to the drug substance(s), mixtures of acids (e.g., citric acid or tartaric acid) and carbonates, and/or sodium bicarbonate. Upon contact with water, these formulations release carbon dioxide, producing the characteristic effervescent action.

HYPODERMIC TABLETS

Molded tablets made from completely and readily water-soluble ingredients; formerly intended for use in making preparations for hypodermic injection. They may be administered orally or sublingually when rapid drug substance availability is required.

MODIFIED-RELEASE TABLETS

There are two categories of modified-release tablet formulations recognized by USP.

Delayed-release tablets: Tablets are sometimes formulated with acid-resistant or enteric (also called "gastro-resistant") coatings to protect acid-labile drug substances from the gastric environment or to prevent adverse events such as irritation.

Extended-release tablets: Extended-release tablets are formulated in such a manner as to make the drug substance available over an extended period of time following ingestion. ■■1S *(USP41)* Requirements for dissolution (see ⟨711⟩) are typically specified in the individual monographs.

ORALLY DISINTEGRATING TABLETS

Orally disintegrating tablets are intended to disintegrate rapidly within the mouth to provide a dispersion before the patient swallows the resulting slurry where the drug substance is intended for gastrointestinal delivery and/or absorption. Some of these dosage forms have been formulated to facilitate rapid disintegration and are manufactured by conventional means or by using lyophilization or molding processes. Further details may be found in the CDER *Guidance for Industry: Orally Disintegrating Tablets*.

SUBLINGUAL TABLETS

Sublingual tablets are intended to be inserted beneath the tongue, where the drug substance is absorbed directly through the oral mucosa. As with buccal tablets, few drug substances are extensively absorbed in this way, and much of the drug substance is swallowed and is available for gastrointestinal absorption.

TABLETS FOR ORAL SOLUTION

Before administration, tablets for oral solution are intended to be solubilized in a liquid diluent. In some cases, tablets for oral solution may also be chewed or swallowed.

TABLETS FOR ORAL SUSPENSION

Tablets for oral suspension are intended to be dispersed in a liquid before administration as a suspension. The dosage form is tablets for oral suspension when either the drug substance or the excipients do not dissolve when dispersed in a liquid. In some cases, tablets for oral suspension may also be chewed or swallowed.

TABLET TRITURATES

Small, usually cylindrical, molded or compacted tablets. Tablet triturates traditionally were used as dispensing tablets in order to provide a convenient, measured quantity of a potent drug substance for compounding purposes, but they are rarely used today.

PREPARATION

Most compacted (compressed) tablets consist of the drug substance(s) and a number of excipients. These excipients may include fillers (diluents), binders, disintegrating agents, lubricants, and glidants. Approved FD&C and D&C dyes or lakes, flavors, and sweetening agents may also be present.

Fillers or diluents are added when the quantity of drug substance(s) is too small or the properties of the drug substance do not allow satisfactory compaction in the absence of other ingredients. Binders impart adhesiveness to the powder blend and promote tablet formation and maintenance of drug substance uniformity in the tableting mixture. Disintegrating agents facilitate reduction of the tablet into small particles upon contact with water or biological fluids. Lubricants reduce friction during the compaction and ejection cycles. Glidants improve powder fluidity, powder handling properties, and tablet weight control. Colorants are often added to tablet formulations for aesthetic value or for product identification.

Tablets are prepared from formulations that have been processed by one of three general methods: wet granulation, dry granulation (roll compaction or slugging), and direct compression.

Wet granulation: Involves the mixing of dry powders with a granulating liquid to form a moist granular mass that is dried and sized prior to compression. It is particularly useful in achieving uniform blends of low-dose drug substances and facilitating the wetting and dissolution of poorly soluble, hydrophobic drug substances.

Dry granulations: Can be produced by passing powders between rollers at elevated pressure (roll compaction). Alternatively, dry granulation can also be carried out by the compaction of powders at high pressures on tablet presses, a process also known as slugging. In either case, the compacts are sized before compression. Dry granulation improves the flow and handling properties of the powder formulation without involving moisture in the processing.

Direct compression: Tablet processing involves dry blending of the drug substance(s) and excipients followed by compression. The simplest manufacturing technique, direct compression is acceptable only when the drug substance and excipients possess acceptable flow and compression properties without prior process steps.

Tablets may be coated to protect the ingredients from air, moisture, or light; to mask unpleasant tastes and odors; to improve tablet appearance; and to reduce dustiness. In addition, coating may be used to protect the drug substance from acidic pH values associated with gastric fluids or to control the rate of drug release in the gastrointestinal tract.

The most common coating in use today is a thin film coating composed of a polymer that is derived from cellulose. Sugar coating is an alternative, less common approach. Sugar-coated tablets have considerably thicker coatings that are primarily sucrose with a number of inorganic diluents. A variety of film-coating polymers are available and enable the development of specialized release profiles. These formulations are used to protect acid-labile drug substances from the acidic stomach environment as well as to prolong the release of the drug substance to reduce dosing frequency (see ⟨711⟩ or ⟨701⟩).

Tapes

A tape is a dosage form suitable for delivering drug substances to the skin. It consists of a drug substance(s) impregnated into a durable yet flexible woven fabric or extruded synthetic material that is coated with an adhesive agent. Typically the impregnated drug substance is present in the dry state. The adhesive layer is designed to hold the tape securely in place without the aid of additional bandaging. Unlike transdermal systems, tapes are not designed to control the release rate of the drug substance. The term "tape" is not preferred and should not be used for new ■official article■₁₅ ₍USP41₎ titles.

The drug substance content of tapes is expressed as amount per surface area with respect to the tape surface exposed to the skin. The use of an occlusive dressing with the tape enhances the rate and extent of delivery of the drug substance to deeper layers of the skin and may result in greater systemic absorption of the drug substance.

Change to read:

GLOSSARY

This glossary provides definitions for terms in use in medicine and serves as a source of official ■titles■₁₅ ₍USP41₎ for official articles, except when the definition specifically states that the term is not to be used in drug product titles. Examples of general nomenclature forms for the more frequently encountered categories of dosage forms appear in ⟨1121⟩. In an attempt to be comprehensive, this glossary was compiled without the limits imposed by current preferred nomenclature conventions. To clearly identify/distinguish preferred from not preferred terms, entries indicate when a term is not preferred and generally direct the user to the current preferred term. ■Descriptive terms or attributes are used to identify a specialized presentation or characteristic of a dosage form. For example, the descriptive term "chewable" may be used with the dosage form "tablets" to identify a specific type of tablet that must be chewed prior to swallowing.■₁₅ ₍USP41₎ When a term is described ■in this glossary■₁₅ *(USP41)* as an attribute of a dosage form, it is generally intended to distinguish ■that■₁₅ *(USP41)* term from those used for ■official■₁₅ *(USP41)* dosage form titles. ■■₁₅ *(USP41)*

Aerosol: A dosage form consisting of a liquid or solid preparation packaged under pressure and intended for administration as a fine mist. The descriptive term "aerosol" also refers to the fine mist of small droplets or solid particles that are emitted from the product.

Aromatic water (■■₁₅ *(USP41)* see *Solution*):   A clear, saturated, aqueous solution of volatile oils or other aromatic or volatile substances. ■The term is not used in official article titles.■₁₅ *(USP41)*

Aural (Auricular) (■■₁₅ *(USP41)* see *Otic*):   For administration into, or by way of, the ear. ■The term is not used in official article titles.■₁₅ *(USP41)*

Bead (■■₁₅ *(USP41)* see *Pellets*):   A solid dosage form in the shape of a small sphere. In most products a unit dose consists of multiple beads. ■The term is not used in official article titles.■₁₅ *(USP41)*

Bolus (not preferred; see *Tablet*):   A large tablet intended for administration to large animals. Occasionally, the term "bolus" is used to describe a method of administration.

Buccal: Administration directed toward the cheek, generally from within the mouth.

Caplet (■■₁₅ *(USP41)* see *Tablet*):   Tablet dosage form in the shape of a capsule. ■The term is not used in official article titles.■₁₅ *(USP41)*

Capsule: A solid dosage form in which the drug substance, with or without other ingredients, is filled into either a hard or soft shell or coated on the capsule shell. Most capsule shells are composed mainly of gelatin.

Chewable: Attribute of a solid dosage form that is intended to be chewed or crushed before swallowing.

■Chewable Gel: Formed or molded oral gel dosage forms that maintain their shape, are elastic, and yield to mastication. Chewable gels are also known as "gummies" but that term is not used for official article titles.■₁₅ *(USP41)*

Coating: Attribute (coated) of a solid dosage form that involves covering with an outer solid. The outer deposit is referred to as a coating or film. The term is used as an attribute when applied to solid oral dosage forms. Coatings are applied for functional or aesthetic purposes such as taste masking, stability, modifying release characteristics, product identification, and appearance.

Collodion (not preferred; see *Solution*):   A preparation that is a solution dosage form composed of pyroxilin dissolved in a solvent mixture of alcohol and ether, and applied externally.

Colloidal dispersion: An attribute of a preparation or formulation in which particles of colloidal dimension (i.e., typically between 1 nm and 1 µm) are distributed uniformly throughout a liquid.

Concentrate (not a preferred term for human or veterinary drug products):   The current use is for drug substances that are not intended for direct administration to humans or animals. The use in drug product nomenclature is being phased out (see ⟨1121⟩ and *Nomenclature Guidelines*[3]).

Conventional-release (■■₁₅ *(USP41)* see *Immediate-release*):   Descriptive term for a dosage form in which no deliberate effort has been made to modify the release rate of the drug substance. In the case of capsules and tablets, the inclusion or exclusion of a disintegrating agent is not interpreted as a modification. ■The term is not used in official article titles.■₁₅ *(USP41)*

Cough drop (■■₁₅ *(USP41)* see *Lozenge*):   ■The term is not used in official article titles.■₁₅ *(USP41)*

Cream: A semisolid emulsion dosage form often containing more than 20% water and volatiles, and/or containing less than 50% hydrocarbons, waxes, or polyols as the vehicle for the drug substance. Creams are generally intended for external application to the skin or mucous membranes.

Delayed-release: A type of modified-release dosage form. A descriptive term for a dosage form deliberately ■formulated■₁₅ *(USP41)* to delay release of the drug substance for some period of time after initial administration. For ■oral products, expressions such as "enteric-coated" or "gastro-resistant" have been used where release of the drug substance is prevented in the gastric environment but promoted in the intestinal environment. However, the term "delayed-release" is used for official article titles.■₁₅ *(USP41)*

Dental: Descriptive term for a preparation that is applied to the teeth for localized action.

Dermal: A topical route of administration where the drug product is intended to reach or be applied to the dermis.

Dip (not preferred; see *Immersion*)

Dispersible tablet (■■₁₅ *(USP41)* see *Tablet, Tablet for oral suspension*, or *Tablet for oral solution*):   ■The term is not used in official article titles.■₁₅ *(USP41)*

Disintegrating tablet (■■₁₅ *(USP41)* see *Tablet, Tablet for oral suspension*, or *Tablet for oral solution*; see also *Orally disintegrating*):   ■The term is not used in official article titles.■₁₅ *(USP41)*

Dosage form: A combination of drug substance(s) and/or excipient(s) in quantities and physical form designed to allow the accurate and efficient administration of the drug substance to the human or animal patient. The term is not used in ■official article■₁₅ *(USP41)* titles.

Dry powder inhaler: A device used to administer an inhalation powder in a finely divided state suitable for oral inhalation by the patient. This term is not used in ■official article■₁₅ *(USP41)* titles.

Effervescent: Attribute of an oral dosage form, frequently tablets or granules, containing ingredients that, when in contact with water, rapidly release carbon dioxide. The dosage form is dissolved or dispersed in water to initiate the effervescence prior to ingestion.

Elixir (not preferred; see *Solution*):   A preparation that typically is a clear, flavored, sweetened hydroalcoholic solution intended for oral use. The term should not be used for new drug products in *USP–NF* but is commonly encountered in compounding pharmacy practice.

Emollient: Attribute of a cream or ointment indicating an increase in the moisture content of the skin following application of bland, fatty, or oleaginous substances. This term should not be used in ■official article■₁ₛ *(USP41)* titles.

Emulsion: A dosage form consisting of a two-phase system composed of at least two immiscible liquids, one of which is dispersed as droplets (internal or dispersed phase) within the other liquid (external or continuous phase), generally stabilized with one or more emulsifying agents. Emulsion is not used as a dosage form term if a more specific term is applicable (e.g., *Cream, Lotion,* or *Ointment*).

Enteric-coated (not preferred; see *Delayed-release*):   Descriptive term for a solid dosage form in which a polymer coating has been applied to prevent the release of the drug substance in the gastric environment.

Excipient: An ingredient of a dosage form other than a drug substance. This term is not used in ■official article■₁ₛ *(USP41)* titles. The term "excipient" is synonymous with inactive ingredient.

Extended-release: Descriptive term for a dosage form that is deliberately ■formulated to prolong the release■₁ₛ *(USP41)* of the drug substance compared to that observed for an immediate-release dosage form. ■Expressions such as "prolonged release", "repeat action", "controlled release", "long acting", and "sustained release" have also been used to describe such dosage forms. However, the term "extended-release" is used for official article titles.■₁ₛ *(USP41)*

Film: A term used to describe a thin sheet of material, usually composed of a polymer. Films are used in various routes of administration including as a means of oral administration of material in a rapidly dissolving form.

Foam: A dosage form containing gas bubbles dispersed in a liquid. Medicated foams have a semisolid consistency and can be formulated to quickly break down into a liquid or to remain as foam to ensure prolonged contact.

Gas: One of the states of matter having no definite shape or volume and occupying the entire container when confined.

Gastro-resistant (■₁ₛ *(USP41)* see *Delayed-release*):   Descriptive term for a solid dosage form in which a polymer coating has been applied to prevent the release in the gastric environment. ■The term is not used in official article titles.■₁ₛ *(USP41)*

Gel: A dosage form that is a semisolid dispersion of small particles or a solution of large molecules interpenetrated by a solution containing a gelling agent to provide stiffness.

■**Gelcap:**   A capsule that is coated is sometimes referred to as a gelcap. Gelcap is not a term used in official article titles.

Geltab/Filmtab: A tablet that is coated is sometimes referred to as a geltab or filmtab. Geltab and filmtab are not terms used in official article titles.■₁ₛ *(USP41)*

Granules: A dosage form composed of dry aggregates of powder particles that may contain one or more drug substances, with or without other ingredients. They may be swallowed as such, dispersed in food, or dissolved in water. Granules are frequently compacted into tablets or filled into capsules, with or without additional ingredients. More commonly, granules are reconstituted as suspensions.

Gum: A dosage form in which the base consists of a pliable material that, when chewed, releases the drug substance into the oral cavity.

■**Gummies** (see *Chewable Gel*):   The term is not used in official article titles.■₁ₛ *(USP41)*

Hard-shell capsule (not preferred; see *Capsules*):   A type of capsule in which one or more drug substances, with or without other ingredients, are filled into a two-piece shell. Most hard-shell capsules are composed mainly of gelatin and are fabricated prior to the filling operation.

Immediate-release: Descriptive term for a dosage form in which no deliberate effort has been made to modify the drug substance release rate. ■The term is not used in official article titles.■₁ₛ *(USP41)*

Immersion: A veterinary route of administration via partial or complete submersion in a specified environment such as liquid or air.

Implant: A dosage form that is a solid or semisolid material containing the drug substance that is inserted into the body. The insertion process is invasive, and the material is intended to reside at the site for a period consistent with the design release kinetics or profile of the drug substance(s).

Inhalation (by inhalation):   A route of administration for aerosols characterized by dispersion of the drug substance into the airways during inspiration.

Injection (by injection):   A route of administration of a liquid or semisolid deposited into a body cavity, fluid, or tissue by use of a needle.

Injection: Liquid preparations that may contain drug substances and/or excipients or solutions thereof. The term "for injection" indicates dry solids that, upon the addition of a suitable vehicle, yield solutions conforming in all respects to the requirements for injections.

Injectable emulsion: Liquid preparations of drug substances dissolved or dispersed in a suitable emulsion medium.

Injectable suspension: Liquid preparations of solids suspended in a liquid medium. The term "for injectable suspension" indicates dry solids that, upon the addition of a suitable vehicle, yield preparations conforming in all respects to the requirements for injectable suspensions.

Injectable suspension, extended-release: Liquid preparations of solids suspended in a suitable vehicle and formulated to allow the drug substance to be available over an extended period of time. The term "for extended-release injectable suspension" indicates dry solids that, upon the addition of a suitable vehicle, yield a preparation that conforms in all respects to the requirements for extended-release injectable suspensions.

Insert: A solid dosage form that is inserted into a naturally occurring (nonsurgical) body cavity other than the mouth or rectum. It should be noted that a suppository is intended for application into the rectum and is not classified as an insert (see *Suppository*).

Intraocular: A route of administration to deliver a sterile preparation within the eye.

Irrigation: A sterile solution or liquid intended to bathe or flush open wounds or body cavities.

Jelly (not preferred; see *Gel*):   A semisolid dispersion of small particles or a solution of large organic molecules interpenetrated by a solution containing a gelling agent to promote stiffness.

Liposomes: Attribute for preparations of amphiphilic lipids that have low water solubility (see ⟨1⟩).

Liquid: A dosage form consisting of a pure chemical in its liquid state. This dosage form term should not be applied to solutions. The term is not used in ■official article■₁S (USP41) titles. When "liquid" is used as a descriptive term, it indicates a material that is pourable and conforms to its container at room temperature.

Lotion: An emulsion liquid dosage form applied to the outer surface of the body. Historically, this term was applied to topical suspensions and topical emulsions. The current definition of a lotion is restricted to an emulsion.

Lozenge: A solid dosage form intended to disintegrate or dissolve slowly in the mouth.

Modified-release: A descriptive term for a dosage form with a drug substance release pattern that has been deliberately changed from that observed for the immediate-release dosage form of the same drug substance. The two types of modified-release are extended-release and delayed-release. The term "modified-release" is not used in ■official article■₁S (USP41) titles.

Molded tablet: A tablet that has been formed by dampening the ingredients and pressing into a mold, then removing and drying the resulting solid mass. This term is not used in ■official article■₁S (USP41) titles.

Mouthwash (■■₁S (USP41) see *Rinse*):   Term applied to a solution preparation used to rinse the oral cavity. ■The term is not used in official article titles.■₁S (USP41)

Nasal: Route of administration (mucosal) characterized by administration to the nose or by way of the nose for local or systemic effect.

Ocular (not preferred; see *Intraocular*):   Route of administration indicating deposition of the drug substance within the eye.

Ointment: A semisolid dosage form, usually containing less than 20% water and volatiles and more than 50% hydrocarbons, waxes, or polyols as the vehicle. This dosage form generally is for external application to the skin or mucous membranes.

Ophthalmic: A route of administration characterized by application of a sterile preparation to the external parts of the eye.

Oral: Route of administration characterized by application to the mouth or delivery to the gastrointestinal tract through the mouth.

Orally disintegrating: A descriptive term for a solid oral dosage form that disintegrates rapidly in the mouth prior to swallowing. The drug substance is intended for gastrointestinal delivery and/or absorption. See also CDER *Guidance for Industry, Orally Disintegrating Tablets*.

Orodispersible (■■₁S (USP41) see *Orally disintegrating*):   ■The term is not used in official article titles.■₁S (USP41)

Oro-pharyngeal: A route of administration characterized by deposition of a preparation into the oral cavity and/or pharyngeal region to exert a local or systemic effect.

Otic: A route of administration characterized by deposition of a preparation into, or by way of, the ear. Sometimes referred to as *Aural* (*Aural* not preferred).

Parenteral: General route of administration which is characterized by injection through the skin or other external boundary tissue or implantation within the body. Specific parenteral routes include intravenous, intraventricular, intra-arterial, intra-articular, subcutaneous, intramuscular, intrathecal, intracisternal, and intraocular (see ⟨1⟩).

Paste: A semisolid dosage form containing a high percentage (20%–50%) of finely dispersed solids with a stiff consistency. This dosage form is intended for application to the skin, oral cavity, or mucous membranes.

Pastille (■■₁S (USP41) see *Lozenge*):   ■The term is not used in official article titles.■₁S (USP41)

Patch (not preferred; see *System*):   Frequently incorrectly used to describe a *System*.

Pellet: A small solid dosage form of uniform, often spherical, shape intended for direct administration as a pellet. Spherical pellets are sometimes referred to as *Beads*. Pellets intended as implants must be sterile. The use of the term "pellet" for implantable dosage forms is no longer preferred (see *Implants*).

Periodontal: Descriptive term for a preparation that is applied around a tooth for localized action.

Pill: A solid, spherical dosage form usually prepared by a wet massing, piping, and molding technique. This term is frequently incorrectly used as a general term to describe solid oral dosage forms such as tablets or capsules.

Plaster (not preferred):   A dosage form containing a semisolid composition supplied on a support material for external application. Plasters are applied for prolonged periods of time to provide protection, support, or occlusion (for macerating action).

Powder: A dosage form composed of a solid or mixture of solids reduced to a finely divided state and intended for internal or external use.

Powder, inhalation: A powder containing a drug substance for oral inhalation. The powder is used with a device that aerosolizes and delivers an accurately metered amount.

Premix (not preferred; see *Animal Drugs for Use in Animal Feeds* ⟨1152⟩, *Scope, Type A Medicated Articles* and *Type B Medicated Feeds*)

Prolonged-release (■■₁S (USP41) see *Extended-release*):   ■The term is not used in official article titles.■₁S (USP41)

Rectal: A route of administration characterized by deposition into the rectum to provide local or systemic effect.

Rinse (see *Solution*):   A liquid preparation used to cleanse by flushing. A rinse is used to swish in the mouth and then expectorated. The nonpreferred term "mouthwash" has sometimes been used for "rinse".

Semisolid: Attribute of a material that exhibits plastic flow behavior. A semisolid material is not pourable, does not readily conform to its container at room temperature, and does not flow at low shear stress. This term is not used in ■official article■15 (USP41) titles.

Shampoo: A solution, emulsion, or suspension dosage form used to clean the hair and scalp. May contain a drug substance intended for topical application to the scalp.

Soap: The alkali salt(s) of a fatty acid or mixture of fatty acids used to cleanse the skin. Soaps used as dosage forms may contain a drug substance intended for topical application to the skin. Soaps have also been used as liniments and enemas.

Soft gel capsule (not preferred; see *Capsule*):   A specific capsule type characterized by increased levels of plasticizers producing a more pliable and thicker-walled material than hard gelatin capsules. Soft gel capsules are further distinguished because they are single-piece sealed dosages. Frequently used for delivering liquid compositions.

Soluble tablet (■15 (USP41) see *Tablet* and *Tablet for oral solution*):   ■The term is not used in official article titles.■15 (USP41)

Solution: A clear, homogeneous liquid dosage form that contains one or more chemical substances dissolved in a solvent or mixture of mutually miscible solvents.

Spirit (not preferred; see *Solution*):   A liquid dosage form composed of an alcoholic or hydroalcoholic solution of volatile substances.

Spot on (pour on):   A method of delivering liquid veterinary drug products by administering them onto the animal's skin, usually between the shoulder blades (spot on) or down the back (pour on).

Spray: A spray is a dosage form that contains drug substance(s) in the liquid state, either as a solution or as a suspension, and is intended for administration as a mist. Sprays are distinguished from aerosols in that spray containers are not pressurized. Most of the sprays are generated by manually squeezing a flexible container or actuation of a pump that generates the mist by discharging the contents through a nozzle.

As an attribute, spray describes the generation of droplets of a liquid or solution to facilitate application to the intended area.

Stent, drug-eluting: A specialized form of implant used for extended local delivery of the drug substance to the immediate location of stent placement.

Strip (only used for diagnostic products, otherwise not preferred; see *Film*):   A dosage form or device in the shape of a long, narrow, thin, absorbent, solid material such as filter paper.

Sublingual: A route of administration characterized by placement underneath the tongue and for release of the drug substance for absorption in that region.

Suppository: A solid dosage form in which one or more drug substances are dispersed in a suitable base and molded or otherwise formed into a suitable shape for insertion into the rectum to provide local or systemic effect.

Suspension: A liquid dosage form that consists of solid particles dispersed throughout a liquid phase.

Syrup (not preferred; see *Solution*):   A solution containing high concentrations of sucrose or other sugars. This term is commonly used in compounding pharmacy.

System: A preparation of drug substance(s) in a carrier device that is applied topically or inserted into a body cavity. The drug substance is designed to be released in a controlled manner over a specified period of time or the drug substance is released based on its concentration in the formulation. Unless otherwise stated in the labeling, the carrier device is removed after use.

Tablet: A solid dosage form prepared from powders or granules by compaction.

Tablet for oral solution: A tablet that is intended to be dispersed in a liquid before administration. When dispersed in the liquid, a solution results.

Tablet for oral suspension: A tablet that is intended to be dispersed in a liquid before administration. When dispersed in the liquid, a suspension results.

Tape (not preferred):   A dosage form or device composed of a woven fabric or synthetic material onto which a drug substance is placed, usually with an adhesive on one or both sides to facilitate topical application. The rate of release of the drug substance is not controlled.

Tincture (not preferred; see *Solution*):   An alcoholic or hydroalcoholic solution prepared from vegetable materials or from chemical substances.

Topical: A route of administration characterized by application to the outer surface of the body.

Transdermal: A route of administration through the dermal layer of the skin to the systemic circulation.

Troche (■15 (USP41) see *Lozenge*):   A solid dosage form intended to disintegrate or dissolve slowly in the mouth and usually prepared by compaction in a manner similar to that used for tablets. ■The term is not used in official article titles.■15 (USP41)

Urethral: A route of administration characterized by deposition into the urethra.

Vaginal: A route of administration characterized by deposition into the vagina.

Vehicle: A term commonly encountered in compounding pharmacy that refers to a component for internal or external use that is used as a carrier or diluent in which liquids, semisolids, or solids are dissolved or suspended. Examples include water, syrups, elixirs, oleaginous liquids, solid and semisolid carriers, and proprietary products (see *Excipient*). This term is not used in ■official article■15 (USP41) titles.

Veterinary: Descriptive term for dosage forms intended for nonhuman use.

〈1231〉 WATER FOR PHARMACEUTICAL PURPOSES

TABLE OF CONTENTS

1. INTRODUCTION

Water is widely used as a raw material, inactive ingredient, medicinal vehicle, and solvent in the processing, formulation, and manufacture of pharmaceutical products (dosage forms), active pharmaceutical ingredients (APIs), API intermediates, compendial articles, and analytical reagents as well as in cleaning applications.

This is an informational chapter on pharmaceutical water topics and includes some of the chemical and microbiological concerns unique to water and its preparation and uses. The chapter provides information about water quality attributes (that may or may not be included within a water monograph) and processing techniques that can be used to improve water quality. It also discusses water system validation and gives a description of minimum water quality standards that should be considered when selecting a water source including sampling and system controls. It is equally important for water systems to be operated and maintained in a state of control to provide assurance of operational stability and therefore the capability to provide water that meets established water quality standards.

This informational chapter is intended to be educational, and the user should also refer to existing regulations or guidelines that cover U.S. and international [International Council for Harmonisation of Technical Requirements for Pharmaceuticals for Human Use (ICH) or World Health Organization (WHO)] good manufacturing practice (GMP) issues, as well as operational and engineering guides and/or other regulatory guidance for water [e.g., from the Food and Drug Administration (FDA), Environmental Protection Agency (EPA), or WHO]. This chapter is not, and should not be considered, an all-inclusive document on pharmaceutical waters. It contains basic information and points to be considered for the processing, holding, monitoring, and use of water. It is the user's responsibility to ensure that:

1. The selection of the type and specifications of water is appropriate for its intended use.
2. Water production and quality meet applicable governmental regulations and guidance.
3. The pharmacopeial specifications for the types of water used in monographed articles are met.
4. Water used in the preparation of reagents for analysis or the performance of required tests meets USP requirements.

Control and monitoring of the chemical and endotoxin purity of waters are important for complying with the requirements of the monographs in this compendium. Attributes listed in *USP* monographs should be considered the "minimum" requirements. More stringent requirements may be needed for some applications to ensure suitability for particular uses. Basic guidance on the appropriate applications of waters can be found in the monographs and is also discussed further in this chapter.

Control of the microbiological quality of water is also important for many of its uses. This attribute is intentionally not specified in most water monographs. Microbiological control is discussed throughout this chapter, but especially in sections *4. Validation and Qualification of Water Purification, Storage, and Distribution Systems, 5. Design and Operation of Purified Water and Water for Injection Systems, 6. Sampling, 8. Microbial Evaluations,* and *9. Alert and Action Levels and Specifications.*

This chapter contains various chemical, microbiological, processing, and engineering concepts of importance to users of water. Water system validation, process control levels, and specifications are also presented later in this chapter.

2. SOURCE WATER CONSIDERATIONS

Source water is the water that enters the facility. The origin of this source water can be from natural surface waters like rivers and reservoirs, deep-bed well waters, sea waters, or some combination of these, potentially including multiple locations of each type of source water. Thus, source water can be supplied from these various origins (public or private), from municipalities' on-site water sourcing, or by external delivery such as a truck. It is possible that source water may not be potable and safe to drink. Such water may require pretreatment to ensure that it meets drinking water standards. It is the responsibility of the users of any source water to ensure that the water used in the production of drug substances (API), as well as water for indirect drug product contact or for purification system feed water purposes meets, at a minimum, drinking (potable) water standards as defined by the requirements of the National Primary Drinking Water Regulations (NPDWR) (40 CFR 141) issued by the U.S. EPA or the drinking water regulations of the European Union (EU) or Japan, or the WHO drinking water guidelines (see *3.3.1*

Drinking Water). These regulations establish limits on the types and quantities of certain chemical and microbiological contaminants and ensure that the water will contain safe quantities of chemical and microbial species.

Where water supplies are from regulated water utility companies, less stringent monitoring may be possible because the attributes may be tested regularly and ensured by the supplier (see *9.4.5 Source Water Control*). Water being withdrawn from a nonregulated supply should be sampled and tested appropriately at a suitable frequency that takes into account local environmental and seasonal changes and other quality fluctuations. Testing should ensure conformance with one of the drinking water standards discussed above.

The use of water complying with one of these designated drinking waters as a source water allows water pretreatment systems to only be challenged to remove small quantities of potentially difficult-to-remove chemicals. Control of objectionable chemical contaminants at the source water stage eliminates the need to specifically test for some of them [e.g., trihalomethanes and elemental impurities (see *Elemental Impurities—Limits* ⟨232⟩)] after the water has been further purified, assuming there is no opportunity for recontamination.

Source waters can be used for nonproduct contact purposes such as for non-contact cooling systems. Such water may not normally be required to meet drinking water standards. Under such circumstances, the quality standards for this water when used in a pharmaceutical facility should be subject to quality standards established by the user and defensible to regulatory agencies.

Change to read:

3. WATERS USED FOR PHARMACEUTICAL MANUFACTURING AND TESTING PURPOSES

There are many different grades of water used for pharmaceutical purposes. Several are described in *USP* monographs that specify uses, acceptable methods of preparation, and quality attributes. These waters can be divided into two general types: bulk waters, which are typically produced on-site where they are used; and sterile waters, which are produced, packaged, and sterilized to preserve microbial quality throughout their packaged shelf life. There are several specialized types of sterile waters that differ in their designated applications, packaging limitations, and other quality attributes. Monographed waters must meet the quality attributes as specified in the related monographs, and any *Notes* appearing in those monographs should be considered and addressed.

With the exception of Bacteriostatic Water for Injection, the monographed bulk and sterile waters have a statement indicating that there are no added substances, or no added antimicrobial agents. In the case of antimicrobial agents, the purpose is to ensure that the sterile water product is rendered sterile based solely on its preparation, packaging, and storage. In the case of the more general statement, "no added substances", this requirement is intended to mean "no added substances that aren't sufficiently removed". Two specific examples support this intention, but there are many examples. First, the use of softeners is commonplace. A softener replaces calcium and magnesium ions ■(also known as hardness ions)■1S (USP41) with sodium, so technically you are adding two sodium ions for each hard ion. The purpose of sodium displacement is to protect downstream equipment from the hard water. The sodium ions are eventually removed sufficiently, and this is proven when the water sample passes the test in *Water Conductivity* ⟨645⟩. Another specific example is the use of ozone as a sanitant that is added to the storage tank for microbial control. This could be considered an added substance, unless the ozone is destroyed before use, as is normally the case. Other notable examples include the addition of chlorine to kill bacteria in the pretreatment system, use of bisulfite to chemically reduce chlorine to chloride and protect downstream equipment, and use of a nitrogen blanket for protection from atmospheric contamination.

There are also other types of water for which there are no monographs. These are waters with names given for descriptive purposes only. Many of these waters are used in specific analytical methods. The descriptive titles may imply certain quality attributes or modes of preparation, but these nonmonographed waters may not necessarily adhere strictly to the stated or implied modes of preparation or specified attributes. Waters produced by other means or controlled by other test attributes, or even a monographed water, may equally satisfy the intended uses for these waters. It is the user's responsibility to ensure that such waters, even if produced and controlled exactly as stated, are suitable for their intended use. Wherever the term "water" is used within this compendium without other descriptive adjectives or clauses, the intent is that water of no less purity than USP *Purified Water* be used (see *3.1.1 Purified Water*). A brief description of the various types of waters commonly associated with pharmaceutical applications and their significant uses or attributes follows.

Figure 1 may be helpful in understanding some of the various types of waters, their preparation, and uses.

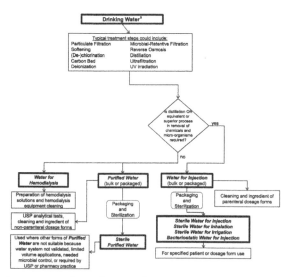

Figure 1. Water for pharmaceutical purposes. ªComplying with U.S. EPA NPDWR or the drinking water regulations of EU or Japan or WHO.

3.1 Bulk Monographed Waters and Steam

The following waters are generally produced in large volumes using a multiple-unit operation water system. These waters are typically distributed in a piping system for use at the same site.

3.1.1 PURIFIED WATER

Purified Water (see the *USP* monograph) is used as an excipient in the production of nonparenteral preparations and in other pharmaceutical applications, such as the cleaning of nonparenteral product-contact components and equipment. Unless otherwise specified, *Purified Water* is also to be used as the minimum water quality for all tests and assays in which "water" is indicated (see *General Notices, 8.230.30 Water in a Compendial Procedure*). This applies regardless of the font and letter case used in its spelling.

The minimal quality of source water for the production of Purified Water is Drinking Water whose attributes are prescribed by the U.S. EPA, EU, Japan, or WHO. This source water may be purified using unit operations that include deionization, distillation, ion exchange, reverse osmosis, filtration, or other suitable purification procedures. Purified Water must meet the requirements for ionic and organic chemical purity and must be protected from microbial contamination. Purified Water systems must be validated to reliably and consistently produce and distribute water of acceptable chemical and microbiological quality. Purified Water systems that function under ambient conditions are particularly susceptible to the establishment of biofilms of microorganisms, which can be the source of undesirable levels of viable microorganisms or endotoxins in the water. These ambient Purified Water systems require frequent sanitization and microbiological monitoring to ensure that the water reaching the points of use has appropriate microbiological quality.

The *Purified Water* monograph also allows bulk packaging for commercial use elsewhere. In contrast to Sterile Purified Water, packaged Purified Water is not required to be sterile. Because there is potential for microbial contamination and other quality changes in this packaged nonsterile water, this form of Purified Water should be prepared and stored in a manner that limits microbial growth, and/or should be used in a timely fashion before microbial proliferation renders it unsuitable for its intended use. Also, depending on the material used for packaging, extractable compounds could be leaching into the water from the packaging. Although this article is required to meet the same chemical purity standards as the bulk water, extractables from the packaging will likely render the packaged water less chemically pure than the bulk water. The nature of these impurities may even render the water an inappropriate choice for some applications. It is the user's responsibility to ensure fitness for use of this packaged article when it is used in manufacturing, clinical, or analytical applications where the purer bulk form of the water is indicated.

3.1.2 WATER FOR INJECTION

Water for Injection (see the *USP* monograph) is used as an excipient in the production of parenteral and other preparations where product endotoxin content must be controlled, and in other pharmaceutical applications, such as the cleaning of certain equipment and parenteral product-contact components.

The minimal quality of source water for the production of Water for Injection is Drinking Water whose attributes are prescribed by the U.S. EPA, EU, Japan, or WHO. This source water may be treated to render it suitable for subsequent final purification steps, such as distillation (or whatever other validated process is used, according to the monograph). The finished water must meet all of the chemical requirements specified in the monograph, as well as an additional bacterial endotoxin specification. Because endotoxins are produced by the kinds of microorganisms that are prone to inhabit water systems, the equipment and procedures used by the system to purify, store, and distribute Water for Injection should be designed to control microbial contamination and must be designed to remove incoming endotoxins from the source water. Water for Injection systems must be validated to reliably and consistently produce and distribute this quality of water.

The *Water for Injection* monograph also allows bulk packaging for commercial use. In contrast to Sterile Water for Injection, packaged Water for Injection is not required to be sterile. However, to preclude significant changes in its microbial and endotoxins content during storage, this form of Water for Injection should be prepared and stored in a manner that limits microbial introduction and growth and/or should be used in a timely fashion before microbial proliferation renders it unsuitable for its intended use. Also, depending on the material used for packaging, extractable compounds could be leaching into the water from the packaging. Although this article is required to meet the same chemical purity standards as the bulk water, extractables from the packaging will likely render the packaged water less chemically pure than the bulk water. The nature of these impurities may even render the water an inappropriate choice for some applications. It is the user's responsibility to ensure fitness for use of this packaged article when it is used in manufacturing, clinical, or analytical applications where the purer bulk form of the water is indicated.

3.1.3 WATER FOR HEMODIALYSIS

Water for Hemodialysis (see the *USP* monograph) is used for hemodialysis applications, primarily the dilution of hemodialysis concentrate solutions. The minimal quality of source water for the production of Water for Hemodialysis is Drinking Water whose attributes are prescribed by the U.S. EPA, EU, Japan, or WHO. Water for Hemodialysis has been further purified to reduce chemical and microbiological components, and it is produced and used on site. This water contains no added antimicrobial agents, and it is not intended for injection. Water for Hemodialysis must meet all of the chemical requirements specified in the monograph as well as an additional bacterial endotoxin specification. The microbial limits attribute for this water is unique among the "bulk" water monographs, but is justified on the basis of this water's specific application, which has microbial content requirements related to its safe use. The bacterial endotoxins attribute is likewise established at a level related to its safe use.

3.1.4 PURE STEAM

Pure Steam (see the *USP* monograph) is also sometimes referred to as "clean steam". It is used where the steam or its condensate would directly contact official articles or article-contact surfaces, such as during their preparation, sterilization, or cleaning where no subsequent processing step is used to remove any impurity residues. These Pure Steam applications include, but are not limited to, porous load sterilization processes, product or cleaning solutions heated by direct steam injection, or humidification of processes where steam injection is used to control the humidity inside processing vessels where the official articles or their in-process forms are exposed. The primary intent of using this quality of steam is to ensure that official articles or article-contact surfaces exposed to it are not contaminated by residues within the steam.

The minimal quality of source water for the production of Pure Steam is Drinking Water whose attributes are prescribed by the U.S. EPA, EU, Japan, or WHO, and which has been suitably treated. The water is then vaporized with suitable mist elimination, and distributed under pressure. The sources of undesirable contaminants within Pure Steam could arise from entrained source water droplets, anticorrosion steam additives, or residues from the steam production and distribution system itself. The chemical tests in the *Pure Steam* monograph should detect most of the contaminants that could arise from these sources. If an official article is exposed to Pure Steam and it is intended for parenteral use or other applications where the pyrogenic content must be controlled, the Pure Steam must additionally meet the specification for *Bacterial Endotoxins Test* 〈85〉.

These purity attributes are measured in the condensate of the article, rather than the article itself. This, of course, imparts great importance to the cleanliness of the process for Pure Steam condensate generation and collection, because it must not adversely impact the quality of the resulting condensed fluid.

Other steam attributes not detailed in the monograph, particularly the presence of even small quantities of noncondensable gases or the existence of a superheated or dry state, may also be important for applications such as sterilization. The large release of energy (latent heat of condensation) as water changes from the gaseous to the liquid state is the key to steam's sterilization efficacy and its efficiency, in general, as a heat transfer agent. If this phase change (condensation) is not allowed to happen because the steam is extremely hot and is in a persistent superheated, dry state, then its usefulness could be seriously compromised. Noncondensable gases in steam tend to stratify or collect in certain areas of a steam sterilization chamber or its load. These surfaces would thereby be at least partially insulated from the steam condensation phenomenon, preventing them from experiencing the full energy of the sterilizing conditions. Therefore, control of these kinds of steam attributes, in addition to its chemical purity, may also be important for certain Pure Steam applications. However, because these additional attributes are use-specific, they are not mentioned in the *Pure Steam* monograph.

Note that lower-purity "plant steam" may be used in the following applications: 1) for steam sterilization of nonproduct-contact nonporous loads, 2) for general cleaning of nonproduct-contact equipment, 3) as a nonproduct-contact heat-exchange medium, and 4) in all compatible applications involved in bulk pharmaceutical chemical and API manufacture.

Finally, because Pure Steam is lethal to microbes, monitoring of microbial control within a steam system is unnecessary, as is microbial analysis of the steam condensate.

3.2 Sterile Monographed Waters

The following monographed waters are packaged forms of either Purified Water or Water for Injection that have been sterilized to preserve their microbiological properties. These waters may have specific intended uses as indicated by their names, and may also have restrictions on the packaging configurations related to those uses. In general, these sterile waters may be used in a variety of applications in lieu of the bulk forms of water from which they were derived. However, there is a substantial difference between the acceptance criteria for the chemical purities of these bulk waters versus sterile waters. The specifications for sterile waters differ from those of bulk waters to accommodate a wide variety of packaging types, properties, volumes, and uses. As a result, the inorganic and organic impurity specifications are not equivalent for bulk and packaged waters. The packaging materials and elastomeric closures are the primary sources of these impurities, which tend to increase over the shelf life of these packaged articles. Therefore, due consideration must be given to the chemical purity suitability at the time of use of the sterile forms of water when used in manufacturing, analytical, and cleaning applications in lieu of the bulk waters from which these waters were derived. It is the user's responsibility to ensure fitness for use of these sterile packaged waters in these applications. Nevertheless, for the applications discussed below for each sterile water, their respective purities and packaging restrictions generally render them suitable by definition.

3.2.1 STERILE PURIFIED WATER

Sterile Purified Water (see the *USP* monograph) is Purified Water, packaged and rendered sterile. It can be used in the preparation of nonparenteral compendial dosage forms or in analytical applications requiring Purified Water where 1) access to a validated Purified Water system is not practical, 2) only a relatively small quantity is needed, 3) Sterile Purified Water is required by specific monograph or pharmacy practice, or 4) bulk packaged Purified Water is not suitably controlled for the microbiological quality for its intended use.

3.2.2 STERILE WATER FOR INJECTION

Sterile Water for Injection (see the *USP* monograph) is Water for Injection packaged and rendered sterile. It is used for extemporaneous prescription compounding and as a sterile diluent for parenteral products. It may also be used for other applications where bulk Water for Injection or Purified Water is indicated but access to a validated water system is not practical, or where only a relatively small quantity is needed. Sterile Water for Injection is packaged in single-dose containers not larger than 1 L.

3.2.3 BACTERIOSTATIC WATER FOR INJECTION

Bacteriostatic Water for Injection (see the *USP* monograph) is Water for Injection, packaged and rendered sterile, to which has been added one or more suitable antimicrobial preservatives. It is intended to be used as a diluent in the preparation of parenteral products, most typically for multi-dose products that require repeated content withdrawals. It may be packaged in single-dose or multiple-dose containers not larger than 30 mL.

3.2.4 STERILE WATER FOR IRRIGATION

Sterile Water for Irrigation (see the *USP* monograph) is Water for Injection packaged and sterilized in single-dose containers that may be larger than 1 L and allow rapid delivery of their contents. Due to its usage, Sterile Water for Irrigation is not required to meet *Particulate Matter in Injections* ⟨788⟩. It may also be used in other applications that do not have particulate matter specifications, where bulk Water for Injection or Purified Water is indicated but where access to a validated water system is not practical, or where somewhat larger quantities are needed than are provided as Sterile Water for Injection.

3.2.5 STERILE WATER FOR INHALATION

Sterile Water for Inhalation (see the *USP* monograph) is Water for Injection that is packaged and rendered sterile and is intended for use in inhalators and in the preparation of inhalation solutions. This monograph has no requirement to meet ⟨788⟩; it carries a less stringent specification for bacterial endotoxins than Sterile Water for Injection, and therefore is not suitable for parenteral applications.

3.3 Nonmonographed Waters

In addition to the bulk monographed waters described above, nonmonographed waters can also be used in pharmaceutical processing steps such as cleaning and synthetic steps, and also as a starting material for further purification or testing purposes. Unless otherwise specified in the compendium, the minimum quality of water is *Purified Water*. [NOTE—The information in this chapter is not an all-inclusive discussion of all nonmonographed waters identified in the *USP–NF*.]

3.3.1 DRINKING WATER

Drinking Water can be referred to as Potable Water (meaning drinkable or fit to drink), National Primary Drinking Water, Primary Drinking Water, or EPA Drinking Water. Except where a singular drinking water specification is stated (such as the U.S. EPA's NPDWR, as cited in 40 CFR Part 141), this water must comply with the quality attributes of either the NPDWR or the drinking water regulations of the EU or Japan, or the *WHO Guidelines for Drinking-Water Quality*. Drinking Water may originate from a variety of sources including a public water supply, a private water supply (e.g., a well), or a combination of these sources (see *2. Source Water Considerations*).

Drinking Water may be used in the early stages of cleaning pharmaceutical manufacturing equipment and product-contact components. Drinking Water is also the minimum quality of water that should be used for the preparation of official substances and other bulk pharmaceutical ingredients. Where compatible with the processes, the contaminant levels allowed in Drinking Water are generally considered safe for use in preparing official substances and other drug substances. However, where required by the processing of the materials to achieve their required final purity, higher qualities of water may be needed for these manufacturing steps, perhaps even water as pure as Water for Injection or Purified Water. Such higher-purity waters, however, might require only selected attributes to be of higher purity than Drinking Water (see *Figure 2a* and *Figure 2b*). Drinking Water is the prescribed source or feed water for the production of bulk monographed pharmaceutical waters. The use of Drinking Water specifications establishes a reasonable set of maximum allowable levels of chemical and microbiological contaminants with which a water purification system will be challenged. Because seasonal variations in the quality attributes of the Drinking Water supply can occur, it is important to give due consideration to its uses. The processing steps in the production of pharmaceutical waters must be designed to accommodate this variability.

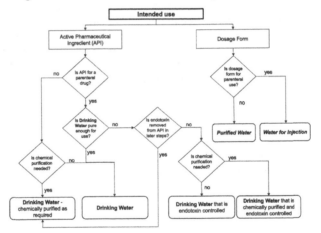

Figure 2a. Selection of water for pharmaceutical purposes: APIs and dosage forms.

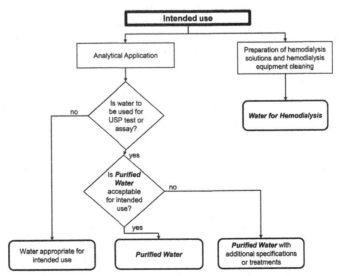

Figure 2b. Selection of water for pharmaceutical purposes: Analytical reagents.

3.3.2 OTHER NONMONOGRAPHED WATERS

In addition to Drinking Water, this compendium discusses waters with various other designations. These include waters of various quality levels for special uses such as, but not limited to, cleaning and testing purposes.

Both *General Notices and Requirements* (see *General Notices, 8.230.30 Water in a Compendial Procedure*) and *Reagents, Indicators, and Solutions* clearly state that where the term "water" is indicated for use in analyses without grammatical qualification or other specification, the quality of the water must be *Purified Water*. However, numerous such qualifications do exist. Some of these qualifications involve adjectives describing methods of preparation, ranging from specifying the primary purification step to specifying additional purification. Other qualifications call for specific attribute "absences" to be met that might otherwise interfere with analytical processes. In most of these cases, the required attribute absences are not specifically tested. Sometimes, a further "purification process" is specified that ostensibly allows the water to adequately meet this required "absence attribute".

However, preparation instructions for many reagents were carried forward from the innovator's laboratories to the originally introduced monograph for a particular *USP–NF* article or general test chapter. The quality of the reagent water described in these tests may reflect the water quality designation of the innovator's laboratory. These specific water designations may have originated without the innovator's awareness of the requirement for *Purified Water* in *USP–NF* tests. Regardless of the original reason for the creation of these numerous special analytical waters, it is possible that the attributes of these special waters could now be met by the basic preparation steps and current specifications of *Purified Water*. In some cases, however, some of the cited post-processing steps are still necessary to reliably achieve the required attributes.

Users are not obligated to utilize specific and perhaps archaically generated forms of analytical water where alternatives with equal or better quality, availability, or analytical performance may exist. The consistency and reliability of operations for producing these alternative analytical waters should be verified so that the desired attributes are produced. In addition, any alternative analytical water must be evaluated on an application-by-application basis by the user to ensure its suitability. The following is a summary of the various types of nonmonographed analytical waters that are cited in the *USP–NF*. This is not an exhaustive listing. Those listed below are used in multiple locations. Several nonmonographed analytical waters are not included below because they are only found in one or perhaps two locations within this compendium.

Note that the names of many of the waters below imply a very low chemical impurity level. For example, "deionized water" implies that all the ions have been removed. However, in most cases discussed below, exposure of the water to air will result in the ingress of carbon dioxide (CO_2), leading to the formation of bicarbonate and hydrogen ions. Therefore, the removal of ions cannot be completely maintained for most analytical applications.

3.3.3 AMMONIA-FREE WATER

From a functional standpoint, Ammonia-Free Water must have a negligible ammonia concentration to avoid interference in tests sensitive for or to ammonia. Due to the nature of the uses of this water, *Purified Water* could be a reasonable alternative for these applications.

3.3.4 CARBON DIOXIDE-FREE WATER

Carbon dioxide-free water is defined in the *Reagents, Indicators, and Solutions* section of *USP–NF* as Purified Water that has been vigorously boiled for NLT 5 min, then cooled and protected from absorption of atmospheric carbon dioxide. Alternatively, this could be *Purified Water* that has a resistivity of NLT 18 megohm-cm at 25°.

Because the absorption of atmospheric carbon dioxide lowers the pH of high-purity waters, most of the uses of Carbon Dioxide-Free Water are either associated as a solvent in pH-related or pH-sensitive determinations or as a solvent in bicarbonate-sensitive reagents or determinations.

The term "Carbon Dioxide-Free Water" is sometimes used improperly. Besides its use for pH or acidity/alkalinity tests, the purpose for using this water is not always clear. The intention could be to use water that was deaerated (free of dissolved air) or deionized (free of extraneous ions), or even Purified Water with an additional boiling step. Although boiling is highly effective for removing carbon dioxide as well as all other dissolved gasses, these gases are readily re-absorbed unless the water is protected. Even with protection, such as use of a stoppered container, re-absorption will occur over time as air will readily transmit through seals and diffuse through most materials. Deionization is also an efficient process for removing dissolved carbon dioxide. Carbon dioxide forms ionic bicarbonate in water, and will be subsequently removed by ion-exchange resins. However, the same problem of carbon dioxide re-absorption will occur after the deionized water is exposed to air. Also, the deionization approach for creating Carbon Dioxide-Free Water does not deaerate the water or remove other dissolved gases such as oxygen (O_2); it only removes carbon dioxide and other ions.

Depending on the application, Purified Water may meet the requirements where Carbon Dioxide-Free Water is called for. This could also include pH or acidity or alkalinity tests. The pH of a sample of pure Deionized Water is, by definition, 7.0. When that same sample is exposed to typical environmental atmospheric conditions, the water sample will absorb carbon dioxide and result in a pH range of approximately 5.4–6.2 ([H^+] is in the range of 4.0×10^{-6} M to 6.3×10^{-7} M). The added acidity caused by carbon dioxide absorption may be insignificant compared to the material being analyzed.

3.3.5 DISTILLED WATER

Distilled Water is produced by vaporizing Drinking Water or a higher quality of water and condensing it into a purer state. It is used primarily as a solvent for reagent preparation, and it is also specified in the execution of other aspects of tests, such as for rinsing an analyte, transferring a test material as a slurry, as a calibration standard or analytical blank, and for test apparatus cleaning. Distilled Water is also cited as the starting water to be used for making High-Purity Water (see *3.3.10 High-Purity Water*). Because none of the cited uses of this water imply a need for a particular purity attribute that can only be derived by distillation, water meeting the requirements for *Purified Water* derived by other means of purification or *Water for Injection* could be equally suitable where Distilled Water is specified. It is the user's responsibility to verify the suitability of Purified Water or Water for Injection.

3.3.6 FRESHLY DISTILLED WATER

Freshly Distilled Water or "recently distilled water" is produced in the same manner as Distilled Water and should be used soon after its generation. This implies the need to avoid endotoxin contamination, as well as any other forms of contamination from the air or containers, that could arise with prolonged storage. Freshly Distilled Water is used for preparing solutions for subcutaneous test-animal injections and for a reagent solvent in tests for which there appears to be no particularly high water purity needed that could be ascribable to being "freshly distilled". In the test-animal application, the term "freshly distilled" and its testing use imply a chemical, endotoxin, and microbiological purity that could be equally satisfied by *Water for Injection* (although no reference is made to these chemical, endotoxin, or microbial attributes or specific protection from recontamination). For non-animal uses, water meeting the requirements for *Purified Water* derived by other means of purification and/or storage periods could be equally suitable where "recently distilled water" or Freshly Distilled Water is specified. It is the user's responsibility to verify the suitability of Purified Water or Water for Injection.

3.3.7 DEIONIZED WATER

Deionized Water can be produced by starting with either Drinking Water or Purified Water, depending upon monograph or testing procedures defined in the compendia. Deionized Water is produced by an ion-exchange process in which the cations and anions are replaced with $H+$ and $OH-$ ions by use of ion-exchange resins. Similar to Distilled Water, Deionized Water is used primarily as a solvent for reagent preparation, but it is also specified in the execution of other aspects of tests, such as for transferring an analyte within a test procedure, as a calibration standard or analytical blank, and for test apparatus cleaning. Also, none of the cited uses of this water imply any needed purity attribute that can only be achieved by deionization. Therefore, water meeting the requirements for *Purified Water* that is derived by other means of purification could be equally suitable where Deionized Water is specified. It is the user's responsibility to verify the suitability of Purified Water.

3.3.8 DEIONIZED DISTILLED WATER

Deionized Distilled Water is produced by deionizing (see *3.3.7 Deionized Water*) Distilled Water. This water is used as a reagent in a liquid chromatography test that requires a low ionic or organic impurity level. Because of the importance of this high purity, water that meets the requirements for *Purified Water* may not be acceptable. High-Purity Water (see *3.3.10 High-Purity Water*) could be a reasonable alternative to this water. It is the user's responsibility to verify the suitability of the alternative water used.

3.3.9 FILTERED WATER

Filtered Water is Purified Water that has been filtered to remove particles that could interfere with the analysis where this water is specified. It is sometimes used synonymously with Particle-Free Water and Ultra-Filtered Water and is cited in some monographs and general chapters as well as in *Reagents, Indicators, and Solutions*. Depending on its referenced location in *USP–NF*, it is variously defined as water that has been passed through filters rated as 1.2, 0.2, or 0.22 µm, or unspecified porosity rating. Even though the water names and the filter ratings used to produce these waters are defined inconsistently, the use of 0.2-µm or 0.22-µm filtered *Purified Water* should be universally acceptable for all applications where Particle-Free Water, Filtered Water, or Ultra-Filtered Water are specified.

3.3.10 HIGH-PURITY WATER

High-Purity Water may be prepared by deionizing previously distilled water and then filtering it through a 0.45-µm rated membrane. This water must have an in-line conductivity of NMT 0.15 µS/cm (NLT 6.67 megohm-cm) at 25°. If the water of this purity contacts the atmosphere even briefly as it is being used or drawn from its purification system, its conductivity will immediately increase by as much as about 1.0 µS/cm ■at 25°■1S (USP41) as atmospheric carbon dioxide dissolves in the water and equilibrates to hydrogen and bicarbonate ions. Therefore, if the analytical use requires that water conductivity remains as low as possible or the bicarbonate/carbon dioxide levels be as low as possible, the water should be protected from atmospheric exposure. High-Purity Water is used as a reagent, as a solvent for reagent preparation, and for test apparatus cleaning where less stringent water specifications would not be considered acceptable. However, if a user's routinely available *Purified Water* is filtered and meets or exceeds the conductivity specifications of High-Purity Water, it could be used in lieu of High-Purity Water.

3.3.11 DEAERATED WATER

Deaerated Water or "degassed water" is Purified Water that has been treated to reduce the content of dissolved air by "suitable means" such as boiling, sonication, and/or stirring during the application of a partial vacuum, followed by immediate use or protection from air reabsorption.

3.3.12 OXYGEN-FREE WATER

Oxygen-Free Water is Purified Water that has been treated to remove or reduce dissolved oxygen. Such treatment could involve deaerating by boiling or sparging with an inert gas such as nitrogen or helium, followed by inert gas blanketing to prevent oxygen reabsorption. Any procedure used for removing oxygen should be verified as reliably producing water that is fit for use.

3.3.13 WATER FOR BACTERIAL ENDOTOXINS TEST

Water for Bacterial Endotoxins Test (BET) is also referred to as Limulus Amebocyte Lysate (LAL) Reagent Water. This type of water is often Water for Injection, which may have been sterilized. It is free from a level of endotoxin that would yield any detectable reaction or interference with the LAL reagent used in the BET (see ⟨85⟩).

Change to read:

4. VALIDATION AND QUALIFICATION OF WATER PURIFICATION, STORAGE, AND DISTRIBUTION SYSTEMS

4.1 Validation Requirement

Establishing the reliability of pharmaceutical water purification, storage, and distribution systems requires demonstrating control of the process through an appropriate period of monitoring and observation. Finished water is typically continuously produced and used, while product and process attributes may only be periodically assessed. The quality of bulk finished water cannot be established by only testing monograph attributes. The unit operations in the pharmaceutical water system need to demonstrate that they are in control through monitoring of the process parameters and water quality. The advent of using conductivity and total organic carbon (TOC) to define chemical purity allows the user to more quantitatively assess the water's chemical purity and its variability as a function of routine treatment system maintenance and regeneration. Treatment processes must also demonstrate control of microbial attributes within the overall system. Some unit operations that are needed for chemical treatment may significantly increase microbial and bacterial endotoxin levels. These are later controlled by downstream unit operations. Knowledge of the treatment system processes and the effectiveness of control measures is needed to ensure that the pharmaceutical waters are acceptable for use.

Efficacy of the design, operation, sanitization, and control of the pharmaceutical water system is demonstrated through the monitoring of chemical and microbial attributes. A typical water system validation program involves an initial increased frequency of monitoring of the treatment system process parameters and sampling and testing of major process points to demonstrate the ability to produce the acceptable water and to characterize the operation of the system. This is followed by a life cycle approach of validation maintenance and monitoring.

4.2 Validation Approach

Validation is the program of documenting, to a high level of assurance, that a specific process is capable of consistently delivering product conforming to an established set of quality attributes. A validation program qualifies and documents the design, installation, operation, and performance of the system. A graphical representation of a typical water system validation life cycle is shown in *Figure 3*.

The validation protocol should be based on the boundaries of the water system and the critical water quality and process attributes needed to maintain consistent performance. The system boundary may stop at the point of use or may include the water transfer process. If the transfer process from the distribution system outlets to the water use locations (typically either with hoses or hard-piped equipment connections) is defined as outside the water system boundary, then this transfer process still needs to be validated to not adversely affect the quality of the water as it is delivered for use. Because routine quality control (QC) microbial monitoring is performed for the same transfer process and components (e.g., hoses and heat exchangers) as that of routine water use (see *6.1.2 QC Sampling*), there is some logic to include this water transfer process within the distribution system validation.

4.2.1 VALIDATION ELEMENTS

Validation is accomplished through the use of a structured, documented process. The phases of this process include Design Qualification (DQ), Installation Qualification (IQ), Operational Qualification (OQ), Performance Qualification (PQ), and Validation Maintenance. The process is documented in a validation protocol. The elements may be in individual protocols for each phase, or integrated into variations of a DQ/IQ/OQ/PQ combined document format. The protocols are formally approved quality documents. Factory Acceptance Testing (FAT), Site Acceptance Testing (SAT), and commissioning testing of the system may supplement qualification tests for IQ or OQ provided that they are properly documented and reviewed; and if it can be shown that the system functionality is not affected by the transport and installation.

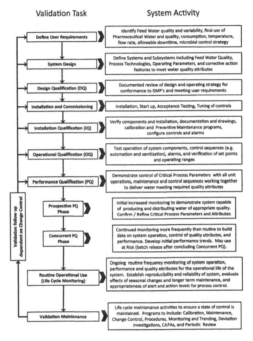

Figure 3. Water system validation life cycle.

4.2.2 USER REQUIREMENTS SPECIFICATION AND DESIGN QUALIFICATION

The user requirements for the water system should identify the design, operation, maintenance, and quality elements needed to produce the desired water type from the available source water, including its anticipated attribute variability. The essential elements of quality need to be built in at this stage and any GMP risks mitigated to an acceptable level.

The review of the specifications, system design, components, functions, and operation should be performed to demonstrate that the system complies with GMPs and verify that the design meets the user requirements. This documented review may be performed as part of the overall design process or as a separate DQ.

4.2.3 IQ

An IQ protocol for a water system confirms that the system has been properly installed and documented. This may include verification of components, piping, installation, and weld quality; documentation of the specifications for all system components present; inspections to verify that the drawings accurately depict the final configuration of the water system and, where necessary, special tests to verify that the installation meets the design requirements. Additionally, the water system is readied for operational testing, including calibration of instruments, configuration of alarm levels and adjustment of operating parameters (e.g., flow rate, pressure).

4.2.4 OQ

The OQ phase consisting of tests and inspections to verify that the equipment, system alerts, and controls are operating reliably and that appropriate Alert and Action Levels are established (this phase of qualification may overlap with aspects of IQ and PQ). During this phase of validation specific testing is performed for alarms, verifying control sequences, equipment functional checks, and verification of operating ranges. SOPs for all aspects of water system operation, maintenance, water use, water sampling, and testing, etc. should be in place and operator training completed. At the completion of the OQ, the water system has demonstrated that the components are operational and the system is producing suitable water.

4.2.5 PQ

The prospective PQ stage considers two aspects of the water system: critical process parameters and critical water attribute parameters. These are evaluated in parallel by monitoring the water quality and demonstrating acceptable quality attributes while demonstrating control of the process parameters (see *6.3 Validation Sampling Plans*). The initial PQ stage may result in refinement of process parameters to yield appropriate water quality. This PQ stage includes an increased frequency of monitoring for approximately 2–4 weeks, or sufficient time to generate adequate data to demonstrate that water meeting the appropriate quality attributes is produced and distributed. One of the reasons for this duration is that biofilm, the source of planktonic organisms in water samples, takes time to develop and to determine if the sanitization unit operations and processes are adequate to control microbial proliferation. The chemical control program adequacy is typically apparent in less time than it takes to see microbial control adequacy. However, chemical purification can be compromised by poor microbial control and, to a lesser degree, vice versa.

Once a level of control of microbial and chemical attributes has been demonstrated, the next phase of PQ is to continue the frequency of monitoring for approximately 2–4 weeks at a somewhat reduced level that will still give adequate data on system performance while using the pharmaceutical water. The water may be used for manufacturing at risk, and the associated products may be released only after water quality attributes have been determined to be acceptable and this validation phase has been completed. At the completion of the second phase, the data should be formally reviewed and the system approved for operational use.

4.3 Operational Use

When the water system has been placed into operational use, monitoring of the water quality attributes and the system process parameters is performed at a routine frequency (see *6.4 Routine Sampling Plans*) to ensure that they remain with a state of control during long-term variability from seasonal variations in source water quality, unit operation maintenance, system sanitization processes, and earlier-established Alert and Action Levels.

The water system should continue to be monitored and evaluated on an on-going basis following a life cycle approach using online instruments or samples for laboratory-based testing. The use of online instruments and process automation technology, such as conductivity, TOC, temperature, flow rate, and pressure can facilitate improved operational control of the attributes and parameters and for process release. Manual observation of operating parameters and laboratory-based testing is also appropriate and acceptable for monitoring and trend evaluation.

4.3.1 MONITORING

The frequency of routine monitoring should be based on the criticality of the finished water, capabilities of the process, and ability to maintain product water quality trends. Monitoring may be adjusted from the initial validation monitoring program when there is sufficient data to support a change (see *6.4 Routine Sampling Plans*).

4.3.2 VALIDATION MAINTENANCE

Maintaining the validated state of control requires a life cycle approach. After the completion of the PQ and release of the water system for use, ongoing activities and programs have to be in place to maintain the validated state of control after the system has been validated and placed into service (see *5.4 Operation, Maintenance, and Control*). This includes unit operation, calibration, corrective maintenance, preventive maintenance, procedures, manuals and drawings, standardization of instruments, process parameter and quality attribute trending, change control, deviations, corrective and preventive actions (CAPA), training, records retention, logbooks, etc.

4.3.3 CHANGE CONTROL

Identification and control of changes made to unit operations and other system components, operation parameters, system sanitization, and laboratory processes or procedures need to be established. Not all changes will require validation follow up, but even minor ones, such as gasket elastomer changes could have an impact on quality attributes. The impact of the change on process parameters and quality attributes must be identified, evaluated and remediated. This may result in a selective validation activity to demonstrate the ongoing state of control for the system and ability to maintain water quality attributes.

Certain calibration and preventive maintenance activities may be considered routine tasks if they do not impact on system operation or water quality. Replacement of components needs to be carefully evaluated. Replacement of components using exact parts generally does not affect system operation or control. Replacement of components with ones that ■are not exact parts but have■₁₅ ₍USP41₎ similar functional specifications can be performed at risk with the critical specifications (e.g., material of construction, dimensions, flow rate, response factors) having been evaluated and the differences determined to be acceptable and documented within the change control system.

4.3.4 PERIODIC REVIEW

The water system qualification, maintenance history, calibration records, quality and process data, issues with the unit operations and any process variability, change control, and other validation maintenance data should be assessed periodically to determine impact on the state of control.

The review may result in adjustments to operating or sanitization processes, calibration or maintenance plans, or monitoring plans. This may also result in additional testing or repeating certain qualification tasks (re-qualification).

Change to read:

5. DESIGN AND OPERATION OF PURIFIED WATER AND WATER FOR INJECTION SYSTEMS

The design, installation, and operation of systems to produce Purified Water and Water for Injection include similar components, control techniques, and procedures. The quality attributes of the two waters differ in their bioburden expectation, the presence of a bacterial endotoxin requirement for Water for Injection, and in their methods of preparation. The similarities in the quality attributes provide considerable common ground in the design of water systems to meet either requirement. The critical difference is the degree of control of the system and the final purification steps needed to ensure removal of bacteria and bacterial endotoxins and reductions in opportunities for biofilm re-development within those purification steps that could become in situ sources of bacteria and endotoxin in the finished water.

Many aspects of system design and operation relate to control and elimination of biofilm. Unit operations can cause the deterioration of water microbial attributes and the formation of biofilm on unit operation surfaces, even when properly maintained (see *8.2 Biofilm Formation in Water Systems*).

Production of pharmaceutical water involves sequential unit operations (processing steps) that address specific water quality attributes and protect the operation of subsequent treatment steps. A typical evaluation process for selecting an appropriate water quality for a particular pharmaceutical purpose is shown in the decision trees in *Figure 2a* and *Figure 2b*. This diagram may be used to assist in defining requirements for specific water uses and in the selection of unit operations. The final unit operation used to produce Water for Injection is limited to distillation or other processes equivalent or superior to distillation in the removal of chemical impurities as well as microorganisms and their components, such as bacterial endotoxins. Distillation coupled with suitable pretreatment technologies has a long history of generally reliable performance (though not completely infallible) and can be validated as a unit operation for the production of Water for Injection. Other combinations of purification technologies may also be suitable in the production of Water for Injection if they can be shown through validation to be as effective and reliable as distillation in the removal of chemicals and microorganisms. The development of new designs and materials of construction for other technologies (such as reverse osmosis, electrodeionization, and ultrafiltration) that allow intermittent or continuous operation at hot bactericidal conditions show promise for a valid use in producing Water for Injection.

5.1 Unit Operations Considerations

To achieve the quality attributes for pharmaceutical waters, multiple-unit operations are required. The design of the water purification system needs to take into consideration different aspects, including the source water quality, sanitization, pharmaceutical water quality attributes, uses of the water, and maintenance programs. Each unit operation contributes specific purification attributes associated with chemical and microbiological parameters.

The following is a brief description of selected unit operations and the design, installation, operation, maintenance, and monitoring parameter considerations associated with them. Not all unit operations are discussed, nor are all potential shortcomings addressed.

5.1.1 PREFILTRATION

The purpose of prefiltration—also referred to as initial, coarse, particulate, or depth filtration—is to remove solid contaminants from the incoming source water supply and protect downstream system components from particulates that can inhibit equipment performance and shorten their effective life. This coarse filtration technology primarily uses sieving effects for particle capture and a depth of filtration medium that has a high "dirt load" capacity. Such filtration units are available in a wide range of designs and for various applications. Removal efficiencies and capacities differ significantly, from granular bed filters such as multimedia or sand for larger water systems, to depth cartridges for smaller water systems. Unit and system configurations vary widely in the type of filtering media and the location in the process. Granular or cartridge prefilters are often situated at the beginning of the water purification system prior to unit operations designed to remove the source water disinfectants. Cartridge-type coarse filters may also be used to capture fines released from granular beds such as activated carbon and deionization beds. These locations, however, do not preclude the need for periodic microbial evaluation.

Design and operational issues that may impact the performance of depth filters include channeling of the filtering media, blockage from silt, microbial growth, and filtering-media loss during improper backwashing. Control methods involve pressure and flow monitoring during use and backwashing, sanitizing, and replacing filtering media. An important design concern is sizing of the filter to prevent channeling or media loss resulting from inappropriate water flow rates as well as proper sizing to minimize excessively frequent or infrequent backwashing or cartridge filter replacement.

5.1.2 ACTIVATED CARBON

Activated carbon beds, depending on the type and placement, are used to adsorb low-molecular-weight organic material, bacterial endotoxins, and oxidizing additives such as chlorine and chloramine compounds, removing them from the water. They are used to achieve certain quality attributes and to protect against reactions with downstream unit operations, stainless steel surfaces, resins, and membranes.

The chief operating concerns regarding activated carbon beds include the propensity to support bacterial growth, the potential for hydraulic channeling, the organic adsorption capacity, and insufficient contact time. Operation deficiencies may result in the release of bacteria, endotoxins, organic chemicals, and fine carbon particles.

Control measures may involve monitoring water flow rates and differential pressures, sanitizing with hot water or steam, backwashing, testing for adsorption capacity, and frequent replacement of the carbon bed. Monitoring of carbon bed unit operation may also include microbial loading, disinfectant chemical reduction, and TOC if used for TOC reduction. The use of hot water or steam for carbon bed sanitization is ineffective if there is channeling rather than even permeation through the bed. Channeling can be mitigated through design and proper flow rates during sanitization.

Microbial biofilm development on the surface of the granular carbon particles can cause adjacent bed granules to agglomerate. This may result in ineffective removal of trapped debris and fragile biofilm during backwashing, and ineffective sanitization.

Alternative technologies to activated carbon beds can be used to avoid their microbial challenges. These include disinfectant-neutralizing chemical additives and intense ultraviolet (UV) light for removal of chlorine, and regenerable organic scavenging deionizing resins for removal of organics.

5.1.3 ADDITIVES

Chemical additives are used in water systems 1) to control microorganisms by use of sanitizing agents, such as chlorine compounds and ozone; 2) to enhance the removal of suspended solids by use of flocculating agents; 3) to remove chlorine compounds; 4) to avoid scaling on reverse osmosis membranes; and 5) to adjust pH for more effective removal of carbonate and ammonia compounds by reverse osmosis. These additives do not constitute "added substances" as long as they are either removed by subsequent processing steps or are otherwise absent from the finished water. Control of additives to ensure a continuously effective concentration and subsequent monitoring to ensure their removal should be designed into the system and included in the monitoring program.

5.1.4 ORGANIC SCAVENGERS

Organic scavenging devices use macroreticular, weakly basic anion-exchange resins capable of removing negatively charged organic material and endotoxins from the water. Organic scavenger resins can be regenerated with appropriate biocidal caustic brine solutions. Operating concerns are associated with organic scavenging capacity; particulate, chemical, and microbiological fouling of the reactive resin surface; flow rate; regeneration frequency; and shedding of fines from the fragile resins. Control measures include TOC testing of influent and effluent, backwashing, monitoring hydraulic performance, and using downstream filters to remove resin fines.

5.1.5 SOFTENERS

Water softeners may be located either upstream or downstream of disinfectant removal units. They utilize sodium-based cation-exchange resins to remove water-hardness ions, such as calcium and magnesium, that could foul or interfere with the performance of downstream processing equipment such as reverse osmosis membranes, deionization devices, and distillation units. Water softeners can also be used to remove other lower affinity cations, such as the ammonium ion, that may be released from chloramine disinfectants commonly used in drinking water. If ammonium removal is one of its purposes, the softener must be located downstream of the disinfectant removal operation. Water softener resin beds are regenerated with concentrated sodium chloride solution (brine).

Concerns include microorganism proliferation, channeling, appropriate water flow rates and contact time, ion-exchange capacity, organic and particulate resin fouling, organic leaching from new resins, fracture of the resin beads, resin degradation by excessively chlorinated water, and contamination from the brine solution used for regeneration.

Control measures involve recirculation of water during periods of low water use; periodic sanitization of the resin and brine system; use of microbial control devices (e.g., UV light and chlorine); locating the unit upstream of the disinfectant removal step (if used only for softening); appropriate regeneration frequency; effluent chemical monitoring (e.g., hardness ions and possibly ammonium); and downstream filtration to remove resin fines. If a softener is used for ammonium removal from chloramine-containing source water, then the capacity, contact time, resin surface fouling, pH, and regeneration frequency are very important.

5.1.6 DEIONIZATION

Deionization (DI) and continuous electrodeionization (CEDI) are effective methods of improving the chemical quality attributes of water by removing cations and anions. DI systems have charged resins that require periodic regeneration with an acid and base. Typically, cation resins are regenerated with either hydrochloric or sulfuric acid, which replace the captured positive ions with hydrogen ions. Anion resins are regenerated with sodium hydroxide or potassium hydroxide, which replace captured negative ions with hydroxide ions. Because free endotoxin is negatively charged, some removal of endotoxin is achieved by the anion resin. The system can be designed so that the cation and anion resins are in separate or "twin" beds, or they can be blended together to form a "mixed" bed.

The CEDI system uses a combination of ion-exchange materials such as resins or grafted material, selectively permeable membranes, and an electric charge, providing continuous flow (of product and waste concentrate) and continuous regeneration. Water enters both the resin section and the waste (concentrate) section. The resin acts as a conductor, enabling the electrical potential to drive the captured cations and anions through the resin and appropriate membranes for concentration and removal in the waste water stream. As the water passes through the resin, it is deionized to become product water. The electrical potential also separates the water in the resin (product) section into hydrogen and hydroxide ions. This permits continuous regeneration of the resin without the need for regenerant additives. However, unlike conventional deionization, CEDI units must start with water that is already partially purified because they generally cannot achieve the conductivity attribute of Purified Water when starting with the heavier ion load of source water.

Concerns for all forms of DI units include microbial and endotoxin control; chemical additive impact on resins and membranes; and loss, degradation, and fouling of resin. Issues of concern specific to DI units include regeneration frequency and completeness; channeling caused by biofilm agglomeration of resin particles; organic leaching from new resins; complete resin separation for mixed bed regeneration; and bed fluidization air contamination (mixed beds).

Control measures may include continuous recirculation loops, effluent microbial control by UV light, conductivity monitoring, resin testing, microporous filtration of bed fluidization air, microbial monitoring, frequent regeneration to minimize and control microorganism growth, sizing the equipment for suitable water flow and contact time, and use of elevated temperatures. Internal distributor and regeneration piping for DI bed units should be configured to ensure that regeneration chemicals contact all internal bed and piping surfaces and resins.

Rechargeable canisters can be the source of contamination and should be carefully monitored. Full knowledge of previous resin use, minimum storage time between regeneration and use, and appropriate sanitizing procedures are critical factors for ensuring proper performance.

5.1.7 REVERSE OSMOSIS

Reverse osmosis (RO) units use semipermeable membranes. The "pores" of RO membranes are intersegmental spaces among the polymer molecules. They are big enough for permeation of water molecules, but they limit the passage of hydrated chemical ions, organic compounds, and microorganisms. RO membranes can achieve chemical, microbial, and endotoxin quality improvement. Many factors, including pH, temperature, source water hardness, permeate and reject flow rate, and differential pressure across the membrane, affect the selectivity and effectiveness of this permeation. The process streams consist of supply water, product water (permeate), and waste water (reject). Depending on the source water, pretreatment and system configuration variations and chemical additives may be necessary to achieve the desired performance and reliability. For most source waters, a single stage of RO filtration is usually not enough to meet Purified Water conductivity specifications. A second pass of this permeate water through another RO stage usually achieves the necessary permeate purity if other factors such as pH and temperature have been appropriately adjusted and the ammonia from source water that has been previously treated with chloramines is removed.

Concerns associated with the design and operation of RO units include membrane materials that are sensitive to sanitizing agents and to particulate, chemical, and microbial membrane fouling; membrane and seal integrity; and the passage of dissolved gases, such as carbon dioxide and ammonia. Failure of membrane or seal integrity will result in product water contamination. Methods of control involve suitable pretreatment of the influent water stream; appropriate membrane material selection; membrane design and heat tolerance; periodic sanitization; and monitoring of differential pressures, conductivity, microbial levels, and TOC.

The development of RO units that can tolerate sanitizing water temperatures and also operate efficiently and continuously at elevated temperatures has added greatly to their microbial control ability and to the avoidance of biofouling. RO units can be used alone or in combination with DI and CEDI units, as well as ultrafiltration, for operational and quality enhancements.

5.1.8 ULTRAFILTRATION

Ultrafiltration is a technology that is often used near the end of a pharmaceutical water purification system for removing endotoxins from a water stream though upstream uses are possible. Ultrafiltration can use semipermeable membranes, but unlike RO, these typically use polysulfone membranes with intersegmental "pores" that have been purposefully enlarged. Membranes with differing molecular weight "cutoffs" can be created to preferentially reject molecules with molecular weights above these ratings.

Ceramic ultrafilters are another molecular sieving technology. Ceramic ultrafilters are self-supporting and extremely durable; they can be backwashed, chemically cleaned, and steam sterilized. However, they may require higher operating pressures than do membrane-type ultrafilters.

All ultrafiltration devices work primarily by a molecular sieving principle. Ultrafilters with molecular weight cutoff ratings in the range of 10,000–20,000 Da are typically used in water systems for removing endotoxins. This technology may be appropriate as an intermediate or final purification step. As with RO, successful performance is dependent upon pretreatment of the water by upstream unit operations.

Issues of concern for ultrafilters include compatibility of membrane material with heat and sanitizing agents, membrane integrity, fouling by particles and microorganisms, and seal integrity. Control measures involve filter membrane composition, sanitization, flow design (dead end vs. tangential), cartridge replacement, elevated feed water temperature, and monitoring TOC and differential pressure.

5.1.9 MICROBIAL-RETENTIVE FILTRATION

Microbial-retentive membrane filters have a larger effective "pore size" than ultrafilters and are intended to prevent the passage of microorganisms and similarly sized particles without unduly restricting flow. This type of filtration is widely employed within water systems for filtering the bacteria out of both water and compressed gases as well as for vent filters on tanks and stills and other unit operations.

In water systems, a filter's microbial retention characteristics exhibit different phenomena than in other aseptic filtration applications.

The following factors interact to create the retention phenomena for water system microorganisms: the variability in the range and average pore sizes created by the various membrane fabrication processes; the variability of the surface chemistry and three-dimensional structure related to the different polymers used in these filter matrices; and the size and surface properties of the microorganism intended to be retained by the filters. ▪₁S (USP41) In some situations, the appearance of water system microorganisms on the downstream sides of some 0.2- to 0.22-μm rated filters after a ▪₁S (USP41) period of use (days to weeks) seems to support the idea that ▪water-borne microorganisms can penetrate the 0.2- to 0.22-μm rated filters.▪₁S (USP41) It is not known whether this downstream appearance is caused by ▪exceeding the retentive capabilities of the filters due to high prefiltration bioburden levels of water-borne microorganisms and extended filtration times. These conditions can lead to a "pass-through" phenomenon resulting from tiny cells or less cell "stickiness", or perhaps by a "grow-through" phenomenon in which cells hypothetically replicate their way through the pores to the downstream side.▪₁S (USP41) Whatever the penetration mechanism, 0.2- to 0.22-μm rated membranes may not be the best choice for some water system uses (see ●*Sterility Assurance* ⟨1211⟩).● (CN 1-May-2018)

Nevertheless, microbial retention success in water systems has been reported with the use of filters rated as 0.2 or 0.1 μm. There is general agreement that, for a given manufacturer, their 0.1-μm rated filters are tighter than their 0.2- to 0.22-μm rated filters. However, comparably rated filters from different manufacturers may not have equivalent performance in water filtration applications because of the different filter materials, different fabrication processes, and nonstandardized microbial retention challenge processes currently used for defining the 0.1-μm filter rating. It should be noted that filters with a 0.1-μm rating may result in a lower flow rate compared to 0.2- to 0.22-μm filters, so whatever filters are chosen for a water system application, the user must verify that they are suitable for their intended application, use period, and use process, including flow rate.

For microbial retentive gas filtrations, the same sieving and adsorptive retention phenomena are at work as in liquid filtration, but the adsorptive phenomenon is enhanced by additional electrostatic interactions between the particles and filter matrix. These electrostatic interactions are so strong, particle retention for a given filter rating is significantly more efficient in gas filtration than in water or product-solution filtrations. These additional adsorptive interactions render filters rated at 0.2–0.22 μm unquestionably suitable for microbial retentive gas filtrations. When microbial retentive filters are used in these applications, the membrane surface is typically hydrophobic (non-wettable by water). A significant area of concern for gas filtration is blockage of tank vents by condensed water vapor, which can cause mechanical damage to the tank. Control measures include electrical or steam tracing and a self-draining orientation of vent filter housings to prevent accumulation of vapor condensate. However, a continuously high filter temperature will take an oxidative toll on polypropylene components of the filter, so sterilization of the unit prior to initial use, and periodically thereafter, as well as regular visual inspections, integrity tests, and filter cartridge changes are recommended control methods.

In water applications, microbial retentive filters may be used downstream of unit operations that tend to release microorganisms or upstream of unit operations that are sensitive to microorganisms. Microbial retentive filters may also be used to filter water feeding the distribution system. It should be noted that regulatory authorities allow the use of microbial retentive filters within distribution systems or even at use points if they have been properly validated and are appropriately maintained. A point-of-use filter should only be intended to "polish" the microbial quality of an otherwise well-maintained system and not to serve as the primary microbial control device. The efficacy of system microbial control measures can only be assessed by sampling the water upstream of the filters. As an added measure of protection, in-line UV lamps, appropriately sized for the flow rate (see *5.3 Sanitization*), may be used just upstream of microbial retentive filters to inactivate microorganisms prior to their capture by the filter. This tandem approach tends to greatly delay potential microbial penetration phenomena and can substantially extend filter service life.

5.1.10 ULTRAVIOLET LIGHT

The use of low-pressure UV lights that emit a 254-nm wavelength for microbial control is discussed in *5.3 Sanitization*, but the application of UV light in chemical purification is also emerging. This 254-nm wavelength is also useful in the destruction of ozone. At wavelengths around 185 nm (as well as at 254 nm), medium-pressure UV lights have demonstrated utility in the destruction of the chlorine-containing disinfectants used in source water as well as for interim stages of water pretreatment. High intensities of ■185 nm alone or 254 nm■₁ₛ ₍USP41₎ in combination with other oxidizing sanitants, such as hydrogen peroxide, have been used to lower TOC levels in recirculating distribution systems. The organics are typically converted to carbon dioxide, which equilibrates to bicarbonate, and incompletely oxidized carboxylic acids, both of which can easily be removed by polishing ion-exchange resins.

Areas of concern include inadequate UV intensity and residence time, gradual loss of UV emissivity with bulb age, gradual formation of a UV-absorbing film at the water contact surface, incomplete photodegradation during unforeseen source water hyperchlorination, release of ammonia from chloramine photodegradation, unapparent UV bulb failure, and conductivity degradation in distribution systems using 185-nm UV lights.

Control measures include regular inspection or emissivity alarms to detect bulb failures or film occlusions, regular UV bulb sleeve cleaning and wiping, downstream chlorine detectors (when used for dechlorination), downstream polishing deionizers (when used for TOC reduction), and regular (approximately yearly) bulb replacement. UV lamps generate heat during operation, which can cause failure of the lamps or increase the temperature of the water. Precautions should be in place to ensure that water flow is present to control excessive temperature increase.

5.1.11 DISTILLATION

Distillation units provide chemical and microbial purification via thermal vaporization, mist elimination, and water vapor condensation. A variety of designs is available, including single effect, multiple effect, and vapor compression. The latter two configurations are normally used in larger systems because of their generating capacity and efficiency. Source water controls must provide for the removal of hardness and silica impurities that may foul or corrode the heat transfer surfaces, as well as the removal of those impurities that could volatize and condense along with the water vapor. In spite of general perceptions, even the best distillation process does not ensure absolute removal of contaminating ions, organics, and endotoxins. Most stills are recognized as being able to accomplish at least a 3–4 log reduction in these impurity concentrations. They are highly effective in sterilizing the feed water.

Areas of concern include carryover of volatile organic impurities such as trihalomethanes (see *2. Source Water Considerations*) and gaseous impurities such as ammonia and carbon dioxide, faulty mist elimination, evaporator flooding, inadequate blow down, stagnant water in condensers and evaporators, pump and compressor seal design, pinhole evaporator and condenser leaks, and conductivity (quality) variations during start-up and operation.

Methods of control may involve the following: preliminary steps to remove both dissolved carbon dioxide and other volatile or noncondensable impurities; reliable mist elimination to minimize feed water droplet entrainment; visual or automated high-water-level indication to detect boiler flooding and boil over; use of sanitary pumps and compressors to minimize microbial and lubricant contamination of feed water and condensate; proper drainage during inactive periods to minimize microbial growth and accumulation of associated endotoxin in boiler water; blow down control to limit the impurity concentration effect in the boiler to manageable levels; on-line conductivity sensing with automated diversion to waste to prevent unacceptable water upon still start-up or still malfunction from getting into the finished water distribution system; and periodic testing for pinhole leaks to routinely ensure that condensate is not compromised by nonvolatized source water contaminants.

5.1.12 STORAGE TANKS

Storage tanks are included in water distribution systems to optimize processing equipment capacity. Storage also allows for routine maintenance within the purification system while maintaining continuous supply to meet manufacturing needs. Design and operation considerations are needed to prevent or minimize the development of biofilm, to minimize corrosion, to aid in the use of chemical sanitization of the tanks, and to safeguard mechanical integrity.

Areas of concern include microbial growth or corrosion due to irregular or incomplete sanitization and microbial contamination from unalarmed rupture disk failures caused by condensate-occluded vent filters.

Control considerations may include using closed tanks with smooth interiors, the ability to spray the tank headspace using spray balls on recirculating loop returns, and the use of heated, jacketed/insulated tanks. This minimizes corrosion and biofilm development and aids in thermal or chemical sanitization. Storage tanks require venting to compensate for the dynamics of changing water levels. This can be accomplished with a properly oriented and heat-traced filter housing fitted with a hydrophobic microbial retentive membrane filter affixed to an atmospheric vent. Alternatively, an automatic membrane-filtered compressed gas blanketing system may be used. In both cases, rupture disks equipped with a rupture alarm device should be used as a further safeguard for the mechanical integrity of the tank.

5.1.13 DISTRIBUTION SYSTEMS

Distribution system configuration should allow for the continuous flow of water in the piping by means of recirculation. Use of no recirculating, dead-end, or one-way systems or system segments should be avoided whenever possible. If not possible, these systems should be flushed periodically and monitored more closely. Experience has shown that continuously recirculated systems are easier to maintain. Pumps should be designed to deliver fully turbulent flow conditions to facilitate thorough heat distribution (for hot-water sanitized systems) as well as thorough chemical sanitant distribution. Turbulent flow also appears to either retard the development of biofilms or reduce the tendency of those biofilms to shed bacteria into the water. If redundant components, such as pumps or filters, are used, they should be configured and used to avoid microbial contamination of the system.

Components and distribution lines should be sloped and fitted with drain points so that the system can be completely drained. In distribution systems, dead legs and low-flow conditions should be avoided, and valved tie-in points should have length-to-diameter ratios of six or less. In systems that operate at self-sanitizing temperatures, precautions should be taken to avoid cool points where biofilm development could occur. If drainage of components or distribution lines is intended as a microbial control strategy, they should also be configured to be dried completely using dry compressed gas because drained but still moist surfaces will still support microbial proliferation. Water exiting from the distribution system should not be returned to the system without first passing through all or a portion of the purification system.

The distribution design should include the placement of sampling valves in the storage tank and at other locations, such as in the return line of the recirculating water system. Direct connections to processes or auxiliary equipment should be designed to prevent reverse flow into the controlled water system. Hoses and heat exchangers that are attached to points of use to deliver water must not chemically or microbiologically degrade the water quality. The distribution system should permit sanitization for microorganism control. The system may be continuously operated at sanitizing conditions or sanitized periodically.

5.1.14 NOVEL/EMERGING TECHNOLOGIES

New water treatment technologies are being developed continuously. Before these technologies are utilized in pharmaceutical water systems, they should be evaluated for acceptable use in a GMP environment. Other considerations should include the treatment process, reliability and robustness, use of added substances, materials of construction, and ability to validate. Consideration should be given to recognize the areas of concern during the evaluation and to identify control measures for the technology. This should include impact on chemical and microbial attributes.

5.2 Installation, Materials of Construction, and Component Selection

Installation techniques are important because they can affect the mechanical, corrosive, and sanitary integrity of the system. Valve installation should promote gravity drainage. Pipe supports should provide appropriate slopes for drainage and should be designed to support the piping adequately under worst-case thermal and flow conditions. The methods of connecting system components—including units of operation, tanks, and distribution piping—require careful attention to preclude potential operational and microbial problems.

Stainless steel welds should provide reliable joints that are internally smooth and corrosion-free. Low-carbon stainless steel, compatible wire filler where necessary, inert gas, automatic welding machines, and regular inspection and documentation help to ensure acceptable weld quality. Follow-up cleaning and passivation of metal surfaces after installation are important for removing contamination and corrosion products and to re-establish the passive corrosion-resistant surface.

Plastic materials can be fused (welded) in some cases, and also require smooth, uniform internal surfaces. Adhesive glues and solvents should be avoided due to the potential for voids and organic extractables. Mechanical methods of joining, such as flange fittings, require care to avoid the creation of offsets, gaps, penetrations, and voids. Use of plastic materials may contribute to TOC levels.

Control measures include good alignment, properly sized gaskets, appropriate spacing, uniform sealing force, and the avoidance of threaded fittings.

Materials of construction should be selected to be compatible with control measures such as sanitizing, cleaning, or passivation. Temperature rating is a critical factor in choosing appropriate materials because surfaces may be required to handle elevated operating and sanitization temperatures. If chemicals or additives will be used to clean, passivate, or sanitize the system, materials resistant to these chemicals or additives must be utilized. Materials should be capable of handling turbulent flow and elevated velocities without erosion of the corrosion-resistant film (such as the passive chromium oxide surface of stainless steel) or reduction in wall thickness for plastics. The finish on metallic materials such as stainless steel, whether it is a refined mill finish, polished to a specific grit, or an electropolished treatment, should complement the system design and provide satisfactory corrosion and microbial activity resistance. The finish should also be a material that can be chemically sanitized. Auxiliary equipment and fittings that require seals, gaskets, diaphragms, filter media, and membranes should exclude materials that permit the possibility of extractables, shedding, and microbial activity. Insulating materials exposed to stainless steel surfaces should be free of chlorides to avoid the phenomenon of stress corrosion cracking that can lead to system contamination and the destruction of tanks and critical system components.

Specifications are important to ensure proper selection of materials and to serve as a reference for system qualification and maintenance. Information such as the manufacturer's metallurgical reports for stainless steel and reports of composition, ratings, and material-handling capabilities for nonmetallic substances should be reviewed for suitability and retained for reference. Component (auxiliary equipment) selection should be made with assurance that it does not create a source of contamination intrusion. Heat exchangers should be constructed to prevent leakage of heat transfer medium into the pharmaceutical water and, for heat exchanger designs where prevention may fail, there should be a means to detect leakage. Pumps should be of sanitary design with seals that prevent contamination of the water. Valves should have smooth internal surfaces with the seat and closing device exposed to the flushing action of water, such as occurs in diaphragm valves. Valves with pocket areas or closing devices (e.g., ball, plug, gate, globe) that move into and out of the flow area should be avoided.

5.3 Sanitization

Microbial control in water systems is achieved primarily through sanitization practices. Systems can be sanitized using either thermal or (photo-)chemical means.

5.3.1 THERMAL SANITIZATION

Thermal approaches to system sanitization include periodic or continuously circulating hot water and the use of steam. Temperatures of 65°–80° are most commonly used for thermal sanitization. Continuously recirculating water of at least 65° at the coldest location in the distribution system has also been used effectively in stainless steel distribution systems when attention is paid to uniformity and distribution of such self-sanitizing temperatures. These techniques are limited to systems that are compatible with the higher temperatures needed to achieve sanitization. Frequent use of thermal sanitization at appropriate temperatures should eliminate the need for other sanitization methods.

The use of thermal methods at temperatures above 80° is contraindicated because it does not add to microbial control of the system or reduction of biofilm. Some methods (e.g., steam sanitizing, hot water circulation at temperatures ≥100°) can be less effective or even destructive because of the need to eliminate condensate or manipulate system components, stress materials of construction, deform filters, and its adverse impact on instrumentation.

Although thermal methods control biofilm development by either continuously inhibiting its growth or, in intermittent applications, by killing the microorganisms within developing biofilms, they are not effective in removing established biofilms. Killed but intact biofilms can become a nutrient source for rapid biofilm regrowth after the sanitizing conditions are removed or halted. In cases of infrequent thermal sanitizations that allow biofilm development between treatments, a combination of routine thermal treatment and periodic supplementation with chemical sanitization may be more effective. The more frequent the thermal sanitization, the more likely it is that biofilm re-development can be eliminated.

5.3.2 CHEMICAL SANITIZATION

Chemical methods, where compatible, can be used on a wider variety of construction materials. These methods typically use oxidizing agents such as ozone, hydrogen peroxide, peracetic acid, or combinations thereof. Halogenated compounds can be effective sanitizers but are less aggressive oxidizing agents and may be difficult to flush from the system. Chemical agents may not penetrate the full biofilm matrix or extend into all biofilm locations (such as crevices at gasketed fittings) and may leave biofilms incompletely inactivated. Compounds such as ozone, hydrogen peroxide, and peracetic acid oxidize bacteria and biofilms with reactive peroxides and by forming very reactive free radicals (notably hydroxyl radicals). The short half-life of ozone in particular, and its limitation on achievable concentrations, require that it be added continuously during the sanitization process. Hydrogen peroxide and ozone rapidly degrade to water and/or oxygen, and peracetic acid degrades to oxygen and acetic acid. The ease of degradation of ozone to oxygen using 254-nm UV lights in circulating loops allows it to be used effectively on a continuously sanitizing basis in holding tanks and on an intermittent basis (e.g., daily or weekly) in the distribution loops. The highly reactive nature of ozone requires the use of system materials and components that are even more oxidation resistant than those typically used with the other oxidizing agents.

It is important to note that microorganisms in a well-developed biofilm can be extremely difficult to kill, even by using aggressive oxidizing chemicals. The less developed and therefore thinner the biofilm, the more effective the biofilm inactivation. Therefore, optimal microbial control is achieved by using oxidizing chemicals at a frequency that does not permit significant biofilm development between treatments.

Validation of chemical sanitization requires demonstration of adequate chemical concentrations throughout the system, exposure to all wetted surfaces including the body of use point valves, and complete removal of the sanitant from the system at the completion of treatment. Methods validation for the detection and quantification of residues of the sanitant or its objectionable degradants is an essential part of the validation program.

5.3.3 UV SANITIZATION

In-line UV light at a wavelength of 254 nm can also be used to continuously "sanitize" only the water circulating in the system, but these devices must be properly sized for the water flow. Such devices inactivate a high percentage (but not 100%) of microorganisms that flow through the device but cannot be used to directly control existing biofilm upstream or downstream of the device. However, when coupled with conventional thermal or chemical sanitization technologies or located immediately upstream of a microbially retentive filter, UV light is most effective and can prolong the interval between needed system re-sanitizations.

5.3.4 SANITIZATION PROCEDURES

Sanitization steps require validation to demonstrate the ability to reduce and hold microbial contamination at acceptable levels. Validation of thermal methods should include a heat distribution study to demonstrate that sanitization temperatures are achieved throughout the system, including the body of use point valves; sampling ports; instrument side branches; and fittings, couplings, and adapters, relying on water convection and thermal conduction through system materials for heat transfer to wetted surfaces.

The routine frequency of sanitization should be supported by the results of system microbial monitoring. Conclusions derived from trend analysis of the microbiological data should be used as the alert mechanism for the need for extraordinary maintenance. The routine frequency of sanitization should be established in such a way that the system operates in a state of microbiological control and does not regularly exceed Alert and Action Levels (see *9.4 Defining Alert and Action Levels and Specifications*).

5.4 Operation, Maintenance, and Control

A preventive maintenance program should be established to ensure that the water system remains in a state of control. The program should include 1) procedures for operating the system, 2) monitoring programs for critical quality attributes and operating conditions including calibration of critical instruments, 3) schedule for periodic sanitization, 4) preventive maintenance of components, and 5) control of changes to the mechanical system and to operating conditions.

5.4.1 OPERATING PROCEDURES

Operating procedures for the water system and for performing routine maintenance and corrective action should be written, and they should also define the point when action is required. The procedures should be well documented, and should detail the function of each job, assign who is responsible for performing the work, describe how the job is to be done, and identify acceptable operating parameters. The effectiveness of these procedures should be assessed during water system validation.

5.4.2 PROCESS MONITORING PROGRAM

A process-monitoring program should establish the critical quality attributes and operating parameters that are documented and monitored. The program may include a combination of in-line sensors and/or automated instruments (e.g., for temperature, TOC conductivity, hardness, and chlorine), automated or manual documentation of operational parameters (e.g., flow rates or pressure drop across a carbon bed, filter, or RO unit), and laboratory tests (e.g., total microbial counts). The frequency of sampling, the requirement for evaluating test results, and the necessity of initiating corrective action should be included.

5.4.3 ROUTINE MICROBIAL CONTROL

Sanitization may be integral to operation and maintenance, and necessary on a routine basis, depending on system design and the selected units of operation, to maintain the system in a state of microbial control. Technologies for sanitization are described above in more detail in *5.3 Sanitization*.

5.4.4 PREVENTIVE MAINTENANCE

A preventive maintenance program should be in effect. The program should establish what preventive maintenance is to be performed, the frequency of maintenance work, and how the work should be documented.

5.4.5 CHANGE CONTROL

The mechanical configuration, operating conditions, and maintenance activities of the water system must be controlled. Proposed changes should be evaluated for their impact on the whole system. The need to requalify the system after changes are made should be determined. After a decision is made to modify a water system, the affected drawings, manuals, and procedures should be revised. Portions or operations of the water system that are affected by the modification should be tested to demonstrate a continued state of control. The extent and duration of testing should be related to the risk impact of the change to the system.

Change to read:

6. SAMPLING

The testing of water samples from a water system is critical to the ongoing control of the system and assessment of the quality of the water being used. If improperly collected, a sample could yield a test result that is unrepresentative of the sample's purpose. This could lead to inaction when remediation is needed or to unnecessary remediation when none is necessary. It could also lead to misinterpretations of product impact. Therefore, properly collecting water samples, understanding their purpose, and establishing appropriate water system sampling plans are essential to water quality control and system control.

6.1 Purposes and Procedures

To assess a particular water ■₁S (USP41) attribute, a sample of the water usually must be removed from a water system for specific ■₁S (USP41) attribute testing. ■The sample needs to be obtained from specific locations that are representative for the purpose being monitored.■₁S (USP41) This sample may be analyzed by in-line/on-line instruments or it may be completely removed from the system as a "grab sample" in a container for off-line testing. In-line/on-line testing avoids the exogenous contamination potential of grab samples that could lead to artifactually variable data trends and incorrect decisions on system performance, maintenance, and utilized ■water,■₁S (USP41) as well as initiating fruitless causative investigations. ■Grab samples may be appropriate where the water in the system is not homogeneous for certain attributes.■₁S (USP41)

The data from water testing are generally used for one of two purposes: for process control (PC) of the water purification and distribution system or for ■release or■₁S (USP41) QC of the water being drawn from the system for some application or use. In many cases, depending on the sampling location and sampling process, the resulting data can be used for both PC and QC purposes.

6.1.1 PC SAMPLING

Because PC sampling is intended to reflect the quality of the water behind the valve and within the distribution system, coming from the purification system, or between its purification steps, efforts should be made to avoid contaminating the water as it ■is■₁S (USP41) drawn from the system so that its test results accurately reflect the water quality within the system at that location. This may require the use of strategically located sampling ports, in addition to points of use.

If microbial testing is needed for PC purposes, the sampling valve should have a properly installed, sanitary design that uses vigorous pre-sampling flushing. This flushing shears off fragile biofilm structures growing on surfaces within the valve and water path before the sample is collected. This avoids biasing the microbial count of perhaps pristine water in the system behind that valve. A fully open valve flush (at >8 ft/s velocity within the valve and connector) for at least 30 s typically provides sufficient shear forces to adequately remove any fragile biofilm structures. Additional control measures for preventing sample contamination could also include stringent pre- and post-sampling outlet sanitation, the use of sterile hoses and gaskets or other connectors to direct the water flow, and other measures.

The data from PC sampling indicate how well the system is maintaining the water quality at that sampling location. These data are subsequently used to signal when some extraordinary intervention might be needed, in addition to normal maintenance and system sanitization operations, to restore the system to the expected level of purity.

PC sampling can only be used to indicate the quality of the water being delivered to the points of use (for QC purposes) if it has been shown to be representative of that point-of-use quality. This may be possible with chemical attributes that are typically not affected by the fluid path of the water delivery process, but is generally not possible with microbial attributes, which can be greatly affected by localized biofilms along that fluid path. If this fluid path is not utilized for PC sampling, then the resulting data typically cannot be used for QC purposes.

6.1.2 QC SAMPLING

QC sampling is intended to reflect the quality of water that is being used. These samples should be collected at the true point of use; that is, where the water is delivered for use, not where it leaves the water system. QC sampling must utilize that same delivery path and components utilized for a water transfer during actual water use. This includes the same valves, hoses, heat exchangers, flow totalizers, hard-piped connections, and other components utilized during water use.

In addition to the water transfer components, QC sampling must also use the same water transfer process employed during water use, including the same pre-use outlet and delivery path flushing procedure and the same outlet, fitting, and hose sanitization practices employed during actual water use. The water delivery process and components used for QC sampling must be identical to manufacturing practices at every system outlet for the QC sample to mimic the quality of water being used by accumulating the same chemical and microbial contaminant levels it would during actual use from that outlet location.

Where permanent connections from the water system to equipment are present, accommodation should be made in the design to collect samples from locations as close to the equipment as possible. For example, samples can be collected from special sample ports or other valves near the equipment connection that allow the collected water sample to accurately reflect the water quality that is used. Where the water transfer conduit is designed and/or definitively treated to eliminate all contaminating influences prior to water transfer through that conduit, PC sampling locations within the distribution system can reflect the quality of the water that is actually used for QC purposes at those permanent connections. However, the success of the design and treatments intended to eliminate these contaminating influences must be verified. This is typically done during water system validation.

Where routine water use practices involve contamination-prone activities, such as no pre-use flushing or poor hose storage/sanitization/replacement practices, these water use practices should be improved to reduce the potential for delivering contaminated water from the water system and for unacceptable QC sample testing results that reflect that same contamination.

6.2 Attributes and Sampling Locations

The tests being performed on the samples are relevant to the sampling location and purpose of the sample. In-process monitoring of nonmonograph attributes may be indicated for specific unit operations. For instance, before and after a softener, it may be important to determine water hardness to verify softener efficacy. Before and after an activated carbon bed/filter, it may be important to verify chlorine or TOC removal and/or reduction or test for an increase in microbial count. Before a distillation unit, it may be important to quantitate the incoming bacterial endotoxin level to ensure that the still is not being overchallenged beyond its typical 3–4 log purification capability. However, once the water is in the distribution system, the compendial attributes of importance typically include at least conductivity, TOC, and microbial count. In Water for Injection systems and other systems or system locations where bacterial endotoxin control is important, endotoxin is also assayed. Other tests may be necessary depending on the intended uses of the water.

6.2.1 CHEMICAL ATTRIBUTES

Dissolved chemical contaminants detected by conductivity or TOC testing tend to be uniformly distributed in the water throughout the water system. However, there are exceptions where localized chemical contamination sources can occur, such as from a coolant-leaking heat exchanger in a sub-loop, or at a point of use, or within a dead leg. These chemical contaminants may only be seen at the associated outlets and not systemically. However, in the absence of localized contamination influences, chemical attributes are candidates for on-line testing at fixed strategic locations within the distribution system, such as near a circulating loop return, and are generally reflective of the same chemical quality at all locations and points of use within the distribution system. Nevertheless, the suitability of the on-line locations of these instruments for QC release purposes must be verified as being representative of the use-point water quality. This is usually done during water system validation.

6.2.2 MICROBIAL ATTRIBUTES

The same uniformity scenario cannot be assumed for microbial attributes. Planktonic organisms in a water sample could have originated from biofilms in the purification or distribution systems releasing more or less uniform levels of planktonic organisms into the circulating water, as detectable in samples from all outlets. However, a local biofilm developing within a water delivery conduit (such as a use-point outlet valve and transfer hose) in an otherwise pristine biofilm-free water system could release planktonic organisms detectable only in water delivered through that conduit. Therefore, QC release samples for assessing the quality of water that is delivered by the system during water use must be collected after the water has traversed the same fluid conduit (including the same preparatory activities such as outlet sanitization and pre-flushing) from the water distribution system to the specific locations where the water is used.

On-line microbial water sampling/testing has value in pharmaceutical water systems only for PC purposes unless the water is taken from the point of use in the same manner as routine water usage, in which case the data can also have a QC release purpose. Microbial counts detected from strategic sampling ports continue to have PC and investigational value, but generally cannot be substituted for QC release testing except in certain scenarios, as described in *6.1.2 QC Sampling*.

6.3 Validation Sampling Plans

The initial sampling plan for a pharmaceutical water system is usually developed for a validation program (see *4. Validation and Qualification of Water Purification, Storage, and Distribution Systems*). This strategy is for characterization of the system's ability to purify, distribute, and deliver pharmaceutical water. Typically, the initial validation sampling is for a short duration (e.g., at least 2–4 weeks) at a high sampling frequency to generate a significant body of data that will allow detection of short-term or localized chemical or microbial quality deviations from all outlets. These data provide an initial assessment of system performance to guide decisions about using the water for operational purposes.

The initial validation sampling plan is re-evaluated when the pharmaceutical water is placed into operation, typically to reduce the amount of data being generated while not compromising the ability to identify anomalous operations/events, especially during the early life cycle of the water system. In the absence of such quality deviations during the initial sampling period, the sampling frequency can be lessened for a period of time (e.g., at least 2–4 additional weeks) to ensure that somewhat longer-term adverse quality trends are not apparent. During this second period of time, the water may be considered for at-risk routine use, pending the acceptable completion of the second validation sampling period. After successful completion, monitoring can eventually be lessened again to what will become the routine sampling plan.

Periodic review of the water system operation and monitoring needs to be performed to assess seasonal source water variability, effectiveness of sanitization, and routine maintenance events. Periodic review should be performed during the complete life cycle of the water system, typically annually, for evidence of longer-term data trends and quality deviations.

The routine sampling plan should be re-evaluated periodically based on the available data to determine the appropriate frequency and sample locations. This review offers an opportunity to improve data evaluation and reduce workloads based on what that data indicate relative to process and quality control. The routine sampling plan should have a rationale for the frequency and locations that are selected to justify how the resulting data will be used to characterize the overall operation of the system and the release of the water for use.

6.4 Routine Sampling Plans

6.4.1 SOURCE WATER SAMPLING

As mentioned in earlier sections, the source water for pharmaceutical water systems must comply with the standards for one of the Drinking Waters listed in the associated compendial water monograph or in *General Notices*. When a municipality or other water authority is providing this Drinking Water, they are required to comply with the local Drinking Water Regulations for the water supplied to a drinking or potable water distribution piping grid for that region. The quality of that water by the time it reaches the pharmaceutical user is dependent on a number of factors including distance from the input source, duration of travel within the piping, and condition of the piping in that potable water distribution grid, any of which could have adversely affected some of its initial chemical and/or microbial attributes. Based on a risk assessment, it may be prudent to verify full compliance with regulations using water collected from sample ports prior to the pretreatment system, or other equivalent Drinking Water outlets within the facility. If the water complies, then continued assurance of compliance could be verified using Drinking Water Regulation test results provided by the water authority or by periodic retesting of selected or all the Drinking Water attributes by the user or by both the user and the water authority. If private sourced water is utilized, it is the user's responsibility to demonstrate full Drinking Water regulation compliance, using water samples from such sampling ports on a periodic basis as determined by a risk analysis.

These pre-pretreatment sampling ports could, at the user's discretion, be used to periodically monitor other source water attributes that could affect specific pretreatment or purification unit operations. Depending on the user's source water quality consistency and a risk assessment of its potential impact on the purification process, the periodically monitored attributes could include microbial count, absence of coliforms, bacterial endotoxin levels, conductivity, TOC, pH, hardness, chlorine, silica, turbidity or silt density index, and others. These data could be useful in investigations and for operational adjustments to critical unit operation parameters and maintenance procedures, or for feedback to the potable water provider if unusual trends are observed.

6.4.2 PRETREATMENT AND PURIFICATION SYSTEM SAMPLING

The location and frequency of sampling from ports within the pretreatment and purification systems may be selected based on a risk analysis of unit operation purpose. The purpose of this sampling is primarily for PC, for example, to ensure maintenance of acceptable unit operation performance, to assess maintenance procedure efficacy, and to investigate the need for remedial action. Quality deviations in the early portions of the purification process can affect unit operation efficiency but usually do not impact the finished water quality or acceptable use.

6.4.3 PURIFIED WATER DISTRIBUTION SYSTEM SAMPLING

Purified Water distribution system sampling is intended to provide continuing assurance of ongoing PC and compliance with the user's finished water chemical and microbiological requirements. Generally, the locations for that sampling and the frequency of testing the specific attributes are a matter of process and quality control consistency, as well as risk tolerance in the event of a deviation.

Depending on the water system design, the chemical attributes of a water system tend to be relatively constant and more uniformly distributed than the microbiological attributes. Therefore, less frequent sampling at only selected locations could be justified for chemical testing based on familiarity with system design and the existence of historically consistent operational data. However, with some purification system designs, the chemical quality could change dramatically in a short period of time (such as from the exhaustion of deionization beds), so frequent or even continuous in-line/on-line monitoring of the chemical attributes would be advisable to be able to recognize and correct the cause of the problem before non-compliant water is produced and used.

For microbial testing, all use points and critical sample ports in a distribution system are typically sampled routinely, including those that are infrequently used by manufacturing. There is no prescribed sampling frequency for Purified Water system outlets, so typical outlet sampling frequencies vary from daily to monthly, with sampling occurring somewhere in the system at least at weekly intervals.

A risk analysis is suggested for determining the sampling plan for a Purified Water system. Factors in this analysis could include (but are not limited to) the test result history for the entire water system as well as specific outlets, the criticality of specific outlets to manufacturing, the usefulness of selected sample ports as indicators of ongoing system control, and the scope of impact on products and activities should an unfavorable test result occur. For the scope of impact, the less frequent the sampling, the more products and processes will be impacted by an unfavorable test result.

6.4.4 WATER FOR INJECTION DISTRIBUTION SYSTEM SAMPLING

The sampling plans for Water for Injection distribution systems (as well as any water system where some level of bacterial endotoxin control is needed) utilize the same general sampling approaches as do Purified Water systems. However, the regulatory expectations for Water for Injection distribution system sampling plans are more prescriptive because microbial control must be much more stringent as it is related to the bacterial endotoxin attribute. In general, water sampling for microbial and bacterial endotoxin testing is expected to occur daily somewhere in the system, with each outlet being sampled periodically, based on a risk assessment, to characterize the quality of the water.

6.5 Non-Routine Sampling

Non-routine sampling can also be performed on the water system for episodic events or reasons for which the routine sampling plans are insufficient to capture the needed information. Examples include change control purposes such as evaluating potential changes to sampling, testing, maintenance procedures, or system design; data or event excursion investigation purposes; or simply for long-term informational purposes and establishing baselines for future investigational value. The purpose of the non-routine sampling dictates the sampling procedures to be used, the attributes to be tested, and the location and repeating occurrence (if any) of that testing. It should also be noted that such non-routine sampling may be done from sampling ports that may or may not be routinely tested. Sampling ports can be positioned in a water system purely for investigational, non-routine sampling, and as such, they do not need to be part of a routine sampling plan.

Change to read:

7. CHEMICAL EVALUATIONS

7.1 Chemical Tests for Bulk Waters

The chemical attributes of *Purified Water* and *Water for Injection* that were in effect prior to *USP 23* were specified by a series of chemistry tests for various specific and nonspecific attributes with the intent of detecting chemical species indicative of incomplete or inadequate purification. Although these methods could have been considered barely adequate to control the quality of these waters, they nevertheless stood the test of time. This was partly because the operation of water systems was, and still is, based on on-line conductivity measurements and specifications generally thought to preclude the failure of these archaic chemistry attribute tests.

In 1996, USP moved away from these chemical attribute tests, switching to contemporary analytical technologies for the bulk waters Purified Water and Water for Injection. The intent was to upgrade the analytical technologies without tightening the quality requirements. The two contemporary analytical technologies employed were TOC and conductivity. The TOC test replaced the test for *Oxidizable Substances* that primarily targeted organic contaminants. A multi-staged conductivity test that detects ionic (mostly inorganic) contaminants replaced, with the exception of the test for *Heavy Metals*, all of the inorganic chemical tests (i.e., *Ammonia, Calcium, Carbon Dioxide, Chloride, Sulfate*).

Replacing the heavy metals attribute was considered unnecessary because 1) the source water specifications (found in the U.S. EPA's NPDWR) for individual heavy metals were tighter than the approximate limit of detection of the *Heavy Metals* test for *USP XXII* Water for Injection and Purified Water (approximately 0.1 ppm), 2) contemporary water system construction materials do not leach heavy metal contaminants, and 3) test results for this attribute have uniformly been negative; there has not been a confirmed occurrence of a singular test failure (failure of only the *Heavy Metals* test with all other attributes passing) since the current heavy metal drinking water standards have been in place.

Total Solids and *pH* were the only tests not covered by conductivity testing. The test for *Total Solids* was considered redundant because the nonselective tests of conductivity and TOC could detect most chemical species other than silica, which could remain undetected in its colloidal form. Colloidal silica in Purified Water and Water for Injection is easily removed by most water pretreatment steps, and even if present in the water, it constitutes no medical or functional hazard except in extreme and rare situations. In such extreme situations, other attribute extremes are also likely to be detected. It is, however, the user's responsibility to ensure fitness for use. If silica is a significant component in the source water, and the purification unit operations could fail and selectively allow silica to be released into the finished water (in the absence of co-contaminants detectable by conductivity), then either silica-specific testing or a total-solids type testing should be utilized to monitor for and control this rare problem.

The *pH* attribute was eventually recognized to be redundant to the conductivity test (which included *pH* as an aspect of the test and specification); therefore, *pH* was discontinued as a separate attribute test.

The rationale used by USP to establish its Purified Water and Water for Injection conductivity specifications took into consideration the conductivity contributed by the two least-conductive former attributes of *Chloride* and *Ammonia*, thereby precluding their failure had those wet chemistry tests been performed. In essence, the *Stage 3* conductivity specifications (see *Water Conductivity* ⟨645⟩, *Bulk Water, Procedure, Stage 3*) were established from the sum of the conductivities of the limit concentrations of chloride ions (from pH 5.0 to 6.2) and ammonia ions (from pH 6.3 to 7.0), plus the unavoidable contribution of other conductivity-contributing ions from water (H^+ and OH^-), dissolved atmospheric carbon dioxide (as HCO_3^-), and an electro-balancing quantity of either sodium (Na^+) or chlorine (Cl^-), depending on the pH-induced ionic imbalance (see *Table 1*). The *Stage 2* conductivity specification is the lowest value in this table, 2.1 µS/cm. The *Stage 1* specifications, designed primarily for on-line measurements, were derived by essentially summing the lowest values in ∎individual (H^+, OH^-, HCO_3^-) and group (Cl^-, Na^+, NH_4^+) of∎₁ₛ ₍USP41₎ contributing ion columns for each of a series of tables similar to *Table 1*, created for each 5° increment between 0° and 100°. For example purposes, the italicized values in *Table 1*, the conductivity data table for 25°, were summed to yield a conservative value of 1.3 µS/cm, the *Stage 1* specification for a nontemperature-compensated, nonatmosphere-equilibrated water sample that actually had a measured temperature of 25°–29°. Each 5° increment in the table was similarly treated to yield the individual values listed in the table of *Stage 1* specifications (see *Water Conductivity* ⟨645⟩, *Bulk Water*).

**Table 1. Contributing Ion Conductivities of the Chloride-Ammonia Model as a Function of pH
(in atmosphere-equilibrated water at 25°)**

	Conductivity (µS/cm)							
pH	H+	OH−	HCO₃−	Cl−	Na+	NH₄+	Combined Conductivities	Stage 3 Limit
5.0	*3.49*	*0*	*0.02*	*1.01*	*0.19*	*0*	4.71	4.7
5.1	2.77	0	0.02	1.01	0.29	0	4.09	4.1
5.2	2.20	0	0.03	1.01	0.38	0	3.62	3.6
5.3	1.75	0	0.04	1.01	0.46	0	3.26	3.3
5.4	1.39	0	0.05	1.01	0.52	0	2.97	3.0
5.5	1.10	0	0.06	1.01	0.58	0	2.75	2.8
5.6	0.88	0	0.08	1.01	0.63	0	2.60	2.6
5.7	0.70	0	0.10	1.01	0.68	0	2.49	2.5
5.8	0.55	0	0.12	1.01	0.73	0	2.41	2.4
5.9	0.44	0	0.16	1.01	0.78	0	2.39	2.4
6.0	0.35	0	0.20	1.01	0.84	0	2.40	2.4
6.1	0.28	0	0.25	1.01	0.90	0	2.44	2.4
6.2	0.22	0	0.31	1.01	0.99	0	2.53	2.5
6.3	0.18	0	0.39	0.63	0	1.22	2.42	2.4
6.4	0.14	0.01	0.49	0.45	0	1.22	2.31	2.3
6.5	0.11	0.01	0.62	0.22	0	1.22	2.18	2.2
6.6	0.09	0.01	0.78	0	0.04	1.22	2.14	2.1
6.7	0.07	0.01	0.99	0	0.27	1.22	2.56	2.6
6.8	0.06	0.01	1.24	0	0.56	1.22	3.09	3.1
6.9	0.04	0.02	1.56	0	0.93	1.22	3.77	3.8
7.0	*0.03*	0.02	1.97	0	1.39	1.22	4.63	4.6

As stated above, this rather radical change to utilizing a conductivity attribute as well as the inclusion of a TOC attribute allowed for on-line measurements. This was a major philosophical change and allowed industry to realize substantial savings. The TOC and conductivity tests can also be performed off-line in the laboratories using collected samples, although sample collection tends to introduce opportunities for adventitious contamination that can cause false high readings. The collection of on-line data is not, however, without challenges. The continuous readings tend to create voluminous amounts of data, where previously only a single data point was available. As stated in *6. Sampling*, continuous in-process data are excellent for understanding how a water system performs during all of its various usage and maintenance events in real time, but this is too much data for QC purposes. Therefore, for example, one can use a justifiable portion of the data (at a designated daily time or at the time of batch manufacturing) or the highest value in a given period as a worst case representation of the overall water quality for that period. Data averaging is generally discouraged because of its ability to obscure short-lived extreme quality events.

7.2 Chemical Tests for Sterile Waters

Packaged/sterile waters present a particular dilemma relative to the attributes of conductivity and TOC. The package itself is the major source of chemicals (inorganics and organics) that leach over time into the packaged water and can easily be detected by the conductivity and TOC tests. The irony of organic leaching from plastic packaging is that before the advent of bulk water TOC testing, when the *Oxidizable Substances* test was the only "organic purity" test for both bulk and packaged/sterile water monographs in *USP*, the insensitivity of that test to many of the organic leachables from plastic and elastomeric packaging materials was largely unrecognized, allowing organic levels in packaged/sterile water to be quite high (possibly many times the TOC specification for bulk water).

Similarly, glass containers can also leach inorganics, such as sodium, which are easily detected by conductivity but poorly detected by the former wet chemistry attribute tests. Most of these leachables are considered harmless based on current perceptions and standards at the rather significant concentrations present. Nevertheless, they effectively degrade the quality of the high-purity waters placed into these packaging systems. Some packaging materials contain more leachables than others and may not be as suitable for holding water and maintaining its purity.

The attributes of conductivity and TOC tend to reveal more about the packaging leachables than they do about the water's original purity. These currently "allowed" leachables could render the sterile packaged versions of originally equivalent bulk water essentially unsuitable for many uses where the bulk waters are perfectly adequate.

Therefore, to better control the ionic packaging leachables, ⟨645⟩ is divided into two sections. The first, *Water Conductivity* ⟨645⟩, *Bulk Water*, applies to *Purified Water*, *Water for Injection*, *Water for Hemodialysis*, and *Pure Steam*, and includes the three-stage conductivity testing instructions and specifications. The second, *Water Conductivity* ⟨645⟩, *Sterile Water*, applies to *Sterile Purified Water*, *Sterile Water for Injection*, *Sterile Water for Inhalation*, and *Sterile Water for Irrigation*. The *Sterile Water* section includes conductivity specifications similar to the *Water Conductivity* ⟨645⟩, *Bulk Water, Procedure, Stage 2* testing approach because it is intended as a laboratory test, and these sterile waters were made from bulk water that already complied with the three-stage conductivity test. In essence, packaging leachables are the primary target analytes of the conductivity specifications in *Water Conductivity* ⟨645⟩, *Sterile Water*. The effect on potential leachables from different container sizes is the rationale for having two different specifications, one for small packages containing nominal volumes of 10 mL or less and another for larger packages. These conductivity specifications are harmonized with the *European Pharmacopoeia* conductivity specifications for Sterile Water for Injection. All monographed waters, except *Bacteriostatic Water for Injection*, have a conductivity specification that directs the user to either the *Bulk Water* or the *Sterile Water* section. For the sterile packaged water monographs, this water conductivity specification replaces the redundant wet chemistry limit tests intended for inorganic contaminants that had previously been specified in these monographs.

Controlling the organic purity of these sterile packaged waters, particularly those in plastic packaging, is more challenging. Although the TOC test can better detect these impurities and therefore can be better used to monitor and control these impurities than the current *Oxidizable Substances* test, the latter has a history of use for many decades and has the flexibility to test a variety of packaging types and volumes that are applicable to these sterile packaged waters. Nevertheless, TOC testing of these currently allowed sterile, plastic-packaged waters reveals substantial levels of plastic-derived organic leachables that render the water perhaps orders of magnitude less organically pure than is typically achieved with bulk waters. Therefore, usage of these packaged waters for analytical, manufacturing, and cleaning applications should only be exercised after the purity of the water for the application has been confirmed as suitable.

▪7.3 Storage and Hold Times for Chemical Tests

Due to the homogeneous nature of chemical impurities in water, unlike the challenges of microbial impurities, the storage requirements and impact of holding times are very practically determined. In general, the chemical purity of high-purity water samples can only degrade over time, possibly generating a failed result of the sample that would have passed if it were tested immediately or on-line. The general fact is that the longer samples are stored, the greater the potential to be adversely impacted by containers or conditions.

For off-line chemical tests or waters, there are no compendial requirements for storage time and conditions. However, the general recommendation is to perform testing as soon as practical to avoid false adverse results. Where possible, store cool and measure as quickly as practical. This reduces the chances that a water sample gets contaminated over time, and this would reduce unwarranted and unnecessary investigations of false positives.

7.3.1 CONTAINERS

When sampling water for off-line analysis, the selection and cleanliness of the container play a significant part in obtaining accurate data. For samples to be tested for chemical impurities according to ⟨645⟩ and *Total Organic Carbon* ⟨643⟩, the proper container should be one that does not contaminate the sample during the storage/hold time. For example, the use and preparation of glass containers could be very acceptable for storing samples for TOC testing, but some glass containers do leach ions over time (hours and days), and they can adversely impact a conductivity test by creating a false positive result—if the storage time is too long. Likewise, there are some polymer materials that can adversely impact the TOC chemical impurity in water. However, many polymer materials are very inert.

In any case, cleanliness of the container is crucial because trace quantities of soaps and fingerprints will adversely impact the chemical purity of the water. Properly cleaned containers are acceptable because chemical impurities are easily rinsed away. Extensive chemical cleaning methods such as acid or caustic rinsing should never be needed. If they are needed, consider replacing the containers.

7.3.2 STORAGE TIME AND CONDITIONS

There are no specific recommendations for storage of samples for water analyses. If there is some trace interaction of the container and water, then generally colder and shorter storage times are better than warmer and longer storage times. Chemical dissolution and reactivity are usually enhanced by increased temperature. Furthermore, time is always an element because the water sample can only get worse in a container, and it never gets better with time.

7.4 Elemental Impurities in Pharmaceutical Waters

Elemental impurities (EI) have the most restrictive limits for Water for Injection used in manufacturing parenterals, in particular large-volume injections (see *Injections and Implanted Drug Products* ⟨1⟩ for a definition of large-volume injections) because of the large dose. The most restrictive permissible daily exposure (PDE) of EI resides with lead, mercury, cadmium, and arsenic. Other EI listed in ⟨232⟩ permit a substantially higher PDE, and are therefore less restrictive.

Water that meets U.S. EPA National Primary Drinking Water Regulations or WHO Drinking Water Guidelines that has been purified by conventional technologies used to produce Water for Injection can comply with ⟨232⟩ for parenterals.

Table 2 shows that source water that meets US EPA NPDWR or WHO Drinking Water Guidelines has maximum contaminant levels (concentration) for lead, mercury, cadmium, and arsenic that are NMT 10 times (1-log) higher than the EI limits for parenterals, based on a daily dose of 2000 mL. For a smaller volume injection, the allowed parenteral daily dose of EI is correspondingly higher. The purification technologies needed to produce Water for Injection that reduce the impurities by a factor of 100 to 1000 will assure compliance with ⟨232⟩, provided there are no elemental impurities added during processing, packaging, delivery, or storage.

Table 2. Elemental Impurity Limits for Drug Products and their Water Components per ⟨232⟩

Element	Parenteral PDE (µg/day)	Parenteral Daily Dose (µg/mL[a])	U.S. EPA National Primary Drinking Water Regulations (µg/mL[b])	WHO Drinking Water Guidelines (µg/mL[b])	Result of 2-Log Reduction of EI Concentration for WFI (µg/mL[c])
Cadmium	2	0.001	0.005	0.003	0.00005
Lead	5	0.0025	0.015	0.01	0.00015
Inorganic arsenic	15	0.0075	0.01	0.01	0.0001
Inorganic mercury	3	0.0015	0.002	0.006	0.00006

[a] Concentration based on a daily dose of 2000 mL, and all drug product elemental impurities coming from the water component.
[b] Drinking Water Regulations state these Maximum Contaminant Levels (MCLs) as mg/L, which equals µg/mL or ppm.
[c] Determined from the greater of the US EPA Regulations column and WHO Guidelines column for each element, then divided by 100 (2–log).

Chemical purification technologies for Purified Water are similarly efficient in removing EI as those for Water for Injection production. Because all sterile waters are prepared from Purified Water or Water for Injection, the assurance of compliance to ⟨232⟩ extends to sterile waters, provided there are no elemental impurities added during processing, packaging, delivery, or storage.

Further discussion can be found in *Pharmacopeial Forum* [see Bevilacqua A, Soli TC, USP Chemical Analysis Expert Committee. Elemental impurities in pharmaceutical waters. *Pharm Forum.* 2013;39(1)].■1S (USP41)

Change to read:

8. MICROBIAL EVALUATIONS

This section of the chapter presents a discussion about the types and sources of microorganisms and whether certain microbes are prone to colonize pharmaceutical water systems. This section also addresses microbiological examination of water samples, including a discussion on recovery methods.

8.1 Microorganism Types

Microorganisms are ubiquitous and their natural habitats are extremely diverse. Based on comparative ribosomal RNA sequencing, the phylogenetic tree of life consists of three domains: Bacteria and Archaea (both prokaryotes), and Eukarya (eukaryotes). Most microorganisms that contaminate pharmaceutical products are prokaryotic bacteria and eukaryotic fungi (yeasts and molds). These microbes are typical isolates from pharmaceutical environments, including the associated personnel, and a few are frank or opportunistic pathogens. Contamination with viruses is a concern in bioprocessing that uses animal cells.

8.1.1 ARCHAEANS

Microbes from the domain Archaea are phylogenetically related to prokaryotes but are distinct from bacteria. Many are extremophiles, with some species capable of growing at very high temperatures (hyperthermophiles) or in other extreme environments beyond the tolerance of any other life form. In general, most extremophiles are anaerobic or microaerophilic chemolithoautotrophs. Because of their unique habitats, metabolism, and nutritional requirements, Archaeans are not known to be frank or opportunistic pathogens, and they are not capable of colonizing a pharmaceutical water system.

8.1.2 BACTERIA

Bacteria are of immense importance because of their rapid growth, mutation rates, and ability to exist under diverse and adverse conditions; ▪some of them are human pathogens.▪1S (USP41) Some are very small and can pass through 0.2-μm rated filters. Others form spores, which are not part of their reproductive cycle. Bacterial spore formation is a complex developmental process that allows the organisms to produce a dormant and highly resistant cell in times of extreme stress. Bacterial endospores can survive high temperatures, strong UV irradiation, desiccation, chemical damage, and enzymatic destruction, which would normally kill vegetative bacteria.

Using a traditional cellular staining technique based on cell wall compositional differences, bacteria are categorized into Gram positive and Gram negative, although many sub-groups exist within each category based on genomic similarities and differences.

8.1.2.1 Gram-positive bacteria: Gram-positive bacteria are common in a pharmaceutical manufacturing environment but not in water systems. This is because they are generally not suited to surviving in a liquid environment that has the chemical purity of a pharmaceutical-grade water system. Gram-positive bacteria include the spore-forming bacteria from the genus *Bacillus*, which are common soil and dust ▪microorganisms,▪1S (USP41) and the non-sporulating bacteria from the genera *Staphylococcus*, *Streptococcus*, and *Micrococcus*, which normally colonize human skin and mucous membranes. Other types of Gram-positive bacterial ▪microorganisms▪1S (USP41) include organisms from the genera *Corynebacterium*, *Mycobacterium*, *Arthrobacter*, *Propionibacterium*, *Streptomyces*, and *Actinomyces*. This latter group of microbes can be found in various natural habitats including the human skin and soil.

Although Gram-positive bacteria can be detected in pharmaceutical water samples, their recovery is often associated with faulty aseptic technique during sampling or testing, or associated with exogenous contamination sources. Although these non-aquatic microorganisms could be present in source water and could, in rare circumstances, make their way into the early stages of a water purification unit operation, Gram-positive bacteria are not known to colonize water systems. In addition, these microbes will likely be removed by one or more of the purification unit operations prior to the ultimate creation of the pharmaceutical-grade water.

8.1.2.2 Gram-negative bacteria: These types of bacteria are found in soil, water, plants, and animals. Gram-negative bacteria are ▪relevant▪1S (USP41) to pharmaceutical manufacturers, primarily due to their production of endotoxins ▪as well as their ability to populate water systems,▪1S (USP41) a topic discussed in *8.4 Endotoxin*. Some Gram-negative bacteria prefer aquatic habitats and tend to colonize water systems and other wet environments as biofilms, a topic discussed in *8.2 Biofilm Formation in Water Systems*.

8.1.2.3 Mycoplasma: Organisms from the genus Mycoplasma are the smallest of the bacteria. Unlike other bacteria, these organisms do not have a cell wall and many exist as intracellular or animal▪/plant▪1S (USP41) parasites. Mycoplasmas also ▪may ▪1S (USP41) require specific nutrients for survival, including ▪sterols,▪1S (USP41) and they cannot survive in a hypotonic environment such as pure water. Based on these facts, this type of bacteria is not a concern for pharmaceutical-grade water systems.

8.1.3 FUNGI

Fungi are mainly aerobic mesophilic microbes. They exist as unicellular (yeast) and multicellular filamentous (mold) organisms. Molds are often found in wet/moist but usually non-aquatic environments, such as soil and decaying vegetation. ▪Yeasts are often associated with humans and vegetation, and both yeasts and molds also can be found in pharmaceutical environment.▪1S (USP41) As mold matures it develops spores, which, unlike bacterial spores, are part of its reproductive cycle and are less resistant to adverse conditions. Mold spores are easily spread through air and materials, and could contaminate water samples.
▪1S (USP41)

Neither yeasts nor molds are suited for colonization or survival in pharmaceutical water systems. Their recovery is often associated with faulty aseptic technique during sampling or testing, or associated with exogenous contamination sources. These non-aquatic microorganisms, if present in source water, could make their way into the early stages of a water purification system; however, they will likely be removed by one or more of the purification unit operations.

8.1.4 VIRUSES

A virus is a small infectious agent unlike eukaryotes and prokaryotes. This is because viruses have no metabolic abilities of their own. Viruses are genetic elements containing either DNA or RNA that replicate within host cells. Human pathogenic viruses, especially those of fecal origin, could be present in source water. However, they are easily neutralized by typical water purification treatments, such as chlorination. Therefore, it is unlikely that ■human pathogenic■₁S (USP41) viruses will be present or will proliferate (due to the absence of host cells) in pharmaceutical-grade waters.

8.1.5 THERMOPHILES

Thermophiles are heat-loving organisms and can be either bacteria or molds. Thermophilic and hyperthermophilic aquatic microorganisms (see *8.1.1 Archaeans*) require unique environmental and nutritional conditions to survive ■(e.g., presence of specific inorganic or organic nutrients and their concentrations, extreme pH, presence or absence of oxygen).■₁S (USP41) These conditions do not exist in the high-purity water of pharmaceutical water systems, whether ambient or hot, to support their growth. Bacteria that are able to inhabit hot pharmaceutical water systems are invariably found in much cooler locations within these hot systems; for example, within infrequently used outlets, ambient subloops off of hot loops, use-point and sub-loop cooling heat exchangers, transfer hoses and connecting pipes, or dead legs. These bacterial contaminants are the same mesophilic (moderate temperature-loving) types found in ambient water systems and are not thermophiles. Based on these facts, thermophilic bacteria are not a concern for hot pharmaceutical-grade water systems.

8.2 Biofilm Formation in Water Systems

A biofilm is a three-dimensional structured community of sessile microbial cells embedded in a matrix of extracellular polymeric substances (EPS). Biofilms form when bacteria attach to surfaces in moist environments and produce a slimy, glue-like substance, the EPS matrix, while proliferating at that location. This slimy matrix facilitates biofilm adhesion to surfaces as well as the attachment of additional planktonic cells to form a microbial community.

The EPS matrix of biofilms that colonize water systems also facilitates adsorption and concentration of nutrients from the water and retains the metabolites and waste products produced by the embedded biofilm cells, which can serve as nutrients for other biofilm community members.

This EPS matrix is also largely responsible for biofilm's resistance to chemical sanitizers, which must penetrate completely through the matrix to contact and kill the biofilm cells within the matrix. Heat sanitization approaches do not generally have these EPS matrix penetration difficulties, so they are usually considered superior to chemicals in killing biofilms where materials of construction allow.

The three-dimensional structure of a well-developed biofilm, as well as the biofilm's creation and release of small, motile "pioneer cells" for further colonization, are facilitated through gene expression modulating "quorum sensing" chemicals released in tiny amounts by individual biofilm cells and concentrated to a functional level within this same EPS matrix. So, the EPS matrix of biofilms is primarily responsible for the biofilm's success in colonizing and proliferating in very low nutrient-containing high-purity water systems. The EPS matrix also explains the difficulty in killing and/or removing biofilms from water purification and distribution system surfaces.

8.2.1 BIOFILM-FORMING BACTERIA IN WATER SYSTEMS

Common microorganisms recovered from water system samples include Gram-negative bacteria from the genera *Pseudomonas, Ralstonia, Burkholderia, Stenotrophomonas, Comamonas, Methylobacterium,* and many other types of *Pseudomonas*-like organisms known collectively as pseudomonads ■(members of the family *Pseudomonadaceae*).■₁S (USP41) These types of microbes, found in soil and source water, tend to colonize all water system distribution and purification system surfaces including activated carbon beds, deionizing resin beds, RO systems, membrane filtration modules, connecting piping, hoses, and valves. If not controlled, they can compromise the functionality of purification steps in the system and spread downstream, possibly forming biofilms on the distribution system surfaces such as tanks, piping, valves, hoses, and other surfaces, from where they can be sheared or otherwise released into the finished water used in processes and products.

Some of the biofilm pseudomonads are opportunistic human pathogens and may possess resistance to commonly used pharmaceutical product preservatives, particularly when embedded in EPS matrix flocs sheared from water system biofilms. Several pseudomonads are also capable of utilizing a wide variety of carbon sources as nutrients, allowing them to colonize austere, adventitious nutrient environments such as water systems. This nutritional diversity also makes them capable of growing to very high numbers in some pharmaceutical products and raw materials, thus leading to product adulteration and potential risk to patient health. Given that these bacteria are commonly found in aqueous environments, endotoxin control for Water for Injection systems (and some Purified Water systems) through biofilm control becomes critical.

8.2.2 NON-BIOFILM-FORMING BACTERIA IN WATER SYSTEMS

Other types of non-pseudomonad Gram-negative bacteria, ■such as■₁ₛ ₍ᵤₛₚ₄₁₎ the genera *Escherichia*, *Salmonella*, *Shigella*, *Serratia*, *Proteus*, *Enterobacter*, and *Klebsiella*, are used as indicators of fecal contamination. Although some of these bacteria ■are also plant pathogens, others■₁ₛ ₍ᵤₛₚ₄₁₎ can be human enteric pathogens, ■and can contaminate potable water supplies.■₁ₛ ₍ᵤₛₚ₄₁₎ These non-pseudomonads are not suited to colonizing or surviving in pharmaceutical water systems owing to the water's chemical purity. In fact, non-pseudomonad enteric bacteria are extremely unlikely contaminants of pharmaceutical water systems unless local sewage and source water controls are not in place. Such controls are required in order to comply with the source water requirements for making USP-grade waters as described in their respective monographs.

8.3 Microorganism Sources

8.3.1 EXOGENOUS CONTAMINATION

Exogenous microbial contamination of bulk pharmaceutical water comes from numerous possible sources, including source water. At a minimum, source water should meet the microbial quality attributes of Drinking Water, which is the absence of fecal coliforms (*E. coli*). A wide variety of other types of microorganisms, chiefly Gram-negative bacteria, may be present in the incoming water. If appropriate steps are not taken to reduce their numbers or eliminate them, these microorganisms may compromise subsequent water purification steps.

Exogenous microbial contamination can also arise from maintenance operations, equipment design, and the process of monitoring, including:
- Unprotected, faulty, or absent vent filters or rupture disks
- Backflow from interconnected equipment
- Non-sanitized distribution system openings for component replacements, inspections, repairs, and expansions
- Inadequate drain air-breaks
- Innate bioburden of activated carbon, ion-exchange resins, regenerant chemicals, and chlorine-neutralizing chemicals
- Inappropriate rinsing water quality after regeneration or sanitization
- Poor sanitization of use points, hard-piped equipment connectors, and other water transfer devices such as hoses
- Deficient techniques for use, sampling, and operation

The exogenous contaminants may not be normal aquatic bacteria but rather microorganisms of soil, air, or even human origin. The detection of non-aquatic microorganisms may be an indication of sampling or testing contamination or a system component failure, which should trigger investigation and remediation. Sufficient care should be given to sampling, testing, system design, and maintenance to minimize microbial contamination from exogenous sources.

8.3.2 ENDOGENOUS CONTAMINATION

Endogenous sources of microbial contamination can arise from unit operations in a water purification system that is not properly maintained and operated. Microorganisms present in source water may adsorb to carbon bed media, ion-exchange resins, filter membranes, and other equipment surfaces, and initiate the formation of biofilms.

Downstream colonization can occur when microorganisms are shed from existing biofilm-colonized surfaces and carried to other areas of the water system. Microorganisms may also attach to suspended particles such as carbon bed fines or fractured resin particles. When the microorganisms become planktonic, they serve as a source of contamination to subsequent purification equipment and to distribution systems.

Another source of endogenous microbial contamination is the distribution system itself. Microorganisms can colonize pipe surfaces, rough welds, misaligned flanges, valves, and dead legs, where they proliferate and form biofilms. Once formed, biofilms can become a continuous source of microbial contamination, which is very difficult to eradicate. Therefore, biofilm development must be managed by methods such as frequent cleaning and sanitization, as well as process and equipment design.

8.4 Endotoxin

■Bacterial endotoxin is a lipopolysaccharide (LPS) that is a component of the outer cell membrane of Gram-negative bacteria. Endotoxins may occur as collections of LPS molecules associated with living microorganisms, fragments of dead microorganisms, the EPS matrix surrounding biofilm bacteria, or free molecular clusters or micelles containing many lipopolysaccharide molecules. The monomeric form of the endotoxin molecule does not exist in high-purity water because of the molecule's amphipathic nature.■₁ₛ ₍ᵤₛₚ₄₁₎ Some grades of pharmaceutical waters, such as those used in parenteral applications (e.g., Water for Injection, Water for Hemodialysis, and the sterilized packaged waters made from Water for Injection) strictly limit the amount of endotoxins that may be present because these compounds are pyrogenic.

8.4.1 SOURCES

■1S (USP41) Endotoxins may be introduced into the system from the source water or may be released from cell surfaces of bacteria ■in water system biofilms.■1S (USP41) For example, a spike in endotoxin may occur following sanitization as a result of endotoxin release from killed cells. Endotoxin quantitation in water samples is not a good indicator of the level of biofilm development in a water system because of the multiplicity of endotoxin sources.

8.4.2 REMOVAL AND CONTROL

To control endotoxin levels in water systems, it is important to control all potential sources of contamination with Gram-negative bacteria as well as free endotoxin in the water. Contamination control includes the use of upstream unit operations to reduce bioburden from incoming water, as well as engineering controls (e.g., heat sanitization, equipment design, UV sanitizers, filters, material surface, and flow velocity) to minimize biofilm development on piping surfaces and to reduce re-inoculation of the system with free-floating bacteria.

Endotoxin remediation may be accomplished through the normal exclusion or removal action afforded by various unit operations within the treatment system. Examples of endotoxin removal steps in a water purification train include RO, deionization, ultrafilters, ■distillation,■1S (USP41) and endotoxin-adsorptive filters.

8.5 Test Methods

Microbes in water systems can be detected as exampled in this section or by methods adapted from *Microbial Enumeration Tests* ⟨61⟩, *Tests for Specified Microorganisms* ⟨62⟩, or the current edition of *Standard Methods for the Examination of Water and Wastewater* by the American Public Health Association. This section describes classical culture approaches to bioburden testing, with a brief discussion on rapid microbiological methods.

Every water system has a unique microbiome. It is the user's responsibility to perform method validation studies to demonstrate the suitability of the chosen test media and incubation conditions for bioburden recovery. In general, users should select the method that recovers the highest planktonic microbial counts in the shortest time, thus allowing for timely investigations and remediation. Such studies are usually performed before or during system validation. ■1S (USP41)

The steady state condition can take months or even years to be achieved, and can be affected by a change in source water quality, changes in finished water purity by using modified or increasingly inefficient purification processes, changes in finished water use patterns and volumes, changes in routine and preventative maintenance or sanitization procedures and frequencies, or any type of system intrusion (e.g., component replacement, removal, or addition).

8.5.1 MICROBIAL ENUMERATION CONSIDERATIONS

Most microbial contaminants in water systems are found primarily as biofilms on surfaces, with only a very small percentage of the microbiome suspended in the water, or planktonic, at any given time. Although it would seem logical to directly monitor biofilm development on surfaces, current technology for surface evaluations in an operating water system makes this impractical in a GMP environment. Therefore, an indirect approach must be used: the detection and enumeration of planktonic microorganisms that have been released from biofilms. This planktonic microbiome will impact the processes or products where the water is used.

The detection and enumeration of the planktonic microbiome can be accomplished by collecting samples from water system outlets. Planktonic organisms are associated with the presence of biofilms as well as free-floating bacteria introduced into the system (pioneer cells), which may eventually form new biofilms. Therefore, by enumerating the microorganisms in water ■1S (USP41) samples, the overall state of control over biofilm development can be assessed. This assessment has historically been accomplished with classical cultural techniques, which are viewed as the traditional method. However, nutritional limitations of the growth media may not satisfy growth requirements of organisms present in the water system that originated from a biofilm. As a result, traditional cultural methods may only detect a fraction of the biofilm bacteria present in the water sample. Other options are available, such as rapid microbiological methods.

There is no ideal cultural enumeration method that will detect all microorganisms in a water sample, although some media or incubation temperatures may be better than others. However, from a PC perspective, this limitation is acceptable because it is the relative changes in the trends for water sample microbial counts that indicate the state of PC.

■Consideration should also be given to the timeliness of microbial testing after sample collection. The number of detectable organisms in a sample collected in a sterile, scrupulously clean sample container will usually decrease as time passes. The organisms within the sample may die or adhere to the container walls, reducing the number that can be withdrawn from the sample for testing. The opposite effect can also occur if the sample container is not scrupulously clean and contains a low concentration of nutrients that could promote microbial growth. Because the number of organisms in the water can change over time after sample collection, it is best to test the samples as soon as possible. If it is not possible to test the sample within 2 h of collection, the sample should be held at refrigerated temperatures (2°–8°) and tested within 24 h. In situations where even 24 h is not possible (such as when using off-site contract laboratories), it is particularly important to qualify the microbiological

sample hold times and storage conditions to avoid significant changes in the microbial population during sample storage.
■1S *(USP41)*

8.5.2 THE CLASSICAL CULTURAL APPROACH

Classical cultural approaches for microbial testing of water include but are not limited to pour plates, spread plates, membrane filtration, and most probable number (MPN) tests. These methods are generally easy to perform, and provide excellent sample processing throughput. Method sensitivity can be increased via the use of larger sample sizes. This strategy is used in the membrane filtration method. Cultural approaches are further defined by the type of medium used in combination with the incubation temperature and duration. This combination should be selected according to the monitoring needs of a specific water system and its ability to recover the microorganisms of interest, i.e., those that could have a detrimental effect on the products manufactured or process uses, as well as those that reflect the microbial control status of the system.

8.5.2.1 Growth media: The traditional categorization is that there are two basic forms of media available: "high nutrient" and "low nutrient". Those media traditionally categorized as high-nutrient include Plate Count Agar (TGYA), Soybean Casein Digest Agar (SCDA or TSA), and m-HPC Agar (formerly m-SPC Agar). These media are intended for the general isolation and enumeration of heterotrophic or copiotrophic bacteria. Low-nutrient media, such as R2A Agar and NWRI Agar (HPCA), have a larger variety of nutrients than the high-nutrient media. These low-nutrient media were developed for use with potable water due to their ability to recover a more nutritionally diverse population of microorganisms found in these environments. The use of R2A may not be the best choice for high-purity water systems. Even though high-purity water creates an oligotrophic environment, it has been shown empirically that in many high-purity compendial waters, the microbial count disparity between low- and high-nutrient media is dramatically less to nil, compared to potable water. Nevertheless, using the medium that has been demonstrated ■as acceptable through comparative media analysis is recommended.■1S *(USP41)*

8.5.2.2 Incubation conditions: Duration and temperature of incubation are also critical aspects of microbiological testing. Classical compendial methods (e.g., ⟨61⟩) specify the use of high-nutrient media, typically incubated at 30°–35° for NLT 48 h. Given the types of microbes found in many water systems, incubation at lower temperatures (e.g., ranges of 20°–25° or 25°–30°) for longer periods (at least 4 days) could recover higher microbial counts than classical compendial methods. Low-nutrient media typically require longer incubation conditions (at least 5 days) because the lower nutrient concentrations promote slower growth. Even high-nutrient media can sometimes yield higher microbial recovery with longer and cooler incubation conditions.

■**8.5.2.3 Selection of method conditions:**   The decision to test a particular system using high- or low-nutrient media, higher or lower incubation temperatures, and longer or shorter incubation times should be based on comparative cultivation studies using the native microbiome of the water system. The decision to use media requiring longer incubation periods to recover higher counts also should be balanced with the timeliness of results. Detection of marginally higher counts at the expense of a significantly longer incubation period may not be the best approach for monitoring water systems, particularly when the slow growers are not new species but the same as those recovered within shorter incubation times. Some cultural conditions using low-nutrient media lead to the development of microbial colonies that are much less differentiated in colonial appearance, an attribute that microbiologists rely on when selecting representative microbial types for further characterization. The nature of some of the slow growers and the extended incubation times needed for their development into visible colonies also may lead to those colonies becoming dysgonic and difficult to subculture. That could limit their further characterization, depending on the microbial identification technology used. The selection of method parameters should provide conditions that adequately recover microorganisms from the water system, including those that are objectionable for the intended water use.■1S *(USP41)*

8.5.3 SUGGESTED CLASSICAL CULTURAL METHODS

■Example methods are presented in *Table 3.*■1S *(USP41)*

Table ■3.■1S *(USP41)* **Example Culture Methods**

Drinking Water	Pour plate method or membrane filtration method[a]
	Suggested sample volume: 1.0 mL[b]
	Growth medium: ■Plate Count Agar■1S *(USP41)*[c]
	Incubation time: 48–72 h[d]
	Incubation temperature: 30°–35°[e]

[a] A membrane filter with a rating of 0.45 μm is generally considered preferable to smaller porosity membranes.

[b] Sample size must be appropriate for the expected microbial count of the water in order to derive statistically valid colony counts.

[c] For optimum recovery, an alternative medium may be more appropriate (e.g., m-HPC, TSA/SCDA, R2A).

[d] For optimum recovery, alternative incubation times may be needed.

[e] For optimum recovery, alternative incubation temperatures may be needed.

Table ■3.■1S (USP41) **Example Culture Methods** (Continued)

Purified Water	Pour plate method or membrane filtration method[b]
	Suggested sample volume: 1.0 mL for pour plate or ■up to■1S (USP41) 100 mL for membrane filtration[b]
	Growth medium: ■Plate Count Agar■1S (USP41)[c]
	Incubation time: 48–72 h[d]
	Incubation temperature: 30°–35°[e]
Water for Injection	Membrane filtration method[a]
	Suggested sample volume: 200 mL[b]
	Growth medium: ■Plate Count Agar■1S (USP41)[c]
	Incubation time: 48–72 h[d]
	Incubation temperature: 30°–35°[e]

[a] A membrane filter with a rating of 0.45 μm is generally considered preferable to smaller porosity membranes.
[b] Sample size must be appropriate for the expected microbial count of the water in order to derive statistically valid colony counts.
[c] For optimum recovery, an alternative medium may be more appropriate (e.g., m-HPC, TSA/SCDA, R2A).
[d] For optimum recovery, alternative incubation times may be needed.
[e] For optimum recovery, alternative incubation temperatures may be needed.

For media growth promotion, use at a minimum *Pseudomonas aeruginosa* ATCC 9027 and *Bacillus subtilis* ATCC 6633. Additional organisms should be used to represent those that are considered objectionable and/or typically isolated from the water system (house isolates).

8.5.4 MICROBIAL IDENTIFICATION

In addition to the enumeration of the bioburden in the water, there is a need to identify and/or select certain microbial species that could be detrimental to products or processes. Some bacteria may also be resistant to preservatives and other antimicrobial chemicals used in ■nonsterile■1S (USP41) liquid and semi-solid products, thus leading to potential product spoilage. For example, *Pseudomonas aeruginosa* and *Burkholderia cepacia*, as well as some other pseudomonads, are known opportunistic pathogens ■under certain conditions.■1S (USP41) As such, it may be appropriate to consider these species as objectionable microorganisms for the type of water used to manufacture ■nonsterile■1S (USP41) liquid and semi-solid products. There is a higher risk of infection if these organisms are found in products targeted for susceptible patient populations (e.g., the very young, the very old, and the immunocompromised) or products contacting highly susceptible tissues (e.g., inhaled products or some topical products). However, if the product where the water is used carries an absence specification for a particular pathogenic species that is not capable of living in a high-purity water system ■(e.g., *Staphylococcus aureus* or *Escherichia coli*),■1S (USP41) then these non-aquatic species should not be candidates for routine ■recovery testing from water samples.■1S (USP41) For more information, see *Microbiological Examination of Nonsterile Products: Acceptance Criteria for Pharmaceutical Preparations and Substances for Pharmaceutical Use* ⟨1111⟩, *Microbial Characterization, Identification, and Strain Typing* ⟨1113⟩, and *Microbiological Best Laboratory Practices* ⟨1117⟩.

For PC and QC, it is valuable to know the microbial species present in the normal microbiome of a water system, even if they are not specifically objectionable. If a new species is detected, it may be an indication of a subtle process change or an exogenous intrusion. The identity of the microorganism may be a clue as to its origin and can help with implementation of corrective or preventive action. Therefore, it is industry practice to identify the microorganisms in samples that yield results exceeding established Alert and Action Levels. It is also of value to periodically identify the normal microbiome in a water system, even if counts are below established Alert Levels. This information can provide perspective on the species recoveries from Alert and Action Level excursion samples, indicating whether they are new species or just higher levels of the normal microbiome. Water system isolates may be incorporated into a company culture collection for use in tests such as antimicrobial effectiveness tests, microbial method validation/suitability testing, and media growth promotion. The decision to use ■water isolates in these studies should be risk-based because many such isolates may not grow well on the high-nutrient media required. And because once adapted to laboratory media, they may not perform like their wild type progenitors.■1S (USP41)

8.5.5 RAPID MICROBIOLOGICAL METHODS

In recent years, new technologies that enhance microbial detection and the timeliness of test results have been adopted by pharmaceutical QC testing labs. Rapid Microbiological Methods (RMM) are divided into four categories: Growth-Based, Viability-Based, ■Metabolite-Based,■1S (USP41) and Nucleic Acid-Based. Examples of RMM used for the evaluation of microbial quality of water systems include:

- Microscopic visual epifluorescence membrane counting techniques
- Automated laser scanning membrane counting approaches
- Early colony detection methods based on autofluorescence, adenosine triphosphate (ATP) bioluminescence, or vital staining
- Genetic-based detection/quantitation

See *Validation of Alternative Microbiological Methods* ⟨1223⟩ for further information on rapid microbiological methods.

Change to read:

9. ALERT AND ACTION LEVELS AND SPECIFICATIONS

9.1 Introduction

Establishment of Alert and Action Levels for any manufacturing process facilitates appropriate and timely control. In the case of a pharmaceutical water system, the key PC parameters can be specific chemical, physical, and microbiological attributes of the water produced. Typically, most chemical attributes can be determined in real time or in the lab within a few minutes after sample collection. Physical attributes such as the pressure drop across a filter, temperature, and flow rate—which are sometimes considered critical for operation or sanitization of the water system—must be measured in situ during operation. Obtaining timely microbial data is more challenging compared to chemical and physical attributes, often taking several days. This limits the ability to control microbial attributes in a timely manner, and therefore requires a more challenging evaluation of the test results and conservative implementation of PC levels. This section provides guidance on the establishment and use of Alert and Action Levels, as well as Specifications to assess the suitability of the water and the water system for use in production.

9.2 Examples of Critical Parameter Measurements

Examples of measurements and parameters that are important to water system processes and products are described below. The list, which is not intended to be exhaustive or required, contains some examples of parameters that could be measured to demonstrate that the system is in a state of control.

Examples of measurements that could be critical to the purification or sanitization process include:
- Temperature, for thermally sanitized systems
- Percent rejection of an RO system
- Endotoxin levels of feed water to a distillation system
- Chlorine presence immediately prior to an RO system

Examples of measurements that could be critical to the water distribution process include:
- Return/end-of-loop line pressure, to forewarn of ▪the potential to aspirate air or fluids because of▪1S (USP41) simultaneous use of too many outlets
- ▪Temperature to assure the self-sanitizing conditions are maintained for a hot water system▪1S (USP41)
- Flow rate, to ensure that sufficient water is available for operations

Examples of measurements that could be critical to final water quality include:
- Conductivity
- TOC
- Endotoxin—for Water for Injection systems
- ▪▪1S (USP41)
- Bioburden
- Ozone or other chemicals—for chemically sanitized systems

9.3 Purpose of the Measurements

Although the purpose of each measurement varies, the results can be used to provide system performance feedback, often immediately, serving as ongoing PC and product quality indicators. At the same time, the results provide information necessary for making decisions regarding the immediate processing and usability of the water (see *6.1 Purposes and Procedures*). However, some attributes may not be monitored continuously or may have a long delay in data availability (e.g., microbial data). Regardless, both real-time data and data with longer cycle times can be used to properly establish Alert and Action Levels, which can serve as an early warning or indication of a potentially approaching quality shift.

As PC indicators, Alert and Action Levels are trigger points for the potential need for investigation and/or remedial action, to prevent a system from deviating from normal conditions and producing water unsuitable for its intended use. This "intended use" minimum quality is sometimes referred to as a "Specification" or "Limit", and may include limits for conductivity and TOC listed in water monographs, or other specifications required for these waters that have been defined by the user internally.

In all cases, the validity of the data should be verified to ensure that the data are accurate and consistently representative of the water quality in the system, regardless of whether the sample was collected from a sampling port or use point. The resulting data must not be unduly biased, positively or negatively, due to the sampling method, the environment in the vicinity of the sampling location, the test procedure, instrumentation, or other artifacts that could obscure or misrepresent the true quality of the water intended by the purpose of the sampling, i.e., for PC or for QC.

9.4 Defining Alert and Action Levels and Specifications

Data generated from routine water system monitoring should be trended to ensure that the system operates in a state of chemical and microbiological control. To assist with the evaluation of system performance, companies should establish in-process control levels based on historical data or a fraction of the water Specifications (as long as this latter approach yields values with relevance to process performance).

When establishing Alert and Action Levels and Specifications, a two- or three-tier approach is typically used. In a three-tier approach, the typical structure is to establish in-process controls using "Alert Level", "Action Level", and "Specifications". Alert and Action Levels are used as proactive approaches to system management prior to exceeding Specifications. The criteria for defining and reacting to adverse trends should be set by the user. These levels should be set at values that allow companies to take action to prevent the system from producing water that is unfit for use. Water Specifications or Limits represent the suitability for use of the water.

In a two-tier approach, a combination of the above terminology is used, depending on the parameter to be monitored. For example, if the attribute does have a monograph specification, the two tiers are Alert Level (or Action Level) and Specification. If the attribute does not have a limit/specification, the two tiers are usually Alert Level and Action Level.

A single-tier approach is possible, but this is risky and difficult to manage. With this approach, where the water/system is either acceptable or not acceptable, the single-tier method does not allow for any adjustment, correction, or investigation prior to stopping production.

However, certain sampling locations, such as sampling ports that are not used for manufacturing products or processes, do not represent the finished water quality where a Specification could be applied. In these locations, a two-tier approach (Alert and Action Levels only) could be applied. In some sampling locations, a single PC level might possibly be appropriate, depending on the attribute.

9.4.1 ALERT LEVEL

An Alert Level for a measurement or parameter should be derived from the normal operating range of the water system. Specifically, Alert Levels are based on the historical operating performance under production conditions, and then are established at levels that are just beyond the majority of the normal historical data. The Alert Level for a parameter is often a single value or a range of values, such as:
- Higher than typical conductivity or TOC
- Higher than typical microbial count
- Higher than typical endotoxin level
- Low temperature during thermal sanitization
- pH range control prior to an RO
- Ozone concentration in a storage tank

Various methods, tools, and statistical approaches are available for establishing Alert Levels, and the user needs to determine the approaches that work for their application. Some numerical examples are two or three standard deviations ■■1S *(USP41)* (or more) in excess of the mean value, or some percentage above the mean value but below a Specification. An event-based example could be the appearance of a new microorganism or a non-zero microbial count where zero is the norm.

When an Alert Level is exceeded, this indicates that a process or product may have drifted from its normal operating condition or range. Alert Level excursions represent a warning and do not necessarily require a corrective action. However, Alert Level excursions may warrant notification of personnel involved in water system operation, as well as the quality assurance (QA) personnel. Alert Level excursions may also lead to additional monitoring, with more intense scrutiny of the resulting and neighboring data as well as other process indicators.

9.4.2 ACTION LEVEL

An Action Level is also based on the same historical data, but the levels are established at values (or ranges) that exceed the Alert Levels. The values/ranges are determined using the same types of numerical or event-based tools as the Alert Levels, but at different values■/ranges.■1S *(USP41)*

In a three-tier approach, it is good practice to select an Action Level that is more than the Alert Level, but less than the Specification to allow the user to make corrective actions before the water would go out of compliance.

Exceeding a quantitative Action Level indicates that the process has allowed the product quality or other critical parameter to drift outside of its normal operating range. An Action Level can also be event-based. In addition to exceeding quantitative Action Levels, some examples of event-based Action Level excursions include, but are not limited to:
- Exceeding an Alert Level repeatedly
- Exceeding an Alert Level in multiple locations simultaneously
- The recovery of specific objectionable microorganisms
- A repeating non-zero microbial count where zero is the norm

If an Action Level is exceeded, this should prompt immediate notification of both QA staff and the personnel involved in water system operations and use, so that corrective actions can be taken to restore the system back to its normal operating range. Such remedial actions should also include investigative efforts to understand what happened and eliminate or reduce the probability of recurrence. Depending on the nature of the Action Level excursion, it may be necessary to evaluate its impact on the water uses during the period between the previous acceptable test result and the next acceptable test result.

9.4.3 SPECIAL ALERT AND ACTION LEVEL SITUATIONS

In new or significantly altered water systems, where there is limited or no historical data from which to derive trends, it is common to establish initial Alert and Action Levels based on equipment design capabilities. These initial levels should be within the process and product Specifications where water is used. It is also common for new water systems, especially ambient water systems, to undergo changes, both chemically and microbiologically, over time as various unit operations (such as RO membranes) exhibit the effects of aging. This type of system aging effect is most common during the first year of use. As the system ages, a steady state ■microbiome■₁ₛ ₍USP41₎ (microorganism types and levels) may develop due to the collective effects of system design, source water, maintenance, and operation, including the frequency of re-bedding, backwashing, regeneration, and sanitization. This established or mature ■microbiome■₁ₛ ₍USP41₎ may be higher than the one detected when the water system was new. Therefore, there is cause for the impurity levels to increase over this maturation period and eventually stabilize.

Some water systems are so well controlled microbially—such as continuously or intermittently hot Water for Injection distribution systems—that microbial counts and endotoxin levels are essentially nil or below the limit of reasonable detectability. This common scenario often coincides with a very low Specification that is poorly quantifiable due to imprecision (as much as two-fold variability) of the test methods that may be near their limits of detection. In such systems, quantitative data trending has little value, and therefore, quantitative PC levels also have little value. The non-zero values in such systems could be due to sporadic sampling issues and not indicative of a water system PC deviation; however, if these non-zero values occur repeatedly, they could be indicative of process problems. So, an alternative approach for establishing Alert and Action Levels with these data could be the use of the incident rate of non-zero values, with the occasional single non-zero "hit" perhaps being an Alert Level (regardless of its quantitative value), and multiple or sequential "hits" being an Action Level. Depending on the attribute, perhaps single hits may not even warrant being considered an Alert Level, so only a multiple-hit situation would be considered actionable. It is up to the user to decide on their approach for system control, i.e., whether to use one, two, or three levels of controls for a given water system and sampling location, and whether to establish Alert and Action Levels as quantitative or qualitative hit-frequency values.

9.4.4 SPECIFICATIONS

Water Specifications or Limits are set based on direct potential product and/or process impact and they represent the suitability for use of the water. The various bulk water monographs contain tests for *Conductivity*, *TOC*, and *Bacterial Endotoxins* (for *Water for Injection*). Aside from the monographs for *Water for Hemodialysis* and multiple sterile waters, microbial specifications for the bulk waters are intentionally not included in their monograph tests.

The need for microbial specifications for bulk waters (*Purified Water* and *Water for Injection*) depends on the water use(s), some of which may require strict control (e.g., very low bioburden, absence of objectionable organisms, or low ionic strength) while others may require no specification due to the lack of impact. For example, microbial specifications are appropriate and typically expected for water that is used in product formulations and final equipment rinses. ■Where the water is used for analytical reagent preparations and the analytical method is not affected by microbial contaminants,■₁ₛ ₍USP41₎ or for cleaning processes that conclude with a final antimicrobial heat drying or solvent rinsing step, the microbial quality of the water is likely less of a concern. The decision to establish microbial Specifications for bulk pharmaceutical waters should be based on a formal risk assessment of its uses and justified by scientific rationale.

It is very important to understand the chemical and microbial quality of the water in its final form as it is delivered from a water system to the locations where it is used in manufacturing activities and other points of use. The quality of the water within the water system could be compromised if it picks up chemical or microbial contaminants during its delivery from the system to the points of use. These points of use, where cumulative contamination could be present, are the locations where compliance with all the water Specifications is mandated.

As discussed above, compliance with chemical Specifications can be confirmed periodically between uses, immediately prior to use, or even while the water is being utilized in product manufacturing. While the use of RMM may provide for timely microbial data, the use of conventional cultivative microbiological testing usually delays confirmation of microbial compliance until after the water has been used. However, for some applications, this logistical limitation should not eliminate the need for establishing microbial Specifications for this very important raw material.

The manufacturing risk imposed by these logistics accentuates the value of validated microbial control for a water system. It also emphasizes the value of ■unbiased sampling for microbial monitoring (e.g., influences from technique, hoses, flushing)■₁ₛ ₍USP41₎ of samples collected from pertinent locations, with evaluation of the resulting data against well-chosen, preferably trend-derived Alert and Action Levels, which can facilitate remedial PC to preclude Specification excursions.

Users should establish their own quantitative microbial Specifications suited to their water uses. But these values should not be greater than 100 cfu/mL for *Purified Water* or 10 cfu/100 mL for *Water for Injection* unless specifically justified, because these values generally represent the highest microbial levels for pharmaceutical water that are still suitable for manufacturing use.

A Specification excursion should prompt an out-of-specification (OOS) investigation. The investigation is performed to determine 1) the root cause of the excursion so that CAPA may be taken for remediation purposes, and 2) assess the impact on affected processes and finished products where the water was used. Product disposition decisions must be made and are dependent on factors that could include:

- Role of water in the product or in-process material
- Chemical or microbial nature of the attribute whose Specification value was exceeded
- Level of product contamination by the water
- Presence of objectionable microorganisms
- Any downstream processing of affected in-process materials that could mitigate the OOS attribute
- Physical and chemical properties of the finished product where the water was used that could mitigate the OOS attribute
- Product administration routes and potentially sensitive/susceptible users

9.4.5 SOURCE WATER CONTROL

The chemical and microbial attributes of the starting source water are important to the ability of the water system to remove or reduce these impurities to meet the finished water Specifications (see *2. Source Water Considerations*). Using the example microbial enumeration methods in *Table* ■3,■1S (USP41) a reasonable maximum bacterial Action Level for source water is 500 cfu/mL. This number is derived from U.S. EPA NPDWR where it is used as an Action Level for the water authority indicating the need for improving disinfection and water filtration to avoid the penetration of viral, bacterial, and protozoal pathogens into the finished Drinking Water. It is not, however, a U.S. EPA heterotrophic plate count Specification or Maximum Contaminant Level (MCL) for Drinking Water.

Nevertheless, of particular importance could be the microbial and chemical quality of this starting water because the water is often delivered to the facility at a great distance from its source and in a condition over which the user has little or no control. High microbial and chemical levels in source water may indicate a municipal potable water system upset, a change in the supply or original water source, a broken water main, or inadequate disinfection, and therefore, potentially contaminated water with objectionable or new microorganisms or coincidental chemical contaminants.

Considering the potential concern about objectionable microorganisms and chemical contaminants in the source water, contacting the water provider about the problem should be an immediate first step. In-house remedial actions could also be needed, including performance of additional testing on the incoming water (as well as the finished water in some cases) or pretreating the water with additional microbial and chemical purification operations (see *5.1 Unit Operations Considerations*).

Dietary Supplements

General Chapters Information

⟨2040⟩ DISINTEGRATION AND DISSOLUTION OF DIETARY SUPPLEMENTS

INTRODUCTION

This general chapter is provided to determine compliance with the disintegration and dissolution standards for dietary supplements where stated in the individual monographs.

For the purposes of this chapter, dietary supplement dosage forms have been divided into three categories: *Vitamin–Mineral Dosage Forms, Botanical Dosage Forms,* and *Dietary Supplements Other Than Vitamin–Mineral and Botanical Dosage Forms. Vitamin–Mineral Dosage Forms* include articles prepared with vitamins, minerals, or combinations of these dietary ingredients, as described in *Table 1. Botanical Dosage Forms* comprise formulations containing ingredients of botanical origin, including plant materials and extracts. *Dietary Supplements Other Than Vitamin–Mineral and Botanical Dosage Forms* encompass dietary supplements formulated with lawfully recognized dietary ingredients that are different from those pertaining to the two foregoing categories (e.g., amino acids, chondroitin, and glucosamine).

Where a dietary supplement represents a combination of the categories mentioned above, and there is a difference between the requirements for the individual categories, the more stringent requirement applies. [NOTE—"More stringent requirement" means stricter acceptance criteria and/or milder operational conditions.]

Disintegration and dissolution tests as described in this chapter are quality-control tools to assess performance characteristics of dietary supplement finished dosage forms. These performance standards are intended to detect problems that may arise due to use or misuse, or changes in coatings, lubricants, disintegrants, and other components. These performance tests are also intended to detect manufacturing process issues, such as overcompression and overdrying, that would affect the release characteristics of the final dosage forms. These tests are not intended to be used as a demonstration or as a surrogate for in vivo absorption, bioavailability, or effectiveness, unless an in vitro–in vivo correlation (IVIVC) has been established.

DISINTEGRATION

This test is provided to determine whether dietary supplement capsules or tablets disintegrate within the prescribed time when placed in a liquid medium at the experimental conditions presented below. Compliance with the limits on *Disintegration* stated in the individual monographs for dietary supplements is required, except where the label states that the products are intended for use as troches, are to be chewed, or are designed as extended-release dosage forms. Dietary supplements claiming to be extended-release dosage forms must comply with standards other than disintegration to verify that the release of the dietary ingredients from the dosage form is for a defined period of time. Dietary supplements claiming to be extended-release dosage forms must not be labeled as in compliance with USP unless a *USP* monograph exists for such product. Determine the type of dosage form under test from the labeling and from observation, and apply the appropriate procedure to 6 or more units.

For purposes of this test, disintegration does not imply complete solution of the unit or even of its active constituent. Complete disintegration is defined as that state in which any residue of the unit, except fragments of insoluble coating or capsule shell, remaining on the screen of the test apparatus or adhering to the lower surface of the disk (if used) is a soft mass having no palpably firm core.

• **APPARATUS**

Apparatus A: Use the *Apparatus* described in *Disintegration* ⟨701⟩, *Apparatus* for capsules or tablets that are NMT 18 mm long. For larger capsules or tablets, use *Apparatus B.*

Apparatus B: The apparatus consists of a basket-rack assembly, a 1000-mL low-form beaker for the immersion fluid, a thermostatic arrangement for heating the fluid between 35° and 39°, and a device for raising and lowering the basket in the immersion fluid at a constant frequency rate between 29 and 32 cycles/min through a distance of 53–57 mm. The volume of the fluid in the vessel is such that at the highest point of the upward stroke, the wire mesh remains at least 15 mm below the surface of the fluid and descends to NLT 25 mm from the bottom of the vessel on the downward stroke. At no time should the top of the basket-rack assembly become submerged. The time required for the upward stroke is equal to the time required for the downward stroke, and the change in stroke direction is a smooth transition rather than an abrupt reversal of motion. The basket-rack assembly moves vertically along its axis. There is no appreciable horizontal motion or movement of the axis from the vertical.

Basket-rack assembly: The basket-rack assembly (see *Figure 1*) consists of three open-ended transparent tubes, each 77.5 ± 2.5 mm long and having an inside diameter of 32.0–34.6 mm and a wall 2.0–3.0 mm in thickness; the tubes are held in a vertical position by two plastic plates, each 97 ± 2 mm in diameter and 7.5–10.5 mm in thickness, with three holes, 36.0–40.6 mm in diameter, equidistant from the center of the plate and equally spaced from one another. Attached to the undersurface of the lower plate is 10-mesh No. 23 (0.025-inch) W- and M-gauge woven stainless-steel wire cloth having a plain square weave. The parts of the apparatus are assembled and rigidly held by means of three bolts passing through the two plastic plates. A suitable means is provided to suspend the basket-rack assembly from the raising and lowering device, using a point on its axis. The design of the basket-rack assembly may be varied somewhat, provided that the specifications for the glass tubes and the screen mesh size are maintained.

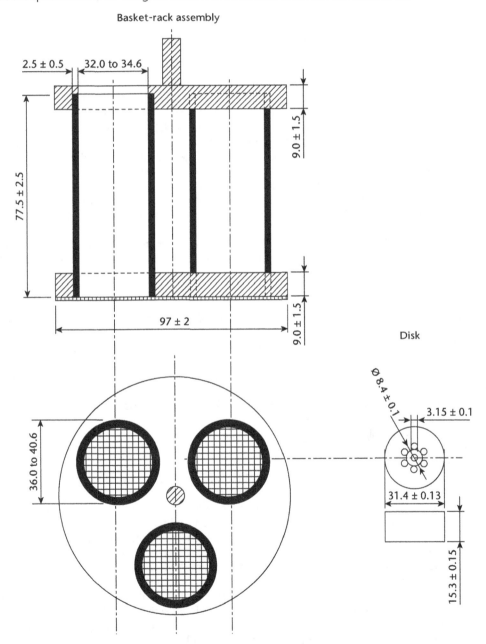

Figure 1. Basket-rack assembly, *Disintegration, Apparatus B* (dimensions in mm).

Beaker: Low form, 1000 mL; the difference between the diameter of the plastic plates, which hold the tubes in a vertical position, and the inside diameter of the beaker should be NMT 6 mm.[1]

---

[1] 1000-mL low-form beakers, designed in compliance with the current ASTM E 960 Type I or Type II or ISO 3819 specifications, meet the size requirements.

Disks: Each tube is provided with a perforated cylindrical disk 15.3 ± 0.15 mm in thickness and 31.4 ± 0.13 mm in diameter. The disk is made of a suitable, transparent plastic material having a specific gravity of between 1.18 and 1.20. Seven holes 3.15 ± 0.1 mm in diameter extend between the ends of the cylinder, one of the holes being in the center and the other six parallel to it and spaced equally tangent to a circle with a radius of 4.2 mm from the center of the disk. All surfaces of the disk are smooth.[2]

- **PROCEDURE:** Test 6 dosage units as described below for each type of dosage form. [NOTE—Two basket arrangements for a total of six tubes are necessary for *Apparatus B*.] If 1 or 2 dosage units fail to disintegrate completely, repeat the test on 12 additional dosage units.

  Uncoated tablets: Place 1 tablet in each of the tubes of the basket and, if prescribed, add a disk to each tube. Operate the apparatus, using water or the specified medium as the immersion fluid, maintained at 37 ± 2°. At the end of 30 min, lift the basket from the fluid and observe the tablets.

  Plain-coated tablets: Place 1 tablet in each of the tubes of the basket and, if the tablet has a soluble external sugar coating, immerse the basket in water at room temperature for 5 min. Then, if prescribed, add a disk to each tube and operate the apparatus, using water or the specified medium as the immersion fluid, maintained at 37 ± 2°. At the end of 30 min, lift the basket from the fluid and observe the tablets.

  Delayed-release (enteric-coated) tablets: Omit the use of a disk. Place 1 tablet in each of the six tubes of the basket, and if the tablet has a soluble external sugar coating, immerse the basket in water at room temperature for 5 min. Then operate the apparatus using simulated gastric fluid TS, maintained at 37 ± 2°, as the immersion fluid. After 1 h of operation in simulated gastric fluid TS, lift the basket from the fluid and observe the tablets: the tablets show no evidence of disintegration, cracking, or softening. Operate the apparatus using simulated intestinal fluid TS, maintained at 37 ± 2°, as the immersion fluid for the time specified in the monograph. Lift the basket from the fluid and observe the tablets.

  Delayed-release (enteric-coated) soft-shell capsules: Place 1 softgel capsule in each of the six tubes of the basket. Omit the use of a disk. Operate the apparatus using simulated gastric fluid TS, maintained at 37 ± 2°, as the immersion fluid. After 1 h of operation in simulated gastric fluid TS, lift the basket from the fluid and observe the softgels: the softgels show no evidence of disintegration or rupture that would permit the escape of the contents. Operate the apparatus with disks using simulated intestinal fluid TS, maintained at 37 ± 2°, as the immersion fluid for NMT 60 min. Lift the basket from the fluid and observe the capsules.

  Hard-shell capsules: Apply the test for *Uncoated tablets* using, as the immersion fluid, maintained at 37 ± 2°, a 0.05 M acetate buffer prepared by mixing 2.99 g of sodium acetate trihydrate and 1.66 mL of glacial acetic acid with water to obtain a 1000-mL solution with a pH of 4.50 ± 0.05. Attach a removable wire cloth, as described in *Basket-rack assembly*, to the surface of the upper plate of the basket-rack assembly. At the end of 30 min, lift the basket from the fluid and observe the capsules.

  Soft-shell capsules: Proceed as directed in the *Rupture Test for Soft-Shell Capsules*.

- **USE OF DISKS**

  Vitamin–mineral dosage forms: Add a disk to each tube unless otherwise specified in the *Procedure* above or in the individual monograph.

  Botanical dosage forms: Omit the use of disks unless otherwise specified in the *Procedure* above or in the individual monograph.

  Dietary supplements other than vitamin–mineral and botanical dosage forms: Omit the use of disks unless otherwise specified above or in the individual monograph.

- **TOLERANCES:** All of the 6 dosage units initially tested or NLT 16 of a total of 18 dosage units tested disintegrate completely.

RUPTURE TEST FOR SOFT-SHELL CAPSULES

Medium: Water; 500 mL

Apparatus: Use *Apparatus 2* as described in *Dissolution* ⟨711⟩, *Apparatus*, operating at 50 rpm.

Time: 15 min

- **PROCEDURE:** Place 1 capsule in each vessel, and allow the capsule to sink to the bottom of the vessel before starting rotation of the blade. Use sinkers if the capsules float. Observe the capsules throughout the test and at the end of the test. The capsule shell is considered ruptured if breached, exposing or allowing the fill contents to escape.

- **TOLERANCES:** The requirements are met if all of the capsules tested rupture in NMT 15 min. If 1 or 2 of the capsules rupture in >15 min but NMT 30 min, repeat the test on 12 additional capsules: NMT 2 of the total of 18 capsules tested rupture in >15 min but NMT 30 min. For soft gelatin capsules that do not conform to the above rupture test acceptance criteria, repeat the test with the addition of papain to the *Medium* in the amount that results in an activity of NMT 550,000 units/L of *Medium* or with the addition of bromelain in the amount that results in an activity of NMT 30 gelatin-digesting units (GDU)/L of *Medium*. [NOTE—Determine papain activity using the *Assay* in the monograph for *Papain* and bromelain activity using the procedure in bromelain, in the *Reagent Specifications* section.]

---

[2] The use of automatic detection using modified disks is permitted where the use of disks is specified or allowed. Such disks must comply with the requirements for density and dimensions given in this chapter.

Change to read:

DISSOLUTION

This test is provided to determine compliance with the *Dissolution* requirements where stated in the individual monographs for dietary supplements. The operative assumption inherent in this test is that if the index vitamin or mineral or marker compound(s) for a botanical is dissolved within the time frame and under conditions specified, the dosage form does not suffer from formulation- or manufacturing-related problems affecting the adequate release of the active ingredients.

- **FOR DOSAGE FORMS CONTAINING OR COATED WITH GELATIN**

    For hard or soft gelatin capsules and gelatin-coated tablets that do not conform to the dissolution specification because of the presence of cross-linking, the dissolution procedure should be repeated with the addition of enzymes to the medium, as described below.

    Dissolution medium with pH ≤4.0
    Enzyme: Pepsin, activity determined by the procedure in pepsin, in the *Reagent Specifications* section
    Amount: A quantity of pepsin that results in an activity of NMT 750,000 units/L of dissolution medium

    Dissolution medium with pH >4.0 and <6.8
    Enzyme: Papain, activity determined by the *Assay* in the monograph for *Papain*; or bromelain, activity determined by the procedure in bromelain, in the *Reagent Specifications* section
    Amount: A quantity of papain that results in an activity of NMT 550,000 units/L of dissolution medium, or a quantity of bromelain that results in an activity of NMT 30 GDU/L of dissolution medium

    Dissolution medium with pH ≥6.8
    Enzyme: Pancreatin, protease activity determined by the procedure in *Assay for protease activity* (*Casein digestive powder*) in the monograph for *Pancreatin*
    Amount: A quantity of pancreatin that results in a protease activity of NMT 2,000 units/L of dissolution medium

    Dissolution medium containing surfactants or other components known to denature the enzyme: If the dissolution medium contains surfactants or other components known to denature the enzyme to be used, a pretreatment step should be applied. The pretreatment step is performed under the same dissolution conditions (apparatus, rotation, and flow rate), except to use a medium with the corresponding amount of enzyme as directed in the preceding section and without the surfactant or component known to denature the enzyme. To achieve the final specified volume of medium, the pretreatment step may be conducted with a smaller volume of medium without the surfactant or component in such a manner that the final specified volume is achieved after the addition of the surfactant or component at the end of the pretreatment step. Perform the pretreatment step until capsule rupture, but for NMT one-half of the total dissolution time specified in the procedure. The pretreatment time is included in the total dissolution time specified in the procedure.

- **APPARATUS:** See ⟨711⟩ for a description of the apparatus used, apparatus suitability test, and other related information. Where the procedure specifies the use of a stationary basket, use the quadrangular basket of stainless steel wire gauze as shown in *Figure 2a* and *Figure 2b*.

    The capsule is placed in a basket, soldered in one of its upper, narrow sides to the end of a steel rod (see *Figure 2a*). The capsule cover is placed in the horizontal diagonal of the basket. The rod assembly is inserted vertically through the cover of the dissolution vessel, and fixed by means of two teflon nuts, 3.2 cm from the center of the vessel, or by any other appropriate means. The lower edge of the bottom of the basket is adjusted to about 1 cm above the top of the paddle blade (see *Figure 2b*).

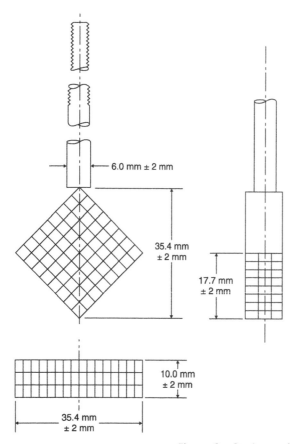

NOTES

1. Rod and Basket with a Capsule cover placed in the horizontal diagonal of the basket

2. Basket and capsule cover material; stainless steel

3. Basket gauze wire size: 8 mesh

6.0 mm ± 2 mm

35.4 mm ± 2 mm

17.7 mm ± 2 mm

10.0 mm ± 2 mm

35.4 mm ± 2 mm

Figure 2a. Stationary basket.

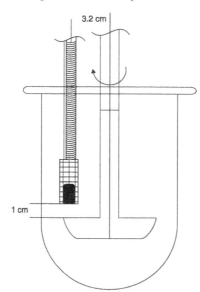

3.2 cm

1 cm

Figure 2b. Stationary basket configuration diagram.

Of the types of apparatus described in ⟨711⟩, use the one specified in the individual monograph.

- **VITAMIN–MINERAL DOSAGE FORMS**

All dietary supplement ■capsules, tablets, or chewable gels■₁ₛ ₍USP41₎ containing folic acid are subject to the dissolution test and criteria for folic acid described in this chapter. This test is required because of the importance of the relationship between folate deficiency and the risk of neural tube defects. Dietary supplement ■capsules, tablets, or chewable gels ■₁ₛ ₍USP41₎ containing water-soluble vitamins, minerals, or their combination are subject to the dissolution test and criteria for index vitamins, index minerals, or both, described in this chapter. Dietary supplement tablets, ■chewable gels,■₁ₛ ₍USP41₎ and hard-shell capsules with solid content dosage forms containing vitamin A are subject to the dissolution test and criteria for vitamin A described in this chapter. Dissolution standards were not established and therefore are not applicable to vitamin A in dietary supplement soft-shell capsules filled with liquids. *Table 1* summarizes the dissolution requirements for the assigned USP classes of dietary supplements. Vitamin–mineral combinations that do not belong to any of the USP classes listed in *Table 1* are subject to the *Dissolution* test and criteria specified in the individual monographs.

Table 1. Dietary Supplements—Vitamin–Mineral Dosage Forms

USP Class	Ingredients	Dissolution Requirements for Tablets, ■Chewable Gels, ■1S *(USP41)* and Hard-Shell Capsules with Solid Contents	Dissolution Requirements for Soft-Shell Capsules Filled with Liquids
I	Oil-soluble vitamins	Vitamin A (if present)	Not applicable
II	Water-soluble vitamins	One index water-soluble vitamin and folic acid (if present)	One index water-soluble vitamin and folic acid (if present)
III	Water-soluble vitamins with minerals	One index water-soluble vitamin, one index element, and folic acid (if present)	One index water-soluble vitamin, one index element, and folic acid (if present)
IV	Oil- and water-soluble vitamins	Vitamin A (if present), one index water-soluble vitamin, and folic acid (if present)	One index water-soluble vitamin and folic acid (if present)
V	Oil- and water-soluble vitamins with minerals	Vitamin A (if present), one index water-soluble vitamin, one index element, and folic acid (if present)	One index water-soluble vitamin, one index element, and folic acid (if present)
VI	Minerals	One index element	One index element
VII	Oil-soluble vitamins with minerals	Vitamin A (if present) and one index element	One index element

Selection of index water-soluble vitamins and index elements: Compliance with the dissolution requirements for dietary supplements representing combinations of water-soluble vitamins and combinations of oil- and water-soluble vitamins is determined by measuring the dissolution of a single index vitamin from the water-soluble vitamins present. Riboflavin is the index vitamin when present in the formulation. For formulations that do not contain riboflavin, pyridoxine is the index vitamin. If neither riboflavin nor pyridoxine is present in the formulation, the index vitamin is niacinamide (or niacin), and in the absence of niacinamide (or niacin), the index vitamin is thiamine. If none of these four water-soluble vitamins are present in the formulation, the index vitamin is ascorbic acid.

Compliance with the dissolution requirements for dietary supplements representing combinations of minerals is determined by measuring the dissolution of only one index element. Iron is the index element when present in the formulation. For formulations that do not contain iron, the index element is calcium. If neither iron nor calcium is present, the index element is zinc. In the absence of all three of these elements, magnesium is the index element.

Compliance with the dissolution requirements for dietary supplements representing combinations of water-soluble vitamins and minerals and combinations of oil- and water-soluble vitamins and minerals is determined by measuring the dissolution of one index water-soluble vitamin and one index element, designated according to the respective hierarchies described above.

Dissolution conditions for vitamin A: [NOTE—Perform this test under light conditions that minimize photodegradation.]
  Medium: 1% (w/v) sodium ascorbate and 1% (w/v) octoxynol 9 in 0.05 M phosphate buffer, pH 6.8; 900 mL
  Apparatus 2: 75 rpm
  Time: 45 min

Dissolution conditions for folic acid: [NOTE—Perform this test under light conditions that minimize photodegradation.]
  Test 1
  Medium: Water; 900 mL
  Apparatus 1: 100 rpm, for capsules
  Apparatus 2: 75 rpm, for tablets
  Time: 1 h
  If the units tested do not meet the requirements for dissolution in water, use the following conditions:
  Buffer: Mix 95 mL of 0.1 M citric acid monohydrate and 405 mL of 0.1 M sodium citrate dihydrate, dilute with water to 1000 mL, mix, and adjust to a pH of 6.0 by using either 0.1 M hydrochloric acid or 0.1 M sodium hydroxide solution.
  Medium: Buffer; 900 mL
  Apparatus 1: 100 rpm, for capsules
  Apparatus 2: 75 rpm, for tablets
  Time: 1 h
  Test 2 (for lipid-filled soft-shell capsules): Proceed as directed for *Test 2* under *Dissolution conditions for index water-soluble vitamins and index minerals*. If the article complies with this test, the labeling indicates that it meets USP *Dissolution Test 2*.

Test 3 (for lipid-filled soft-shell capsules):   Proceed as directed for *Test 3* under *Dissolution conditions for index water-soluble vitamins and index minerals*. If the article complies with this test, the labeling indicates that it meets USP *Dissolution Test 3*.

[NOTE—Compliance with the dissolution requirements for folic acid does not exempt the article from compliance with the dissolution requirements of the pertinent index vitamin or the corresponding index mineral.]

Dissolution conditions for index water-soluble vitamins and index minerals

Test 1
 Medium: 0.1 N hydrochloric acid; 900 mL
 Apparatus 1:   100 rpm, for capsules
 Apparatus 2:   75 rpm, for tablets
 Time: 1 h
 For formulations containing 25 mg or more of the index vitamin, riboflavin, use the following conditions:
 Medium: 0.1 N hydrochloric acid; 1800 mL
 Apparatus 1:   100 rpm, for capsules
 Apparatus 2:   75 rpm, for tablets
 Time: 1 h

Test 2 (for lipid-filled soft-shell capsules):   If the article complies with this test, the labeling indicates that it meets USP *Dissolution Test 2*.
 Medium: 0.25% (w/v) octoxynol 9, 0.02% (w/v) ascorbic acid, and 0.04% (w/v) simethicone in simulated gastric fluid TS; ■250 mL■₁ₛ ₍USP41₎
 Apparatus 3:   15 dpm
 Screen (top and bottom):   20-mesh
 Time: 1 h

Test 3 (for lipid-filled soft-shell capsules):   If the article complies with this test, the labeling indicates that it meets USP *Dissolution Test 3*.
 Medium: 0.25% (w/v) octoxynol 9 and 0.02% (w/v) ascorbic acid in simulated gastric fluid TS; 500 mL
 Apparatus 2:   125 rpm; dosage unit placed in stationary basket (*Figure 2a* and *Figure 2b*)
 Time: 1 h

[NOTE—Compliance with dissolution requirements for the pertinent index vitamin or index mineral does not exempt the article from compliance with the dissolution requirements for folic acid, if present.]

Procedures: In the following procedures, combine equal volumes of the filtered solutions of the six individual specimens withdrawn, and use the pooled sample as the test specimen. Determine the average amount of vitamin A, folic acid, or the index vitamin or element dissolved in the pooled sample. Make any necessary modifications, including concentration of the analyte in the volume of *Sample solution* taken. Use the *Medium* for preparation of the *Standard solution* and dilution, if necessary, of the *Sample solution*.

Vitamin A: Determine the percentage of retinyl acetate or retinyl palmitate dissolved by using the following procedure.
 Standard solution: Dissolve a suitable amount of USP Retinyl Acetate RS or USP Retinyl Palmitate RS in isopropyl alcohol, and dilute with *Medium* to obtain a concentration similar to that expected in the *Sample solution*. [NOTE—The amount of isopropyl alcohol should be 5%–10%.]
 Sample solution: Withdraw a portion of the solution under test, pass through a suitable filter of 0.45-μm pore size, and use the pooled sample as the test specimen.
 Solution A: Methanol and water (90:10)
 Solution B: Methanol and isopropyl alcohol (55:45)
 Mobile phase: See *Table 2*.

Table 2

Time (min)	Solution A (%)	Solution B (%)
0	100	0
8	0	100
13	0	100
13.1	100	0
15	100	0

Chromatographic system
 (See *Chromatography* ⟨621⟩, *System Suitability*.)
 Mode: LC
 Detector: UV 325 nm
 Column: 4.6-mm × 10-cm; 3-μm packing L1
 Flow rate: 1.0 mL/min
 Injection volume: 50 μL

System suitability
  Sample: *Standard solution*
  Suitability requirements
    Tailing factor: NMT 1.5 for retinyl acetate; NMT 2.0 for retinyl palmitate
    Relative standard deviation: NMT 2.0%
Analysis
  Samples: Appropriate *Standard solution* and *Sample solution*

$$\text{Result} = (r_U/r_S) \times (C_S \times V/L) \times 100$$

r_U	= peak area of the all-*trans*-retinyl ester from the *Sample solution*
r_S	= peak area of the all-*trans*-retinyl ester from the appropriate *Standard solution*
C_S	= concentration of retinol in the appropriate *Standard solution* (μg/mL)
V	= volume of *Medium*, 900 mL
L	= label claim of vitamin A, as retinol (μg/tablet)

Folic acid: Determine the amount of folic acid ($C_{19}H_{19}N_7O_6$) dissolved by using the procedure set forth in the assay for folic acid in the individual monograph. Make any necessary modifications.

Niacin or niacinamide, pyridoxine, riboflavin, and thiamine: Determine the amount of the designated index vitamin dissolved by using the procedure set forth in the assay for niacin or niacinamide, pyridoxine hydrochloride, riboflavin, and thiamine in the individual monographs. Make any necessary modifications.

Ascorbic acid: Determine the amount of ascorbic acid ($C_6H_8O_6$) dissolved by using the procedure set forth in the assay for ascorbic acid in the individual monograph. Make any necessary modifications.

Iron, calcium, magnesium, and zinc: Determine the amount of the designated index element dissolved by using the procedure set forth in the appropriate assay in the individual monographs. Make any necessary modifications.

Tolerances: The requirements are met if NLT 75% of the labeled content of vitamin A, NLT 75% of the labeled content of folic acid, and NLT 75% of the labeled content of the index vitamin or the index element from the units tested is dissolved.

- **BOTANICAL DOSAGE FORMS**

  Compliance with dissolution requirements necessitates the testing of 6 dosage units individually, or testing 2 or more dosage units in each of the six vessels of the dissolution apparatus, and measuring the dissolution of one or more index/marker compound(s) or the extract specified in the individual monograph.

  Procedures: Combine equal volumes of the filtered solutions of the six or more individual specimens withdrawn, and use the pooled sample as the *Sample solution*. Determine the average amount of index or marker compound(s) or the extract dissolved in the pooled sample by the procedure specified in the individual monograph. Make any necessary modifications, including concentration of the analyte in the volume of the *Sample solution* taken. Use the *Medium* for preparation of the *Standard solution* and dilution, if necessary, of the *Sample solution*.

  Tolerances: Unless otherwise specified in the individual monograph, the requirements are met if NLT 75% of the labeled content of the index or marker compound(s) or the extract from the units tested is dissolved in 1 h.

- **DIETARY SUPPLEMENTS OTHER THAN VITAMIN–MINERAL AND BOTANICAL DOSAGE FORMS**

  Unless otherwise stated in the individual monographs for dietary supplement dosage forms in this category, compliance requires the testing of 6 individual units, measuring the dissolution of the dietary ingredient as the average of the 6 units tested.

  Procedures: Combine equal volumes of the filtered solutions of the six specimens withdrawn, and use the pooled sample as the *Sample solution*. Determine the average amount of the dietary ingredient dissolved in the pooled sample by the procedure specified in the individual monograph. Make any necessary modifications, including concentration of the analyte in the volume of the *Sample solution* taken. Use the *Medium* for preparation of the *Standard solution* and for dilution, if necessary, of the *Sample solution*.

  Tolerances: Because of the diversity of chemical characteristics and solubilities of dietary ingredients pertaining to this category, general tolerances cannot be established. See individual monographs for *Tolerances*.

Combined Index to USP 41 and NF 36, Volumes 1–5, including First Supplement

Page citations refer to the pages of Volumes 1, 2, 3, 4 and 5 of USP 41–NF 36 and its First Supplement. This index is repeated in its entirety in each volume.

Numbers in angle brackets such as ⟨421⟩ refer to chapter numbers in the General Chapters section.

Anhydrous

Capsules

Cream

Dietary supplements

Elixir

Esomeprazole strontium, 1596
Estazolam, 1598
  tablets, 1599
Estradiol, 1600
  vaginal cream, 1601
  vaginal inserts, 1602
  transdermal system, 1604
  tablets, 1607
  benzoate, 1611, 8334
  cypionate, 1612
  cypionate injection, 1614
  and norethindrone acetate tablets, 1608
  valerate, 1614
  valerate injection, 1615
Estriol, 1616
Estrogens
  conjugated, 1617
  esterified, 1622
  tablets, conjugated, 1619
  tablets, esterified, 1623
Estrone, 1624
  injectable suspension, 1625
Estropipate, 1625
  tablets, 1627
  vaginal cream, 1626
Eszopiclone, 1628
  tablets, 1629, 8335
Ethacrynate sodium for injection, 1631
Ethacrynic acid, 1632
  tablets, 1632
Ethambutol hydrochloride, 1633
  rifampin, isoniazid, and pyrazinamide
    tablets, 3614
  Compounded oral suspension, 1634
  tablets, 1635
Ethanesulfonic acid, 5694
Ethchlorvynol, 1636
  capsules, 1637
Ether, 1638, 5694
  absolute, 5664, 5694
  diphenyl, 5694
  isopropyl, 5694
  nonyl phenyl polyethylene glycol, 5694
  peroxide-free, 5694
Ethidium bromide, 5694
Ethinyl estradiol, 1639
  and desogestrel tablets, 1186
  and drospirenone tablets, 1447
  and ethynodiol diacetate tablets, 1649
  and levonorgestrel tablets, 2402
  and norethindrone acetate tablets, 2975
  and norethindrone tablets, 2970
  and norgestimate tablets, 2981
  and norgestrel tablets, 2983
  tablets, 1639
Ethiodized oil injection, 1641
Ethionamide, 1642
  tablets, 1642
Ethopabate, 1643
Ethosuximide, 1643
  capsules, 1644
  oral solution, 1645
Ethotoin, 1646
  tablets, 1647
4'-Ethoxyacetophenone, 5694
2-Ethoxyethanol, 5694, 5695
Ethyl
  acetate, 5336, 5694
  acrylate, 5694
  acrylate and methacrylic acid copolymer,
    5442
  acrylate and methacrylic acid copolymer,
    partially-neutralized, 5446
  acrylate and methyl methacrylate
    copolymer dispersion, 5337

alcohol, 5694
arachidate, 5694
benzoate, 5694
chloride, 1648
cyanoacetate, 5694
ether, 5694
ether, anhydrous, 5664, 5694
maltol, 5339
oleate, 5339
salicylate, 5694
vanillin, 5340
2-Ethylaminopropiophenone hydrochloride,
  5695
4-Ethylbenzaldehyde, 5695
Ethylbenzene, 5695
Ethylcellulose, 5341, 8485
  aqueous dispersion, 5342
  dispersion type b, 5343
Ethylene
  dichloride, 5688, 5695
  glycol, 5695
  glycol, diethylene glycol, and triethylene
    glycol in ethoxylated substances ⟨469⟩,
    6237
  glycol monoethyl ether, 5695
  glycol stearates, 5348
  glycol and vinyl alcohol graft copolymer,
    5346
  oxide and dioxane ⟨228⟩, 6142
  oxide in methylene chloride (50 mg/mL),
    5695
Ethylenediamine, 1648, 5695
2-Ethylhexanoic acid, 8500
N-Ethylmaleimide, 5695
2-Ethyl-2-methylsuccinic acid, 5695
Ethylparaben, 5349, 5695
Ethylparaben sodium, 5350
1-Ethylquinaldinium iodide, 5695
Ethynodiol diacetate, 1648
  and ethinyl estradiol tablets, 1649
  and mestranol tablets, 1650
Etidronate disodium, 1651
  tablets, 1652
Etodolac, 1654
  capsules, 1655
  tablets, 1655
  extended-release tablets, 1656
Etomidate, 1658
  injection, 1659
Etoposide, 1660
  capsules, 1662
  injection, 1663
Eucalyptol, 1665
Eucalyptus oil, 5351
Eugenol, 1665
Evaluation of plastic packaging systems and
  their materials of construction with respect
  to their user safety impact ⟨1661⟩, 7902
Evaluation of the inner surface durability of
  glass containers ⟨1660⟩, 7897
Evening primrose oil, 4605
  capsules, 4606
Excipient biological safety evaluation
  guidelines ⟨1074⟩, 7095
Excipient performance ⟨1059⟩, 7011
Excipients
  USP and NF, listed by category, 5169,
    8475
Exemestane, 1666
Exenatide, 1667
Expert committees (2015–2020), xii, 8236
  Food Chemicals Codex, xvii, 8242
  National Formulary, xvi, 8240
  United States Pharmacopeia, xii, 8236

United States Pharmacopeia and the *Dietary
  Supplements Compendium*, xvi, 8241
United States Pharmacopeia and *USP on
  Compounding*, xviii, 8242
Expert Panels for the Council of Experts
  Executive Committee, xii, 8236
Extended release tablets
  nevirapine, 2915

Extract

Andrographis, powdered, 4433
Ashwagandha root, powdered, 4439
Astragalus root, dry, 4452
Aztec Marigold Zeaxanthin Extract, 4454
Bacillus subtilis subsp. *subtilis*
  menaquinone-7, 4765
Bacopa, powdered, 4459
Banaba leaf, dry, 4464
Beef, 5672
Belladonna, 458
Belladonna tablets, 459
Bilberry, powdered, 4472
Black cohosh, powdered, 4478
Black pepper, powdered, 4487
Boswellia serrata, 4491
Cascara fluidextract, aromatic, 738
Cascara sagrada, 736
Cascara sagrada fluidextract, 738
Cat's claw, powdered, 4509
Centella asiatica, powdered, 4516
Chaste tree, powdered, 4524
Clover, red, powdered, 4817
coffee fruit dry, 8455
Echinacea angustifolia, powdered, 4571
Echinacea pallida, powdered, 4578
Echinacea purpurea, powdered, 4587
Eleuthero, powdered, 4599
Fenugreek seed, powdered, 4612
Garcinia hydroxycitrate, powdered, 4638
Garlic, powdered, 4646
Garlic fluidextract, 4647
Ginkgo, powdered, 4660
Ginseng, American, powdered, 4425
Ginseng, Asian, powdered, 4444
Goldenseal, powdered, 4684
Green tea, decaffeinated, powdered, 4687
Guggul, native, 4690
Guggul, purified, 4691
Gymnema, native, 4696
Gymnema, purified, 4697
Holy basil leaf powdered, 4708
Horse chestnut, powdered, 4529
Japanese honeysuckle flower, dry, 4712
Licorice, powdered, 4737
Licorice fluidextract, 5422
Malabar-nut-tree, leaf, powdered, 4754
Maritime pine, 4757
Milk thistle, powdered, 4773
Northern schisandra fruit, dry, 4866
Olive leaf dry, 4794
Powdered *Rhodiola rosea*, 4828
Pygeum, 4807
Pyrethrum, 3522
Red clover aerial parts isoflavone
  aglycones, dry, 4814
Rhodiola crenulata root and rhizome dry,
  4822
Salix species bark dry, 4852, 8467
Saw palmetto, 4860
Senna fluidextract, 3741
Soy isoflavones, powdered, 4877
Stinging nettle, powdered, 4892

G

General chapters

General chapters

Inhalation

Inhalation and nasal drug products: aerosols, sprays, and powders—performance quality tests ⟨601⟩, 6327
Inhalation and nasal drug products general information and product quality tests ⟨5⟩, 5938

Injection

Acepromazine maleate, 33
Acetazolamide for, 66
Acyclovir for, 81
Adenosine, 90
Alcohol, dehydrated, 107
Alcohol in dextrose, 107
Alfentanil, 113
Alprostadil, 140
Alteplase for, 144
Amifostine for, 199
Amikacin sulfate, 203
Aminocaproic acid, 218
Aminohippurate sodium, 222
Aminopentamide sulfate, 225
Aminophylline, 228
Amiodarone hydrochloride, 243
Amitriptyline hydrochloride, 249, 8269
Ammonium chloride, 265
Ammonium molybdate, 268
Amobarbital sodium for, 269
Amphotericin B for, 291
Ampicillin for, 300
Ampicillin and sulbactam for, 305
Anileridine, 316
Aprotinin, 345
Arginine hydrochloride, 350
Articaine hydrochloride and epinephrine, 358
Ascorbic acid, 360
Atenolol, 384
Atracurium besylate, 403
Atropine sulfate, 406
Azaperone, 413
Azathioprine sodium for, 418
Azithromycin for, 425
Aztreonam, 433
Aztreonam for, 434
Bacitracin for, 437
Bacteriostatic sodium chloride, 3784
Bacteriostatic water for, 4346
Benztropine mesylate, 493
Benzylpenicilloyl polylysine, 497
Betamethasone sodium phosphate, 512
Bethanechol chloride, 522
Bleomycin for, 546
Bretylium tosylate, 548
Bretylium tosylate in dextrose, 548
Brompheniramine maleate, 558
Bumetanide, 563
Bupivacaine hydrochloride, 566
Bupivacaine hydrochloride in dextrose, 567
Bupivacaine hydrochloride and epinephrine, 567
Butorphanol tartrate, 607
Caffeine citrate, 612
Caffeine and sodium benzoate, 614
Calcitonin salmon, 623
Calcitriol, 626
Calcium chloride, 639
Calcium gluceptate, 642
Calcium gluconate, 645
Calcium levulinate, 651

Capreomycin for, 671
Carbenicillin for, 690
Carboplatin for, 709
Carboprost tromethamine, 711
Carmustine for, 722
Cefamandole nafate for, 755
Cefazolin, 758
Cefazolin for, 759
Cefepime for, 770
Cefmenoxime for, 776
Cefmetazole, 778
Cefmetazole for, 779
Cefonicid for, 780
Cefoperazone, 781
Cefoperazone for, 782
Ceforanide for, 784
Cefotaxime, 785
Cefotaxime for, 786
Cefotetan, 791
Cefotetan for, 791
Cefotiam for, 794
Cefoxitin, 796
Cefoxitin for, 797
Cefpiramide for, 799
Ceftazidime, 809
Ceftazidime for, 810
Ceftizoxime, 817
Ceftizoxime for, 818
Ceftriaxone, 818
Ceftriaxone for, 819
Cefuroxime, 822
Cefuroxime for, 823
Cephalothin, 837
Cephalothin for, 838
Cephapirin for, 839
Cephradine for, 844
Chloramphenicol, 863
Chloramphenicol sodium succinate for, 870
Chloroprocaine hydrochloride, 889
Chloroquine hydrochloride, 890
Chlorothiazide sodium for, 897
Chlorpheniramine maleate, 902
Chlorpromazine hydrochloride, 907
Chorionic gonadotropin for, 1982
Chromic chloride, 920
Chromium Cr 51 edetate, 922
Cimetidine, 935
Cimetidine in sodium chloride, 937
Ciprofloxacin, 942
Cisapride compounded, veterinary, 953
Cisatracurium besylate, 957
Cisplatin for, 961
Cladribine, 974
Clavulanic acid and ticarcillin, 4081
Clindamycin, 990
Clindamycin for, 991
Cloprostenol, 1036
Codeine phosphate, 1063
Colchicine, 1070
Colistimethate for, 1074
Corticotropin, 1094
Corticotropin for, 1095
Corticotropin, repository, 1097
Cr 51, sodium chromate, 921
Cupric chloride, 1111
Cupric sulfate, 1112
Cyanocobalamin, 1114
Cyclophosphamide for, 1126
Cyclosporine, 1131
Cysteine hydrochloride, 1140
Cytarabine for, 1142
Dacarbazine for, 1143
Dactinomycin for, 1145
Dantrolene sodium for, 1155

Daunorubicin hydrochloride for, 1159
Deferoxamine mesylate for, 1162
Dehydrated alcohol, 107
Deslanoside, 1176
Desmopressin acetate, 1183
Dexamethasone, 1196
Dexamethasone sodium phosphate, 1204
Dexamethasone sodium phosphate compounded, 1205
Dexmedetomidine, 1215
Dextran 40 in dextrose, 1222
Dextran 40 in sodium chloride, 1223
Dextran 70 in dextrose, 1226
Dextran 70 in sodium chloride, 1227
Dextrose, 1234
Dextrose and sodium chloride, 1235
Diatrizoate meglumine, 1236
Diatrizoate meglumine and diatrizoate sodium, 1237
Diatrizoate sodium, 1240
Diazepam, 1245
Diazoxide, 1247
Dibucaine hydrochloride, 1251
Dicyclomine hydrochloride, 1269
Diethylstilbestrol, 1280
Digitoxin, 1289
Digoxin, 1292
Dihydroergotamine mesylate, 1296
Dihydrostreptomycin, 1297
Dimenhydrinate, 1313
Dimercaprol, 1316
Dinoprost tromethamine, 1320
Diphenhydramine hydrochloride, 1330
Dipyridamole, 1346
Dobutamine, 1367
Dobutamine for, 1368
Dobutamine in dextrose, 1369
Docetaxel, 1373
Dopamine hydrochloride, 1393
Dopamine hydrochloride and dextrose, 1394
Doxapram hydrochloride, 1401
Doxorubicin hydrochloride, 1411
Doxorubicin hydrochloride for, 1413
Doxycycline for, 1420
Droperidol, 1443
Dyphylline, 1460
Edetate calcium disodium, 1470
Edetate disodium, 1472
Edrophonium chloride, 1472
Electrolytes and dextrose type 1, multiple, 1485
Electrolytes and dextrose type 2, multiple, 1488
Electrolytes and dextrose type 3, multiple, 1492
Electrolytes type 1, multiple, 1480
Electrolytes type 2, multiple, 1482
Elements, trace, 1494
Emetine hydrochloride, 1498
Enalaprilat, 1506
Enoxaparin sodium, 1512
Ephedrine sulfate, 1527
Epinephrine, 1530
Epirubicin hydrochloride, 1537
Ergonovine maleate, 1555
Ergotamine tartrate, 1559
Erythromycin, 1568
Erythromycin ethylsuccinate, 1577
Erythromycin lactobionate for, 1581
Estradiol cypionate, 1614
Estradiol valerate, 1615
Ethacrynate sodium for, 1631
Ethiodized oil, 1641
Etomidate, 1659

Injection *(continued)*

Etoposide, 1663
Famotidine, 1680
Fenoldopam mesylate, 1703
Fentanyl citrate, 1709
Ferumoxides, 1722
Floxuridine for, 1753
Fluconazole, 1755
Fluconazole in dextrose, 1758
Fluconazole in sodium chloride, 1760
Fludarabine phosphate, 1770
Fludarabine phosphate for, 1771
Fludeoxyglucose F18, 1794
Flumazenil, 1776
Flunixin meglumine, 1782
Fluorescein, 1789
F 18, sodium fluoride, 1795
Fluorouracil, 1802
Fluphenazine decanoate, 1812
Fluphenazine enanthate, 1814
Fluphenazine hydrochloride, 1816
Folic acid, 1866
Fondaparinux sodium, 1872
Fosphenytoin sodium, 1885
Fructose, 1887
Fructose and sodium chloride, 1888
Furosemide, 1893
Gadodiamide, 1902
Gadopentetate dimeglumine, 1904
Gadoteridol, 1908
Gadoversetamide, 1911
Gallamine triethiodide, 1924
Gallium citrate Ga 67, 1924
Ganciclovir for, 1926
Gemcitabine for, 1931
Gentamicin, 1935
Glucagon for, 1957
Glycopyrrolate, 1973
Gold sodium thiomalate, 1976
Gonadorelin for, 1976
Gonadotropin, chorionic for, 1982
Granisetron hydrochloride, 1992
Guaifenesin for, 2002
Haloperidol, 2020
Heparin sodium, 2031
Histamine phosphate, 2036
Hyaluronidase, 2042
Hyaluronidase for, 2042
Hydralazine hydrochloride, 2045
Hydrochloric acid, 2047
Hydrocortisone sodium phosphate, 2069
Hydrocortisone sodium succinate for, 2071
Hydromorphone hydrochloride, 2079
Hydroxocobalamin, 2084
Hydroxyprogesterone caproate, 2087
Hydroxyzine hydrochloride, 2092
Hyoscyamine sulfate, 2103
I 123, iobenguane, 2189
I 123, iodohippurate sodium, 2191
I 125, iothalamate sodium, 2194
I 125, albumin, iodinated, 2193
I 131, iobenguane, 2190
I 131, iodohippurate sodium, 2195
I 131, rose bengal sodium, 2196
I 131, albumin, iodinated, 2194
I 131, albumin aggregated, iodinated, 2195
Idarubicin hydrochloride, 2118
Idarubicin hydrochloride for, 2117
Ifosfamide for, 2122
Imipenem and cilastatin for, 2124
Imipramine hydrochloride, 2127
Inamrinone, 2137
Indigotindisulfonate sodium, 2141
Indium In 111 capromab pendetide, 2143

Indium In 111 ibritumomab tiuxetan, 2145
Indium In 111 pentetate, 2147
Indium In 111 pentetreotide, 2147
Indium In 111 satumomab pendetide, 2148
Indocyanine green for, 2149
Indomethacin for, 2155
injection, 930
Insulin, 2163
Insulin aspart, 2166
Insulin glargine, 2169
Insulin human, 2173
Insulin, human, and human insulin isophane suspension, 2174
Insulin lispro, 2180
Inulin in sodium chloride, 2186
Invert sugar, 3846
Iodipamide meglumine, 2198
Iodixanol, 2202
Iohexol, 2209
Iopamidol, 2211
Iopromide, 2215
Iothalamate meglumine, 2216
Iothalamate meglumine and iothalamate sodium, 2216
Ioversol, 2219
Ioxaglate meglumine and ioxaglate sodium, 2220
Ioxilan, 2223
Irinotecan hydrochloride, 2237
Iron dextran, 2239
Iron sorbitex, 2241
Iron sucrose, 2241
Isoniazid, 2253
Isoproterenol hydrochloride, 2260
Isoxsuprine hydrochloride, 2286
Ivermectin, 2293
Ivermectin and clorsulon, 2297
Kanamycin, 2304
Ketamine hydrochloride, 2308
Ketorolac tromethamine, 2316
Labetalol hydrochloride, 2321
Leucovorin calcium, 2361
Levetiracetam, 2389
Levocarnitine, 2387
Levorphanol tartrate, 2403
Lidocaine hydrochloride, 2413
Lidocaine hydrochloride and dextrose, 2417
Lidocaine hydrochloride and epinephrine, 2417
Lincomycin, 2420
Lorazepam, 2471
Magnesium sulfate, 2519
Magnesium sulfate in dextrose, 2519
Manganese chloride, 2524
Manganese sulfate, 2526
Mannitol, 2529
Mannitol in sodium chloride, 2529
Mechlorethamine hydrochloride for, 2541
Menadiol sodium diphosphate, 2570
Menadione, 2572
Meperidine hydrochloride, 2575
Mepivacaine hydrochloride, 2581
Mepivacaine hydrochloride and levonordefrin, 2582
Meropenem for, 2592
Mesoridazine besylate, 2602
Metaraminol bitartrate, 2610
Methadone hydrochloride, 2628
Methocarbamol, 2645
Methohexital sodium for, 2648
Methotrexate, 2651, 8352
Methotrexate for, 2652
Methotrimeprazine, 2653

Methyldopate hydrochloride, 2672
Methylene blue, 2673
Methylene blue, veterinary, 2675
Methylergonovine maleate, 2677
Methylprednisolone sodium succinate for, 2694
Metoclopramide, 2700
Metoprolol tartrate, 2713
Metronidazole, 2724
Mezlocillin for, 2734
Miconazole, 2737
Midazolam, 2741
Milrinone lactate, 2748
Minocycline for, 2751
Mitomycin for, 2772
Mitoxantrone, 2774
Morphine sulfate, 2812
Morphine sulfate compounded, 2813
Morrhuate sodium, 2815
Mycophenolate mofetil for, 2831
N 13, ammonia, 2955
Nafcillin, 2847
Nafcillin for, 2848
Nalorphine hydrochloride, 2855
Naloxone hydrochloride, 2856
Nandrolone decanoate, 2860
Neomycin for, 2882
Neostigmine methylsulfate, 2909
Netilmicin sulfate, 2910
Niacin, 2918
Niacinamide, 2924
Nicardipine hydrochloride, 2927
Nitroglycerin, 2957
Norepinephrine bitartrate, 2967
Ondansetron, 3031
Orphenadrine citrate, 3049
Oxacillin, 3061
Oxacillin for, 3062
Oxaliplatin, 3067
Oxaliplatin for, 3069
Oxymorphone hydrochloride, 3117
Oxytetracycline, 3125
Oxytetracycline for, 3128
Oxytocin, 3133
Paclitaxel, 3136
Pamidronate disodium for, 3144
Pancuronium bromide, 3152
Papaverine hydrochloride, 3163
Paricalcitol, 3171
Particulate matter in injections ⟨788⟩, 6537
Pemetrexed, 3186
Penicillin G potassium, 3199
Penicillin G potassium for, 3200
Penicillin G sodium for, 3212
Pentazocine, 3225
Pentobarbital sodium, 3229
Perphenazine, 3246, 8396
Phenobarbital sodium, 3262
Phentolamine mesylate for, 3271
Phenylbutazone, 3274
Phenylephrine hydrochloride, 3279
Phenytoin sodium, 3293
Physostigmine salicylate, 3296
Phytonadione injectable emulsion, 3298
Piperacillin for, 3324
Piperacillin and tazobactam for, 3325
Polymyxin B for, 3349
Potassium acetate, 3354
Potassium chloride concentrate for, 3361
Potassium chloride in dextrose, 3364
Potassium chloride in dextrose and sodium chloride, 3365
Potassium chloride in lactated ringer's and dextrose, 3367

Lotion

M

O

Oil

Ointment

Ophthalmic ointment

Ophthalmic solution

Ophthalmic suspension

Orally inhaled and nasal drug products
〈1664.1〉, 7937

Oral powder

Containing at least three of the
following—acetaminophen and (salts of)
chlorpheniramine, dextromethorphan,
and pseudoephedrine, 47
Levothyroxine sodium, 2407
Sodium bicarbonate, 3779

Oral solution

Abacavir, 19
Acacia syrup, 5179
Acetaminophen, 37
Containing at least three of the
following—acetaminophen and (salts of)
chlorpheniramine, dextromethorphan,
and pseudoephedrine, 49
Acetaminophen and codeine phosphate,
56
Acetaminophen, dextromethorphan
hydrobromide, doxylamine succinate,
and pseudoephedrine hydrochloride, 60
Acetaminophen for effervescent, 37
Amantadine hydrochloride, 196
Aminobenzoate potassium for, 212
Aminocaproic acid, 219
Aminophylline, 229
Amprolium, 307
Aromatic elixir, 5206
Ascorbic acid, 361
Ascorbic acid compounded, 361
Aspirin effervescent tablets for, 371
Atenolol, 385
Beclomethasone dipropionate
compounded, 456
Benzaldehyde elixir, compound, 5215
Betamethasone, 503
Bethanechol chloride, 523
Bromodiphenhydramine hydrochloride,
555
Bromodiphenhydramine hydrochloride and
codeine phosphate, 556
Brompheniramine maleate, 558
Brompheniramine maleate and
pseudoephedrine sulfate, 559
Butabarbital sodium, 593
Caffeine citrate, 613
Calcium glubionate syrup, 641
Captopril, 678
C 13 for, urea, 706
Cetirizine hydrochloride, 848
Cherry syrup, 5289
Chloral hydrate, 860
Chloramphenicol, 865
Chlorpheniramine maleate, 902
Chlorpheniramine maleate and
pseudoephedrine hydrochloride, 904
Chlorpromazine hydrochloride syrup, 908
Chocolate syrup, 5296
Citalopram, 963
Clindamycin hydrochloride, 994
Clindamycin palmitate hydrochloride for,
995
Cloxacillin sodium for, 1052
Cyanocobalamin Co 57, 1056
Codeine phosphate, 1064
Codeine sulfate, 1066

Cyclosporine, 1133
Cyproheptadine hydrochloride, 1136
Dexamethasone, 1198
Dexamethasone elixir, 1196
Dexbrompheniramine maleate and
pseudoephedrine sulfate, 1209
Dexchlorpheniramine maleate, 1211
Dextromethorphan hydrobromide, 1232
Dicyclomine hydrochloride, 1270
Didanosine for, 1275
Digoxin, 1292
Dihydrotachysterol, 1299
Diltiazem hydrochloride, 1309
Dimenhydrinate, 1314
Diphenhydramine hydrochloride, 1331
Diphenoxylate hydrochloride and atropine
sulfate, 1339
Docusate sodium syrup, 1380
Dolasetron mesylate, 1384
Doxepin hydrochloride, 1407
Doxylamine succinate, 1438
Dyphylline, 1461
Dyphylline and guaifenesin, 1462
Ephedrine sulfate, 1529
Ergocalciferol, 1549
Ergoloid mesylates, 1552
Escitalopram, 1584
Ethosuximide, 1645
Ferric ammonium citrate for, 266
Ferrous gluconate, 1717
Ferrous sulfate, 1720
Ferrous sulfate syrup, 1720
Fluoxetine, 1806
Fluphenazine hydrochloride, 1817
Fluphenazine hydrochloride elixir, 1815
Folic acid, compounded, 1866
Furosemide, 1893
Galantamine, 1917
Glycerin, 1969
Guaifenesin, 2003
Guaifenesin and codeine phosphate, 2004
Haloperidol, 2021
Hydralazine hydrochloride, 2045
Hydromorphone hydrochloride, 2079
Hydroxyzine hydrochloride, 2092
Hyoscyamine sulfate, 2104
Hyoscyamine sulfate elixir, 2103
Ipecac, 2226
Isoniazid, 2254
Isosorbide, 2267
Lamivudine, 2328
Leucovorin calcium compounded, 2361
Levetiracetam, 2373
Levocarnitine, 2388
Levofloxacin, 2397
Lincomycin, 2421
Lithium, 2436
Loperamide hydrochloride, 2448
Lopinavir and ritonavir, 2453
Loratadine, 2464
Magnesium carbonate, citric acid, and
potassium citrate for, 2503
Magnesium carbonate and citric acid for,
2502
Manganese chloride for, 2524
Magnesium citrate, 2506
Magnesium citrate for, 2507
Meperidine hydrochloride, 2575
Mesoridazine besylate, 2602
Metaproterenol sulfate, 2608
Methadone hydrochloride, 2629
Methdilazine hydrochloride, 2634
Methenamine, 2636
Methenamine mandelate for, 2639
Methylcellulose, 2666

Metoclopramide, 2701
Metoprolol tartrate, 2714
Mibolerone, 2735
Nafcillin sodium for, 2850
Neomycin sulfate, 2884
Nortriptyline hydrochloride, 2986
Ondansetron, 3032
Orange syrup, 5476
Oxacillin sodium for, 3062
Oxtriphylline, 3090
Oxybutynin chloride, 3094
Oxycodone hydrochloride, 3103
Paromomycin, 3173
Penicillin G potassium for, 3201
Penicillin V potassium for, 3217
Perphenazine, 3246, 8396
Phenobarbital, 3260
Piperazine citrate syrup, 3334
Polyethylene glycol 3350 and electrolytes
for, 3345
Potassium bicarbonate effervescent tablets
for, 3355
Potassium bicarbonate and potassium
chloride for effervescent, 3356
Potassium bicarbonate and potassium
chloride effervescent tablets for, 3356
Potassium bicarbonate, potassium chloride,
and potassium citrate effervescent
tablets for, 3367
Potassium bromide, veterinary, 3359
Potassium chloride, 3362
Potassium chloride for, 3363
Potassium citrate and citric acid, 3375
Potassium gluconate, 3377
Potassium gluconate and potassium
chloride, 3378
Potassium gluconate and potassium
chloride for, 3379
Potassium gluconate and potassium citrate,
3380
Potassium gluconate, potassium citrate,
and ammonium chloride, 3380
Potassium iodide, 3382
Potassium and sodium bicarbonates and
citric acid effervescent tablets for, 3357
Prednisolone, 3412
Prednisolone sodium phosphate
compounded, 3418
Prednisone, 3422
Prochlorperazine, 3448
Promazine hydrochloride, 3462
Promazine hydrochloride syrup, 3463
Promethazine and phenylephrine
hydrochloride, 3470
Promethazine and phenylephrine
hydrochloride and codeine phosphate,
3473
Promethazine hydrochloride, 3466
Pseudoephedrine hydrochloride, 3508
Pseudoephedrine hydrochloride,
carbinoxamine maleate, and
dextromethorphan hydrobromide, 3511
Pyridostigmine bromide, 3524
Ranitidine, 3580
Risperidone, 3639
Ritonavir, 3651
Saccharin sodium, 3691
Senna, 3743
Sertraline hydrochloride, 3749
Sodium bromide, veterinary, 3780
Sodium citrate and citric acid, 3787
Sodium fluoride, 3790, 8422
Sodium phosphates, 3807
Stavudine for, 3836
Sulfaquinoxaline, 3880

Oral suspension

Powder

Powdered

Q

R

Radiopharmaceuticals

Sodium *(continued)*
 phosphate, dibasic, heptahydrate, 5731
 phosphate, dibasic, TS, 5760
 phosphate, monobasic, 3805, 5709, 5731
 phosphate, monobasic, anhydrous, 5731
 phosphate, monobasic, dihydrate, 5732
 phosphate P 32 solution, 3295
 phosphates injection, 3805
 phosphates oral solution, 3807
 phosphates rectal solution, 3807
 phosphate, tribasic, 5574, 5732
 phosphite pentahydrate, 5732
 phosphotungstate TS, 5760
 picosulfate, 3807
 polystyrene sulfonate, 3809
 polystyrene sulfonate suspension, 3809
 and potassium bicarbonates and citric acid
  effervescent tablets for oral solution,
  3357
 propionate, 5575
 pyrophosphate, 5732
 pyruvate, 5732
 rabeprazole, 3562
 salicylate, 3810, 5732
 salicylate tablets, 3811
 selenite, 5732
 starch glycolate, 5575
 stearate, 5577
 stearyl fumarate, 5578
 sulfate, 3812, 5732
 sulfate, anhydrous, 5669, 5732
 sulfate decahydrate, 5732
 sulfate injection, 3813
 sulfide, 3813, 5732
 sulfide topical gel, 3813
 sulfide TS, 5760
 sulfite, 5580, 5732
 sulfite, anhydrous, 5669, 5732
 p-sulfophenylazochromotropate, 5732
 tartrate, 5581, 5733
 tartrate TS, 5760
 tetraphenylborate, 5733
 tetraphenylboron, 5733
 tetraphenylboron, fiftieth-molar (0.02 M),
  5771
 tetraphenylboron TS, 5760
 thioglycolate, 5733
 thioglycolate TS, 5760
 thiosulfate, 3814, 5733
 thiosulfate injection, 3814
 thiosulfate, tenth-normal (0.1 N), 5760,
  5771
 thiosulfate TS, 5760
 L-thyroxine, 5733
 3-(trimethylsilyl)-1-propane sulfonate,
  5729, 5733
 tungstate, 5733
Sodium bicarbonate
 compounded injection, 3778
Sodium chloride
 0.5 M TS, 5759
0.1 N Sodium chloride
 TS, 8502
Sodium 1-dodecanesulfonate, 5729
Sodium ferrous citrate, 4876
Sodium hydroxide
 0.0025 N TS, 5759
 0.2 N, TS, 5759
 0.02 N TS, 5759
 10 N TS, 5759
 2.5 N TS, 5759
 2 N TS, 5759
 5 N, TS, 5759
 0.1 N VS, 5770
 0.01 N VS, 5770

 0.5 N VS, 5770
Sodium phenylbutyrate, 3801
Sodium phosphate, 8502
Sodium phosphates
 compounded injection, 3806
Sodium succinate, 5579
Sodium thiosulfate
 0.01 M VS, 5772, 8503
Solubilities, 5851
Soluble starch, 5733

Solution

Acetaminophen and codeine phosphate
 oral, 56
Acetaminophen, dextromethorphan
 hydrobromide, doxylamine succinate,
 and pseudoephedrine hydrochloride
 oral, 60
Acetaminophen for effervescent oral, 37
Acetaminophen oral, 37
Acetic acid otic, 70
Acetylcholine chloride for ophthalmic, 73
Acetylcysteine, 74
Acidulated phosphate and sodium fluoride
 topical, 3791, 8423
Aluminum acetate topical, 163
Aluminum chlorohydrate, 165
Aluminum dichlorohydrate, 168
Aluminum sesquichlorohydrate, 173
Aluminum subacetate topical, 175
Aluminum sulfate and calcium acetate for
 topical, 176
Aluminum sulfate and calcium acetate
 tablets for topical, 177
Aluminum zirconium octachlorohydrate,
 179
Aluminum zirconium octachlorohydrex gly,
 181
Aluminum zirconium pentachlorohydrate,
 183
Aluminum zirconium pentachlorohydrex
 gly, 185
Aluminum zirconium tetrachlorohydrate,
 187
Aluminum zirconium tetrachlorohydrex
 gly, 189
Aluminum zirconium trichlorohydrate, 191
Aluminum zirconium trichlorohydrex gly,
 193
Amantadine hydrochloride oral, 196
Aminobenzoate potassium for oral, 212
Aminobenzoic acid topical, 217
Aminocaproic acid oral, 219
Aminophylline oral, 229
Aminophylline rectal, 231
Ammonia, diluted, 5668
Ammonia, strong, 5197
Amprolium oral, 307
Anticoagulant citrate dextrose, 324
Anticoagulant citrate phosphate dextrose,
 326
Anticoagulant citrate phosphate dextrose
 adenine, 327
Anticoagulant heparin, 2025
Anticoagulant sodium citrate, 329
Antipyrine and benzocaine otic, 332
Antipyrine, benzocaine, and phenylephrine
 hydrochloride otic, 333
Apraclonidine ophthalmic, 338
Aromatic elixir, 5206
Ascorbic acid oral, 361
Aspirin effervescent tablets for oral, 371

Atenolol oral, 385
Atropine sulfate ophthalmic, 408
Benoxinate hydrochloride ophthalmic, 466
Benzaldehyde elixir, compound, 5215
Benzalkonium chloride, 5217
Benzethonium chloride topical, 467
Benzocaine, butamben, and tetracaine
 hydrochloride topical, 483
Benzocaine otic, 476
Benzocaine topical, 478
Betamethasone oral, 503
Betaxolol ophthalmic, 519
Bethanechol chloride oral, 523
Bromodiphenhydramine hydrochloride and
 codeine phosphate oral, 556
Bromodiphenhydramine hydrochloride
 oral, 555
Brompheniramine maleate and
 pseudoephedrine sulfate oral, 559
Brompheniramine maleate oral, 558
Buprenorphine compounded buccal,
 veterinary, 570
Butabarbital sodium oral, 593
Caffeine citrate oral, 613
Calcitonin salmon nasal, 624
Calcium hydroxide topical, 647
Captopril oral, 678
Carbachol intraocular, 682
Carbachol ophthalmic, 683
Carbamide peroxide topical, 690
Carbol-fuchsin topical, 704
C 13 for oral, urea, 706
Carteolol hydrochloride ophthalmic, 727
Cefazolin ophthalmic, 760
Cetylpyridinium chloride topical, 858
Chloral hydrate oral, 860
Chloramphenicol for ophthalmic, 865
Chloramphenicol ophthalmic, 864
Chloramphenicol oral, 865
Chloramphenicol otic, 865
Chlorhexidine gluconate, 881
Chlorpheniramine maleate and
 pseudoephedrine hydrochloride oral,
 904
Chlorpheniramine maleate oral, 902
Cholecalciferol, 917
Chymotrypsin for ophthalmic, 924, 8311
Ciprofloxacin ophthalmic, 944
Clindamycin hydrochloride oral, 994
Clindamycin palmitate hydrochloride for
 oral, 995
Clindamycin phosphate topical, 999
Clobetasol propionate topical, 1008
Clotrimazole topical, 1044
Cloxacillin sodium for oral, 1052
Coal tar topical, 1055
Cyanocobalamin Co 57 oral, 1056
Cocaine hydrochloride tablets for topical,
 1058
Cocaine and tetracaine hydrochlorides and
 epinephrine topical, 1059
Codeine sulfate oral, 1066
Cromolyn sodium ophthalmic, 1107
Cupriethylenediamine hydroxide, 1.0 M,
 5685
Cyclopentolate hydrochloride ophthalmic,
 1123
Cyclosporine oral, 1133
Cyproheptadine hydrochloride oral, 1136
Demecarium bromide ophthalmic, 1165
Dexamethasone elixir, 1196
Dexamethasone oral, 1198
Dexamethasone sodium phosphate
 ophthalmic, 1207

Suppositories

Suppositories (continued)
  Progesterone vaginal, 3457
  Promethazine hydrochloride, 3467
  Thiethylperazine maleate, 4052

Suprofen, 3900
  ophthalmic solution, 3900

Suspension

Acetaminophen and codeine phosphate
  oral, 57
Acetaminophen oral, 39, 8264
Acetazolamide oral, 68
Acyclovir oral, 83
Albendazole oral, 93
Allopurinol oral, 123
Alprazolam oral, 131
Alumina, magnesia, and calcium carbonate
  oral, 151
Alumina and magnesia oral, 149
Alumina, magnesia, and simethicone oral,
  155
Alumina and magnesium carbonate oral,
  158
Alumina and magnesium trisilicate oral,
  161
Amoxicillin and clavulanate potassium for
  oral, 284
Amoxicillin for oral, 280
Amoxicillin for injectable, 279
Amoxicillin oral, 279
Amoxicillin tablets for oral, 283
Ampicillin for injectable, 301
Ampicillin for oral, 301
Ampicillin and probenecid for oral, 303
Atenolol compounded oral, 386
Atenolol compounded oral, veterinary, 386
Atovaquone oral, 400
Aurothioglucose injectable, 411
Azathioprine oral, 417
Azithromycin for oral, 428
Baclofen oral, 444
Barium sulfate, 452
Barium sulfate for, 453
Benazepril hydrochloride compounded
  oral, veterinary, 463
Betamethasone sodium phosphate and
  betamethasone acetate injectable, 512
Bethanechol chloride oral, 523
Bisacodyl rectal, 532
Bismuth subsalicylate oral, 540
Brinzolamide ophthalmic, 550
Calamine topical, 615
Calamine topical, phenolated, 616
Calcium carbonate oral, 633
Calcium and magnesium carbonates oral,
  637
Captopril oral, 679
Carbamazepine oral, 685
Cefaclor for oral, 744
Cefadroxil for oral, 752
Cefdinir for oral, 767
Cefixime for oral, 775
Cefpodoxime proxetil for oral, 801
Cefprozil for oral, 806
Cefuroxime axetil for oral, 825
Cellulose sodium phosphate for oral, 832
Cephalexin for oral, 834
Cephradine for oral, 845

Chloramphenicol and hydrocortisone
  acetate for ophthalmic, 866
Chloramphenicol palmitate oral, 868
Chlorothiazide oral, 895
Cholestyramine for oral, 919
Chromic phosphate P 32, 3295
Ciclopirox olamine topical, 928
Ciprofloxacin and dexamethasone otic,
  951
Clarithromycin for oral, 977
Clavulanate potassium and amoxicillin for
  oral, 284
Clindamycin phosphate topical, 999
Clonazepam oral, 1021
Clopidogrel compounded oral, 1033
Colestipol hydrochloride for oral, 1072
Colistin and neomycin sulfates and
  hydrocortisone acetate otic, 1075
Colistin sulfate for oral, 1075
Cortisone acetate injectable, 1100, 8315
Demeclocycline oral, 1166
Desoxycorticosterone pivalate injectable,
  1194
Dexamethasone acetate injectable, 1200
Dexamethasone ophthalmic, 1197
Diazoxide oral, 1248
Dicloxacillin sodium for oral, 1267
Didanosine tablets for oral, 1275
Diltiazem hydrochloride oral, 1310
Dipyridamole oral, 1347
Dolasetron mesylate oral, 1385
Doxycycline calcium oral, 1425
Doxycycline compounded oral, veterinary,
  1427
Doxycycline for oral, 1421
Enalapril maleate compounded oral,
  veterinary, 1501
Erythromycin estolate for oral, 1574
Erythromycin estolate oral, 1574
Erythromycin estolate and sulfisoxazole
  acetyl oral, 1575
Erythromycin ethylsuccinate for oral, 1578
Erythromycin ethylsuccinate oral, 1578
Erythromycin ethylsuccinate and
  sulfisoxazole acetyl for oral, 1580
Estrone injectable, 1625
Famotidine for oral, 1682
Ferumoxsil oral, 1724
Flucytosine oral, 1767
Fluorometholone ophthalmic, 1798
Furazolidone oral, 1891
Ganciclovir oral, 1927
Gentamicin and prednisolone acetate
  ophthalmic, 1943
Griseofulvin oral, 1998
Hydrocortisone rectal, 2060
Hydroxyzine pamoate oral, 2099, 8339
Ibuprofen oral, 2110
Imipenem and cilastatin for injectable,
  2125
Indomethacin oral, 2158
Isophane insulin human, 2177
Human insulin isophane and human insulin
  injection, 2174
Isophane insulin, 2176
Insulin zinc, 2181
Insulin zinc, extended, 2182
Insulin zinc, prompt, 2184
Isoflupredone acetate injectable, 2247
Ketoconazole oral, 2310
Labetalol hydrochloride oral, 2321
Lamotrigine compounded oral, 2342
Lansoprazole compounded oral, 2351
Loracarbef for oral, 2461
Magaldrate and simethicone oral, 2498

Magaldrate oral, 2497
Magnesium carbonate and sodium
  bicarbonate for oral, 2504
Mebendazole oral, 2535
Medroxyprogesterone acetate injectable,
  2548
Megestrol acetate oral, 2554
Meloxicam oral, 2560, 8349
Meprobamate oral, 2585
Mesalamine rectal, 2597
Methacycline hydrochloride oral, 2626
Methadone hydrochloride tablets for oral,
  2630
Methenamine mandelate oral, 2640
Methyldopa oral, 2667
Methylprednisolone acetate injectable,
  2691
Metolazone oral, 2705
Metoprolol tartrate oral, 2714
Metronidazole benzoate compounded oral,
  2722
Minocycline hydrochloride oral, 2754
Nalidixic acid oral, 2853
Naproxen oral, 2864
Natamycin ophthalmic, 2876
Neomycin and polymyxin B sulfates and
  dexamethasone ophthalmic, 2901
Neomycin and polymyxin B sulfates and
  hydrocortisone otic, 2903
Neomycin and polymyxin B sulfates and
  hydrocortisone acetate ophthalmic, 2904
Neomycin and polymyxin B sulfates and
  hydrocortisone ophthalmic, 2903
Neomycin and polymyxin B sulfates and
  prednisolone acetate ophthalmic, 2906
Neomycin sulfate and hydrocortisone otic,
  2889
Neomycin sulfate and hydrocortisone
  acetate ophthalmic, 2890
Neomycin sulfate and prednisolone acetate
  ophthalmic, 2907
Nevirapine oral, 2912
Nitrofurantoin oral, 2951
Nystatin for oral, 2990
Nystatin oral, 2990
Ondansetron hydrochloride oral, 3033
Oxfendazole oral, 3087
Oxytetracycline and nystatin for oral, 3126
Oxytetracycline calcium oral, 3127
Oxytetracycline hydrochloride and
  hydrocortisone acetate ophthalmic, 3129
Pantoprazole oral, 3154
Penicillin G benzathine injectable, 3195
Penicillin G benzathine and penicillin G
  procaine injectable, 3196
Penicillin G benzathine oral, 3196
Penicillin G, neomycin, polymyxin B,
  hydrocortisone acetate, and
  hydrocortisone sodium succinate topical,
  3193
Penicillin G procaine, dihydrostreptomycin
  sulfate, chlorpheniramine maleate, and
  dexamethasone injectable, 3207
Penicillin G procaine and
  dihydrostreptomycin sulfate injectable,
  3207
Penicillin G procaine, dihydrostreptomycin
  sulfate, and prednisolone injectable,
  3209
Penicillin G procaine, neomycin and
  polymyxin B sulfates, and hydrocortisone
  acetate topical, 3210
Penicillin G procaine injectable, 3205
Penicillin G procaine for injectable, 3205
Penicillin V benzathine oral, 3216

Syrup

T

Tablets

Tincture

Topical solution

U

V

Vaccine

Veterinary

W

Water

X

Y

Z